BLACKBOARD®

The next big thing in digital education!

Ingredients

1 Single sign-on with Blackboard Learn

1 Deeply integrated McGraw-Hill content and tools

1 Automatic Roster/Gradebook synchronization

1 Company—first to use Learning Technology Interoperability (LTI) Standards

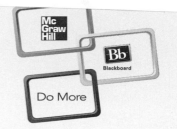

Directions

1. Go to **www.domorenow.com**.

2. Customize and integrate McGraw-Hill content and ground-breaking learning tools into your Bb courses.

3. Increase student retention and satisfaction.

4. Less building and managing. More teaching!

5. More integration on the way—ask us about the LMS used on your campus.

McGRAW-HILL CREATE™

Customize your perfect course solution!

Ingredients

1 New, self-service website that allows you to quickly and easily create custom course materials with McGraw-Hill's comprehensive, cross-disciplinary content and other third party resources

1 Place to create, edit, view, and purchase customized products

1 eBook or print text—you choose the best format for your students

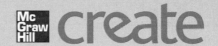

Directions

1. Go to **www.mcgrawhillcreate.com**.

2. Select, then arrange the content in a way that makes sense for your course.

3. Combine material from different sources and even upload your own content.

4. Edit and update your course materials as often as you'd like.

5. Receive your pdf review copy in minutes!

6. Create what you've only imagined!

McGRAW-HILL TEGRITY®

Students can focus on your lectures with digital lecture capture!

Ingredients

1 Ability to record from anywhere, anytime, with or without an Internet connection

1 Key word search allows students to search for exactly what they need to review

1 Highly personalized learning environment makes study time incredibly efficient

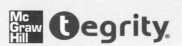

Directions

1. You need nothing more than a computer and microphone to quickly and easily record lectures.

2. Tegrity captures synchronized audio, video, and computer screen activity with the click of a button.

3. View recordings on a PC, Mac, or mobile device 24/7. Tegrity's intuitive interface with a detailed timeline and associated thumbnails makes it easy to find exactly what you're looking for.

4. Help students retain more and achieve higher levels of performance!

Tip: Learn more at **www.tegrity.com**

Nutrition

FOR HEALTHY LIVING Third Edition

Wendy J. Schiff M.S., R.D.

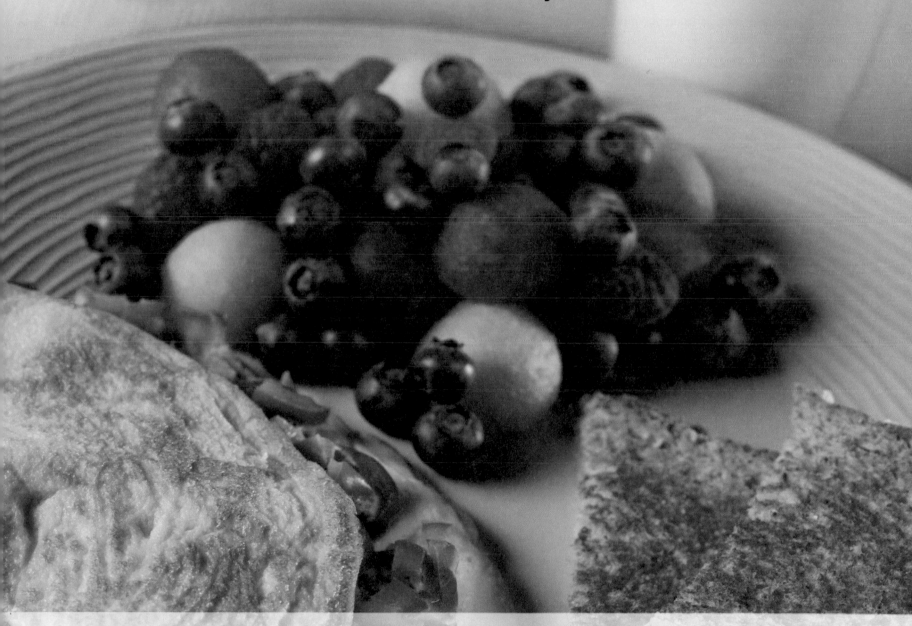

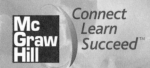
Mc Graw Hill

Connect Learn Succeed™

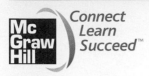

NUTRITION FOR HEALTHY LIVING, THIRD EDITION

Published by McGraw-Hill, a business unit of The McGraw-Hill Companies, Inc., 1221 Avenue of the Americas, New York, NY 10020. Copyright © 2013 by The McGraw-Hill Companies, Inc. All rights reserved. Printed in the United States of America. Previous editions © 2011 and 2009. No part of this publication may be reproduced or distributed in any form or by any means, or stored in a database or retrieval system, without the prior written consent of The McGraw-Hill Companies, Inc., including, but not limited to, in any network or other electronic storage or transmission, or broadcast for distance learning.

Some ancillaries, including electronic and print components, may not be available to customers outside the United States.

This book is printed on acid-free paper.

5 6 7 8 9 0 DOW/DOW 1 0 9 8 7 6 5 4

ISBN 978–0–07–352275–3
MHID 0–07–352275–9

Vice President, Editor-in-Chief: *Marty Lange*
Vice President, EDP: *Kimberly Meriwether David*
Senior Director of Development: *Kristine Tibbetts*
Publisher: *Michael S. Hackett*
Sponsoring Editor: *Lynn M. Breithaupt*
Director of Digital Content Development: *Barbekka Hurtt, Ph.D.*
Senior Developmental Editor: *Rose M. Koos*
Marketing Manager: *Amy L. Reed*
Senior Project Manager: *April R. Southwood*
Senior Buyer: *Sherry L. Kane*
Senior Media Project Manager: *Tammy Juran*
Manager, Creative Services: *Michelle D. Whitaker*
Cover Designer: *Ellen Pettengell*
Interior Designer: *Greg Nettles/Squarecrow Creative*
Cover Image: *(front)* © *The McGraw-Hill Companies, Inc., Kevin May Photography;*
(back) blueberries: © *PhotoAlto/PunchStock*
Senior Photo Research Coordinator: *John C. Leland*
Photo Research: *Jerry Marshall/pictureresearching.com*
Art Studio and Compositor: *Electronic Publishing Services Inc., NYC*
Typeface: *10/12 Giovanni*
Printer: *R. R. Donnelley*

All credits appearing on page or at the end of the book are considered to be an extension of the copyright page.

Library of Congress Cataloging-in-Publication Data

Schiff, Wendy.
    Nutrition for healthy living / Wendy J. Schiff. — 3rd ed.
        p. cm.
    Includes index.
    ISBN 978–0–07–352275–3 — ISBN 0–07–352275–9 (hard copy : alk. paper)   1. Human nutrition—Textbooks.   I. Title.
    QP141.S3435 2013
    612.3—dc22

                        2011039188

www.mhhe.com

To my mother and late father.

Brief Contents

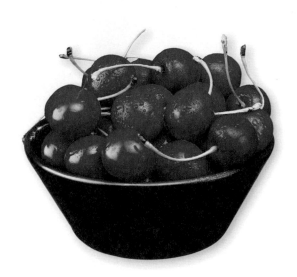

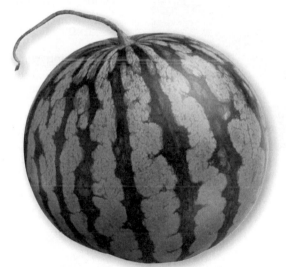

Meet the Author

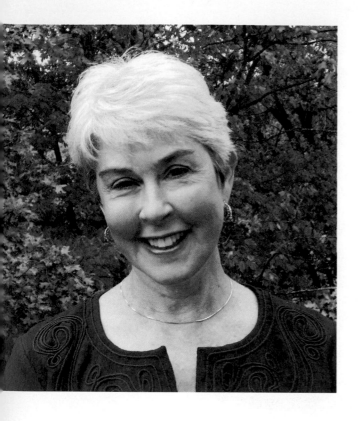

Wendy J. Schiff, M.S., R.D. received her B.S. in biological health/medical dietetics and M.S. in human nutrition from The Pennsylvania State University. She has taught introductory food and nutrition courses at the University of Missouri–Columbia as well as nutrition, human biology, and personal health courses at St. Louis Community College–Meramec. She has worked as a public health nutritionist at the Allegheny County Health Department (Pittsburgh, Pennsylvania) and State Food and Nutrition Specialist for Missouri Extension at Lincoln University in Jefferson City, Missouri. In addition to authoring *Nutrition for Healthy Living*, Wendy has coauthored a college-level personal health textbook and authored many other nutrition-related educational materials. She is a registered dietitian and a member of the Academy of Nutrition and Dietetics.

Welcome to the Third Edition of Nutrition for Healthy Living

We think of ourselves as consumers when we purchase homes, cars, computers, and food. We are also consumers of nutrition-related information. Nearly every day, we are literally bombarded with messages in media and from acquaintances concerning nutrition, foods, and health. Much of this information is unreliable, and often it is intended to promote sales of products or services. Nevertheless, we may use the information when making decisions about which foods or nutrition-related products to buy. Why? Many consumers lack the knowledge and skills needed to analyze such information critically and decide whether or not to apply it to their decision-making process.

Helping students become better-informed consumers, particularly as this relates to food and nutrition, is the foundation of *Nutrition for Healthy Living*. This major theme flows throughout the textbook by providing students with practical information, critical thinking skills, and the scientific foundation needed to make better-informed choices about their diet and health. By reading *Nutrition for Healthy Living*, not only will students learn basic principles of nutrition, they will also be able to evaluate various sources of nutrition information critically and to apply sound nutrition practices to improve their lives.

Wendy J. Schiff

Instructors

Connect via Customization

Presentation Tools
allow you to customize your lectures.

Enhanced Lecture Presentations contain lecture outlines, art, photos, tables, and animations. Fully customizable, complete, and ready to use—these presentations will streamline your work and let you spend less time preparing for lecture!

Editable Art   Fully editable (labels and leaders) line art from the text.

Animations   Over 50 animations bring key concepts to life, available for instructors *and* students.

Animation PPTs   Animations are truly embedded in PowerPoint® for ultimate ease of use! Just copy and paste into your custom slideshow and you're done!

Take your course online—*easily and quickly*—
with one-click Digital Lecture Capture.

McGraw-Hill Tegrity® records and delivers your lectures with just a click of a button. Students can view them anytime, anywhere via computer or mobile device. Tegrity records and indexes your slideshow presentations, and anything shown on your computer, so students can use keywords to find exactly what they want to study.

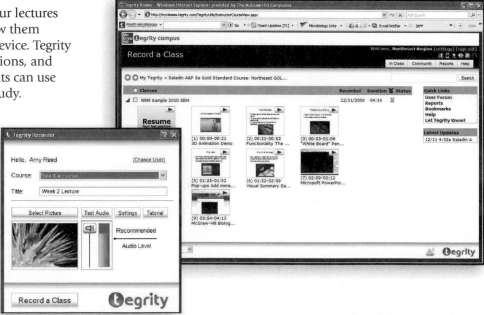

Access content anywhere, anytime, with a customizable, interactive eBook.

McGraw-Hill ConnectPlus® eBook takes digital texts beyond a simple PDF. With the same content as the printed book, but optimized for the screen, ConnectPlus has embedded animations and videos, which bring concepts to life and provide "just in time" learning for students. Fully integrated self-study questions allow students to interact with the questions in the text and determine if they're gaining mastery of the content.

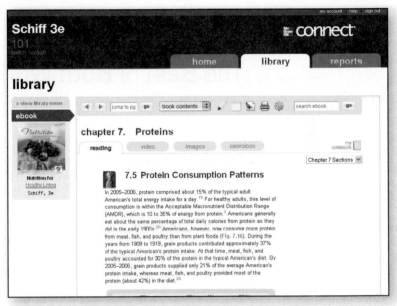

> "Use of technology, especially LEARN-SMART, assisted greatly in keeping on track and keeping up with the material."
>
> —student, Triton College

McGraw-Hill LearnSmart™ A Diagnostic, Adaptive Learning System

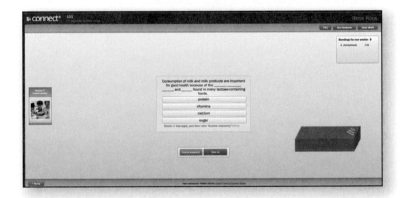

McGraw-Hill LearnSmart™ is an adaptive learning system designed to help students learn faster, study more efficiently, and retain more knowledge for greater success.

LearnSmart effectively assesses students' skill levels to determine which topics students have mastered and which require further practice. A personalized learning path based upon student strengths and weaknesses gives students exactly the help they need, when they need it.

> "I love LearnSmart. Without it, I would not be doing as well."
>
> —student, Triton College

Self-study resources are also available at www.mhhe.com/schiff3.

Connecting Instructors to Students

**McGraw-Hill Higher Education and Blackboard® have teamed up!
What does this mean for you?**

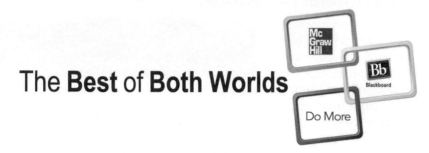

The **Best** of **Both Worlds**

Your life, simplified. Now you and your students can access McGraw-Hill Connect®
and Create™ right from within your Blackboard course—all with one single sign on! Say
goodbye to the days of logging in to multiple applications.

Deep integration of content and tools. Not only do you get single sign on with Connect and Create, you also get deep integration of McGraw-Hill content and content
engines right in Blackboard. Whether you're choosing a book for your course or building
Connect assignments, all the tools you need are right where you want them—inside of
Blackboard.

Seamless gradebooks. Are you tired of keeping multiple gradebooks and manually syn-
chronizing grades into Blackboard? We thought so. When a student completes an integrated Connect assignment, the grade for that assignment automatically (and instantly)
feeds your Blackboard grade center.

A solution for everyone. Whether your institution is already using Blackboard or you
just want to try Blackboard on your own, we have a solution for you. McGraw-Hill and
Blackboard can now offer you easy access to industry leading technology and content,
whether your campus hosts it, or we do. Be sure to ask your local McGraw-Hill represen-
tative for details.

and Students to Course Concepts

Introducing McGraw-Hill ConnectPlus® Nutrition

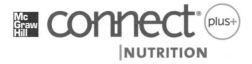

McGraw-Hill Connect® is a web-based assignment and assessment platform that gives students the means to better connect with coursework, instructors, and important concepts that they will need to know for success now and in the future. Connect Nutrition includes high-quality interactive questions and tutorials, Learn-Smart, digital lecture capture, eBook, and more!

Save time with auto-graded assessments and tutorials.

You can easily create customized assessments that will be automatically graded. All Connect content is created by nutrition instructors so it is pedagogical, instructional, and at the appropriate level. Interactive questions using high-quality art from the textbook, and animations and videos from a variety of sources, take you way beyond multiple choice.

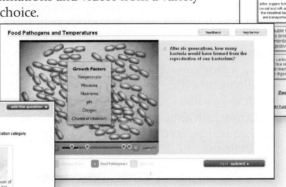

Connect Assessment: Labeling Interactive

Connect Assessment: Animation Tutorial

Connect Assessment: Classification Interactive

"… I and my adjuncts have reduced the time we spend on grading by 90 percent and student test scores have risen, on average, 10 points since we began using Connect!"

—William Hoover, Bunker Hill Community College

Gather assessment information

All Connect questions are tagged to a learning outcome, specific topic, and level of difficulty, and allow you to tag your own learning outcomes—so you can easily track assessment data!

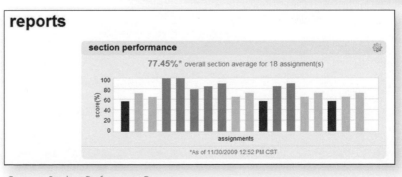

Connect: Student Performance Report

The ABCs of Nutrition

Who Was *Nutrition for Healthy Living* Written for?

Writing a nutrition textbook is not an easy task, but throughout the process I relied on my experience in teaching nutrition, foods, biology, and personal health classes at both the university and the community college level to develop a vision for a fresh approach to presenting basic information about nutrition. My teaching experiences also provided valuable insights into the diversity, as well as the needs, interests, and capabilities, of today's students. In addition, manuscript reviews and introductory nutrition syllabi provided by colleagues helped define the shared goals of those who teach the course, which in turn helped shape the content of this textbook.

Nutrition for Healthy Living is intended for students who are interested in learning about nutrition for personal reasons, as well as students considering majoring in nutrition, nursing, or other health- and science-related fields. Students from a wide variety of academic backgrounds often enroll in introductory nutrition courses, and in many instances, they have not taken college-level science courses prior to this nutrition course. With this in mind, I wrote the textbook with the understanding that an introductory textbook must appeal to students who represent a broad range of interests and academic backgrounds—English majors as well as nursing majors. My hope is that this introductory course, along with my textbook, can spark students' interest in adopting healthier dietary practices and possibly even inspire some students to consider nutrition as their major.

The *Nutrition for Healthy Living* Difference Is *ABC*

When I began to write this textbook, I felt strongly that I wanted to craft an alternative to established nutrition textbooks, while maintaining a focus on concepts that are fundamental to introductory nutrition courses. By building upon my experiences as coauthor of a college-level personal health textbook, I sought to develop a nutrition textbook that not only was scientifically up to date but also included consumer-oriented content and features. I wanted to create a textbook that would be visually appealing and fun to read, engage students' interest, be well organized, and have features that contribute to the pedagogy without being distracting. As my developmental editor gathered feedback from numerous instructors, the advantages that the new textbook would offer took shape—what my team at McGraw-Hill and I refer to as the **"ABCs of *Nutrition for Healthy Living*."**

"I don't think I've read a better written introductory nutrition text. It is informative, has a nice flow, and is easy to understand. The examples are engaging and clear."

Danita Kelley
Western Kentucky University

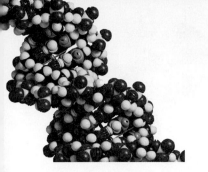

A = Accessible Science

Nutrition is an "offspring" science that requires a basic understanding of certain chemical and physiological concepts and terms. Ignorance about chemistry and physiology contributes to food faddism and health quackery. By providing a solid scientific foundation, nutrition educators can more easily dispel commonly held but inaccurate beliefs, such as "When you're inactive, muscle turns into fat," and "Cellulite is a special type of body fat."

Becoming knowledgeable about nutrition involves a certain level of understanding of basic scientific principles. *Nutrition for Healthy Living* recognizes the importance of introducing such principles in a manner that every college student can understand. As my primary goal for students who use this textbook, I want students to acquire a basic understanding of nutritional science so that they can make intelligent, practical choices that can result in improved nutrition and health.

Chapter 4 (Body Basics) presents basic principles of chemistry and human physiology as they apply to the study of nutrition, but at a level that students can easily understand. This chapter, for example, introduces and defines terms that relate to nutrition and foods, such as "acid," "basic," "enzyme," and "solvent." Because students and courses vary in the depth of scientific foundation required, this chapter features some flexibility. The chapter is divided into two main sections, chemistry and human physiology, so professors can choose to skip the chemistry section if they prefer.

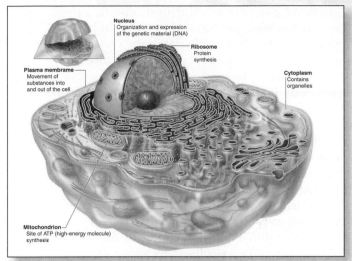

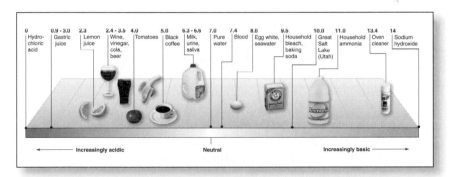

"The text is at a very good level. Not too simple that it will insult those with a strong science background, but easy enough for those with weak science backgrounds."

Janet Colson
Middle Tennessee State University

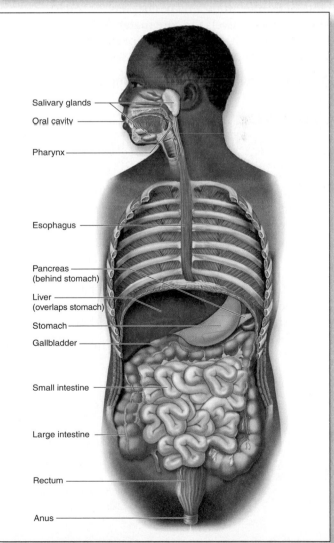

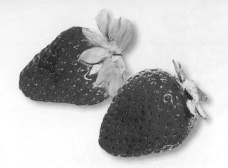

B = Brief Organization

In developing the structure of this book, a new approach emerged; instructors often do not have the time to cover all the material in their textbooks. Based upon their feedback, I chose to organize the core content into 13 chapters. I believe this organization makes teaching introductory nutrition more manageable and fits the time frame of most courses better than textbooks that include 15 or more chapters. Furthermore, basic information concerning world nutrition, diet and cancer, and dietary supplements is incorporated where it is relevant throughout the book.

Although some topics were important to cover, they did not warrant using a full chapter. Thus, topics such as global nutrition concerns, alcohol and alcohol abuse, and eating disorders are presented in Highlight features at the end of chapters. *Nutrition for Healthy Living* covers the core material instructors need in a format that is logical and practical for nearly all introductory nutrition courses:

- Chapter 1 introduces students to nutrition and nutrients, and presents 10 key nutrition concepts, such as "Most naturally occurring foods are mixtures of nutrients" and "Eating a variety of foods can help ensure the nutritional adequacy of a diet."
- Chapter 2 presents basic information about scientific methodology as it relates to nutrition research and provides tips for becoming a more wary consumer of nutrition- and health-related information.
- Chapter 3 discusses dietary standards and guidelines, food groups and guides, and how to use information provided on nutrient labels.
- Chapter 4 introduces basic chemical and physiological concepts and key terms that relate to the science of nutrition.

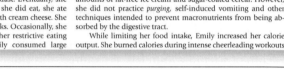

Chapter 10 Highlight

EATING DISORDERS: OVER THE DEEP EDGE

By the time she was a junior in high school, Emily Manoff was on top of her world. She had been freshman class president, captain of the cheerleading squad, and a homecoming "maid." Although she was academically and socially successful, Emily sensed that her peers were jealous of her. Also, she was concerned about her weight—130 pounds. At 5'2", she had a BMI (23.8) within the healthy range. Nevertheless, Emily began an effort to lose some weight after she overheard a teacher commenting that her cheerleading uniform was too tight.

At first, Emily's food choices were healthy, but soon she began skipping breakfast. Eventually, she stopped eating every other day, and when she did eat, she ate mostly fruit, vegetables, and some bagels with cream cheese. She avoided milk but drank lots of diet soft drinks. Occasionally, she would *binge eat*, that is, lose control over her restrictive eating practices. During such food binges, Emily consumed large amounts of fat-free ice cream and sugar-coated cereal. However, she did not practice *purging*, self-induced vomiting and other techniques intended to prevent macronutrients from being absorbed by the digestive tract.

While limiting her food intake, Emily increased her calorie output. She burned calories during intense cheerleading workouts

- Chapters 5, 6, 7, 8, and 9 present basic and practical information about the nutrients, such as their major functions in the body, food sources, and roles in health.
- Chapters 10, 11, 12, and 13 focus on applying basic nutrition information for special needs or important concerns. Chapter 10, for example, covers weight management; Chapter 11 presents information relating to physical fitness; Chapter 12 features information about food-borne illness; and Chapter 13 discusses nutrition during the life span.

"The Table of Contents . . . is arranged in a logical sequence. It has the chapters that I really teach. I never have time to include all the chapters in my current book."

Anne Marietta
Southeast Missouri State University

Nutrition for Healthy Living follows a more traditional approach to the study of nutrition, in that the textbook's organization focuses on nutrients rather than certain functions, tissues, or diseases. Additionally, the textbook integrates health information, particularly diet-related chronic diseases, within each chapter where it is appropriate, rather than relegate it to a single chapter near the end of the textbook. For example, the chapters that discuss nutrients provide fundamental information first and then present applications, including the nutrient-related health effects of certain lifestyle practices, particularly dietary choices. Additionally, the quantity and length of boxed features in the chapters are limited, as they tend to disrupt the flow of content and students often skip reading them.

Chapter Highlights

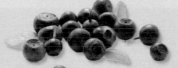

C = Consumer Focus

Regardless of their backgrounds, students are consumers of nutrition information from a wide variety of sources, including popular magazines, friends, diet books, infomercials, and the Internet. Oftentimes these students arrive in class with many misconceptions about their diet and health. As nutrition educators, we seek to identify these beliefs and to impart sound, reliable nutrition and health information. We also strive to equip our students with the tools they need to make intelligent, informed food- and nutrition-related decisions beyond the classroom. Chapter 2 (Evaluating Nutrition Information) presents a practical introduction to becoming an informed consumer of nutrition and nutrition-related information. This book is unique among nutrition textbooks in its inclusion of this chapter, which provides basic information concerning scientific research and a thorough discussion of how to evaluate nutrition- and health-related sources and messages.

In addition to devoting an entire chapter to the topic of evaluating nutrition-related information and ways of becoming a more wary consumer of nutrition information, the consumer emphasis is integrated throughout the book.

> "I absolutely loved Chapter 2 (Evaluating Nutrition Information). This is a concise way of presenting much needed information that is too brief in many textbooks, including the one I currently use. The author did an excellent job producing a practical, consumer-oriented approach to this necessary information for all introductory students."
>
> **Lorri Kanauss**
> Western Illinois University

Food & Nutrition *tip*

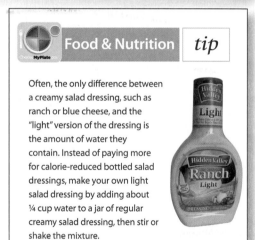

Often, the only difference between a creamy salad dressing, such as ranch or blue cheese, and the "light" version of the dressing is the amount of water they contain. Instead of paying more for calorie-reduced bottled salad dressings, make your own light salad dressing by adding about ¼ cup water to a jar of regular creamy salad dressing, then stir or shake the mixture.

- **Food & Nutrition Tips** present practical suggestions that apply material discussed in a section. These tips provide information students can use every day—and for the rest of their lives. Such features include tips for selecting fresh foods, managing energy intake, and keeping foods safe to eat.

- **Real People, Real Stories** feature information about people who actually have recovered from or are currently living with nutrition-related conditions such as celiac disease, type 1 diabetes, eating disorders, and hypertension. This feature is designed to help students recognize the daily challenges people with such conditions face and the role diet and physical activity play in managing health.

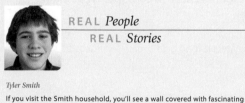

REAL *People*
REAL *Stories*

Tyler Smith

If you visit the Smith household, you'll see a wall covered with fascinating photographs—two that are especially attention grabbing. One photo shows a teenage boy holding a record-breaking 20-pound peacock bass and another photo is of the same teenager kneeling proudly next to a slain wild boar. Tyler Smith, the teenager in the photos, is only 18 years old, but he's done a lot of amazing things that most 18-year-olds don't even dream about doing. Tyler has taken two fishing trips on the Amazon River in South America. On one of those trips, he caught the huge bass. While on a hunting trip in Florida, Tyler shot the wild boar. Closer to home, Tyler enjoys hunting quail and pheasant. Aside from his enthusiasm for hunting, the young man is an Eagle Scout and serious NASCAR fan; he's often in the stands watching one of the races. Tyler has other interests. Since he was 2 years old, he has helped raise money for his local branch of the American Diabetes Association. For the past several years, the Association has honored Tyler for being the number one individual fundraiser in his area. The money that's collected by the American Diabetes Association is used to fund research efforts to find a cure for diabetes and support summer camps for children with the disorder. While attending one of those camps as a young child, Tyler learned how to give himself insulin injections. Why? Since he was 14 months old, Tyler has had type 1 diabetes.

As you can tell from Tyler's busy lifestyle, he doesn't let diabetes interfere with his life. Today, he doesn't need to take insulin injections four times a day; he wears an external insulin pump on his belt that is programmed to deliver tiny amounts of the hormone into his body continuously. If Tyler needs extra insulin, he can push a button and the device provides an additional dose of the hormone. Although using an insulin pump has made Tyler's ability to manage diabetes easier, he still watches his diet. He avoids consuming foods that contain high amounts of simple sugars, such as candy bars and regular soft drinks. According to Tyler, "Sometimes, when I order a diet soft drink, the restaurant worker asks, 'Why? You don't look like you need a diet drink.'" Tyler responds by informing the person, "I have to; I'm a diabetic."

Tyler's friends don't give him any special treatment, but they're aware of the signs of hyperglycemia and hypoglycemia. According to Tyler, "My friends know when my blood sugar is too high and I need insulin because I'm really thirsty and I have to go to the bathroom [urinate] a lot. When I'm hypoglycemic, I get agitated and shaky, and I have trouble concentrating on what I'm doing. Then my friends know to get me something with sugar in it."

- **Recipes for Healthy Living** is a practical application of nutrition and food information that will appeal to most college students. Each chapter features one or more easy-to-make, kitchen-tested recipes that help bring the chapter's content to life (e.g., high-fiber waffles). In addition to the pie graph for macronutrient content and a bar chart to illustrate % Daily Value for energy and key nutrients in a serving of the food, this feature also indicates which MyPlate food groups the major ingredients in the dish represent. This feature demonstrates that preparing nutritious foods can be fun and economical. By trying the recipes, students can develop basic food preparation skills and may be inspired to cook more foods "from scratch." As a result, they may rely less on vending machines and fast-food outlets.

Recipes for Healthy Living

Mango Lassi

Lassi (*luh-see*) is a simple yogurt-based beverage that originated in India. Lassi is usually made and served before a meal, but the drink can also be a refreshing, nutritious snack. This recipe makes about four ½-cup servings. Each serving supplies approximately 85 kcal, 4 g protein, 17 g carbohydrate, 0 g fat, 3.7 g fiber, 130 mg calcium, and 14 mg vitamin C.

INGREDIENTS:

1 ripe mango
1 cup plain, fat-free yogurt
1 Tbsp sugar
6 ice cubes

PREPARATION STEPS:

1. Wash and peel mango. Remove fruit pulp from mango and discard large seed and peel.
2. Dice mango pulp and place in blender.
3. Add yogurt, sugar, and ice cubes to the blender.
4. Blend ingredients until smooth.
5. Serve immediately or refrigerate for up to 24 hours.

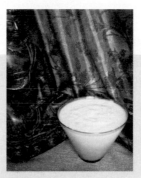

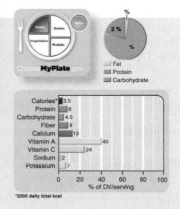

- **Did You Know?** This margin feature notes interesting nutrition-related tidbits that relate to information presented in that section of the chapter. Some of these features dispel commonly held beliefs about food and nutrition that are inaccurate.

Did You Know?

Have you heard of the "Freshman 15," the popular belief that college students gain 15 pounds during their freshman year? Results of scientific studies confirm that freshmen are likely to gain weight, but the increase is much less than 15 pounds—only 3 pounds on average.[26] In one study, 290 college students were weighed at the beginning of their freshman year and again at the completion of their sophomore year. During their first two years in college, 70% of the students participating in the study gained weight, on average, about 9 pounds.[27]

Assessment and Evaluation of Learning

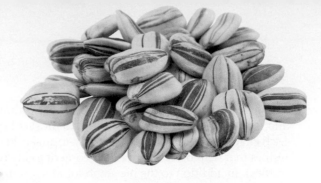

One of our primary goals as nutrition educators is to ensure that our students leave the introductory nutrition course with a better understanding of the nutrition principles and concepts needed to improve their diet and health. In order to assess how well faculty are achieving that goal, many colleges and universities are implementing Student Learning Outcomes as a way to measure what students have learned upon completing an introductory nutrition course. Student Learning Outcomes can also be used to help instructors identify content areas that need more refined teaching methods. *Nutrition for Healthy Living* has been developed around the following coursewide outcomes.

Student Learning Outcomes

1. Identify functions and sources of nutrients.
2. Demonstrate basic knowledge of digestion, absorption, and metabolism.
3. Apply current dietary guidelines and nutrition recommendations.
4. Analyze and evaluate nutrition information scientifically.
5. Relate roles of nutrients in good health, optimal fitness, and chronic diseases.
6. Summarize basic concepts of nutrition throughout the life span.
7. Evaluate a personal diet record using a computer database.

Additionally, each chapter opens with a list of chapter-specific learning outcomes that build upon the broader coursewide outcomes. The "Chapter Learning Outcomes" help students prepare for reading the chapter and also clarify major concepts they are expected to learn. These measurable outcomes are further supported by assessment methods and study aids found within the chapters and on McGraw-Hill's Connect®.

Quiz Yourself

This pretest, comprised of five true-or-false questions, appears at the beginning of each chapter; answers to the quiz are provided at the end of the chapter. The purpose of "Quiz Yourself" is to stimulate interest in reading the chapter. By taking the quiz, students may be surprised to learn how little or how much they know about the chapter's contents.

Practice Test

Each chapter ends with a series of 10 or more multiple-choice questions that test students' comprehension and recall of information presented in the chapter. Answers to the test questions are in Appendix H. The multiple-choice questions prepare students for classroom exams, because they are similar in type and format to those in the test bank. In many instances, the test questions are correlated to the coursewide Student Learning Outcomes and Chapter Learning Outcomes.

> "I was very impressed with this area. I liked the study tools. It is great to have quizzes at the beginning of the chapters to see how much a student knows."
>
> Jennifer L. Fuller
> Bluegrass Community and Technical College

Chapter Learning Outcomes

After reading Chapter 2, you should be able to

1. Define terms, including anecdote, variable, epidemiology, placebo, placebo effect, peer review, and quackery.
2. Explain the basic steps of the scientific method.
3. Explain the importance of having controls when performing experiments.
4. Define "research bias."

Quiz *Yourself*

Before reading the rest of Chapter 2, test your knowledge of scientific methods and reliable sources of nutrition information by taking the following quiz. The answers are on page 57.

1. Scientists generally do not raise questions about or criticize the conclusions of their colleagues' research data, even when they disagree with those conclusions. _____ T _____ F
2. Popular health-related magazines typically publish articles that have been peer-reviewed. _____ T _____ F
3. By conducting a prospective epidemiological study, medical

PRACTICE TEST

Select the best answer.
1. Which of the following statements is false?
   a. Lean tissue contains more water than fat tissue.
   b. Water is a major solvent.
   c. Generally, young women have more body water than young men.
   d. Water does not provide energy.
2. If the extracellular fluid has an excess of sodium ions,
   a. sodium ions move into cells.
   b. intracellular fluid moves to the outside of cells.

CRITICAL THINKING

1. Before the advent of refrigeration, salting meat was a common way of preventing microbes from spoiling the food. Explain why salting was effective as a means of food preservation.

2. A friend of yours refuses to drink tap water because she thinks it is contaminated. She drinks only bottled water or well water. If she asked you to explain why you drink tap water, what would you tell her?

Concept **Checkpoint**

8. Explain why people should be careful about taking megadoses of vitamin supplements.
9. List three side effects from taking megadoses of nicotinic acid.
10. Explain why people should avoid taking high doses of vitamin B-6.

SUMMARY

Scientists ask questions about the natural world and follow generally accepted methods to obtain answers to these questions. Nutrition research relies on scientific methods that may involve making observations, asking questions and developing possi-

CHAPTER REFERENCES

See Appendix I.

Thus, breastfed infants should consume a supplement containing 10 mcg (400 IU) of vitamin D per day soon after birth. The adult form of rickets is called **osteomalacia** (*ahs'-tee-o-mah-lay'-she-a*). The bones of people with osteomalacia have normal amounts of *collagen*, the protein that provides structure for the skeleton, but they contain less-than-normal amounts of calcium. The bones are soft and weak, and break easily as a result. Muscle weakness is also a symptom of o

osteomalacia adult rickets; condition characterized by poorly mineralized (soft) bones

alpha-tocopherol vitamin E

Personal *Dietary* Analysis

Using the DRIs

1. Refer to your 3-day food log from the "Personal Dietary Analysis" feature in Chapter 3.

a. Find the RDA/AI values for minerals under your life stage/gender group category in the DRI tables (see the inside back cover of this book). Write those values under the "My RDA/AI" column in the table below.

Critical Thinking

The "Critical Thinking" feature involves higher-level cognitive skills, including applying, analyzing, synthesizing, and evaluating information. This assessment features a series of thought-provoking questions at the end of the chapter. The questions can help students develop higher-level cognitive skills using nutrition-related content. Acquiring and/or sharpening these skills can help students become better consumers of nutrition-related information.

Concept Checkpoint

The "Concept Checkpoint" feature includes review questions, many of which involve critical thinking skills, posed at the end of major headings. Such questions enable students to test their acquisition of information presented in the section. Answers to the questions in each "Concept Checkpoint" are located in Appendix H.

> "I like the . . . Checkpoints; they encourage critical thinking."
>
> Ingrid Lofgren
> University of New Hampshire

End-of-Chapter Summary

This feature provides a brief review of each chapter's main points. Sometimes students have difficulty determining the key points in a chapter; the chapter summary helps them focus on these points.

References

Nutrition for Healthy Living includes in-text citations and extensive lists of references in Appendix I. References provide readers with access to sources of information for more in-depth understanding or for topics that hold particular interest.

Key Terms and Pronunciation Guide

Key terms and definitions are provided in the margins on the same two-page spread where the terms first appear in the chapter. Many unfamiliar terms have pronunciations provided within the text. A glossary of these key terms is at the end of the textbook. These tools facilitate students' recall and understanding of important, and possibly unfamiliar, terminology.

Personal Dietary Analysis

Many chapters include an end-of-chapter activity for analyzing personal eating habits. Most of these activities require the use of a dietary analysis software program, such as McGraw-Hill's NutritionCalc Plus. Students can gain insight into their eating behaviors by completing this activity.

What's New in This Edition?

The first edition of this textbook included beautiful, pedagogically based illustrations and creative page layouts that were designed to facilitate learning. The third edition maintains this energetic and visually appealing design. We have added more photos to help draw students' attention to the written information and relate content to the "real world." It is important to note that the use of products in photos is for example representation only and does not constitute an endorsement.

The third edition of *Nutrition for Healthy Living* has been enhanced in several ways. The content has been undated extensively and some of the illustrations have been modified to increase their clarity. Furthermore, My Diverse Plate, a new feature that reflects the multiethnic, multicultural nature of the United States, has been added to several chapters. My Diverse Plate introduces foods that may be unfamiliar to the average American college student. The "Recipes for Healthy Living" feature at the end of each chapter includes a MyPlate illustration to help students visually relate the recipes to this food guide.

The following list describes key updates to specific chapters:

Chapter 1: The Basics of Nutrition

- Figure 1.3 shows a graph of the 10 leading causes of death in the United States and indicates which causes are related to diet.
- *Healthy People 2020*
- My Diverse Plate focuses on the use of locusts as food.

Chapter 3: Planning Nutritious Diets

The Major Food Groups, Dietary Guidelines, and Dietary Guides sections of the chapter underwent extensive revisions to accommodate updates that were introduced by the government in 2011. Such updates include:

- U.S. Dietary Guidelines, 2010
- MyPlate (www.choosemyplate.gov)

Chapter 5: Carbohydrates

- My Diverse Plate features red lentils.

Chapter 6: Fats and Other Lipids

- My Diverse Plate features ghee.

Chapter 7: Proteins

- My Diverse Plate features miso.

Chapter 8: Vitamins

- My Diverse Plate features guava.

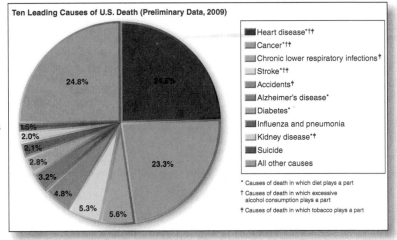

Ten Leading Causes of U.S. Death (Preliminary Data, 2009)

- Heart disease*††
- Cancer*††
- Chronic lower respiratory infections†
- Stroke*††
- Accidents†
- Alzheimer's disease*
- Diabetes*
- Influenza and pneumonia
- Kidney disease*†
- Suicide
- All other causes

24.8%, 24.6%, 23.3%, 1.5%, 2.0%, 2.1%, 2.8%, 3.2%, 4.8%, 5.3%, 5.6%

* Causes of death in which diet plays a part

† Causes of death in which excessive alcohol consumption plays a part

† Causes of death in which tobacco plays a part

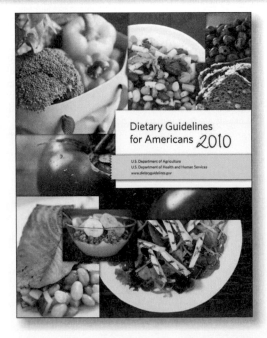

Dietary Guidelines for Americans 2010

U.S. Department of Agriculture
U.S. Department of Health and Human Services
www.dietaryguidelines.gov

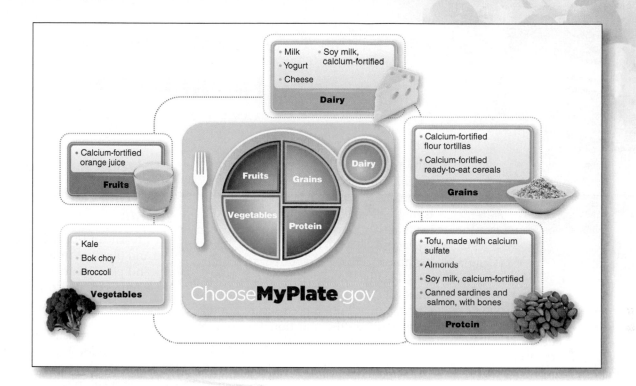

Chapter 9: Water and Minerals

- Many new photos and illustrations, including new MyPlate art for individual minerals, have been included.
- My Diverse Plate features bok choy.

Chapter 10: Energy Balance and Weight Control

- This chapter provides information about visceral fat and brown fat and their roles in health.

Chapter 11: Nutrition for Physically Active Lifestyles

- Table 11.7, which focuses on popular ergogenic supplements and aids, has been updated.

Chapter 13: Nutrition for a Lifetime

- The latest information about childhood obesity has been included.
- "Let's Move" is introduced.

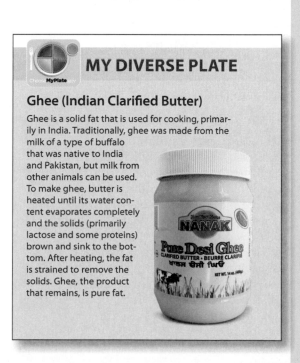

MY DIVERSE PLATE

Ghee (Indian Clarified Butter)

Ghee is a solid fat that is used for cooking, primarily in India. Traditionally, ghee was made from the milk of a type of buffalo that was native to India and Pakistan, but milk from other animals can be used. To make ghee, butter is heated until its water content evaporates completely and the solids (primarily lactose and some proteins) brown and sink to the bottom. After heating, the fat is strained to remove the solids. Ghee, the product that remains, is pure fat.

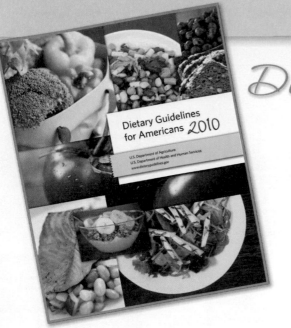

Dietary Guidelines for Americans, 2010
For a Healthier Life

THE *Dietary Guidelines for Americans, 2010* provide nutrition and physical activity advice based on the latest and strongest scientific information to improve the health of all Americans ages two and older. In light of the current epidemic of overweight and obesity—pressing health issues that now affect two-thirds of adults and one-third of children and adolescents—the message of calorie balance is woven throughout this seventh edition of the *Dietary Guidelines for Americans*.

Previous editions of the Dietary Guidelines have targeted healthy Americans, but these latest recommendations also include those at risk of developing chronic diseases. The health of children is highlighted. The new recommendations are also more culturally sensitive to reflect the growing diversity and varied health concerns of the American population. Finally, the new Dietary Guidelines recognize the prevalence of food insecurity and aim to help food insecure populations optimize the nutritional content of meals within their resource constraints.

These recommendations have been issued to guide the development of educational materials, aid policymakers, and serve as the basis for nutrition messages and consumer materials for the general public and specific audiences. Overall, Americans should use this information along with related tools, such as the new MyPlate icon, to form dietary and physical activity patterns that optimize health.

KEY RECOMMENDATIONS
Balancing Calories to Manage Weight

- Prevent and/or reduce overweight and obesity through improved eating and physical activity behaviors.
- Control total calorie intake to manage body weight. For people who are overweight or obese, this will mean consuming fewer calories from foods and beverages.
- Increase physical activity and reduce time spent in sedentary behaviors.
- Maintain appropriate calorie balance during each stage of life—childhood, adolescence, adulthood, pregnancy and breastfeeding, and older age.

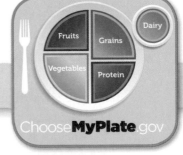

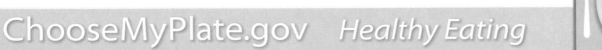

ChooseMyPlate.gov *Healthy Eating*

Many consumers and nutrition professionals found MyPyramid to be difficult to understand because it conveyed too much information. Some argued that the pyramid shape was too abstract a concept to apply to food choices. Now, MyPlate shapes the key recommendations from the Dietary Guidelines into an easily recognizable and universally applicable visual—a place setting. Although it is not intended to stand alone as a source of dietary advice, it serves as a reminder of healthy food choices.

Actionable Health Messages

Consumer research points to the need for simple, actionable health messages to capture the attention of the public and achieve successful behavior change. Accordingly, ChooseMyPlate.gov provides a series of succinct imperatives to help Americans make healthier food choices. Selected messages for consumers include:

Balancing Calories
- Enjoy your food, but eat less.
- Avoid oversized portions.

Foods to Increase
- Make half your plate fruits and vegetables.
- Make at least half your grains whole.
- Switch to skim or 1% milk.

Foods to Reduce
- Compare sodium in foods like soup, bread, and frozen meals—and choose the foods with lower numbers.
- Drink water instead of sugary drinks.

Acknowledgments

The development of an accurate and current manuscript for *Nutrition for Healthy Living,* Third Edition, was facilitated by the input of numerous college instructors and emeriti. These individuals reviewed chapters and contributed encouraging comments and constructive suggestions concerning content and pedagogy. Moreover, certain reviewers contributed additional input on specific sections of the manuscript. Their willingness to provide suggestions for developing content was gratifying.

I offer my sincere thanks to the following colleagues, who provided a wide range of valuable input, including reviewing manuscript, class-testing chapters, serving on our Advisory Board blog, and preparing supplemental materials:

Reviewers

Kwaku Addo
University of Kentucky

Laurie Allen
University of North Carolina at Greensboro

Dawn E. Anderson
Winona State University

Sharon Antonelli
San Jose City College

Richard C. Baybutt
Kansas State University

Valerie Benedix
Clovis Community College

Stephanie F. Beplay
Colorado Community Colleges Online

Alan Bergson
Westchester Community College

Ginny Berkemeier
Ozarks Technical Community College

Shawn Bjerke
Minnesota State Community and Technical College

Patricia B. Brevard
James Madison University

Anne Bridges
University of Alaska Anchorage

Tracey Brigman
University of Georgia

Jim Burkard
Nashville State Community College

Melanie Tracy Burns
Eastern Illinois University

Dorothy A. Byrne
University of Texas–San Antonio

Cindy Cadieux
James Madison University

Janet Colson
Middle Tennessee State University

Karen Dahl
Youngstown State University

Robert T. Davidson
Brigham Young University

Richard P. Dowdy
University of Missouri–Columbia

Beth Fontenot
McNeese State University

Bernard Frye
The University of Texas Arlington

Jennifer L. Fuller
Bluegrass Community and Technical College

Art Gilbert
University of California–Santa Barbara

Melissa Davis Gutschall
Radford University

Charlene G. Harkins
University of Minnesota–Duluth

Nancy G. Harris
East Carolina University

Kimberly Heidal
East Carolina University

Sharon Himmelstein
Central New Mexico Community College

Ann P. Hunter
Wichita State University

Jean Jackson
Bluegrass Community and Technical College

Lorri Kanauss
Western Illinois University

Judy Kaufman
Monroe Community College

Danita Kelley
Western Kentucky University

Alex Kojo Anderson
University of Georgia

Ingrid Lofgren
University of New Hampshire

Mary Lyons
El Camino Community College

Anne B. Marietta
Southeast Missouri State University

Mary Martinez
Central New Mexico Community College

Mark S. Meskin
California State Polytechnic University Pomona

Jeanine L. Mincher
Youngstown State University

Allison Miner
Prince George's Community College

Millicent Owens
College of the Sequoias

Gloria Payne
Middle Tennessee State University

Wanda Perkins
Salisbury University

Wanda Ragland
Macomb Community College

Linda Rankin
Idaho State University

Rebecca Roach
University of Illinois

Anne-Marie Scott
University of North Carolina–Greensboro

Carole A. Sloan
Henry Ford Community College

Anastasia Snelling
American University

LuAnn Soliah
Baylor University

Diana Spillman
Miami Univiersity

Bernice G. Spurlock
Hinds Community College

Tammy J. Stephenson
University of Kentucky

Leeann S. Sticker
Northwestern State University

Stefanie F. Tierney
Central New Mexico Community College

Amy A. Vaughan
Radford University

Priya Venkatesan
Pasadena Area Community College

Vicky I. Walker
California State Polytechnic University

Kelly H. Webber
University of Kentucky

Sally Weerts
University of North Florida

Cynthia B. Wright
Southern Utah University

I would also like to thank Kelly Webber, Carole Sloan, Stacy Hastey, Diana Sloan, Elaine Higgins, and Maureen Reidenauer for developing LearnSmart and Connect content, PowerPoint slides, "Practice Tests," Online Quizzes, Instructor's Manual materials, and Game Show slides.

Additionally, I would like to acknowledge the contributions that Helen Guthrie, Barbara Shannon, the late Dorothy Kolodner, Judith Dodd, Richard Dowdy, and Sandra Alters have made to my personal and professional development and growth. This special group of individuals provided mentoring, encouragement, and friendship that shaped my career as a nutrition and dietetics student, dietitian, and college educator and textbook author.

My very special thanks is necessary to Lisa Gottschalk; Tyler Smith; Anne Buchanan, the mother of the late Jason Reinhardt; Dallas Clasen; Emily Manoff; Justin Steinbruegge; Jill Kohl; Katie Adams; Sarah Haskins; and Jan Haapala. These individuals helped make *Nutrition for Healthy Living* more real and interesting by contributing their stories to chapter openers, "Highlights," and "Real People, Real Stories" features. I also appreciate the assistance of Deborah McEnery for graciously providing her grandfather's baby photo that appears in Chapter 13, and Trip Straub of Straub's Markets for allowing me to take photographs in his stores.

Many McGraw-Hill employees invested a great deal of time and effort into the development and production of *Nutrition for Healthy Living*. My sincerest thanks is extended to all the members of the McGraw-Hill editorial, design, production, and marketing team for their enthusiastic support and encouragement. While I was writing this textbook, the team consulted me when making important decisions that directly affected the textbook's features, layout, design, and pedagogy. It was a pleasure to work with people who were willing to listen to my concerns and incorporate many of my suggestions.

A few members of the team deserve special recognition. Lynn Breithaupt took over the reins as my sponsoring editor around the time that the production of this new edition began. Under her very capable direction, I was able to focus my attention on the preparation of the third edition. I am also grateful to Amy Reed, Marketing Manager, for her work in promoting this third edition. When the first edition was in development, Michelle Whitaker managed the production of the unique and visually stimulating design. The first edition's design won a first place award at the Chicago Book Clinic in 2008. Michelle continued to provide her creative talents to the development of the third edition. April Southwood had the difficult task of managing my chapters as they progressed through production, and she helped convey my wishes concerning the art and layout to the compositor. Michelle and April's efforts were instrumental in the production of a superior textbook.

I also want to thank Marty Lange, Vice-President, and Michael Hackett, Publisher, for being instrumental in making certain that McGraw-Hill provided ample financial support for the production of a superior textbook. Last, but not least, my developmental editor, Rose Koos, deserves my heartfelt gratitude for the hard work, long hours, and extraordinary dedication she invested in the production of *Nutrition for Healthy Living*. While this new edition was in production, Rose's expertise, creativity, and dedication to this project contributed to making my work an enjoyable experience.

Wendy J. Schiff

"I found the chapters to be very well written and engaging. I appreciated how specific examples and personal stories were utilized to capture the reader's attention. The Highlight boxes and supplemental material are also very interesting and current. GREAT job!"

Tammy Stephenson
University of Kentucky

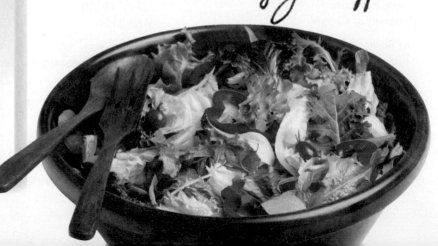

Contents

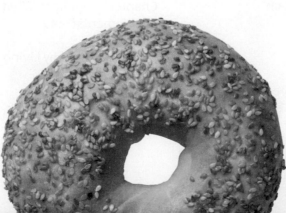

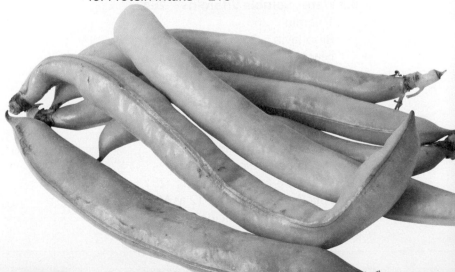

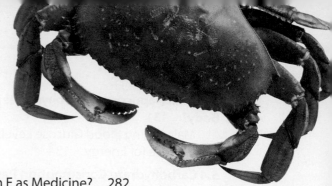

8 Vitamins 240

9 Water and Minerals 296

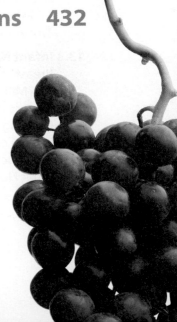

13 Nutrition for a Lifetime   466

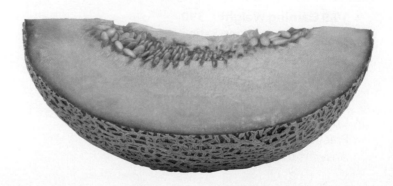

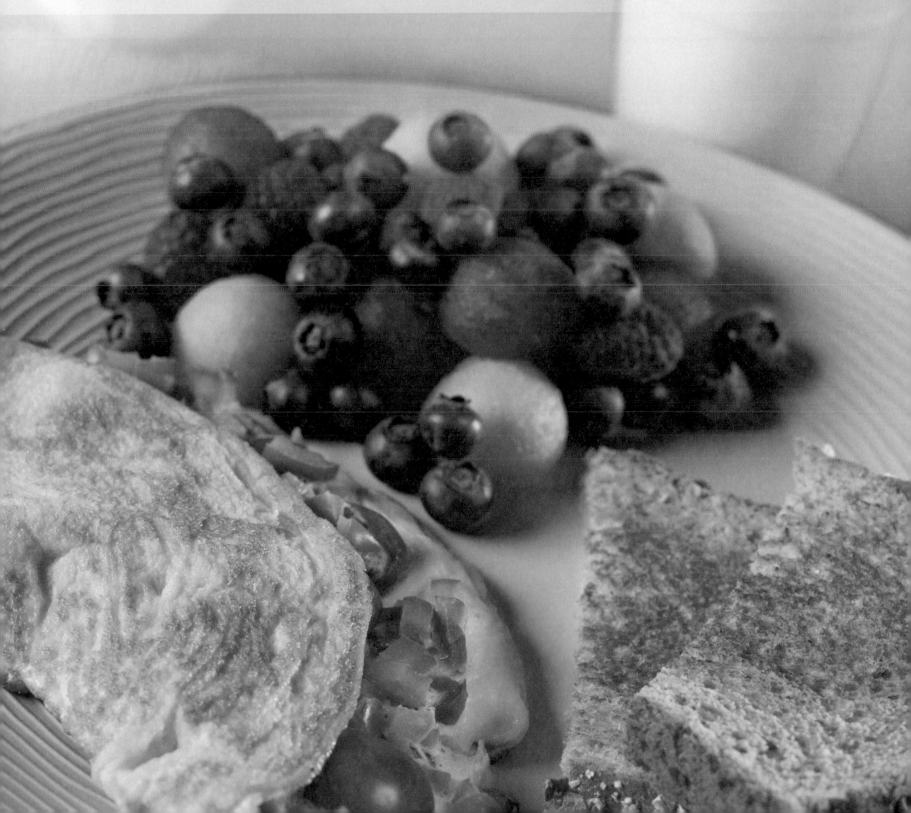

Nutrition
FOR HEALTHY LIVING

CHAPTER 1

The Basics of Nutrition

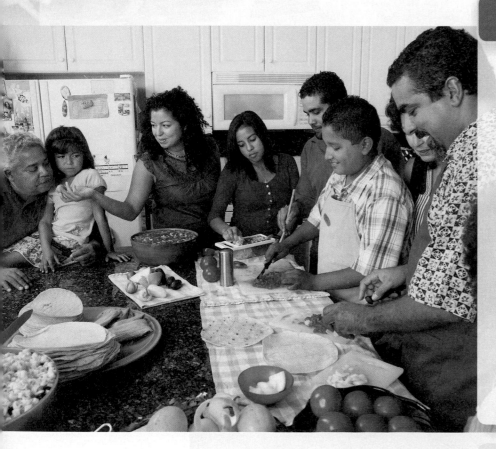

Chapter Learning Outcomes

After reading Chapter 1, you should be able to

1. Define the terms diet, nutrition, nutrient, essential nutrient, macronutrient, micronutrient, kilocalorie, phytochemical, and malnutrition.

2. Identify factors that influence personal food choices.

3. Identify lifestyle factors that contribute to the leading causes of death in the United States.

4. List the six classes of nutrients and identify a major role of each class of nutrient in the body.

5. Identify basic units of the metric system often used in nutrition.

6. Explain the concept of energy density and identify energy-dense foods.

7. Use the caloric values of energy-yielding nutrients to estimate the amount of energy (kcal) in a food.

8. Identify key basic nutrition concepts, such as the importance of eating a variety of foods and that no food supplies all nutrients.

9. Discuss factors that contribute to malnutrition in the world.

10. Identify major federal food assistance programs.

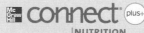

www.mcgrawhillconnect.com

A wealth of proven resources are available on ConnectPlus® Nutrition! Ask your instructor about ConnectPlus, which includes an interactive eBook, an adaptive learning program and much, much more!

WHEN YOU WERE an infant and a young child, your parents or other adult caregivers were the "gatekeepers" of your food; they chose what you ate and prepared it, and you probably ate most of it. If you balked at eating steamed broccoli or baked salmon, they may have told you, "Eat your vegetables if you expect to get dessert," or "Finish that fish. People in Africa are starving!" As you grew older, your **diet,** your usual pattern of food choices, came increasingly under your control. Today, your diet is more likely to be composed of foods that you enjoy as well as can afford, and probably those you can prepare easily or obtain quickly. Your family's ethnic and cultural background may also play a role in determining what you eat regularly. For example, do you eat tamales, tripe, goat, or kim chee because you ate these foods as a child? Numerous other factors influence your food choices, including friends and food advertising, as well as your beliefs and moods (Fig. 1.1).

Food is a basic human need for survival. You become hungry and search for something to eat when your body needs **nutrients,** the life-sustaining substances in food. Nutrients are necessary for the growth, maintenance, and repair of your body's cells. However, you have no instinctual drive that enables you to select the appropriate mix of nutrients your body requires for proper functioning. To eat well, you need to learn about the nutritional value of foods and the effects that your diet can have on your health.

Simply having information about nutrients and foods and their effects on health may not be enough for people to change ingrained food-related behaviors—a person must be motivated to make such changes. Some people become motivated to improve their diets because they want to lose or gain weight. Others are so concerned about their health, they are motivated to change their eating habits in specific ways, such as by eating fewer salty or fatty foods. Many people, however, could not care less if the food they eat is beneficial or harmful to their health. According to results of a national survey conducted in 2000, 70% of adult Americans eat "pretty much whatever they want."[1]

Why should you care about your diet? In the United States, poor eating habits contribute to several leading causes of death, including heart disease, some types of cancer, stroke, and type 2 diabetes. According to results of one national study, premature deaths from any cause in American men and women, about 16% and 9%, respectively, could be eliminated if the population adopted recommended dietary behaviors.[2] Consuming more fruits, vegetables, unsalted nuts, fat-free or low-fat dairy products, and whole-grain cereals, as well as exercising regularly, may reduce your chances of developing serious diseases that contribute to premature deaths, such as heart disease, type 2 diabetes, and excess body fat.[3] On the other hand, a poor diet, physical inactivity, and excess alcohol consumption may increase your risks of these health problems and dying prematurely as a result.

(continued)

Quiz *Yourself*

Take the following quiz to test your basic nutrition knowledge; the answers are on page 29.

1. There are four classes of nutrients: proteins, lipids, sugars, and vitamins. _____T _____F
2. Proteins are the most essential class of nutrients. _____T _____F
3. All nutrients must be supplied by the diet, because they cannot be made by the body. _____T _____F
4. Vitamins are a source of energy. _____T _____F
5. Milk, carrots, and bananas are examples of "perfect" foods that contain all nutrients. _____T _____F

diet usual pattern of food choices

nutrients chemicals necessary for proper body functioning

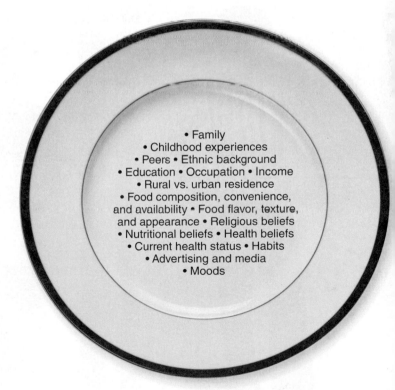

- Family
- Childhood experiences
- Peers • Ethnic background
- Education • Occupation • Income
- Rural vs. urban residence
- Food composition, convenience, and availability • Food flavor, texture, and appearance • Religious beliefs
- Nutritional beliefs • Health beliefs
- Current health status • Habits
- Advertising and media
- Moods

Figure 1.1 What influences your eating practices? Numerous factors influence food choices, including food advertising, peers, income, moods, and personal beliefs.

Are you concerned about the nutritional quality of your diet? The fact that you are taking this course indicates you have a strong interest in nutrition and a desire to learn more about the topic. A major objective of this textbook is to provide you with the basic information you need to better understand how your diet can influence your health. Managing your diet is your responsibility. We will not tell you what to eat to guarantee optimal health—no one can make that promise. After reading this textbook and learning about foods and the nutrients they contain, you can use the information to make informed decisions concerning the foods you eat. Furthermore, you will be able to evaluate your diet and decide if it needs to be changed.

Each chapter of this textbook begins with "Quiz Yourself," a brief true-or-false quiz to test your knowledge of the material covered in the chapter. At the end of each chapter, you will find the answers to this quiz, as well as a group of multiple-choice questions that test your understanding of the material in the chapter. The answers to those questions are also provided in Appendix H. References for information cited in chapters are in Appendix I.

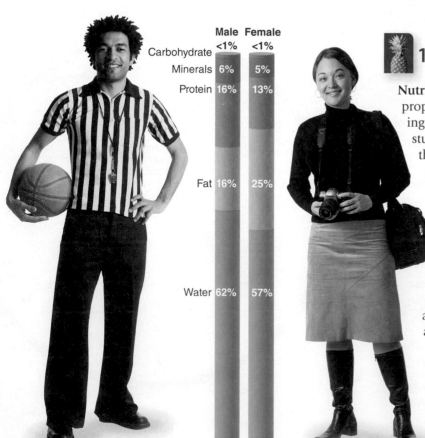

Figure 1.2 Comparing composition. These illustrations present the approximate percentages of nutrients that comprise the bodies of a healthy young man and woman. Note that the amount of vitamins in the human body is so small, it is not shown.

	Male	Female
Carbohydrate	<1%	<1%
Minerals	6%	5%
Protein	16%	13%
Fat	16%	25%
Water	62%	57%

1.1 Nutrition: The Basics

Nutrition is the scientific study of nutrients, chemicals necessary for proper body functioning, and how the body uses them. Understanding nutrition requires learning about chemistry. **Chemistry** is the study of the composition and characteristics of matter, and changes that can occur to it. Matter is anything that takes up space and has mass or weight (on Earth). The air you breathe, this textbook, and even your body consist of chemicals and are forms of matter. "There are chemicals in our food!" This statement may sound frightening, but it is true. Food is matter; therefore, it contains chemicals, some of which are nutrients.

There are six classes of nutrients: carbohydrates, fats and other lipids, proteins, vitamins, minerals, and water. Your body is comprised of these nutrients (Fig. 1.2). Although an average healthy young man and woman have similar amounts of vitamins, minerals, and carbohydrates in their bodies, the young woman has less water and protein, and considerably more fat.

Table 1.1 presents major roles of nutrients in your body. In general, your body uses certain nutrients for energy, growth and development, and regulation of processes, including the repair and maintenance of cells. A **cell** is the smallest living functional unit in an organism, such as a human being. There are hundreds of different types of cells in your body. Cells do not need food to survive, but they need the nutrients in food to carry out their metabolic activities. **Metabolism** is the total of all chemical processes that occur in living cells, including chemical reactions (changes) involved in generating energy, making proteins, and eliminating waste products.

TABLE 1.1 *Major Functions of Nutrients in the Body*

Nutrient	Major Functions
Carbohydrates	Energy (most forms)
Lipids	Energy (fat)
	Cellular development, physical growth and development
	Regulation of body processes (certain chemical messengers, for example)
	Absorption of certain vitamins
Proteins	Production of structural components, such as cell membranes, and functional components, such as enzymes
	Cellular development, growth, and maintenance
	Regulation of body processes (certain chemical messengers, for example)
	Energy
Vitamins	Regulation of body processes, including cell metabolism
	Maintenance of immune function, production and maintenance of tissues, and protection against agents that can damage cellular components
Minerals	Regulation of body processes, including fluid balance and metabolism; formation of certain chemical messengers; structural and functional components of various substances and tissues; and necessary for physical growth, maintenance, and development
Water	Maintenance of fluid balance, regulation of body temperature, elimination of wastes, and transportation of substances
	Participant in many chemical reactions

nutrition scientific study of nutrients and how the body uses these substances

chemistry study of the composition and characteristics of matter and changes that can occur to it

cell smallest living functional unit in an organism

metabolism total of all chemical processes that take place in living cells

essential nutrient nutrient that must be supplied by food

deficiency disease state of health that occurs when a nutrient is missing from the diet

Understanding nutrition also involves learning about human *physiology*, the study of how the body functions. Chapter 4 (Body Basics) prepares you for the study of nutrition by presenting basic information about chemistry and human physiology. Chapters 5 (Carbohydrates), 6 (Fats and Other Lipids), 7 (Proteins), 8 (Vitamins), and 9 (Water and Minerals) provide information about the functions of nutrients in the body.

What Is an Essential Nutrient?

The body can *synthesize* (make) many nutrients, such as the lipids cholesterol and fat, but about 50 nutrients are dietary essentials. An **essential nutrient** must be supplied by food, because the body does not synthesize the nutrient or make enough to meet its needs. Water is the most essential nutrient.

There are three key features that help identify an essential nutrient:

- If the nutrient is missing from the diet, a **deficiency disease** occurs as a result. The deficiency disease is a state of health characterized by certain abnormal physiological changes. Visible or measurable changes are referred to as *signs* of disease. Disease signs include rashes, failure to grow properly, and elevated blood pressure. *Symptoms* are subjective complaints of ill health that are difficult to observe and measure, such as dizziness, fatigue, and headache.
- When the missing nutrient is added to the diet, the abnormal physiological changes are corrected. As a result, signs and symptoms of the deficiency disorder resolve as normal functioning is restored and the condition is cured.
- After scientists identify the nutrient's specific roles in the body, they can explain why the abnormalities occurred when the substance was missing from the diet.

If you wanted to test your body's need for vitamin C, for example, you could avoid consuming foods or vitamin supplements that contain the vitamin. When the amount of vitamin C in your cells became too low for them to function normally, you

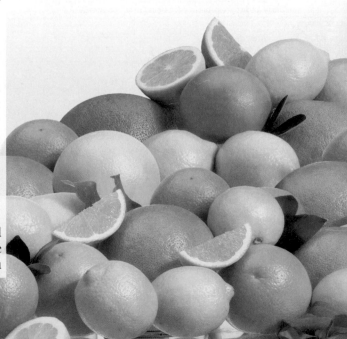

TABLE 1.2 *Essential Nutrients for Humans*

Water	Minerals (continued):
Vitamins:	Magnesium
A	Manganese
B vitamins	Molybdenum
Thiamin	Phosphorus
Riboflavin	Potassium
Niacin	Selenium
Pantothenic acid	Sodium
Biotin	Sulfur
Folic acid (folate)	Zinc
B-6	**Fats that contain linoleic and alpha-linolenic acids**
B-12	
Choline*	
C	**The following amino acids are generally recognized as essential:**
D**	
E	
K	Histidine
Glucose †	Leucine
Minerals:	Isoleucine
Calcium	Lysine
Chloride	Methionine
Chromium	Phenylalanine
Copper	Threonine
Iodine	Tryptophan
Iron	Valine

* The body makes choline but may not make enough to meet needs. Often classified as a *vitamin-like* compound.

**The body makes vitamin D after exposure to sunlight, but a dietary source of the nutrient is often necessary.

† A source of glucose is needed to supply the nervous system with energy and spare protein from being used for energy.

would develop physical signs of *scurvy*, the vitamin C deficiency disease. Early in the course of the deficiency, tiny red spots that are actually signs of bleeding under the skin (bruises) would appear where the elastic bands of your clothing applied pressure. When you brushed your teeth, your gums would bleed from the pressure of the toothbrush. If you cut yourself, the wound would heal slowly or not at all. If you started consuming vitamin C–containing foods again, the deficiency signs and symptoms would disappear within a few days as your body recovered. By reading about vitamin C in Chapter 8, you will learn that one of the physiological roles of vitamin C is maintaining a substance in your body that literally holds cells together. This substance is also needed to produce scar tissue for wound healing. When the vitamin is lacking, the tiniest blood vessels in your skin begin to leak blood where the skin is compressed, and even minor cuts have difficulty healing. Thus, vitamin C meets all the required features of an essential nutrient.

Table 1.2 lists nutrients that are generally considered to be essential. Fortunately, the human body is designed to obtain these substances from a wide variety of foods. The recommended way to obtain all nutrients is to build a core diet comprised of minimally processed foods including whole grains; peas, beans, and nuts; fruits and vegetables; low-fat or fat-free dairy products; lean meats, fish, and poultry; and small amounts of vegetable oils.

What Are Phytochemicals?

Some foods, particularly those from plants, contain substances that are not nutrients, yet they may have healthful benefits. Plants make hundreds of **phytochemicals** (*phyto* = plant). Caffeine, for example, is a phytochemical naturally made by coffee plants that has a stimulating effect on the body. Many phytochemicals are antioxidants that may reduce risks of heart disease and certain cancers. An **antioxidant** protects cells and their components from being damaged or destroyed by exposure to certain environmental and internal factors. Not all phytochemicals, however, have beneficial effects on the body; some are *toxic* (poisonous) or can interfere with the absorption of nutrients. Scientific research that explores the effects of phytochemicals on the body is ongoing. Table 1.3 lists several phytochemicals that are currently under scientific investigation, identifies rich food sources of these compounds, and indicates their biological effects on the body, including possible health benefits.

Dietary Supplements

Many Americans purchase dietary supplements such as vitamin pills and herbal extracts to improve their health. The Dietary Supplement and Health Education Act of 1994 (DSHEA) allows manufacturers to classify nutrient supplements and certain herbal products as foods.[4] According to the DSHEA, a **dietary supplement** is a product (excluding tobacco) that contains a vitamin, a mineral, an herb or other plant product, an amino acid, or a dietary substance that supplements the diet by increasing total intake. According to scientific evidence, some dietary supplements, such as vitamins and certain herbs, can have beneficial effects on health. However, results of scientific testing also indicate that many popular dietary supplements are not helpful and may even be harmful. The Highlight in Chapter 2 ("What Are Dietary Supplements?") discusses dietary supplements. Information about specific dietary supplements is also woven into chapters where it is appropriate.

Concept **Checkpoint**

1. Identify at least two of the 10 leading causes of death that are diet related.
2. Identify at least four factors that influence your eating habits.
3. List the six major classes of nutrients.
4. What is the smallest living functional unit in the body?
5. What are three key factors that determine whether a substance is an essential nutrient?
6. What is a phytochemical?
7. Define "dietary supplement."

phytochemicals compounds made by plants that are not nutrients

antioxidant substance that protects other compounds from being damaged or destroyed by certain factors

dietary supplements nutrient preparations, certain hormones, and herbal products

TABLE 1.3 *Phytochemicals of Scientific Interest*

Classification and Examples	Rich Food Sources	Biological Effects/Possible Health Benefits
Carotenoids		
Alpha-carotene, beta-carotene, lutein, lycopene, zeaxanthin	Orange, red, yellow fruits and vegetables; egg yolks	May reduce risk of certain cancers, may reduce risk of macular degeneration (cause of blindness)
Phenolics		
Quercetin	Apples, tea, red wine, onions, olives, raspberries, cocoa	Antioxidant activity, may inhibit cancer growth, may reduce risk of heart disease
Catechins	Green and black tea, chocolate, plums, apples, berries, pecans	
Naringenin, hesperitin	Citrus fruits	
Anthocyanins	Red, blue, or purple fruits and vegetables	
Resveratrol	Red wine, purple grapes and grape juice, dark chocolate, cocoa	
Isoflavonoids	Soybeans and other legumes	
Lignans	Flaxseed, berries, whole grains, bran, nuts	
Tannins	Tea, coffee, chocolate, blueberries, grapes, persimmons	
Ellagic acid	Raspberries, strawberries, cranberries, walnuts, pecans, pomegranates	
Monterpenes	Oranges, lemons, grapefruit, cherries	
Organosulfides		
Isothiocyanates, indoles, allylic sulfur compounds	Garlic, onions, leeks, cruciferous vegetables (broccoli, cauliflower, cabbage, kale, bok choy, collard and mustard greens)	Antioxidant effects; may improve immune system functioning and reduce the risk of heart disease
Alkaloids		
Caffeine	Coffee, tea, kola nuts, cocoa	Stimulant effects
Glycosides		
Saponins	Chickpeas, beans, oats, grapes, olives, spinach, garlic, quinoa	May kill certain microbes, inhibit certain cancers, and reduce risk of heart disease
Capsaicinoids		
Capsaicin	Chili peppers	May provide some pain relief
Fructooligosaccharides		
	Onions, bananas, asparagus, wheat	May stimulate the growth of beneficial bacteria in the human intestinal tract

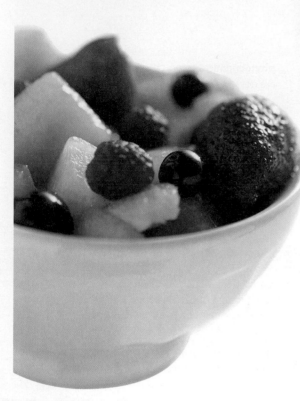

In general, fruits are rich sources of phytochemicals.

1.2 Factors That Influence Your Health

As mentioned in the opener of this chapter, poor eating habits contribute to several of the leading causes of death in the United States. The graph shown in Figure 1.3 illustrates the 10 leading causes of deaths and the percentages of deaths that were attributed to each of them in 2009. Note that heart disease is the leading cause of death for all Americans, and cancer is the second leading cause of death. In 2009, these two diseases accounted for almost 50% of all deaths.[5]

Conditions such as heart disease and cancer are *chronic* diseases. Chronic diseases usually take many years to develop and have complex causes. A **risk factor** is a personal characteristic that increases your chances of developing a chronic disease. For example, genetic background or family history is an important risk factor for heart disease. If your father's father had a heart attack before he was 55 years old and your mother is being treated for having a high blood cholesterol level (a risk factor for heart disease), your family history indicates you have a higher-than-average risk of having a heart attack. For many people, however, having a family history of a chronic disease does not mean that they definitely will develop the condition. Other risk factors that contribute to health are age, environmental conditions, psychological factors, access to health care, and lifestyle practices.

Lifestyle is a person's way of living that includes dietary practices, physical activity habits, use of drugs such as tobacco and alcohol, and other typical patterns of behavior. Your lifestyle may increase or reduce your chances of developing a chronic disease or delay its occurrence for years, even decades. Poor diet, cigarette smoking, and excess alcohol consumption, for example, are risk factors that increase the likelihood of heart disease, stroke, and many forms of cancer (see Fig. 1.3). Cigarette smoking is the primary cause of preventable cancer deaths, but dietary habits and physical activity patterns also contribute to the development of certain cancers.[6,7] Additionally, poor diet and lack of physical activity can result in *obesity*, a condition characterized by the accumulation of too much body fat. Obesity is a risk factor for numerous health problems, including heart disease, certain cancers, type 2 diabetes, and *hypertension* (chronic high blood pressure).

Americans may dramatically reduce their risk of heart disease, cancer, and many other serious chronic diseases by exercising regularly, maintaining a healthy body weight, avoiding tobacco exposure, limiting alcohol intake, and eating fruits, vegetables, and

risk factor personal characteristic that increases a person's chances of developing a disease

lifestyle way of living

Figure 1.3 Ten leading causes of U.S. deaths (preliminary data, 2009). Lifestyle factors contribute to many of the 10 leading causes of death in the United States.

Ten Leading Causes of U.S. Death (Preliminary Data, 2009)

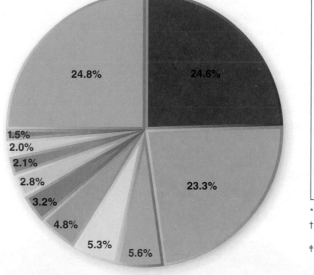

24.8% · 24.6% · 23.3% · 1.5% · 2.0% · 2.1% · 2.8% · 3.2% · 4.8% · 5.3% · 5.6%

- Heart disease*†‡
- Cancer*†‡
- Chronic lower respiratory infections‡
- Stroke*†‡
- Accidents†
- Alzheimer's disease*
- Diabetes*
- Influenza and pneumonia
- Kidney disease*†
- Suicide
- All other causes

* Causes of death in which diet plays a part

† Causes of death in which excessive alcohol consumption plays a part

‡ Causes of death in which tobacco plays a part

whole-grain cereals. Chapter 5 discusses diabetes, and Chapter 6 explains the role of diet and other lifestyle factors in the development of heart disease and hypertension. The Chapter 8 Highlight takes a closer look at the diet and cancer connection. Chapter 10 (Energy Balance and Weight Control) provides information about obesity.

Our Changing Eating Habits

Americans' diets have changed considerably over the past 40 years.[1] Today, we eat less red meat and eggs, and more fish and poultry, than in 1970. Our diet supplies more grain and cereal products than in 1970, but *refined* grain foods, especially white bread, corn chips, and pasta, make up the majority of these products. In general, the more refined a food is, the more processing it has undergone before it reaches your plate, and as a result, the food has lost vitamins, minerals, and other beneficial natural substances. Compared to past years, Americans are eating additional servings of fruit, but many people do not consume enough to meet recommended amounts. Despite the wide variety of fruit available throughout the year, we generally limit our choices to orange juice, bananas, and apples. Today, Americans eat higher amounts of vegetables than in the past, but our choices also tend to lack variety. Almost 50% of the typical American's daily vegetable intake is from iceberg lettuce, French fries, fresh potatoes, potato chips, and canned tomatoes.

Over the past 60 years, our per capita milk and carbonated soft drink consumption patterns have changed dramatically (Table 1.4). In 1947, Americans drank over three and a half times more milk than carbonated soft drinks.[8] By 2008–2009, our milk consumption had declined by over 60% and our soft drink consumption had increased by over 300%.[8,9] Sugar-sweetened soft drinks may contribute to unwanted weight gain[10] and replace more nutrient-rich beverages in diets.

Today, the typical American consumes more fat, sugar, and total food energy than in 1970.[11] If a person's energy intake is more than needed, especially for physical activity, his or her body fat increases. Nationwide surveys indicate that Americans are fatter than in previous decades. Dietary practices, however, should not receive all the blame for this unhealthy finding; during the same period, we have become increasingly dependent on various labor-saving gadgets and machines that make our lives easier but also reduce the amount of energy we need to expend. Chapter 10 examines weight management in detail.

Healthy People

Since the late 1970s, health promotion and disease prevention have been the focus of public health efforts in the United States. A primary focus of such efforts is developing educational programs that can help people prevent chronic and infectious diseases, birth defects, and other serious health problems. In many instances, it is more practical and less expensive to prevent a serious health condition than to treat it.

Healthy People 2010, a report issued in 2000 by the U.S. Department of Health and Human Services (DHHS), included 467 specific national health promotion and disease prevention objectives that were to be met by 2010. The main goals of **Healthy People 2010** were to promote healthful lifestyles and reduce preventable death and disability among Americans.

In early 2011, the U.S. Department of Health and Human Services (DHHS) issued *Healthy People 2020*, a report that includes national health promotion and disease prevention objectives to be met by 2020. The "vision" of *Healthy People 2020* is "A society in

Did You Know?

Your genetic makeup influences the effects of diet on your health as well as disease susceptibility. *Nutritional genomics* or *nutrigenomics* is a relatively new area of nutrition research that explores complex interactions among gene functioning, diet and other lifestyle choices, and the environment.

TABLE 1.4 *Milk and Carbonated Soft Drink Consumption: Then and Now*

	1970 Gallons/Person	2008–2009 Gallons/Person
Milk	39.9	14.6
Carbonated soft drinks	11.0	46.0

Did You Know?

Overall, the health status of minorities lags behind that of the rest of the U.S. population. Efforts to improve the health of minorities is a major focus of *Healthy People 2020* nutrition-related programs.

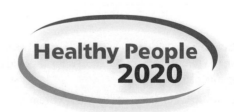

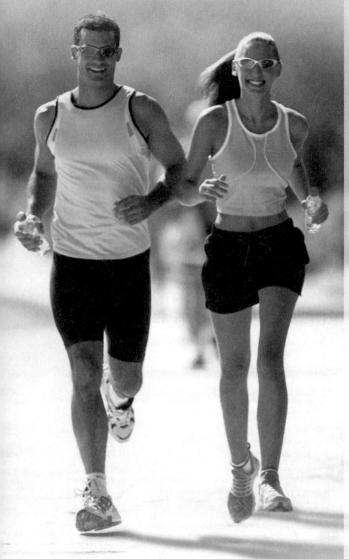

 TABLE 1.5 *Some Healthy People 2020 Objectives: Nutrition and Weight Status (NWS)*

Goal: Promote health and reduce chronic disease associated with diet and weight.

Goal Number	Objective's Short Title
NWS 8	Healthy weight in adults
NWS 9	Obesity in adults
NWS 10	Obesity in children and adolescents
NWS 14	Fruit intake
NWS 15	Vegetable intake
NWS 16	Whole grain intake
NWS 17	Solid fat and added sugar intake
NWS 18	Saturated fat intake
NWS 19	Sodium intake
NWS 20	Calcium intake
NWS 21	Iron deficiency in young children and in females of childbearing age
NWS 22	Iron deficiency in pregnant females

which all people live long, healthy lives."[12] *Healthy People 2020* goals encourage Americans to:

- Attain higher quality, longer lives that are free of preventable disease, disability, injury, and premature death
- Achieve health equity by eliminating disparities to improve the health of all groups
- Create social and physical environments that promote good health for all
- Promote quality of life, healthy development, and healthy behaviors across all life stages.

Healthy People 2020 has several major nutrition-related objectives, some of which are listed in Table 1.5. You can access more information about these objectives at the government's website (http://www.healthypeople.gov/2020/topicsobjectives2020/default.aspx).

Did You Know?

The average daily energy intake of individual adult Americans increased from 1803 Calories in 1977–1978 to 2374 Calories in 2003–2006.[13] This change represents about a 32% increase in the average person's daily energy intake.

Concept **Checkpoint**

8. What is a risk factor?
9. Explain how your lifestyle can affect your health.
10. Discuss how Americans' eating habits have changed since the mid-1900s.
11. Identify at least one main objective of *Healthy People 2020*.

kilocalorie or **Calorie** heat energy needed to raise the temperature of 1 liter of water 1° Celsius; measure of food energy

macronutrients nutrients needed in gram amounts daily and that provide energy; carbohydrates, proteins, and fats

micronutrients vitamins and minerals

 ## 1.3 Metrics for Nutrition

Scientists classify specific nutrients according to their chemical composition and major functions in the body. Nutrients can also be classified based on how much of them are in food. Americans usually refer to length in terms of inches and feet, weight in pounds, and amounts of food in familiar household measures (e.g., teaspoons, tablespoons, cups). Scientists, however, generally use metric values to report length (*meter*), weight (*gram*), and volume (*liter*). The following section provides a basic review of the metric system. Appendix A provides common English-to-metric and metric-to-household unit conversions.

Metric Basics

The metric prefixes *micro-*, *milli-*, *deci-*, *centi-*, and *kilo-* indicate whether a measurement is a fraction or a multiple of a meter (m), gram (g), or liter (l or L) (Table 1.6).

There are approximately 2.54 centimeters (cm) per inch. To obtain your approximate height in centimeters, multiply your height in inches by 2.54. For example, a person who is 5′5″ in height (65″) measures about 165 cm (65 × 2.54) in length. There are approximately 28 g in an ounce and 454 g in a pound. A kilogram (*kilo* = 1000) equals 1000 g or about 2.2 pounds. To determine your weight in kilograms (kg), divide your weight in pounds by 2.2. A person who weighs 130 pounds, for example, weighs about 59 kg.

Assume that a small raisin weighs 1 gram. If you cut this raisin into 1000 equal pieces, then each piece weighs 1 milligram (*milli* = 1000). Thus, 1000 milligrams (mg) equal 1 gram (g). Imagine cutting a small raisin into 1 million equal pieces. Each piece of raisin would weigh 1-millionth of a gram, or a microgram (mcg or μg). Amounts of nutrients in blood are often reported as the number of milligrams or micrograms of the substance per deciliter of blood. For example, a normal blood glucose level for a healthy fasting person is 90 milligrams/deciliter (90 mg/dl).

What's a Calorie?

Running, sitting, studying—your body uses energy even while sleeping. Every cell in your body needs energy to carry out its various activities. As long as you are alive, you are constantly using energy. You are probably familiar with the term *calorie*, the unit that describes the energy content of food. A calorie is the heat energy necessary to raise the temperature of 1 g (1 ml) of water 1° Celsius (C). A calorie is such a small unit of measurement, the amount of energy in food is reported in 1000-calorie units called kilocalories or Calories. Thus, a **kilocalorie** (kcal) or **Calorie** is the heat energy needed to raise the temperature of 1000 g (a liter) of water 1° Celsius (C). A small apple, for example, supplies 40,000 calories or 40 kcal or 40 Calories. If no number of kilocalories is specified, it is appropriate to use "calories." In this textbook, the term "kilocalories" (kcal) is interchangeable with "food energy" or simply "energy."

A gram of carbohydrate and a gram of protein each supply about 4 kcal; a gram of fat provides about 9 kcal (Fig. 1.4). Although alcohol is not a nutrient, it does provide energy; a gram of pure alcohol furnishes 7 kcal. If you know how many grams of carbohydrate, protein, fat, and/or alcohol are in a food, you can estimate the number of kilocalories it provides. For example, if a serving of food contains 10 g of carbohydrate and 5 g of fat, multiply 10 by 4 (the number of kcal each gram of carbohydrate supplies). Then multiply 5 by 9 (the number of kcal each gram of fat supplies). By adding the two values (40 kcal from carbohydrate and 45 kcal from fat), you will determine that this food provides 85 kcal/serving.

Macronutrients and Micronutrients

Carbohydrates, fats, and proteins are referred to as **macronutrients** because the body needs relatively large amounts (grams) of these nutrients daily. Vitamins and minerals are **micronutrients**, because the body needs very small amounts (milligrams or micrograms) of them to function properly. In general, a serving of food supplies grams of carbohydrate, fat, and protein and milligram or microgram quantities of vitamins and minerals. It is important to understand that macronutrients supply energy for cells, whereas micronutrients do not. Although the body requires large amounts of water, this nutrient provides no energy and is not usually classified as a macronutrient.

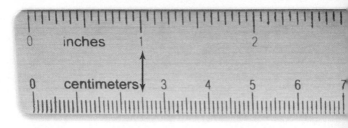

TABLE 1.6 *Common Metric Prefixes in Nutrition*

kilo- (k) = one thousand	
deci- (d) = one-tenth (0.1)	
centi- (c) = one-hundredth (0.01)	
milli- (m) = one-thousandth (0.001)	
micro- (mc or μ) = one-millionth	

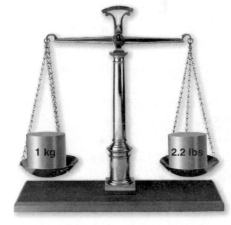

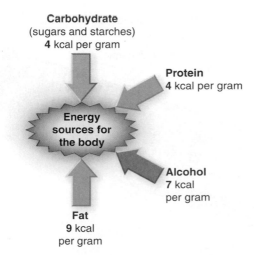

Carbohydrate
(sugars and starches)
4 kcal per gram

Protein
4 kcal per gram

Energy sources for the body

Alcohol
7 kcal per gram

Fat
9 kcal per gram

Figure 1.4 Energy sources for the body. Most forms of carbohydrate supply 4 kcal/g; protein also provides 4 kcal/g. Fat supplies 9 kcal/g, and alcohol (a nonnutrient) provides 7 kcal/g.

Amounts of nutrients present in different foods vary widely, and even the same food from the same source can contain different amounts of nutrients. Therefore, food composition tables and nutrient analysis software generally indicate average amounts of nutrients in foods. By using these tools, however, you can obtain approximate values for each nutrient measured and estimate your nutrient intake.

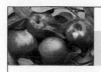

Concept **Checkpoint**

12. Scientists generally use which metric values to report volume, weight, and length?
13. A person weighs 154 pounds. How many kilograms does this person weigh?
14. A slice of whole-wheat bread supplies approximately 13 g of carbohydrate, 1 g of fat, 3 g of protein, and 11 g of water. Based on this information, estimate the number of kilocalories this food provides.
15. Which nutrients are classified as macronutrients? Which are classified as micronutrients?

1.4 Key Nutrition Concepts

Before learning about the nutrients and their roles in health, it is important to grasp some key basic nutrition concepts (Table 1.7). The content in the chapters that follow will build upon these key concepts and can help you make more informed choices concerning your dietary practices.

Concept 1: Most Naturally Occurring Foods Are Mixtures of Nutrients

Which foods do you think of when you hear the words "protein" or "carbohydrate"? You probably identify meat, milk, and eggs as sources of protein; and potatoes, bread, and candy as sources of carbohydrate. Most naturally occurring foods, however, are mixtures of nutrients. In many instances, water is the major nutrient in foods. For example, an 8-fluid-ounce serving of fat-free milk is about 91% water by weight, but it is an excellent source of protein and supplies carbohydrate, very little fat, and several vitamins and minerals. A 6-ounce plain white potato baked in its skin is 75% water and only about 23% carbohydrate by weight. The baked potato also supplies iron and potassium (minerals) and vitamins C and niacin. About half the weight of a slice of whole-wheat bread is carbohydrate, but slightly over one-third of its weight is water. The bread also contains protein, fat, and some vitamins and minerals.

You may be surprised to learn that many sweet snacks are sources of nutrients other than sugar, a carbohydrate. Although sugar comprises about 44% of the weight of a chocolate with almonds candy bar, over one-third of the sweet snack's energy is from fat. The candy bar also contains small amounts of protein, iron, calcium, vitamin A, and the B-vitamin riboflavin. Figure 1.5 compares the energy, water, protein, carbohydrate, fat, and calcium contents of a 6-ounce baked potato, a slice of whole-wheat bread, 8 ounces of fat-free milk, and a 1.45-ounce chocolate and almond candy bar. If you have access to the Internet, you can find information about the energy and nutrient contents of foods by using "What's in the Foods You Eat Search Tool" at the U.S. Department of Agriculture's website: www.ars.usda.gov/Services/docs.htm?docid=17032.

Concept 2: Balance and Variety Can Help Ensure the Nutritional Adequacy of a Diet

No natural food is "perfect" in that it contains all nutrients in amounts that are needed by the body. To help ensure the nutritional adequacy of your diet, choose a *balanced*

TABLE 1.7

Key Basic Nutrition Concepts

- Most naturally occurring foods are mixtures of nutrients.
- Balance and variety can help ensure the nutritional adequacy of a diet.
- There are no "good" or "bad" foods.
- Enjoy eating all foods in moderation.
- For each nutrient, there is a range of safe intake.
- Food is the best source of nutrients and phytochemicals.
- There is no "one size fits all" approach to planning a nutritionally adequate diet.
- Foods and the nutrients they contain are not cure-alls.
- Malnutrition includes *under*nutrition as well as *over*nutrition.
- Nutrition is a dynamic science.

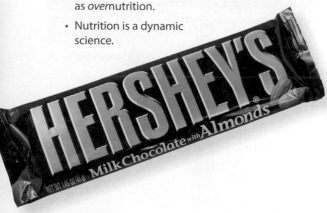

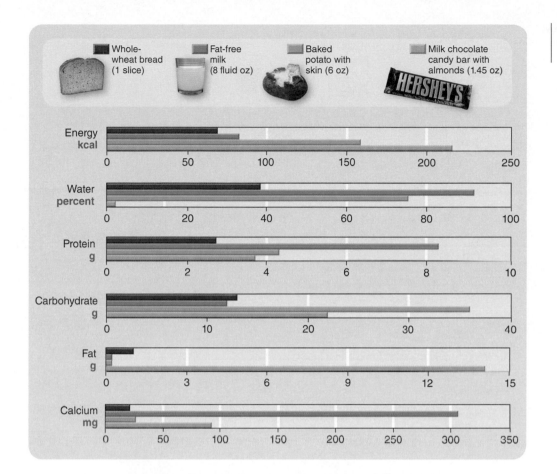

Figure 1.5 Energy and nutrient comparison. These foods contribute very different amounts of energy, water, protein, carbohydrate, fat, and calcium to diets.

diet that contains foods from each food group, including fruits, low-fat or fat-free dairy products, and whole grains. Furthermore, select a *variety* of foods from each food group. To make menu planning more interesting and dishes more appealing, try unfamiliar foods and new recipes for preparing your usual fare. Chapter 3 (Planning Nutritious Diets) provides information about the food groups and practical menu planning tools, such as the MyPlate plan. MyPlate is a personalized approach to menu planning that can help you incorporate a variety of foods from all food groups into your daily diet.

Concept 3: There Are No "Good" or "Bad" Foods

Are some foods "good" and others "bad" for your body? If you think there are such foods, which ones are good and which are bad? Do you sometimes feel guilty about eating "junk foods"? What is a junk food? Should pizza, chips, candy, doughnuts, ice cream, and sugar-sweetened soft drinks be classified as junk food?

No food deserves the label of "bad" or "junk," because all foods have nutritional value. For example, many people think pumpkin pie is a junk food. Pumpkin pie, however, is a good source of protein, the mineral iron, and the phytochemical beta-carotene that the body can convert to vitamin A. Even sugar-sweetened soft drinks provide water and the carbohydrate sugar, a source of energy. Although pies, doughnuts, and ice cream contain a lot of fat and sugar, these foods also supply small amounts of protein, vitamins, and minerals to diets.

Some foods and beverages, such as bacon, candy, pastries, snack chips, and alcoholic or sugar-sweetened drinks, are described as sources of "empty calories." An **empty-calorie** food contributes a large portion of its energy from *solid fat, added sugar,* and/or alcohol in relation to its supply of micronutrients. People should limit their intake of empty-calorie foods. Consuming too much food energy in relation to one's needs can result in depositing excess body fat. Furthermore, eating too many empty-calorie foods may displace more nutritious foods from the diet. Chapter 3 provides more information about empty-calorie foods.

empty-calorie describes food or beverage that is a poor source of micronutrients in relation to its energy value

Pumpkin pie is a good source of beta-carotene, a substance the body can convert to vitamin A. Because the pie is made with eggs and milk, this holiday favorite is also a good source of protein.

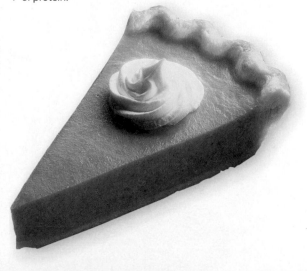

Figure 1.6 Comparing foods. This graph compares energy contents and amounts of key nutrients in 8-fluid-ounce servings of fat-free milk and sugar-sweetened soft drink. Although the two beverages have similar calorie contents, milk contains vitamins A and riboflavin, considerably more protein, and the minerals calcium and phosphorus.

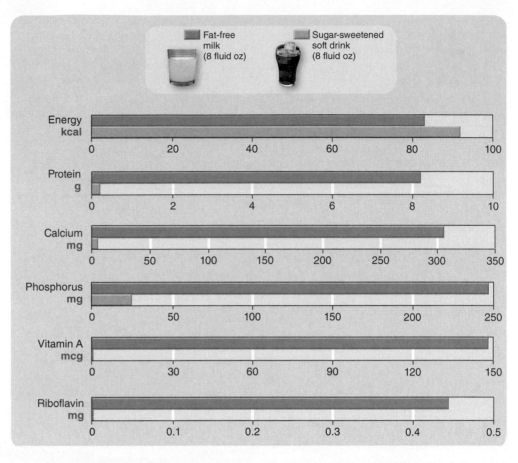

nutrient-dense describes food or beverage that has more vitamins and minerals in relation to its energy value

Certain foods are more nutritious than others. A **nutrient-dense** food contains more vitamins and minerals in relation to its fat, sugar, and/or alcohol contents. Broccoli, leafy greens, fat-free milk, orange juice, lean meats, and whole-grain cereals are examples of nutrient-dense foods. Figure 1.6 compares the nutritional values of 8-fluid-ounce servings of a cola-type soft drink and fat-free milk. Note that milk supplies water, protein, and certain vitamins and minerals, whereas cola supplies water and carbohydrate but is a poor source of protein and micronutrients. A nutritionally balanced diet contains a variety of nutrient-dense foods. Therefore, you should focus on eating nutrient-dense foods to improve the nutrient content of your diet.

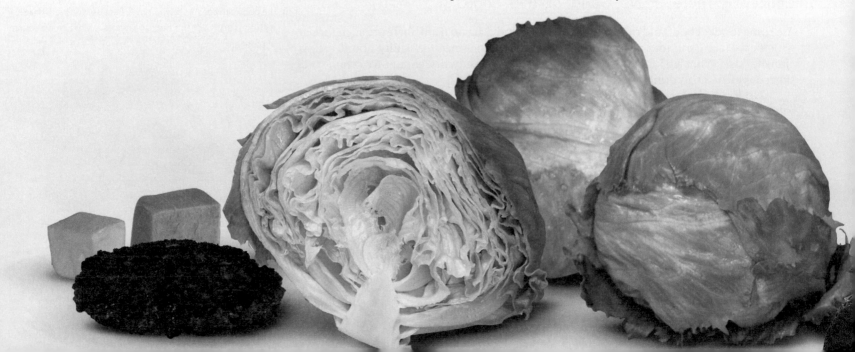

Energy density describes the energy value of a food in relation to the food's weight. For example, a chocolate, cake-type frosted doughnut that weighs about 2 ounces provides 242 kcal; 5 medium strawberries also weigh about 2 ounces, but they provide only 19 kcal. You would have to eat nearly 64 of the strawberries to obtain the same amount of food energy that is in the chocolate doughnut. Therefore, the doughnut is an energy-dense food in comparison to the berries. In general, high-fat foods such as doughnuts are energy dense because they are concentrated sources of energy. Most fruits are not energy dense, because they contain far more water than fat.

Figure 1.7 compares a group of foods that supply similar amounts of calories but differ in their energy densities. It is important to note that not all energy-dense foods are empty-calorie foods. Nuts, for example, are high in fat and, therefore, energy dense. However, nuts are also nutrient dense because they contribute protein, vitamins, minerals, and fiber to diets. Most forms of fiber are classified as carbohydrates.

A food *is* bad for you if it contains toxic substances or is contaminated with bacteria, viruses, or microscopic animals that cause food-borne illness. You have probably suffered from a food-borne illness at least once. The abdominal cramps, nausea, vomiting, and diarrhea that usually accompany a food-borne illness occur within a few hours or days after eating the contaminated food. Chapter 12 (Food Safety Concerns) focuses on food safety concerns, including major types of food-borne illnesses and how to prevent them.

Concept 4: Enjoy Eating All Foods in Moderation

Dietary **moderation** involves obtaining enough nutrients from food to meet one's needs while avoiding excessive amounts and balancing calorie intake with calorie expenditure, primarily by physical activity. This can be accomplished by choosing nutrient-dense foods, limiting serving sizes, and incorporating moderate- to vigorous-intensity physical activities into your daily routine. Although moderation requires planning meals and setting aside time for physical activity daily, it can help you achieve your health and fitness goals. If, for example, you overeat during a meal or snack, you can regain dietary moderation and balance by eating less food and exercising more intensely during the next 24 hours.

The diets of many Americans contain excessive amounts of empty-calorie foods in relation to nutrient-dense foods. However, eliminating all empty-calorie foods from your diet is not generally recommended or necessary. If your core diet is comprised primarily of nutrient-dense foods and meets your nutritional needs, including some empty-calorie items adds enjoyment to living when they are consumed in moderation. Physically active individuals, such as athletes in training programs, often find it difficult to consume enough energy from foods to sustain healthy body weights, unless they include some empty-calorie items in their diets.

Concept 5: For Each Nutrient, There Is a Range of Safe Intake

By eating a variety of nutrient-dense foods, you are likely to obtain adequate and safe amounts of each nutrient. The **physiological dose** of a nutrient is the amount that is within the range of safe intake and enables the body to function optimally. Consuming

energy density energy value of a food in relation to the food's weight

moderation obtaining adequate amounts of nutrients while balancing calorie intake with calorie expenditure

physiological dose amount of a nutrient that is within the range of safe intake and enables the body to function optimally

When a diet meets nutritional needs, including some empty-calorie items adds enjoyment when such foods are consumed in moderation.

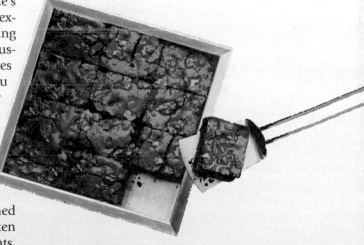

Figure 1.7 Energy density. Although each of these portions of food supplies about 200 kcal, they differ in their energy densities. For example, you would need to eat over 4 cups of whole strawberries to consume the same amount of energy in a 3-ounce hamburger patty.

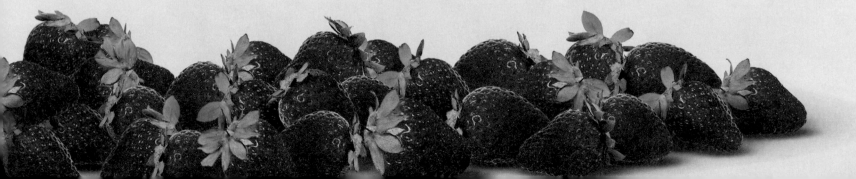

megadose generally defined as 10 times the recommended amount of a vitamin or mineral

Figure 1.8 Intake continuum. For each nutrient, there is a range of safe intake.

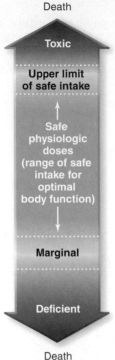

Death

Toxic

Upper limit of safe intake

Safe physiologic doses (range of safe intake for optimal body function)

Marginal

Deficient

Death

less than the physiological dose can result in marginal nutritional status. In other words, the person's body has just enough of the nutrient to function adequately, but that amount is not sufficient to overcome the added stress of infection or injury. If a person's nutrient intake falls below the marginal level, the individual is at risk of developing the nutrient's deficiency disease. For example, the recommended amounts of the B-vitamin niacin are 16 mg for men and 14 mg for women. People whose diets contain little or no niacin are at risk of developing *pellagra*, the vitamin's deficiency disease.

Most people require physiological amounts of micronutrients. A **megadose** is generally defined as an amount of a vitamin or mineral that is at least 10 times the recommended amount of the nutrient.[14] When taken in high amounts, many vitamins behave like drugs and can produce unpleasant and even toxic side effects. For example, physicians sometimes use megadoses of the B-vitamin niacin to treat high blood cholesterol levels, but such amounts may cause painful facial flushing and liver damage. Megadoses of vitamin C can cause intestinal upsets and diarrhea; consuming extremely high amounts of vitamin A can even be deadly. Minerals have very narrow ranges of safe intakes.

Many consumers take megadoses of vitamin and/or mineral supplements without consulting physicians, because they think the micronutrients will prevent or treat ailments such as the common cold or heart disease. For most people, consuming amounts of nutrients that exceed what is necessary for good health is economically wasteful and could be harmful to the body. "More is not always better," when it relates to optimal nutrition.

In their natural states, most commonly eaten foods do not contain toxic levels of vitamins and minerals. You probably do not need to worry about consuming toxic levels of micronutrients, unless you are taking megadoses of vitamin/mineral supplements or eating large amounts of foods that are fortified with these nutrients regularly. The diagram shown in Figure 1.8 illustrates the general concept of deficient, safe, and toxic intake ranges for nutrients such as vitamins and minerals. Chapters 8 and 9 provide more information about micronutrients, including deficiencies and toxicities.

Concept 6: Food Is the Best Source of Nutrients and Phytochemicals

The most natural, reliable, and economical way to obtain nutrients and beneficial phytochemicals is to base your diet on a variety of "whole" and minimally processed foods. Plant foods naturally contain a variety of nutrients and phytochemicals, but processing the foods often removes some of the most healthful parts. For example, a whole-wheat kernel is stripped of its germ and outer hull (bran) during refinement into white flour (Fig. 1.9). Wheat germ is a rich source of vitamin E and beneficial lipids. Wheat bran contains fiber and certain phytochemicals, and it is a concentrated source of micronutrients. The endosperm that remains is primarily *starch* (a form of carbohydrate) with some

Figure 1.9 What is white flour? During refinement, a wheat kernel is stripped of its nutrient-rich germ and bran. The endosperm (white flour) that remains is mostly starch.

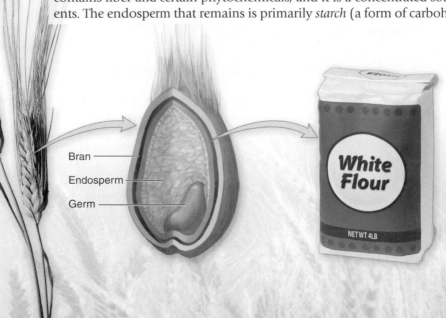

Bran

Endosperm

Germ

White Flour

NET WT 4LB

protein and very small amounts of micronutrients and fiber. By replacing refined grain products, such as white bread, with whole-grain products, you can increase the likelihood of obtaining a wide variety of nutrients and phytochemicals.

In addition to eating food, many people take nutrient supplements in the form of pills, powders, bars, wafers, or beverages. The human body, however, is designed to obtain nutrients from foods, not supplements. In some instances, nutrients from food are more available, that is, more easily digested and absorbed, than those in supplements.

It is important to understand that nutrient supplements do not contain everything one needs for optimal nutrition. For example, they do not contain the wide variety of phytochemicals found in plant foods. Although supplements that contain phytochemicals are available, they may not provide the same healthful benefits as consuming the plants that contain these compounds. Why? Nutrients and phytochemicals may need to be consumed together to provide the desirable effects in the body. Food naturally contains combinations of these chemicals in very small amounts and certain proportions. There is nothing "natural" about gulping down handfuls of supplements.

A few individuals have inherited defects that increase their needs for certain nutrients, particularly vitamins. People who have chronic illnesses, digestive disorders that interfere with nutrient absorption, and certain inherited disorders may also require supplemental nutrients. Additionally, many older adults may need higher amounts of vitamins and other nutrients than those found in food. Because it is often difficult to plan and eat nutritious menus each day, taking a supplement that contains a variety of vitamins may be advisable, even for healthy adults.[15] In general, there appears to be little danger in taking a *multivitamin/multimineral supplement* that provides 100% of recommended amounts of the micronutrients daily.[16] However, healthy adults should consider taking such supplements as an "insurance policy" and not a substitute for eating a variety of nutrient-dense foods.

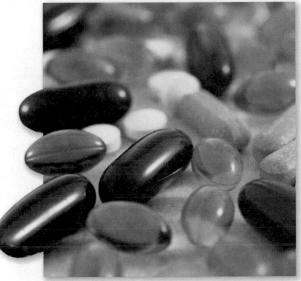

Dietary supplements should not be considered substitutes for nutrient-dense food.

Concept 7: There Is No "One Size Fits All" Approach to Planning a Nutritionally Adequate Diet

By using food guides presented in Chapter 3, you can individualize your diet so that it is nutritionally adequate and suits your food likes and dislikes, budget, and lifestyle. Individualizing a diet does not mean only eating foods that "match" your blood type, hair color, personality, or shoe size. If someone promotes a diet based on such personal traits, steer clear of the diet and the promoter. Consider this: Human beings would not have survived as a species for thousands of years if their diets had to be matched to physical characteristics or personalities.

Physicians often prescribe special diets, sometimes referred to as *medical nutrition therapies*, for people with chronic health conditions such as diabetes. Even the nutritional needs of healthy people vary during different stages of their lives. Chapter 13 (Nutrition for a Lifetime) provides information about the importance of diet during pregnancy, childhood, and other stages of the life cycle.

Concept 8: Foods and the Nutrients They Contain Are Not Cure-Alls

Although specific nutrient deficiency diseases, such as scurvy, can be cured by eating foods that contain the nutrient that is missing or in short supply, nutrients do not "cure" other ailments. Diet is only one aspect of a person that influences his or her health. By making certain dietary changes, however, a person may be able to prevent or forestall the development of certain diseases, or possibly lessen their severity if they occur.

Although there is no legal definition for "*functional foods*," such products have health-related purposes.[17] Functional foods are often manufactured to boost nutrient intakes or help manage specific health problems. For example, consumers who want to increase their calcium intake can purchase orange juice that has the mineral added to it. Certain margarine substitutes contain phytochemicals that interfere with the body's ability to absorb

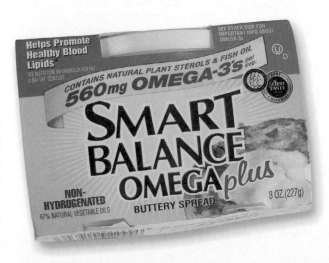

cholesterol from food and, as a result, may lower the risk of heart disease. Many yogurt products contain specific forms of live bacteria that may relieve diarrhea. These bacteria are *probiotics*, that is, microorganisms that can benefit human health. Although some functional foods can help Americans improve their health, more research is needed to determine their benefits as well as possible harmful effects.

Concept 9: Malnutrition Includes *Under*nutrition as Well as *Over*nutrition

Malnutrition is a state of health that occurs when the body is improperly nourished. Everyone must consume food and water to stay alive, yet despite the abundance and variety of nutritious foods, many Americans consume nutritionally poor diets and suffer from malnutrition as a result. Some people select nutritionally inadequate diets because they lack knowledge about nutritious foods or the importance of nutrition to health. Low-income people, however, are at risk for malnutrition because they have limited financial resources for making wise food purchases. Other people who are at risk of malnutrition include those who have severe eating disorders, are addicted to drugs such as alcohol, or have certain serious medical problems. The Chapter 1 Highlight discusses the international problem of *under*nutrition.

Although many people associate malnutrition with undernutrition and starvation, *over*nutrition, the long-term excess of energy or nutrient intake, is also a form of malnutrition. Overnutrition is often characterized by obesity. You may be surprised to learn that overnutrition is more common in the United States than undernutrition (Fig. 1.10). Obesity is widespread in countries where most people have the financial means to buy food, have an ample food supply, and obtain little exercise. Chapter 10 provides information about obesity.

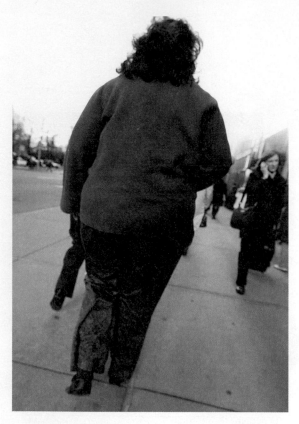

Figure 1.10 Obesity. Obesity is a prevalent nutrition-related health problem in many nations.

malnutrition state of health that occurs when the body is improperly nourished

MY DIVERSE PLATE

Locusts

In parts of Africa, Cambodia, and the Philippines, many people eat locusts, especially when the insects are plentiful. Popular ways to cook locusts include removing the wings and legs before frying with seasonings or placing locusts on skewers and roasting them over hot embers. The legs and wings are removed from the grilled insects before they are cooked or eaten. Over 60% of the dry weight of a locust is protein, so the insect is an excellent source of the macronutrient.
Source: Food and Agricultural Organization, http://www.fao.org/ag/locusts/en/info/info/faq/

Concept 10: Nutrition Is a Dynamic Science

As researchers continue to explore the complex relationships between diets and health, nutrition information constantly evolves. As a result, dietary practices and recommendations undergo revision as new scientific evidence becomes available and is reviewed and accepted by nutrition experts. Unfortunately such changes can be confusing to the general public, who expect medical researchers to provide definite answers to their nutrition-related questions and rigid advice concerning optimal dietary practices.

Even nutrition educators find it difficult to keep up with the vast amount of research articles published in scientific journals. Chapter 2 explains how nutrition research is conducted using scientific methods. Furthermore, Chapter 2 provides information to help you become a better consumer of nutrition and health information that appears in popular sources such as magazines, infomercials, and the Internet.

Concept **Checkpoint**

16. Identify at least five of the key nutrition-related concepts presented in this section.
17. What is the difference between an empty-calorie and a nutrient-dense food?
18. What is the difference between a physiological dose and a megadose of a nutrient?

MALNUTRITION: A WORLDWIDE CONCERN

Malnutrition is a state of health that results from improper nourishment. Chronic undernutrition occurs when long-term energy and nutrient intakes are insufficient to meet an individual's needs. Hunger, the physiological need for food, usually accompanies undernutrition. Throughout the world, social, environmental, economic, political, and other factors contribute to undernutrition (Fig. 1.11). However, undernutrition is a serious problem, particularly in sub-Saharan Africa and certain regions of Asia, where decades of civil unrest, wars, and the AIDS epidemic have left millions of people impoverished and living in uncertainty. Many developing nations in these regions owe large sums of money to wealthy countries. Having high national debts often causes government leaders to reduce or eliminate basic services, including health care and education programs. Furthermore, undernutrition is common among impoverished people in developing countries where food production and supplies are inadequate.

Undernutrition

The world's population is estimated to be over 6.5 billion people. If the present rate of population growth does not slow, an estimated 9 billion people will be living on Earth in 2050.[18] Most of the explosive population growth is occurring in developing countries, where economic growth is unable to keep pace with the rapidly increasing number of people.

In 2009, an estimated 1 billion people were on the brink of starvation.[19] Regional food shortages can result from traditional dietary practices, crop failures, local warfare, and political instability and corruption. Poverty and undernutrition are commonplace in many developing countries. Impoverished people must also cope with infectious diseases, parasitic infestations, overcrowded and unsafe housing conditions, and polluted water supplies. In developing countries, poor sanitation practices and lack of clean cooking and drinking water cause the majority of all diseases and more than one-third of all deaths (Fig. 1.12).

In undernourished children, nutrient deficiencies are responsible for stunted physical growth, delayed physical development, blindness, impaired intellectual development, and premature death. Chronic un-

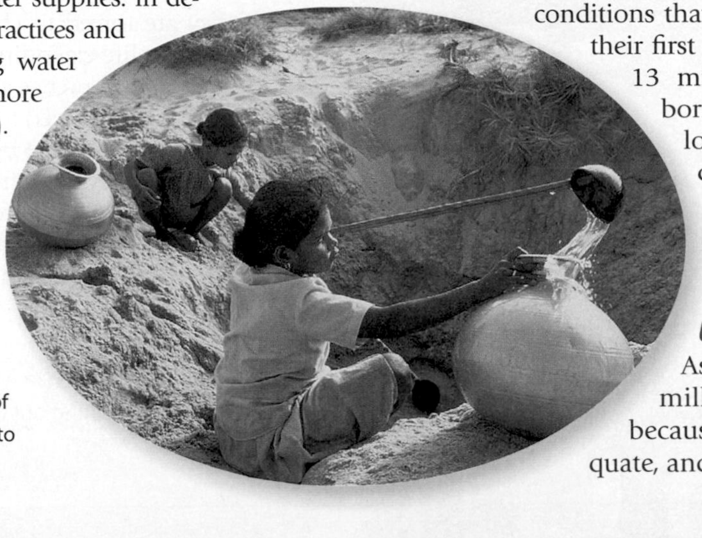

Figure 1.12 Poor sanitation. In developing countries, poor sanitation practices and lack of clean cooking and drinking water contribute to the spread of infectious diseases.

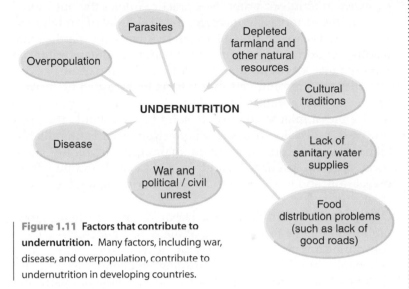

Figure 1.11 Factors that contribute to undernutrition. Many factors, including war, disease, and overpopulation, contribute to undernutrition in developing countries.

dernutrition depresses the body's immune functioning, increasing the risk of death from infectious diseases, such as measles, especially in childhood. Each year, maternal and child undernutrition contribute to 3.5 million deaths; nutrition-related factors such as undernutrition and vitamin A deficiency are responsible for 35% of deaths in children under 5 years of age.[20] The vast majority of childhood deaths associated with undernutrition occur among poor populations in developing countries, particularly in Africa and Southeast Asia.[21]

Undernutrition During Pregnancy Undernutrition can be very harmful when it occurs during periods of rapid growth, such as pregnancy, infancy, and childhood. Women who are undernourished during pregnancy are more likely to die while giving birth than pregnant women who are adequately nourished. Furthermore, malnourished pregnant women have a high risk of giving birth to infants that are born too soon. These babies often suffer from breathing problems and have low birth weights—conditions that increase their risk of dying during their first year of life. Each year, an estimated 13 million low-birth-weight infants are born in the world.[22] The vast majority of low-birth-weight infants are born in developing countries. Chapter 13 provides more information about the importance of adequate nutrition during pregnancy.

Undernutrition During Infancy As explained in Chapter 13, breast milk is the best food for young infants because it is sanitary, is nutritionally adequate, and provides babies with immunity to some infectious diseases. In developing countries, many new mothers do not exclusively breastfeed their babies for more than a few weeks.[20] Infant formulas are nutritious substitutes for breast milk, but they are generally more expensive. To extend infant formulas, poor parents in developing countries often add excessive amounts of water. This practice dilutes the nutritional value of the formula and increases the likelihood of contaminating it with disease-causing microbes. In infants, the diarrhea that results from drinking formula mixed with unsanitary water can rapidly cause loss of body water (*dehydration*) and death.

Dietitians recommend that infants be breastfed exclusively for the first six months of life. Ideally, babies should continue to receive breast milk in addition to solid foods well into their second year, especially in places where clean water is unavailable. Signs and symptoms of protein malnutrition typically occur soon after impoverished children are weaned abruptly from breast milk and introduced to far less nourishing solid foods.

Undernutrition During the Preschool Years The brain grows rapidly during the first five years of life. When undernutrition occurs during this period, the effects can be devastating to the child's brain and result in permanent learning disabilities. Additionally, chronically undernourished children do not grow normally and tend to be shorter if they survive to adulthood (Fig. 1.13). In the United States and other developed countries, children are usually well nourished and vaccinated against common childhood diseases such as measles. In poorer nations, however, many children are malnourished and not protected from the virus that causes measles. Measles often is a life-threatening illness for malnourished children because their immune systems do not function normally.

Undernutrition in the United States

Undernutrition also occurs in wealthy, developed nations such as the United States. In some instances, undernutrition is not due to

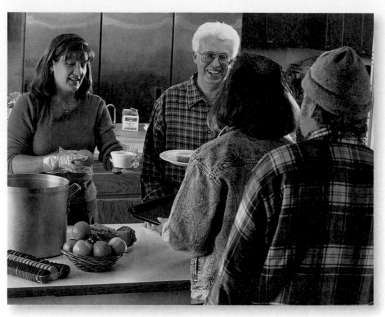

Figure 1.14 Feeding the hungry. In many cities, charities and churches operate food pantries and "soup kitchens" to feed food-insecure people.

poverty in these countries. For example, many people suffering from anorexia nervosa and chronic alcoholism are undernourished despite having the financial resources to purchase food. Nevertheless, Americans with low incomes have a higher risk of malnutrition than members of the population who are in higher income categories. In 2009, about 44 million Americans, or about 14.3% of the population, were living at or below the U.S. Department of Health and Human Services *poverty guideline*.[23] In 2009, this guideline was $21,954 for a family of four. In 2011, the poverty guideline was $22,350 for a family of four.[24] Most American households are *food secure*, which means the people in those households have access to and can purchase sufficient food to lead healthy, active lives. In 2009, **food insecurity** was reported in almost 15% of all households in the United States.[25] Food insecurity describes individuals or families who are concerned about running out of food or not having enough money to buy more food. People who are unemployed, work in low-paying jobs, or have excessive medical and housing expenses often experience food insecurity. Food insecurity may also affect elderly Americans who live on fixed incomes, especially if they are forced to choose between purchasing nutritious food and buying life-extending medications.

Charities and churches in many cities operate food pantries and "soup kitchens" to feed food-insecure people (Fig. 1.14). In addition to the help provided by the private sector, low-income individuals can obtain food aid from federal food assistance programs. Although not every eligible food-insecure person has access to or takes advantage of the aid, federal food assistance programs protect most American children from hunger and undernutrition.

Figure 1.13 Chronic undernutrition. This photograph shows a group of undernourished children outside a Nigerian orphanage during the late 1960s.

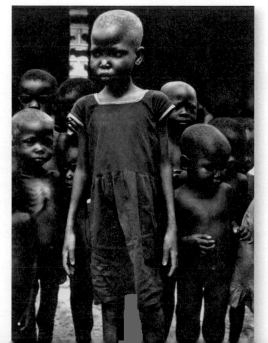

food insecurity situation in which individuals or families are concerned about running out of food or not having enough money to buy more food

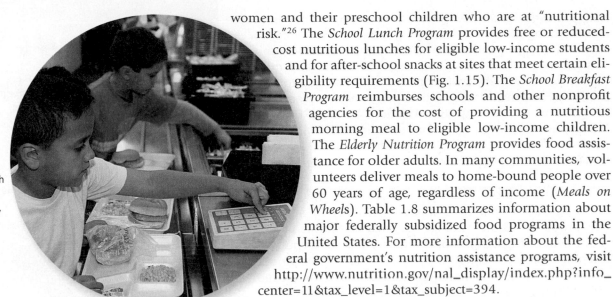

Figure 1.15 School Lunch Program. Any child who attends a school that participates in the School Lunch Program can purchase a nutritious lunch. After selecting from the menu, the child enters his or her personal identification number (PIN) into the device shown in the photo. The device records the purchase and debits the child's school lunch account. By using this system, the program protects the identity of children who receive free or reduced-price lunches.

women and their preschool children who are at "nutritional risk."[26] The *School Lunch Program* provides free or reduced-cost nutritious lunches for eligible low-income students and for after-school snacks at sites that meet certain eligibility requirements (Fig. 1.15). The *School Breakfast Program* reimburses schools and other nonprofit agencies for the cost of providing a nutritious morning meal to eligible low-income children. The *Elderly Nutrition Program* provides food assistance for older adults. In many communities, volunteers deliver meals to home-bound people over 60 years of age, regardless of income (*Meals on Wheels*). Table 1.8 summarizes information about major federally subsidized food programs in the United States. For more information about the federal government's nutrition assistance programs, visit http://www.nutrition.gov/nal_display/index.php?info_center=11&tax_level=1&tax_subject=394.

Major U.S. Food Assistance Programs

The *Supplemental Nutrition Assistance Program* (*SNAP*), formerly known as the Food Stamp Program, enables eligible low-income participants to use a special debit card to purchase food and garden seeds at authorized stores. The *Women, Infants, and Children* program (*WIC*) provides nutrition education and checks or vouchers to purchase specific foods for low-income pregnant and breastfeeding

World Food Crisis: Finding Solutions

Reducing hunger through food aid programs is a major goal of the United Nations. The World Food Program and United Nations Children's Fund (UNICEF) are agencies within the United Nations that provide high-quality food for undernourished populations. UNICEF also supports the development and distribution of

TABLE 1.8 *Major Federally Subsidized Food Programs in the United States*

Program	General Eligibility Requirements	Description
Supplemental Nutrition Assistance Program (SNAP)	Low-income individuals and families	Participants use an electronic benefit transfer (debit) card to purchase allowable food items.
Commodity Distribution Program	Certain low-income groups, including pregnant women, preschool-age children, and the elderly	In some states, state agencies distribute USDA surplus foods to eligible people.
Women, Infants, and Children (WIC)	Low-income pregnant or breastfeeding women, infants, and children under 5 years of age who are at nutritional risk	Participants receive checks or vouchers to purchase milk, cheese, fruit juice, certain cereals, infant formula, and other specific food items at grocery stores. Nutrition education is also provided.
School Lunch and School Breakfast Programs	Low-income children of school age	Certain schools receive subsidies from the government to provide free or reduced-price nutritionally balanced lunches and breakfasts.
Elderly Nutrition Program	Age 60 or older (no income guidelines)	Provides grants for sites to provide nutritious congregate and home-delivered meals.
Child and Adult Care Food Program	Children enrolled in organized childcare programs and seniors in adult care programs	Site receives reimbursement for nutritious meals and snacks supplied to participants.
Food Distribution Program on Indian Reservations	Low-income American Indian or non-Indian households on reservations; members of federally recognized Native American tribes	Distribution of monthly food packages. This program is an alternative to SNAP and includes a nutrition education component.

ready-to-use therapeutic food (*RUTF*) to treat severe undernutrition among young children in developing countries. *Plumpy'nut*, for example, is an energy and nutrient-dense paste made from a mixture of peanuts, powdered milk, oil, sugar, vitamins, and minerals. During processing, the paste is placed in foil packets to keep the food clean and make it easy to transport to remote places without refrigeration. According to United Nations officials, RUTFs such as Plumpy'nut are the "best weapon" to fight severe childhood malnutrition.[27] In 2010, UNICEF supplied nearly 23,000 tons of RUTFs to feed starving children in developing nations.[28]

The Promise of Biotechnology   *Biotechnology* involves the use of living things—plants, animals, microbes—to manufacture new products.[29] Biotechnology in agriculture has led to the development of crops that supply higher yields, resist pests, or are tolerant of drought conditions. By increasing food production or modifying the nutritional content of foods, biotechnology offers another way of alleviating the world food crisis.

Genetic modification methods, such as *genetic engineering*, involve scientific methods that alter an animal or plant's hereditary material (*genes* or DNA). For example, genes that produce a desirable trait are transferred from one organism into the DNA of a second organism, altering its genes. Most of the soybeans and about 40% of the corn grown in the United States are from seeds that were genetically modified (Fig. 1.16). Although these *genetically modified organisms* or *GMOs* are used for feeding livestock, many processed foods manufactured for human consumption also contain ingredients from GMOs.

According to Dr. J. Craig Venter, geneticist and founder of the Institute for Genomic Research, the safety of genetically engineered crops destined for human consumption has been tested extensively.[30] In 2004, a committee of scientists with the National Research Council reported that there was no documented evidence that genetic engineering resulted in human health problems.[29] Some scientists, however, have raised concerns that GMOs introduce new proteins into the food chain, creating the potential for environmental harm. Moreover, certain people who consume foods that contain the new proteins might experience unexpected side effects, such as allergic responses, as a result. Despite these concerns, experts at the U.S. Food and Drug Administration (FDA) think currently approved varieties of genetically engineered foods are safe for human consumption. Nevertheless, more research is needed to determine the long-term safety of GMOs.[29]

In the near future, farmers may find it difficult to sustain a high degree of agricultural productivity as crops and livestock reach their maximum capacity to produce food, particularly as water for irrigation becomes scarce and farmland is used for other purposes, such as housing for the ever-expanding population. Biotechnological advances in agriculture may help reduce the prevalence of undernutrition by increasing livestock production and crop yields in many parts of the world.

genetic modification techniques that alter an organism's DNA

Figure 1.16 Genetically modified corn. This seed corn is the result of genetic engineering.

Taking Action   Poverty and hunger have always plagued humankind; the causes of poverty and hunger are complex and, therefore, difficult to eliminate. Nevertheless, certain social, political, economic, and agricultural changes can reduce the number of people who are chronically hungry. In the short run, wealthy countries can provide food aid to keep impoverished people from starving to death. Families and small farmers in underdeveloped nations need to learn new and more efficient methods of growing, processing, preserving, and distributing nutritious regional food products. Additionally, governments can support programs that encourage breastfeeding and fortify locally grown or commonly consumed foods with vitamins and minerals that are often deficient in local diets.

In the long run, population control is critical for preserving the earth's resources for future generations. Impoverished parents in poor countries often have many children because they expect only a few to survive and reach adulthood. When people are financially secure, adequately nourished, and well educated, they tend to have fewer, healthier children. Thus, long-term ways to slow population growth include providing well-paying jobs, improving public education, and increasing access to health care services.

Although waging a battle against worldwide hunger may seem like a daunting prospect, there are actions you can take to help relieve the problem in your community. You can stimulate student interest by researching the extent of food insecurity in the area and then writing an article about the situation for the campus newspaper. You can help food-insecure people directly by volunteering to prepare or serve food at a soup kitchen or homeless shelter in your community. You can also initiate and coordinate a canned food drive on your campus to benefit a local food pantry.

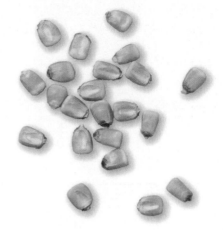

CHAPTER REFERENCES

See Appendix I.

SUMMARY

Lifestyle choices, including poor eating habits and lack of physical activity, contribute to the development of many of the leading causes of premature deaths for American adults, including heart disease, cancer, stroke, and diabetes. However, you may be able to extend your life span and improve your quality of life by applying what you learn about nutrition and the role of diet and health.

There are six classes of nutrients: carbohydrates, lipids, proteins, vitamins, minerals, and water. The body needs certain nutrients for energy, growth and development, and regulation of processes, including the repair and maintenance of cells. The human body can synthesize many nutrients, but about 50 nutrients are dietary essentials that must be supplied by food, because the body does not synthesize the nutrient or make enough to meet its needs.

Plant foods naturally contain a variety of phytochemicals, substances that are not classified as nutrients yet may have healthful benefits. Many phytochemicals are antioxidants that protect cells from being damaged or destroyed by exposure to certain environmental factors. However, some phytochemicals are toxic. The Dietary Supplement Health and Education Act of 1994 (DSHEA) allows manufacturers to classify herbal products and nutrient supplements, including vitamins, minerals, and protein or amino acid preparations, as dietary supplements.

Heart disease is the leading cause of death for all Americans. Chronic diseases, such as heart disease, are complex conditions that have multiple risk factors. A risk factor is a personal characteristic such as family history and lifestyle practices that increases a person's chances of developing diseases. In many instances, people can live longer and healthier by modifying their diets, increasing their physical activity, and altering other aspects of their lifestyles. Objectives to improve the status of Americans' health, including nutrition-related programs, are an important focus of *Healthy People 2020*.

Scientists generally use metric values when measuring volume, weight, and length. The metric prefixes micro-, milli-, deci-, centi-, and kilo- indicate whether a measurement is a fraction or a multiple of a meter, gram, or liter. Approximately 28 g are in an ounce and 454 g are in a pound; a kilogram equals 1000 grams or about 2.2 pounds. Each gram equals 1000 milligrams or 1 million micrograms.

Every cell needs energy. A Calorie is the heat energy needed to raise the temperature of 1 liter of water 1° Celsius (C). Calories or kilocalories (kcal) are used to indicate

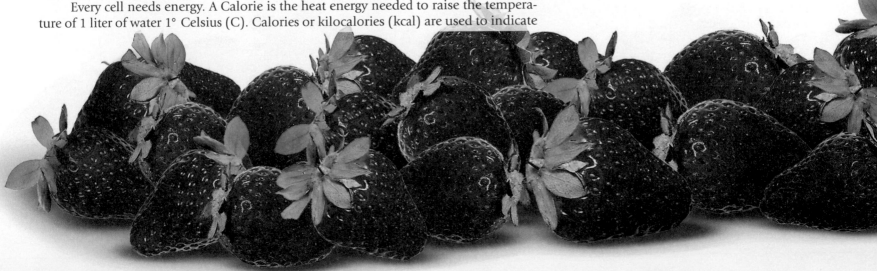

the energy value in food. If no number of kilocalories is specified, it is appropriate to use "calories." A gram of carbohydrate and a gram of protein each supply about 4 kcal; a gram of fat provides about 9 kcal. Although alcohol is not a nutrient, a gram of pure alcohol furnishes 7 kcal.

Carbohydrates, fats, and proteins are referred to as macronutrients because the body needs relatively large amounts of these nutrients daily. Vitamins and minerals are micronutrients, because the body needs very small amounts. Although the body requires large amounts of water, this nutrient provides no energy and is not usually classified as a macronutrient.

There are several key points to understanding nutrition. Most naturally occurring foods are mixtures of nutrients, but no food contains all the nutrients needed for optimal health. Thus, nutritionally adequate diets include a variety of foods from all food groups. Instead of classifying foods as "good" or "bad," people can focus on eating all foods in moderation and limit empty-calorie foods. For each nutrient, there is a range of safe intake. Healthy people should rely on eating a variety of foods to meet their nutrient needs instead of taking dietary supplements. Although nutrients are vital to good health, foods and the nutrients they contain are not cure-alls. There is no "one size fits all" approach to planning a nutritionally adequate diet. Malnutrition is not simply starvation; the term includes overnutrition as well as undernutrition. Finally, nutrition is a dynamic science; new scientific information about nutrients and their roles in health is constantly emerging. Therefore, ways the science of nutrition is applied, such as dietary recommendations, also change.

Poverty and undernutrition are commonplace in many developing countries. Impoverished people must often cope with infectious diseases, parasitic infestations, overcrowded and unsafe housing conditions, and polluted water supplies. In developing countries, poor sanitation practices and lack of clean cooking and drinking water cause the majority of all diseases and more than one-third of all deaths. In undernourished children, nutrient deficiencies are responsible for stunted physical growth, delayed physical development, blindness, impaired intellectual development, and premature death. Chronic undernutrition depresses the body's immune functioning, increasing the risk of death from infectious diseases, such as measles, especially in childhood. The vast majority of childhood deaths associated with undernutrition occur among poor populations in developing countries, particularly in Africa and Southeast Asia. When undernutrition occurs during the first five years of life, the effects can be devastating to the child's brain and result in permanent learning disabilities. Additionally, chronically undernourished children do not grow normally and tend to be shorter if they survive to adulthood.

Reducing hunger through food aid programs is a major goal of the United Nations. Biotechnological advances in agriculture have led to the development of crops that supply higher yields, resist pests, or are tolerant of drought conditions. By increasing food production or modifying the nutritional content of foods, biotechnology offers another way of alleviating the world food crisis.

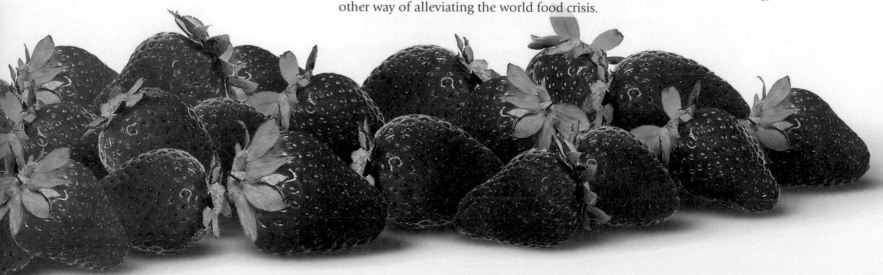

Recipes for Healthy Living

Food Preparation Basics (Yes, You *Can* Cook!)

By learning how to prepare dishes, experiment with recipe ingredients, and use a variety of spices and herbs as seasonings, you can make home-cooked meals that are more tasty, more appealing, and lower in fat, sugar, salt, and calories than the usual choices at fast-food restaurants. Additionally, you can save money by making your meals and snacks instead of purchasing them from restaurants and vending machines. At the end of each chapter, you will find the "Recipes for Healthy Living," a collection of nutritious, easy-to-prepare recipes. Each recipe includes a list of ingredients, instructions, and some information concerning the energy and selected nutrient contents in a serving of the product. You will also see the "MyPlate" icon that indicates which of the U.S. Department of Agriculture's food groups are represented in the recipe (Fig. 1.17).

Even if you've had little or no cooking experience, you can learn the basics of preparing foods. Some cooks don't measure ingredients; they know from experience how to estimate amounts of foods and seasonings to add when preparing dishes. Until you feel confident with your food preparation skills, it is best to follow recipes and measure ingredients carefully.

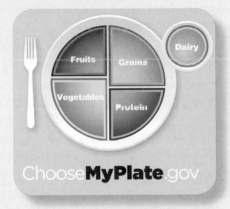

Figure 1.17 MyPlate. In 2011, the U.S. Department of Agriculture introduced a guide for planning nutritious and balanced menus. For more information about MyPlate, see Chapter 3.

You'll need some basic food preparation equipment to get started. You don't have to spend a lot of money, but buy well-made stainless steel (rustproof) cooking utensils and mixing bowls that will last for decades. Baking pans should also be stainless steel. A square or rectangular tempered-glass baking dish can be used for a variety of cooking needs, including heating foods in a toaster oven or microwave oven.

Understanding how to use household measurements is a good place to begin when learning how to cook. Purchase a set of metal measuring spoons that include ⅛ teaspoon (tsp), ¼ tsp, ½ tsp, 1 tsp, and 1 tablespoon (Tbsp) measures. You'll also need a set of plastic or metal measuring cups that include the following measures: ¼ cup, ⅓ cup, ½ cup, and 1 cup. These cups are used to measure dry ingredients such as flour or sugar. Finally, purchase a 2-cup glass or clear plastic measuring pitcher that is marked to indicate fluid ounces. This pitcher is used for measuring liquid ingredients such as water, milk, and oil.

To measure dry ingredients, fill the appropriate measuring cup or spoon to the top, and skim off the excess with the straight edge of a knife. To measure liquid ingredients, use a liquid measuring pitcher. Fill the pitcher to the desired amount, and place it on a level surface. Kneel down so you are eye level with the fluid's level, and then carefully add more or remove some fluid if necessary.

Household Units

Common household units often used for measuring food ingredients and their commonly used abbreviations are listed below. Ounces (oz) are a measure of weight; *fluid* ounces are a measure of volume. Appendix A provides information about English-to-metric and metric-to-household unit conversions.

Common Household Units for Measuring Food Ingredients

3 tsp = 1 Tbsp	1 cup = 8 fluid ounces (oz)
4 Tbsp = ¼ cup	1 cup = ½ pint
5 Tbsp + 1 tsp = ⅓ cup	2 cups = 1 pint
8 Tbsp = ½ cup	4 cups or 2 pints = 1 quart
16 Tbsp = 1 cup	4 quarts = 1 gallon

Low-Fat Applesauce Oatmeal Muffins

The following muffin recipe is simple and will give you an opportunity to practice measuring dry and liquid ingredients. This recipe makes 12 small muffins, so you'll need a muffin tin with 12 muffin cups.
Each muffin supplies about 195 kcal, 5.0 g fat, 32.0 g carbohydrate, 5.5 g protein, 3.0 g fiber, and 1.7 mg iron.

INGREDIENTS:
1 ½ cups quick oats, uncooked
1 ¼ cups all-purpose flour
1 tsp baking powder
¾ tsp baking soda
1 tsp ground cinnamon
¼ tsp ground nutmeg
1 cup applesauce
  (see recipe in Chapter 13)
½ cup fat-free milk
½ cup brown sugar
3 Tbsp vegetable oil
1 medium egg
vegetable oil cooking spray

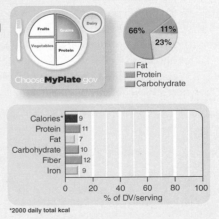

*2000 daily total kcal

PREPARATION STEPS:

1. Preheat oven to 400° F. Spray vegetable oil spray lightly on the bottom of each cup of the muffin tin.

2. Combine oats, flour, baking powder, baking soda, and spices in a large bowl. Stir until well mixed. By using a large spoon, form a depressed area (a "well") in the center of the dry ingredients.

3. In another bowl, break egg and use a fork to beat the egg to blend the white and yolk into a yellow mixture.

4. Add applesauce, milk, brown sugar, and oil to the beaten egg, and stir with a large spoon until ingredients are well mixed.

5. Pour the applesauce-containing mixture into the "well" of dry ingredients in the first bowl. Stir gently and just until the dry ingredients have been moistened by the applesauce mixture. Do not be concerned if small lumps of dry ingredients are in the batter. Do not beat or overmix the ingredients; otherwise the muffins will form air tunnels and have peaked rather than rounded tops.

6. Spoon batter into muffin cups, until the cup is half full of batter.

7. Bake 20 minutes or until muffins are golden brown. Use pot holders to protect your hands when taking the muffin tin out of the oven. Cool muffins for about 5 minutes before removing them from the tin. Muffins can be stored in a closed container in the refrigerator for up to a week. Before eating, warm each muffin in a microwave oven for about 15 seconds.

Tip: For easier cleanup, soak the bowl that contained the batter in cold, soapy water.

Sunflower Seed Cookies

When you want a sweet snack, instead of grabbing a chocolate chip or cream-filled sandwich cookie, have a healthier choice— a cookie made with sunflower seeds and quick-cooking oats. These fiber-rich cookies are easy to make, and if you are a novice at preparing foods "from scratch," the recipe will give you another chance to practice your dry ingredient–measuring skills.

This recipe makes about three dozen cookies. Each cookie supplies about 75 kcal, 3.0 g fat, 10.5 g carbohydrate, 1.6 g protein, and 1 g fiber.

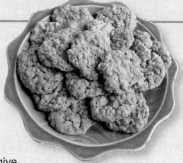

PREPARATION STEPS:

1. Preheat oven to 350° F (175° C). Lightly spray cookie sheet with nonstick vegetable oil.

2. In a large bowl, mix oil and sugars together until the mixture is smooth.

3. Beat egg into oil and sugar mixture; add vanilla extract and milk to the mixture and set aside.

4. In another large bowl, combine flour, cinnamon, baking powder, soda, oats, and sunflower seeds (dry ingredients). Stir until ingredients are well blended together.

5. Add dry ingredients slowly to other ingredients, stirring with a large spoon until dry ingredients are fully moistened and form a sticky, stiff dough.

6. Using a teaspoon, form cookies by scooping about 1 tsp of dough and place them on the lightly oiled cookie sheet. Cookies should have about an inch of space between them to allow for spreading.

7. Bake for 11 minutes or until the edges of the cookies turn golden brown. Remove the sheet of cookies from the oven and allow them to cool for a few minutes before removing them with a flat, sturdy spatula. Repeat steps 6 and 7 with any remaining cookie dough.

8. To maintain freshness, store cookies in a metal or plastic container.

INGREDIENTS:

¼ cup white sugar
½ cup brown sugar
¼ cup vegetable oil
1 large egg
½ tsp vanilla extract
2 Tbsp fat-free milk
1 cup all-purpose white flour
¼ tsp ground cinnamon
¼ tsp baking powder
½ tsp baking soda
1 cup quick-cooking oats, uncooked
½ cup dry roasted, unsalted sunflower seeds
non-stick vegetable oil spray

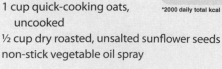

Personal *Dietary* Analysis

1. For a week, keep grocery and convenience store receipts.
   a. How much money did you spend on foods purchased at these markets?
   b. Which foods were the most expensive items purchased?
   c. How much money did you spend on empty-calorie foods and beverages such as salty snacks, cookies, soft drinks, and candy? _____
   d. What percentage of your food dollars were spent on empty-calorie foods? _____ (Divide the amount of money spent on empty-calorie foods by the total cost of food for the week. Move the decimal point over 2 places to the right and place a percent sign after the number.)
   e. How much money did you spend on nutrient-dense foods such as whole-grain products, fruits, and vegetables? _____
   f. What percentage of your food dollars were spent on nutrient-dense foods? _____ (Divide the amount of money spent on nutrient-dense foods by the total cost of food for the week. Move the decimal point over 2 places to the right and place a percent sign after the number.)

2. For one week, keep a detailed log of your usual vending machine purchases, including the item(s) purchased and amount of money spent for each purchase.
   a. What types of foods and beverages did you buy from the machines?
   b. How many soft drinks did you consume each day? _____
   c. How much money did you spend on vending machine foods and beverages? _____
   d. Based on this week's vending machine expenditures, estimate how much money you spend on such purchases in a year. _____

3. For one week, keep a detailed log of your usual fast-food consumption practices, including fast-food purchases at convenience stores. List the types of food and beverages you purchased and amount of money you spent.
   a. According to your weekly record, how often do you buy food from fast-food places and convenience stores? _____
   b. What types of foods did you usually buy?
   c. How much money did you spend on fast foods? _____
   d. Based on this week's expenditures, estimate how much money you spend on fast-food purchases in a year. _____

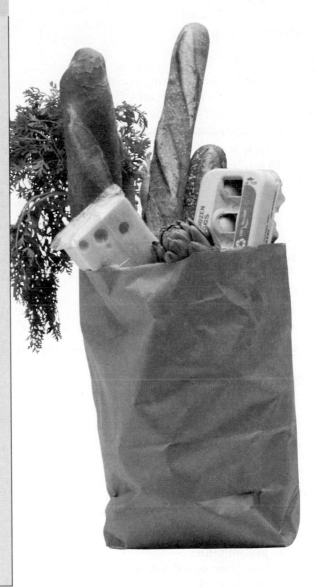

CRITICAL THINKING

1. Identify at least six factors that influence your food and beverage selections. Which of these factors is the most important? Explain why.

2. Consider your current eating habits. Explain why you think your diet is or is not nutritionally adequate.

3. "Everything in moderation." Explain what this statement means in terms of your diet.

4. If you were at risk of developing a chronic health condition that could be prevented by changing your diet, would you make the necessary changes? Explain why or why not.

5. Have you ever used certain foods or dietary supplements, such as vitamins, to treat or prevent illnesses? If you have, describe the situations and discuss which foods or supplements were used.

6. What actions have you taken or can you take to help hungry or food-insecure people obtain adequate nutrition?

PRACTICE TEST

Select the best answer.

1. Diet is a
   a. practice of restricting energy intake.
   b. pattern of food choices.
   c. method of reducing portion sizes.
   d. technique to reduce carbohydrate intake.

2. Which of the following conditions is not one of the 10 leading causes of death in the United States?
   a. tuberculosis
   b. cancer
   c. heart disease
   d. stroke

3. The nutrients that provide energy are
   a. carbohydrates, vitamins, and lipids.
   b. lipids, proteins, and minerals.
   c. vitamins, minerals, and proteins.
   d. proteins, fats, and carbohydrates.

4. _____ refers to all chemical processes that occur in living cells.
   a. Physiology
   b. Catabolism
   c. Anatomy
   d. Metabolism

5. Phytochemicals
   a. are essential nutrients.
   b. may have healthful benefits.
   c. should be avoided.
   d. are in animal sources of food.

6. Which of the following foods is energy and nutrient dense?
   a. peanut butter
   b. sugar-sweetened soft drink
   c. fat-free milk
   d. iceberg lettuce

7. Which of the following foods is a rich source of phytochemicals?
   a. hamburger
   b. fish
   c. peaches
   d. chicken

8. Which of the following conditions is a chronic disease?
   a. heart disease
   b. stroke
   c. cancer
   d. All of the above are correct.

9. In the United States, the primary cause of preventable cancer deaths is
   a. physical inactivity.
   b. tobacco use.
   c. high-fat diet.
   d. excessive alcohol intake.

10. Compared to 40 years ago, the typical American
    a. eats less fruit.
    b. drinks more milk.
    c. drinks more carbonated soft drinks.
    d. eats more eggs.

11. Lena weighs 165 pounds. What is her weight in kilograms?
    a. 75 kg
    b. 7.5 kg
    c. 82 kg
    d. 8.2 kg

12. A serving of food contains 10 g carbohydrate, 2 g protein, and 4 g fat. Based on this information, a serving of this food supplies ____ kcal.
    a. 64
    b. 74
    c. 84
    d. 94

13. A serving of food supplies 20 g carbohydrate, 4 g protein, 10 g fat, and 50 g water. Which of the following statements is true about a serving of the food?
    a. Fat provides the most food energy.
    b. Carbohydrate provides the most food energy.
    c. Water provides the most food energy.
    d. Fat provides about 25% of total calories.

14. Which of the following foods is the most nutrient dense?
    a. potato chips
    b. broccoli
    c. butter
    d. chocolate chip cookie

15. Which of the following statements is false?
    a. A megadose is 10 times the recommended amount of a nutrient.
    b. Megadoses of nutrients may behave like drugs in the body.
    c. In general, megadoses of nutrients are safe to consume.
    d. A physiological dose of a vitamin is less than a megadose of the vitamin.

16. The _____ Program enables eligible low-income participants to use a special debit card to purchase food at authorized stores.
    a. Nutritious Food Purchase
    b. Supplemental Nutrition Assistance
    c. Healthy Diets for All
    d. Eat Better for Less

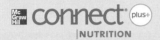

Additional resources related to the features of this book are available on ConnectPlus® Nutrition. Ask your instructor how to get access.

Answers to Chapter 1 **Quiz** *Yourself*

1. There are four classes of nutrients: proteins, lipids, sugars, and vitamins. **False** (p. 4)

2. Proteins are the most essential class of nutrients. **False** (p. 5)

3. All nutrients must be supplied by the diet, because they cannot be made by the body.
   False (p. 5)

4. Vitamins are a source of energy. **False** (p. 11)

5. Milk, carrots, and bananas are examples of "perfect" foods that contain all nutrients. **False** (p. 12)

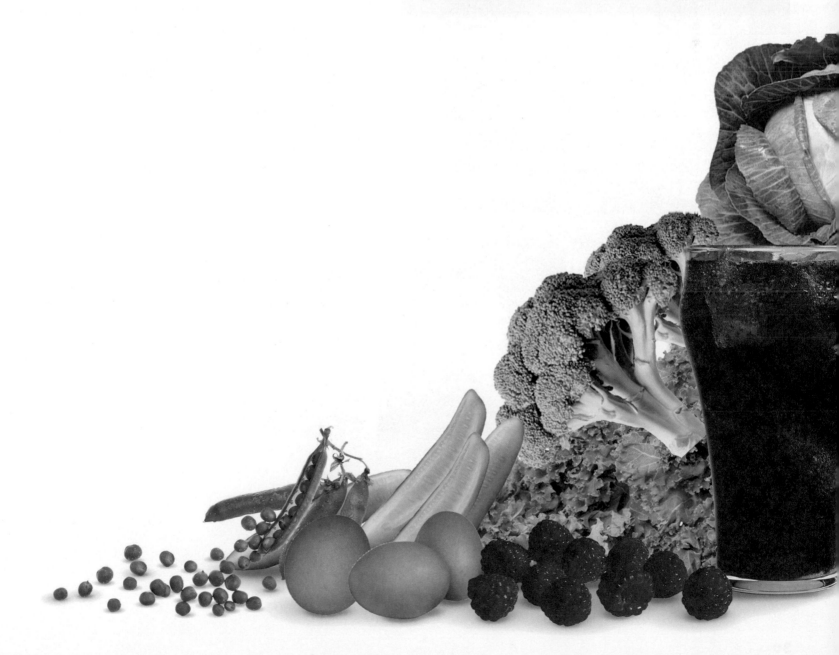

Evaluating Nutrition Information

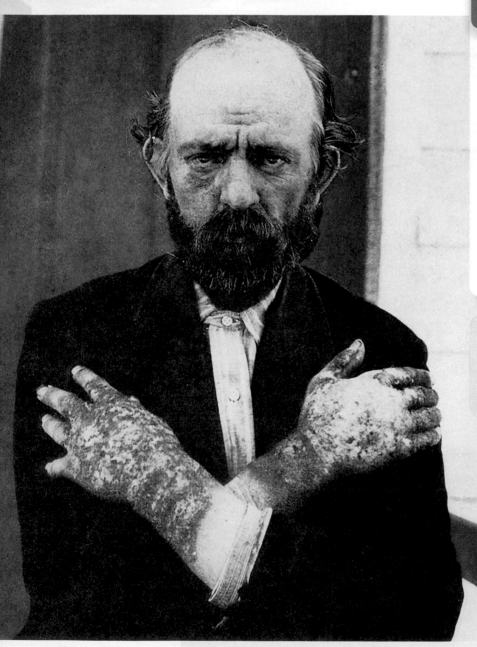

Chapter Learning Outcomes

After reading Chapter 2, you should be able to

1. Define terms, including anecdote, variable, epidemiology, placebo, placebo effect, peer review, and quackery.

2. Explain the basic steps of the scientific method.

3. Explain the importance of having controls when performing experiments.

4. Define "research bias."

5. Describe how to identify questionable sources of nutrition information.

6. Identify reliable sources of nutrition information.

7. Define "dietary supplement" and provide examples of different types of these products.

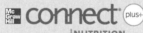

Mc Graw Hill **connect** plus+
|NUTRITION   **www.mcgrawhillconnect.com**

A wealth of proven resources are available on ConnectPlus® Nutrition!
Ask your instructor about ConnectPlus, which includes an interactive
eBook, an adaptive learning program and much, much more!

IN THE EARLY 1900s, the disease *pellagra* was widespread in the United States, especially in southern states. Individuals with pellagra were weak, and they developed diarrhea, a skin rash, and mental confusion. Each year, thousands of Americans died from this dreaded illness.

In 1914, the U.S. surgeon general assigned Joseph Goldberger, a physician who worked in a federal government laboratory, to study pellagra. Most medical experts thought pellagra was an infectious disease because it often occurred where people lived in close quarters, such as prisons, orphanages, and mental health institutions. Goldberger knew from his previous research that infectious diseases usually spread through a population by close physical contact. While investigating factors associated with pellagra, Goldberger observed that not everyone who was exposed to people suffering from pellagra developed the condition. For example, many prisoners had pellagra, but none of their guards or prison administrators suffered from the disease, even though they associated closely with the affected inmates. Based on his observations, Goldberger rejected the medical establishment's notion that pellagra was an infectious disease.

Dr. Goldberger also noted that prisoners ate a diet that was typically eaten by other people with pellagra. The diet emphasized corn bread, hominy grits (a corn product), molasses, potatoes, cabbage, and rice. At the time, this monotonous low-protein diet was associated with poverty throughout the southern United States. He also observed that people who did not develop pellagra had higher incomes and ate more meat, milk, and fresh vegetables. Goldberger developed the hypothesis that pellagra resulted from the lack of something in poor people's diet. A **hypothesis** is a possible explanation for an observation that guides scientific research. Goldberger hypothesized that the missing dietary factor was in meat, milk, and other foods eaten regularly by people with high incomes. To test his hypothesis, Goldberger gave these foods to children in two Mississippi orphanages and patients in a Georgia mental institution who were suffering from pellagra, and they were cured of the disease. Despite the results of Goldberger's experiment, many members of the medical establishment rejected his finding that a poor diet was the cause of pellagra, and they continued to think pellagra was an infectious disease.

To satisfy his critics, Goldberger enrolled a group of healthy Mississippi prison inmates in an

(continued)

Quiz *Yourself*

Before reading the rest of Chapter 2, test your knowledge of scientific methods and reliable sources of nutrition information by taking the following quiz. The answers are on page 57.

1. Scientists generally do not raise questions about or criticize the conclusions of their colleagues' research data, even when they disagree with those conclusions. _____T _____F

2. Popular health-related magazines typically publish articles that have been peer-reviewed. _____T_____F

3. By conducting a prospective epidemiological study, medical researchers can determine risk factors that may influence health. _____T _____F

4. Dietary supplements include vitamin pills as well as products that contain echinacea, ginseng, and garlic. _____T _____F

5. In general, registered dietitians are reliable sources of food and nutrition information. _____T _____F

hypothesis possible explanation about an observation that guides scientific research

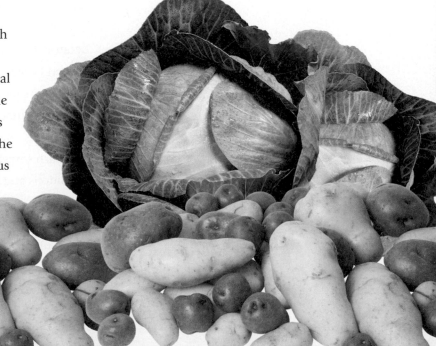

experiment that involved consuming the corn- and molasses-based diet commonly eaten in the southern states at the time. After a few months, more than half of the inmates developed cases of pellagra, confirmed by medical experts who were not associated with Goldberger. Once again, however, many of Goldberger's critics rejected his finding that poor diet was the cause of pellagra.

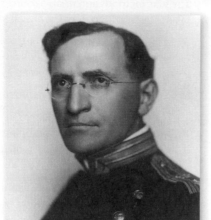

Dr. Joseph Goldberger

In 1916, Dr. Goldberger decided to end the controversy by experimenting on himself and some volunteers during what they called a "filth party." The group applied secretions taken from inside the nose and throat of a patient with pellagra into their noses and throats; they also swallowed pills made with flakes of skin scraped from the rashes of people with the disease. Additionally, Goldberger and one of his colleagues gave each other an injection of blood from a person who had pellagra. If pellagra were infectious, filth party participants should have contracted the disease—but none of them did. Despite the results of Dr. Goldberger's extraordinary experiment, a few physicians still resisted the idea that pellagra was associated with diet.[1]

Dr. Goldberger died in 1929—eight years before Dr. Conrad Elvehjem and his team of scientists at the University of Wisconsin isolated a form of the vitamin niacin from liver extracts. Elvehjem and his colleagues discovered niacin cured "black tongue," a condition affecting dogs that was similar to pellagra.[2] Not long after Elvehjem's findings were published, niacin was determined to be effective in treating pellagra, and the medical establishment finally accepted the fact that the disease was the result of a dietary deficiency.

Today, the idea that something missing in diets can cause a nutrient deficiency disease is widely accepted. A hundred years ago, however, it was a novel idea that most medical experts dismissed because they thought only "germs" caused disease. It is interesting to note that raw corn actually contains niacin, but it is in a form the body cannot digest. Furthermore, consuming meat and milk helps prevent pellagra because these foods contain tryptophan, a component of proteins that the body can convert to niacin.

A more recent example of the time and effort it takes to gain support for a medical hypothesis that opposes established beliefs is the case of the mysterious microbe. In the mid–1950s, the medical community generally accepted the cause of peptic ulcers (stomach sores) as stress and poor diet. Monkeys and rodents living under stressful conditions and humans recovering from severe burns often developed such ulcers. In 1982, Australian physicians Barry Marshall and Robin Warren isolated a type of bacteria from the stomachs of patients with gastritis, inflammation of the stomach lining that can result in peptic ulcers.[3] Marshall and Warren hypothesized that this microbe might be related to the development of gastritis and peptic ulcers, and they suggested treating the conditions with antibiotics. Initially, other physicians were skeptical about Marshall and Warren's hypothesis because it challenged traditional medical beliefs and treatment practices. Traditional treatment for gastritis and peptic ulcers generally included antacids and a bland diet, not antibiotics. To provide support for his idea, Marshall actually swallowed some of the bacteria and developed severe stomach inflammation as a result. Then other researchers published articles that confirmed the presence of a type of bacteria that was capable of living in human stomachs and likely responsible for certain chronic stomach ailments. Within a few years, the medical profession accepted the idea that the bacterium (*Helicobacter pylori* or *H. pylori*) was a primary cause of gastritis and peptic ulcers (Fig. 2.1). Today people with peptic ulcers who test positive for *H. pylori* in their stomachs are treated with antibiotics that kill the bacterium. In 2005, Marshall and Warren received the Nobel Prize in medicine for their groundbreaking research and scientific contribution to medical care.

These experiences are just two of many fascinating examples that illustrate how researchers use scientific methods to solve medical mysteries relating to nutrition and health. As in these cases, it is not unusual for scientists to refrain from making quick judgments about a novel nutrition hypothesis until it undergoes repeated testing. Thus it often takes many years before a scientific discovery becomes widely accepted by other experts in the nutrition field.

How do nutrition scientists determine facts about foods, nutrients, and diets? Why do nutrition scientists seem to contradict themselves so much? How can you evaluate the reliability of nutrition information? Where can you obtain up-to-date, accurate nutrition information? Chapter 2 will provide answers to these questions and help you become a more critical and careful consumer.

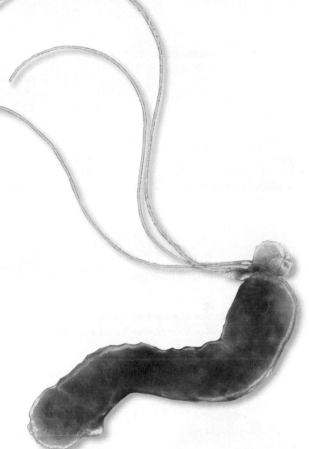

Figure 2.1 *H. pylori.* Infection with the bacterium *H. pylori* (shown in colorized micrograph above) is a primary cause of gastritis and peptic ulcers. Today, people with peptic ulcers who test positive for *H. pylori* are treated with antibiotics that kill the bacterium.

2.1 Understanding the Scientific Method

Scientists ask questions about the natural world and follow generally accepted, standardized methods to obtain answers to these questions. In the past, nutrition facts and dietary practices were often based on intuition, common sense, "conventional wisdom" (tradition), or **anecdotes** (reports of personal experiences). Today, *registered dietitians* and other nutrition experts discard conventional beliefs, explanations, and practices when the results of current scientific research no longer support them.

Nutrition researchers rely on scientific methods that may involve making observations, asking questions and developing hypotheses, performing tests, and collecting and analyzing data (information) to find relationships between variables. A **variable** is a factor such as a person's age, weight, or environment that can change and influence an outcome. After analyzing *data* (information), researchers draw conclusions from the data and report on the findings. Other scientists can test the findings to support or refute them. Figure 2.2 presents the general steps nutrition researchers take when conducting scientific investigations. The following sections take a closer look at some common methods that scientists use to collect nutrition information and establish nutrition facts.

anecdotes reports of personal experiences

variable personal characteristic or other factor that changes and can influence an outcome

1. Make observations that generate questions

2. Formulate hypotheses to explain events

SCIENTIFIC METHOD

6. Conduct more research, the results of which may confirm or refute previous findings

3. Design studies, perform tests, and collect data

5. Share results with peers (report findings)

4. Analyze data and draw conclusions based on the results

Figure 2.2 Nutrition science: Scientific method. Nutrition scientists generally follow these steps when conducting research.

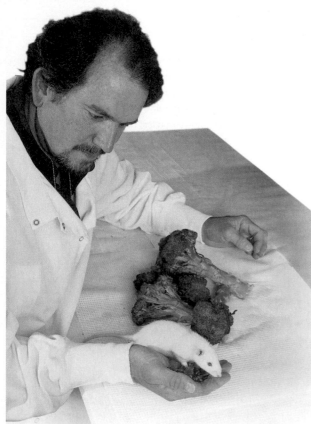

Figure 2.3 Rodents for research. Nutrition scientists often conduct in vivo experiments on small rodents that are raised for experimentation purposes. USDA nutritionist John Finley holds a laboratory rat and a sample of broccoli that is fortified with the mineral selenium.

Laboratory Experiments

An *experiment* is a systematic way of testing a hypothesis. Because of safety and ethical concerns, nutrition scientists often conduct experiments on small mammals before performing similar research on humans. Certain kinds of mice and rats are raised for experimentation purposes (Fig. 2.3). These rodents are inexpensive to house in laboratories, and their food and other living conditions can be carefully controlled. An experiment that uses whole living organisms, such as mice, is called an *in vivo* experiment. Nutrition researchers also perform controlled laboratory experiments on cells or other components derived from living organisms. These studies are *in vitro* or "test tube" experiments.

Experiments generally involve the basic steps shown in Figure 2.2. A team of nutrition scientists, for example, makes observations and generates questions that result in the development of a hypothesis. According to their hypothesis, consuming "chemical X" in charcoal-grilled meat is harmful. To test this hypothesis, the scientists divide 100 genetically similar 3-week old mice into two groups of 50 mice. One group (**treatment group**) is fed a certain amount of chemical X daily for 52 weeks; the second group (**control group**) does not receive the treatment during the period (Fig. 2.4). Why is a control group necessary? Having a control group enables scientists to compare results between the two study groups to determine whether the treatment had any effect. Many variables can influence the outcome of an experimental study. Therefore, scientists who want to determine the effect or effects of a single variable, such as chemical X intake, need to control the influence of other variables. Therefore, all other conditions, including availability of water and room temperature, must be the same for both groups of mice. If researchers design an experiment in which they fail to control variables that are not being tested, their findings are likely to be unclear or inaccurate.

For the duration of this study, the scientists examine the mice regularly for signs of health problems and record their results. If the mice in the treatment group are as healthy as the mice in the control group at the end of this experiment, the researchers may conclude that mice can safely consume the amount of chemical X used in the study on a daily basis for a year.

Medical researchers must be careful when applying the results of in vivo animal studies to people, because of the physiological differences between humans and other animals. Nevertheless, scientists are often able to determine the safety and effectiveness of treatments by conducting research on laboratory animals before engaging in similar testing on humans.

Researchers are also cautious when drawing conclusions from results of in vitro experiments, because components removed from a living thing may not function the same way they do when they are in the entire life form.

Human Research: Epidemiological Studies

For decades, medical researchers have noted differences in rates of chronic diseases and causes of death among various populations. The most common type of diabetes, for example, occurs more frequently among Native-American, Hispanic, and non-Hispanic African-American adults than among non-Hispanic, white American adults.[4] Additionally, breast cancer is more common among non-Hispanic, white females than among females who are members of other American racial or ethnic groups.[5] To understand why these differences exist, medical researchers rely on the findings of epidemiological studies. **Epidemiology** (*ehp-e-dee-me-all'-uh-jee*) is the study of the occurrence, distribution, and causes of health problems in populations.[6] Epidemiologists often use physical

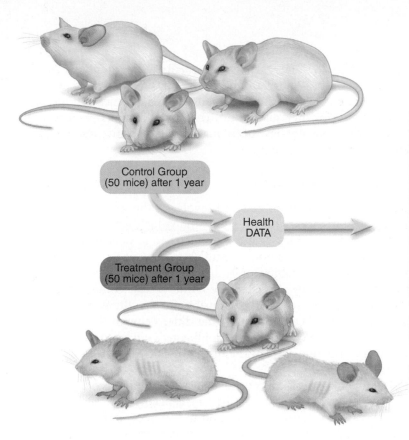

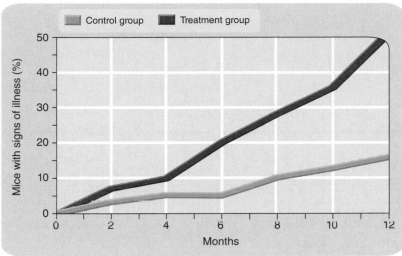

Figure 2.4 An experiment. Based on the findings shown in the graph, is it safe for mice to consume chemical X daily for a year?

examinations of people to obtain health data (Fig. 2.5). Additionally, they may collect information by conducting surveys. Such surveys question people about their personal and family medical histories, environmental exposures, health practices, and attitudes. Two types of epidemiological research are *experimental* (intervention) studies and *observational* studies. Such investigations can provide nutritional epidemiologists with clues about the causes, progression, and prevention of diet-related diseases.

Experimental (Intervention) Epidemiological Studies

Nutrition scientists often conduct experimental epidemiological studies to obtain information about health conditions (*outcomes*) that may result from specific dietary practices. When conducting an experimental study involving human subjects, researchers usually divide a large group of people into treatment and control groups. Then the scientists provide all study participants with the same instructions and a form of intervention, such as a dietary supplement or experimental food. However, only members of the treatment group actually receive the treatment. Subjects in the control group are given a **placebo.** Placebos are not simply "sugar pills"; they are a fake treatment, such as a sham pill, injection, or medical procedure. The placebo mimics the treatment. For example, a placebo dietary supplement pill looks, tastes, and smells like the supplement pill with an active ingredient that is given subjects in the treatment group. The placebo pill, however, has *inert* ingredients, that is, the pill contains substances that do not produce any measurable physical changes. Providing placebos to members of the control group enables scientists to compare the extent of the treatment's response with that of the placebo.

What Is the Placebo Effect? People may report positive or negative reactions to a treatment even though they received the placebo. If a patient believes a medical treatment will improve his or her health, the patient is more likely to report positive results for the therapy. Such wishful thinking is called the **placebo effect.**

People who take certain herbal products or use other unconventional medical therapies to prevent or treat diseases are often convinced the products and treatments are effective, despite the general lack of scientific evidence to support their beliefs. Such personal findings may be examples of the placebo effect. However, placebos can produce

treatment group group being studied that receives a treatment

control group group being studied that does not receive a treatment

epidemiology study of the occurrence, distribution, and causes of health problems in populations

placebo fake treatment, such as a sham pill, injection, or medical procedure

placebo effect response to a placebo

Figure 2.5 Collecting nutrition-related information. Epidemiologists and dietitians often rely on physical examinations of people to obtain health data. In the photo below, USDA nutrition expert Pat Wiggins prepares to weigh a 1-year-old boy while his mother watches.

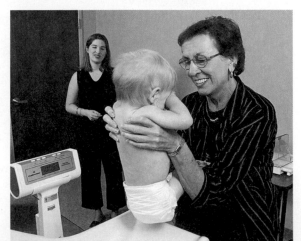

beneficial physiological and psychological changes, particularly in conditions that involve pain.[7] Because subjects in the control group believe they are receiving a real treatment, their faith in the "treatment" can stimulate the release of chemicals in the brain that alter pain perception, reducing their discomfort. Therefore, when people report that a treatment was beneficial, they may not have been imagining the positive response, even when they were taking a placebo.

Observational Epidemiological Studies

Most epidemiological research is observational and involves either *case-control study* or *cohort study* designs (Fig. 2.6). In a **case-control study,** individuals with a health condition (cases) such as heart disease or breast cancer are matched to persons with similar characteristics who do not have the condition (controls). Information such as personal and family medical histories, eating habits, and other lifestyle behaviors are collected from each participant in the study. By analyzing the results of case-control studies, researchers identify factors that may have been responsible for the illness. Scientists, for example, may be able to identify dietary practices that differ between the two groups, such as long-term fruit and vegetable intakes. Dr. Goldberger's efforts to determine the cause of pellagra involved comparing cases of the disease with people who lived in the same area but were healthy.

In a **cohort study,** epidemiologists collect and analyze various kinds of information about a large group of people over time. The scientists are generally interested in making associations between exposure to a specific factor and the subsequent development of health conditions. Cohort studies can be *retrospective* or *prospective*. Retrospective means "to look back" and prospective means "to look forward" in time. (See Figure 2.6.) In a retrospective cohort study, researchers collect information about a group's past exposures and identify current health outcomes. For example, nutritional epidemiologists might examine whether a group of people who have stomach cancer consumed more charcoal-broiled meat (the exposure) in the past than a group of people with similar characteristics who do not have stomach cancer. In a prospective cohort study, a group of healthy people are followed over a time period and any diseases that eventually develop are recorded. Scientists then try to identify links between exposures and diseases that occurred between the beginning and end of the study period.

The Framingham Heart Study that began in 1949 in Framingham, Massachusetts, is one of the most well-known prospective studies. At the beginning of the study, the over 5200 healthy participants (men and women) underwent extensive physical examinations and questioning about their family and personal medical histories as well as their lifestyle practices. Over the following years, a group of medical researchers periodically collected data concerning each participant's health and, if the person died, cause of death. The scientists analyzed this information and found relationships between a variety of personal characteristics and health outcomes. Findings from the Framingham Heart Study identified numerous risk factors for heart disease, including elevated blood cholesterol levels, cigarette smoking, and hypertension. Today, medical researchers are still collecting information from the original Framingham Heart Study participants as well as their descendants.

Limitations of Epidemiological Studies

Epidemiological studies cannot establish *causation*, that is, whether a practice is responsible for an effect. When two different natural events occur simultaneously within a population, it does not necessarily mean they are correlated. A **correlation** is a relationship between variables. A correlation occurs when two variables change

EPIDEMIOLOGICAL STUDIES

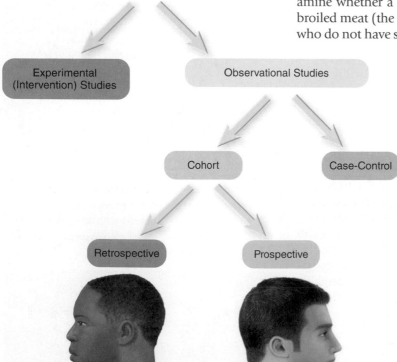

Figure 2.6 Epidemiological studies. Most epidemiological research involves observational studies that have a case-control or cohort design. Cohort studies can be retrospective or prospective.

over the same period; for example, when a population's intake of sugar-sweetened soft drinks increases, the percentage of overweight people in the population also increases (Fig. 2.7a). In this case, the correlation is *direct* or *positive* because the two variables—body weight and regular soft drink consumption—are changing in the same direction; they are both increasing. An *inverse* or *negative* correlation occurs when one variable increases and the other one decreases. An example of an inverse correlation is the relationship between fruit intake and hypertension; as a population's fruit consumption increases, the percentage of people with hypertension in that population decreases (Fig. 2.7b).

What appears to be a correlation between a behavior and an outcome could be a coincidence, that is, a chance happening, and not an indication of a *cause-and-effect* relationship between the two variables. For example, in a survey of lemonade consumption in Colorado over a 10-year period, we might observe that fewer people drank lemonade during the winter than during the summer months. In a survey of snow skiing accidents in Colorado during the same 10-year period, we might also find that snow skiing accidents were more likely to occur during the winter than in the summer. Thus, as lemonade consumption declined, snow skiing accidents increased. Does this mean lemonade consumption is inversely correlated to skiing accidents, and people who do not drink lemonade have a greater risk of having a skiing accident at this time of year? It is more likely that the relationship between snow skiing and lemonade drinking is coincidental, because both activities are associated with seasonal weather conditions. Although this example is obviously far-fetched, it illustrates the problems scientists can have when analyzing results of epidemiological studies.

> **case-control study** study in which individuals who have a health condition are compared with individuals with similar characteristics who do not have the condition
>
> **cohort study** study that measures variables of a group of people over time
>
> **correlation** relationship between two variables

Elements of an Experimental Epidemiological Study

Scientific studies can have very complicated designs and involve several years and thousands of dollars to plan and conduct. However, most nutrition-related research involving human subjects incorporates some basic steps—*reviewing* scientific literature, *developing* a

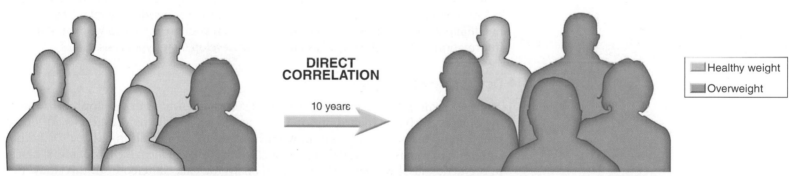

a. As a population's intake of sugar-sweetened soft drinks increases (↑), the percentage of overweight people in that population increases (↑.

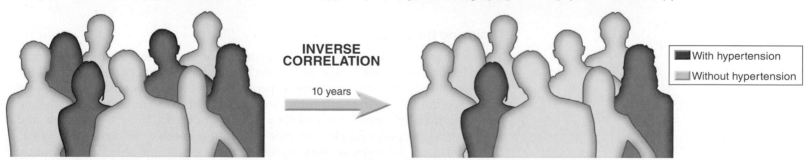

b. As a population's fruit intake increases (↑), the percentage of people in that population with hypertension decreases (↓).

Figure 2.7 Examples of direct and inverse correlations. (*a*) Direct (positive) correlation: As a population's intake of sugar-sweetened soft drinks increases (↑), the percentage of overweight people in that population increases (↑). (*b*) Inverse (negative) correlation: As a population's fruit intake increases (↑), the percentage of people in that population with hypertension declines (↓).

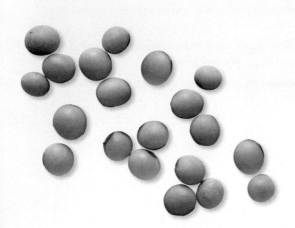

hypothesis, *designing* the study, *conducting* the research, *analyzing* results, *reporting* the results, and possibly, conducting another study that is related to the original research findings.

By conducting studies that explore differences in dietary practices and disease occurrences among populations, nutritional epidemiologists may learn much about the influence of diet on health. If one group of people is more likely to develop a certain health disorder than another group and the two populations consume very different diets, scientists can speculate about the role diet plays in this difference. For example, results of several epidemiological studies indicate that the incidence of breast cancer is generally higher among women in Western countries than women in Asian countries, and Western women typically have lower intakes of soy products than Asian women.[8,9] Based on this information, you might conclude that eating a soy-rich diet prevents breast cancer—but is your conclusion valid? To answer this question, scientists would conduct an experimental epidemiological study such as the one described in the following sections.

Reviewing the Scientific Literature

Before nutrition scientists conduct studies, they perform a review of literature that involves a search of scientific articles previously published on their topic of interest. For example, a team of scientists plans to conduct a 5-year intervention study to determine the effects of adding 25 grams of soy/day to the diets of American women who are *premenopausal* (they can become pregnant) and have higher-than-average risks of breast cancer. The scientists prepare for their study by reading articles about research that examined the effects of soy intake on breast cancer risk. The findings and conclusions of the previous research may raise questions that can be explored in a new study.

In cases involving chronic diseases such as breast cancer, it is difficult to determine a single variable that is responsible for the development of the condition. Multiple factors, including a person's *genetic susceptibility* (inherited proneness) to develop the disease, usually influence whether the chronic disease occurs. For example, many environmental, physiological, and lifestyle variables are responsible for the development of breast cancer in women. By conducting a review of scientific articles, the researchers learn that body weight, alcohol consumption, and age are some of the variables that influence a woman's risk of breast cancer.[10] Therefore, it is possible that variables besides soy intake account for the different rates of breast cancer observed between Western and Asian women. With this information in mind, the scientists are ready to develop their hypothesis.

Developing a Hypothesis

After performing the literature review, our team of scientists can develop one or more hypotheses, such as: "Increasing soy intake to 25 grams daily reduces the risk of breast cancer in premenopausal American women." Another hypothesis might be: "Daily consumption of wafers that provide a total of 25 grams of soy reduces the risk of breast cancer in premenopausal women." The results of analyzing data gathered from this study may support or refute each hypothesis.

Designing the Study

The findings of experimental research involving human subjects are more likely to be generalized to other people, but conducting human experiments can be costly and often involves ethical concerns. Furthermore, people are not likely to enroll in *clinical studies* that may require living in tightly controlled settings such as the nutrition research unit of a major university's medical school for a few days or weeks. Such participation would likely restrict people's lifestyles too much. Nutrition scientists recognize that valuable information can be collected from recruiting subjects who are able to go about their usual routines. Thus, researchers often design studies to allow subjects to maintain their lifestyle practices, except for the variable being studied.

Our team of scientists decides to recruit a large group of healthy premenopausal women who have been told they have high risk of breast cancer by their physicians. The researchers will *randomly* assign the women to treatment and control groups. For example, every other woman who enrolls in the study is placed in the treatment group. The remaining women become control group members. Random assignment helps ensure that the members of the treatment and control groups have similar variables, such as age and other characteristics. All subjects will be instructed to maintain their usual lifestyle during the duration of the 5-year study, except for the activities required by their participation in the research.

Double-Blind Studies Human experimental studies are usually **double-blind**—that is, neither the investigators nor the subjects are aware of the subjects' group assignments. Codes are used to identify a subject's group membership, and this information is not revealed until the end of the study. Maintaining such secrecy is important during the course of a human study involving placebos, because researchers and subjects may try to predict group assignments based on their expectations. If the investigators who interview the participants are aware of their individual group assignments during the study, they may unwittingly convey clues to each subject, perhaps in the form of body language, that could influence the subject's belief about being in the experimental or control group. Subjects who suspect they are in the control group and taking a placebo may report no changes in their condition, because they expect a placebo should have no effect on them. On the other hand, subjects who think they are in the treatment group could insist that they feel better or have more stamina as a result of the treatment, even though the treatment may not have produced any measurable changes in their bodies. Ideally, subjects should not be able to figure out their group assignment while researchers are collecting information from them.

Reviewing Human Subjects Research Designs Scientists must follow U.S. government guidelines when performing research involving human subjects. Before conducting this type of research, scientists must have the study design scrutinized and approved by their institution's human subjects review committee. To pass the review, a study generally should avoid causing physical and psychological harm or discomfort to subjects beyond that which may be encountered in daily life or during a routine physical examination. Furthermore, the study should treat each subject fairly and protect subjects' privacy. Before participating in the study, adult subjects must provide legally obtained informed consent indicating they are aware of the benefits and risks of the research effort and are willing participants.

> **double-blind study** experimental design in which neither the participants nor the researchers are aware of each participant's group assignment

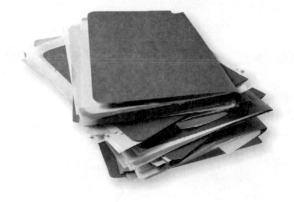

Conducting Human Research

To reduce the likelihood that the results of the soy study occur by chance, the researchers enroll in the study a large group of premenopausal women (800, for example) who are healthy but have higher-than-average risks of breast cancer. Subjects are randomly assigned into two groups; 400 are in the treatment group and 400 are in the control group.

The investigative team provides a supply of wafers to the treatment group's participants and instructions concerning their daily consumption. By following these instructions, each treatment group member will consume 25 grams of soy/day. Members of the control group are also given a supply of wafers, but their wafers are the placebos that do not contain soy. Both groups are given the same instructions concerning their food intake, dietary record keeping, health care reporting, and lifestyle for the duration of the study.

Analyzing Data, Drawing Conclusions, and Reporting Findings

Nutrition researchers use a variety of statistical methods to analyze data collected from observations and experiments. These methods may enable the researchers to find relationships between the variables and health outcomes that were studied. As a result, scientists can determine whether their hypotheses are supported by the data. According to results of our example study investigating the effects of soy intake on breast cancer risk,

peer review expert critical analysis of a research article before it is published

the rate of new cases of breast cancer was 10/400 among members of the experimental group and 45/400 among the members of the control group. Based on their analyses, the scientists concluded that eating at least 25 grams of soy daily for 5 years may reduce the risk of breast cancer in premenopausal women who have high risk of the disease.

When an experiment or study is completed and the results analyzed, researchers summarize the findings and seek to publish articles with information about their investigation in scientific journals. Before articles are accepted for publication, they undergo **peer review,** a critical analysis conducted by a group of "peers." Peers are investigators who were not part of the study but are experts involved in related research. If peers agree that a study was well conducted, its results are fairly represented, and the research is of interest to the journal's readers, these scientists are likely to recommend that the journal's editors publish the article. Examples of peer-reviewed medical and nutrition journals include the *Journal of Nutrition, American Journal of Clinical Nutrition, The New England Journal of Medicine, Journal of the American Medical Association,* and *Nutrition Reviews.*

Research Bias Scientists expect other researchers to avoid relying on their personal attitudes and biases ("points of view") when collecting and analyzing data, and to evaluate and report their results objectively and honestly. This process is important because much of the scientific research that is conducted in the United States is supported financially by the federal government, nonprofit foundations, and drug companies and other private industries. Some funding sources can have certain expectations or biases about research outcomes, and as a result, they are likely to finance studies of scientists whose research efforts support their interests. The beef industry, for example, might not fund scientific investigations to find connections between high intakes of beef and the risk of certain cancers. On the other hand, the beef industry might be interested in supporting a team of scientists whose research indicates that a high-protein diet that contains plenty of beef is useful for people who are trying to lose weight.

Peer-reviewed journals usually require authors of articles to disclose their affiliations and sources of financial support. Such disclosures may appear on the first page or at the end of the article. By having this information, readers can decide on the reliability of the findings. Although peer review helps ensure that the scientists are as ethical and objective as possible, it is impossible to eliminate all research bias.

Spreading the News

After the results of a study are published in a nutrition-related journal or reported to health professionals attending a meeting of a nutrition or medical society, the media (e.g., newspapers, magazines, Internet news sources) may receive notice of the findings. If the information is simplistic and sensational, such as a finding that drinking green tea can result in weight loss, it is more likely to be reported in the popular press. In many instances, you learn about the study's results when they are reported in a television or radio news broadcast as a 15- or 30-second "sound bite." Such sources generally provide very little information concerning the way the study was conducted or how the data were collected and analyzed.

Popular sources of nutrition information, such as magazines and the Internet, generally do not subject articles or blogs to peer review or other scientific scrutiny, and as a result, they may feature faulty, biased information. For example, a health news column in a popular magazine may report findings from a few nutrition journal articles that support the use of garlic supplements for reducing blood cholesterol levels. However, you may conclude that the column is biased if it excludes results of other studies that do not indicate such benefits. You can often distinguish a peer-reviewed scientific journal from a popular magazine simply by looking at their covers and skimming their pages. Compared to scientific journals, magazines typically have more colorful, attractive covers and photographs, and their articles are shorter and easier for the average person to read (Fig. 2.8).

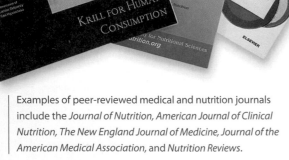

Examples of peer-reviewed medical and nutrition journals include the *Journal of Nutrition, American Journal of Clinical Nutrition, The New England Journal of Medicine, Journal of the American Medical Association,* and *Nutrition Reviews.*

It is important to keep in mind that sensational media coverage of a medical "break-through" is not necessarily an indication of the value or quality of research that resulted in the news story or magazine article. More research is often necessary for scientists to determine whether the results of a widely reported study are valid and can be generalized to other populations.

Following Up with More Research

The results of one study are rarely enough to gain widespread acceptance for new or unusual findings or to provide a basis for nutritional recommendations. Thus, the findings obtained by one research team must be supported by those generated in other studies. If the results of several scientific investigations conducted under similar conditions confirm the original researchers' conclusions, then these findings are more likely to be accepted by other nutrition scientists.

Confusion and Conflict

One day the news highlights dramatic health benefits from eating garlic, dark chocolate, brown rice, or cherries. A few weeks later, the news includes reports of more recent scientific investigations that do not support the earlier findings. When consumers become aware of conflicting results generated by nutrition studies, they often become confused and disappointed. As a result, some people may mistrust the scientific community and think nutrition scientists do not know what they are doing.

Consumers need to recognize that conflicting findings often result from differences in the ways various studies are designed. Even when investigating the same question, different groups of scientists often conduct their studies and analyze the results differently. For example, the numbers, ages, and physical conditions of subjects; the type and length of the study; the amount of the treatment provided; and the statistical tests used to analyze results typically vary among studies. Additionally, individual genetic differences often contribute to a person's response to a treatment. Not only are people genetically different, they also have different lifestyles, and they typically recall dietary information and follow instructions concerning health care practices differently. These and other factors can influence the results of nutrition research involving human subjects.

The science of nutrition is constantly evolving; old beliefs and practices are discarded when they are not supported by more recent scientific evidence, and new principles and practices emerge from the new findings. By now you should understand that science involves asking questions, developing and testing hypotheses, gathering and analyzing data, drawing conclusions from data, and sometimes, accepting change.

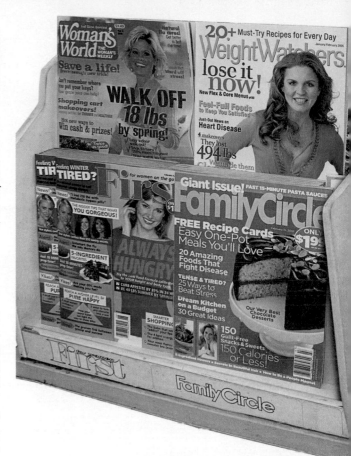

Figure 2.8 Judging by the cover. Consumers can be trained to look for features, such as covers, that distinguish peer-reviewed scientific journals from popular magazines.

Concept **Checkpoint**

1. What is epidemiology?
2. Explain the importance of having a control group when conducting experimental research.
3. What is the major difference between a prospective study and a retrospective study?
4. What is a "placebo"? Why are placebos often used in studies involving human subjects?
5. What is a "double-blind study"?
6. What is a "peer-reviewed" article?
7. Explain why results of similar studies may provide different findings.

2.2 Nutrition Information: Fact or Fiction

While "channel surfing" one afternoon, you stop and watch the host of a televised home shopping program promote FatMegaMelter, his company's brand of a dietary supplement for losing weight. According to the host, the supplement contains a chemical derived from a plant that grows naturally in South Africa. This amazing chemical reduces the appetite for fattening foods, enabling an overweight person taking FatMegaMelter to lose up to 30 pounds in 30 days, without the need to exercise more or eat less. The host interviews an attractive young actress who claims to have lost a lot of weight after she started taking FatMegaMelter pills. A few days later, a friend mentions that she has lost three pounds since she began taking this product a week ago. You would like to lose a few pounds without resorting to restricting your food intake or exercising. Should you take FatMegaMelter? The supplement helped the actress and your friend; will it help you?

Although the actress's health history appears to be compelling evidence that the weight-loss supplement is effective, her information is a **testimonial**, a personal endorsement of a product. People are usually paid to provide their testimonials for advertisements, therefore their remarks may be biased in favor of the product. Your friend's experience with taking the same weight-loss product is intriguing, but it is an anecdote and not *proof* that FatMegaMelter promotes weight loss. When your source of nutrition information is a testimonial, anecdote, or advertisement, you cannot be sure that the information is based on scientific facts and, therefore, reliable.

testimonial personal endorsement of a product

pseudoscience presentation of information masquerading as factual and obtained by scientific methods

Be Skeptical of Claims

People may think they have learned facts about nutrition by reading popular magazine articles or best-selling books; visiting Internet websites; or watching television news, infomercials, or home shopping network programs. In many instances, however, they have been misinformed. To be a careful consumer, do not assume that all nutrition information presented in the popular media is reliable. The First Amendment to the U.S. Constitution guarantees freedom of the press and freedom of speech, so people can provide nutrition information that is not true. Thus, the First Amendment does not protect consumers with freedom from nutrition misinformation or false nutrition claims.

The U.S. Food and Drug Administration (FDA) can regulate nutrition- and health-related claims on product labels, but the agency cannot prevent the spread of health and nutrition misinformation published in books or pamphlets or presented in television or radio programs. As a consumer, you are responsible for questioning and researching the accuracy of nutrition information as well as the credentials of the people making nutrition-related claims.

Promoters of worthless nutrition products and services often use sophisticated marketing methods to lure consumers. For example, some promoters of dietary supplements claim their products

Be wary of ads for nutrition-related products that rely on testimonials and anecdotes.

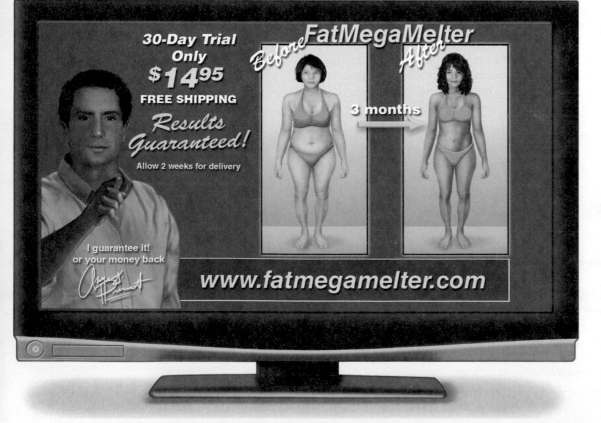

are "scientifically tested" or they include citations to what appear to be scientific journal articles in their ads or articles. Consumers, however, cannot be certain the information is true. Few dietary supplements have been thoroughly evaluated by reputable scientists. In some instances, these products have been scientifically tested, but the bulk of the research has shown that most dietary supplements, other than vitamins and minerals, provide little or no measurable health benefits. Nevertheless, promoters of nonnutrient dietary supplements usually ignore the scientific evidence and continue to sell their goods to an unsuspecting, trusting public. The Highlight at the end of this chapter focuses on dietary supplements.

Consumers also need to be alert for promoters' use of **pseudoscience,** the presentation of information masquerading as factual and obtained by scientific methods. In many instances, pseudoscientific nutrition or physiology information is presented with complex scientific-sounding terms, such as "enzymatic therapy" or "colloidal extract." Such terms are designed to convince people without science backgrounds that the nutrition-related information is true. Often, promoters of nutrition misinformation try to confuse people by weaving false information with facts into their claims, making the untrue material seem credible too.

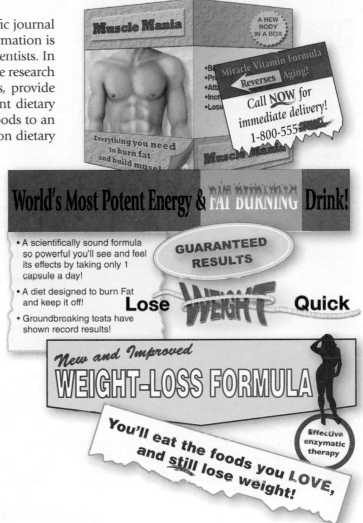

Although people's lives have improved as a result of scientific advancements in medicine, the general public tends to mistrust scientists, medical professionals, and the pharmaceutical industry. Promoters of nutrition misinformation exploit this mistrust to sell their products and services. For example, they may tell consumers that physicians rely on costly diagnostic methods and treatments for serious diseases because they are more interested in making money than doing what is best for their patients, such as recommending a dietary supplement. Are physicians driven by the desire to make money from their patients' illnesses, and do they hide information about natural cures from them? Do pharmaceutical companies promote the use of their expensive medications instead of dietary supplements because the active ingredients in medications can be patented, and as a result, be highly profitable?

It is true that physicians need incomes to support themselves and their families and drug companies strive to make profits and recover the large amounts of money they spend on testing new drugs for safety and usefulness. However, people who tell you that the "medical/scientific establishment and drug companies are hiding information about natural cures from you just to make money from your misery" are using *scare tactics* to build mistrust in the medical establishment. Over the past 100 years, people's lives have been greatly improved by contributions of medical researchers, such as physicians Salk and Sabin, who developed vaccines for preventing polio (Fig. 2.9), and Marshall and Warren, who determined that a bacterium was responsible for most peptic ulcers. By discovering effective ways to prevent or treat serious diseases, medical researchers are likely to enjoy considerable positive worldwide recognition for their efforts, such as the Nobel Prize in medicine.

As a group, physicians are dedicated to improving their patients' health and saving lives. Physicians have nothing to gain from concealing a cure from the public. They strive to diagnose and treat diseases using scientifically tested and approved techniques. Moreover, a physician may face a malpractice lawsuit if he or she fails to diagnose and treat a condition

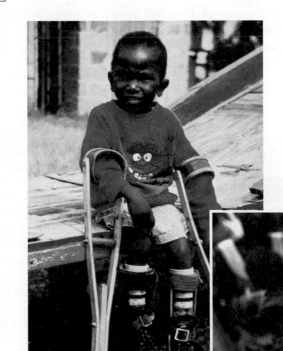
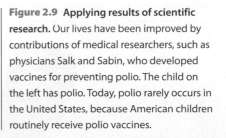

Figure 2.9 Applying results of scientific research. Our lives have been improved by contributions of medical researchers, such as physicians Salk and Sabin, who developed vaccines for preventing polio. The child on the left has polio. Today, polio rarely occurs in the United States, because American children routinely receive polio vaccines.

quackery promotion of useless medical treatments

If this person appeared on a television show or in a magazine advertisement, would you consider him to be a reliable source of nutrition information? Explain why you would or would not trust his nutrition-related advice.

effectively. Additionally, physicians have much to gain from treating their patients kindly and effectively. Consider this: If you follow a physician's advice and have positive results, are you likely to be that doctor's patient for a long time and recommend the practitioner to others?

If your car is not functioning properly, you probably would want people who have the best training, tools, and equipment to determine the problem and repair it. If you think something is wrong with your body, it is prudent to seek information and opinions from medical professionals who have the best training and experience to diagnose and treat health disorders.

Ask Questions

If you are like most people, you do not want to waste your money on things you do not need or that are useless or potentially harmful. How can you become a more careful, critical consumer of nutrition-related information or products? The following questions should help you evaluate various sources of nutrition information:

- *What motivates the authors, promoters, or sponsors to provide the information? Do you think they are more interested in your health and well-being or in selling their products?* Salespeople often have favorable biases toward the things they sell, and therefore, they may not be reliable sources of information about these products. A clerk in a dietary supplements outlet store, for example, may wear a white lab coat to look as though he or she has a science or medical educational background, but you should keep in mind that the clerk was hired to sell dietary supplements and may have little or no scientific training. Furthermore, salespeople who work in such outlets may be unwilling to inform customers about the potential health hazards of taking certain products, particularly when they earn a commission from each sale.

- *Is the source scientific, such as an article from a peer-reviewed nutrition journal?* In general, popular sources of nutrition information, such as best-selling books and articles in magazines, are not peer-reviewed by scientists. Additionally, radio or TV programs that promote nutrition information may actually be sophisticated advertisements for nutrition-related products.

- *If a study is cited, how was the research conducted? Did the study involve humans or animals? If people participated in the study, how many subjects were involved in the research? Who sponsored the study?* As mentioned earlier in this chapter, epidemiological studies are not useful for finding cause-and-effect relationships. Additionally, the results of studies involving large numbers of human subjects are more reliable than studies of animals. Sponsors may influence the outcomes of the studies they fund.

- *To provide scientific support for claims, does the source cite respected nutrition or medical journals or mention reliable experts?* Be careful if you see citations in popular nutrition or health books and magazines. Promoters of nutrition misinformation may refer to scientific-appearing citations from phony medical journals to convince people that their information is reliable. Furthermore, be wary of nutrition experts introduced or identified as "Doctor" because they may not be physicians or scientists. Furthermore, a so-called nutrition expert who is referred to as "Doctor" may not have a doctorate degree (Ph.D.) in human nutrition from an accredited university. Such experts may have obtained their degrees simply by purchasing them on the Internet or through a mail-order outlet, without having taken appropriate coursework or graduated from an accredited university or college.

Practicing medicine without the proper training and licensing is illegal. However, providing nutrition information and advice without the proper training and licensing is legal. **Quackery** involves promoting useless medical treatments, such as copper bracelets to treat arthritis.

To obtain information about a nutrition expert's credentials, enter the person's name at an Internet search engine and evaluate the results. For example, is the person associated with an accredited school of higher education or a government agency such as the U.S. Department of Agriculture? You can also visit www.quackwatch.org and submit an "Ask a Question" e-mail requesting information about a person's credentials from the site's sponsors.

Look for Red Flags

To become a skeptical consumer of nutrition information, you need to be aware of "red flags," clues that indicate a source of information is unreliable. Common red flags include the following:

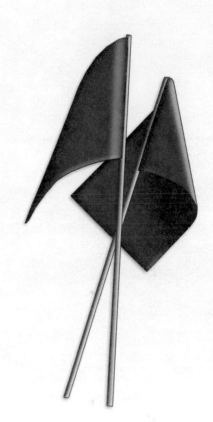

1. **Promises of quick and easy remedies for complex health-related problems:** "Our product helps you lose weight *without* exercising or dieting," "Eating yogurt prevents gastrointestinal diseases," or "Garlic cures heart disease."

2. **Claims that sound too good to be true:** "Our all-natural product blocks fat and calories from being absorbed, so you can eat everything you like and still lose weight," or "Why eat food when you'll get all the nutrients you need by taking our supplements?" These claims are rarely true. Remember, if the claim sounds too good to be true, it probably is not true.

3. **Scare tactics that include sensational, frightening, false, or misleading statements about a food, dietary practice, or health condition:** "Dairy products cause cancer," or "Children who eat meat and drink milk mature too early because of the hormones and chemical additives in these foods," or "Eating sugar causes hyperactivity."

4. **Personal attacks on the motives and ethical standards of registered dietitians or conventional scientists:** "Dietitians and medical researchers don't want you to know the facts about natural cures for cancer, diabetes, and heart disease because it will dry up their funding." Such statements indicate unsubstantiated biases against bona fide nutrition experts and the scientific community.

5. **Statements about the superiority of certain dietary supplements or unconventional medical practices:** "Russian scientists have discovered the countless health benefits of taking Siberian ginseng," or "Colon cleansing with herbs is the only cure for intestinal cancer."

6. **Testimonials and anecdotes as evidence of effectiveness:** "I lost 50 pounds in 30 days using this product," or "I rubbed this vitamin E–containing lotion on my scar and it disappeared in days."As mentioned earlier, these sources of information are unreliable. Reliable nutrition information is based on scientific evidence.

7. **Information that promotes a product's benefits while overlooking its risks:** "Our all-natural supplement boosts your metabolism naturally so it won't harm your system," or "One hundred percent of the people who used our product to treat diabetes had excellent results." Anything you consume, even water, can be toxic in high doses. Beware of any source of information that fails to mention the possible side effects of using a dietary supplement or nutrition-related treatment.

8. **Vague, meaningless, or scientific-sounding terms to impress or confuse consumers:** "Our *all-natural, clinically tested, patented, chelated* dietary supplement works best," or "The typical vegetable grown in the United States lacks high-grade nutrients because conventional farming methods have *devitalized* the soil."

9. **Sensational statements with incomplete references of sources:** "Clinical research performed at a major university and published in a distinguished medical journal indicates food manufacturers have added ingredients to products that make you hungry and fat," or "Millions of Americans suffer from various nutritional deficiencies." Which "major university" and "distinguished medical journal"? What study reported that "millions of Americans" are deficient in nutrients?

10. **Recommendations based on a single study:** "Research conducted at our private health facility proves coffee enemas can cure cancer."

11. **Information concerning nutrients or human physiology that is not supported by reliable scientific evidence:** "This book explains how to combine certain foods based on your blood type," or "Most diseases are caused by undigested food that gets stuck in your guts," or "People with alkaline bodies don't develop cancer."

12. **Dramatic generalizations:** "Our revolutionary new dietary supplement cured Mary's diabetes; it can cure you too."

13. **Results disclaimers, usually in small or difficult-to-read print:** "Results may vary," or "Results not typical" (Fig. 2.10). Disclaimers are clues that the product probably will not live up to your expectations or the manufacturer's claims.

Using the Internet Wisely

You can find abundant sources of information about nutrition and the benefits of dietary supplements on the Internet. However, you must be careful and consider the sources. Who or what organization sponsors the site? Is the information intended to promote sales? Be wary if the site discusses benefits of dietary supplements and enables you to purchase these products online. Furthermore, a site is likely to be unreliable if it includes comprehensive disclaimers such as, "The manufacturer is not responsible or obligated to verify statements," or "The FDA has not evaluated this website. This product is not intended to diagnose, cure, or prevent any disease." Also avoid sites that publish disclaimers such as, "The nutrition and health information at this site is provided for educational purposes only and not as a substitute for the advice of a physician or dietitian. The author and owner of this site are not liable for personal actions taken as a result of the site's contents."

Be wary of websites that are authored or sponsored by one person, or sites that promote or sell products for profit (*.com) because such sources of information may be biased. In general, websites sponsored by nationally recognized health associations such as the Academy of Nutrition and Dietetics, formerly the American Dietetic Association (www.eatright.org) and nonprofit organizations such as the National Osteoporosis Foundation (www.nof.org) are reliable sources of nutrition information. Government agencies (*.gov) and nationally accredited colleges and universities (*.edu) are also excellent sources of credible nutrition information. Table 2.1 presents some tips for using the Internet to obtain reliable nutrition information.

The Federal Trade Commission (FTC) enforces consumer protection laws and investigates complaints about false or misleading health claims that appear on the Internet. For information to help you evaluate nutrition and health-related claims, visit the agency's website (www.ftc.gov/bcp/edu/pubs/consumer/health/hea07.shtm). To complain about a product, you can complete and submit the FTC's complaint form at the website or call the agency's toll-free line (1-877-382-4357).

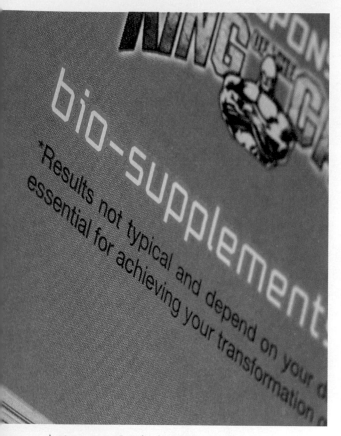

Figure 2.10 Results disclaimer. This disclaimer may be a red flag indicating the product has limited effectiveness, despite its promoter's claims.

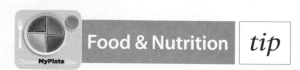

Food & Nutrition *tip*

If you are looking for a recipe for guacamole, cranberry chutney, or sweet and sour cabbage, simply use the Internet—it is like having a cookbook at your fingertips. Recipes for nearly every food and from various countries and ethnic groups are available on the Internet, and you can also find menu planning and cooking tips from this vast resource.

When searching the Web for recipes, you need to recognize that many food manufacturers use the sites to promote their products in recipes. If the brand name of a product is mentioned in the recipe, you can usually substitute another company's product. Additionally, recipes do not always provide accurate information about the nutrients and calories in a serving of food, and you cannot be certain that the recipes have been tested for quality. Therefore, it is a good idea to check more than one site for a recipe and compare the information.

Concept **Checkpoint**

8. What is the difference between a testimonial and an anecdote?
9. List at least three "red flags" that may indicate a questionable source of nutrition information.
10. List at least three tips for using the Internet as a reliable source of nutrition information.

TABLE 2.1 *Tips for Searching Nutrition Information on the Internet*

To be a careful consumer of Internet sources of information:

1. Use multiple sites, especially government sites, such as the Centers for Disease Control and Prevention (www.cdc.gov) and the Food and Drug Administration (www.fda.gov) as well as the sites of nationally recognized nutrition- or health-related associations such as the Academy of Nutrition and Dietetics (www.eatright.org) and the American Heart Association (www.americanheart.org).

2. Be wary of sites that have surveys for you to complete, advertisements for diet-related products, and promotions in pop-up windows.

3. Rely primarily on sites that are managed or reviewed by a group of qualified health professionals. Blogs might be fun and interesting to read, but they are not necessarily reliable.

4. Look for the Health on the Net symbol at the bottom of the main page of the website. The Health on the Net Foundation is a nonprofit, international organization that promotes the HONcode, a set of principles for standardizing the reliability of health information on the Internet. Currently, website sponsors are not required to follow HONcode standards. For more information about HONcode, you can visit the organization's website (www.hon.ch/).

5. Do not trust information at a site that does not indicate valid sources, such as well-respected peer-reviewed scientific journals or nationally recognized universities or medical centers. Contributing authors and their credentials should be identified; when they are, perform an online search of the scientific journals, as well as the authors' names and credentials to determine their validity.

6. Do not trust a site that includes attacks on the trustworthiness of the medical or scientific establishment.

7. Avoid sites that provide online diagnoses and treatments.

8. Be wary of commercial sites (*.com) with links to government sites or the sites of well-known medical, nutrition, or scientific associations. An unreliable *.com site can be linked to reliable sites without having received their endorsements.

9. Avoid providing your personal information at the site because its confidentiality may not be protected.

For more tips, visit: http://ods.od.nih.gov/Health_Information/How_To_Evaluate_Health_Information_on_the_Internet_Questions_and_Answers.aspx.

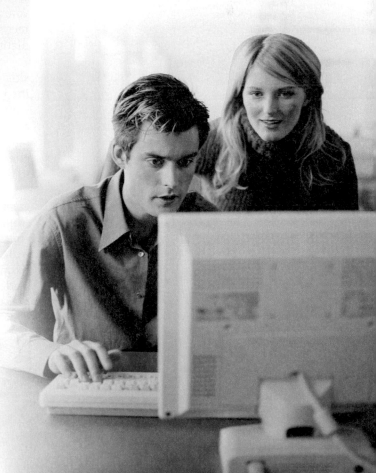

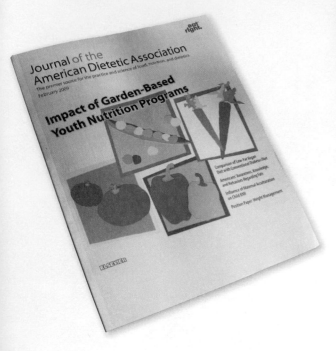

 ## 2.3 Reliable Nutrition Experts

If you have questions about food or nutrition, where do you find factual answers? Although some states regulate and license people who call themselves nutritionists, you cannot always rely on someone who refers to him- or herself as a "nutritionist" or "nutritionalist" for reliable nutrition information, because there are no standard legal definitions for these descriptors. Should you ask a physician for nutrition advice? Physicians are not necessarily the best sources of nutrition information, because most doctors do not have extensive college coursework in the subject.

If your university or college has a nutrition or dietetics department, you are likely to find nutrition experts, including professors and registered dietitians, who are faculty members. A *registered dietitian* is a college-trained health care professional who has extensive knowledge of foods, nutrition, and *dietetics*, the application of nutrition and food information to treat many health-related conditions. The title "registered dietitian" is legally protected.

You can also locate registered dietitians by consulting the yellow pages of telephone directories, contacting your local dietetic association or dietary department of a local hospital, or visiting the Academy of Nutrition and Dietetics website (www.eatright.org) or the Dietitians of Canada's website (www.dietitians.ca).

Becoming a Registered Dietitian

Are you interested in science? Would you like to learn how diets can be altered to treat disease? Would you like a challenging career as a health professional? If you answered "yes" to each of these questions, you may want to consider becoming a registered dietitian (R.D.). There are three major professional divisions for registered dietitians—clinical dietetics, community nutrition, and food service systems management. Clinical dietitians can work as members of medical teams in hospitals or clinics. Clinical dietitians can also work as community nutritionists in public health settings or as dietary counselors in private practice or with wellness programs. Food service systems management dietitians direct food systems in hospitals, schools, or other settings. Although most registered dietitians work in health care settings, some are educators or researchers.

An R.D. has completed a baccalaureate degree program approved by the Commission on Accreditation for Dietetics Education of the Academy of Nutrition and Dietetics, the largest organization of dietitians in the United States. As undergraduate students, dietetics majors are required to take a wide variety of college-level courses, including food and nutrition sciences, organic chemistry, biochemistry, biology, physiology, microbiology, food service systems management, business, and communications classes. If you are attending a major university, you can check the course or program catalog at your school to determine whether an accredited dietetics program is offered.

There are two pathways students can take to become dietitians. A *Coordinated Program (CP)* combines classroom instruction with at least 900 hours of supervised professional practice experience. A *Didactic Program in Dietetics (DPD)* provides classroom courses, and after graduation, students need to complete a dietetic internship program, which provides at least 900 hours of supervised practice experience and generally takes six months to a year to complete. After completing a CP or dietetic internship program, students are eligible to take the national examination to become registered dietitians. To maintain their certification, registered dietitians must continually update their knowledge in the field of dietetics and obtain continuing education credits.

Concept **Checkpoint**

11. What is the difference between a nutritionist and a registered dietitian?

12. List three ways of locating reliable nutrition experts.

Chapter 2 Highlight

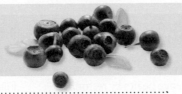

WHAT ARE DIETARY SUPPLEMENTS?

Do you take a daily multivitamin/multimineral pill because you are concerned about the nutritional quality of your diet? Do you use herbal pills or extracts to strengthen your immune system, boost your memory, or treat illnesses such as the common cold? If you follow any of these practices, you are not alone. According to results of surveys, about 20% to 50% of adult Americans used these and other dietary supplements during the period 1999–2002.[12,13,14]

According to the Dietary Supplement and Health Education Act of 1994 (DSHEA), a dietary supplement is a product (other than tobacco) that

- adds to a person's dietary intake and contains one or more dietary ingredients, including nutrients or *botanicals* (herbs or other plant material)
- is taken by mouth
- is not promoted as a conventional food or the only item of a meal or diet[15]

Dietary supplements include nutrient pills, protein powders, and herbal extracts, as well as energy bars and drinks. Many dietary supplements are often referred to as "nutraceuticals," but there is no legal definition for this term.

In the United States, the most commonly used dietary supplements are *multivitamin/multimineral* (*MVMM*) products that typically contain several vitamins and minerals.[16] Among American adults, the most popular nonvitamin, nonmineral dietary supplements are fish oil or "omega 3," glucosamine, echinacea, and flaxseed oil and pills.[17] Some people use dietary supplements, particularly those containing nutrients, because the products are recommended by their physicians or dietitians. Physicians, for example, may prescribe a prenatal MVMM supplement for their pregnant patients. Most dietary supplements are available without the need for prescriptions, so people can take them without their doctors' knowledge and approval. When researchers asked a group of people why they used dietary supplements, subjects gave a variety of reasons, including to boost their nutrient intakes, to prevent certain diseases, to obtain more energy, to enhance good health, and to treat existing ailments.[18]

Table 2.2 provides information about some non-micronutrient dietary supplements that are popular among adult Americans. Benefits and risks of supplementing diets with micronutrients are discussed in Chapters 8 and 9.

What Is Complementary and Alternative Medicine?

The use of herbal products and other dietary supplements to treat disease or promote good health is an aspect of *complementary and alternative medicine* (*CAM*). CAM includes a variety of health care practices and products that are not accepted by the majority of physicians and other conventional health care providers. In 2007, approximately 38% of American adults and 12% of American children used CAM therapies, including chiropractic manipulations, homeopathy, naturopathy, and massage therapy.[17] Among American adults, taking nonvitamin, nonmineral natural products was the most popular form of CAM therapy. However, there is little scientific evidence that supports the usefulness as well as the safety of taking most nonnutrient dietary supplements, including botanicals.[17]

A few types of CAM are gaining acceptance among conventional medical practitioners, primarily because there is sufficient scientific support for the practices. For example, species of "unfriendly" bacteria can overpopulate the large intestine when a person takes an antibiotic for infection. The overgrowth of these bacteria can cause cramping and diarrhea. Some physicians recommend probiotics in yogurt or tablet form for patients who are taking antibiotics. Research has shown that certain probiotics can help prevent or limit diarrhea that results from antibiotic use.[19]

The practice of using CAM with conventional medicine is called *integrative medicine*. The National Center for Complementary and Alternative Medicine (NCCAM), an agency within the National Institutes of Health, funds research intended to increase scientific evidence about the usefulness and safety of CAM practices. To learn more about CAM, visit the National Center for Complementary and Alternative Medicine website at http://nccam.nih.gov.

How Are Dietary Supplements Regulated?

The U.S. Food and Drug Administration (FDA) is the federal agency that is responsible for ensuring the safety and effectiveness of medications and other health-related products. The FDA strictly regulates the development, production, and marketing of new medications (drugs). A drug is a substance, natural or human-made, that alters body functions. As a result, drugs can produce beneficial as well as harmful effects on the body. Before marketing a new drug, the manufacturer must submit evidence to the FDA indicating that the product has been tested extensively and is safe and effective. If FDA experts have serious concerns about a medication's side effects or question its usefulness, the agency may reject the manufacturer's petition to sell the product.

TABLE 2.2 *Some Popular Dietary Supplements*

Dietary Supplement	Major Claims	Known Health Effects*	
		Benefits	**Risks**
Acidophilus	Live bacterial culture reduces risk of harmful bacterial overgrowth in large intestine	May improve health by restoring the balance of beneficial to harmful bacteria in the intestinal tract	Infectious complications can occur when probiotics are used by people with inflammation of the pancreas (pancreatitis)
Beta carotene	Antioxidant Reduces risk of cancer and heart disease	Source of vitamin A Antioxidant	Excess may stimulate cancer cell growth
Chondroitin	Relieves joint damage associated with arthritis	Some scientific evidence supports health benefit claims, but more research is needed Often combined with glucosamine	None identified
Coenzyme Q-10	Increases exercise tolerance Prevents heart disease and cancer Reverses signs of aging and disease	Antioxidant made by the body and involved in energy metabolism Insufficient scientific evidence to support most claims	May reduce elevated blood pressure, but more research is needed Low toxicity but long-term safety is unknown
Echinacea	Boosts immune system Prevents the common cold and reduces cold symptoms	Mixed scientific evidence to support common cold prevention claims, but research is ongoing	Generally safe but may provoke allergic response or intestinal upset
Evening primrose oil	Treats eczema (a common skin condition) Relieves arthritis and postmenopausal symptoms	May relieve eczema Little scientific evidence to support other health benefit claims	None identified
Fish oil	Prevents heart disease and stroke Cures rheumatoid arthritis Reduces depression and risk of Alzheimer's disease	Source of omega-3 fatty acids Reduces inflammation and lowers elevated blood triglyceride (fat) levels, but more research is needed to determine other health benefits	May interfere with blood clotting, increasing the risk of hemorrhagic stroke Cod liver oil contains vitamin A, which is toxic when taken in large doses
Flaxseed and flaxseed oil	Acts as a laxative (flaxseed) Reduces blood cholesterol levels	Nonanimal source of omega-3 fatty acids Seeds have laxative effects May benefit people with heart disease, but more research is needed	Generally safe
Garlic	Lowers blood cholesterol levels	Does not lower cholesterol consistently May reduce elevated blood pressure	Can cause allergic reaction, unpleasant body odor, and interfere with prescription blood thinners
Ginger	Treats "morning sickness" and other forms of nausea Relieves stomach upsets	Can safely treat morning sickness and may reduce other forms of nausea Lack of scientific evidence to support other health benefit claims	None identified
Gingko biloba	Improves memory Reduces the risk of Alzheimer's disease and other forms of dementia	Lack of scientific evidence to support health benefit claims	May increase the risk of bleeding and cause allergic reactions, headaches, intestinal upsets, and nausea Gingko seeds are toxic

TABLE 2.2 *Some Popular Dietary Supplements (continued)*

Dietary Supplement	Major Claims	Known Health Effects*	
		Benefits	**Risks**
Ginseng (Asian)	Boosts overall health Treats erectile dysfunction (male impotence)	May lower elevated blood glucose levels and benefit immune system Lack of scientific evidence to support other health benefit claims	May cause headaches, sleep disturbances, allergic responses, and gastrointestinal upsets Long-term use may increase risk of toxicity
Glucosamine	Relieves joint damage associated with arthritis	Some scientific evidence supports health benefit claims, but more research is needed (frequently used with chondroitin)	None identified
Green tea	Prevents or treats cancer Promotes weight loss Reduces blood cholesterol levels	Results of some laboratory studies indicate green tea protects against cancer or reduces cancer cell growth, but results of human studies are not conclusive Lack of reliable evidence to support other health benefit claims	Green tea extracts may damage the liver Caffeine content may cause sleep disturbances, irritability, and digestive upset
Kava	Reduces stress	Potential harm of using kava outweighs any benefit	Toxic—can damage the liver May cause abnormal muscle movements, yellowed skin, and sleepiness
Lysine	Prevents recurrence of genital herpes outbreaks	Amino acid (component of proteins) Lack of scientific evidence that supports health benefit claims	None identified
Melatonin	Treats some sleep disorders Prevents jet lag	May be effective for treating certain sleep disorders and preventing jet lag	Questions about long-term safety
Red yeast rice	Lowers blood cholesterol, reducing risk of heart disease	May be useful, especially for people who cannot take prescription medications to lower blood cholesterol	Long-term safety is unknown
St. John's wort	Reduces depression	May be effective in treating mild-to-moderate depression	May interact with other herbal products and certain medications, including prescription antidepressants and oral contraceptives
Valerian	Promotes relaxation Treats sleep disorders	Evidence to support claims is inconsistent	Dizziness, headache, stomach upset Questions about long-term safety

* Sources: Office of Dietary Supplements http://ods.od.nih.gov/factsheets/list-Botanicals/; National Center for Complementary and Alternative Medicine *http://nccam.nih.gov/health/coenzyme.htm*; and http://nccam.nih.gov/health/herbsataglance.htm
Accessed: July 4, 2011

When consumed, many dietary supplements act as drugs in the body. However, the FDA regulates dietary supplements as foods, not medications.[20] As a result, dietary supplement manufacturers can bypass most of the strict regulations that the FDA applies to the introduction of new medications into the marketplace. Supplement manufacturers, for example, generally do not need FDA approval before manufacturing or marketing their products. Additionally, the manufacturers are not required to provide the FDA with scientific evidence indicating their products provide measurable health benefits. Manufacturers, however, must notify the FDA and provide the agency with information about the safety of any supplement that contains dietary ingredients that were not marketed in dietary supplements prior to 1994, unless the substance had been used in foods.

The FDA regulates the labeling of dietary supplements, including the kinds of claims that are permitted on labels. The "Food and Dietary Supplement Labels" section of Chapter 3 provides information about supplement labeling.

The FDA's role in regulating dietary supplements generally begins after products enter the marketplace.[21] Supplement manufacturers are required to keep records concerning reports they receive about serious adverse (negative) health effects that may have been caused by their products.[22] Furthermore, the manufacturers must also inform the FDA about such reports. Consumers and health care professionals can also report health problems that are possibly associated with supplement use directly to the FDA.

When the FDA determines that a particular supplement presents a significant or unreasonable risk of harm, the agency alerts consumers about the risk and seeks to recall the product, that is, initiates efforts to have it removed from the market. In most instances, the manufacturer voluntarily recalls the product after determining there is a problem with it or being notified by the FDA about the problem.[23] In some cases, however, the FDA requests a recall.

If the FDA determines that the manufacturer's response to the recall is inadequate, the agency can take enforcement steps, such as initiating legal action against the company to seize products or stop producing the items. In every recall case, the FDA oversees the manufacturer's handling of the recall and assesses whether the steps taken to remove the product were adequate.[23]

Recalls of dietary supplements occur when the products are

- contaminated with dangerous microbes, pesticides, or metals
- labeled improperly, such as missing a substance that is in the list of ingredients
- not legitimate dietary supplements, such as a product that includes ingredients referred to as "vitamins," when these substances are not vitamins[24]

Using Dietary Supplements Wisely

When used properly, many dietary supplements, particularly micronutrient products, are generally safe. Herbal supplements, however, are made from plants that may have toxic parts. Comfrey, pennyroyal, sassafras, kava, lobelia, and ma huang are among the plants known to be highly toxic or cancer-causing. Products containing material from these plants should be avoided. The use of botanical products can also evoke allergic or inflammatory responses that often result in skin, sinus, or respiratory signs and symptoms. Herbal teas may contain pollens and other parts of plants that can cause allergies, particularly in people who are sensitive to the herbs or their related species. Echinacea (purple cone flower) is related to ragweed, a plant that is often associated with seasonal respiratory allergies.[25] When people who are allergic to ragweed pollen take supplements that contain echinacea, they may develop allergic responses that mimic symptoms of the common cold (watery eyes, runny nose, and sneezing). In some instances, inflammatory responses, such as asthma attacks, can occur after exposure to echinacea or other plants. Asthma can be a

life-threatening condition. Therefore, people who have asthma or allergies should be very careful when using botanical supplements.

Consumers also need to be aware that medicinal herbs may contain substances that interact with prescription or over-the-counter medications as well as other herbs. Such responses can produce unwanted and even dangerous side effects (see Table 2.2). Ginkgo biloba, for example, can interact with aspirin, increasing the risk of bleeding. Garlic, ginseng, and vitamin E supplements can also increase bleeding. Kava and valerian act as sedatives (calming agents) and can amplify the effects of anesthetics and other medications used during surgery. Therefore, consult a physician or pharmacist before using any dietary supplement or giving such products to your children. Additionally, treat dietary supplements as drugs: store them away from children and provide your physicians and other health care professionals with a list of the ones you are taking.

If you use or are thinking about using one or more dietary supplements:

- Determine whether the supplement is necessary. Some people have medical reasons for taking dietary supplements that contain one or more micronutrients, such as folic acid, calcium, or vitamin D. Discuss your need for the supplement with your physician or a dietitian before you purchase or use the product. This action is particularly important if you are pregnant, are breastfeeding a baby, or have a chronic medical condition such as diabetes or heart disease.
- Consult a physician as soon as you develop signs and symptoms of a serious illness. Using supplements to treat serious diseases instead of seeking conventional medical care that has proven effectiveness is a risky practice. In these instances, delaying or forgoing useful medical treatment may result in the worsening of the condition or even be life threatening.
- Be wary of claims made about a supplement's benefits and investigate the claims used to promote the product. The following government websites provide reliable information about dietary supplements:
  U.S. National Library of Medicine www.nlm.nih.gov/medlineplus/herbalmedicine.html
  Food and Drug Adminstration www.fda.gov/Food/DietarySupplements/default.htm
  National Institutes of Health, National Center for Complementary and Alternative Medicine http://nccam.nih.gov/health/herbsataglance.htm
  Office of Dietary Supplements http://ods.od.nih.gov/factsheets/dietarysupplements/.
- Determine hazards associated with taking the supplement. Information about the risks and benefits of various dietary supplements can be found at the **Office of Dietary Supplements'** website: http://ods.od.nih.gov/factsheets/dietarysupplements/.
- Avoid using dietary supplements as substitutes for nutritious foods. Plant foods provide a wide array of phytochemicals, many of which may have health benefits when taken in their

natural forms—foods. When these substances are isolated from plants and manufactured into supplements, they may lose their beneficial properties.

If you experience negative side effects after using a particular dietary supplement, it is a good idea to be examined by a physician immediately. Furthermore, you as well as your physician should report the problem to the FDA's MedWatch program by calling (800) FDA-1088 or visiting the agency's website: http://www.fda.gov/Safety/MedWatch/HowToReport/default.htm.

It is important to recognize that the manufacturing of dietary supplements is a profitable industry in the United States. In 2010, Americans spent almost $29 billion on such products.[26] In many instances, however, people do not need dietary supplements, and they are wasting their money by purchasing them—money that could be better spent on natural sources of nutrients and phyto chemicals, particularly fruits, vegetables, and whole-grain cereals.[27]

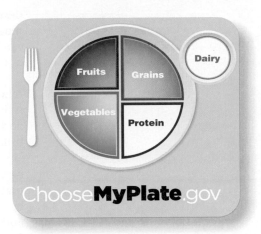

CHAPTER REFERENCES

See Appendix I.

SUMMARY

Scientists ask questions about the natural world and follow generally accepted methods to obtain answers to these questions. Nutrition research relies on scientific methods that may involve making observations, asking questions and developing possible explanations, performing tests, collecting and analyzing data, drawing conclusions from data, and reporting on the findings. Other scientists can test the findings to confirm or reject them.

Epidemiology is the study of the occurrence, distribution, and causes of health problems in populations. By studying differences in dietary practices and disease occurrences among populations, epidemiologists can suggest nutrition-related hypotheses for the prevalence of certain diseases. Epidemiologists often conduct observational studies to provide clues about the causes, progression, and prevention of the diseases. Epidemiological studies, however, cannot indicate whether two variables are correlated, because the relationship could be a coincidence.

When an experiment or study is completed and the results analyzed, researchers summarize the findings and seek to publish articles with information about their investigations in scientific journals. Before articles are accepted for publication, they undergo peer review. Scientists generally do not accept a hypothesis or the results of a study until they are supported by considerable research evidence. Thus, researchers often face stiff criticism and rejection from members of the medical establishment when their hypotheses or findings contradict accepted nutrition principles. Media coverage of a medical breakthrough is not necessarily an indication of the value or quality of research that resulted in the news story. More research is often necessary for scientists to determine whether the results are valid and can be generalized.

Consumers may think scientists do not know what they are doing when conflicting research findings are reported in the media. However, consumers need to recognize that conflicting findings often result because different teams of researchers use different study

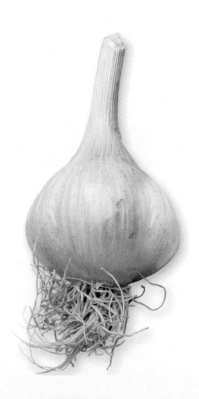

designs when investigating the same hypothesis. Furthermore, each team of scientists may analyze the results differently. Other factors, such as genetic and lifestyle differences, can also influence the results of nutrition research involving human subjects. The science of nutrition is constantly evolving.

Although testimonials and anecdotes are often used to promote nutrition-related products and services, consumers cannot be sure that this information is reliable or based on scientific facts. Personal observations are not evidence of a cause-and-effect relationship because many factors, such as lifestyle and environment, can influence outcomes.

Popular magazine articles, best-selling trade books, Internet websites, television news reports, and other forms of media are often unreliable sources of nutrition information. Consumers need to be skeptical and question the reliability of such sources, because the First Amendment to the U.S. Constitution guarantees freedom of the press and freedom of speech. People who promote nutrition misinformation often benefit from these freedoms.

Consumers need to become more knowledgeable about the basics of human nutrition and physiology, and they need to be skeptical about the reliability of the nutrition information that is so readily available in the press, in magazines, and on the Internet. To determine whether a source of information is reliable, consumers need to ask questions to determine the author's reasons for promoting the information. Consumers should also look for red flags, such as scare tactics and claims that sound too good to be true.

Much of the nutrition information that is on the Internet is unreliable and intended to promote sales. Websites sponsored by nonprofit organizations, nationally recognized health associations, government agencies, and nationally accredited colleges and universities are generally reliable sources of information.

Although some states regulate and license nutritionists, there is no standard legal definition for "nutritionist" in the United States. For reliable food, nutrition, and dietary information, consumers can consult persons with degrees in human nutrition from accredited institutions of higher learning, such as nutrition instructors and registered dietitians. Registered dietitians also can be located by consulting local yellow pages of telephone directories, contacting local dietetic associations, calling the dietary departments of local hospitals, or visiting the Academy of Nutrition and Dietetics website.

A dietary supplement is a product (other than tobacco) that adds to a person's dietary intake, contains one or more dietary ingredients, is taken by mouth in tablet or other forms, and is not promoted as a conventional food or the only item of a meal or diet.

Dietary supplements include nutrient pills, protein powders, and herbal extracts, as well as energy bars and drinks. Some people have medical reasons for taking dietary supplements that contain one or more micronutrients, but in many instances, people do not need dietary supplements. Healthy people should focus on obtaining nutrients and phytochemicals from foods, particularly fruits, vegetables, and whole-grain cereals. Before taking a dietary supplement, discuss the matter with your physician.

Recipes for Healthy Living

Grandma's Chicken Soup

Long before the advent of over-the-counter antihistamines and cough syrups, there was chicken soup. Sometimes referred to as "Jewish penicillin," chicken soup has been used as a cold remedy for over 1000 years. Chicken soup is not a cure for the common cold. However, results of a laboratory study indicated chicken soup contains substances that can subdue the body's inflammatory response to upper respiratory tract infections. This inflammatory response typically results in common cold symptoms such as cough and excess nasal discharge. Although the soup's specific actions on cold-causing microbes still need to be determined, consuming a soothing, warm bowl of chicken soup contributes to the sick person's fluid and other nutrient intake at a time when he or she may not feel like eating anything else. Even if you don't have a cold, the following chicken soup recipe is delicious and easy to make. You can freeze the soup in small covered plastic containers for future meals.

Source: Rennard BO and others: Chicken soup inhibits neutrophil chemotaxis in vitro. *Chest* 118(4):1, 2000.

This recipe makes approximately 6 to 8 cups of soup. A 1-cup serving of the soup supplies approximately 90 kcal, 6 g of protein, 3 g fat, 340 mg sodium, 250 mg potassium, and 3.8 mg niacin.

INGREDIENTS:

1 package of raw chicken wings, approx. 3 to 4 lbs
1 large onion, cut in wedges
4 large carrots, cleaned and cut into 3-inch lengths
⅛ tsp black pepper
1 chicken bouillon cube
3 celery stalks, cleaned and cut into 3-inch lengths
⅛ tsp paprika
⅛ tsp thyme
⅛ tsp curry seasoning
few parsley sprigs (optional)

PREPARATION STEPS:

1. Place the raw chicken in a large cooking pot and add enough cold water to cover chicken, approximately 2 quarts of water.

2. Add onion, carrots, celery, pepper, bouillon cube, and spices to chicken and water; turn burner on high. When mixture comes to a boil, reduce heat to medium and cover the pot with a lid. Soup should boil for at least an hour.

3. Turn off the heat, remove chicken wings from the soup, and place them in a bowl. Cover and refrigerate.

4. Cover soup and refrigerate for 12 hours.

5. Skim chicken fat from top of soup. Remove skin from the wings, separate the meat from the bones, and add the meat to the soup. Reheat soup before eating; sprinkle with parsley sprigs, if desired.

6. Cover and store leftover soup in refrigerator for up to 3 days, or freeze.

   Note: When you reheat the soup, you can also add your favorite soup ingredients, such as frozen vegetables, broccoli florets, whole-wheat noodles, or cooked brown rice.

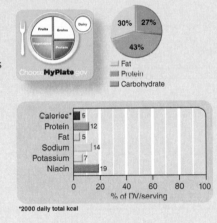

30% 27%
43%
☐ Fat
▨ Protein
☐ Carbohydrate

	% of DV/serving
Calories*	5
Protein	12
Fat	5
Sodium	14
Potassium	7
Niacin	19

*2000 daily total kcal

Ginger Green Tea

Plain tea is a source of beneficial antioxidants that provides 0 kcal/fl oz. Commercially bottled black and green teas are available in supermarkets and from vending machines. However, commercial teas that are sugar-sweetened contain 15 or more grams of sugar/serving. You can save a lot of money and avoid extra calories by making your own teas. The following ginger tea recipe is flavored with raw gingerroot from which the spice ground ginger is made. Like tea, ginger is also a source of antioxidants. This recipe makes 16 fl oz of tea. Each 8 fl oz serving provides about 40 kcal, 10 g carbohydrate, 2.5 mg vitamin C, and 80 mg potassium. (Omit the honey to consume a calorie-free drink.)

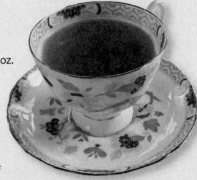

INGREDIENTS:

2 cups water
2 green tea bags
Gingerroot (1" piece)
2 Tbsp lemon juice
1 Tbsp honey

PREPARATION STEPS:

1. Wash and peel the gingerroot. Slice the peeled root into thin "coins."

2. Boil water.

3. Pour boiled water into a tea pot and dangle green tea bags into the water. Add gingerroot and steep in the hot water for 10 minutes.

4. Remove the tea bags and use a slotted spoon to remove gingerroot. Add lemon juice and if desired, honey.

100%
☐ Fat
▨ Protein
☐ Carbohydrate

	% of DV/serving
Calories*	2
Carbohydrate	3
Vitamin C	4
Potassium	2

*2000 daily total kcal

CRITICAL THINKING

1. A news broadcaster reports the results of a study in which people who took fish oil and vitamin E supplements daily did not reduce their risk of heart attack. Moreover, the researchers stopped the study when they determined the supplements increased the subjects' risk of stroke! Explain how you would determine whether this information is reliable.

2. Explain how you can verify the reliability of advice about dietary supplements provided at an Internet website.

3. Design a study that involves observing a nutrition-related practice of college students, such as vending machine choices or fast-food preferences, and share your idea with the class. Your study should be designed so that it is ethical and does not harm subjects physically or psychologically.

4. Results from one scientific study often suggest a new set of questions for researchers to investigate. Chapter 2 described current research that suggests a relationship between soy foods and the risk of breast cancer. Think of two questions this finding is likely to generate that could be answered by further scientific investigation.

5. Browse through popular health-related magazines to find an article or advertisement that relates to nutrition, and make a copy of the article or advertisement. Analyze each sentence or line of the article or advertisement for signs of unreliability. Is the article or advertisement a reliable source of information? Explain why it is or why it is not.

PRACTICE TEST

Select the best answer.

1. The first step of the scientific method usually involves

   a. gathering data.
   b. developing a hypothesis.
   c. identifying relationships between variables.
   d. making observations.

2. A group of scientists observe a group of college students over 4 years to determine which of their characteristics leads to weight gain. This study is an example of

   a. a case-control study.
   b. a prospective study.
   c. a retrospective study.
   d. an experimental study.

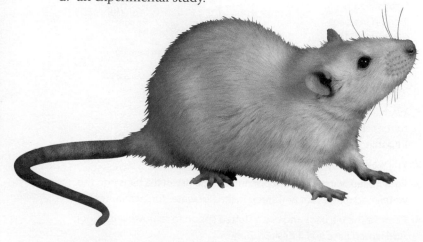

3. An aspect of _____ involves studying causes of health problems in a population.

   a. epidemiology
   b. technobiology
   c. diseasiology
   d. censusology

4. Comparing individuals with iron-deficiency anemia to individuals who have very similar characteristics but are healthy would be an example of

   a. a prospective study.
   b. an anecdotal study.
   c. a retrospective study.
   d. a case-control study.

5. Generally, epidemiological studies

   a. establish causation.
   b. prove correlations.
   c. cannot determine cause-and-effect relationships.
   d. are experimental-based research efforts that examine two variables.

6. Which of the following journals does not have peer-reviewed articles?

   a. *Journal of the American Medical Association*
   b. *American Journal of Clinical Nutrition*
   c. *Journal of Nutrition Association*
   d. None of the above is correct.

7. The government agency that enforces consumer protection laws by investigating false or misleading health-related claims is the

   a. Federal Trade Commission (FTC).
   b. Environmental Protection Agency (EPA).
   c. Agricultural Research Service (ARS).
   d. Centers for Disease Control and Prevention (CDC).

8. A testimonial is

   a. an unbiased report about a product's value.
   b. a scientifically valid claim.
   c. a personal endorsement of a product.
   d. a form of scientific evidence.

9. Which of the following websites is most likely to provide biased and unreliable nutrition information?

   a. the site of a nationally recognized health association (*.org)
   b. a site that promotes or sells dietary supplements (*.com)
   c. the site of a U.S. government agency (*.gov)
   d. an accredited college or university's site (*.edu)

10. A fake treatment is a(n)

    a. anecdote.
    b. double-blind study.
    c. pseudoscience experiment.
    d. placebo.

11. Which of the following substances would be classified as a dietary supplement according to the Dietary Supplement and Health Education Act of 1994?

    a. tobacco
    b. aspirin
    c. ginseng
    d. All of the above are correct.

12. The _____ is the federal agency that tries to ensure the safety and effectiveness of health-related products.

    a. FDA
    b. FTC
    c. EPA
    d. USGS

Answers to Chapter 2 Quiz *Yourself*

1. Scientists generally do not raise questions about or criticize the conclusions of their colleagues' research data, even when they disagree with these conclusions. **False.** (p. 40)

2. Popular health-related magazines typically publish articles that have been peer-reviewed. **False.** (p. 40)

3. By conducting a prospective epidemiological study, medical researchers can determine risk factors that may influence health. **True.** (p. 36)

4. Dietary supplements include vitamin pills as well as products that contain echinacea, ginseng, and garlic. **True.** (p. 49)

5. In general, registered dietitians are reliable sources of food and nutrition information. **True.** (p. 48)

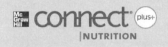 Additional resources related to the features of this book are available on ConnectPlus® Nutrition. Ask your instructor how to get access.

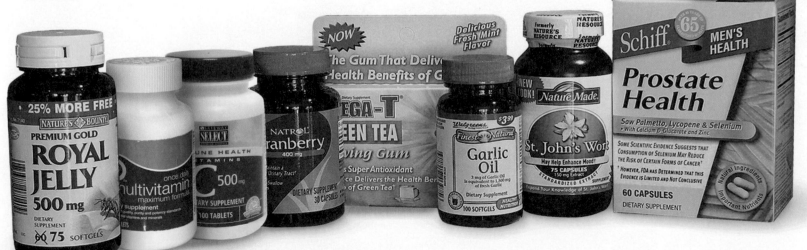

Planning Nutritious Diets

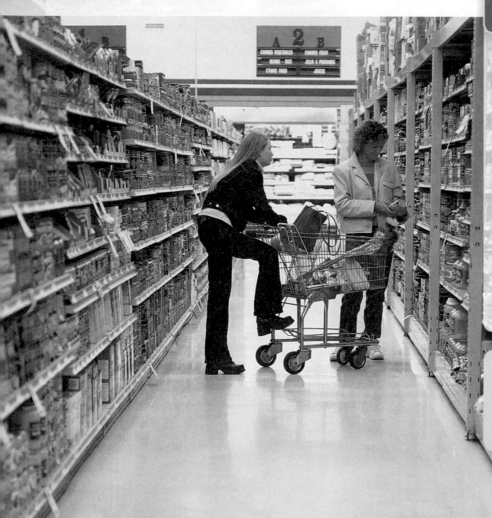

Chapter Learning Outcomes

After reading Chapter 3, you should be able to

1. Identify the various dietary standards of the Dietary Reference Intakes and explain how they can be used.

2. List the five key components of the *Dietary Guidelines, 2010.*

3. List major food groups and identify foods that are typically classified in each group.

4. Use www.choosemyplate.gov to develop nutritionally adequate daily menus.

5. Use the Nutrition Facts panel to make more nutritious food choices.

6. Identify nutrition-related claims the FDA allows on food and dietary supplement labels.

7. Discuss how ethnic and religious groups influence Americans' food choices.

McGraw Hill **connect** plus+
|NUTRITION **www.mcgrawhillconnect.com**
A wealth of proven resources are available on ConnectPlus® Nutrition! Ask your instructor about ConnectPlus, which includes an interactive eBook, an adaptive learning program and much, much more!

WHEN YOU SHOP for groceries, do you sometimes feel overwhelmed by the vast array of foods that are available? If your answer is "yes," your response is not surprising, considering the average supermarket offered nearly 39,000 items in 2010.[1] Every time you enter a supermarket, you are likely to find food items that were not on the shelves during your last visit to the store. In 2009, for example, over 19,000 new food and beverage products were introduced into the marketplace.[2]

Chapter 1 introduced some key nutrition concepts, including the need for dietary adequacy, moderation, balance, and a variety of foods. Chapter 2 described how you can become a more careful consumer of nutrition information. However, you are also a consumer of food. With so many grocery items from which to choose, what are the primary factors that influence your food purchases? Do you select foods simply because they taste good, are reasonably priced, or are easy to prepare? Do you ever consider the effects certain foods may have on your health before you purchase them?

Your lifestyle reflects your health-related behaviors, including your dietary practices and physical activity habits. Americans of all ages may reduce their risk of chronic disease by adopting nutritious diets and engaging in regular physical activity. However, consumers need practical advice to help them make decisions that can promote more healthy lifestyles.

Chapter 3 discusses dietary standards, including how the standards are established and used. The information in this chapter also presents practical ways to plan a nutritionally adequate, well-balanced diet using tools such as the Dietary Guidelines and MyPlate. Furthermore, a section of Chapter 3 explains how to interpret and use nutrition-related information that appears on food and dietary supplement labels.

Quiz *Yourself*

Before reading the rest of Chapter 3, test your knowledge of dietary standards, recommendations, and guides, as well as nutrient labels, by taking the following quiz. The answers are found on page 91.

1. According to the latest U.S. Department of Agriculture food guide, fruits and vegetables are combined into one food group. _____ T _____ F

2. According to the recommendations of the *Dietary Guidelines for Americans, 2010,* it is acceptable for certain adults to consume moderate amounts of alcoholic beverages. _____ T _____ F

3. Last week, Colin didn't consume the recommended amount of vitamin C for a couple of days. Nevertheless, he is unlikely to develop scurvy, the vitamin C deficiency disease. _____ T _____ F

4. The Food and Drug Administration develops Dietary Guidelines for Americans. _____ T _____ F

5. The Nutrition Facts panel on a food label provides information concerning amounts of energy, fiber, and cholesterol that are in a serving of the food. _____ T _____ F

3.1 From Requirements to Standards

By using research methods discussed in Chapter 2, scientists have been able to estimate the amount of many nutrients required by the body. A **requirement** can be defined as the smallest amount of a nutrient that maintains a defined level of nutritional health.[3] In general, this amount saturates (fills) certain cells with the nutrient or prevents the nutrient's deficiency disease. The requirement for a particular nutrient varies to some degree from person to person. Your age, sex, general health status, physical activity level, and use of medications and drugs are among factors that influence your nutrient requirements.

Simply consuming required amounts of nutrients does not result in optimal nutritional status. If your intake of a nutrient just meets the required amount, your body has no extra supply available to use in case your diet becomes limited. Many nutrients are stored in the body, and for optimal nutrition, you need to consume enough of those nutrients to maintain storage levels. Your body uses its nutrient stores much like you can use a savings account to help manage your money. When you have some extra cash, it is wise to place the money in a savings account, so you can withdraw some of the reserves to meet future needs without going into debt. When your consumption of

requirement smallest amount of a nutrient that maintains a defined level of nutritional health

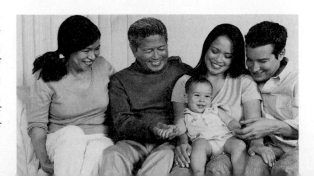

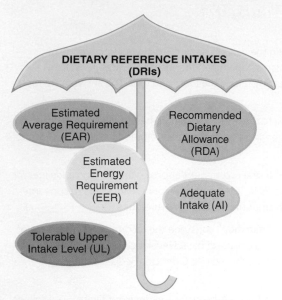

Figure 3.1 Dietary Reference Intakes. The Dietary Reference Intakes (DRIs) encompass a variety of terms that represent standards for energy and nutrient recommendations.

Dietary Reference Intakes (DRIs) various energy and nutrient intake standards for Americans

Food and Nutrition Board (FNB) group of nutrition scientists who develop DRIs

Estimated Average Requirement (EAR) amount of a nutrient that meets the needs of 50% of healthy people in a life stage/gender group

Estimated Energy Requirement (EER) average daily energy intake that meets the needs of a healthy person maintaining his or her weight

Recommended Dietary Allowances (RDAs) standards for recommending daily intakes of several nutrients

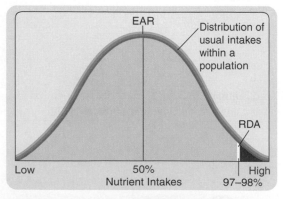

Figure 3.2 Establishing RDAs. To set an RDA, scientists add a margin of safety amount to the Estimated Average Requirement (EAR) that allows for individual variations in nutrient needs and helps maintain tissue stores. As a result, a nutrient's RDA is high enough to meet or exceed the requirements of 97–98% of the population for the nutrient. In other words, about 98% of the population will have their needs for the nutrient met by just consuming the RDA amount.

certain nutrients is more than enough to meet your needs, the body stores the excess, primarily in the liver, body fat, and/or bones. When your intake of a stored nutrient is low or needs for this nutrient become increased, such as during recovery from illness, your body withdraws some from storage. As a result of having optimal levels of stored nutrients, you may avoid or delay developing deficiencies of those nutrients.

Dietary Reference Intakes

Dietary Reference Intakes (DRIs) encompass a variety of energy and nutrient intake standards that nutrition experts in the United States use as references when making dietary recommendations. DRIs are intended to help people reduce their risk of nutrient deficiencies and excesses, prevent disease, and achieve optimal health.[4] The standards (Fig. 3.1) are the Estimated Average Requirement (EAR), which includes Estimated Energy Requirement (EER); Recommended Dietary Allowance (RDA), Adequate Intake (AI), and Tolerable Upper Intake Level (UL).

A group of nutrition scientists, the **Food and Nutrition Board (FNB)** of the Institute of Medicine, develop DRIs. Periodically, members of the Board adjust DRIs as new information concerning human nutritional needs and dietary adequacy becomes available. You can find tables for the latest DRIs in the inside back cover. The following sections provide basic information about the various DRI standards. It is important to become familiar with these terms, because we refer to them in this and other chapters.

Estimated Average Requirement

An **Estimated Average Requirement (EAR)** is the amount of the nutrient that should meet the needs of 50% of healthy people who are in a particular *life stage/gender group*.[4] Life stage/gender groups classify people according to age, sex, and whether females are pregnant or breastfeeding. A typical 20-year-old female college student, for example, would be classified as a female, between 19 and 30 years old, and not pregnant or breastfeeding.

To establish an EAR for a nutrient, the Food and Nutrition Board identifies a *physiological marker*, a substance in the body that reflects proper functioning and can be measured. This marker indicates whether the level of a nutrient in the body is adequate. A marker for vitamin C, for example, is the amount of the vitamin in certain blood cells. When these cells contain nearly all the vitamin C they can hold, the body has an optimal supply of the vitamin. Thus, a physician can diagnose whether a patient is vitamin C deficient by taking a blood sample from the person and measuring the vitamin C content of certain blood cells.

Estimated Energy Requirement The **Estimated Energy Requirement (EER)** is the average daily energy intake that meets the needs of a healthy person who is maintaining his or her weight. Dietitians can use EERs to evaluate an individual's energy intake. The EER takes into account the person's physical activity level, height, and weight, as well as sex and life stage. Because the EER is an average figure, some people have energy needs that are higher or lower. Chapter 10 provides formulas for calculating your EER.

Recommended Dietary Allowances

The **Recommended Dietary Allowances (RDAs)** are standards for recommending daily intakes of several nutrients. RDAs meet the nutrient needs of nearly all healthy individuals (97–98%) in a particular life stage/gender group. To establish an RDA for a nutrient, nutrition scientists first determine its EAR. Then scientists add a "margin of safety" amount to the EAR that allows for individual variations in nutrient needs and helps maintain tissue stores (Fig. 3.2). For example, the adult EAR for vitamin C is 60 mg for women who are not pregnant or breastfeeding, and 75 mg for men.[3]

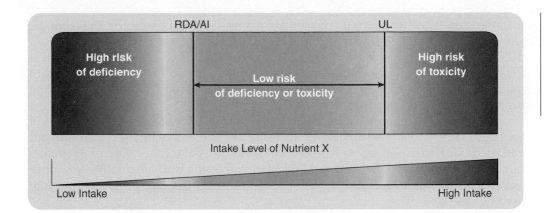

RDA/AI   UL

**High risk
of deficiency**

**Low risk
of deficiency or toxicity**

**High risk
of toxicity**

Intake Level of Nutrient X

Low Intake   High Intake

Figure 3.3 Adequate Intakes and Upper Limits.
Consuming too much or not enough of a nutrient can cause health problems. Nutrition scientists set an Adequate Intake (AI) for a nutrient if there is not enough information to determine an RDA. The Tolerable Upper Intake Level (UL) is the highest average amount of a nutrient that is unlikely to harm most people when the amount is consumed daily.

However, the adult RDA for vitamin C is 15 mg higher than the EAR—75 mg for women who are not pregnant or breastfeeding, and 90 mg for men. Thus, the margin of safety for vitamin C is 15 mg. Because smoking cigarettes increases the need for vitamin C, smokers should add 30 mg to their RDA for the nutrient.

Adequate Intakes

In some instances, nutrition scientists are unable to develop RDAs for nutrients because there is not enough information to determine human requirements. Until such information becomes available, scientists set **Adequate Intakes (AIs)** for these nutrients. To establish an AI, scientists record eating patterns of a group of healthy people and estimate the group's average daily intake of the nutrient. If the population under observation shows no evidence of the nutrient's deficiency disorder, the researchers conclude that the average level of intake must be adequate and use that value as the AI (Fig. 3.3). Vitamin K and the mineral potassium are among the nutrients that have AIs instead of RDAs.

Tolerable Upper Intake Level

Nutrition scientists also establish a **Tolerable Upper Intake Level (Upper Level** or **UL)** for many vitamins and minerals. The UL is the highest average amount of a nutrient that is unlikely to harm most people when the amount is consumed daily (see Fig. 3.3).[4] The risk of a toxicity disorder increases when a person regularly consumes amounts of a nutrient that exceed its UL. The UL for vitamin C, for example, is 2000 mg/day for adults.

Acceptable Macronutrient Distribution Ranges   The results of scientific research suggest that food energy sources (macronutrients) are associated with risk of certain diet-related chronic diseases, such as heart disease. **Acceptable Macronutrient Distribution Ranges (AMDRs)** indicate ranges of carbohydrate, fat, and protein intakes that provide adequate amounts of vitamins and minerals and may reduce the risk of diet-related chronic diseases.[4] The AMDR for carbohydrates, for example, is 45 to 65% of total energy intake. Table 3.1 lists adult AMDRs.

Applying Nutrient Standards

Dietitians refer to DRIs as standards for planning nutritious diets for groups of people and evaluating the nutritional adequacy of a population's diet. Nevertheless, RDAs and AIs are often used to evaluate an individual's dietary practices.[4,5] Your diet is likely to be nutritionally adequate if your average daily intake for each nutrient meets the nutrient's RDA or AI value. If your diet consistently supplies less than the EAR for a nutrient, you may be at risk of eventually developing the nutrient's deficiency

Adequate Intakes (AIs) dietary recommendations that assume a population's average daily nutrient intakes are adequate because no deficiency diseases are present

Tolerable Upper Intake Level (Upper Level or UL) standard representing the highest average amount of a nutrient that is unlikely to be harmful when consumed daily

Acceptable Macronutrient Distribution Ranges (AMDRs) macronutrient intake ranges that are nutritionally adequate and may reduce the risk of diet-related chronic diseases

TABLE 3.1 *Acceptable Macronutrient Distribution Ranges: Adults*

Macronutrient	AMDR (% of total energy intake)
Carbohydrate	45–65
Protein	10–35
*Fat**	20–35

* Fat intake should include essential fatty acids (see Chapter 6).

disorder. On the other hand, if your intake of a nutrient is consistently above its UL, you are at risk of developing that nutrient's toxicity disorder. Nutrient toxicity disorders are more likely to occur when people take high doses of individual nutrient supplements, particularly vitamins and minerals. If you do not take large doses of nutrient supplements and you eat reasonable amounts of food, your risk of developing a nutrient toxicity disorder is low.

Nutritional standards have a variety of commercial applications. Pharmaceutical companies refer to DRIs when developing formulas that replace breast milk for infants and special formulas for people who cannot consume regular foods. As a result, babies can thrive on commercially prepared formulas, and adults who are unable to swallow can survive for years on formula feedings administered through tubes inserted into their bodies.

For nutrition labeling purposes, the Food and Drug Administration (FDA) uses RDAs to develop a set of standards called *Daily Values (DVs)*. For adults, DVs are based on a standard diet that supplies 2000 kcal/day and certain dietary recommendations. Consumers may find DVs useful for comparing the nutritional contents of similar foods. The "Food and Dietary Supplement Labels" section of Chapter 3 provides more information about nutritional labeling, including DVs.

If you review the DRI tables, you are likely to be overwhelmed with the number of tables and confusing array of values. The information provided by DRIs is complex and not in a form that is practical for consumers to use when planning menus. To overcome these hurdles, nutrition experts develop dietary guides to help people make healthier food choices. As menu-planning tools, such food guides are not perfect, but they can help consumers add interest and variety to their diets while ensuring nutritional balance and adequacy. The "Dietary Guides" section of Chapter 3 discusses dietary guides.

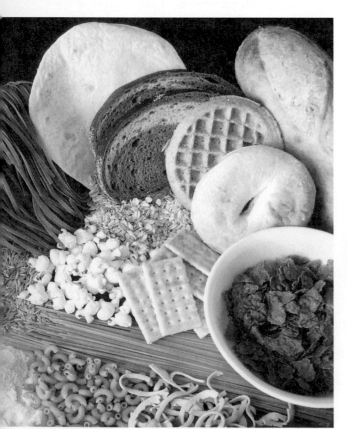

Grains include products made from wheat, rice, corn, barley, and oats.

Concept **Checkpoint**

1. What is the difference between an RDA and an AI?
2. Describe how scientists establish the RDA for a nutrient.
3. Explain how an EER differs from an RDA or AI.
4. Discuss how dietitians, pharmaceutical companies, and the FDA use nutrient standards.

 3.2 Major Food Groups

Foods can be classified into major food groups according to their natural origins and key nutrients. Major food groups are usually grains, dairy products, fruits, vegetables, and protein-rich foods. In most instances, dietary guides also provide recommendations concerning amounts of foods from each group that should be eaten daily. The following points identify major food groups and summarize key features of each group.

- *Grains* include products made from wheat, rice, and oats. Pasta, noodles, and flour tortillas are members of this group because wheat flour is their main ingredient. In general, 1 ounce of a grain food is equivalent to 1 slice of bread, 1 cup of ready-to-eat cereal, or ½ cup of cooked rice, pasta, or cereal such as oatmeal. Although corn is a type of grain, it is often used as a vegetable in meals. Cornmeal and popcorn, however, are usually grouped with grain products.

Carbohydrate (starch) and protein are the primary macronutrients in grains. In the United States, refined grain products can also be good sources of several vitamins and minerals when they have undergone enrichment or fortification. **Enrichment** is the addition of iron and certain B vitamins to cereal grain products such as flour and rice. In general, enrichment replaces some of the nutrients that were lost during processing. **Fortification** is the addition of nutrients to food, such as adding calcium to orange juice, vitamins A and D to milk, and numerous vitamins and minerals to ready-to-eat breakfast cereals.

Dietary guides generally recommend choosing foods made with whole grains instead of refined grains. According to FDA, whole grains are the intact, ground, cracked, or flaked seeds of cereal grains, such as wheat, buckwheat, oats, corn, rice, wild rice, rye, and barley.[6] Compared to refined grain products, foods made from whole grains naturally contain more fiber as well as micronutrients that are not replaced during enrichment.

- *Dairy foods* include milk and products made from milk that retain their calcium content, such as yogurt and hard cheeses. Dairy foods are also excellent sources of protein, phosphorus (a mineral), and riboflavin (a B vitamin). Additionally, most of the milk sold in the United States is fortified with vitamins A and D. Ice cream, pudding, frozen yogurt, and ice milk are often grouped with dairy foods, even though they often have high sugar and fat contents. Although cream cheese, cream, and butter are dairy foods, they are not included in this group, because they have little or no calcium and are high in fat.

Most dietary guides recommend choosing dairy products that have most of the fat removed, such as fat-free or low-fat milk. (Fat-free milk may also be referred to as nonfat or skim milk.) Compared to whole milk, which is about 3.25% fat by weight, low-fat milk contains only 1% fat by weight and is often called "1% milk."

In general, 1 cup of milk is equivalent to 1 cup of plain yogurt, frozen yogurt, or pudding; 2 cups of cottage cheese; 1 ½ ounces of natural cheese such as Swiss or cheddar; or 2 ounces of processed cheese. To obtain about the same amount of calcium and protein as in 1 cup of fat-free milk, you would have to eat almost 1⅔ cups of vanilla ice cream. This amount of ice cream provides 470 kcal and about 26 g of fat, whereas the same amount of fat-free milk supplies only 135 kcal and less than 1 g of fat.

- *Protein-rich foods* include beef, pork, lamb, fish, shellfish, liver, and poultry. Beans, eggs, nuts, and seeds are included with this group because these protein-rich foods can substitute for meats. One ounce of food from this group generally equals 1 ounce of meat, poultry, or fish; ¼ cup cooked dry beans or peas; 1 egg; 1 tablespoon of peanut butter; or ½ ounce of nuts or seeds. *Tofu*, a food made from soybeans, is a good source of protein. One-fourth cup of regular tofu is equivalent to 1 ounce of meat.

Foods in the protein group are rich sources of micronutrients, especially iron, zinc, and B vitamins. In general, the body absorbs minerals, such as iron and zinc, more easily from animal foods than from plants. However, animal foods often contain a lot of saturated fat and cholesterol. Diets that supply high amounts of these lipids are associated with increased risk of heart and blood vessel diseases (*cardiovascular disease* or *CVD*).

Some dietary guides use fat content to categorize meats and other protein-rich foods. According to these guides, low-fat cottage cheese and the white meat of turkey are very lean meats; ground beef that is not more than 15% fat by weight and tuna are lean meats. Pork sausage, bacon, regular cheeses, and hot dogs are examples of high-fat meats.

- *Fruits* include fresh, dried, frozen, sauced, and canned fruit, as well as 100% fruit juice. In general, 1 cup of food from this group equals 1 cup of fruit or fruit juice,

enrichment addition of iron and certain B vitamins to cereal grain products

fortification addition of nutrients to food

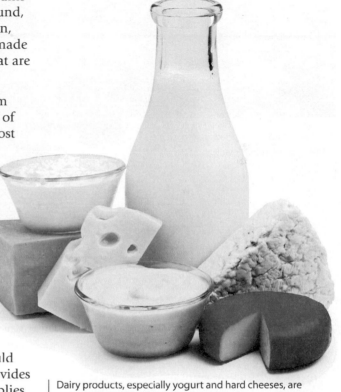

Dairy products, especially yogurt and hard cheeses, are excellent sources of calcium, protein, phosphorus, and riboflavin. Additionally, milk is often fortified with vitamins A and D.

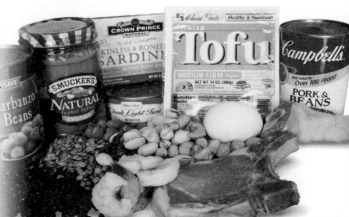

Dry beans, peas, eggs, nuts, and seeds are protein-rich foods that can substitute for meat.

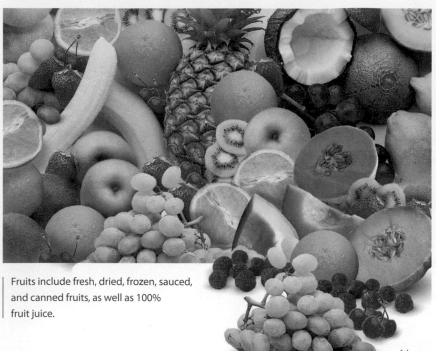

Fruits include fresh, dried, frozen, sauced, and canned fruits, as well as 100% fruit juice.

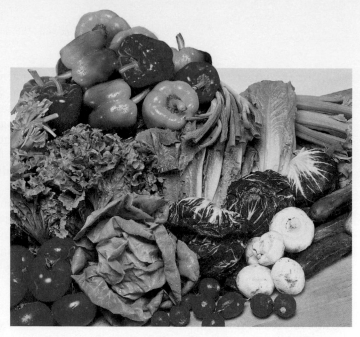

Vegetables include raw, cooked, canned, frozen, and dried/dehydrated vegetables, and 100% vegetable juice.

or ½ cup of dried fruit, such as raisins or apricots.[7] Most fruits are low in fat and good sources of phytochemicals and micronutrients, especially the mineral potassium and vitamins C and folate. Additionally, whole or cut-up fruit is a good source of fiber. Although 100% juice is a source of phytochemicals and can count toward your fruit intake, the majority of your choices from this group should be whole or cut-up fruits.[8] Whole or cut-up fruits are healthier options than juices because they contain more dietary fiber.

• *Vegetables* include fresh, cooked, canned, frozen, and dried/dehydrated vegetables, and 100% vegetable juice. Vegetables may be further grouped into dark green, orange, and starchy categories. Some guides include dried beans and peas in the vegetable group as well as in the meat and meat substitutes group. In general, 1 cup of food from this group equals 1 cup of raw or cooked vegetables, 1 cup vegetable juice, or 2 cups of uncooked leafy greens, such as salad greens. Many vegetables are good sources of micronutrients, fiber, and phytochemicals. Furthermore, many vegetables are naturally low in fat and energy.

Other Foods

Dietary guides may include an oils group and a group for empty-calorie foods or beverages. Oils include canola, corn, and olive oils, as well as other fats that are liquid at room temperature. Certain spreadable foods made from vegetable oils, such as mayonnaise, margarine, and salad dressing, are also classified as oils. Because nuts, olives, avocados, and some types of fish have high fat contents, a dietary guide may group these foods with oils.[9] Oils are often good sources of fat soluble vitamins and may be sources of "healthy" fats.

Empty-calorie foods generally add a lot of sugar, alcohol, and/or solid fat to diets. Sugary foods ("sweets") include candy, regular soft drinks, jelly, and other foods that contain high amounts of sugar added during processing or preparation. Sugary foods and alcoholic beverages typically supply energy but few or no micronutrients. Solid fats, such as beef fat, butter, lard (pork fat), and shortening, are fairly hard at room temperature. Solid fats are often grouped with sweets and alcoholic beverages, because diets that contain high amounts of these fats are associated with increased risk of CVD. Cream, cream cheese, and sour cream are liquid or soft at room temperature, but these foods are usually classified as solid fats. Chapter 6 discusses how dietary fats can affect health.

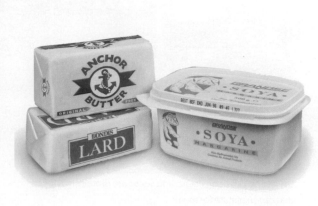

It is important to note that the nutritional content of foods within each group often varies widely. For example, 3.5 ounces of fresh sliced apples and 3.5 ounces of fresh orange slices each supply about 50 kcal. However, the apples contribute about 4 mg of vitamin C, whereas oranges supply about 46 mg of the vitamin to diets (Fig. 3.4). Therefore, dietary guides generally recommend that people choose a variety of foods from each food group when planning daily meals and snacks.

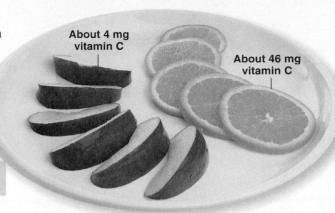

About 4 mg vitamin C

About 46 mg vitamin C

Concept **Checkpoint**

5. List at least three foods that are generally classified as grain products.
6. What is the difference between nutrient fortification and nutrient enrichment?
7. List at least four foods that are generally classified as dairy products.
8. Why are dry beans often classified with meat?
9. According to the information in this section of Chapter 3, how many cups of dried apricots are nutritionally equivalent to 2 cups of fresh apricots?
10. Most dietary guides classify eggs and nuts with meat. Why?
11. Identify at least two foods that are classified as solid fat.

Figure 3.4 Comparing apples to oranges. The nutritional content of foods within each group often varies widely. For example, ounce per ounce, oranges supply more vitamin C than apples. Therefore, dietary guides generally recommend that people eat a variety of foods from each food group daily.

3.3 Dietary Guidelines

Heart disease, cancer, hypertension (chronically elevated blood pressure), and diabetes mellitus (commonly referred to as *diabetes*) are among the leading causes of disability and death among Americans. According to a considerable amount of scientific evidence, risk of these diseases is strongly linked with certain lifestyles, particularly poor dietary choices and lack of regular physical activity. As required by law, the U.S. Department of Health and Human Services (USDHHS) and the U.S. Department of Agriculture (USDA) publish the *Dietary Guidelines for Americans* (Dietary Guidelines), a set of general nutrition-related lifestyle recommendations that are intended for healthy people over 2 years of age.[10] The Dietary Guidelines are designed to promote adequate nutritional status and good health, and to reduce the risk of major nutrition-related chronic health conditions, such as obesity and cardiovascular disease. These guidelines are updated every 5 years.

The most recent version of the guidelines, *Dietary Guidelines for Americans, 2010*, was introduced in 2011. Table 3.2 indicates the overarching concepts of the guidelines, which focus on improving the nutritional quality of the population's food intake and reducing the prevalence of obesity. Table 3.3 lists the key components of the Dietary Guidelines. These components form the foundation for the following key recommendations:[10]

Balancing Calories to Manage Weight

- Prevent and/or reduce overweight and obesity through improved eating and physical activity behaviors.

- Control total caloric intake to manage body weight. For people who are overweight or obese, this means consuming fewer calories from foods and beverages.

- Increase physical activity and reduce time spend in sedentary behaviors.

- Maintain appropriate calorie balance during each stage of life—childhood, adolescence, adulthood, pregnancy and breastfeeding, and older age.

Foods and Food Components to Reduce

- Reduce daily sodium intake to less than 2300 mg. African Americans and people who are 51 years of age and older or those who have hypertension, diabetes, or chronic kidney disease should reduce their daily sodium intake to 1500 mg.

TABLE 3.2 *Dietary Guidelines for Americans, 2010: Overarching Concepts*

- Maintain caloric balance over time to achieve and sustain a healthy weight

- Focus on consuming nutrient-dense foods and beverages

TABLE 3.3 *Key Components of the Dietary Guidelines, 2010*

- Balancing calories to manage weight

- Foods and food components to reduce

- Foods and nutrients to increase

- Building healthy eating patterns

- Helping Americans make healthy choices

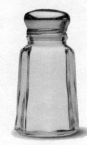

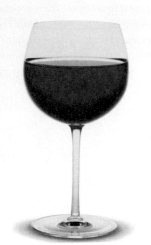

- Consume less than 10% of calories from saturated fat by replacing them with unsaturated fat (see Chapter 6).
- Consume less than 300 mg of cholesterol per day.
- Keep *trans* fat intake as low as possible by limiting foods that are sources of synthetic *trans* fats, such as partially hydrogenated oils, and by limiting intake of other solid fats.
- Reduce the intake of foods that contain refined grains, especially foods that contain solid fats, added sugars, and sodium.
- If alcohol is consumed, it should be consumed in moderation (see the "Highlight" in Chapter 6) and only by adults of legal drinking age.

Foods and Nutrients to Increase

Individuals should meet the following recommendations as part of a healthy eating pattern while staying within their caloric needs.

- Increase fruit and vegetable intake.
- Eat a variety of vegetables, especially dark green, red, and orange vegetables; beans; and peas.
- Consume at least half of all grains as whole grains. Increase whole-grain intake by replacing refined grains with whole grains.
- Increase intake of fat-free or low-fat milk and milk products, such as milk, yogurt, cheese, or fortified soy beverages.
- Choose a variety of protein foods, which include seafood, lean meat and poultry, eggs, beans and peas, soy products, and unsalted nuts and seeds.
- Increase the amount and variety of seafood consumed by choosing seafood in place of some meat and poultry.
- Replace protein foods that are higher in solid fats with choices that are low in solid fats and/or are sources of oils.
- Use oils to replace solid fats where possible.
- Choose foods that provide more potassium, dietary fiber, calcium, and vitamin D, which are "nutrients of concern" that Americans tend to consume in limited amounts.

Recommendations for Specific Population Groups

Women who are capable of becoming pregnant:
- Choose foods that contain iron, particularly heme iron, which is more readily absorbed than nonheme iron. Also choose foods that enhance iron absorption such as vitamin C–rich foods.
- Consume 400 mcg of folic acid/day (from fortified foods and/or supplements) in addition to folate from the diet.

Women who are pregnant or breastfeeding:
- Consume 8 to 12 ounces of seafood per week from a variety of seafood types.
- Limit white (albacore) tuna to 6 ounces per week and do not eat tilefish, shark, swordfish, and king mackerel because of their high methylmercury content.
- If pregnant, take an iron supplement as recommended by your health care provider.

Individuals ages 50 years and older:
- Consume foods fortified with vitamin B12, such as fortified cereals, or take dietary supplements that contain the vitamin.

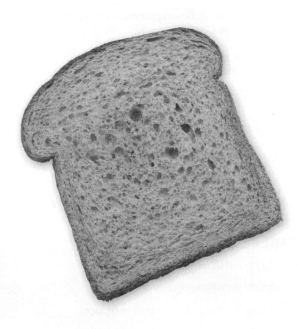

Building Healthy Eating Patterns

- Select an eating pattern that meets nutrient needs over time at an appropriate calorie level.
- Account for all foods and beverages consumed and assess how they fit within a total healthy eating pattern.
- Follow food safety recommendations when preparing and eating foods to reduce the risk of foodborne illnesses.

Helping Americans Make Healthy Choices

Educators, health professionals, businesses, policy makers, and other groups that influence Americans' food and physical activity environment can help individuals make positive health-related choices. This "call to action" has three guiding principles:

- Ensure that all Americans have access to nutritious foods and opportunities for physical activity.
- Support positive behavioral changes through environmental strategies, such as implementing the U.S. National Physical Activity Plan, which strives to reduce inactivity.
- Set the stage for lifelong healthy eating, physical activity, and weight management behaviors.

Applying the Dietary Guidelines

The Dietary Guidelines include seven selected food and nutrition-related messages for consumers, such as "Make half your plate fruits and vegetables" (Table 3.4). Table 3.5 suggests practical ways you can apply the Dietary Guidelines' recommendations to your

TABLE 3.4 *Selected Messages for Consumers*

- Enjoy your food, but eat less.
- Avoid oversized portions.
- Make half your plate fruits and vegetables.
- Make at least half your grains whole grains.
- Switch to fat-free or low-fat (1%) milk
- Compare sodium in foods and choose the foods with the lowest sodium content.
- Drink water instead of sugary drinks.

TABLE 3.5 *Applying the Dietary Guidelines to Your Usual Food Choices*

If You Usually Eat:	Consider Replacing With:
White bread and rolls	Whole-wheat bread and rolls
Sugary breakfast cereals	Low-sugar high-fiber cereal sweetened with berries, bananas, peaches, or other fruit
Cheeseburger, French fries, and a regular (sugar-sweetened) soft drink	Roasted chicken or turkey sandwich, baked beans, fat-free or low-fat milk, or soy milk
Potato salad or cole slaw	Leafy greens or three-bean salad
Doughnuts, chips, or salty snack foods	Small bran muffin or whole-wheat bagel topped with peanut butter or soy nut butter, unsalted nuts, and dried fruit
Regular soft drinks	Water, fat-free or low-fat milk, or 100% fruit juice
Boiled vegetables	Raw or steamed vegetables (often retain more nutrients than boiled)
Canned vegetables	Frozen vegetables (retain more nutrients during processing)
Breaded and fried meat, fish, or poultry	Broiled or roasted meat, fish, or poultry
Fatty meats such as barbecued ribs, sausage, and hot dogs	Chicken, turkey, or fish; lean meats such as ground round
Whole or 2% milk, cottage cheese with 4% fat, or yogurt made from whole milk	1% or fat-free milk, low-fat cottage cheese (1% fat), or low-fat yogurt
Ice cream	Frozen yogurt or ice milk
Cream cheese	Low-fat cottage cheese (mashed) or reduced-fat cream cheese
Creamy salad dressings or dips made with mayonnaise or sour cream	Oil and vinegar dressing, reduced-fat salad dressings, or dips made from low-fat sour cream or plain yogurt
Chocolate chip or cream-filled cookies	Fruit-filled bars, oatmeal cookies, or fresh fruit
Salt added to season foods	Herbs, spices, or lemon juice

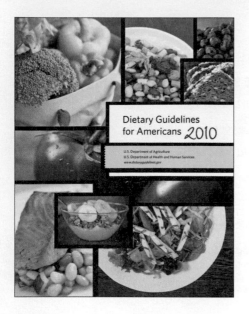

usual food choices. However, making recommended dietary and other lifestyle changes does not always reduce risk factors for disease. For example, a man who has hypertension may find that his blood pressure remains dangerously elevated after several months of exercising, limiting his salt intake, and maintaining a healthy weight for his height. In this case, genetic factors may be influencing the man's health more than his lifestyle, and medication may be necessary to reduce his blood pressure.

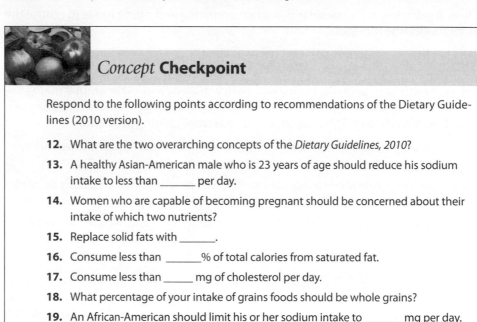

Concept **Checkpoint**

Respond to the following points according to recommendations of the Dietary Guidelines (2010 version).

12. What are the two overarching concepts of the *Dietary Guidelines, 2010*?

13. A healthy Asian-American male who is 23 years of age should reduce his sodium intake to less than _____ per day.

14. Women who are capable of becoming pregnant should be concerned about their intake of which two nutrients?

15. Replace solid fats with _____.

16. Consume less than _____% of total calories from saturated fat.

17. Consume less than _____ mg of cholesterol per day.

18. What percentage of your intake of grains foods should be whole grains?

19. An African-American should limit his or her sodium intake to _____ mg per day.

20. For adults who drink alcohol, how many alcoholic beverages per day are permitted?

21. Which nutrients are "of concern" in the American diet?

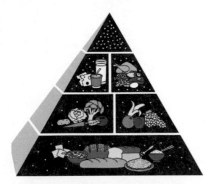

Figure 3.5 Food Guide Pyramid. In 1992, the USDA introduced the Food Guide Pyramid. This food guide ranked food groups according to their emphasis in menu planning.

3.4 Dietary Guides

For over 100 years, the USDA has issued specific dietary recommendations for Americans. In 1943, the USDA issued the first food guide based on RDAs for the general public to use. The guide grouped foods into seven categories. This guide was designed to help Americans plan nutritious menus despite shortages of certain foods that often occurred during World War II. By the mid–1950s, the USDA simplified the original food guide to include only four food groups: milk, meat, fruit and vegetable, and bread and cereal. The recommendations of the "Basic Four" provided the foundation for an adequate diet while supplying about 1200 to 1400 kcal/day. Extra servings of food could be added to the basic diet plan for people who had higher energy needs. In 1979, the USDA issued the "Hassle-Free Guide to a Better Diet" that was similar to the "Basic Four." The "Hassle-Free Guide," however, included a fifth food group for fats, sweets, and alcoholic beverages. Furthermore, the Hassle-Free Guide provided basic information about calories, physical activity, and fiber.[11]

In 1992, the USDA introduced the Food Guide Pyramid, a completely revamped version of the Hassle-Free Guide (Fig. 3.5). Unlike earlier dietary guides, the Food Guide Pyramid incorporated knowledge about the health benefits and risks associated with certain foods and ranked food groups according to their emphasis in menu planning. The Food Guide Pyramid displayed the groups in a layered format with grain products at the base to establish the foundation for a healthy diet. Fruit and vegetable groups occupied the next layer of the Food Guide Pyramid, followed by a layer shared by the milk and milk products and meat and meat substitutes groups. Fatty and sugary foods formed the small peak of the Pyramid, a visual reminder that people should limit their intake of these foods.

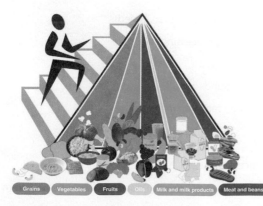

Figure 3.6 MyPyramid Plan. The MyPyramid Plan (2005–2011) was an interactive menu planning and physical activity guide developed by the USDA.

Although the Food Guide Pyramid became a familiar feature on many packaged foods, the USDA released the *MyPyramid Plan* in 2005 (Fig. 3.6). The MyPyramid Plan was a *food guidance system,* which was based on *Dietary Guidelines for Americans, 2005.* In addition to providing foods and nutrition information, the MyPyramid.gov website emphasized the importance of physical activity and enabled consumers to monitor their activity levels. In 2011, the USDA replaced the MyPyramid Plan with *MyPlate,* another interactive dietary and menu planning guide accessible at a website.

MyPlate

MyPlate (www.choosemyplate.gov) includes a variety of food, nutrition, and physical activity resources for consumers that are based on the recommendations of the *Dietary Guidelines for Americans, 2010.* MyPlate differs from the two previous USDA food guides in that it no longer has six food groups depicted by boxes or stripes within a pyramid (Fig. 3.7). MyPlate focuses on 5 different food groups: fruits, vegetables, protein foods, grains, and dairy.[12] According to the USDA, "oils" is not a food group.[9] The government agency, however, notes the need for some fat in the diet as well as limited amounts of "empty calories." In the previous guide (MyPyramid), oils formed a food group and empty calories were referred to as "discretionary calories."

To learn more about MyPlate's five food groups, visit http://www.choosemyplate.gov/ and click on "MyPlate" in the menu bar to obtain a list of food groups. Click on each food group to find practical information about foods in the group, including how much food should be eaten, scientifically supported health benefits of foods, and helpful food-related tips. Information about physical activity can be accessed at http://www.choosemyplate.gov/physical-activity.html.

Choosemyplate.gov also has useful interactive tools such as "Food-A-Pedia," which provides information about specific foods, and "SuperTracker" for accessing the energy and nutrient content of your daily food choices. SuperTracker allows you to record and monitor your daily diet and physical activity habits.

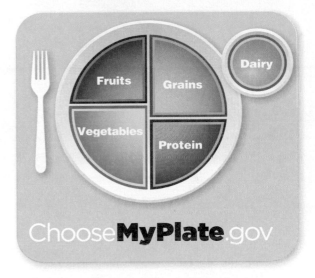

Figure 3.7 MyPlate. In 2011, the USDA introduced MyPlate as its latest interactive menu planning guide.

What Are Limits for Empty Calories?

Empty calories include energy from alcoholic beverages and foods that contain high amounts of added sugars and/or solid fats. Many commonly eaten foods include various amounts of empty calories. According to the USDA, the foods and beverages that supply the most empty calories in Americans' diets are:

- Cakes, cookies, pastries, and donuts
- Sugar-sweetened soft drinks, sports drinks, and fruit drinks
- Cheese (source of solid fat)
- Pizza (source of solid fat)
- Ice cream[12]

MyPlate dietary patterns allow some empty calories, based on a person's total energy needs. The **empty calorie allowance** is the amount of energy that remains after a person consumes recommended amounts of foods that contain little or no solid fats and added sugars from the major food groups. The 2000 kcal dietary pattern, for example, allows only 260 empty calories, which is less than the energy in a cup of ice cream or two 12-ounce sugar-sweetened soft drinks.

You can use up your empty calorie allowance by choosing foods that contain a lot of solid fat and added sugars. For example, you could eat high-fat meats instead of lean meats, add cream cheese to your bagel instead of eating it plain, or eat a sugary breakfast cereal instead of unsweetened cooked oatmeal. On the other hand, you could spend your empty calorie allowance on more nutrient-dense foods, such as fresh fruits, vegetables, nuts, or minimally processed grain products.

MyPlate USDA's interactive Internet dietary and menu planning guide

empty calorie allowance daily amount of energy remaining after a person consumes recommended amounts of foods that contain little or no solid fats and added sugars from the major food groups

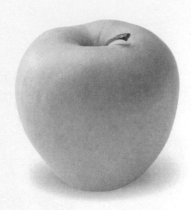

Tips for "Building a Better Plate"

The "Tips & Resources" page of the choosemyplate.gov website includes some helpful information and tips to help consumers make healthier food selections:

- Make at least ½ of your grains foods whole grains.
- Vary vegetable choices.
- Make ½ of your plate fruits and vegetables.
- Focus on fruit.
- Consume sources of calcium.
- Choose lean protein sources.
- Find your balance between food and physical activity.
- Keep food safe to eat.

Using MyPlate for Menu Planning

To use MyPlate as a personalized menu planning guide, visit www.choosemyplate.gov/myplate/index.aspx and click on "Daily Food Plan." Fill in boxes that request information, including your age, sex, weight, height, and estimated level of physical activity. After you provide this information, MyPlate estimates your daily energy needs and indicates how much food you should eat from each of the food groups daily to meet your recommended energy level. Table 3.6 indicates MyPlate's food intake recommendations for average healthy young adults who consume 1800 to 3200 kilocalories per day.

Overall, MyPlate can be helpful for planning menus because it promotes food variety, nutritional adequacy, and moderation. You can also use MyPlate to evaluate the nutritional quality of your daily diet by recording your food and beverage choices, classifying your choices into food groups, and estimating your intake of servings from each food group.

A computer and Internet access are necessary to use the program. Many people, particularly older adults, are unfamiliar with personal computers and may find the interactive www.choosemyplate.gov website challenging and frustrating to use. You may encounter some difficulties when using MyPlate to evaluate your diet's adequacy. How

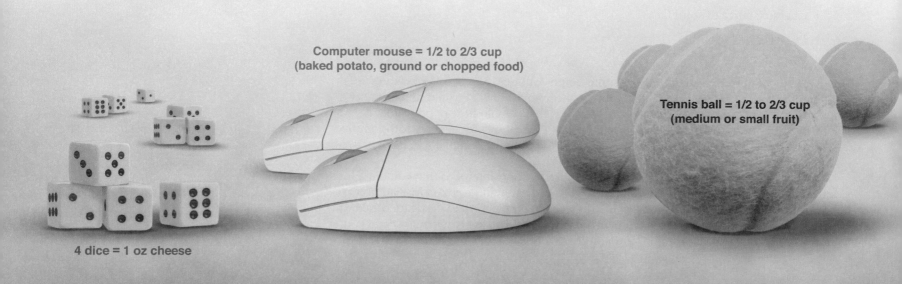

Computer mouse = 1/2 to 2/3 cup
(baked potato, ground or chopped food)

Tennis ball = 1/2 to 2/3 cup
(medium or small fruit)

4 dice = 1 oz cheese

TABLE 3.6 *MyPlate: Recommendations for Average, Healthy 20-Year-Old Young Adults*

MyPlate Guidelines (Daily)	Women	Men
Kilocalories	1800–2400	2600–3200
Fruit	2 cups	2–2.5 cups
Vegetable	2.5–3 cups	3.5–4.0 cups
Grains	6–8 oz	9–10 oz
Protein foods	5.0–6.5 oz	6.5–7 oz
Dairy	3 cups	3 cups
Oils	5–7 tsp	8–11 tsp
Empty calories	160–330 kcal	360–600 kcal

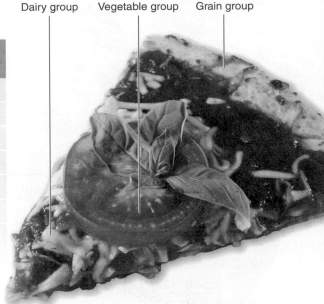

Dairy group   Vegetable group   Grain group

Classifying foods that combine ingredients from different food groups is challenging. This slice of pizza, for example, has crust (grains), tomato sauce and tomatoes (vegetable), and cheese (dairy).

do you classify menu items that combine small amounts of foods from more than one group, such as pizza, sandwiches, and casseroles? A slice of pizza, for example, has thin crust made with wheat flour (grains), tomato sauce (vegetable), and cheese (dairy). The first step is to determine the ingredients and classify each into an appropriate food group. Estimate the number of cups or ounces of each ingredient and record the amounts contributed from a particular food group. The slice of pizza may provide ¼ cup of a vegetable, 2 ounces of grains, and ¼ cup of dairy. Another problem you may have when using MyPlate is judging portion sizes without keeping handy a battery of measuring cups and a scale for weighing foods. Figure 3.8 provides convenient ways to estimate typical portions using familiar objects, including a tennis ball and bar of soap.

The USDA has also developed MyPlate menu planning tools for children and pregnant or breastfeeding women. These guides can also be accessed at www.choosemyplate .gov/. For information about MyPlate guides for various life stages, see Chapter 13.

Figure 3.8 Estimating portion sizes. You can use familiar items such as these to estimate portion sizes.

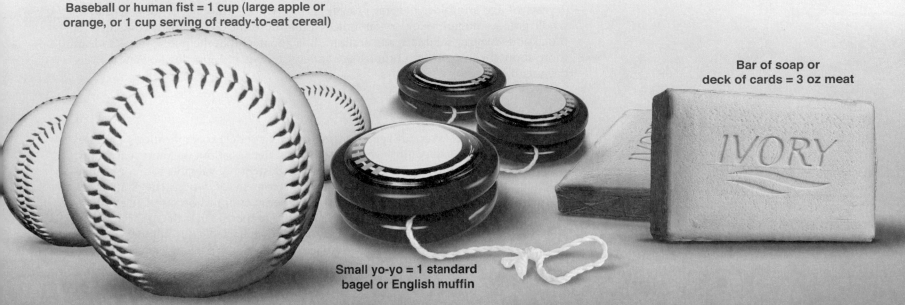

Baseball or human fist = 1 cup (large apple or orange, or 1 cup serving of ready-to-eat cereal)

Small yo-yo = 1 standard bagel or English muffin

Bar of soap or deck of cards = 3 oz meat

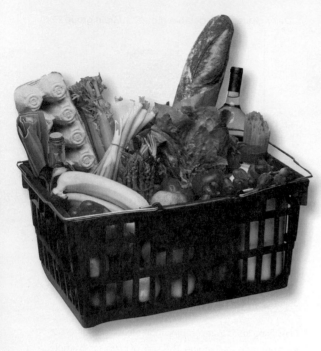

MyPlate for Losing Weight

The "Steps to a Healthier weight" page (http://www.choosemyplate.gov/STEPS/stepstoahealthierweight.html) provides information about "energy balance" and planning nutritionally adequate diets for persons who are trying to lose weight. If you would like to lose weight, start by obtaining your personalized daily food plan (http://www.choosemyplate.gov/myplate/index.aspx). In the box for "Weight," fill in your present weight; in the box for height, fill in your height. If you are too heavy for your height, the program will let you know and provide a food plan that will help you reach a healthy weight for your height (see Chapter 10). One way to reduce your calorie intake without sacrificing the nutritional adequacy of your diet is to eat smaller amounts of foods included in the empty-calorie allowance or eliminate them altogether. Additionally, you can increase the amount of time that you are physically active each day.

MyPlate: Physical Activity   Although you may be busy while performing daily activities, you may not be moving your body enough to strengthen your muscles and prevent unwanted weight gain. To obtain important health benefits, you should engage in moderate or vigorous physical activity every day.[13] Choosemyplate.gov includes some information about physical activity, including examples of activities that are moderate or vigorous (http://www.choosemyplate.gov/foodgroups/physicalactivity_tips.html). Chapter 11 provides more information about physical activity and the importance of a physically active lifestyle.

Other Dietary Guides

The USDA's original Food Guide Pyramid inspired the development of other food pyramids for people who follow cultural and ethnic food traditions that differ from the mainstream American ("Western") diet. The Highlight at the end of Chapter 3 discusses various cultural, ethnic, and religious influences on American dietary practices. The Highlight also includes illustrations of the traditional Mediterranean Diet Pyramid (see Fig. 3.15) and the Asian Diet Pyramid (see Fig. 3.16). Health Canada, the federal agency responsible for helping Canadians achieve better health, also has a dietary guide, "Eating Well with Canada's Food Guide" (see Appendix B). To use this interactive guide, go to this website: www.hc-sc.gc.ca/fn-an/food-guide-aliment/index_e.html.

Do Americans Follow Dietary Recommendations?

Analysis of government food consumption data indicates that most Americans do not follow the USDA's dietary advice.[14] In 2003–2004, the typical diet of Americans who were 2 years of age and older did not provide recommended amounts of fruit, vegetables, whole grains, and fat-free or low-fat milk. Furthermore, the diet generally contained too much added sugar, solid fats, and sodium. It is apparent that the public needs to learn more about the importance of choosing a variety of foods and applying MyPlate to everyday menu planning.

What Is the Exchange System?

Many chronic diseases require special diets to prevent or delay complications. Diabetes, for example, is easier to control when the person's diet has about the same macronutrient composition from day to day. The **Exchange System** is a valuable tool for estimating the energy, protein, carbohydrate, and fat content of foods. The System was originally developed by a committee of the Academy of Nutrition and Dietetics (formerly the American Dietetic Association) and American Diabetic Association for planning diets of people with diabetes, a condition characterized by abnormal carbohydrate metabolism. Because the Exchange System makes it relatively easy to plan nutritious calorie-reduced meals and snacks, it is also useful for people who are trying to lose weight.

Exchange System method of classifying foods into numerous lists based on macronutrient composition

The Exchange System categorizes foods into three broad groups: carbohydrates, meat and meat substitutes, and fats.[15] The foods within each group have similar macronutrient composition, regardless of whether the food is from a plant or animal. For example, the carbohydrate group includes fruits, vegetables, and grains, as well as milk products. Nuts and seeds are grouped with fats. Meats and meat substitutes are grouped according to their fat content. Cheeses are in the meat and meat substitutes group because of their high protein and fat content. Thus, the Exchange System classifies foods differently than MyPlate does.

Within each of the three major food groups, the Exchange System provides *exchange lists* of specific types of foods. The specified amount of a food listed in an exchange list provides about the same amount of macronutrients and calories as each of the other specified amounts of foods in that list. According to the fruit list, for example, an orange is equivalent to a small apple, a kiwifruit, one-half of a fresh pear, or one-half of a large grapefruit. This equality allows people to plan a wide variety of nutritious menus by exchanging one food for another within each list. For more information about the Exchange System, you can visit the Academy of Nutrition and Dietetics' website (www .eatright.org) to order easy-to-read publications such as *Eating Healthy with Diabetes* or the *ADA Guide to Eating Right When You Have Diabetes*.

Counting carbohydrates ("counting carbs") is another meal planning technique that people with diabetes can use to control their blood sugar levels. The American Diabetes Association offers information about counting carbohydrates (http://www .diabetes.org/food-and-fitness/food/planning-meals/carb-counting/). You will learn more about diabetes in the section of Chapter 5 that discusses this serious disease in detail.

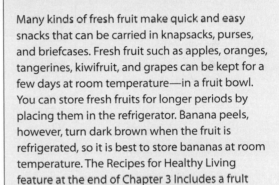

Did You Know?

Many kinds of fresh fruit make quick and easy snacks that can be carried in knapsacks, purses, and briefcases. Fresh fruit such as apples, oranges, tangerines, kiwifruit, and grapes can be kept for a few days at room temperature—in a fruit bowl. You can store fresh fruits for longer periods by placing them in the refrigerator. Banana peels, however, turn dark brown when the fruit is refrigerated, so it is best to store bananas at room temperature. The Recipes for Healthy Living feature at the end of Chapter 3 Includes a fruit salad that is easy to prepare.

Concept **Checkpoint**

22. List five tips for "building a better plate," according to www.choosemyplate.gov.
23. Explain how to use www.choosemyplate.gov to evaluate the nutritional adequacy of an individual's daily food choices.
24. What is an empty-calorie food, according to www.choosemyplate.gov?
25. Describe how the Exchange System differs from MyPlate.

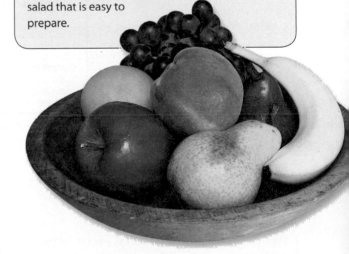

 ## 3.5 Food and Dietary Supplement Labels

Consumers can use information on food labels to determine ingredients and to compare energy and nutrient contents of packaged foods and beverages. In the United States, the FDA regulates and monitors information that can be placed on food labels, including claims about the health benefits of ingredients. Today, nearly all foods and beverages sold in grocery stores must have labels that provide the product's name, manufacturer's name and address, and amount of product in the package. Producers and sellers of fresh and frozen fruits and vegetables; fresh meats, poultry, fish, and shellfish; and a few other food items must declare the product's *country of origin* either on the packaging or where the product is located in stores. Furthermore, products that have more than one ingredient must display a list of the ingredients in descending order according to weight. The product shown in Figure 3.9, for example, has whole-wheat flour, water, and brown sugar as the first three ingredients. Thus, this food probably contains higher amounts of whole-wheat flour, water, and brown sugar than of the remaining ingredients listed.

Serving size is shown in household units and grams.

% Daily Values relate to 2000 Kcal/day diet.

To reduce risk of heart disease, choose foods that are low in saturated fat, trans fat, cholesterol, and sodium.

There is no % Daily Value for sugar, but limit your intake of foods with **added** sugars included among the first few items in the ingredients list.

Consume adequate amounts of fiber and these micronutrients.

Ingredients are listed in descending order by weight.

Nutrition Facts

Serving Size 1 cup (38 g)
Servings Per Container 18

Amount Per Serving

Calories 100
Calories from Fat 20

	% Daily Value*
Total Fat 2g	**3%**
Saturated Fat 0g	**0%**
Trans Fat 0g	
Cholesterol 0mg	**0%**
Sodium 160mg	**7%**
Total Carbohydrate 17g	**6%**
Dietary Fiber 2g	**8%**
Sugars 3g	
Protein 4g	

Vitamin A	**10%**
Vitamin C	**0%**
Calcium	**10%**
Iron	**8%**

* Percent Daily Values are based on a 2,000 calorie diet. Your daily values may be higher or lower, depending on your calorie needs:

	Calories	2,000	2,500
Total Fat	Less than	65g	80g
Sat Fat	Less than	20g	25g
Cholesterol	Less than	300mg	300mg
Sodium	Less than	2,400mg	2,400mg
Total Carbohydrate		300g	375g
Dietary Fiber		25g	30g

INGREDIENTS: Whole wheat flour, Water, Brown sugar, Wheat gluten, Cracked wheat, Wheat bran, Yeast, Salt, Molasses, Soybean oil, Calcium propionate (preservative), Mono–and diglycerides, Lecithin, Reduced fat milk

Figure 3.9 What's in a food? You can learn about the nutrient content and ingredients of a packaged food by reading the Nutrition Facts panel and ingredients list. When the FDA introduces the new format for the Nutrition Facts panel, some of these features may change.

Nutrition Facts

The FDA requires food manufacturers to use a special format, the *Nutrition Facts* panel, to display information about the energy and nutrient contents of products (see Fig. 3.9).[16] The Nutrition Facts panel indicates the amount of a serving size, in household units as well as grams, and the number of servings in the entire container. Serving sizes must be consistent among similar foods—for example, all brands of ice cream must use the same serving size (½ cup) in the Nutrition Facts panel to describe the product's nutritional content. The panel also must display the total amount of energy and energy from fat, indicated as numbers of calories, in a serving. The panel uses grams (g) and milligrams (mg) to indicate amounts of fiber and nutrients in a serving of food.

The Nutrition Facts panel must provide information about the food's total fat, saturated fat, trans fat, cholesterol, sodium, total carbohydrate, fiber, sugars, protein, vitamin A, vitamin C, calcium, and iron contents. Food manufacturers can also include amounts of polyunsaturated and monounsaturated fats, as well as potassium and other micronutrients in the Nutrition Facts panel. Listing these particular food components is required, if the manufacturer has fortified the food with the nutrients or made claims about their health benefits. The FDA plans to introduce a new format for the Nutrition Facts panel in 2012, so some of these features may change.

Foods such as fresh fruits and vegetables, fish, and shellfish are not required to have Nutrition Facts labels. However, many food suppliers and supermarket chains provide consumers with information about their products' nutritional content on posters or shelf tags displayed near the foods.

What About Restaurant and Vending Machine Foods?

A section of the *Patient Protection and Affordable Care Act of 2010* requires restaurants and similar retail food establishments with 20 or more locations to list calorie content information for standard menu items on restaurant menus and menu boards.[17] Information about total calories, fat, saturated fat, cholesterol, sodium, total carbohydrates, sugars, fiber, and total protein contents of menu items must be available in writing when the customer requests it. According to this act, companies that maintain 20 or more food vending machines must disclose calorie contents of certain items. The FDA is responsible for developing the rules for providing the nutrition information.

Information about the calorie contents of restaurant foods can help consumers make healthier menu selections. However, the accuracy of the caloric values listed by restaurants can vary.[18] The displayed or published nutrition information may give a close estimate of the food's actual energy and nutrient values, but portions are not exactly the same every time a food is served. Therefore, calorie levels posted at restaurants should be used by consumers as a rough guide for making healthier food choices.

Daily Values

Nutrient standards such as the RDA and AI are gender-, age-, and life stage–specific. For example, the RDA for vitamin C is 75 mg/day and 65 mg/day for nonsmoking 18-year-old males and females, respectively. The vitamin's RDA increases to 80 mg/day for 18-year-old pregnant females. Because the RDAs and AIs are so specific, it is not practical to provide nutrient information on food labels that refers to these complex standards. To help consumers evaluate the nutritional content of food products, FDA developed the **Daily Values (DVs)** for labeling purposes. Compared to the RDAs, the DVs are a more simplified and practical set of nutrient standards. The adult DV for a nutrient is based on a standard diet that supplies 2000 kcal/day. Not all nutrients have DVs, but they have been established for total fat, cholesterol, total carbohydrate, fiber, and several vitamins and minerals. There are no DVs for sugars or trans fat.

Appendix C lists DVs. A set of DVs that applies to people over 4 years of age is used for foods and beverages that adults consume. Three other sets of DVs are used on labels of foods intended for infants, children between 1 and 4 years of age, and pregnant or breastfeeding women.

Although DVs are often the highest RDA or AI for a particular nutrient, in many instances, they are based on recommendations of public health experts. For example, the RDA for carbohydrate is 130 g/day for people over 1 year of age. The DV for carbohydrate, however, is 300 g/day. This amount reflects the general dietary recommendations that carbohydrate can contribute 60% of a person's total energy intake, or 1200 kcal (300 g × 4 kcal/g of carbohydrate) of a 2000 kcal/day diet. For people older than 1 year of age, no RDA or AI has been set for daily fat intake. However, the DV for fat is 65 g/day. This amount meets the general recommendation that fat intake can be about 30% of a person's total energy intake for a 2000 kcal/day diet.

The %DVs can be confusing to use. When evaluating or planning nutritious menus, your goal is to obtain at least 100% of the DVs for fiber, vitamins, and minerals each day. On the other hand, you may need to limit your intake of foods that have high %DVs of total fat, cholesterol, and sodium. High intakes of these nutrients may have negative effects on your health. Thus, your goal is to consume less than 100% of the DV for total fat, cholesterol, and sodium each day. The general rule of thumb: A food that supplies 5%DV or less of a nutrient is a low source of the nutrient; a food that provides 20%DV or more is a high source of the nutrient.[16]

Percents of DVs are designed to help consumers compare nutrient contents of packaged foods to make more healthful choices. However, most people do not eat just packaged foods. Fresh fruits and vegetables, as well as most restaurant meals, do not have labels or menus with information about %DVs per serving. Therefore, many consumers will underestimate their nutrient intakes, if they do not consider the contribution that unlabeled foods make to their diets.

It is important to note the description of a serving size and the number of servings per container when using nutritional labeling information to estimate your intakes of energy, fiber, and nutrients in the food. A common mistake people make when using a Nutrition Facts panel is assuming the information applies to the entire package. For example, the Nutrition Facts panel on a package of food indicates there are four servings in the container. If you eat all the container's contents, you must multiply the information concerning calories, fat, and other food components by four. Why? Because you ate four servings and the nutritional information on the Nutrition Facts panel applies to only *one* serving.

Make Your Calories Count, an interactive program developed by the FDA, helps consumers use Nutrition Facts on food labels to plan nutritionally adequate diets while managing calorie intake. You can access the program by visiting the website: http://www.fda.gov/Food/ResourcesForYou/Consumers/NFLPM/ucm275438.htm and downloading

Daily Values (DVs) set of nutrient intake standards developed for labeling purposes

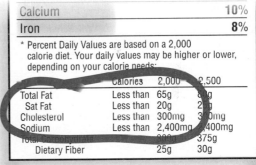

High intakes of solid fat, cholesterol, and sodium can have negative effects on your health. Therefore, consider consuming no more than 65 g total fat, 300 mg cholesterol, and 2400 mg sodium daily (2000 Calories).

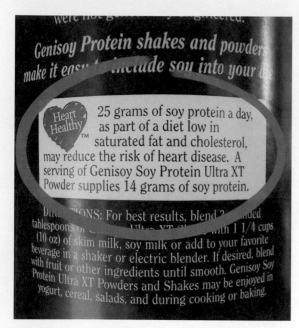

Figure 3.10 Label claims. The FDA permits food manufacturers to include certain health claims on food labels.

"Make Your Calories Count," an interactive training module. The FDA also provides "The Food Label and You," a video that you can watch at http://www.fda.gov/Food/ResourcesForYou/Consumers/NFLPM/ucm275409.htm.

Health Claims

To make their foods more appealing to consumers, manufacturers often promote products as having certain health benefits or high amounts of nutrients. A health claim describes the relationship between a food, food ingredient, or dietary supplement and the reduced risk of a nutrition-related condition. The FDA permits food manufacturers to include certain health claims on food labels (Fig. 3.10). For example, an allowable health claim may state, "Diets low in saturated fat and cholesterol may reduce the risk of heart disease."

For the FDA to allow a health claim on a product label, the claim should:

- Indicate that the product has health benefits only when it is part of a daily diet.
- Be complete, easy to understand, honest, and not misleading.
- Refer to a product that contains 10% or more of the DV for vitamins A and C, calcium, iron, fiber, or protein, *before* being fortified with nutrients. (This condition does not apply to dietary supplements.)
- Be for a product intended for people who are 2 years of age or older.
- Use "may" or "might" to describe the relationship between the product and disease. For example, "Diets containing foods that are good sources of potassium and that are low in sodium may reduce the risk of high blood pressure and stroke" is an allowable claim. However, the claim "Reduces the risk of stroke" would not be permitted on a label.
- Not quantify any degree of risk reduction. For example, a claim that states, "Reduces risk of cancer by 41%" would not be allowed because it specifies the degree of risk reduction.
- Indicate that many factors influence disease.

The FDA requires specific wording for certain health claims that are allowed on labels. For example, a claim that a whole-grain product may reduce the risk of heart disease and certain cancers must state: "Diets rich in whole grains and other plant foods and low in total fat, saturated fat, and cholesterol may reduce the risk of heart disease and some cancers." Table 3.7 lists some permissible health claims that can be used for labeling purposes. For more information, visit FDA's website at www.cfsan.fda.gov and search for "qualified health claims."

The FDA will not approve health claims for foods that contain more than 13 g of fat, 4 g of saturated fat, 60 mg of cholesterol, or 480 mg of sodium per serving. For example, calcium

TABLE 3.7 *Examples of Permissible Health Claims for Food Labels*

Dietary Factor/Health Condition	Example of Permissible Health Claim
Certain lipids and heart disease	"While many factors affect heart disease, diets low in saturated fat and cholesterol may reduce the risk of this disease."
Diet and heart disease	"Diets low in saturated fat and cholesterol and rich in fruits, vegetables, and grain products that contain some types of dietary fiber, particularly soluble fiber, may reduce the risk of heart disease, a disease associated with many factors."
Calcium, exercise, and osteoporosis (a disease that weakens bones)	"Regular exercise and a healthy diet with enough calcium help teen and young adult white and Asian women maintain good bone health and may reduce their high risk of osteoporosis."
Sodium (a mineral) and high blood pressure	"Diets low in sodium may reduce the risk of high blood pressure, a disease associated with many factors."
Folate (a B vitamin) and neural tube defects (conditions in which the skull and spinal bones do not form properly before birth)	"Healthful diets with adequate folate may reduce a woman's risk of having a child with a brain or spinal cord defect."
Fruits and vegetables and risk of cancer	"Foods that are low in fat and contain dietary fiber, vitamin A, or vitamin C may reduce the risk of some types of cancer, a disease associated with many factors. Broccoli is high in vitamins A and C, and it is a good source of dietary fiber."

Source: U.S. Food and Drug Administration, Center for Food Safety and Applied Nutrition. *A food labeling guide.* 1994; revised 1999 and 2000; updated 2006. www.cfsan.fda.gov/~dms/flg-6c.html Accessed: December 19, 2006

is a mineral that strengthens bones and protects them from *osteoporosis*, a condition in which bones become brittle and break easily. Whole milk is a rich source of calcium. Nevertheless, the label on a carton of whole milk cannot include a health claim about calcium and osteoporosis, because the milk contains more than 4 g of saturated fat per serving. In addition, the product must meet specific conditions that relate to the health claim. For example, a claim regarding the benefits of eating a low-fat diet is allowed only if the product contains 3 g or less of fat per serving, which is the FDA's standard definition of a low-fat food.

Structure/Function Claims

A *structure/function* claim describes the role a nutrient or dietary supplement plays in maintaining a structure, such as bone, or promoting a normal function, such as digestion. The FDA allows structure/function claims such as "calcium builds strong bones" or "fiber maintains bowel regularity" (Fig. 3.11). Structure/function statements cannot claim that a nutrient, food, or dietary supplement can be used to prevent or treat a serious health condition. For example, the FDA would not permit a claim that a product "promotes low blood pressure," because that claim implies the product has druglike effects and can treat high blood pressure.

Nutrient Content Claims

The FDA permits labels to include claims about levels of nutrients in packaged foods. Nutrient content claims can use terms such as "free," "high," or "low" to describe how much of a nutrient is in the product. Additionally, nutrient content claims can use terms such as "more" or "reduced" to compare amounts of nutrients in a product to those in a similar product. This claim is often used for an item that substitutes for a *reference food*, a similar and more familiar food. For example, a "reduced-fat" salad dressing has considerably less fat than its reference food, regular salad dressing.

Table 3.8 lists some legal definitions for common nutrient content claims that were allowed on labels in 2011. Note that a product may contain a small amount of a nutrient such as fat or sugar, yet the Nutrition Facts panel can indicate the amount as "0 g." For example, the Nutrition Facts panel may indicate that a serving of food supplies "0" grams of trans fat, even though the food actually supplies less than 0.5 g of trans fat. As a result, it is possible to consume some trans fats from processed foods even though labels indicate a serving of each food does not contain this type of fat. When the FDA introduces the new labeling format, specific amounts of such ingredients, such as trans fat, may need to be shown. To learn more about the FDA's regulations concerning nutrient claims, visit the

Figure 3.11 Structure/function claim. The FDA allows structure/function claims such as "calcium builds strong bones" or "helps naturally regulate your digestive system." Structure/function statements cannot claim that a nutrient, food, or dietary supplement can be used to prevent or treat a serious health condition.

TABLE 3.8 *Legal Definitions for Common Nutrient Content Claims (2011)*

Sugar	• **Sugar free:** The product provides less than 0.5 g of sugar per serving.
	• **Reduced sugar:** The food contains at least 25% less sugar per serving than the reference food.
Calories	• **Calorie free:** The food provides fewer than 5 kcal per serving.
	• **Low calorie:** The food supplies 40 kcal or less per serving.
	• **Reduced or fewer calories:** The food contains at least 25% fewer kcal per serving than the reference food.
Fat	• **Fat free:** The food provides less than 0.5 g of fat per serving.
	• **Low fat:** The food contains 3 g or less fat per serving. Two percent milk is not "low fat," because it has more than 3 g of fat per serving. The term *reduced fat* can be used to describe 2% milk.
	• **Reduced or less fat:** The food supplies less than 25% of the fat per serving than the reference food.
Cholesterol	• **Cholesterol free:** The food contains less than 2 mg of cholesterol and 2 g or less of saturated fat per serving.
Fiber	• **High fiber:** The food contains 5g or more fiber per serving. Foods that include high-fiber claims on the label must also meet the definition for low fat.
	• **Good source of fiber:** The food supplies 2.5 to 4.9 g of fiber per serving.
Meat and poultry products regulated by USDA	• **Extra lean:** The food provides less than 5 g of fat, 2 g of saturated fat, and 95 mg of cholesterol per serving.
	• **Lean:** The food contains less than 10 g of fat, 4.5 g of saturated fat, and 95 mg of cholesterol per serving.

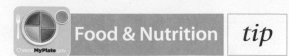

Often, the only difference between a creamy salad dressing, such as ranch or blue cheese, and the "light" version of the dressing is the amount of water they contain. Instead of paying more for calorie-reduced bottled salad dressings, make your own light salad dressing by adding about ¼ cup water to a jar of regular creamy salad dressing, then stir or shake the mixture.

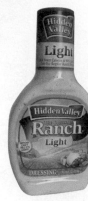

agency's website (http://www.fda.gov/Food/GuidanceComplianceRegulatoryInformation/default.htm).

Other Descriptive Labeling Terms

According to the FDA, a *light* or *lite* food has at least one-third fewer kilocalories or half the fat of the reference food. For example, a tablespoon of lite pancake syrup has one-third fewer kcal than a tablespoon of regular pancake syrup, and a tablespoon of light mayonnaise has less than half the fat of regular mayonnaise. The term *light* may also describe such properties as texture and color, as long as the label explains the intent—for example, "light brown sugar." To include the term "natural" on the label, the food must not contain food coloring agents, synthetic flavors, or other unnatural substances.

Dietary Supplement Labels

According to federal law, every dietary supplement container must be properly labeled (Fig. 3.12). The label must include the term "dietary supplement" or a similar term that describes the product's particular ingredient, such as "herbal supplement" or "vitamin C supplement." Dietary supplement labels are also required to display the list of ingredients, manufacturer's address, and suggested dosage. Furthermore, the label must include facts about the product's contents in a special format—the "Supplement Facts" panel (see Fig. 3.12). The panel provides information about the serving size; amount per serving; and percent Daily Value (%DV) for ingredients, if one has been established. Daily Values (DVs) are standard desirable or maximum intakes for several nutrients, but DVs have not been established for nonnutrient products.

According to the FDA, dietary supplements are not intended to treat, diagnose, cure, or alleviate the effects of diseases. Therefore, the agency does not permit manufacturers to market a dietary supplement product as a treatment or cure for a disease, or to relieve signs or symptoms of a disease. Although such products generally cannot prevent diseases, some can improve health or reduce the risk of certain diseases or conditions. Thus, the FDA allows supplement manufacturers to display structure/function claims on labels. Manufacturers of iron supplements, for example, may have a claim on the label that

Figure 3.12 Supplement Facts label. A nutrient supplement label must list the product's ingredient(s), serving size, amount(s) per serving, suggested use, manufacturer and the company's address, and %DV, if one has been established. If a health claim appears on the supplement's label, the claim must be followed by the FDA disclaimer.

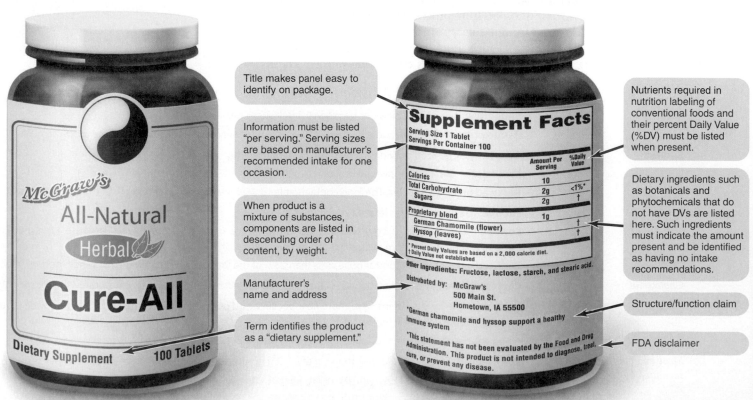

states: "Iron is necessary for healthy red blood cell formation." If the FDA has not reviewed a claim, the label must include the FDA's disclaimer indicating that the claim has not been evaluated by the agency (Fig. 3.13).

The FDA does not require dietary supplement manufacturers or sellers to provide evidence that labeling claims are accurate or truthful before they appear on product containers. However, manufacturers that include structure/function claims on labels must notify the FDA about the claims within 30 days after introducing the products into the marketplace. If FDA officials question the safety of a dietary supplement or the truthfulness of claims that appear on supplement labels, manufacturers are responsible for providing the agency with evidence that their products are safe and the claims on labels are honest and not misleading.

In 2007, the FDA issued rules that required dietary supplement manufacturers to evaluate the purity, quality, strength, and composition of their products before marketing them. The regulations are designed to result in the production of supplements that contain the ingredients listed on the label, are wholesome, contain standard amounts of ingredients per dose, and are properly packaged and accurately labeled.

Organic Food

By the late twentieth century, emphasis on increasing agricultural production resulted in an inexpensive and abundant food supply in the United States. However, the rise of agribusiness also resulted in social, economic, and environmental costs. Rural agricultural communities experienced a dramatic decline in the number of small farms, as the farms' owners could not compete with the production capabilities and financial resources of large commercially run farms.

Instead of producing a variety of crops, big farms often focus on growing corn, soybeans, or wheat. These crops require conventional farming methods that include heavy use of fertilizers and products to control pests (*pesticides*). In some parts of the country, large farms also need considerable amounts of water for irrigating crops. As a result, underground water supplies are being depleted in these regions.

The rise in agribusiness helped fuel interest in sustainable agriculture. *Sustainable agriculture* focuses on producing adequate amounts of food without reducing natural resources and harming the environment.[19] Such agricultural methods promote crop variety, soil and water conservation, and recycling of plant nutrients. Additionally, sustainable agriculture can support small farms, particularly *organic* farms.

Technically, organic substances have the element carbon bonded to hydrogen (another element) in their chemical structures. Therefore, all foods are organic because they contain substances comprised of carbon bonded with hydrogen. The term "organic," however, also refers to certain agricultural methods that can promote sustainability. Organic farming and the production of **organic foods** do not rely on the use of antibiotics, hormones, synthetic fertilizers and pesticides, genetic improvements, or ionizing radiation.[20] Table 3.9 compares organic and nonorganic agricultural systems. Although organic farming techniques can benefit the environment, crop yields are typically lower than yields of similar crops grown conventionally.[21]

Over the past 40 years, the popularity of organic foods has increased in the United States as many Americans have become concerned about the environment and the safety and nutritional value of the food supply. Sales of organic foods have increased steadily since the 1990s, even though these products are usually more expensive than the same foods produced by conventional farming methods.[23] According to the Food Marketing Institute, Americans spent $25 billion on organic foods and beverages in 2009.[24]

People who purchase organically grown foods often think the products are better for their health and more nutritious than conventionally produced foods. Few well-designed studies have compared nutrient and phytochemical contents of organically grown foods to their conventionally grown counterparts. Nevertheless, some general trends have been determined. In general, organic food crops are not more nutritious than conventionally grown food crops.[26] Organic crops, however, may contain fewer pesticides than conventionally grown crops.[27] Nevertheless, more research is needed to determine whether there are health advantages to eating organic foods.

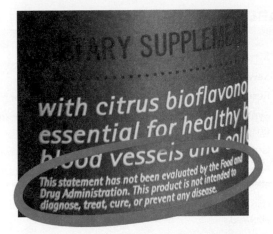

Figure 3.13 Label disclaimer. The FDA permits dietary supplement manufacturers to include certain health-related claims on their product labels. However, the label of products bearing such claims also must display this disclaimer.

organic foods foods produced without the use of antibiotics, hormones, synthetic fertilizers and pesticides, genetic improvements, or spoilage-killing radiation

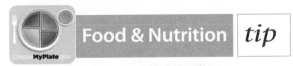

Food & Nutrition *tip*

According to the Environmental Protection Agency, you can reduce your exposure to pesticides in food by:

- Washing and scrubbing all fresh fruits and vegetables under running water. However, not all pesticide residues can be removed by washing.

- Peeling and trimming fruits and vegetables before eating them.

- Trimming fat from meat and skin of poultry and fish, because some pesticide residues accumulate in fat.

- Eating a variety of foods; this reduces the likelihood of exposure to a single pesticide.

- Eating organically grown foods.[22]

Did You Know?

In January 2008, FDA scientists issued documents indicating that meat and milk from certain cloned animals and the offspring of any cloned animal were safe to consume.[25] A cloned animal is a genetic copy of a donor animal. Cloning is not the same process as genetic engineering, because cloning does not involve altering an animal's DNA. Because many consumers are likely to be wary of foods from cloned animals, such items may not be commercially available for several years.

TABLE 3.9 *Comparing Organic and Nonorganic Farming Systems*

Organic	Nonorganic
Synthetic fertilizers are not allowed.	Limited restrictions on fertilizers
Sewage sludge products are not allowed.	Sludge products may be used on some fields.
Restrictions on use of raw manure on fields used for food crops	Few restrictions on raw manure use for edible crop fields
Synthetic pesticides are not allowed; natural pest management practices are encouraged.	Any government-approved pesticide may be used according to label instructions. Natural pest management practices may also be used.
Genetically modified organisms (GMOs) are not allowed.	Government-approved GMOs are permitted.
Feeding livestock mammal and poultry by-products and manure is not allowed.	Certain mammal and poultry by-products are allowed in livestock feed.
Use of growth hormones and antibiotics in livestock production is not allowed.	Government-approved hormone and antibiotic treatments are permitted.
Food irradiation (a food safety method) is not allowed.	Food irradiation may be used.
Detailed record keeping and site inspections by regulators are required.	Some records are required, but no on-site checks by regulators are necessary.

Labeling Organic Foods

To protect consumers, the USDA developed and implemented rules for the organic food industry. A food product cannot be labeled "organic" unless its production meets strict national standards. For labeling purposes, organic food manufacturers can use the circular "USDA Organic" symbol on the package (Fig. 3.14). This symbol indicates the products meet USDA's standards for organic food. According to the USDA, there are three organic labeling categories (Table 3.10). Note that certain foods can have the organic symbol on the package, yet they may contain small amounts of nonorganic ingredients. For more information about the government's organic food standards, visit the USDA's National Organic Program's website (http://www.ams.usda.gov/AMSv1.0/nop).

TABLE 3.10 *Organic Labeling Categories*

"100% Organic" (may use USDA seal)	100% organic ingredients, including processing aids
"Organic" (may use USDA seal)	Contains at least 95% organic ingredients. Remaining 5% of ingredients are on USDA's allowable list of allowed ingredients.
"Made with organic ingredients"	Contains 70 to 95% organic ingredients

Source: Robinson B: Value through verification: USDA National Organic Program. http://www.ams.usda.gov/AMSv1.0/getfile?dDocName=STELDEV3049688&acct=noppub

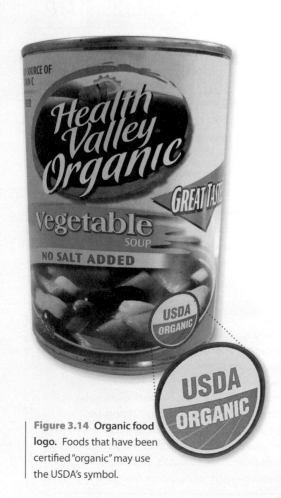

Figure 3.14 Organic food logo. Foods that have been certified "organic" may use the USDA's symbol.

Concept **Checkpoint**

26. Identify at least one limitation of using %DVs to determine your nutrient intakes.
27. Explain how you can use nutritional information provided on food and dietary supplement labels to become a more careful consumer.
28. What is the difference between a health claim and a structure/function claim? What is a nutrient content claim? Give an example of each type of claim.
29. Discuss the role of the FDA in protecting consumers from false nutrition and health claims on food and dietary supplement labels.
30. Explain how organic food production methods differ from conventional food production methods.

3.6 Using Dietary Analysis Software

How much selenium, magnesium, and niacin are in an ounce of Swiss cheese? Have you ever wanted information about nutrients in a food that are not listed on the Nutrition Facts panel? In the past, people relied on food composition tables, lists of commonly eaten foods that provide amounts of energy, fiber, macronutrients, and several micronutrients. Today, people can determine the energy and nutrient contents of their food choices by using a dietary analysis software program. Furthermore, people with Internet access can obtain the information from certain websites.

Dietary analysis software and websites can be quick and easy tools for determining nutrient and energy contents of a specific food. However, the values provided by these resources are not necessarily exact amounts. The same type of plant food may vary in nutrient content depending on hereditary factors, age, growing conditions, and production methods. Therefore, scientists generally analyze several samples of a particular food to determine their nutrient contents, and then the researchers average the results. For example, if the amount of energy in three Valencia oranges that each weigh about 4 ounces (120 g) were 55, 60, and 62 kcal, respectively, the value listed in the food composition table for a Valencia orange weighing 4 ounces would be 59 kcal, the average of the three. In many instances, values for certain nutrients are missing. This occurs when accurate data concerning the complete nutrient analysis of the food are unavailable.

The following section discusses some government-sponsored websites that provide practical tools for evaluating food intakes and physical activity habits. The Personal Dietary Analysis feature at the end of Chapter 3 provides an opportunity for you to practice using dietary analysis software.

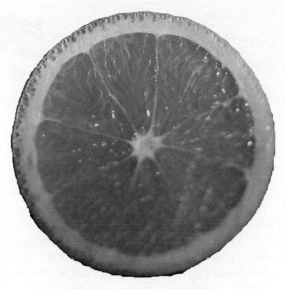

Valencia oranges and other produce may vary in nutrient content depending on numerous factors, including growing conditions.

Government-Sponsored Dietary Analysis Websites

In addition to www.choosemyplate.gov, the USDA sponsors other websites to help you assess the energy and nutrient contents of your food intake. The "What's in the Food You Eat *Search Tool*" (www.ars.usda.gov/Services/docs.htm?docid=17032) is one such site. Another USDA-sponsored site that provides extensive information regarding the energy and nutrient content of food is the National Nutrient Database for Standard Reference. You can access this nutrient database by visiting www.nal.usda.gov/fnic/foodcomp/search/. To keep current, USDA-sponsored websites are updated regularly to provide information about new products and serving sizes.

Concept **Checkpoint**

31. Identify at least two reliable sources of information about the energy and nutrient contents of foods and beverages.

Chapter 3 Highlight

THE MELTING POT

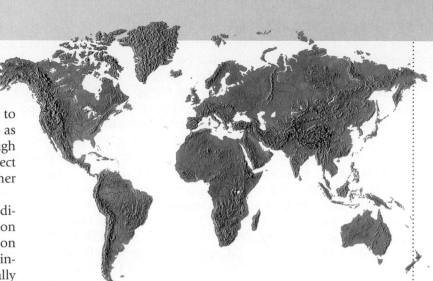

Wherever you live or travel in the United States, you're likely to find restaurants that serve a wide variety of ethnic fare, such as Italian, Thai, Vietnamese, or Middle Eastern dishes. Although your primary food selection and cooking habits probably reflect your cultural/ethnic heritage, you likely enjoy foods from other cultures and ethnic groups.

The Chapter 3 Highlight examines the influences that the dietary practices of certain cultures and ethnic groups have had on the American diet and the possible effects of these practices on health. Traditional ethnic diets are often based on dishes containing small amounts of animal foods and larger amounts of locally grown fruits, vegetables, and unrefined grains. However, these foods are typically the first to be abandoned as immigrants *assimilate*, that is, blend into the general population over time. After an immigrant population has assimilated fully, the prevalence of chronic diseases such as cardiovascular disease (CVD), type 2 diabetes, and high blood pressure often increases among them, partly as a result of adopting less healthy eating practices.

Northwestern European Influences

Immigrants from northwestern European regions or countries such as the United Kingdom, Scandinavia, and Germany established the familiar "meat-and-potatoes" diet that features a large portion of beef or pork served with a smaller portion of potatoes. In the past, the potatoes were either boiled or mashed; today, they are usually fried. This mainstream American diet, often referred to as a "Western" diet, provides large amounts of animal protein and fat, and lacks fruits, whole grains, and a variety of green vegetables. Such diets are associated with high rates of serious chronic diseases, particularly CVD and type 2 diabetes, which are discussed in later chapters of this textbook.

Hispanic Influences

The Hispanic (people with Spanish ancestry) population is now the largest minority group in the United States. Many Hispanic-Americans migrated to the United States from Mexico. The traditional Mexican diet included corn, beans, chili peppers, avocados, papayas, and pineapples. Many supermarkets in the United States sell other plant foods that are often incorporated into Mexican meals, such as fresh chayote, cherimoya, jicama, plantains, and cactus leaves and fruit. Such fruits and vegetables add fiber and a variety of nutrients, phytochemicals, vivid colors, and interesting flavors to Mexican dishes.

Authentic Mexican meals are based primarily on rice, tortillas, and beans, depending on the region. However, many non-Hispanic Americans do not like to eat meals limited to these inexpensive yet nutritious plant foods. To appeal to people with more Western food preferences, "Mexican" fast-food restaurants in the United States often serve dishes that contain large portions of high-fat beef topped with sour cream and cheese. Diets that contain high amounts of these fatty foods are associated with excess body fat, CVD, and type 2 diabetes.

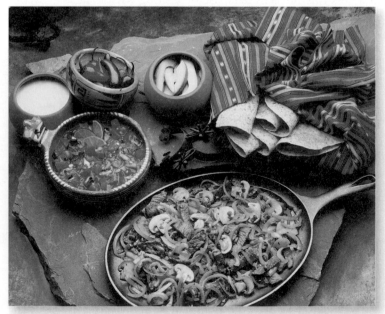

| Fresh fruits and vegetables add flavor, color, and micronutrients to Mexican meals.

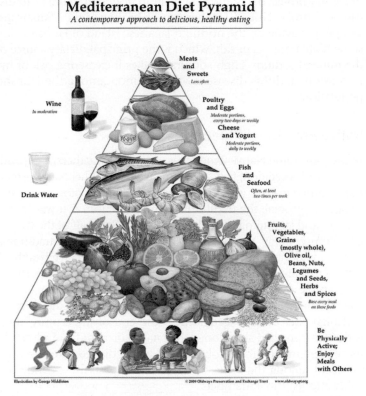

Figure 3.15 Mediterranean Diet Pyramid. The Mediterranean Diet Pyramid is based on traditional dietary practices of Greece, southern Italy, and the island of Crete.

Italian and Other Mediterranean Influences

The traditional Italian diet of pasta and other grain products, olive oil, fish, nuts, fruits, and vegetables is healthier than the Western diet. Pasta, a product made from wheat flour and water, is the core of the traditional Italian diet. To the typical American, *pasta* is spaghetti topped with tomato sauce, meatballs, and grated Parmesan cheese. However, Italians eat a variety of different forms of pasta, such as penne, linguini, acini de pepe, and rotini, along with sauces that are often meatless. Pizza, a dish from southern Italy, is one of the most frequently consumed foods in the United States. Unlike traditional Italian pizza that has a thin crust and is lightly covered with tomatoes, basil (a leafy herb), and mozzarella cheese, many Americans choose thick-crust pizza topped with tomato sauce, plenty of shredded mozzarella cheese, and dotted with fatty pork sausage or pepperoni.

Dietary pyramids or plans developed by governmental agencies or private organizations have plant foods as the core of a healthy diet. The Mediterranean Diet Pyramid shown in Figure 3.15 is based on traditional dietary practices of Greece, southern Italy, and the island of Crete. Grains, fruits, and vegetables, particularly beans and potatoes, form the foundation of this diet. Red meat is rarely eaten. Main dishes often include seafood and poultry, and wine may be included with meals. Although the Mediterranean Diet Pyramid allows as much as 35% of total calories as fat in the diet, much of the fat is from olive oil. Olive oil is a rich source of a type of fat that reduces rather than increases the risk of CVD. Chapter 6 provides more information about oils and fats and their roles in health. For more information about ethnic diet pyramids, visit www.oldwayspt.org/.

African Influences

The people who were forced to migrate from West Africa as slaves brought traditional foods such as sweet potatoes, okra, and peanuts from their homelands. West African dietary practices easily blended with Native American, Spanish, and French food traditions, creating Cajun and Creole cuisines associated with Louisiana and the Gulf Coast today. African-American "soul foods" include sweet potato pie, fried chicken, black-eyed peas, and "*greens*," the nutritious leafy parts of plants such as kale, collards, mustard, turnip, and dandelion. To add flavor, greens are usually cooked with small pieces of smoked pork.

Traditional African-American cuisine has both health benefits and deficits. Although fruit, beans, and leafy vegetables provide fiber and a variety of vitamins and minerals, salt-cured pork products contribute undesirable levels of fat and sodium to the diet. Reliance on frying foods also increases fat intakes. High-fat diets are associated with obesity, and high-sodium diets raise the risk of hypertension. Obesity and hypertension are quite prevalent among African-Americans. You will learn more about diet and blood pressure in Chapters 6 and 9.

Asian Influences

Traditional Asian foods, such as Chinese, Japanese, Vietnamese, Thai, and Korean cuisines, are similar and generally feature large amounts of vegetables, rice, or noodles combined with small amounts of meat, fish, or shellfish. The variety of vegetables used in Asian dishes adds color, flavor, texture, phytochemicals, and nutrients to meals. Additionally, Asian dishes often include flavorful sauces and seasonings made from plants, such as soy sauce, rice wine, gingerroot, garlic, scallions, peppers, and sesame seeds. The Asian Diet Pyramid, shown in Figure 3.16, illustrates the traditional Asian dietary pattern, which generally provides inadequate amounts of calcium from milk and milk products. However, using calcium-rich or calcium-fortified foods can add the mineral to diets.

Chinese foods are popular among Americans. Many Americans, however, do not favor dishes that feature seafood and contain large portions of vegetables and grains, because they believe meat should form the basis of a meal. Thus, North American Chinese restaurants that specialize in Cantonese, Szechwan, or Mandarin cuisines typically offer menu items that contain much larger portions of animal foods such as beef and chicken than authentic dishes. Furthermore, American-Chinese foods are often prepared with far greater amounts of fat than are used in true Chinese cooking.

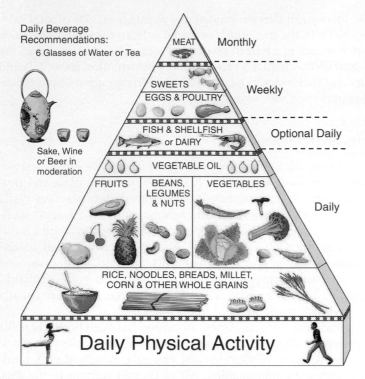

Figure 3.16 Asian Diet Pyramid. The Asian Diet Pyramid dietary pattern generally provides inadequate amounts of calcium from milk and milk products.

Traditional Chinese food preparation methods, particularly steaming and stir-frying, tend to preserve the vitamins and minerals in fresh vegetables. Stir-frying involves cooking foods in a lightly oiled, very hot pan for a short period of time. Unlike Western methods of deep-fat frying or boiling vegetables, stir-frying vegetables keeps them crisp and colorful.

Rice is the staple food in the traditional Japanese diet. Additionally, fish, poultry, pork, and foods made from soybeans provide protein in this diet. The Japanese people eat sushi, small pieces of raw fish or shellfish that are usually served rolled in or pressed into rice and served with vegetables and seaweed. American-Japanese restaurants often feature sushi, and many non-Japanese Americans like to order the exotic dish.

Some of the longest-lived, healthiest people in the world reside on Okinawa, a tiny island south of the main Japanese islands. The traditional diet of fresh vegetables, minimal amounts of salt and animal protein (mainly from pork and fish), and moderate amounts of fat may protect the island's population from premature heart disease and stroke. Not all Japanese are as healthy as the Okinawans. The people living on the northern Japanese island of Honshu consume high amounts of salt, which is the principal dietary source of the mineral sodium. High sodium intakes increase the risk of hypertension, and this disease is very common among the Honshu population.

Native American Influences

In the past, some Native Americans were hunter-gatherers, depending on wild vegetation, fish, and game for food. Other Native Americans learned to grow vegetable crops, including tomatoes, corn, and squash. In general, the traditional Native American diet was low in sodium and fat and high in fiber. During the last half of the twentieth century, many Native Americans abandoned their traditional diets and adopted the typical Western diet. The negative health effects of this lifestyle change have been significant. Before the 1930s, for example, members of the Pima tribe in the southwestern United States primarily ate native foods that included low-fat game animals and high-fiber desert vegetation. By the end of the century, most American Pima had abandoned their native diets and had adopted a more Western diet. Today, obesity and type 2 diabetes are extremely prevalent among the Pima, whereas in the past, these conditions rarely affected tribal members.

The traditional native Alaskan diet was composed of fatty fish and sea mammals, game animals, and a few plants. Alaskan natives who still follow traditional dietary practices have CVD rates that are lower than those in the general North American population, but those who switched to a more Western diet have developed CVD at rates similar to those of the general population.

Religious Influences

Many religions require members to follow strict food handling and dietary practices that often include the prohibition of certain foods and beverages (see Table 3.11). According to Jewish dietary laws, for example, meat and poultry products must be kept separate from milk products. Milk products are not used to prepare

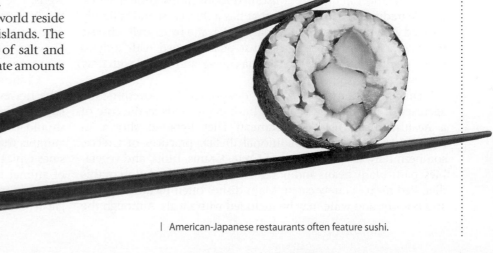

American-Japanese restaurants often feature sushi.

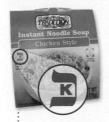

foods that contain meat or poultry, nor are they served with them. A cheeseburger, for example, is not *kosher*. "Kosher" refers to a specific procedure concerning killing, butchering, and preparation activities that makes food acceptable for the religion's followers to eat. Fruits, grains, and vegetables are "neutral" foods that can be eaten with meals that contain either meat or dairy products. However, vegetables cooked with meat become a "meat" food and cannot be served with milk; peaches served with cottage cheese become a "milk" food and cannot be eaten with meat or poultry. Today many American Jews do not follow their religion's complex dietary laws as closely as their ancestors did.

Bagels with smoked salmon (*lox*), pickled herring, cream cheese, dill pickles, corned beef, and pastrami are popular among the Ashkenazi, the predominant group of Jews in America. Although many non-Jews enjoy eating these traditional Ashkenazic foods, such items may be too high in sodium and animal fat to be healthy.

The Role of Diet in Health

Diet is only one aspect of lifestyle that affects the health of a particular population. Physical activity habits also have a major influence on health. Today, most Americans enjoy and depend on a variety of labor-saving devices that make housework, occupations, and leisure time less physically demanding than these activities were 100 years ago. As immigrants and other members of the population become less physically active, they also tend to develop obesity, type 2 diabetes, and hypertension. Current recommendations for reducing the prevalence of these conditions generally include making specific dietary changes as well as increasing physical activity levels. Nevertheless, nutrition researchers need to learn more about the influence that traditional diets can have on the risk of chronic diseases.

TABLE 3.11

Religion	Dietary Practices*
Buddhist	Meat is avoided; vegetarianism is encouraged.
Eastern Orthodox	Meat and fish restrictions; fasting and specific food abstinence during certain holidays
Hindu	Beef is forbidden, but dairy products are "pure" for consumption. Pork may be restricted. Alcohol is avoided. Fasting is often encouraged.
Islam	Pork; birds of prey; reptiles; insects, except locusts; most gelatins; and alcohol are prohibited ("ha-raam"). Ritual killing of animals that are permitted as food ("ha-lal") Stimulant beverages (I.e., coffee and tea) are avoided. Fasting from all food and drink (daytime) during month of Ramadan and certain other religious holidays
Jewish	Only kosher foods are acceptable. "Tref" (*trayf*) refers to prohibited foods. Pork and shellfish are prohibited. Eating meat with dairy is prohibited. Consuming blood is forbidden. Raw meat is soaked in cold water to remove blood, salted for one hour, and then rinsed. Eggs, fruits, and vegetables can be eaten with either meat or dairy foods. Eggs, however, are inspected to make sure they do not contain blood specks. Only fish with fins and scales can be eaten. Only land animals that have split hooves and chew their cud can be eaten, and only the front half of the cud-chewing animal is used. Ritual killing of certain animals is required. Fasting and specific food restrictions for certain holidays
Mormon	Beverages containing alcohol or caffeine are prohibited. Fasting is practiced occasionally.
Roman Catholic	Fasting before communion; fasting and specific food abstinence during certain holidays
Seventh Day Adventist	Animal product consumption generally limited to milk, milk products, and eggs (lacto-ovo vegetarianism) Alcohol and beverages containing stimulants are prohibited.

* Some religions have extensive rules governing food-related practices, but many people do not follow their religion's dietary guidelines fully or at all.

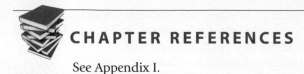

CHAPTER REFERENCES

See Appendix I.

SUMMARY

A requirement is the smallest amount of a nutrient that maintains a defined level of health. Numerous factors influence nutrient requirements. Scientists use information about nutrient requirements and storage capabilities to establish specific dietary recommendations. The Dietary Reference Intakes (DRIs) are various energy and nutrient intake standards for Americans. An Estimated Average Requirement (EAR) is the amount of the nutrient that meets the needs of 50% of healthy people in a particular life stage/gender group. The Estimated Energy Requirement (EER) is used to evaluate a person's energy intake. The Recommended Dietary Allowances (RDAs) meet the needs of nearly all healthy individuals (97 to 98%) in a particular life stage/gender group. When nutrition scientists are unable to determine an RDA for a nutrient, they establish an Adequate Intake (AI) value. The Tolerable Upper Intake Level (UL) is the highest average amount of a nutrient that is unlikely to harm most people when the amount is consumed daily.

DRIs can be used for planning nutritious diets for groups of people and evaluating the nutritional adequacy of a population's diet. RDAs and AIs are often used to evaluate an individual's dietary practices. For nutrition labeling purposes, FDA uses RDAs to develop Daily Values (DVs).

Dietary guides generally classify foods into groups according to their natural origins and key nutrients. Such guides usually feature major food groups. Some dietary guides also include groups for oils and empty-calorie foods or beverages. The Dietary Guidelines is a set of general nutrition-related lifestyle recommendations designed to promote adequate nutritional status and good health, and to reduce the risk of major chronic health conditions. Choosemyplate.gov is an online, interactive food intake and physical activity guide that is based on Dietary Guidelines. Most Americans do not follow the government's dietary recommendations.

The Exchange System, a tool for estimating the calorie and macronutrient contents of foods, categorizes foods into three broad groups. The foods within each group have similar macronutrient composition. A specified amount of food in an exchange list provides about the same amount of macronutrients and calories as each of the other specified amounts of foods in that list. Carbohydrate counting is a method that people can use for planning menus.

Consumers can use information on food labels to determine ingredients and compare nutrient contents of packaged foods and beverages. The FDA regulates and monitors information that can be placed on food labels, including claims about the product's health benefits. Nearly all foods and beverages sold in supermarkets must be labeled with the product's name, manufacturer's name and address, amount of product in the package, and ingredients listed in descending order by weight. Furthermore, food labels must use a special format for listing specific information on the Nutrition Facts panel.

The Daily Values (DVs) are a practical set of nutrient standards for labeling purposes. The nutrient content in a serving of food is listed on the label as a percentage of the DV (%DV). Not all nutrients have DVs. A dietary goal is to obtain at least 100% of the DVs for fiber, vitamins, and minerals (except sodium) each day.

The FDA permits food manufacturers to include certain health claims on food labels. However, the agency requires that health claims meet certain guidelines and, in some instances, use specific wording. A structure/function claim describes the role a nutrient plays in the body. Structure/function statements cannot claim that a nutrient or food can be used to prevent or treat a serious health condition.

Organic foods are produced without the use of antibiotics, hormones, synthetic fertilizers and pesticides, genetic improvements, or spoilage-killing radiation. In general, organic food crops are not more nutritious than similar conventionally grown foods. More research is needed to determine whether there are health advantages to eating organic foods. A food product cannot be labeled "organic" unless its production meets strict national standards.

Traditional ethnic diets are often based on dishes containing small amounts of animal foods and larger amounts of locally grown fruits, vegetables, and unrefined grains. However, these foods are typically abandoned as people migrate to other countries and assimilate into the general population. After an immigrant population has assimilated fully, the prevalence of chronic diseases such as cardiovascular disease, type 2 diabetes, and high blood pressure often increases among them, partly as a result of adopting unhealthy eating practices. Many religions require members to follow strict food handling and dietary practices that often include the prohibition of certain foods and beverages.

Recipes for Healthy Living

Mango Lassi

Lassi (*luh-see*) is a simple yogurt-based beverage that originated in India. Lassi is usually made and served before a meal, but the drink can also be a refreshing, nutritious snack. This recipe makes about four ½-cup servings. Each serving supplies approximately 85 kcal, 4 g protein, 17 g carbohydrate, 0 g fat, 3.7 g fiber, 130 mg calcium, and 14 mg vitamin C.

INGREDIENTS:

1 ripe mango
1 cup plain, fat-free yogurt
1 Tbsp sugar
6 ice cubes

PREPARATION STEPS:

1. Wash and peel mango. Remove fruit pulp from mango and discard large seed and peel.
2. Dice mango pulp and place in blender.
3. Add yogurt, sugar, and ice cubes to the blender.
4. Blend ingredients until smooth.
5. Serve immediately or refrigerate for up to 24 hours.

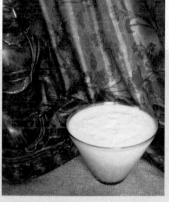

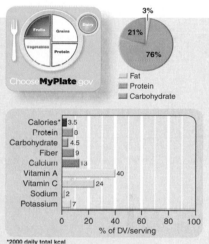

3%
21%
76%

- Fat
- Protein
- Carbohydrate

Calories*	3.5
Protein	0
Carbohydrate	4.5
Fiber	9
Calcium	13
Vitamin A	40
Vitamin C	24
Sodium	2
Potassium	7

0 20 40 60 80 100
% of DV/serving
*2000 daily total kcal

Fresh Fruit Salad

The following recipe is for a colorful fresh fruit salad that is high in antioxidants. Fruits are so versatile, you can invent your own salads by adding different fresh fruits to a basic mixture of bananas, apples, and grapes. When selecting fresh fruit, avoid fruits that are too hard or soft, because they may be underripe or too ripe. If you need help, ask the produce manager to show you how to choose the best-quality fruit.

This recipe makes approximately six 1-cup servings. A serving of this fruit salad supplies about 84 kcal, 1 g protein, 0 g fat, 20 g carbohydrate, 2.3 g fiber, 37 mg vitamin C, 290 mg potassium, and 3 mg sodium.

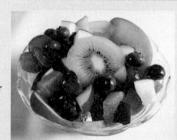

INGREDIENTS:

½ cup blueberries
1 slice of watermelon, about 1" thick
1 cup red or purple seedless grapes
1 medium peach
2 medium kiwifruit, slightly firm
1 medium Jonathan apple, with skin
½ cup orange juice

PREPARATION STEPS:

1. Wash fruit in cool water, including the watermelon peel. Drain blueberries, place in a bowl, and remove and discard stems and damaged berries. Dry other fruit with paper towels.
2. Remove green rind of watermelon and discard. Cut watermelon into cubes and add to the berries.
3. Slice each grape in half and add to watermelon.
4. Slice peach in half and discard seed. Cut into thin wedge-shaped segments and add to fruit.
5. Peel kiwifruit and slice into rounds that are about ¼" thick. Add to fruit mixture.
6. Remove core and seeds from the apple. Cut fruit into small pieces and add to mixture.
7. Add orange juice to mixture and gently stir with a large spoon, coating fruit with juice.
8. Refrigerate.

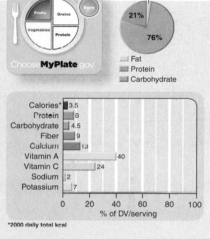

5%
95%

- Fat
- Protein
- Carbohydrate

Calories*	4
Protein	2
Carbohydrate	8
Fiber	9
Vitamin C	62
Potassium	8

0 20 40 60 80 100
% of DV/serving
*2000 daily total kcal

Personal *Dietary* Analysis

I. Record Keeping
 A. 24-Hour Dietary Recall
  1. Recall every food and beverage that you have eaten over the past 24 hours. Recall how much you consumed and how it was prepared.
   a. How easy or difficult was it to recall your food intake?
 B. Three-Day Diet Record
  1. Without changing your usual diet, keep a detailed log of your food and beverage intake for 3 days; one of the days should be Friday or Saturday. Use a separate log for each day.

II. Analysis
Using nutritional analysis software, analyze your daily food intakes and answer questions in Part III of this activity. Keep the record on file for future applications.
 A. Computer-Generated Dietary Analysis
  1. Load the software into the computer, or log on to software website.
  2. Choose the DRIs or related nutrient standard from the inside back cover, based on your life stage, sex, height, and weight.
  3. Enter the information from the 3-day food intake record. Be sure to enter each food and drink and the specific amounts.
  4. The software program will give you the following results:
   a. The appropriate RDA (or related standard) for each nutrient
   b. The total amount of each nutrient and the kilocalories consumed for each day
   c. The percentage intake compared with the standard amount for each nutrient that you consumed each day
  5. Keep this assessment for activities in other chapters.

III. Evaluation of Nutrient Intakes
Remember it is not necessary to consume the maximum of your nutrient recommendations every day. A general standard is meeting at least 70% of the standards averaged over several days. It is best not to exceed the Upper Level (if set) over the long term to avoid potential toxic effects of some nutrients.
 A. For which nutrients did your average intake fall below the recommended amounts, that is, to less than 70% of the RDA/AI?
 B. For which nutrients did your average intake exceed the Upper Level (if a UL has been set)?

IV. MyPlate
This activity determines how your diet stacks up when compared to the amounts of foods from each food group that are recommended in the USDA's www.choosemyplate.gov.
 A. Refer to your 3-day food intake record. Classify each food item in the appropriate food group of MyPlate. For each food group, indicate whether you ate the recommended amount daily for your sex, age, height, weight, and physical activity level. Note that some of your food choices—pizza, for example—may contribute to more than one food group. Enter a minus sign (–) if your total falls below the MyPlate recommendation or a plus sign (+) if it equals or exceeds the daily recommendation for each food group.

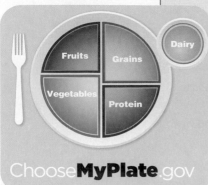

CRITICAL THINKING

1. Your friend takes several dietary supplements daily, and as a result, his vitamin B-6 intake is 50 times higher than the RDA for the vitamin. You would like to convince him to stop taking the supplements. To support your advice, which nutrient standards would you show him? Explain why.

2. Why should consumers use MyPlate to plan menus instead of the DRIs?

3. How do your fiber, sodium, and alcohol intakes compare to the recommendations of the latest Dietary Guidelines?

4. Examine Table 3.5. Which foods in the left-hand column do you eat regularly? Why are those foods listed in that column?

5. The ingredient list on a package of crackers includes vegetable oil. What can you do to learn which type of vegetable oil is in the product?

6. Discuss whether you use or would use one of the menu-planning tools described in Chapter 3 to plan your daily food intake.

7. Visit the USDA's website (www.ars.usda.gov/Services/docs .htm?docid=17032) to access "What's in the Foods You Eat *Search Tool*," a database for searching the nutritional content of foods. To practice using this search tool, find the number of kilocalories and the amounts of fiber, vitamin C, iron, and caffeine in 1 cup of raw jicama, 1 cup of 2% milk with added vitamin A, and 100 g of dry roasted, salt-added sunflower seed kernels.

8. According to a newspaper article, an 8-oz serving of fat-free milk contains 15 mcg of folate (a B vitamin). Another source of nutrition information indicates that an 8-oz serving of fat-free milk contains 12 mcg of folate. Explain why both sources of information can be correct.

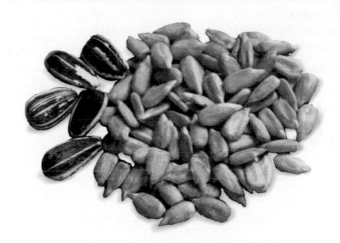

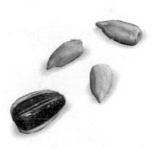

PRACTICE TEST

Select the best answer.

1. The amount of a nutrient that should meet the needs of half of the healthy people in a particular group is the
   a. Estimated Average Requirement (EAR).
   b. Recommended Dietary Allowance (RDA).
   c. Adequate Intake (AI).
   d. Tolerable Upper Intake Level (UL).

2. Which of the following statements is false?
   a. RDAs are standards for daily intakes of certain nutrients.
   b. RDAs meet the nutrient needs of nearly all healthy people.
   c. RDAs contain a margin of safety.
   d. RDAs are requirements for nutrients.

3. The Estimated Energy Requirement (EER)

   a. has a margin of safety.
   b. does not account for a person's height, weight, or physical activity level.
   c. is based on the average daily energy needs of a healthy person.
   d. reflects a person's actual daily energy needs.

4. A diet is likely to be safe and nutritionally adequate if

   a. average daily intakes for nutrients meet RDA or AI values.
   b. intakes of various nutrients are consistently less than EAR amounts.
   c. nutrient intakes are consistently above ULs.
   d. vitamin supplements are included.

5. Nutritional standards, such as the RDAs, are

   a. used to develop formula food products.
   b. the basis for establishing DVs.
   c. used to evaluate the nutritional adequacy of diets.
   d. All of the above are correct.

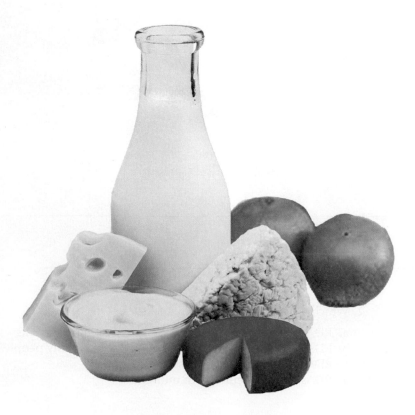

6. According to the MyPlate plan, which of the following foods is grouped with dairy products?

   a. cheese
   b. eggs
   c. butter
   d. All of the above are correct.

7. Protein-rich food sources that also contain saturated fat and cholesterol include

   a. peanut butter.
   b. dry beans.
   c. nuts.
   d. beef.

8. Fruit is generally a good source of all of the following substances, except

   a. fiber.
   b. vitamin C.
   c. phytochemicals.
   d. protein.

9. The *Dietary Guidelines for Americans* is

   a. revised every year.
   b. a set of general nutrition-related recommendations.
   c. published by the Centers for Disease Control and Prevention.
   d. All of the above are correct.

10. Which of the following foods would be classified as "empty calories" by MyPlate?

    a. chocolate syrup
    b. fat-free milk
    c. white bread
    d. corn oil

11. Which of the following statements is true?

    a. According to MyPlate, vegetable oils are grouped into the "Fats and Oils" food group.
    b. The MyPlate menu planning guide cannot be individualized to meet a person's food preferences.
    c. A person can use www.choosemyplate.gov to evaluate his or her diet's nutritional adequacy.
    d. MyPlate was the first food guide developed for Americans.

12. The Exchange System

    a. classifies foods in the same groups as MyPlate.
    b. has exchange lists based on macronutrient contents.
    c. is useful only for people who have diabetes.
    d. incorporates high-protein foods with high-carbohydrate foods.

13. Which of the following information is not provided by the Nutrition Facts panel?

    a. percentage of calories from fat
    b. amount of carbohydrate per serving
    c. serving size
    d. amount of trans fat per serving

14. Daily Values are

    a. for people who consume 1200 to 1500 kilocalorie diets.
    b. based on the lowest RDA or AI for each nutrient.
    c. dietary standards developed for food-labeling purposes.
    d. used to evaluate the nutritional adequacy of a population's diet.

15. Organically grown foods are

    a. nutritionally superior to conventionally produced foods.
    b. produced without the use of antibiotics, pesticides, or genetic improvements.
    c. usually less expensive than conventionally produced foods.
    d. All of the above are correct.

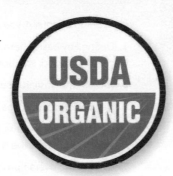

16. People who follow Islamic dietary rules will not consume

    a. pork.
    b. rice.
    c. beef.
    d. milk.

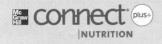

Additional resources related to the features of this book are available on ConnectPlus® Nutrition. Ask your instructor how to get access.

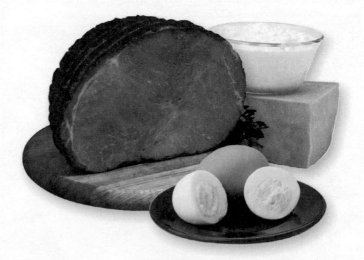

Answers to Chapter 3 Quiz *Yourself*

1. According to the latest U.S. Department of Agriculture food guide, fruits and vegetables are combined into one food group. **False.** (p. 69)

2. According to the recommendations of the *Dietary Guidelines for Americans, 2010*, it is acceptable for certain adults to consume moderate amounts of alcoholic beverages. **True.** (p. 66)

3. Last week, Colin didn't consume the recommended amount of vitamin C for a couple of days. Nevertheless, he is unlikely to develop scurvy, the vitamin C deficiency disease. **True.** (p. 61)

4. The Food and Drug Administration develops Dietary Guidelines for Americans. **False.** (p. 65)

5. The Nutrition Facts panel on a food label provides information concerning amounts of energy, fiber, and cholesterol that are in a serving of the food. **True.** (p. 74)

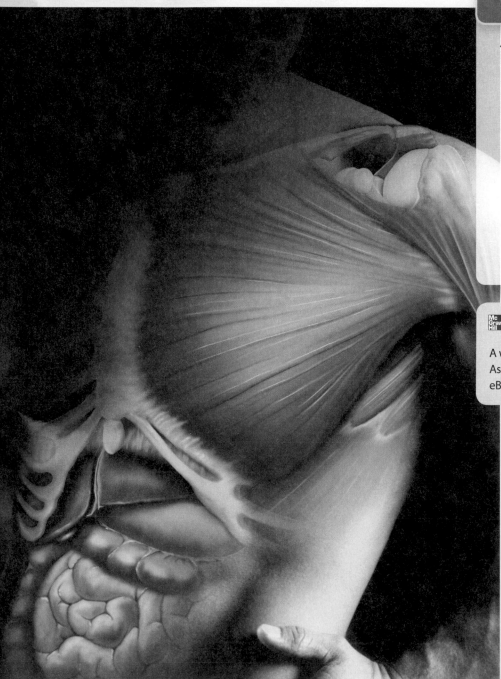

CHAPTER 4

Body Basics

Chapter Learning Outcomes

After reading Chapter 4, you should be able to

1. Define key basic chemistry terms, including atom, element, ion, chemical bond, solution, solvent, solute, acid, base, and enzyme.

2. Explain the basic function of an enzyme.

3. Define cell, tissue, organ, and organ system.

4. List the organ systems, identify major organs or tissues in each system, and describe primary functions of each system.

5. Discuss the overall processes of nutrient digestion, absorption, and transport, and waste elimination.

6. Identify some common gastrointestinal health problems and discuss preventive measures and treatments for these conditions.

THE HUMAN BODY is often compared to a complex machine, such as a car. Like a car, the body has numerous interrelated working parts and requires a source of fuel to operate. Additionally, the body has to be able to cool itself, eliminate waste products, and rely on lubrication to keep operating smoothly. Unlike most machines, however, the human body can make many of its spare parts, enabling the body to repair and maintain itself for long periods. When the body functions properly, this wondrous machine may be taken for granted and expected to perform optimally. Nevertheless, the quality of the fuel that powers the human body can affect performance, much like the quality of gasoline that runs a car.

In Chapter 1, we defined chemistry as the study of the composition and characteristics of matter, and the changes that it can undergo. We also defined human physiology as the study of how the human body functions. Principles of chemistry and human physiology form the foundation for the scientific study of nutrition. The foods you eat and the air you breathe provide nutrients and oxygen, the raw materials (matter) that your cells need to survive and function. By reading Chapter 4, you will learn some basic chemistry concepts to help you understand how the matter in food becomes the raw materials for building, fueling, and sustaining healthy bodies. Additionally, you will learn about body structures and functions so you can understand the roles of nutrients in the body and why these particular chemicals are so important.

If you have taken general biology or human physiology courses in high school or college, much of the information in Chapter 4 will be a review for you. However, many students who enroll in nutrition classes do not have a strong science background, and they are likely to find the chapter's content interesting but possibly more challenging to understand. Parts of this chapter may seem to be filled with unfamiliar terms and their definitions, but learning the meaning of these terms can help you communicate more effectively with physicians and help you become a wiser consumer of health-related information.

4.1 Basic Chemistry Concepts

Do you or does someone you know avoid eating foods that are not labeled organic because they contain chemicals such as additives, hormones, or pesticides? It is true that chemicals are in your food, but they are not necessarily harmful. Chemicals make up food as well as every other aspect of your environment—air, water, rocks, and other forms of matter contain chemicals. In fact, you are a complex collection of chemicals, much of which is organized into cells. The following sections provide basic information about some chemistry concepts that apply to the study of nutrition.

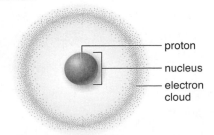

Figure 4.1 An atom. Matter is comprised of atoms that contain particles, including protons and electrons. The nucleus of this hydrogen atom contains one positively charged proton.

From Atoms to Compounds

Matter is comprised of atoms that contain certain particles, including protons and electrons (Fig. 4.1). **Protons** are positively charged particles in the *nucleus*, the central region

protons positively charged particles in the nucleus of an atom

93

electrons small, negatively charged particles that surround the nucleus of an atom

element each type of atom; substance that cannot be separated into simpler substances by ordinary chemical or physical means

minerals elements that are found in the earth's crust

chemical bond attraction that holds atoms together

TABLE 4.1 *Elements in the Body*

Element	Symbol
Hydrogen	H
Oxygen	O
Carbon	C
Nitrogen	N
Calcium	Ca
Phosphorus	P
Potassium	K
Sulfur	S
Sodium	Na
Chloride	Cl
Magnesium	Mg
Iron	Fe
Iodine	I
Copper	Cu
Zinc	Zn
Manganese	Mn
Cobalt	Co
Chromium	Cr
Selenium	Se
Molybdenum	Mo
Fluoride*	F
Tin	Sn
Silicon**	Si
Vanadium**	V
Nickel**	Ni
Boron**	B
Arsenic**	As

* Although fluoride is not essential, the mineral helps strengthen teeth and bones.

** When experimental animals are fed diets that are deficient in these mineral elements, they eventually develop deficiency symptoms. However, there have been no reports of widespread deficiencies of these minerals in human populations. Therefore, scientists have not established human requirements for them.

of an atom. **Electrons** are small negatively charged particles that form a cloud surrounding the nucleus. The number of electrons surrounding the nucleus equals the number of protons within the nucleus. Thus, the negative and positive charges cancel out each other, making an atom neutral, which means it has no electrical charge.

More than 100 different types of atoms exist, and each type is an **element,** a substance that cannot be separated into simpler substances by ordinary chemical or physical means. Elements are the "building blocks" of matter. Table 4.1 lists several elements, most of which are essential for human nutrition. An element is essential if the body cannot function normally without it and the element must be supplied by the diet. Note that chemists use letters as symbols to represent elements. For example, the symbols for carbon, nitrogen, and sodium are C, N, and Na, respectively.

Minerals are elements, such as calcium, iron, and potassium, that are found in the earth's crust. Many minerals are essential nutrients. However, not every mineral is in living things or is necessary for life. Your external environment has natural and human-made forms of matter that may contain elements such as mercury (Hg), aluminum (Al), and cadmium (Cd). The human body does not need these minerals to function properly, and they can be quite toxic. Chapter 9 discusses the importance of various minerals to health.

Molecules

When atoms interact, they may share electrons and rearrange themselves, forming a chemical bond. A **chemical bond** is an attraction that holds atoms together and forms a **molecule.** When illustrating the structure of molecules, chemists often use straight lines to show the bonds (Fig. 4.2a).

Molecules can contain the same element or different elements. For example, an oxygen molecule forms when two oxygen atoms bind together, whereas a water molecule forms when two hydrogen atoms bond to an oxygen atom. To identify a particular molecule without using lines to draw its chemical structure, chemists use a chemical formula. The chemical formula for an oxygen molecule is O_2; the subscript "2" indicates the presence of 2 oxygen atoms. The chemical formula for a water molecule is H_2O. The chemical formula for the simple sugar *glucose* is $C_6H_{12}O_6$. Judging from its formula, how many carbon, hydrogen, and oxygen atoms are in a glucose molecule?

Some atoms form single bonds, but a few atoms can form multiple bonds. Each carbon atom (C) has four bonding sites, and as a result, carbon atoms can bond to each other by single, double (Fig. 4.2b), and even triple bonds (Fig. 4.2c). Carbon's ability to bond to other carbon atoms as well as form multiple bonds with a neighboring carbon atom contributes to the formation of a vast array of organic (carbon-containing) compounds. **Compounds** are molecules that contain two or more different elements in specific proportions.

Solutions

A **solution** is an evenly distributed mixture of two or more compounds. In living things, water is the **solvent,** the primary component of solutions. Your body, for example, is about 60% water. A substance that dissolves in the solvent is a **solute.** Many beverages

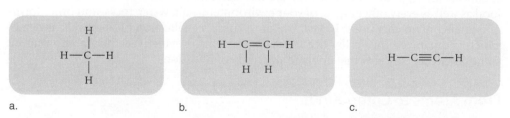

a.   b.   c.

Figure 4.2 Chemical bonds. Some atoms form single bonds (*a*), but a few atoms can form multiple bonds. Carbon atoms can bond to each other by single, double (*b*), and even triple bonds (*c*).

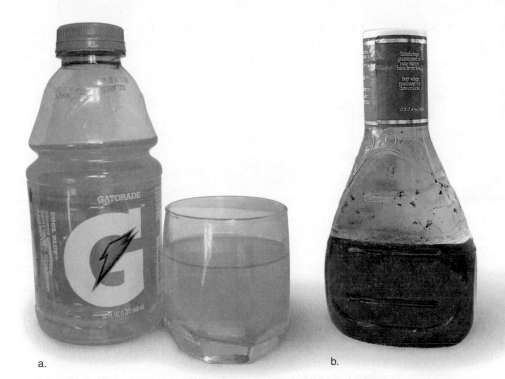

a.   b.

Figure 4.3 Solubility. The solubility of a compound describes how easily it forms a solution in a liquid solvent. Many substances, including table sugar, dissolve in water. (*a*) Sports drinks are beverages in which sugar remains dissolved in water. Other substances, such as fat, are insoluble in water and will not dissolve in it. (*b*) Vinaigrette is an example of a food in which oil and water (balsamic vinegar) do not form a solution. In this particular product, note how the oil separates from the vinegar and forms a layer on top of the darker balsamic vinegar layer.

and foods are solutions that have water as the solvent (Fig. 4.3a). A sports drink, for example, is a solution that is mostly water, the solvent. The drink has relatively small amounts of sugar, minerals, colorings, and flavorings (solutes) dissolved in the water.

The **solubility** of a substance describes how easily it dissolves, that is, forms a solution, in a liquid solvent. Many naturally occurring substances, including simple carbohydrates such as sugar and all mineral elements, dissolve in water. Other substances, such as fat, are insoluble and will not dissolve in water (Fig. 4.3b). Your blood has high water content, a characteristic that makes it easier for the body to transport and eliminate water-soluble substances than water-insoluble materials.

Ions

When an atom (or group of atoms) gains or loses one or more electrons, it has an electrical charge and is called an **ion** (Fig. 4.4). If an atom gains one electron, it becomes an ion with a negative charge, because electrons are negatively charged. If an atom loses an electron, it becomes an ion with a positive charge, because it has an extra proton and protons are positively charged. A negative charge is indicated with a minus sign ($^-$) and a positive charge is indicated with a plus sign ($^+$) after the chemical symbol or formula. For example, a molecule of ammonia is neutral, that is, has no electrical charge, because it has the same number of protons and electrons. If the molecule loses an electron, it becomes the

molecule matter that forms when two or more atoms interact and are held together by a chemical bond

compounds molecules that contain two or more different elements in specific proportions

solution evenly distributed mixture of two or more compounds

solvent primary component of a solution

solute lesser component of a solution that dissolves in solvent

solubility how easily a substance dissolves in a liquid solvent

ion atom or group of atoms that has a positive or negative charge

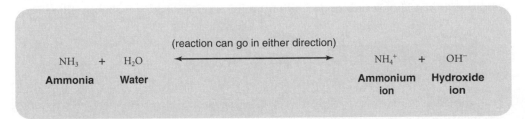

(reaction can go in either direction)

NH_3 + H_2O ⟷ NH_4^+ + OH^-

Ammonia   Water   **Ammonium   Hydroxide
                                            ion   ion**

Figure 4.4 What is an ion? An ion is an atom or group of atoms that loses or gains one or more electrons and, as a result, has an electrical charge. In this reaction, ammonia and water react to form the positively charged ammonium ion and the negatively charged hydroxide ion.

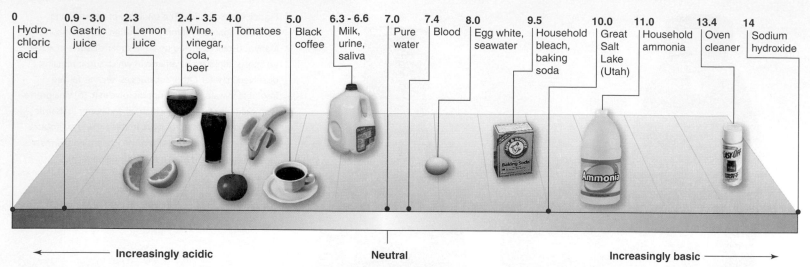

Figure 4.5 pH scale. Chemists measure the concentration of hydrogen ions in a watery solution by using the pH scale. This scale indicates the pH values of some substances, including foods. Substances with low pH values are more acidic than substances with high pH values (bases).

H⁺ hydrogen ion chemical formula

electrolytes ions that conduct electricity when they are dissolved in water

acids substances that donate hydrogen ions

bases substances that accept hydrogen ions

pH measure of the acidity or alkalinity of a solution

positively charged ion, ammonium. The formula for the positively charged *hydrogen ion* is simply **H⁺**.

When most mineral elements, including sodium and potassium, dissolve in water, they form solutions containing ions that can conduct electricity. Thus, sodium and potassium are called **electrolytes**. Electrolytes have many important functions in the body, including helping to maintain proper fluid balance.

What Are Acids and Bases?

Acids are substances that lose H⁺ when dissolved in water; **bases** are substances that remove and accept H⁺ when dissolved in water. Many of the chemicals you encounter daily are either acidic or basic (alkaline). As you can tell by their names, phosphoric acid in soft drinks and ascorbic acid (better known as vitamin C) are acids. Baking soda and sodium hydroxide, an ingredient of many hair removal products, are bases.

Chemists measure the concentration of hydrogen ions (**pH**) in a watery solution by using the pH scale. The scale ranges from 0 to 14. With each whole number increase within the scale, the H⁺ concentration decreases 10 times. Examine the pH scale shown in Figure 4.5. Note that black coffee has a pH of about 5.0 and tomatoes have a pH of about 4.0. Thus, tomatoes are 10 times more acidic than black coffee. Although it may seem confusing, a solution with a pH of 2.0 has a *higher* H⁺ concentration and is *more* acidic than a solution with a pH of 12.0.

Pure water has equal concentrations of H⁺ and OH⁻, so it is neither acidic nor basic. Thus, pure water has a pH of 7 and is neutral. By combining an acid with a base, the pH of a solution can become 7.

Your body must maintain its *acid-base balance* to function properly. Under normal conditions, the pH of your blood ranges from 7.35 to 7.45, which is slightly alkaline. To

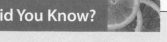

Common household products such as baking soda, household ammonia, and certain oven cleaners are bases.

Did You Know?

Blueberries, raspberries, red cabbage, and strawberries contain the pigment *anthocyanin*. This pigment is used as a natural dye for coloring yarns and can also be used as a crude pH meter. Anthocyanin is red when it is in solutions that have a pH of less than 4; this pigment loses its color at higher pH values. Aside from being an interesting pigment, anthocyanin has antioxidant activity and may provide health benefits as a result (see Table 1.3).

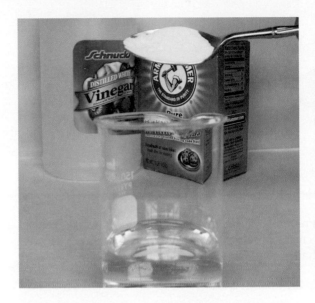
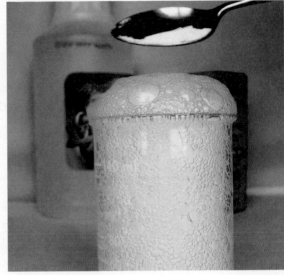

Figure 4.6 Chemical reaction. A chemical reaction occurs when vinegar (an acid) combines with baking soda (a base). This reaction forms sodium acetate (a salt), water, and carbon dioxide.

control its pH within normal limits, blood contains buffers—ions or molecules that accept excess OH^- or H^+ when necessary. Acids form naturally as by-products of cellular activity, but if the pH of blood begins to fall, the excess H^+ must be eliminated to prevent *acidosis,* a condition that can be deadly. The lungs remove excess H^+ from blood by means of chemical reactions that result in the release of carbon dioxide (CO_2) and H_2O in exhaled air. Kidneys also participate in the buffering system by removing excess H^+ from the blood when forming urine. As a result, urine is an acidic fluid.

What Is a Chemical Reaction?

Most molecules can undergo **chemical reactions,** processes that change the arrangement of atoms in the molecules. The elements that comprise the molecules that react are never destroyed, but they combine with other elements to form new molecules or compounds. When elements or compounds combine to form new substances, a synthetic reaction has occurred. The new substances often have physical and chemical characteristics (properties) that are quite different from those of the reactants. Decomposition reactions involve the breaking down of molecules. **Digestion,** the process by which large molecules in food are broken down into smaller ones, requires decomposition reactions.

You can observe a simple chemical reaction by combining the reactants vinegar (an acid) and baking soda (a base). As soon as the vinegar makes contact with the soda, the powdery baking soda disappears and a fizzy liquid forms (Fig. 4.6). This particular reaction produces carbon dioxide gas that forms bubbles in the fizzy liquid and sodium acetate. Thus, carbon dioxide and sodium acetate are two of the products that result when vinegar and baking soda react. Sodium acetate is a **salt,** a substance that forms when an acid reacts with a base. Table salt (sodium chloride) is actually one type of salt. Sodium chloride forms when an acid, such as hydrochloric acid (HCl), reacts with a base, such as sodium hydroxide (NaOH) (Fig. 4.7).

chemical reactions processes that change the atomic arrangements of molecules

digestion process by which large food molecules are mechanically and chemically broken down

salt substance that forms when an acid combines with a base

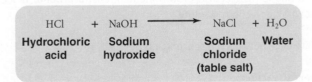

$$HCl + NaOH \longrightarrow NaCl + H_2O$$

| Hydrochloric acid | Sodium hydroxide | Sodium chloride (table salt) | Water |

Figure 4.7 What is a salt? A salt forms when an acid reacts with a base. For example, sodium chloride (NaCl) and H_2O form when hydrochloric acid (HCl) reacts with sodium hydroxide (NaOH).

Figure 4.8 Enzyme action. Enzymes initiate or catalyze chemical reactions. Enzymes are recyclable; they do not become part of the products of a reaction, and as a result, one enzyme molecule can catalyze many reactions. In this reaction, the enzyme sucrase is necessary to break down sucrose into glucose and fructose.

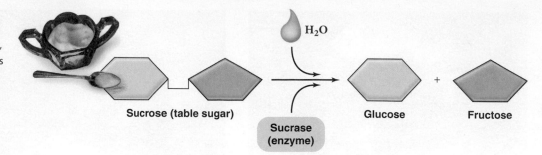

H_2O

Sucrose (table sugar)

Sucrase (enzyme)

Glucose

+

Fructose

metabolism the sum of all chemical reactions occurring in living cells

enzyme protein that speeds the rate of a chemical reaction but is not altered during the process

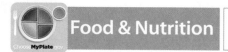

Food & Nutrition *tip*

Gelatin is an animal protein that dissolves in boiled water. As it cools, gelatin holds the water and thickens, forming a gel, a solution that takes the shape of its container. Pineapple, papaya, kiwifruit, and guava naturally contain enzymes that break down gelatin. Therefore, when using gelatin in recipes, don't add fresh or frozen forms of these fruits, because the enzymes will break down gelatin and the mixture will not gel. Heating destroys these enzymes; thus, you can make a molded gelatin salad or dessert that contains canned pineapple. (Foods undergo heating during the canning process.)

In recipes for baked goods that require baking soda, you will find an acid ingredient such as lemon juice, buttermilk, or cream of tartar (tartaric acid) included to react with the soda. The carbon dioxide gas that forms "raises" the mixture, giving it a light, airy structure after baking.

Metabolism

Metabolism refers to the sum of all chemical reactions that occur in living cells. *Catabolic reactions* involve breaking down molecules. Catabolism, for example, occurs during digestion. *Anabolic reactions* involve synthesizing new compounds. Repairing damaged muscle tissue after injury is an example of anabolism.

Enzymes

Living things contain thousands of chemicals, and life depends upon chemical reactions. However, many of these reactions occur slowly or do not occur spontaneously. Living cells produce **enzymes,** proteins that initiate or facilitate (catalyze) chemical reactions. Enzymes are recyclable; they do not become part of the products of a reaction, and as a result, one enzyme molecule can catalyze many reactions. Figure 4.8 illustrates an enzyme's action.

In general, the names of most enzymes end with *-ase*. Sucrase, for example, is the enzyme that catalyzes the reaction that breaks down the carbohydrate sucrose (table sugar) to its component simple sugars, glucose and fructose (see Fig. 4.8). Additionally, each enzyme usually has a specific action. For example, sucrase breaks down sucrose, but the enzyme does not affect lactose, the type of sugar in milk.

Enzymes are sensitive to environmental conditions, including pH, temperature, and the presence of certain vitamins and minerals. If the pH or temperature is too high or too low, the enzyme will not function. Raw food contains enzymes, but cooking food usually destroys them.

Concept **Checkpoint**

1. Define the following terms: electron, proton, element, chemical bond, molecule, compound, solution, solvent, and solute.
2. What is an ion?
3. Explain the difference between an acid and a base.
4. What is pH?
5. What is a chemical reaction?
6. What is an enzyme?
7. What factors can alter an enzyme's activity?

4.2 Basic Physiology Concepts

Anatomy is the scientific study of cells and other body structures; **physiology** is the scientific study of how cells and body structures function. This section provides some basic information about human anatomy and physiology, including the organization of the body into systems. By learning about human anatomy and physiology, you may appreciate the complexity of your body and be amazed at the variety of metabolic activities that occur within you to keep you alive, physically active, mentally alert, and healthy.

The Cell

A cell is the smallest living functional unit in an organism. Your body has about 100 trillion cells that can be classified into numerous cell types. Each type of cell has a specific function. For example, muscle cells are necessary for movement, red blood cells transport oxygen, and certain white blood cells protect the body from disease-causing bacteria and viruses.

Most human cells contain several different types of **organelles,** structures that have specific functions (Fig. 4.9). The nucleus, for example, contains **DNA,** the molecule that provides coded instructions for synthesizing proteins. DNA enables the nucleus to control various cellular activities, including cell division and enzyme production. Mitochondria are organelles that play a major role in the generation of energy. Ribosomes are structures involved in the assembly of proteins. The nucleus, mitochondria, and other organelles are surrounded by a watery fluid called cytoplasm. Many chemical reactions take place in the cytoplasm, including some reactions necessary to make proteins. Each human cell has a plasma membrane that defines the boundaries of the cell and holds the cytoplasm in place. The plasma membrane also controls the passage of materials into and out of the cell.

anatomy scientific study of cells and other body structures

physiology scientific study of the functioning of cells and other body structures

organelles structures in cells that perform specialized functions

DNA molecule that contains coded instructions for synthesizing proteins

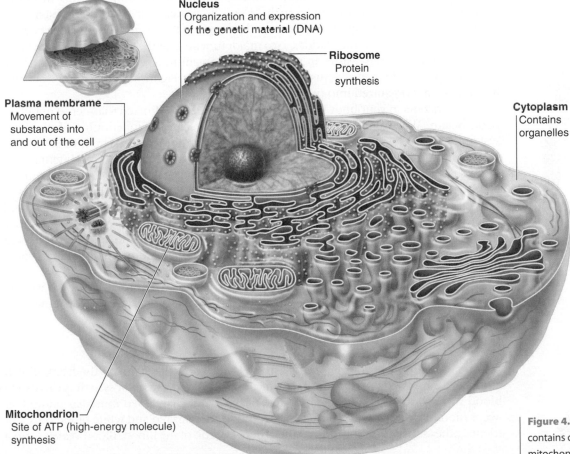

Nucleus
Organization and expression
of the genetic material (DNA)

Ribosome
Protein
synthesis

Plasma membrame
Movement of
substances into
and out of the cell

Cytoplasm
Contains
organelles

Mitochondrion
Site of ATP (high-energy molecule)
synthesis

Figure 4.9 Typical human cell. A typical human cell contains certain structures and various organelles, including mitochondria, ribosomes, and a nucleus.

tissues masses of cells that have similar characteristics and functions

epithelial tissue cells that line every body surface

connective tissue type of cells that hold together, protect, and support organs

organ collection of tissues that function in a related fashion

organ system group of organs that work together for a similar purpose

homeostasis maintenance of an internal chemical and physical environment that is critical for good health and survival

arteries vessels that carry blood away from the heart

capillaries smallest blood vessels

veins vessels that return blood to the heart

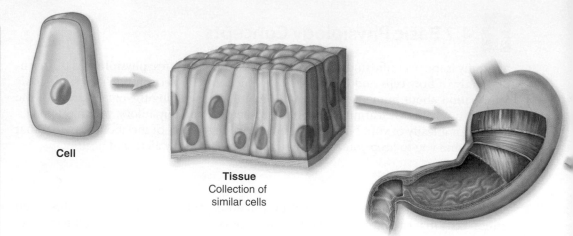

Cell

Tissue
Collection of
similar cells

Organ
Collection of various types of
tissues with related functions

Figure 4.10 Organization of the human body. Cells in the body are organized into tissues, organs, and organ systems. A living organism is a complete individual comprised of organ systems that function together.

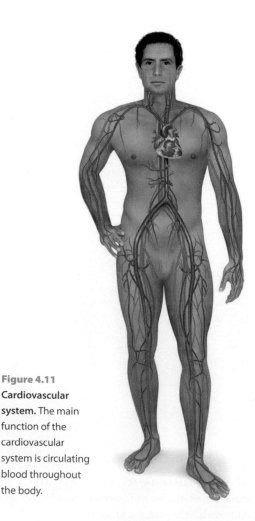

Figure 4.11
Cardiovascular system. The main function of the cardiovascular system is circulating blood throughout the body.

From Cells to Systems

Cells that have similar characteristics and functions are usually joined together into larger masses called **tissues.** The cells that line every body surface, including skin and the inside of blood vessels, are **epithelial tissues.** Fat, bone, and blood are types of **connective tissue.**

An **organ** is composed of various tissues that function in a related fashion. The brain, for example, is an organ because it contains different forms of nervous tissue that work together to interpret information from the environment, find meaning from this information, and signal responses, such as muscle movements. An **organ system** is a group of organs that work together for a similar purpose. The urinary system, for example, includes the kidneys and the bladder. Two major functions of the urinary system are filtering blood and excreting wastes in urine. A living organism is a complete individual life form comprised of organ systems that function together. Figure 4.10 illustrates how cells in the body are organized into tissues, organs, and systems.

All systems in your body must work together in a coordinated manner to maintain good health. When one system fails to function correctly, the functioning of the other systems is soon affected. The body's ability to maintain **homeostasis,** an internal chemical and physical environment that supports life and good health, is critical. Internal conditions such as body temperature and blood pressure normally fluctuate throughout the day, but the body strives to maintain such factors within fairly specific limits. Changes in the cell's internal and external environment can disrupt homeostasis, and sickness and even death can result if the abnormality persists. A healthy body, however, uses various mechanisms to regain its normal internal status. As you read about the nutrients, you will recognize how many play crucial roles in homeostasis, including maintaining proper body temperature, acid-base balance, and tissue fluid levels.

Table 4.2 lists each system's major organs or tissues and summarizes their primary functions. The following sections provide a brief description of each organ system.

Cardiovascular System

The major components of the cardiovascular ("circulatory") system are the heart, blood, and blood vessels (Fig. 4.11). The main function of the cardiovascular system is circulating blood throughout the body. The human heart is a four-chambered muscular pump that keeps blood moving through blood vessels. Blood contains red and white blood cells, nutrients, other substances, and *plasma,* the watery portion of the blood. Blood vessels form a

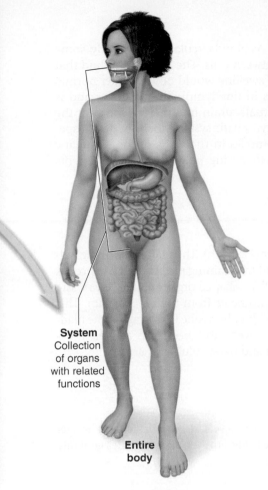

System
Collection
of organs
with related
functions

**Entire
body**

TABLE 4.2 *The Organ Systems of the Human Body*

System	Major Organs or Tissues	Primary Functions
Digestive	Mouth, salivary glands, esophagus, stomach, intestines, pancreas, liver, gallbladder	Digestion and absorption of nutrients
Cardiovascular	Heart, blood vessels, blood	Circulation of blood throughout the body
Respiratory	Nose, pharynx, larynx, trachea, bronchi, lungs	Exchange of oxygen and carbon dioxide
Lymphatic and Immune systems	Lymphatic fluid, white blood cells, lymph vessels and nodes, spleen, thymus	Defense and immunity against infectious agents, fluid balance, white blood cell production, absorption of fat-soluble nutrients from intestinal tract
Urinary	Kidneys, bladder	Elimination of salts, water, and wastes; maintenance of fluid balance
Muscular	Muscles	Movement and stability of the body
Skeletal	Bones, tendons, ligaments	Support, movement, protection, and production of blood cells
Nervous	Brain, spinal cord, nerves, sensory receptors	Thought processes, regulation and coordination of many body activities, detection of changes in external and internal environments
Endocrine	Glands or organs that secrete hormones	Regulation and coordination of many body activities, including growth, nutrient balance, and reproduction
Integumentary	Skin, hair, nails	Protection and immunity, regulation of body temperature, vitamin D synthesis
Reproductive	Gonads and genitals	Procreation

Adapted from: Widmaier EP, and others: *Vander's human physiology,* 10th ed. Boston: McGraw-Hill, 2006.

network of tubes that help circulate blood throughout the body. **Arteries** carry blood away from the heart. Arteries branch into smaller and smaller vessels until they form **capillaries**, a network of tiny blood vessels with walls that are only one cell thick. The thin capillary walls enable nutrients and oxygen to move out of the blood and into cells, and carbon dioxide and other waste products to pass from cells and into the blood. After this exchange occurs, the deoxygenated (oxygen-poor) blood enters **veins** for the return trip to the heart.

After entering the right side of the heart, deoxygenated blood is pumped to the lungs, via the pulmonary arteries (see Fig. 4.11). In the lungs, red blood cells release carbon dioxide, a cellular waste product, and pick up oxygen from inhaled air. Cells need oxygen to obtain energy. Hemoglobin, an iron-containing protein in red blood cells, carries most of the oxygen in blood. The oxygenated (oxygen-rich) blood then returns to the heart via the pulmonary veins, so it can be pumped to the rest of the body's cells.

Respiratory System

Lungs, the primary structures of the respiratory system, enable the body to exchange gases, particularly oxygen and carbon dioxide (Fig. 4.12). As mentioned in the previous section, blood circulates through the lungs, picks up oxygen from inhaled air, and releases carbon dioxide, a waste product that forms when cells obtain energy. By exhaling, you eliminate carbon dioxide from your body.

Lymphatic System

The lymphatic system helps maintain fluid balance, absorb many fat-soluble nutrients, and defend the body against diseases (*immune* function). This system includes a network

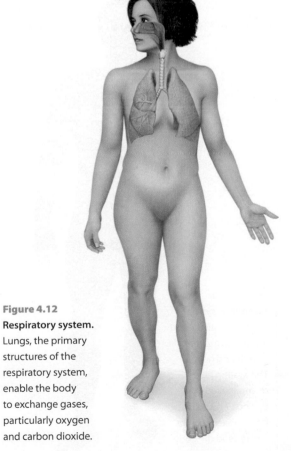

Figure 4.12
Respiratory system.
Lungs, the primary
structures of the
respiratory system,
enable the body
to exchange gases,
particularly oxygen
and carbon dioxide.

lymph fluid in the lymphatic system

of lymphatic vessels and lymph nodes (Fig. 4.13). As blood circulates in the body, some plasma leaks out of capillaries and into spaces between cells. The amount of fluid that surrounds cells must be limited; otherwise, tissue swelling would occur. Under normal conditions, the extra fluid, called **lymph,** collects in tiny lymphatic capillaries and is transported by lymphatic system vessels that eventually drain into major veins near the heart, where it enters the general circulation. The lymphatic system does not have a special organ like the heart that circulates lymph. Muscles in the walls of the lymphatic vessels and skeletal muscle contractions that occur during normal body movements squeeze lymph through the lymphatic system.

Urinary System

The urinary system includes the kidneys and bladder (Fig. 4.14). The major role of the kidneys is filtering unneeded substances from blood and maintaining proper fluid balance. As blood circulates, it passes through the kidneys, two bean-shaped organs that remove waste products as well as excess water and water-soluble nutrients from the bloodstream. This filtration process forms urine that moves from each kidney by a tube for storage in the bladder. Urine is mostly water, but it also contains dissolved substances such as urea, a by-product of protein metabolism, and excess minerals and water-soluble vitamins.

Muscular System

Muscles are the main organs of the muscular system (Fig. 4.15). Muscles enable movement to occur, and they also provide stability for the body. Furthermore, muscles generate heat that helps maintain normal body temperature.

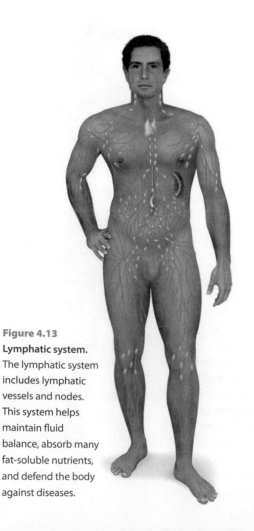

Figure 4.13 Lymphatic system. The lymphatic system includes lymphatic vessels and nodes. This system helps maintain fluid balance, absorb many fat-soluble nutrients, and defend the body against diseases.

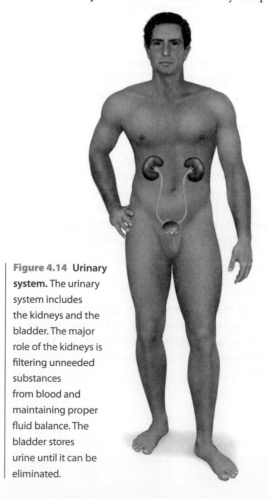

Figure 4.14 Urinary system. The urinary system includes the kidneys and the bladder. The major role of the kidneys is filtering unneeded substances from blood and maintaining proper fluid balance. The bladder stores urine until it can be eliminated.

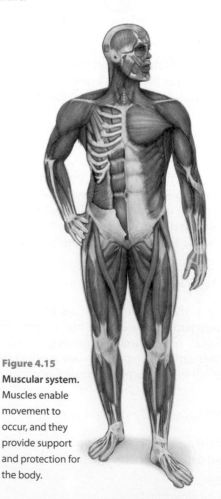

Figure 4.15 Muscular system. Muscles enable movement to occur, and they provide support and protection for the body.

Skeletal System

Bones, tendons, and ligaments are the principal organs of the skeletal system (Fig. 4.16). These structures provide support, movement, and protection for the body. Additionally, bones store excesses of several minerals and produce blood cells.

Nervous System

The brain, spinal cord, and nerves throughout the rest of the body make up the nervous system (Fig. 4.17). The brain produces a variety of intellectual functions and emotional responses, including thoughts, memories, and emotions. The brain also controls and regulates many body functions, including hunger, muscle contractions, and physical responses to danger. Nervous system cells (*neurons*) transmit information and responses by electrical and chemical signals.

Endocrine System

The endocrine system is comprised of organs and tissues, including the thyroid gland and pancreas, that produce a variety of chemical messengers called **hormones** (Fig. 4.18). When released into the bloodstream, a hormone conveys information to cells that are specially equipped to respond (target cells). Hormones regulate a variety of physiological activities, including metabolism, digestion, maintenance of fluid balance, and the maturation of reproductive organs that occurs during puberty.

hormones chemical messengers that convey information to target cells

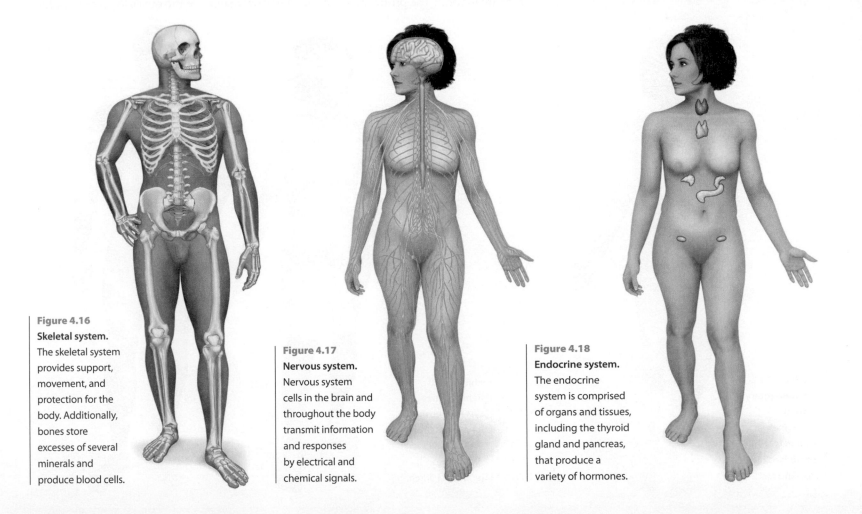

Figure 4.16
Skeletal system.
The skeletal system provides support, movement, and protection for the body. Additionally, bones store excesses of several minerals and produce blood cells.

Figure 4.17
Nervous system.
Nervous system cells in the brain and throughout the body transmit information and responses by electrical and chemical signals.

Figure 4.18
Endocrine system.
The endocrine system is comprised of organs and tissues, including the thyroid gland and pancreas, that produce a variety of hormones.

Integumentary System

Hair, nails, and skin, the largest organ of your body, are structures of the integumentary system (Fig. 4.19). Skin protects against minor injuries and invading disease-causing agents, such as bacteria. Skin also helps maintain body temperature, primarily by perspiration.

Healthy skin needs many nutrients for its maintenance, including vitamin A, several types of B vitamins, and the mineral zinc. Each day, the dead cells that form the outermost layer of skin are shed and new skin cells form that will eventually replace them. Because new skin cells are constantly being produced, skin tissue has a high need for nutrients. Therefore, the early signs of many nutritional deficiency disorders often appear as skin abnormalities such as roughened, dry skin.

Reproductive System

The main function of the reproductive system is to produce children (Fig. 4.20). Adequate nutrition is essential for fertility, healthy pregnancies, and healthy newborns. Compared to women whose diets are nutritionally adequate before and during pregnancy, poorly nourished pregnant women have higher risks of miscarriage and stillbirths (infants who are born dead), as well as of giving birth to babies with birth defects and low birth weights. During their first year of life, severely underweight infants are more likely to die than infants whose weights are normal.

Digestive System

Your cells do not need food to carry out their metabolic activities—they need nutrients that are in food. The primary roles of the digestive system are the breakdown of large food

absorption process by which substances are taken up from the GI tract and enter the bloodstream or the lymph

gastrointestinal (GI) tract muscular tube that extends from the mouth to the anus

bioavailability extent to which the digestive tract absorbs a nutrient and how well the body uses it

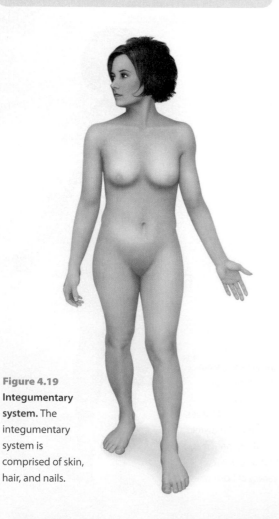

Figure 4.19
Integumentary system. The integumentary system is comprised of skin, hair, and nails.

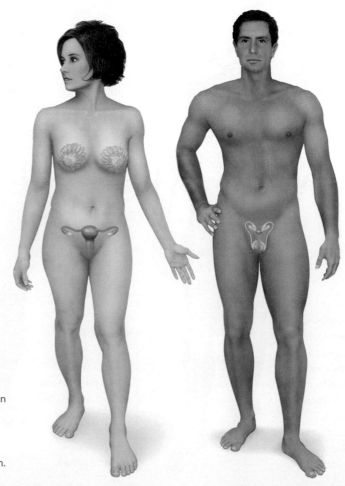

Figure 4.20
Reproductive system. The main function of the reproductive system is to produce children.

molecules into smaller components (nutrients) and the **absorption** of nutrients into the bloodstream or lymphatic system (Fig. 4.21). Section 4.3 focuses on the process of digestion and absorption.

Concept **Checkpoint**

8. Define cell, organelle, DNA, and tissue.
9. Define homeostasis.
10. List at least six of the organ systems that comprise the human body and indicate at least one major function of each organ system listed.

4.3 Digestion, Absorption, Transport, and Elimination

The mouth, esophagus, stomach, and small and large intestines are the major structures of the **gastrointestinal (GI) tract.** In a living person, the GI tract is a hollow, muscular tube that extends approximately 16 feet from the mouth to the anus (see Fig. 4.21).[1] The length is longer in a *cadaver* (dead body), because there is no muscle tone.

It is important to recognize that many foods need to undergo some processing before they are eaten. Although some nutrients can be lost during food preparation, practices such as removing inedible parts or cooking raw foods often make them more digestible and safe to eat. Additionally, cooking food can enhance the absorption of its nutrients. **Bioavailability** refers to the extent to which the digestive tract absorbs a nutrient and how well the body uses it.

The teeth, tongue, salivary glands, liver, gallbladder, and pancreas are *accessory organs* of the digestive system that assist the GI tract in food digestion, nutrient absorption and distribution, and waste elimination. This section of Chapter 4 describes the digestive system, including accessory organs and their basic functions. More detailed information about digestion and absorption can be found in chapters that discuss specific classes of nutrients, such as Chapters 5, 6, and 7.

Mouth

Digestion actually starts in the mouth. The mouth controls the intake of food; teeth begin the *mechanical digestion* of food by biting, tearing, and grinding food into smaller chunks that are easier to swallow. The tongue helps direct food to the back of the mouth where it can be swallowed.

Chemical digestion refers to the chemical breakdown of foods by substances secreted into the GI tract. As you chew, watery saliva from salivary glands mixes with food and lubricates it. Saliva contains the enzymes *salivary amylase* and *lingual lipase*. Salivary amylase enables a minor amount of starch digestion to occur in the mouth. Lingual lipase does not begin to digest fat until the food reaches the stomach. In addition to playing an important role in digestion, the mouth senses the taste and texture of foods.

When food comes in contact with saliva or other watery fluids, certain molecules in the food dissolve. When these chemicals are in solution, they stimulate sensory structures called *taste buds* that are located primarily on the tongue. Taste buds have specialized cells that help you distinguish sweet, sour, salty, bitter, and umami (*ew-mom´-e*) tastes. Taste buds relay information about the chemicals dissolved in saliva to a part of the brain that identifies the particular taste based on past experiences. The entire tongue can detect all five tastes, but certain areas are more sensitive to specific tastes than other tastes.[1] The tip

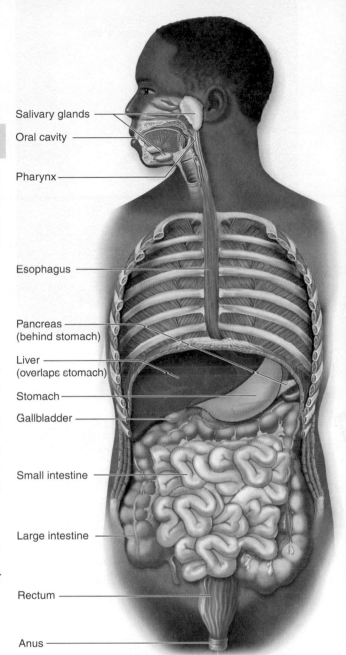

Salivary glands
Oral cavity
Pharynx
Esophagus
Pancreas (behind stomach)
Liver (overlaps stomach)
Stomach
Gallbladder
Small intestine
Large intestine
Rectum
Anus

Figure 4.21 Digestive system. The primary roles of the digestive system are the digestion of food and the absorption of nutrients into the circulatory or lymphatic systems.

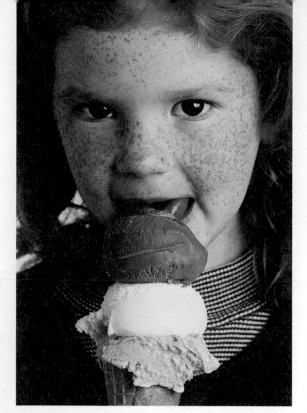

The tongue has regions that are more sensitive to a particular taste.

of the tongue is most likely to detect sweet-tasting foods and beverages; the sides of the tongue are more sensitive to salty and sour items; and the rear portion of the tongue is more likely to detect bitter things than other regions of the organ.

What benefits do you gain from being able to detect various tastes? The sense of taste is important for stimulating appetite and detecting nutrients or toxic substances in substances that enter the mouth. Foods that taste sweet usually contain carbohydrates, major energy sources for your cells. Chemicals that elicit a bitter taste are often poisonous, so you are more likely to eat sweet-tasting foods and reject bitter-tasting ones. The sour taste can indicate the presence of ascorbic acid, more commonly known as vitamin C. You may like foods that taste tart or sour, especially when they are teamed up with sweet ingredients. Sodium ions stimulate your taste buds to detect a salty taste; a food that tastes salty may contain other mineral nutrients as well. The umami or savory taste is often associated with meat and is detected when certain amino acids stimulate taste buds.[1] Foods that produce the umami taste may be protein-rich; protein is another important component of a healthy diet. Recently, scientists have identified a protein in the tongues of rodents that appears to help the animals detect fatty foods. However, researchers have not determined whether human taste buds are capable of sensing the presence of fat in food.[2]

The sense of smell also contributes to your ability to sense the taste of food. As you chew food, it releases chemicals that become airborne and stimulate your nasal passages. Your brain combines such information with taste sensations from your mouth to identify foods' flavors. Thus, favorite foods may seem tasteless and unappealing when you have an upper respiratory tract infection and the inside of your nose is congested.

esophagus tubular structure of the GI tract that connects the pharynx with the stomach

epiglottis flap of tissue that folds down over the windpipe to keep food from entering the respiratory system during swallowing

peristalsis type of muscular contraction of the gastrointestinal tract

gastroesophageal sphincter section of esophagus next to the stomach that controls the opening to the stomach

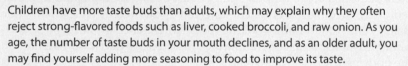
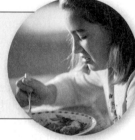

Did You Know?

Children have more taste buds than adults, which may explain why they often reject strong-flavored foods such as liver, cooked broccoli, and raw onion. As you age, the number of taste buds in your mouth declines, and as an older adult, you may find yourself adding more seasoning to food to improve its taste.

Esophagus

The **esophagus** (*e-sof´-ah-gus*) is a muscular tube that extends about 10 inches from the back of the mouth, the pharynx, to the top of the stomach. The primary function of the esophagus is to transfer a mass of swallowed food into the stomach. The entrance to the esophagus is near the voicebox (larynx) and the opening of the windpipe (trachea). The **epiglottis** (*eh-pe-glot´-tis*) is a flap of tough tissue that prevents the food from entering the larynx and trachea (Fig. 4.22). When you swallow, breathing automatically stops and the food normally lands

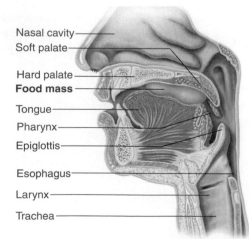
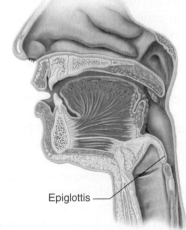
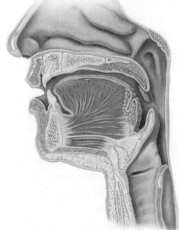

Nasal cavity
Soft palate
Hard palate
Food mass
Tongue
Pharynx
Epiglottis
Esophagus
Larynx
Trachea

Epiglottis

Epiglottis

Figure 4.22 What happens when you swallow? The esophagus transfers food into the stomach. The epiglottis prevents the food from entering the larynx and trachea. When a person swallows, breathing automatically stops, and the food normally lands on the epiglottis, making it cover the opening of the larynx.

on the epiglottis, making it cover the opening of the larynx. These responses keep swallowed food from entering your trachea and choking you. Now you know why it is not a good idea to talk while you are eating!

Swallowing signals the GI tract that food is being eaten and stimulates **peristalsis** (*per´-e-stall´-sis*), waves of muscular activity that help propel material through the digestive tract. In the esophagus, each muscular contraction is followed by a brief period of muscle relaxation. Peristalsis moves small amounts of food and beverage from the esophagus into the stomach (Fig. 4.23). Peristalsis is an involuntary response, which means the movements happen without the need to think about them.

Stomach

The stomach is a muscular sac that can expand and hold about 4 to 6 cups of food after a typical meal.[1] The **gastroesophageal sphincter** (*gas´-tro-e-sof-ah-jee´-al sfink´-ter*) is the section of esophagus that is next to the stomach (Fig. 4.24). After food enters the stomach, the gastroesophageal sphincter constricts, closing the opening between the esophagus and the stomach.

As food enters the stomach, certain cells within the organ secrete *gastric juice*, a watery solution that contains hydrochloric acid (HCl) and some enzymes. HCl helps convert chemically inactive digestive enzymes to their active forms and makes proteins easier to digest. The acid also kills many dangerous disease-causing microorganisms that may be in food.

Stimulated by the presence of food, the stomach's muscular walls respond with waves of muscular contractions ("mixing waves") and peristalsis.[3] The churning movements mix food with gastric juice, and as a result of this mechanical and chemical activity, some of the protein and fat in food breaks down. At this point, the stomach contents are a semisolid liquid called **chyme** (*kime*). Although the stomach absorbs very few nutrients from chyme, a few drugs, including some alcohol, can pass through the organ's walls and enter the bloodstream.

Stomach walls consist of muscle proteins—so how does the stomach avoid digesting itself? Special cells that line the inside of the stomach produce a thick layer of **mucus**. Mucus is a slippery alkaline substance that protects the stomach from its acid and digestive enzymes. If the layer of mucus breaks down, HCl and gastric enzymes can reach the stomach wall, destroying the tissue. Such destruction can cause one or more sores (ulcers) to form. If the gastroesophageal sphincter does not function properly and relaxes while food is still in the stomach, reflux, the backflow of irritating stomach contents into the esophagus, can occur and cause **heartburn.** For more information about factors that increase the risk of gastrointestinal tract ulcers and heartburn, read the "Highlight" at the end of Chapter 4.

The *pyloric* (*pie-lor´-ic*) sphincter, a ring of muscular tissue at the base of the stomach, controls the rate at which chyme is released into the small intestine (see Fig. 4.24). Following a meal, the stomach empties in about 3 to 4 hours, depending on the contents and size of the meal.[3] Watery meals such as soups spend less time in the stomach; fatty meals spend more time there. Obviously, larger meals take longer to empty from the stomach than smaller meals.

Did You Know?

When you eat foods or drink beverages, you swallow some air. Burping expels most of this air before it enters the stomach. If some air manages to enter your stomach and small intestine, it mixes with chyme and bubbles through it, often producing rather loud, gurgling sounds that can be embarrassing.

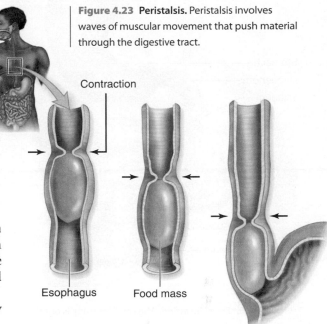

Figure 4.23 Peristalsis. Peristalsis involves waves of muscular movement that push material through the digestive tract.

Contraction

Esophagus   Food mass

chyme mixture of gastric juice and partially digested food

mucus fluid that lubricates and protects certain cells

heartburn backflow of irritating stomach contents into the esophagus

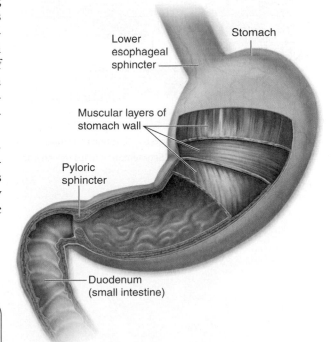

Stomach

Lower esophageal sphincter

Muscular layers of stomach wall

Pyloric sphincter

Duodenum (small intestine)

Figure 4.24 The stomach and duodenum. The gastroesophageal sphincter prevents stomach contents from backing up into the esophagus; the pyloric sphincter helps control the passage of stomach contents into the small intestine.

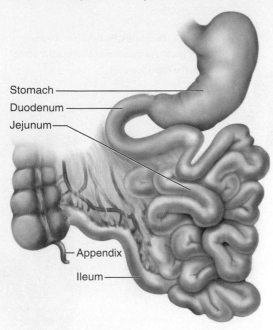

Stomach

Duodenum

Jejunum

Appendix

Ileum

Figure 4.25 **Small intestine.** The small intestine is tightly coiled within the abdominal cavity. The three sections of the small intestine are the duodenum, jejunum, and ileum. Although the appendix may have immune function, you can live without it.

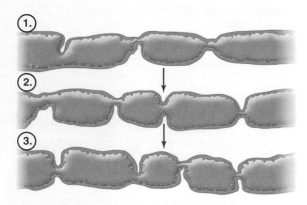

Figure 4.26 **Segmentation.** Segmentation involves ringlike muscular contractions followed by relaxation of a small region of the small intestine. Segmentation helps mix chyme.

Small Intestine

The small intestine is a coiled hollow tube that extends from the stomach to the large intestine. In a living person, the organ measures about 9 to 15 feet long.[1] The small intestine is "small" because the tube's diameter is only about 1 inch, about half the width of the large intestine.

The small intestine has three sections (Fig. 4.25). The first, the **duodenum** (*do-wah-dee´-num*), is only about 10 inches long. Within the duodenum, the acidic stomach contents mix with alkaline fluids secreted by the pancreas and gallbladder. This process neutralizes the acidity of chyme and enables enzymes that function in more alkaline conditions to work. The middle segment of the small intestine is the **jejunum** (*jeh-ju´-num*). The jejunum is about 3 to 5.5 feet in length. Most digestion and nutrient absorption occurs in the upper part of the small intestine, primarily in the jejunum.[2] The last portion of the small intestine, the **ileum** (*il´-lee-um*), is about 5 to 9 feet in length.

A **lumen** is a hollow space in an organ or structure that is surrounded by walls, such as the lumen of the small and large intestines. Each day, the small intestine secretes approximately 1½ quarts (1500 ml) of watery fluids into the lumen. This fluid lubricates the intestinal walls, facilitating the passage of chyme. The cells lining the small intestine also produce mucus that protects the tissue from being damaged by chyme as it moves through the tract.

Many of the major chemical reactions that occur during digestion are *hydrolytic* (*hydro* = water; *lytic* = breakdown), because water molecules are necessary for the reactions to occur. Water in intestinal fluid contributes H^+ and OH^- ions. These ions react with certain nutrients and become part of the products. Sucrose, for example, undergoes hydrolysis in the small intestine (see Fig. 4.8).

The small intestine relies on peristalsis and *segmentation* to help digestion.[3] Segmentation involves regular contractions of ringlike intestinal muscles followed by muscular relaxations to mix chyme within a short portion of the small intestine (Fig. 4.26). The alternating pressure forces chyme to move back and forth within the segment.

As chyme passes through the lumen of the small intestine, enzymes break down the large compounds in chyme and the intestinal cells into smaller fragments and individual nutrients that can be absorbed. The cells also contain enzymes that are added to chyme and contribute to the digestive process. By the time chyme reaches the middle part of the ileum, most of its nutrient contents have been digested and absorbed. It takes about 3 to 5 hours for chyme to move from the duodenum to the end of the ileum.[3]

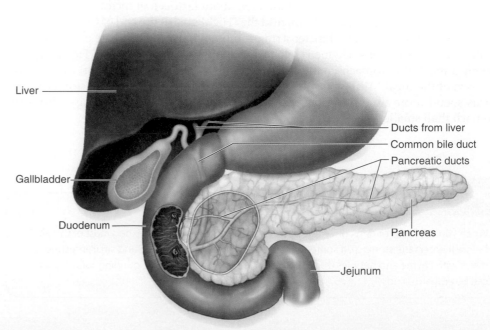

Liver

Ducts from liver

Common bile duct

Pancreatic ducts

Gallbladder

Duodenum

Pancreas

Jejunum

Figure 4.27 **Accessory organs (abdominal).** The liver, gallbladder, and pancreas play important roles in digestion. *Ducts* are small tubes that convey fluids, such as bile or pancreatic juice, from one structure to another.

The Liver, Gallbladder, and Pancreas

The liver, gallbladder, and pancreas play major roles in digestion, even though chyme does not move through them (Fig. 4.27). The liver processes and stores many nutrients. This organ also makes cholesterol and uses this lipid to make bile, a substance that prepares fat and fat-soluble vitamins for absorption. Bile flows from the liver into the gallbladder, where it is stored until needed. When food and, particularly, fat are in the duodenum, the small intestine sends a hormonal signal to the gallbladder, and as a result, the gallbladder contracts, releasing bile into the duodenum. The pancreas produces and secretes most of the enzymes that break down carbohydrates, protein, and fat in the GI tract. Additionally, the pancreas secretes *bicarbonate ions* (HCO_3^-) that neutralize HCl in chyme when it enters the duodenum. This is a critical step in the digestion process because the enzymes that function in the small intestine do not work in acidic conditions.

In the United States, many adults develop gallstones within their gallbladders. Gallstones usually consist of cholesterol; they can be small and grainy, like particles of sand, or as large as a coin (Fig. 4.28). When a gallbladder that contains stones contracts or a gallstone lodges in one of the ducts that carry bile from the gallbladder to the small intestine, it causes considerable pain in the right upper part of the abdomen. If the stone moves out of the duct, the discomfort ends, but in some cases, the duct remains blocked and bile backs up into the liver or pancreas. When this occurs, surgery to remove the diseased gallbladder is necessary to prevent damage to the liver or pancreas. After surgery, bile drips from the liver directly into the small intestine. Having excess body fat increases the risk of gallstones, so keeping your weight at a healthy level can reduce your chances of developing the condition.

When chyme is in the duodenum, its fat and protein content triggers the release of a hormone *cholecystokinin* (*co'-lee-sis'-toe-ky'-nin*) from small intestinal cells. Cholecystokinin enters the bloodstream and circulates to the pancreas, where it stimulates the organ to secrete digestive enzymes into the duodenum. This hormone also signals the gallbladder to

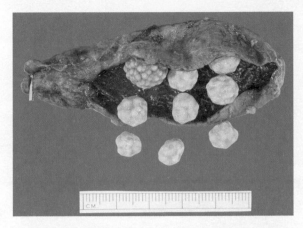

Figure 4.28 Gallstones. Gallstones can form in the gallbladder. The stones usually consist of cholesterol.

duodenum first segment of the small intestine

jejunum middle segment of the small intestine

ileum last segment of the small intestine

lumen open space within a structure such as the small intestine

TABLE 4.3 *Digestive System and Accessory Organs*

Organ	Major Digestive Functions
Mouth	• Intake of food • Sensory responses to food • Minor chemical digestion of starch
Esophagus	• Transfers food from back of mouth to stomach
Stomach	• Mechanical digestion of food • Produces and secretes HCl • Begins chemical digestion of protein and fat • Secretes chemical messengers that regulate digestion
Small intestine	• Digestion and absorption
Large intestine	• Absorption • Elimination of waste
Accessory Organs	
Tongue	• Sensory responses to food, such as taste and texture • Facilitates swallowing
Teeth	• Break food into small pieces
Salivary glands	• Produce saliva
Liver	• Produces and secretes bile • Stores many nutrients
Gallbladder	• Stores and concentrates bile from the liver • Releases bile into duodenum
Pancreas	• Produces and secretes pancreatic juice

Villus

Capillaries
(bloodstream)

Absorptive cells

Small intestine

Lacteal
(lymph vessel)

Muscle
layers

Intestinal absorptive cell

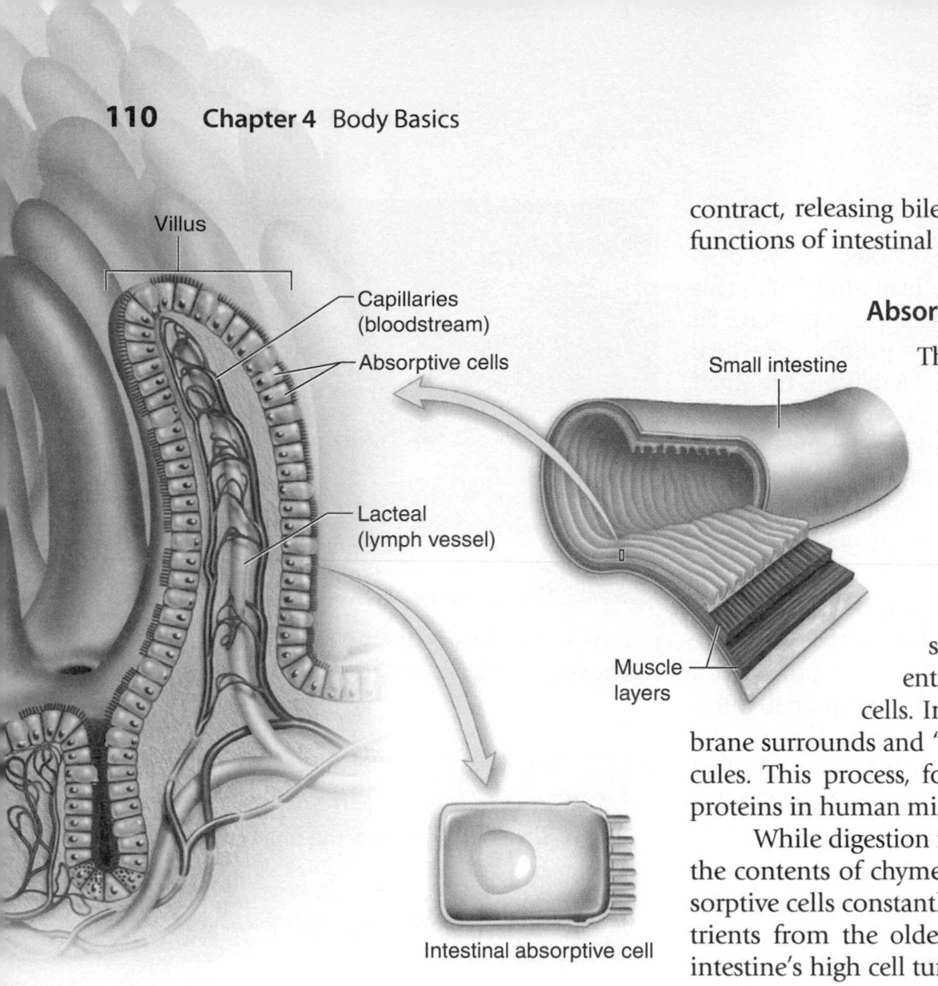

Figure 4.29 Small intestinal absorption. The lining of
the small intestine is covered with villi, and the surface of
each villus is covered with absorptive cells. Absorptive cells
move nutrients from chyme into intestinal blood or lymph
vessels.

contract, releasing bile along with the pancreatic enzymes. Table 4.3 summarizes major
functions of intestinal structures, including the accessory organs.

Absorbing and Transporting Nutrients

The lining of the small intestine is highly folded and covered by tiny,
fingerlike projections called **villi** (singular, villus). Each villus has
an outer layer of epithelial cells called *absorptive cells* (Fig. 4.29).
Absorptive cells complete digestion and remove nutrients from
chyme and transfer them into intestinal blood or lymph vessels.
This process occurs in a variety of ways. Some nutrients require
the help of transport proteins or pumping mechanisms within
the absorptive cell's plasma membrane to enter the cell. Other
kinds of nutrients can simply *diffuse* into these cells. Such diffusion usually happens when the concentration of a particular nutrient is higher in the lumen of the small intestine than in the absorptive
cells. In a few instances, a segment of an absorptive cell's plasma membrane surrounds and "swallows" relatively large substances, such as entire protein molecules. This process, for example, enables an infant's intestinal tract to absorb whole
proteins in human milk that provide immune benefits.

While digestion is occurring, absorptive cells are shed into the lumen and added to
the contents of chyme. The old cells are digested along with chyme. Newly formed absorptive cells constantly replace those that have been shed. The new cells can absorb nutrients from the older cells and recycle some of their contents. However, the small
intestine's high cell turnover rate leads to relatively high nutrient needs for these tissues.

Figure 4.30 Transport to the liver. After being absorbed,
certain water-soluble nutrients move from the intestinal tract
to the liver via the hepatic portal vein. The liver stores various
nutrients, including iron and vitamin B-12.

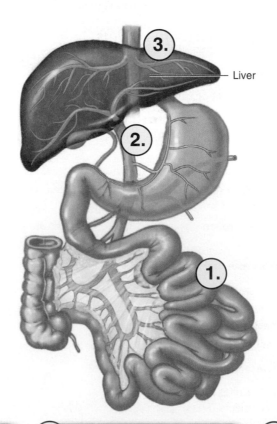

Liver

1. Small intestine absorbs
products of digestion.

2. Certain nutrients travel in
hepatic portal vein to liver.

3. Liver monitors nutrient content of
blood and stores various nutrients.

If the nutrients needed for cell division are lacking, fewer absorptive cells can be replaced, and nutrient *malabsorption* (*mal* = poor) can occur as a result.

After being absorbed, water-soluble nutrients enter the villus's capillary and, eventually, the **hepatic portal vein.** This vein delivers nutrients directly to the liver, where many undergo processing before they enter the general circulation (Fig. 4.30). Most of the absorbed lipids are coated with a layer that contains protein, forming a **chylomicron.** Chylomicrons move into a **lacteal,** a type of lymphatic system structure in each villus (see Fig. 4.29). Chylomicrons are transported by lymph and eventually enter the bloodstream via a vein near the heart.

About 7.6 to 8.5 quarts (8 to 9 liters) of water from ingested foods and beverages and the secretions of intestinal cells enter into the GI tract daily. Most of the water is absorbed along with other nutrients in the small intestine.[3] Any remaining water and the undigested material that reaches the end of the small intestine must pass through another sphincter before entering the large intestine. This sphincter prevents the contents of the large intestine from reentering the small intestine.

Cystic Fibrosis   In the United States, cystic fibrosis (CF) is an inherited incurable disease that is usually diagnosed in early childhood. In CF, certain cells produce thick, sticky mucus that blocks passageways, particularly in the respiratory and digestive systems. People with CF often suffer from serious breathing problems and respiratory infections. The pancreatic ducts of an affected person may also become blocked by thick mucus, which interferes with the organ's ability to deliver digestive enzymes to the small intestine. As a result, the digestion of nutrients, especially fat, is impaired. To overcome the malabsorption problem, patients with cystic fibrosis can take capsules that contain pancreatic enzymes with their meals.

Large Intestine

The large intestine is about 5 feet long (in a cadaver)[1], and its major sections are the *colon* and the *rectum* (Fig. 4.31). Under normal circumstances, very little carbohydrate, protein, and fat escape digestion and absorption in the small intestine and enter the large intestine. However, the large intestine has no villi; therefore, little additional absorption other than water and minerals takes place in this structure. As chyme passes through the large intestine, most of its water content is absorbed. As a result, the residue becomes semisolid and is called *feces*. In addition to containing relatively large amounts of water, feces consist primarily of bacteria that normally live in the large intestine. Feces also contain undigested fiber from plant foods; a small amount of fat; and some protein, mucus, and cells shed from the walls of the intestinal tract. Under normal conditions, the large intestine converts chyme to feces within 18 to 24 hours.[3]

Elimination

Feces remain in the **rectum,** a lower section of the large intestine, until muscular contractions move the material into the anal canal and then out of the body through the anus (see Fig. 4.31). The *external anal sphincter* that allows feces to be expelled is under voluntary control, so a healthy person can determine when to relax the sphincter and have a bowel movement. Young children must reach the stage of physical and emotional maturity in which they are able to relax or tighten their external anal sphincter voluntarily. The timing of this stage varies but generally occurs in healthy children by 4 years of age.

Inflammatory Bowel Disease   Inflammatory bowel disease (IBD) is the general name for a group of diseases that cause inflammation and swelling of the intestines. The inflammation disrupts digestion and nutrient absorption, and damages the intestines. Crohn's disease and ulcerative colitis are the two most common forms of IBD. The "Real People, Real Stories" feature highlights Lisa Gottschalk, a woman who has Crohn's disease.

Did You Know?

Using "high colonics" and other types of enemas to "cleanse" your colon is not necessary because the large intestine does not need to be cleansed. Furthermore, frequent enemas may deplete the body of vital minerals, including sodium and potassium. Check with your physician before trying enema treatments.

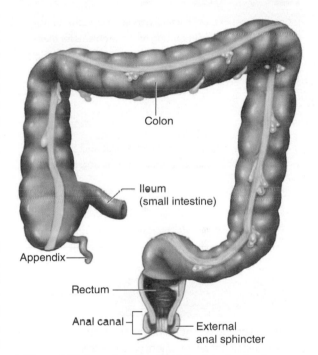

Figure 4.31 Large intestine. The large intestine has two major sections—the colon and the rectum.

villi (singular, villus) tiny, fingerlike projections of the small intestinal lining that participate in digesting and absorbing food

hepatic portal vein vein that collects nutrients from the intestinal tract and delivers them to the liver

chylomicron particle formed by small intestinal cells that transports lipids in the bloodstream

lacteal lymph vessel in villus that absorbs most lipids

rectum lower section of the large intestine

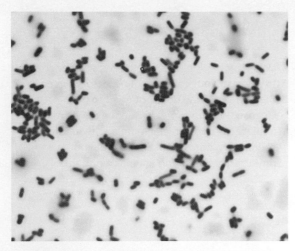

Certain types of *E. coli* bacteria normally live in the human intestinal tract without causing health problems for their host. Infection with one particular type of *E. coli* can be deadly. (See Chapter 12.)

omnivore organism that can digest and absorb nutrients from plants, animals, fungi, and bacteria

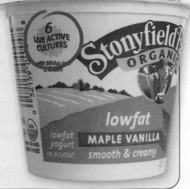
Microbes in Your Digestive Tract

The small intestine of a healthy person usually has few microorganisms residing in its lumen, particularly in the duodenum and jejunum.[4] On the other hand, the large intestine is home to vast numbers of various *species* (types) of bacteria. Under normal conditions, the different bacterial populations maintain a balance with each other that is beneficial to their human hosts. Interestingly, the usual composition of the various bacterial species varies from person to person, because of dietary differences. Starvation, antibiotic use, and excessive emotional stress are among the factors that can upset the normal balance of intestinal bacteria and result in intestinal infections.

Intestinal bacteria can metabolize undigested food, make the vitamins K and biotin, which their human hosts can absorb, and produce substances that colon cells can use for energy. As a result of their metabolic activity, intestinal bacteria also produce gases that are expelled through the anus.

Large numbers of intestinal bacteria eventually become a major component of feces. Some species of these bacteria can be harmful if they enter other parts of the body or contaminate food. People should wash their hands after having bowel movements to reduce the likelihood of spreading dangerous microbes from their intestinal tract to others. Chapter 12 discusses microorganisms that cause common food-borne infections and ways to limit your exposure to them.

Your Adaptable Digestive Tract

Sometimes popular diet "experts" claim that eating certain combinations of foods, such as meats and fruits together, is unhealthy because the food "rots" in the intestinal tract or one type of food interferes with the digestion of another type. Some people claim the human digestive tract is not designed for the consumption of animal foods and the undigested food blocks the intestinal tract. According to some of these sources, the blockages can be the size of a young child, weighing 40 pounds! Such information is simply not true.

A human being is an **omnivore,** an organism that can digest and absorb nutrients from plants, animals, fungi, and even bacteria. Additionally, the healthy human GI tract responds to dietary changes, such as alterations in the nutritional composition or amounts of food consumed, by increasing the production of various digestive enzymes. Consider this: How would people be able to survive in extreme environments, including deserts and permanently frozen regions, if they were unable to digest foods from a wide variety of sources? And finally, a healthy digestive tract does not become blocked by rotted or undigested food, nor does it store large amounts of feces.

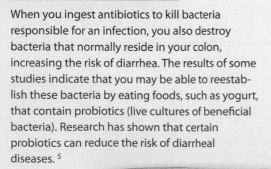

Concept **Checkpoint**

11. Describe what happens to a cheese sandwich after it is eaten and as it moves through the digestive tract.
12. Provide an example of mechanical digestion and chemical digestion.
13. Identify four different tastes.
14. Eliot choked on a piece of hot dog. Explain why choking can occur while eating.
15. Sara takes medication that reduces her stomach's mucus production. Based on this information, what common stomach disorder is she at risk of developing?
16. What functional aspect of a healthy digestive system prevents food from becoming "stuck" in the tract?
17. What keeps stomach contents from reentering the esophagus?
18. List the sections of the small intestine. Where does most digestion and absorption occur?
19. How would removal of the pancreas affect digestion?
20. Describe at least two different ways that nutrients can enter villi.

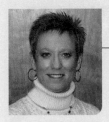

REAL *People*

REAL *Stories*

Lisa Gottschalk

One winter, Lisa Gottschalk began experiencing painful abdominal cramps followed by frequent bouts of diarrhea. It seemed whatever she ate would pass through her digestive tract and be eliminated quickly. When over-the-counter diarrhea remedies didn't work, Lisa sensed her ailment was not a self-limiting intestinal tract infection. Before the illness struck, Lisa weighed 125 pounds—a healthy weight for a 5'2" person. She was physically active and strong. Four weeks after developing the digestive tract problems, she had lost about 12 pounds and become noticeably weaker.

Lisa's physician suspected a form of inflammatory bowel disease (IBD) was responsible for her condition. She was admitted into a local hospital and treated with prednisone, a steroid medication that helps reduce inflammation. When her weight stabilized, her physician prescribed additional medications that are specific for treating IBD. Her special diet included foods that were easily digested. She soon learned which foods she could eat without suffering from diarrhea. For example, she couldn't eat raw carrots, but she could tolerate cooked carrots. Because IBD damaged the ileum, the site for vitamin B-12 absorption, Lisa had to have injections of vitamin B-12 regularly. Within a few weeks, Lisa was well enough to leave the hospital, but she remained on the medication.

About six months after being released from the hospital, Lisa experienced a major setback as her colon became severely inflamed, and she had to be rushed to the hospital by ambulance. While in the hospital, she was given special formula feedings administered through a vein, but she continued to lose weight and her condition deteriorated. At this point, Lisa's physician recommended she obtain treatment at Mayo Clinic in Minnesota.

While Lisa was a patient at Mayo Clinic, her physicians determined she had Crohn's disease, a form of IBD. Medical experts suspect Crohn's disease is an autoimmune disorder, a condition in which the body's immune system does not function properly and begins to attack normal cells. Rheumatoid arthritis and multiple sclerosis (MS) are also autoimmune diseases. In Crohn's disease, certain immune system cells invade the intestinal lining and cause inflammation.

People who have autoimmune disorders often have genes that make them vulnerable to develop such conditions. Lisa eventually learned that she has a gene associated with increased risk of Crohn's disease. However, she was not aware of anyone in her family who also suffered from Crohn's disease or another autoimmune disorder.

The clinic's physicians treated Lisa with a medication specifically used to treat Crohn's disease. Within 2 days of starting treatment, Lisa began to feel better. After several days, her weight had risen to 87 pounds, and her physicians allowed her to return home, but she would need to return to the clinic every few weeks to receive the medication.

Today, Lisa is back at work and back to feeling "normal." She still has to obtain treatment for Crohn's disease, but her local hospital is able to provide the special medication she needs every 8 weeks. Lisa continues to avoid eating certain foods, especially raw vegetables. She recommends that people be aware of autoimmune diseases such as Crohn's, because they are relatively common conditions. Furthermore, she says, "Follow your doctor's advice, take medicines as scheduled, and have an open and honest relationship with your doctor. The key to health and wellness is to listen to your body and keep a positive attitude."

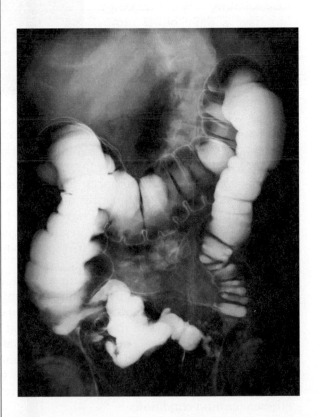

Chapter 4 Highlight

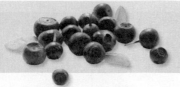

GUT REACTION

Even though you may be healthy, you have probably experienced occasional bouts of constipation, vomiting, diarrhea, or heartburn. After being miserable and uncomfortable for a while, you recovered and returned to your usual routine. This "Highlight" provides general information about common intestinal problems, including peptic ulcers.

Constipation

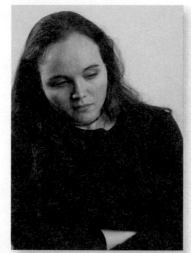

Many Americans, especially older adults, think they are constipated if they do not have a bowel movement at least once a day. According to the American Gastroenterological Association, it is not necessary to have a daily bowel movement. Although the normal frequency of bowel movements varies individually, a healthy person should have a bowel movement at least every three days.[6] When bowel movements occur less frequently and/or are difficult to eliminate, the condition is called constipation.

Many factors influence the frequency of bowel movements. Lack of dietary fiber; low water intake; anxiety, depression, and other psychological disturbances; and changes in your typical routine, such as taking a long trip or having major surgery, can alter your usual pattern of bowel movements. Furthermore, constipation can result when people regularly ignore their normal bowel urges and avoid making a trip to the bathroom when it's not convenient.

Although occasional constipation is a common health problem, *chronic* constipation can cause discomfort and may contribute to the development of hemorrhoids and diverticula. Hemorrhoids are swollen veins in the anal canal that can cause itching and bleeding. Diverticula are tiny pouches that can form in the lining of the large intestine. If diverticula become infected, antibiotics and, sometimes, surgery may be necessary to treat the condition (diverticulitis). Chapter 5 provides more information on these common conditions.

If you feel uncomfortable because your bowel habits have changed or you have hard, dry bowel movements that are difficult to eliminate, discuss the matter with your physician. In many instances, adding more fiber-rich foods to your diet is the first step to becoming more "regular." Chapter 5 provides information about dietary fiber, including rich food sources.

Diarrhea

Diarrhea is a condition characterized by frequent, loose bowel movements. Diarrhea occurs when more water than normal is secreted into the GI tract or the tract absorbs less water than normal. Most cases of diarrhea result from bacterial or viral infections of the intestinal tract. The infectious bacteria or viruses produce irritating or toxic substances that increase the movements (motility) of the GI tract. As a result, the GI tract propels chyme more rapidly through it, absorbing less water than normal in the process. Increased GI motility also enables the large intestine to eliminate the watery feces and the toxic material it contains rapidly.

Loperamide, a medication that is available without a prescription, can be helpful for relieving an occasional bout of mild diarrhea. Cases of severe diarrhea, however, require more immediate medical attention, because frequent watery bowel movements (stools) can deplete the body's fluid volume, causing dehydration and excessive losses of the minerals sodium and potassium. Therefore, treatment of severe diarrhea generally includes drinking replacement fluids that contain sodium, potassium, and simple sugars such as glucose. It's also prudent to avoid eating solid foods until the condition resolves. Prompt treatment of severe diarrhea—within 24 to 48 hours—is especially crucial for infants and the elderly, because they can become dehydrated quickly by the loss of body water. In adults, diarrhea that is accompanied by bloody stools or lasts more than 7 days may be a sign of a serious intestinal disease, and a physician should be consulted.

Vomiting

Not long after eating something toxic or drinking too much alcohol, you begin to feel queasy or "sick to your stomach." You soon become well aware that your body has an effective way of removing the harmful food or beverage—vomiting. Although vomiting is an unpleasant experience, it prevents toxic substances from entering your small intestine, where they can do more harm or be absorbed. Vomiting can also be a response to intense pain or emotional stress, head injury, rotating movements of the head (motion sickness), hormonal changes in pregnancy (morning sickness), and unpleasant odors.[7]

Vomiting occurs when the vomiting center in the brain interprets information from various nervous system receptors concerning the physical and chemical conditions of the stomach, small intestine, and bloodstream. When a toxic chemical is detected, the center initiates vomiting by contracting the abdominal muscles, expelling the contents of the stomach and duodenum forcefully out of the body via the mouth.

Vomiting generally does not last more than 24 hours. Repeated vomiting, however, can result in dehydration, especially if it's accompanied by diarrhea. Treatment includes avoiding solid food until the condition resolves. Additionally, sipping small amounts of water or clear liquids, including noncarbonated soft drinks such as sports drinks, can help prevent dehydration. If the affected person is able to retain small amounts of fluid, then he or she can try to drink increasing amounts of fluid until the vomiting subsides completely.

According to the Cleveland Clinic, adults should contact a physician if their vomiting lasts for more than a day and they have signs of dehydration such as increased thirst, decreased urination, and dry lips and mouth.[7] Contact a physician immediately if the vomit is bloody (looks like coffee grounds) or vomiting is accompanied by other signs and symptoms, such as diarrhea, weakness, confusion, fever, or severe abdominal pain (see Table 4.4). Children who suffer from vomiting and/or diarrhea are likely to develop dehydration more rapidly than adults who are suffering from these conditions. Signs of dehydration in young children include sunken eyes, dry lips and mouth, and decreased urination. Contact a physician if a child who is less than 6 years of age has vomiting and diarrhea that persists for more than a few hours and shows signs of dehydration.

Heartburn

About half of North American adults experience occasional heartburn ("acid indigestion"), a gnawing pain or burning sensation generally felt in the upper chest, under the breastbone. Ten percent of the population has heartburn at least once a week. This discomfort is not the result of a heart problem but is caused by the passage of acidic contents from the stomach into the esophagus. Because the esophageal lining does not produce as much protective mucus as the stomach, the acid quickly destroys the tissue, causing pain and, sometimes, bleeding. Many factors can contribute to heartburn or worsen the condition, including being pregnant; smoking cigarettes; having excess body fat; drinking alcohol; and consuming certain foods.

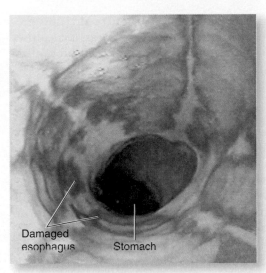

Figure 4.32 Acid reflux damage. An endoscopic view of the esophagus near the opening to the stomach. The reddened areas are signs of damage caused by acid reflux.

Damaged esophagus

Stomach

Although many people think heartburn is a trivial health problem, frequent chronic heartburn can be a symptom of gastroesophageal reflux disease (GERD). Symptoms of GERD include frequent heartburn and may include nausea, gagging, coughing, or hoarseness. If not treated properly, GERD damages the lining of the esophagus and contributes to the development of esophageal ulcers (sores) (Fig. 4.32). Such ulcers can damage blood vessels in the wall of the esophagus, causing bleeding. Signs of bleeding from the esophagus and stomach include black, tarry bowel movements and iron-deficiency anemia. In severe cases, the loss of blood from a bleeding ulcer can be deadly.

People who suffer from GERD have a higher risk of esophageal cancer than people who do not have a history of this condition. If you or someone you know suffers from GERD, typical dietary advice for treating the condition includes consuming smaller, more frequent meals that are low in fat; not overeating at mealtimes; and limiting intake of foods that relax the gastroesophageal sphincter, such as greasy foods, chili powder, onions, garlic, peppermint, caffeine, alcohol, and chocolate.[8] Additionally, you should wait about 2 hours after meals before lying down, because remaining upright reduces the likelihood that stomach contents will push against the gastroesophageal sphincter and move into your esophagus. Table 4.5 lists these and other recommendations for reducing the risk of heartburn and managing GERD. Taking over-the-counter antacids can neutralize excess stomach acid and relieve the discomfort of

TABLE 4.4

Vomiting Danger Signs

Contact a physician when vomiting:

1. Lasts longer than a few hours (children under 6 years of age)
2. Lasts longer than a day (people over 6 years of age)
3. Is accompanied by:
   - blood in vomit (looks like coffee grounds)
   - signs of dehydration
   - diarrhea
   - fever
   - weakness
   - headache or stiff neck
   - severe abdominal pain
   - confusion or decreased alertness

TABLE 4.5

Recommendations to Reduce the Risk of Heartburn

1. If you have too much body fat, lose the excess weight.
2. Do not lie down within 2 hours after eating a meal.
3. Do not overeat at mealtimes.
4. Avoid smoking cigarettes.
5. Elevate the head of your bed 6 inches higher than the foot of the bed.
6. Do not wear tight belts or clothes with tight waistbands.
7. Learn to recognize foods that cause heartburn.

heartburn within minutes, but these products do not prevent heartburn. People suffering from GERD can take other medications that inhibit stomach acid production, preventing heartburn.

Peptic Ulcer

A peptic ulcer is a sore that occurs in the lining of the stomach or the upper small intestine. The typical symptoms of a peptic ulcer are deep, dull upper abdominal pain and a feeling of fullness that occur about 2 hours after eating. The pain results when most of the chyme has left the stomach, and the HCl acid that remains comes in contact with and digests the lining of the organ, forming one or more sores. It is not unusual for the sores to damage the wall of a blood vessel, causing bleeding; thus, untreated gastrointestinal ulcers may result in iron-deficiency anemia. Furthermore, an ulcer may erode through the stomach or intestinal wall and allow GI contents to leak into the body cavities, resulting in a potentially life-threatening infection. Therefore, it is important to recognize ulcer symptoms and obtain treatment early.

Physicians detect peptic ulcers by performing a clinical examination called upper endoscopy.[9] The first step of this procedure involves administering a medication that relaxes the patient. Then the physician inserts a special flexible scope into the mouth, down the esophagus, and into the stomach and upper small intestine. The scope is equipped with a video camera that transmits images of the lining of the esophagus, stomach, and upper small intestine to a screen that the physician views for the presence of ulcers, eroded areas, or cancerous tumors. The scope also enables the physician to use tools to treat areas of bleeding or remove pieces of tissue (biopsy) for microscopic examination.

At one time, medical experts thought excessive emotional stress caused peptic ulcers. By the 1990s, however, researchers determined that *Helicobacter pylori* (*H. pylori*), a type of bacteria that can live in parts of the stomach, was responsible for the development of most stomach ulcers (see Fig. 2.1). *H. pylori* infection makes the lining of the stomach more susceptible to being damaged by stomach acid. In addition to infection with *H. pylori*, other factors are associated with the development of peptic ulcers, particularly smoking cigarettes, heavy consumption of alcohol, and use of NSAIDs (nonsteroidal anti-inflammatory drugs) such as aspirin, ibuprofen, and naproxen. Table 4.6 lists these and other factors that increase a person's risk of peptic ulcers. Note that stress is still considered a risk

TABLE 4.6

Factors That Increase the Risk of Peptic Ulcers

Infection with *H. pylori*
NSAIDs
Alcohol consumption
Genetics
Smoking
Emotional stress
Excess acid production

factor for ulcer formation. People who have difficulty coping with excess emotional stress are more likely to develop peptic ulcers when compared to people who manage their stress better. Having good stress management skills may explain why some people who are infected with *H. pylori* do not develop these ulcers.

Today, a combination of medical approaches is used for ulcer therapy. People infected with *H. pylori* are given antibiotics as well as medications that reduce stomach acid production. This treatment is highly effective for combating *H. pylori* infections and healing peptic ulcers.

Current dietary approaches to treatment simply recommend avoiding foods that increase ulcer symptoms; often such foods vary individually. For example, a man who has a history of peptic ulcer may find peppery foods irritating to his stomach, while his friend who is being treated for an ulcer may be able to tolerate the same foods. Today, the combination of medical treatment and lifestyle changes has minimized the need for peptic ulcer patients to make drastic dietary changes.

Irritable Bowel Syndrome (IBS)

As many as 20% of adult Americans suffer from irritable bowel syndrome (IBS), a condition characterized by intestinal cramps and abnormal bowel function, particularly diarrhea, constipation, or alternating episodes of both.[10] Loose stools are often accompanied with mucus, and after bowel movements, the affected person feels as though elimination of stools was incomplete. For reasons that are unknown, women are more likely than men to suffer from IBS.[10]

The cause of IBS is unknown, but certain foods and beverages as well as emotional stress may trigger severe bouts of the disorder. The intestinal tract muscles of people with IBS may produce stronger contractions that last longer than the GI muscles of people who do not have this condition.[11] Researchers are investigating the role of the nervous system in stimulating these abnormal intestinal tract movements.

Therapy is individualized and may include elimination diets that focus on determining which foods are most likely to contribute to IBS symptoms. Foods often eliminated include dairy products, carbonated beverages, raw fruits, beans, and certain vegetables, especially cabbage and broccoli. Treatment often includes learning stress management strategies, obtaining psychological counseling, and taking antidepressant and other medications. Although irritable bowel syndrome can be uncomfortable and upsetting, the condition does not appear to inflame the tissue of the large intestine or increase the risk of colorectal cancer.[11] For more information about this condition, visit the website www.ibsgroup.org or www.mayoclinic.com.

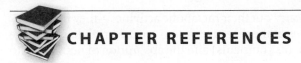

CHAPTER REFERENCES

See Appendix I.

SUMMARY

Matter is composed of chemicals. Over 100 different types of atoms exist, and each type is an element. Atoms of elements may react with each other to form chemical bonds that hold the atoms together in a new arrangement called a molecule. Molecules that contain two or more different elements are called compounds. A solution is an evenly distributed mixture of two compounds. In living things, water is the solvent, the primary compound of a solution.

Ions, acids, and bases play important physiological roles in the body. An ion is an atom or group of atoms that has a positive or negative electrical charge. Electrolytes are ions that can conduct electricity. An acid is a molecule that donates hydrogen ions (H^+); a base is a molecule that accepts H^+. Chemists use the pH scale to describe the H^+ concentration of a watery solution.

Most molecules undergo chemical reactions that change their arrangement of atoms, forming new molecules or compounds. When elements or compounds combine to form new substances, a synthetic reaction has occurred. The new substances often have physical and chemical properties that are quite different from those of the reactants. Decomposition reactions, such as those occurring during digestion, involve the breaking down of molecules. Enzymes are proteins that facilitate or catalyze chemical reactions. Enzymes do not become part of the products of a reaction and, as a result, can catalyze many reactions.

Anatomy is the scientific study of cells and other body structures; physiology is the scientific study of how cells and body structures function. A cell is the smallest functioning unit in a living organism. Cells that have similar characteristics and functions are usually joined together into larger masses called tissues. An organ is composed of various tissues that function in a related fashion. An organ system is a group of organs that work together for a similar purpose.

The cardiovascular system involves the pumping action of the heart to circulate blood in blood vessels throughout the body. Arteries carry blood away from the heart; veins convey blood back to the heart. The thin walls of capillaries allow nutrients and oxygen to move out of the blood and into cells, and carbon dioxide and other waste products to pass from cells and into the blood.

The respiratory system enables the body to obtain oxygen and eliminate carbon dioxide. The lymphatic system helps maintain fluid balance, absorb certain nutrients, and defend the body against infectious disease. The urinary system filters and excretes unneeded substances from blood and maintains proper fluid balance.

The muscular and skeletal systems enable the body to move within its environment and provide support and protection for the body. The nervous system produces intellectual and emotional responses, and controls and regulates many body functions. The endocrine system produces hormones that convey information to target cells; hormones regulate a variety of physiological activities. Hair, nails, and skin are structures of the integumentary system. Skin protects against minor injuries and infectious disease-causing agents, and helps maintain body temperature. The main function of the reproductive organs is to produce children.

To be healthy, all organ systems must work together in a coordinated manner to maintain homeostasis. When homeostasis is disrupted, the body uses various mechanisms to regain its normal internal status, but sickness and even death can result if the abnormality persists.

Your cells do not need food to carry out their metabolic activities—they need nutrients that are in food. The primary roles of the digestive system are the breakdown of large food molecules into smaller components (nutrients) and the absorption of nutrients into the bloodstream.

Digestion is a mechanical and chemical process that breaks down large food components into nutrients that can be absorbed. The mechanical aspects of digestion include the chewing action of teeth as well as involuntary muscular activity, including peristalsis. Chemical digestion includes the actions of enzymes and substances such as hydrochloric acid and bile.

Digestion begins in the mouth with the mechanical action of teeth and some minor chemical action of salivary amylase. The esophagus conveys food from the mouth to the stomach, where it mixes with gastric juice and is referred to as chyme. The chyme moves from the stomach to the duodenum of the small intestine. In the small intestine, enzymes complete the process of digestion. In the small intestine, cells of villi absorb the end products of digestion and transfer them to blood or lymph. Any remaining undigested material, some water, and intestinal bacteria are eliminated from the body as feces.

Common gastrointestinal disorders include constipation, heartburn, peptic ulcer, and irritable bowel syndrome. Chronic constipation can cause discomfort and may contribute to the development of hemorrhoids and diverticula. Frequent chronic heartburn can be a symptom of GERD. People with GERD are at risk of esophageal cancer. Peptic ulcers can cause life-threatening bleeding. In addition to infection with *H. pylori*, smoking cigarettes, heavy consumption of alcohol, and use of nonsteroidal anti-inflammatory drugs increase the risk of peptic ulcer. Although irritable bowel syndrome is common, the condition does not result in inflammation of the large intestine.

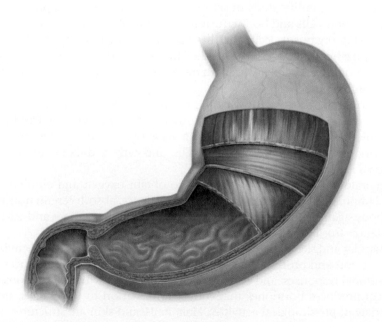

Recipes for Healthy Living

Chopped Chicken Liver Pâté

At some point, you may have sampled calves', beef, or pork liver and decided it would never become one of your favorite foods. You might change your mind when you learn that liver is an excellent source of several vitamins and minerals.

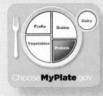

The following recipe for pâté (*pah-tay´*) uses chicken livers, because they are more mild-tasting than beef or other commonly eaten types of liver. Adding onions, hard-cooked eggs, and a sauce made from chili peppers to the liver makes a flavorful nutritious spread for crackers. Although liver is very nutritious, the organ produces cholesterol and contains high amounts of this lipid. If you are concerned about consuming too much cholesterol but you still want to try this recipe, eat small amounts of the pâté as a snack or appetizer.

This recipe makes approximately 8 servings. Each serving supplies 150 kcal, 11 g protein, 11 g fat, 250 g cholesterol, 1892 RAE vitamin A, 11 mg vitamin C, 5.5 mg niacin (a B vitamin), 341 mcg folate (a B vitamin), 223 mg sodium, 5.3 mg iron, and 1.6 mg zinc.

INGREDIENTS:

1 lb raw chicken livers

3 Tbsp vegetable oil

½ cup sweet onion, peeled and coarsely chopped

2 Tbsp lite mayonnaise

2 hard-cooked eggs*, peeled

½ tsp salt

¼ tsp ground black pepper

3 to 5 drops commercially prepared hot pepper sauce (optional)

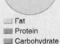

* To hard-cook eggs:

1. Place the eggs in a small saucepan and cover the eggs completely with about 2 inches of water.

2. Heat the saucepan containing the water and eggs to a boil, then cover the saucepan with its lid, and remove it from the heat.

3. Allow the eggs to remain in the hot water for approximately 20 to 25 minutes (large eggs).

4. Remove eggs from the saucepan and cool by immersing in cold water.

5. Prepare a hard-cooked egg for peeling by tapping it on a countertop, cracking the shell as completely as possible.

6. If the shell sticks to the egg white, run cold water over the egg as you peel it. Discard the shells in the garbage.

PREPARATION STEPS:

1. Rinse chicken livers in cool water and drain on paper towels. Cut each liver into thirds.

2. Place oil in a large frying pan and heat at a medium-high temperature for about 45 seconds. Add chopped onion and gently cook in oil (sauté) until translucent.

3. Add liver to the onion mixture. Reduce the heat to medium-low temperature and cook slowly for 7 to 10 minutes, stirring until no pinkness remains within the liver.

4. Drain excess oil from cooked liver and onions, and transfer mixture to the top of a large cutting board.

5. Add peeled eggs. Using a knife, chop the mixture until its texture is coarse. Add salad dressing and seasonings. Mix with a spoon until ingredients are well blended. If you have a food processor or blender, just add the ingredients into the bowl of the machine and blend.

6. Place in a bowl, cover, and refrigerate for several hours.

7. Serve as a spread on whole-grain crackers.

Egg Salad

Like liver, eggs are a nutrient-dense food. Egg salad is an easy-to-make meal or snack. This recipe makes about three ⅓-cup servings. Each serving supplies approximately 131 kcal, 8.5 g protein, 9 g fat, 280 mg cholesterol, and 125 mg sodium.

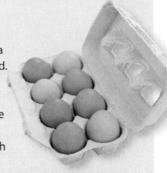

INGREDIENTS:

2 Tbsp peeled, finely chopped yellow onion

4 hard-cooked large eggs

2 Tbsp lite mayonnaise

1 tsp pickle relish

dash of black pepper

PREPARATION STEPS:

1. Place chopped onion in small mixing bowl.

2. Peel hard-cooked eggs and discard peels. Chop eggs on a cutting board.

3. Add chopped eggs to onions.

4. Add lite mayonnaise and pickle relish to the egg and onion mixture. Blend together. Mixture should be moist.

5. Wash a few lettuce leaves. Shake excess water from lettuce and dry by patting with clean paper towels. Arrange lettuce leaves on a plate.

6. Spoon egg salad on lettuce. Serve as a spread on whole-wheat crackers or on rye bread.

7. Egg salad is perishable, so cover any leftover salad and store in the refrigerator for no longer than a day.

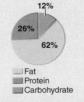

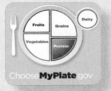

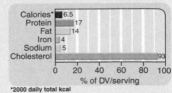

CRITICAL THINKING

1. If you stain your clothes with blueberry juice, what can you do to remove the stain? Explain your answer.

2. Why would a person's stomach feel uncomfortably full several hours after eating a bacon-topped double cheeseburger, a large serving of French fries, and a milkshake?

3. Explain why the label for a multivitamin supplement recommends taking the pill with meals, particularly meals that contain some fat.

4. Taylor had a serious condition that required removal of the upper third of his small intestine. Based on this information, is Taylor at risk for developing multiple nutrient deficiencies? Explain why or why not.

5. Your mother complains of having persistent heartburn, but she does not think her discomfort is serious enough to be investigated by her physician. Do you agree or disagree with her attitude about heartburn? Explain your position.

PRACTICE TEST

Select the best answer.

1. Which of the following substances is insoluble in water?
   a. fat
   b. sugar
   c. calcium
   d. sodium

2. Which of the following substances has the lowest pH?
   a. plain coffee
   b. household ammonia
   c. plain water
   d. gastric juice

3. A _____ is a group of similar cells that perform similar functions.
   a. ribosome
   b. tissue
   c. cytoplasm
   d. system

4. Which of the following organs is an accessory organ of the digestive system?
   a. heart
   b. kidney
   c. liver
   d. bladder

5. Which of the following statements is false?
   a. Arteries carry blood away from the heart.
   b. Hemoglobin carries most of the oxygen in the blood.
   c. Cells need oxygen to obtain energy.
   d. All arteries carry deoxygenated blood.

6. Mechanical digestion begins in the
   a. mouth.
   b. stomach.
   c. small intestine.
   d. liver.

7. Two or more atoms that are held together by a chemical bond form a
   a. pH.
   b. molecule.
   c. proton.
   d. nucleus.

8. A salt forms when an _____ combines with a _____.
   a. electrolyte; proton
   b. acid; base
   c. element; pH
   d. enzyme; mineral

9. Chemical messengers in the body are

   a. enzymes.
   b. cells.
   c. capillaries.
   d. hormones.

10. Tiny, fingerlike projections of the small intestine that absorb nutrients are called

    a. lumen.
    b. villi.
    c. duodenum.
    d. calculi.

11. A lacteal is a

    a. lymph vessel within each villus.
    b. form of carbohydrate in milk.
    c. muscular structure that regulates digestion in the large intestine.
    d. specialized cell.

12. A _____ transports lipids in the bloodstream.

    a. sodium acetate
    b. cholecystokinin
    c. gastrin
    d. chylomicron

13. The stomach secretes

    a. salivary amylase.
    b. hydrochloric acid.
    c. bile.
    d. All of the above are correct.

14. Peristalsis

    a. is a common intestinal infection.
    b. interferes with lipid absorption in the small intestine.
    c. stimulates red blood cell formation in bone marrow.
    d. helps move food/chyme through the digestive tract.

15. Starch digestion begins in the

    a. gastric pouch.
    b. esophagus.
    c. mouth.
    d. gallbladder.

16. Which of the following practices increases the risk of peptic ulcer?

    a. chewing gum
    b. smoking cigarettes
    c. drinking orange juice
    d. eating a low-fiber diet

Answers to Chapter 4 Quiz *Yourself*

1. The atom is the smallest living unit in the body. **False.** (p. 99)
2. The stomach produces hydrochloric acid. **True.** (p. 107)
3. Digestion actually begins in the stomach. **False.** (p. 105)
4. The human intestinal tract cannot digest certain combinations of foods, such as mixtures of simple carbohydrates and proteins. **False.** (p. 112)
5. Undigested food rots in your stomach, causing toxic materials to build up in your tissues. **False.** (p. 112)

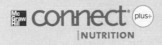

Additional resources related to the features of this book are available on ConnectPlus® Nutrition. Ask your instructor how to get access.

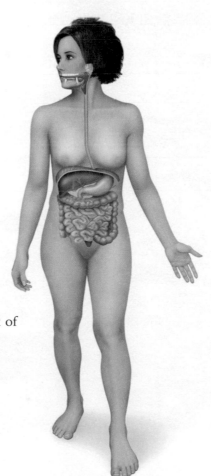

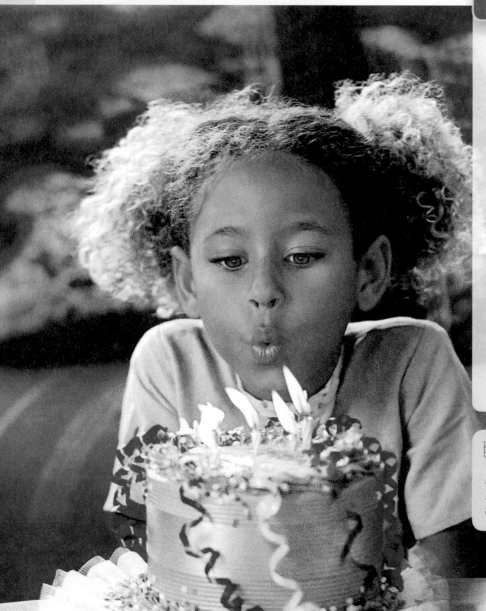

CHAPTER 5

Carbohydrates

WHEN YOU ARE bored, excited, or in a good or bad mood, do you reach for something sweet to eat? Can you imagine celebrating birthdays, weddings, or holidays without cakes, candies, or cookies? If you are like many Americans, you enjoy eating sweets and may even describe yourself as having a "sweet tooth." According to U.S. Department of Agriculture (USDA) estimates, the average American (2 years of age and older) consumed nearly 100 pounds of added caloric sweeteners, such as table sugar and high-fructose corn syrup, in 2008.[1] This amount was almost 15% more than the amount estimated to have been eaten by the average American in 1970.

Why do humans, even newborn infants, prefer foods that taste sweet? The pleasant and sometimes irresistible taste of sugar is a clue that the food contains **carbohydrates,** a major source of energy for cells. Without a steady supply of energy, cells cannot function and they die.

Plants are rich sources of carbohydrates; they make these substances by using the sun's energy to combine carbon, oxygen, and hydrogen atoms from

(continued)

Quiz *Yourself*

Do "carbs" cause diabetes or unwanted weight gain? Would sweetening your cereal with honey be a healthier choice than using table sugar? Should you choose foods according to their *glycemic index*? Check your knowledge of carbohydrates by taking the following quiz. The answers are found on page 155.

1. Compared to table sugar, honey is a natural and far more nutritious sweetener. _____T _____F

2. Ounce per ounce, sugar provides more energy than starch. _____T _____F

3. Eating a high-fiber diet can improve the functioning of your large intestine and reduce your blood cholesterol levels. _____T _____F

4. The average American consumes 80% of his or her energy intake as refined sugars. _____T _____F

5. The results of clinical studies indicate that eating too much sugar makes children hyperactive. _____T _____F

carbohydrates class of nutrients that is a major source of energy for the body

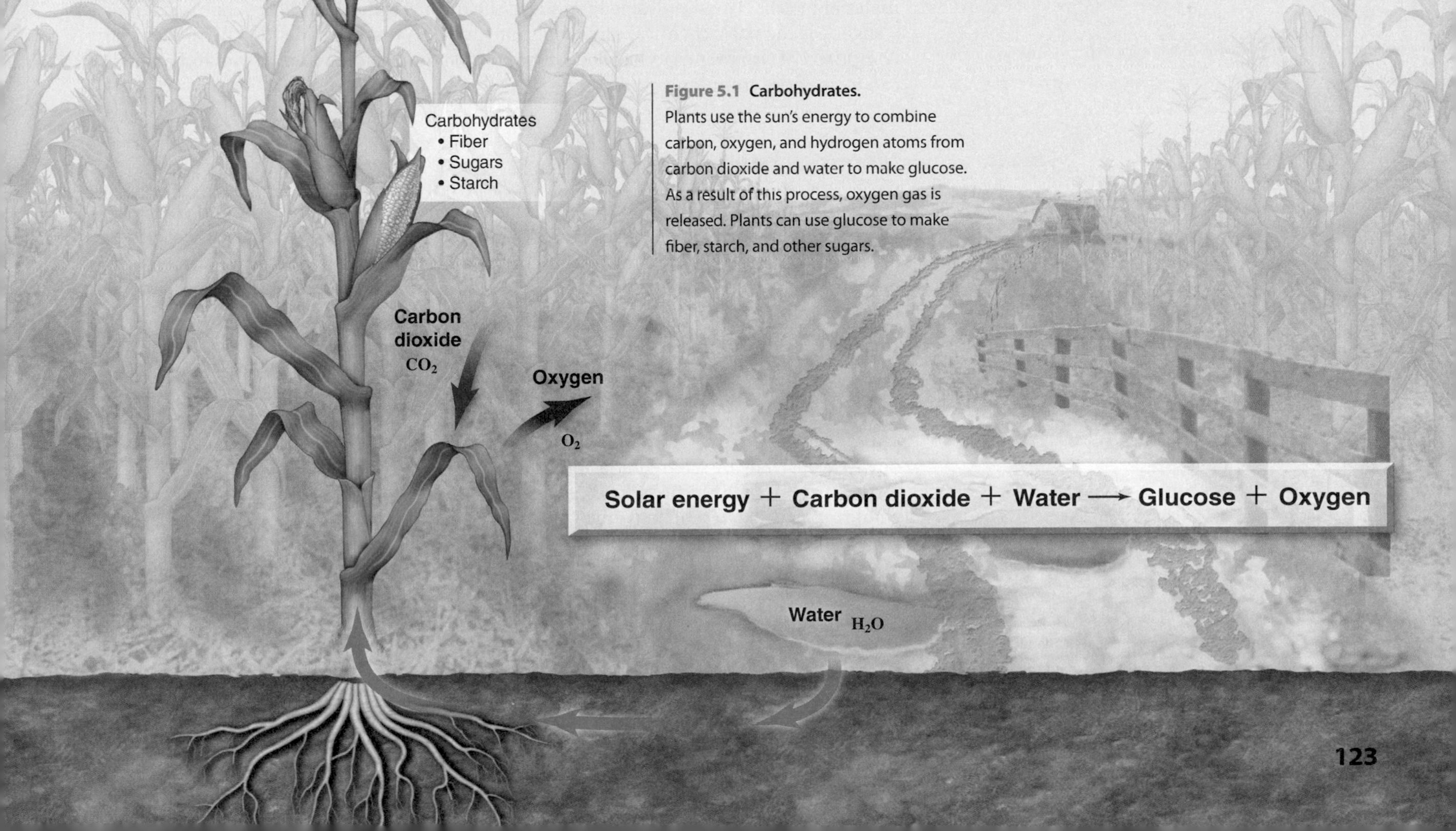

Sunlight

Carbohydrates
• Fiber
• Sugars
• Starch

Figure 5.1 Carbohydrates.
Plants use the sun's energy to combine carbon, oxygen, and hydrogen atoms from carbon dioxide and water to make glucose. As a result of this process, oxygen gas is released. Plants can use glucose to make fiber, starch, and other sugars.

Carbon dioxide CO_2

Oxygen O_2

Water H_2O

Solar energy + Carbon dioxide + Water ⟶ Glucose + Oxygen

123

carbon dioxide and water (Fig. 5.1). Some of the energy from the sun is stored in the bonds that hold the carbon and hydrogen atoms together. Our cells can break down some of those bonds, releasing energy that powers various forms of cellular work, including the energy to contract muscles, make vital compounds, and build bones.

Regardless of whether your goals include becoming a computer programmer, health care professional, or world-class athlete, carbohydrates play an important role in your health. In Chapter 5, you will learn about the major roles of carbohydrates in the body. Additionally, you will learn which foods are rich sources of carbohydrates, including simple sugars and complex carbohydrates.

5.1 Simple Carbohydrates: Sugars

You probably are familiar with sugar as the sweet, white, granulated crystals often sprinkled on cereal or into iced tea, but table sugar is only one type of sugar. You may be unaware that there are different types of sugars in milk, blood, and DNA, the genetic material in cells. The simplest type of sugar, the **monosaccharide** (*mono* = one; *saccharide* = sugar), is the basic chemical unit of carbohydrates. A **disaccharide** (*di* = two) is a sugar comprised of two monosaccharides. By combining monosaccharides, plants and animals can form more complex carbohydrates.

Monosaccharides

The three most important dietary monosaccharides are glucose, fructose, and galactose. Figure 5.2 shows the chemical structures of glucose, fructose, and galactose as well as the geometric symbols used to represent them in this textbook. The chemical names of carbohydrates, particularly sugars, end in *ose*. Gluc*ose*, fruct*ose*, and sucr*ose* are sugars commonly found in foods.

Fruits and vegetables, especially berries, grapes, corn, and carrots, are good food sources of **glucose.** Glucose is the most important monosaccharide in the human body because it is a primary fuel for muscle and other cells. In fact, red blood and nervous system cells, including brain cells, must use glucose for energy under normal conditions. Thus, a healthy body maintains its *blood glucose* levels carefully. Glucose is also called dextrose and may be referred to as blood sugar.

Fructose (fruit sugar or levulose) is naturally found in fruit, honey, and a few vegetables, particularly cabbage, green beans, and asparagus. Since fructose tastes much sweeter than glucose and is easily made from corn, food manufacturers use large amounts of *high-fructose corn syrup* (*HFCS*) as a food additive to satisfy Americans' demand for "regular" soft drinks, candies, and baked goods. The body has little need for fructose; therefore, most fructose is converted into glucose or fat.

Unlike glucose and fructose, **galactose** is not commonly found in foods. Galactose is a component of lactose, the form of carbohydrate in milk. After a woman gives birth, special glands in her breasts convert glucose into galactose, which is necessary for production of lactose in breast milk.

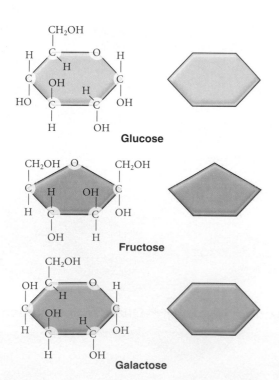

Figure 5.2 Monosaccharides. These chemical symbols for glucose, fructose, and galactose indicate the number and arrangement of carbon, hydrogen, and oxygen atoms. For simplicity, we will omit the atoms and just show the color symbol for each monosaccharide.

Disaccharides

Disaccharides include maltose, sucrose, and lactose. **Maltose** (malt sugar) has two glucose molecules bonded together (Fig. 5.3a). Few foods naturally contain maltose. **Sucrose** (table sugar) consists of a molecule of glucose and one of fructose (Fig. 5.3b). **Lactose** (milk sugar) forms when a galactose molecule bonds to a glucose molecule (Fig. 5.3c). Although most animal foods are not sources of carbohydrate, milk and some products made from milk, such as yogurt and ice cream, contain lactose.

Sucrose

Although sucrose occurs naturally in honey, maple syrup, carrots, and pineapples, much of the sucrose in the American diet is refined from sugar cane and sugar beets. The refining process strips away the small amounts of vitamins and minerals in sugar cane and sugar beets. "Raw sugar," turbinado sugar, and some forms of brown sugar are not as fully processed from sugar cane as white sugar. These sweeteners contain a small amount of molasses, which contributes to their flavor, color, and nutritional value. Since refined sucrose has the reputation of being a "junk food," some manufacturers use creative names, such as "granulated cane juice," to disguise the presence of table sugar in their product's ingredient list.

Some people claim that refined white sugar is poisonous and honey is nutritionally superior to table sugar. However, these claims are not true. Table sugar does not contain toxic substances; in fact, it is almost 100% carbohydrate. Table 5.1 compares the nutritional value of honey with certain forms of sucrose. Note that none of the sweeteners is a good source of protein, vitamins, or minerals. The simple sugars in honey are not superior to those that comprise sucrose, and your body does not distinguish whether glucose or fructose came from sugar or honey.

A tablespoon of white table sugar is almost 100% sucrose; a tablespoon of honey has glucose, fructose, water, and a small amount of sucrose. A tablespoon of honey contains more protein and micronutrients than a tablespoon of white sugar, but the amounts are insignificant. For example, you would have to eat a cup of honey to obtain 1 g of protein, 2 mg of vitamin C, and 1.4 mg of iron. That amount of honey supplies over 1000 kcal! Although honey contains phytochemicals, substances in plant foods that may provide health benefits, the amounts are too small to make this sticky sweetener a valuable source of these compounds. Table sugar and honey are sources of empty calories.

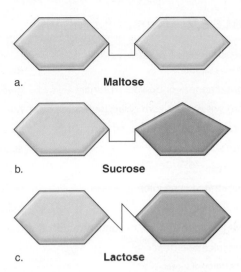

Figure 5.3 Disaccharides. Disaccharides include maltose, sucrose, and lactose. *(a)* Maltose consists of two glucose molecules. *(b)* Sucrose consists of a glucose and a fructose molecule. *(c)* Lactose consists of a galactose and a glucose molecule.

monosaccharide simple sugar that is the basic molecule of carbohydrates

disaccharide simple sugar comprised of two monosaccharides

glucose monosaccharide that is a primary fuel for muscles and other cells; "dextrose" or "blood sugar"

fructose monosaccharide in fruits, honey, and certain vegetables; "levulose" or "fruit sugar"

galactose monosaccharide that is a component of lactose

maltose disaccharide comprised of two glucose molecules; "malt sugar"

sucrose disaccharide comprised of a glucose and a fructose molecule; "table sugar"

lactose disaccharide comprised of a glucose and a galactose molecule; "milk sugar"

Did You Know?

Bees make honey by consuming the sucrose-rich nectar from flowers and digesting most of it into glucose and fructose. The bees regurgitate this material within the beehive, and eventually it is collected by beekeepers for human processing and packaging.

TABLE 5.1 *Nutritional Comparison of Selected Sweeteners*

Sugar/Syrup 1 Tablespoon	Water %	Kcal	Protein g	Carb g	Vit. C mg	Calcium mg	Folate mcg	Potassium mg	Iron mg	Zinc mg
Honey	17	64	0	17	0.1	1	0	11	0.09	0.05
Raw sugar	2	46	0	12	0	10	0.125	42	0.23	0.03
Brown sugar	<1	36	0	9	0	8	0	33	0.18	0.02
White granulated sugar	0	48	0	13	0	0	0	0	0	0

TABLE 5.2 *Names for Sugars*

Sugars Can Be:		
brown sugar	glucose	polydextrose
confectioner's or powdered sugar	granulated cane juice	raw sugar
corn sweeteners, corn syrup, high-fructose	honey	sorbitol*
corn syrup (HFCS), cultured corn syrup	invert sugar	mannitol*
date sugar	lactose	xylitol*
dextrose	maltose, high-maltose corn syrup	table sugar (sucrose)
evaporated cane juice	maltodextrin	turbinado sugar
fructose (levulose)	maple syrup	
fruit juice concentrate or concentrated	molasses	
fruit juice sweetener		

* Alcohol forms of sugars

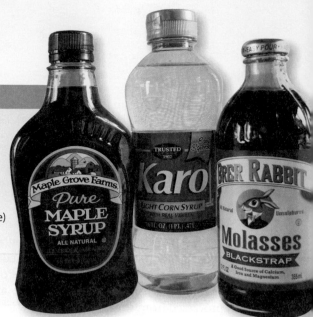

nutritive sweeteners substances that sweeten and contribute energy to foods

added sugars sugars added to foods during processing or preparation

alternative sweeteners substances that sweeten foods while providing few or no kilocalories

nonnutritive sweeteners group of synthetic compounds that are intensely sweet tasting compared to sugar

Nutritive and Nonnutritive Sweeteners

Sugars are **nutritive sweeteners** because they contribute energy to foods. Each gram of a mono- or disaccharide supplies 4 kcal. **Added sugars,** such as sucrose and HFCS, which is chemically similar to sucrose, are often added to foods during processing or preparation. In baked cereal products, added sugars contribute to the browning and tenderness of the food. Sugar also serves as a preservative by inhibiting the growth of molds and bacteria that would otherwise cause food spoilage. If one of the nutritive sweeteners listed in Table 5.2 is the first or second ingredient listed on a product's label, the food probably contains a high amount of added sugar. Table 5.3 indicates the amounts of added sugars that are in typical servings of commonly consumed foods and beverages. The following section provides information about other kinds of sweeteners.

TABLE 5.3 *How Much Added Sugar Is in That Food?*

Food	Serving Size	Kcal	Approximate Teaspoons Added Sugars
Doughnut, cake, plain	3¼" diameter	226	2
Chocolate chip cookies, commercial brand	2 medium (50 g)	239	4
Sugar-frosted cornflakes	¾ cup	114	3
Chocolate-flavored 2% milk	1 cup	158	3
Ice cream, vanilla, light, soft-serve	½ cup	111	2
Chocolate candy bar with almonds	1.76 oz	235	5
Apple pie, double crust	⅛ 8" diameter pie	277	4
Snack sponge cake with cream filling	1 cake (43g)	157	4
Yogurt, vanilla low-fat	8 oz	193	4
Cola, canned	12 fl oz	136	8
Fruit punch drink	12 fl oz	175	10
Chocolate milkshake, fast food	16 fl oz	580	10

Source of data: Krebs-Smith SM: Choose beverages and foods to moderate your intake of sugars: Measurement requires quantification. *Journal of Nutrition* 131:527S, 2006.

Alternative Sweeteners

Some people try to control their caloric intake by reducing their consumption of foods and beverages sweetened with nutritive sweeteners such as sugar. **Alternative sweeteners** (also referred to as sugar replacers, sugar substitutes, or "artificial" sweeteners) are substances added to food that sweeten the item while providing few or no kilocalories. Alternative nutritive sweeteners include sugar alcohols: *sorbitol*, *xylitol*, and *mannitol*. Unlike sugars, sugar alcohols do not promote dental decay. Thus, these compounds are used to replace sucrose in products such as sugar-free chewing gums, breath mints, and "diabetic" candies. Sugar alcohols are not fully absorbed by the intestinal tract, and as a result, they supply an average of 2 kcal/g. However, sugar alcohols may cause diarrhea when consumed in large amounts.

Nonnutritive sweeteners are a group of synthetic compounds that elicit an intensely sweet taste when compared to the same amount of sugar (Table 5.4). Thus, a very small amount of a nonnutritive sweetener is needed to sweeten a food, and they supply no energy per serving. Nonnutritive sweeteners may help people control their energy intake and manage their body weight without increasing their appetite.[4] Consumers, however, need to recognize that most "sugar-free" or "diabetic" foods are not calorie free. Furthermore, results of some studies suggest that artificially sweetened foods and beverages can promote excess calorie consumption. Why? More research is needed, but the taste of products that contain artificial sweeteners may interfere with a person's ability to regulate his or her intake of sugary foods and beverages.[5]

The Food and Drug Administration (FDA) has approved the use of the nonnutritive sweeteners saccharin, aspartame, acesulfame-K, sucralose, neotame, and stevia extracts as additives to sweeten foods as well as other products that may be swallowed, such as mouthwash and toothpaste. Nonnutritive sweeteners do not contribute to dental decay.

In the United States, the safety of nonnutritive sweeteners has been under public and scientific scrutiny for decades. In 1970, the FDA banned the nonnutritive sweetener *cyclamate* after research indicated that the substance caused bladder cancer in mice. In the 1980s, panels of experts at the FDA and the National Academy of Sciences reviewed the scientific evidence and determined that cyclamate did not increase the risk of cancer in humans. Nevertheless, the ban on this food additive continues in the United States. Although *saccharin* has been in use for over 100 years, its safety has also been questioned. Despite the concern, most of the scientific evidence indicates that saccharin is safe when consumed in typical amounts.

Aspartame, better known by its trade names "NutraSweet" or "Equal," consists of phenylalanine and aspartic acid, two amino acids, the molecules that comprise proteins. Some people must avoid aspartame and certain protein-rich foods because they have phenylketonuria (PKU) (*fen'-nul-keet'-en-yur'-e-ah*), a rare inherited disorder that results in abnormal phenylalanine metabolism. If an infant with PKU is not treated with a special diet, phenylalanine and its metabolic by-products accumulate in the child's

Food & Nutrition *tip*

Honey can contain spores, the inactive life stage, of the deadly bacterium *Clostridium botulinum* that resist being destroyed by food preservation methods.[2] These spores can become active within an infant's intestinal tract and produce a poison that is extremely toxic to nerves. According to experts at the Centers for Disease Control and Prevention (CDC), honey should not be fed to children younger than 12 months of age or used to sweeten infant foods because it may cause botulism poisoning.[3] Older children and adults can eat honey without being concerned about botulism, because the mature stomach produces enough acid to destroy the bacterial spores.

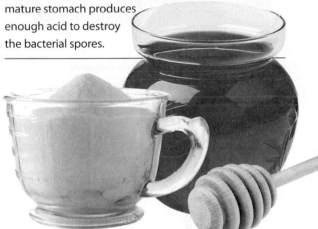

Honey and table sugar have similar nutritional value.

TABLE 5.4 *Comparing Nonnutritive Sweeteners*

Sweetener	Comparison to Sugar	Brand Name	Kilocalories/tsp
Aspartame	200 times sweeter	NutraSweet, Equal	Nearly 0
Saccharin	200 to 700 times sweeter	Sweet'N Low, Sweet Twin, Necta Sweet	0
Acesulfame-K	200 times sweeter	Sunett, Sweet One	0
Neotame	7,000 to 13,000 times sweeter	Neotame	0
Sucralose	600 times sweeter	Splenda	0
Rebiana (Stevia) extracts	200 to 300 times sweeter	Truvia, SweetLeaf	0

Source: Artificial sweeteners: No calories…sweet! *FDA Consumer Magazine*. 2006. www.fda.gov/fdac/features/2006/406_sweeteners.html

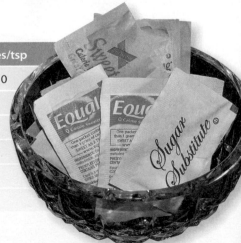

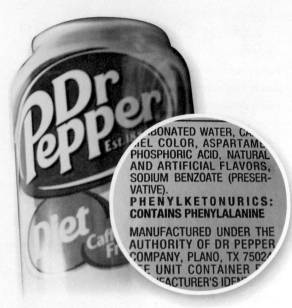

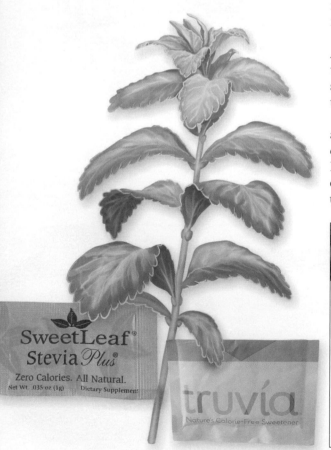

Figure 5.4 **Warning label for people with PKU.** People with PKU need to be concerned about their phenylalanine intake. Artificially sweetened foods that contain aspartame carry this warning on the label because aspartame contains phenylalanine.

TABLE 5.5 *Acceptable Daily Intakes for Nonnutritive Sweeteners*

Food/Beverage	Nonnutritive Sweetener	Amount
diet cola	aspartame	18 to 19 12-oz cans
packets	saccharin	9 to 12 packets
lemon-lime soft drink	acesulfame-K	30 to 32 12-oz cans
diet cola	sucralose	6 12-oz cans

Source: Mattes RD, Popkin BM: Non-nutritive sweetener consumption in humans: Effects on appetite and food intake and their putative mechanisms. *American Journal of Clinical Nutrition* 89(1):1, 2009.

bloodstream and cause severe brain damage. To alert people with PKU about the presence of aspartame in foods, the FDA requires manufacturers of products containing the nonnutritive sweetener to include a warning on the label (Fig. 5.4). The Real People, Real Stories feature in Chapter 7 is about a young person who has PKU.

Since its approval for use as a food additive in 1981, aspartame has been blamed for causing a variety of health problems, including cancer, certain immune system diseases, and chronic headaches. Despite claims to the contrary, no scientifically reliable studies have linked aspartame to any health disorder.[4] In 2006, results of a European study involving rats concluded aspartame increased the risk of cancer in the animals.[6] The European Food Safety Authority challenged the findings of this study when the agency determined the conclusions were not supported by the data. After a review of the data, FDA reported that the safety of aspartame has been studied extensively, and at the present time, no links to cancer have been found.[7]

Sucralose, sold under the brand name "Splenda," is made from a molecule of sucrose that has been chemically modified to escape digestion and absorption. As a result, sucralose sweetens foods and beverages without increasing their caloric value. Since the sweetener is not digested or absorbed by the intestinal tract, it is excreted in feces unchanged. During normal cooking and storage conditions, sucralose resists destruction by heat, a feature that makes it better for sweetening baked products than aspartame.

Some of the newest nonnutritive sweeteners are made from the leaves of the South American shrub *Stevia rebaudiana* Bertoni. For hundreds of years, people have used extracts of stevia leaves as sweeteners. *Rebiana* is the common name for the chemical in stevia leaves that is responsible for their intense sweetness. FDA considers rebiana safe for use as an all-purpose sweetener.

Do nonnutritive sweeteners pose a danger to health? A group of international health and safety organizations, including FDA, have established *Acceptable Daily Intakes* (*ADI*) for certain nonnutritive sweeteners (Table 5.5). According to the Academy of Nutrition and Dietetics, nonnutritive sweeteners are safe when consumed "within acceptable daily intakes, even during pregnancy."[4] Nevertheless, researchers continue to investigate the safety and usefulness of artificial sweeteners.

Concept **Checkpoint**

1. What is the major function of carbohydrate in the body?
2. Identify the three most important dietary monosaccharides.
3. What are the chemical names for blood sugar, table sugar, milk sugar, and malt sugar? Which monosaccharides comprise each molecule of maltose, lactose, and sucrose?
4. What is the difference between a nutritive sweetener and a nonnutritive sweetener?
5. Parents of a child with PKU can give their child either a beverage sweetened with sucralose or one containing aspartame. Which drink should they choose? Explain your answer.

5.2 Complex Carbohydrates

Complex carbohydrates (polysaccharides) are comprised of 10 or more monosaccharides bonded together. Plants and animals use complex carbohydrates to store energy or make certain structural components such as stems and leaves. The most common dietary polysaccharides consist of hundreds of glucose molecules and include digestible and indigestible forms.

Starch and Glycogen

Starch and **glycogen** are polysaccharides that contain hundreds of glucose molecules bound together into large chainlike structures (Fig. 5.5). Plants store glucose as starch, particularly in their seeds, roots, and fleshy underground stems called tubers. Rich food sources of starch include bread and cereal products made from wheat, rice, barley, and oats; vegetables such as corn, squash, beans, and peas; and tubers such as potatoes, yams, taro, cassava, and jicama. Sports drinks and sports or energy bars often include *modified starches* such as maltodextrin and dextrin. Regardless of its source, each gram of starch supplies 4 kcal.

The human body stores limited amounts of glucose as glycogen (see Fig. 5.5c). Muscles and the liver are the major sites for glycogen formation and storage. Although muscles contain glycogen, most animal foods (for example, meat or the flesh of fish and poultry) are not sources of this complex carbohydrate, because muscle glycogen breaks down soon after an animal dies.

Fiber

In addition to storing energy as starch, plants use complex carbohydrates to make supportive structures and protective seed coats that contribute to the fiber content of your diet. Most forms of **dietary fiber (fiber)** are complex carbohydrates comprised of monosaccharides connected by bonds that humans cannot digest. Cellulose, hemicellulose, pectin, gums, and mucilages are carbohydrate forms of fiber; lignin is the only type of fiber that is not carbohydrate. Since fiber is not digested, it moves through the human intestinal tract and contributes to the fecal residue that is eventually eliminated in bowel movements.

There are two types of dietary fiber, **soluble fiber** and **insoluble fiber.** Soluble types of fiber, such as pectins and gums, dissolve or swell in water. Insoluble forms of fiber, such as cellulose and lignin, generally do not dissolve in water. Oat bran and oatmeal, beans, apples, carrots, oranges and other citrus fruits, and psyllium (*sill'-e-um*) seeds are rich sources of soluble fiber; whole-grain products, including brown rice, contain high amounts of insoluble fiber. Table 5.6 provides information about the solubility

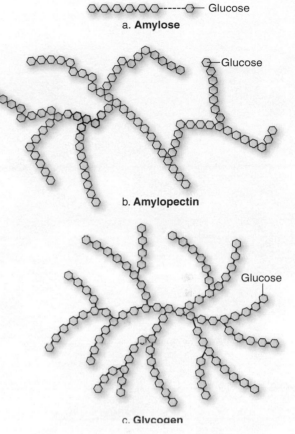

Figure 5.5 Starch and glycogen. Starch and glycogen contain hundreds of glucose molecules bound together into large chainlike structures. *(a) Amylose* and *(b) amylopectin* are forms of starch made by plants. *(c)* The chains of glycogen are more highly branched than those of starch.

TABLE 5.6 *Classifying Fiber*

Type	Component(s)	Physiological Effects	Food Sources
Insoluble	Cellulose, hemi-celluloses	Increases fecal bulk and speeds fecal passage through GI tract	All plants Wheat, rye, brown rice, vegetables
	Lignin	Increases fecal bulk, may ease bowel movements	Whole grains, wheat bran
Soluble	Pectins, gums, mucilages, some hemicelluloses	Delays stomach emptying; slows glucose absorption; can lower blood cholesterol	Apples, bananas, citrus fruits, carrots, oats, barley, psyllium seeds, beans, and thickeners added to foods

complex carbohydrates (polysaccharides) compounds comprised of 10 or more monosaccharides bonded together

starch storage polysaccharide in plants

glycogen storage polysaccharide in animals

dietary fiber (fiber) indigestible plant material; most types are polysaccharides

soluble fiber forms of dietary fiber that dissolve or swell in water

insoluble fiber forms of dietary fiber that generally do not dissolve in water

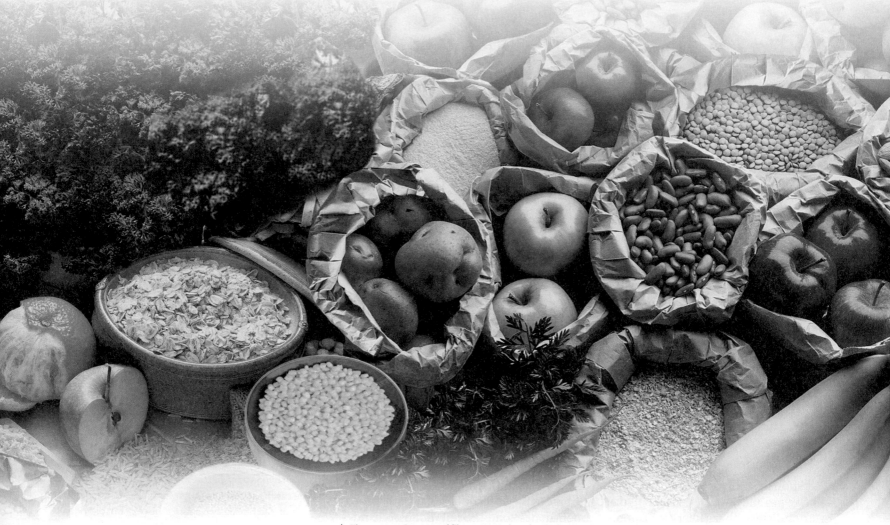

| Figure 5.6 **Sources of fiber.** Most plant foods contain both soluble and insoluble fiber.

of various types of fiber, effects of fiber in the body, and major food sources of soluble and insoluble fiber. Although the foods listed in Table 5.6 are rich sources of either soluble or insoluble fiber, plant foods usually contain both forms (Fig. 5.6).

According to food labeling guidelines issued by the FDA, whole grains are the intact, ground, cracked, or flaked seeds of cereal grains (Fig. 5.7). Such grains may include wheat, buckwheat, oats, corn, rice, wild rice, rye, barley, bulgur, millet, and sorghum. If a "whole-grain" product is made from ground, cracked, or flaked cereal grains, the forms must contain the starchy endosperm, oily germ, and fiber-rich bran seed components in the same relative proportions as they exist in the intact grain.[8] (Figure 1.9 is an illustration of a whole grain kernel that shows the endosperm, germ, and bran components.)

Although fiber is not digested by humans, soluble and insoluble fiber provide important health benefits. Soluble fiber can help reduce blood cholesterol levels, and insoluble fiber may ease bowel movements. The "Carbohydrates and Health" section of Chapter 5 provides information about the benefits of adding more fiber to your diet and practical ways to increase your fiber intake.

Table 5.7 lists common foods that are sources of dietary fiber. Note that only plant foods provide fiber; animal flesh contains muscle fibers, which are digestible proteins.

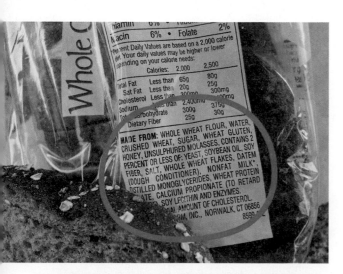

Figure 5.7 Whole grain. According to food labeling guidelines issued by the FDA, whole grains are the intact, ground, cracked, or flaked seeds of cereal grains.

TABLE 5.7 *Dietary Fiber Content of Common Foods*

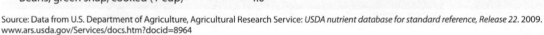

Food	Fiber (g)	Food	Fiber (g)
Split peas, cooked (1 cup)	16.3	Banana, sliced (1 cup)	3.9
Black beans, cooked (1 cup)	15.0	Almonds (24 almonds)	3.5
Kidney beans, canned (1 cup)	13.6	Strawberries, raw, sliced (1 cup)	3.3
Kellogg's All-Bran cereal (⅓ cup)	12.9	Carrots, raw (1 cup)	3.4
Chickpeas, cooked (1 cup)	12.5	Orange, raw (1 orange)	3.1
Dates, chopped (1 cup)	11.8	Baked potato, medium, with skin (approx. 4.5 oz)	3.0
Baked beans, canned (1 cup)	10.4		
Frozen peas, cooked (1 cup)	8.8	Barley, cooked (½ cup)	3.0
Raspberries, raw (1 cup)	8.0	Prunes, dried uncooked (4 prunes)	2.7
Blackberries (1 cup)	7.6	Whole-grain bread (1 slice)	1.9
Kellogg's Raisin Bran (1 cup)	6.5	Romaine lettuce (1 cup)	1.0
Oat bran, ready-to-eat (1 ¼ cup)	5.6	Iceberg lettuce (1 cup)	0.7
Apple, with skin (approx. 6 oz)	4.8	White bread (1 slice)	0.6
Beans, green snap, cooked (1 cup)	4.0		

Source: Data from U.S. Department of Agriculture, Agricultural Research Service: *USDA nutrient database for standard reference, Release 22.* 2009. www.ars.usda.gov/Services/docs.htm?docid=8964

Concept **Checkpoint**

6. What is starch? What is glycogen?
7. What is dietary fiber? Identify at least two food sources of soluble and insoluble fiber.

Did You Know?

The fiber content of different forms of a food can vary widely. For example, an unpeeled raw apple that weighs 6 ounces (about 3 inches in diameter) has 4.4 g of fiber. However, 6 ounces of applesauce contains 2.0 g of fiber, and a 6-ounce serving of apple juice provides only 0.4 g of fiber.

 ## 5.3 What Happens to Carbohydrates in Your Body?

If you eat cooked oatmeal made with milk and sweetened with a little brown sugar for breakfast, what happens to the carbohydrates in these foods? The carbohydrates in oats are primarily starch and fiber; mixing milk and brown sugar with the cereal adds lactose and sucrose. The small intestine is the main site for carbohydrate digestion and absorption, but a minor amount of starch digestion begins in the mouth, as **salivary amylase** converts some of the oat starch molecules into maltose (Fig. 5.8). Starch digestion stops soon after the food enters the acid environment of the stomach.

In the small intestine, an amylase secreted by the pancreas (**pancreatic amylase**) breaks down the remaining polysaccharides in oat starch into maltose molecules. The enzyme maltase digests maltose into glucose molecules. The final products of starch

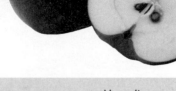

salivary amylase enzyme secreted by salivary glands that begins starch digestion

pancreatic amylase enzyme secreted by pancreas that breaks down starch into maltose molecules

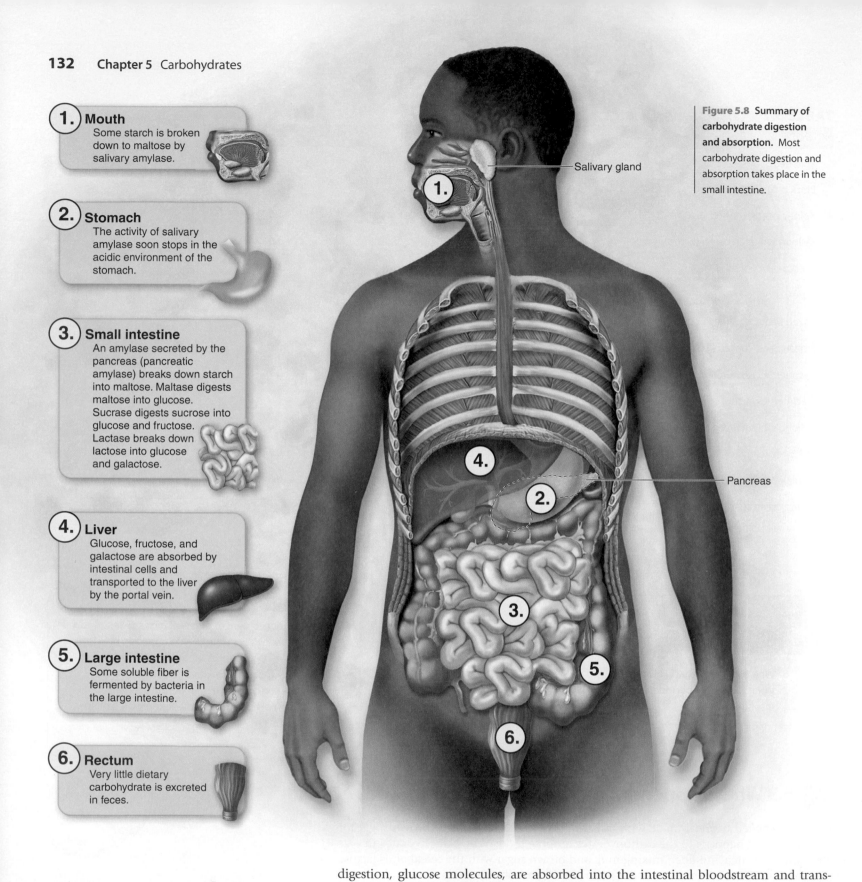

1. Mouth
Some starch is broken down to maltose by salivary amylase.

2. Stomach
The activity of salivary amylase soon stops in the acidic environment of the stomach.

3. Small intestine
An amylase secreted by the pancreas (pancreatic amylase) breaks down starch into maltose. Maltase digests maltose into glucose. Sucrase digests sucrose into glucose and fructose. Lactase breaks down lactose into glucose and galactose.

4. Liver
Glucose, fructose, and galactose are absorbed by intestinal cells and transported to the liver by the portal vein.

5. Large intestine
Some soluble fiber is fermented by bacteria in the large intestine.

6. Rectum
Very little dietary carbohydrate is excreted in feces.

Salivary gland

Pancreas

Figure 5.8 Summary of carbohydrate digestion and absorption. Most carbohydrate digestion and absorption takes place in the small intestine.

digestion, glucose molecules, are absorbed into the intestinal bloodstream and transported to the liver via the hepatic portal vein. Under normal conditions, the process is very efficient and nearly all the starch is digested. The complex carbohydrates that remain are primarily forms of fiber.

The molecules of sucrose in brown sugar and lactose in milk are too large to enter the bloodstream directly from the intestinal tract. The small intestinal enzyme **sucrase** splits each sucrose molecule, forming one glucose and one fructose molecule in the process (see Fig. 5.8). Additionally, the enzyme **lactase** breaks down the lactose from milk into glucose and galactose molecules. Intestinal cells absorb the monosaccharides, and the portal vein

sucrase enzyme that splits sucrose molecule

lactase enzyme that splits lactose molecule

transports them to the liver. The liver can use the simple sugars to make glycogen or fat, but if the body needs energy, the organ releases glucose into the bloodstream.

The fiber in oats is not digested by your small intestine, and it eventually enters the large intestine. The "friendly" intestinal bacteria that reside in the large intestine can break down (ferment) the soluble fiber and metabolize the fermentation products for energy. Soluble fiber is sometimes referred to as *viscous fiber*, because it usually forms a semisolid mass in the intestinal tract that is rapidly fermented by bacterial action. On the other hand, insoluble or fermentation-resistant fiber does not break down completely, and as a result, contributes to softer and easier-to-eliminate bowel movements.[9]

At one time, scientists thought fiber was a nonnutrient because it had no nutritional value. Recent scientific evidence indicates that the body, particularly the cells that line the large intestine, can use by-products produced by the bacterial metabolism of fiber for energy. According to estimates, a gram of fiber adds less than 3 kcal to human diets.[9] The average American consumes only about 15 g of fiber daily; therefore, fiber contributes relatively little to a typical person's energy intake.[10]

Maintaining Blood Glucose Levels

Glucose is such an important cellular fuel, its blood level is carefully maintained by hormones. Hormones are chemicals that convey messages concerning specific responses to target cells. The pancreas, a digestive system organ shown in Figure 4.27 on page 108, contains beta cells, clusters of special cells that produce **insulin,** and groups of alpha cells that produce **glucagon.** These two hormones play key roles in regulating blood glucose levels. Figure 5.9 illustrates the effects of insulin and glucagon on blood glucose levels.

If you are healthy, your body maintains your blood glucose level at between 70 and 100 milligrams per deciliter of blood (mg/dl). If you have not eaten for a while, your blood glucose level begins to fall, you start to feel hungry, and your stomach growls. You may grab an apple or a cheese sandwich to eat, and as the carbohydrates in these foods are digested, the glucose from these foods is absorbed into your bloodstream and transported to the liver. As your blood glucose level begins to rise, your pancreas responds by secreting insulin into the bloodstream (see Fig. 5.9). Insulin helps regulate blood glucose levels because the hormone enables glucose to enter most cells.

Insulin also influences fat and protein metabolism. The hormone enhances energy storage by promoting fat, glycogen, and protein production. Another effect of insulin's action—you feel satisfied with your snack or meal and are no longer hungry.

If you ignore the hunger signals and do not eat, the alpha cells in your pancreas secrete glucagon. Glucagon opposes insulin's effects by promoting the breakdown of glycogen. This

insulin hormone that helps regulate blood glucose levels

glucagon hormone that helps regulate blood glucose levels

glycogenolysis glycogen breakdown

Figure 5.9 Regulating blood glucose. Insulin and glucagon are key hormones in maintaining normal blood glucose concentration. When blood glucose rises above the normal range (1), insulin from the pancreas (2) acts to lower the level (3 and 4), and blood glucose level becomes normal (5). When blood glucose falls below normal (6), glucagon from the pancreas (7) has the opposite effects of insulin (8 and 9), and blood glucose rises to normal levels (10).

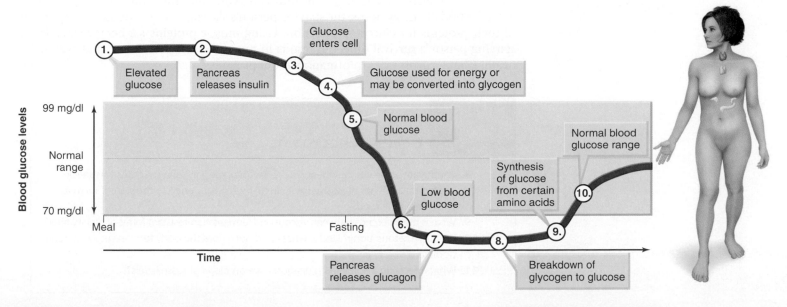

lipolysis fat breakdown

ketone bodies chemicals that result from incomplete fat breakdown

process, called **glycogenolysis** (*lysis* = break down), releases glucose into the bloodstream and as a result, boosts your blood glucose level back to normal (see Fig. 5.9). Glucagon also stimulates liver and kidney cells to produce glucose from certain *amino acids*, the basic molecules that make up proteins. Furthermore, glucagon stimulates **lipolysis** (*lipo* = fat), the breakdown of triglyceride (fat) into *glycerol* and *fatty acids*. As a result, glycerol and fatty acids rapidly enter into the bloodstream. The liver uses glycerol to produce glucose, and most cells, including muscle cells, can metabolize fatty acids for energy. Although the body can convert certain amino acids into glucose, it cannot use fatty acids to make glucose.

What happens to glucose? Its fate depends on the state of your body. If your muscles and other cells that use glucose need energy, glucose enters the cells and is metabolized for energy. When you are well fed and resting, your body stores the extra glucose as glycogen. When glycogen storage reaches maximum capacity, your liver can convert some excess glucose into fat and releases it into the bloodstream. Adipose (*ad'-eh-pose*) (fat) cells remove and store the fat.

Glucose for Energy

Cells metabolize glucose to release the energy stored in the molecule's chemical bonds. As a result of this process, cells form carbon dioxide and water (Fig. 5.10). Glucose is a primary fuel for the body's cells. Furthermore, red blood cells as well as brain and other nervous system cells burn mostly glucose for energy.

Cells need a small amount of glucose to metabolize fat for energy properly. When a person has poorly controlled diabetes, is fasting or starving, or follows a very low-carbohydrate/high-protein diet (the Atkins diet, for example), his or her cells must use greater-than-normal amounts of fat for energy. Under these conditions, there is not enough glucose available for cells to metabolize the fat efficiently, and excessive amounts of *ketone bodies* ("ketones") form as a result. **Ketone bodies** are chemicals that result from the incomplete breakdown of fat. Muscle and brain cells can use ketone bodies for energy, but a condition commonly called *ketosis* occurs when these compounds accumulate in the blood. If not treated, severe ketosis can disrupt the body's ability to maintain normal blood chemistry, resulting in loss of consciousness and even death.

The Recommended Dietary Allowance (RDA) for carbohydrate is 130 g/day.[9] This amount of carbohydrate is enough to prevent ketosis. (The RDAs and other DRIs were discussed in Chapter 3.) To estimate your daily carbohydrate intake, complete the Personal Dietary Analysis at the end of Chapter 5.

Under normal conditions, human cells obtain a small proportion of their energy needs by converting certain amino acids from proteins into glucose. Starvation, however, dramatically alters the body's energy metabolism. Starvation diets lack sources of energy such as glucose and amino acids. The body, however, desperately needs glucose to fuel vital activities such as breathing, transmitting nervous impulses, and pumping blood. To meet the body's energy needs, the starving person's skeletal muscles sacrifice components of their proteins for glucose production. Using muscle proteins for energy extends the starving person's survival time, but results in muscle wasting, weakness, and eventually, death. Chapter 7 provides information about proteins.

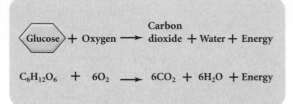

$$\boxed{\text{Glucose} + \text{Oxygen} \longrightarrow \text{Carbon dioxide} + \text{Water} + \text{Energy}}$$

$$C_6H_{12}O_6 + 6O_2 \longrightarrow 6CO_2 + 6H_2O + \text{Energy}$$

Figure 5.10 Releasing energy from glucose. Cells use oxygen to release the energy stored in glucose. As a result of this process, cells produce carbon dioxide and water.

Concept **Checkpoint**

8. Sherita ate some whole-wheat crackers with grape jelly for a snack. As this snack passed through her digestive tract, discuss what happened to the starch, sucrose, and fiber in the food.

9. What is the difference between viscous and fermentation-resistant forms of dietary fiber?

10. What is a ketone body? Under what conditions does the body form excessive ketone bodies?

11. What effects do insulin and glucagon have on blood glucose levels?

5.4 Carbohydrate Consumption Patterns

In developing nations, millions of people rely on diets that supply 70% or more of energy from relatively unprocessed carbohydrates, especially complex carbohydrates from whole grains, beans, potatoes, corn, and other starchy vegetables. In industrialized nations, people tend to eat more highly refined starches and added sugars. Nutritionally adequate diets should provide 45 to 65% of total energy from carbohydrates.[9] The diet of the typical American, 2 years of age and older, supplies about 50% of calories from carbohydrates, much of which is sugars added to foods during processing (Fig. 5.11).

According to MyPlate discussed in Chapter 3, added sugars are grouped with solid fats as empty calories. Most people only have about 100 to 300 empty calories allowed in their personal dietary plans. For example, if your individual dietary plan indicates that you need 2000 kcal daily, then at least 1740 kcal will need to be "spent" consuming foods rich in essential nutrients.[11] The 260 kcal that remain are empty calories, some of which can be used by eating foods with added sugars.

In 2008, the average American consumed about 30 teaspoons of added sugars daily—about 23% of the energy in a diet that supplies 2000 kcal/day.[1] A 12-ounce can of a cola-flavored, sugar-sweetened soft drink contains about 32 g of HFCS, a refined sugar.[12] Each gram of sugar supplies 4 kcal, so this soft drink contributes about 128 kcal to the diet. By drinking only one can of the cola, a person who needs 2000 kcal daily will almost meet one-half of his or her daily limit for the intake of empty calories.

A 12-ounce serving of 100% orange juice supplies about the same amount of sugar as 12 ounces of a sugar-sweetened cola. Because they both contain simple sugars, should you drink regular soft drinks instead of fruit juices? Unlike colas and other soft drinks, 100% fruit juices, such as orange, grapefruit, and cranberry juice, contribute water-soluble vitamins and antioxidant phytochemicals to your diet. According to MyPlate, adults should consume 1½ to 2 cups of fruit or fruit equivalents each day.

Regular soft drinks and energy drinks are major sources of added sugars in Americans' diets.[13] Although energy drink consumption has increased, soft drink consumption has declined since 1999–2000. In 2008, however, the average American drank about 47 gallons of soft drinks, or about 17 fluid ounces of these beverages daily, most of which are sweetened with refined sugars.[14] How many fluid ounces of energy drinks and/or sugar-sweetened soft drinks do you consume each day?

Reducing Your Intake of Refined Carbohydrates

Regular soft drinks, energy drinks, cookies, chips, and many other types of processed snack foods contain large amounts of refined carbohydrates, including added sugars. Such foods may satisfy your hunger and thirst, but they may be crowding out more nutritious items from your diet. If you frequently purchase foods and beverages from vending machines, convenience stores, or fast-food restaurants, you are probably eating unhealthy amounts of refined carbohydrates. Some fast-food restaurants and college cafeterias sell yogurt, fresh fruit, and fat-free or low-fat milk as well as unsweetened fruit juices. With a little advance planning, you can prepare your own portable, tasty, and nutritious snacks. For example, place whole fresh fruit or small plastic containers filled with chunks of fresh fruit and pieces of vegetables into your purse or book bag to eat during the day. At home, keep a bowl of fresh grapes, apples, bananas, or other easy-to-eat fruit available for handy snacks, and eat fresh fruit for dessert. Most fruits contain a variety of antioxidants, and they have less fat and more fiber, vitamins, and minerals than pastries or chips.

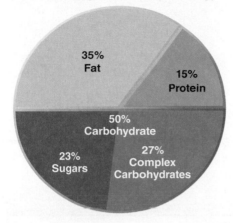

Average Percentage of Calories per Person (One Day)

35% Fat · 15% Protein · 50% Carbohydrate · 23% Sugars · 27% Complex Carbohydrates

Figure 5.11 Average macronutrient intakes. This graph shows the average American's intake of macronutrients as percentages of total kilocalories from macronutrients (2041) on one day in 2007–2008. (Percentage of total energy from alcohol is not included.) *Source: Data from U.S. Department of Agriculture, Agricultural Research Service. Nutrient intakes from food. 2010. http://www.ars.usda.gov/SP2UserFiles/Place/12355000/pdf/0708/Table_1_NIN_GEN_07.pdf*

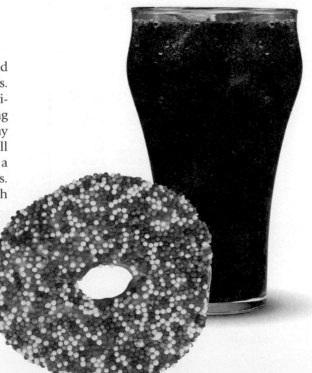

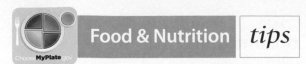

Food & Nutrition | *tips*

- Replace soft drinks with a naturally calorie-free thirst-quencher—plain water.
- Make plain water more interesting to drink by adding to it a slice of lemon or lime, or a few fresh or frozen berries.
- Add 1 part club soda to 1 part orange or other 100% fruit juice to make a refreshing carbonated drink.
- Read the label for information about juice content when selecting a fruit juice product. Fruit "drinks," "punches," "blends," "cocktails," or "ades" often contain added sugars and only 10% fruit juice.
- In addition to water, manufacturers typically use apple or grape juice to dilute more expensive fruit juices, such as cranberry juice. Therefore, beverage descriptors such as "100% juice" or "pure juice" can be misleading. Read the ingredient list on the label to determine the types of juices used to prepare the product.

Concept **Checkpoint**

12. What is the primary source of added sugars in the typical American diet?
13. Instead of drinking orange juice, should you choose a beverage called "Orange-Ade"? Explain why or why not.

5.5 Understanding Nutrient Labeling: Carbohydrates and Fiber

You can learn how much total carbohydrate, sugars, and dietary fiber are in packaged foods and beverages by reading the Nutrition Facts panel of a food label. As you can see in Figure 5.12, total grams of carbohydrate in a slice (one serving) of whole-wheat bread is listed, and under it, grams of fiber and sugar. Food labels for high-fiber products, such as whole-grain cereals, may indicate amounts of soluble and insoluble fiber in a serving of the product. In 2011, information about sugar content did not distinguish between added sugars and sugars naturally present in the food. The new label format may include this information.

According to the label shown in Figure 5.12, 17 g of carbohydrate are in one serving (a slice) of the bread; of this amount, sugar contributes 3 g and fiber supplies 2 g. How can you estimate the grams of starch in the serving of bread? In this example, add the number of grams of sugar with that of fiber and subtract this amount from grams of total carbohydrates, and you will find that starch comprises 12 g of the carbohydrate in the slice of whole-wheat bread. If you are interested in the types of sugars used to make a product, read the ingredient list at the bottom of the panel. In this product, there are three sources of sugar. Can you identify them? Check the nutritive sweeteners listed in Table 5.2 to see if your answers are correct.

Nutrition Facts

Serving Size 1 slice (38 g)
Servings Per Container 18

Amount Per Serving

Calories 100
 Calories from Fat 20

	% Daily Value*
Total Fat 2g	3%
Saturated Fat 0g	0%
Trans Fat 0g	
Polyunsaturated Fat 1g	
Monounsaturated Fat 0g	
Cholesterol 0mg	0%
Sodium 160mg	7%
Total Carbohydrate 17g	6%
Dietary Fiber 2g	8%
Sugars 3g	
Protein 4g	

Vitamin A	10%
Vitamin C	0%
Calcium	10%
Iron	8%

* Percent Daily Values are based on a 2,000 calorie diet. Your daily values may be higher or lower, depending on your calorie needs:

	Calories	2,000	2,500
Total Fat	Less than	65g	80g
Sat Fat	Less than	20g	25g
Cholesterol	Less than	300mg	300mg
Sodium	Less than	2,400mg	2,400mg
Total Carbohydrate		300g	375g
Dietary Fiber		25g	30g

INGREDIENTS: Whole-wheat flour, Water, Brown sugar, Wheat gluten, Cracked wheat, Wheat bran, Yeast, Salt, Molasses, Soybean oil, Calcium propionate (preservative), Mono–and diglycerides, Lecithin, Reduced fat milk

Figure 5.12 Using the Nutrition Facts panel (2011). This Nutrition Facts panel from a package of whole-wheat bread displays carbohydrate content, including amounts of dietary fiber and sugars.

Concept **Checkpoint**

14. According to the Nutrition Facts panel, a serving of ready-to-eat cereal contains 44 g of total carbohydrate, 5 g of dietary fiber, and 10 g of sugars. Estimate the grams of starch in the serving of the cereal.

5.6 Carbohydrates and Health

Carbohydrates seem to get a lot of "bad press." Promoters of low-carbohydrate/high-protein diets often blame sugars and starches for causing obesity and diabetes. Many Americans think consuming sugary foods causes depression and hyperactive behavior. On the other hand, "carbs" are welcomed by athletes as an inexpensive and efficient source of energy. What have scientists learned about the roles of carbohydrates in health?

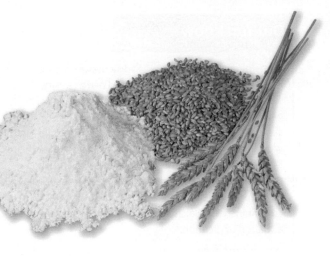

Are Carbohydrates Fattening?

If you are one of millions of overweight Americans who has tried to lose weight recently, you may have followed a fad low-carbohydrate diet, such as the Atkins, Sugar Busters!, or the Zone diet, to shed the extra fat. A fad is a practice that gains widespread popularity rapidly and then loses its appeal quickly when people tire of the behavior or follow a newer trend. Americans are fatter now than they were 20 years ago. Are carbohydrates responsible for the epidemic of excess body fat in the United States?

"Calories do count," because you will gain body fat if your intake of food energy from macronutrients and the nonnutrient alcohol exceeds your output of energy for metabolic, physical activity, and other physiological needs. Regardless of whether you eat a high-carbohydrate, high-fat, or high-protein diet, you will maintain your weight as long as your energy intake matches your energy output. Foods that contain large amounts of refined carbohydrates, however, do not satisfy hunger as well as those that contain more protein or fat. As a result, you may become hungrier sooner after eating a meal or snack that contains a lot of added sugars and refined starches than if you ate a high-protein, high-fat meal or snack. Thus, a person following a high-protein, high-fat diet can lose weight in the short term, because the diet keeps his or her appetite under control by reducing hunger. On the other hand, diets in which carbohydrates supply more than 70% of a person's energy needs also result in weight loss, particularly when the diets include foods that are rich in fiber and contain plenty of unrefined starches.[15] People following such high-carbohydrate diets generally eat less, because fiber-rich foods tend to be more filling than similar amounts of food that contain a lot of refined carbohydrates.[16]

Metabolism plays a major role in the development of obesity. When a person consumes excess carbohydrate, his or her body converts some of the glucose into fat, but much of the excess is "burned" as a biological fuel. As a result, dietary fat is spared from being used as a fuel and stored in fat cells.[17] Thus, eating too much carbohydrate indirectly contributes to excess body fat.

Foods that contain a lot of added sugars and fats tend to be energy dense. Thus, people can reduce their energy intake by eating fewer energy-dense foods.[18] Fats supply 9 kcal/g compared to only 4 kcal/g of carbohydrates, so adding even small amounts of fat to food can dramatically increase its energy content. People, however, tend to blame carbohydrates for their unwanted weight gain because starches and sugars are often combined with hidden fats such as butter, oil, or shortening (a solid fat) in processed foods. Fats make foods taste rich, creamy, and difficult to resist. Moreover, the sweet taste of sugar masks the bland taste of fat. Although you would not consider eating spoonfuls of plain sugar, flour, shortening, or butter, your mouth waters at the sight of candy bars, fruit pies, doughnuts, and other baked or fried foods, and like many people, you probably find it is difficult to resist eating these foods.

During the past 35 years, the percentage of obese Americans rose dramatically. During this same period, Americans substantially increased their consumption of HFCS. Some nutrition scientists think Americans' love of foods and beverages sweetened with HFCS is largely responsible for the population's rising rate of obesity.[19] The rising prevalence of obesity among children is a major public health concern; regular soft drinks are the primary source of added sugar in the diets of American children[20] and high school

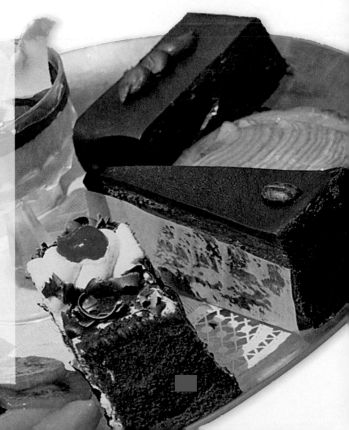

Many people find it difficult to resist foods that contain a lot of sugar and fat, such as cheesecake.

Many people think sucrose is addictive. Addiction is characterized by an uncontrolled need (compulsion) to take a substance and the development of withdrawal signs and symptoms when the substance is not taken.[22] Many people, especially women, report an extreme preference for sweet fatty foods, such as cakes and pastries. However, there is no scientific evidence that people can become addicted to foods, particularly those containing sucrose, as cigarette smokers become addicted to nicotine.[23]

diabetes mellitus (diabetes) group of serious chronic diseases characterized by abnormal glucose, fat, and protein metabolism

hyperglycemia abnormally high blood glucose level

TABLE 5.8 *Classifying Diabetes Mellitus*

Blood Glucose Level (Fasting)	Classification
70 to 99 mg/dl	Normal
100 to 125 mg/dl	Pre-diabetes
126 mg/dl or more	Diabetes

students.[21] School boards in many communities are so concerned about the epidemic of childhood obesity, they have banned empty-calorie foods, including sugar-sweetened soft drinks, from school cafeterias and vending machines. Is there a connection between consumption of regular soft drinks and excess body fat?

The role that regular soft drink consumption plays in the development of obesity is controversial.[19] Findings from some scientific studies suggest that people who drink regular soft drinks do not reduce their energy intake from solid food accordingly.[24] The reasons are unclear, but the fructose in these beverages may not reduce the urge to eat as does solid food. As a result, consumers of regular soft drinks ("liquid candy") are likely to overeat and have excessive energy intakes. If, for example, you begin to drink three 12-ounce cans of a cola-flavored sugar-sweetened soft drink per day, you will obtain about 410 extra kilocalories daily. Unless you increase your daily physical activity level to metabolize the 410 kcal or cut back your food intake by 410 kcal each day, you are likely to gain over 3 pounds of fat in four weeks! By contributing to unwanted weight gain, consumption of regular soft drinks may increase the risk of type 2 diabetes, the most common form of the disease.[25]

Although consumption of regular soft drinks has increased over the past few decades, other dietary changes have occurred during this period. In 2008, the average American consumed about 500 kcal/day more than the typical person did in 1970.[26] Grains, fats and oils, and sugars accounted for 45%, 21%, and 14%, respectively, of the average person's increased energy intake. Therefore, Americans' overall dietary habits, including intakes of pizza, baked goods, and other refined grain products, may be partly to blame for rising rates of obesity among the U.S. population.

What Is Diabetes?

Diabetes mellitus (diabetes) is actually a group of serious chronic diseases characterized by abnormal glucose, fat, and protein metabolism.[27] There are two major types of diabetes mellitus—type 1 and type 2 diabetes. About 5 to 10% of people with diabetes have type 1; in the past, this form of diabetes was called "juvenile diabetes" because it was diagnosed more often in children and young adults. Type 1 diabetes, however, can strike at any age.[28] The majority of people with diabetes have type 2, which used to be called "adult-onset diabetes." As in the case of type 1 diabetes, type 2 can affect any person, regardless of age.

The primary sign of diabetes is **hyperglycemia** (*hyper* = excess; *glycemia* = blood glucose), abnormally elevated blood glucose levels. A person's blood glucose levels are usually measured after he or she has not eaten (has fasted) for about 12 hours. Normal fasting blood glucose levels are 70 to 99 mg/dl (Table 5.8). People with *pre-diabetes* have fasting blood glucose levels that are 100 to 125 mg/dl. Individuals who have fasting blood glucose levels of 126 mg/dl or more have diabetes.

Some people with diabetes experience hyperglycemia because their beta cells do not produce any insulin or do not produce enough to meet their needs. In other cases, the affected person produces some insulin, but his or her body

2010
(18.8)

2005
(15.8)

2000
(12.0)

Estimated number of Americans diagnosed with diabetes (millions)

1995
(8.0)

1990
(6.6)

1985
(6.2)

1980
(5.6)

does not respond properly to the hormone, and hyperglycemia results. Major signs and symptoms of hyperglycemia include excessive thirst, frequent urination, blurred vision, and poor wound healing (Table 5.9). Over time, untreated or poorly controlled hyperglycemia damages nerves, organs, and blood vessels. In fact, poorly controlled diabetes is a major cause of heart disease, kidney failure, blindness, and lower limb amputations. In 2009, diabetes was the seventh leading cause of death in the United States.[28]

In the United States, the prevalence of diabetes is increasing at an alarming rate. In 2010, an estimated 25.8 million Americans had diabetes; 18.8 million of these persons were diagnosed with diabetes, and the remainder did not know they had the disease.[28] According to the Centers for Disease Control and Prevention (CDC), an estimated 79 million Americans had pre-diabetes in 2010. The prevalence of diabetes increases with advancing age; about 27% of Americans who are 65 years of age or older have diabetes.[28] Children also develop diabetes. Public health officials are very concerned about the increasing number of children and adolescents who have diabetes, particularly type 2 diabetes.

Type 1 Diabetes

Type 1 diabetes is an *autoimmune* disease that occurs when certain immune system cells malfunction and do not recognize the body's own beta cells.[29] As a result, the immune system cells attack and destroy the beta cells, and the affected person must obtain insulin regularly. It is not clear why the immune cells of some individuals malfunction, but genetic susceptibility and environmental factors, particularly exposure to certain viral intestinal infections, are associated with the development of type 1 diabetes.[30] Infants who drink cow's milk based formulas may have a greater risk of developing type 1 diabetes than breastfed babies.[31] Nevertheless, the association between type 1 diabetes and consuming cow's milk or infant formulas made from cow's milk is controversial. The role of dietary factors in the development of type 1 diabetes continues to undergo scientific study.

Tyler Smith has type 1 diabetes. You can learn about him and how he manages his health by reading the Real People, Real Stories feature on page 147.

Type 2 Diabetes

The most common form of diabetes is type 2 diabetes. Beta cells of people with type 2 diabetes usually produce insulin, but the hormone's target cells are insulin-resistant cells, which do not respond properly to the hormone and do not allow glucose to enter them. As a result, the level of glucose in the bloodstream becomes abnormally elevated and the signs of diabetes occur.

Over the past 20 years, the number of adults and children with type 2 diabetes has reached epidemic proportions in the United States. Certain people have greater risk of type 2 diabetes than others. Individuals who are physically inactive (sedentary), overweight or obese, and genetically related to a close family member with type 2 diabetes are more likely to develop the disease than persons who do not have these characteristics. Additionally, Americans who have Hispanic, Native American, Asian, African, or Pacific Islander ancestry are more likely to develop type 2 diabetes than Americans who are not members of these racial/ethnic groups.[28] The American Diabetes Association has an online questionnaire that you can take to assess your risk of type 2 diabetes (www.diabetes.org/diabetes-basics/prevention/diabetes-risk-test/).

Gestational Diabetes   Women may develop diabetes during pregnancy (*gestational diabetes*). The fetus of a woman with poorly controlled gestational diabetes receives too much glucose from its hyperglycemic mother. As a result, the fetus gains weight rapidly and can be abnormally heavy at birth, weighing 9 pounds or more. Giving birth to such a large infant is risky for the mother as well as the baby, because the birth process is often prolonged in such cases.[32] Furthermore, women with gestational diabetes are more

TABLE 5.9 *Signs and Symptoms of Diabetes Mellitus*

Signs and Symptoms
Elevated blood glucose levels
Excessive thirst
Frequent urination
Blurry vision
Vaginal yeast infections (adult women)
Foot pain, abdominal pain
Numbness
Impotence (male)
Sores that do not heal
Increased appetite with weight loss*
Breath that smells like fruit*
Fatigues easily*
Confusion*

* Typical symptoms of poorly controlled type 1 rather than type 2 diabetes.

Figure 5.13 Managing diabetes. Nine-year-old Carson Smith was diagnosed with type 1 diabetes when he was 5 years of age. (*a*) Carson checks his blood glucose at least four times a day. (*b*) After obtaining information about Carson's blood glucose level, his parents determine the amount and type of insulin he needs, and Carson uses a special device to inject the insulin into his body.

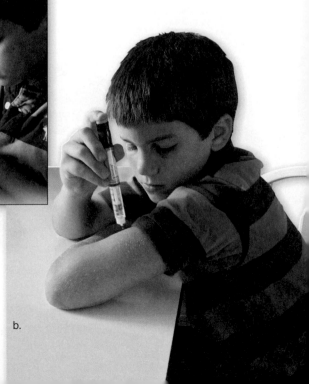

a.

b.

likely to have babies who have difficulty controlling their own blood glucose levels. Some women who have gestational diabetes continue to have diabetes after delivery of their babies. Furthermore, women who recover from gestational diabetes are more likely to develop type 2 diabetes within 5 to 10 years, compared to women who did not develop diabetes during pregnancy.

Controlling Diabetes

To avoid or delay serious health complications, people who have diabetes need to achieve and maintain normal or near-normal blood glucose levels. Many people with diabetes rely on daily blood testing to monitor their blood glucose levels (Fig. 5.13). Physicians can measure *glycated hemoglobin,* also called glycosylated hemoglobin or *hemoglobin A1c* ("HbA1c"), to determine their patients' average blood glucose levels over longer periods. Results of this blood test can provide information about a patient's long-term management of the condition.

Hemoglobin is the compound in red blood cells that carries oxygen. HbA1c is a component of hemoglobin that attracts some glucose that is in blood. About 5% of a healthy person's hemoglobin is HbA1c. A person with poorly controlled diabetes often has blood glucose levels that are much higher than normal. As a result, this individual's hemoglobin will have a higher percentage of HbA1c. People with diabetes should strive to maintain their HbA1c level below 7%. [33]

Proper blood glucose management involves monitoring blood glucose levels regularly and carefully following a special diet that usually includes counting grams of carbohydrate. Including physical activity in one's daily routine is also recommended. People with type 2 diabetes who are overweight can often reduce their insulin resistance by losing small amounts of excess body fat.[34] Additionally, exercise increases glucose uptake by muscles, reducing blood glucose levels and improving the body's insulin response. In some instances, however, people with type 2 diabetes need oral medication to stimulate their bodies' insulin production, or they must receive insulin injections.

Promoters of certain weight reduction diets claim that people can lose weight or control diabetes by following *low glycemic index* diets. However, some medical experts question the value of the glycemic index for predicting the body's blood glucose level after eating. To learn more about the glycemic index and glycemic load, read the "Highlight" on page 148.

Can Diabetes Be Prevented?

There is no way to prevent type 1 diabetes. However, you may reduce your risk of type 2 diabetes by losing excess weight (if necessary), exercising regularly, and eating less fat and fewer total calories.[35] Medical experts refer to these actions as *therapeutic lifestyle changes* (TLC).

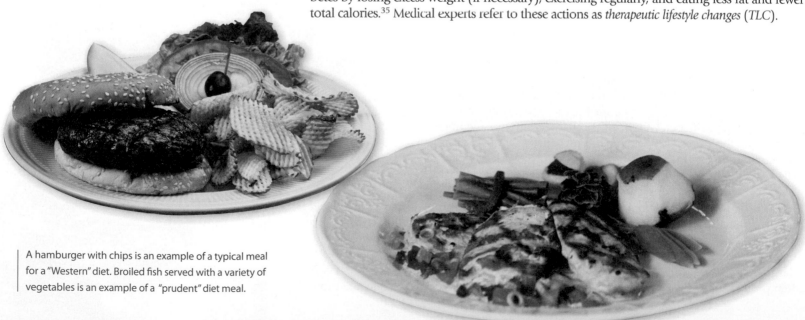

A hamburger with chips is an example of a typical meal for a "Western" diet. Broiled fish served with a variety of vegetables is an example of a "prudent" diet meal.

Certain eating habits may help prevent type 2 diabetes. The typical American diet ("Western diet") contains high amounts of red meat, processed meats, French fries, high-fat dairy foods, and refined sugars and starches. Diets that contain more poultry, fish, and fiber-rich whole grains, fruits, and vegetables than the Western diet are referred to as "prudent diets." People who follow prudent diets have a lower risk of developing type 2 diabetes than people who consume Western diets.[36,37,38] Some medical experts are concerned that diets that contain excess sugar, particularly fructose, may increase the risk for type 2 diabetes and other serious chronic diseases.[39]

Currently, there is no cure for diabetes. Medical researchers, however, are testing promising new treatments, such as transplanting beta cells from a donor pancreas into the pancreas of a person with diabetes. Since it may take several years before a safe and effective therapy is available, at this time, the best "cure" for diabetes is prevention, if possible.

> **hypoglycemia** condition that occurs when the blood glucose level is abnormally low
>
> **epinephrine** hormone produced by adrenal glands; also called adrenalin
>
> **metabolic syndrome** condition that increases risk of type 2 diabetes and CVD
>
> **syndrome** group of signs and symptoms that occur together and indicate a specific health problem

What Is Hypoglycemia?

If you are healthy and have not eaten for a while, your blood glucose levels decline, and you become hungry. Eating a meal or snack raises your blood glucose. **Hypoglycemia** (*hypo* = low) is a condition that occurs when the blood glucose level is too low to provide enough energy for cells.

Hypoglycemia may be diagnosed when the blood glucose level is less than 70 mg/dl.[40] In response to rapidly declining blood glucose levels, the body responds by secreting **epinephrine,** a hormone that is produced by the adrenal glands (see Fig. 4.18 [endocrine system] on page 103). You may be more familiar with epinephrine's common name, *adrenalin*. Like glucagon, epinephrine increases the supply of glucose and fatty acids in the bloodstream, but the hormone can also make a person with hypoglycemia feel irritable, restless, shaky, and sweaty. If the blood glucose level drops too low, the affected person can become confused, and he or she may lose consciousness and die.

Several years ago, popular books and magazine articles warned Americans about the dangers of hypoglycemia and its signs and symptoms. Many people became convinced that they suffered from the condition. Although hypoglycemia is a serious disorder that can affect people with diabetes mellitus and certain tumors of the pancreas, it rarely affects otherwise healthy persons. Some people develop *reactive hypoglycemia* after they eat highly refined carbohydrates because the pancreas responds by releasing too much insulin. However, these individuals generally have normal fasting blood glucose levels. People with reactive hypoglycemia may feel better if they avoid eating large amounts of sugary foods and eat smaller, more frequent meals that contain a mixture of macronutrients.

Metabolic Syndrome

Do you or does someone you know have a "spare tire," "beer belly," "love handles," or an "apple shape"? These popular terms describe a physical condition that has become common among adult Americans as the prevalence of overweight and obesity increases. People who are too fat often have excess abdominal fat, which can be dangerous, especially when it is accompanied by hypertension and elevated blood lipid (triglyceride and cholesterol) levels.

An estimated 47 million Americans have **metabolic syndrome,** a condition characterized by three or more of the signs listed in Table 5.10.[41] A **syndrome** is a group of signs and symptoms that occur together and indicate a specific health problem. Compared to people who do not have metabolic syndrome, individuals with

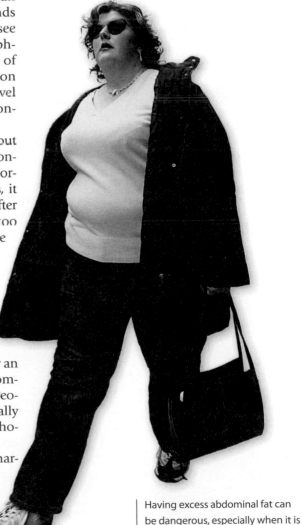

Having excess abdominal fat can be dangerous, especially when it is accompanied by hypertension and elevated blood lipid levels.

TABLE 5.10 *Signs of Metabolic Syndrome*

Sign	Defining Value
*Large waist circumference**	≥ 40 inches (men)
	≥ 35 inches (women)
Chronically elevated blood pressure (hypertension)	≥ 130 mm Hg systolic (upper value)
	or
	≥ 85 mm Hg diastolic (lower value)
	or
	Drug treatment for hypertension
Chronically elevated fasting blood fats (triglycerides)	≥ 150 mg/dl
	or
	Drug treatment for elevated triglycerides
Low fasting high-density lipoprotein cholesterol (HDL cholesterol)	< 40 mg/dl (men)
	< 50 mg/dl (women)
	or
	Drug treatment for reduced HDL
High fasting blood glucose	≥ 100 mg/dl
	or
	Drug treatment for elevated glucose

* To measure your waist circumference, remove clothing from the midsection of your body. Locate the top of your hip bones and place a flexible measuring tape around your abdomen at the top of the bones. Exhale normally and take the measurement. (The measuring tape should fit snugly around your waist without pinching the skin and be parallel to floor.)

Source: Data from Grundy SM and others: Diagnosis and management of the metabolic syndrome: An American Heart Association/National Heart, Lung, and Blood Institute scientific statement: Executive summary. *Circulation* 112:e285, 2005.

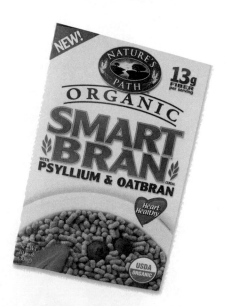

Eating more fiber-rich foods, such as whole-grain cereals, may reduce the risk of metabolic syndrome.

this condition have about five times the risk of type 2 diabetes and almost twice the risk of heart and blood vessel (cardiovascular) disease.[42]

Although genetic factors play a major role in the development of metabolic syndrome, excess abdominal fat and insulin resistance are the primary risk factors for the condition.[43] Poor diet, cigarette smoking, and lack of regular physical activity also contribute to the development of the syndrome. People may lower their likelihood of developing metabolic syndrome by increasing their intake of fruits and vegetables and other fiber-rich foods, such as whole-grain cereals.[44]

Individuals who already have metabolic syndrome may reduce their risk of cardiovascular disease (CVD) by lowering their elevated blood pressure, glucose, insulin, and triglyceride levels. Lifestyle changes that can help manage these levels include losing excess weight, exercising regularly, reducing intakes of salt, saturated fat, cholesterol, and simple sugars,[44] and eating oily fish at least twice a week.[43] If such TLC do not alleviate the condition, medication may be necessary to manage blood pressure and blood lipid levels. Chapter 6 provides more information about cardiovascular disease.

Tooth Decay

Tooth decay is clearly associated with consuming carbohydrates, particularly simple sugars that stick to teeth. If a person does not follow good dental hygiene practices, the debris becomes food for bacteria that live on teeth. As the bacteria metabolize carbohydrate for their energy needs, the acid they produce damages tooth enamel and results in decay.

Infants and young children who drink bedtime bottles of milk, juice, or other beverages that contain sugars are susceptible to "nursing bottle syndrome" (see Fig. 13.10 on page 486). When a sleepy child sucks slowly on the bottle, the carbohydrate-rich solution stays in contact with teeth, increasing the likelihood of dental decay and, eventually, the loss of primary teeth. To reduce the risk of nursing bottle syndrome, offer a young child a bottle of plain water to drink at bedtime.

Lactose Intolerance

Millions of Americans suffer from **lactose intolerance** (also referred to as lactose maldigestion), the inability to digest lactose completely. Lactose-intolerant people do not produce enough lactase, the enzyme that breaks lactose into glucose and galactose. Lactose intolerance is not the same as milk allergy, which is an immune system response to cow's milk proteins. Milk allergy is most likely to occur during infancy; lactose intolerance is more likely to occur in adulthood.[45]

When a lactose-intolerant person consumes lactose, the disaccharide is not completely digested and absorbed by the time it enters the large intestine. Bacteria that reside in the large intestine break down lactose and produce irritating gases and acids as metabolic by-products. As a result, a lactose-intolerant person usually experiences intestinal cramps, bloating, gas, and diarrhea within a couple of hours after consuming milk or other lactose-containing products.

Normally, infants produce lactase, but by the time children are 2 years old, their small intestine begins to produce less of the enzyme. Many older children and adults, particularly those with African, Asian, and Eastern European ancestry, are lactose intolerant and experience some degree of abdominal discomfort after drinking milk.

Milk and milk products are excellent sources of protein, many vitamins, and the minerals calcium and phosphorus. What can people with lactose intolerance do to achieve a nutritionally adequate diet without drinking milk? Lactose-intolerant people are often able to eat hard cheeses and yogurt without experiencing any digestive tract discomfort. Milk loses most of its lactose content when it is processed to make aged cheeses, such as cheddar and Swiss. The bacteria used to make yogurt convert much of the lactose in milk to lactic acid, and the microbes assist with the digestion of the remaining lactose even after the yogurt is eaten.[46]

Some people with lactose intolerance discover through trial and error that they can consume small amounts of milk without experiencing intestinal discomfort. If you suspect you cannot digest lactose, try consuming a smaller-than-usual size serving of milk and note if you have intestinal discomfort within a few hours. People who cannot tolerate even limited amounts of fresh fluid milk can probably drink milk that has been pretreated with lactase to reduce its lactose content. Most large supermarkets sell fresh lactase-treated milk in the dairy food section (Fig. 5.14). Also, lactase-containing solutions and pills are available without prescription. A lactose-intolerant person simply adds a small amount of the solution to fresh milk before drinking the beverage or takes one of the pills with lactose-containing food. People who cannot tolerate lactose can substitute soy milk for cows' milk, because soy milk does not contain lactose.

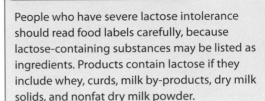

lactose intolerance inability to digest lactose properly

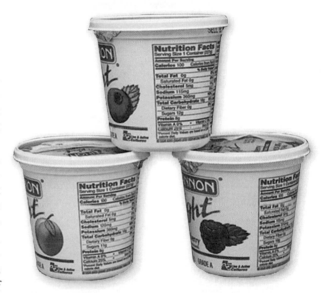

Lactose-intolerant people may be able to eat yogurt without experiencing digestive tract discomfort.

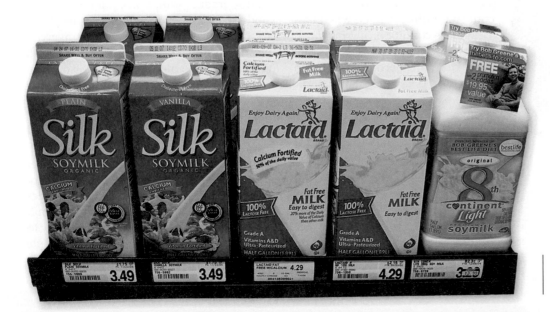

Figure 5.14 Lactase-treated milk. Fresh lactase-treated milk is often available near soy milk in the dairy section of supermarkets.

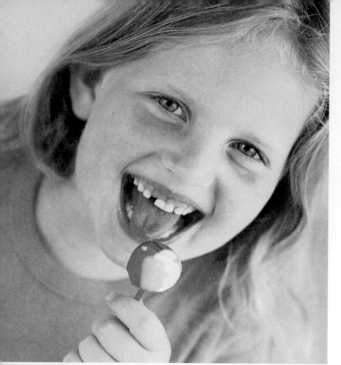

Contrary to popular belief, eating sugary foods does not cause hyperactive behavior.

diverticula abnormal, tiny sacs that form in wall of colon

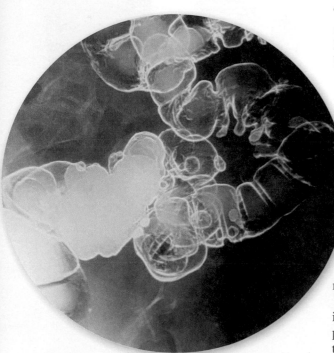

Figure 5.15 Diverticula. Constipation can increase the risk of diverticulosis, a condition characterized by the formation of tiny pouches (*diverticula*) in the lining of the large intestine. In this color-enhanced x-ray, the blue areas are diverticula.

Does Sugar Cause Hyperactivity?

If you have ever been in charge of a 7-year-old child's birthday party or observed third graders preparing for their Halloween celebration, you can understand why people often blame sugary foods for causing unruly and "hyperactive" behavior. Attention deficit hyperactivity disorder (ADHD) is characterized by impulsivity and difficulty controlling behavior and/or paying attention.[47] By 2007, approximately 5.4 million American children had been diagnosed with ADHD at some point in their lives.[48] Although the cause of ADHD is uncertain, it probably involves genetic and environmental factors. Eating sweets can produce pleasurable sensations, but the results of scientific studies do not indicate that sugar increases children's physical activity levels, causes ADHD, or otherwise negatively affects their behavior.[47] Birthday and school parties are exciting and happy occasions that typically involve a radical change from a child's usual routine. In these situations, a youngster's excitement and more active behavior is more likely to be the result of the occasion rather than a particular food.

Fiber and Health

Technically, fiber is not a nutrient, because the human body can live without it. You can live *better*, however, by adding fiber-rich foods to your diet. Eating high-fiber foods may reduce your risk of obesity, diabetes, certain intestinal tract disorders, and cardiovascular disease, which includes heart disease and stroke. The importance of adequate fiber intake to health is so well recognized that information about a food's fiber content can be found on the food labels of most packaged foods. The following information discusses some roles of fiber in health.

Fiber and the Digestive Tract

"Bloated, constipated, or irregular? Feeling sluggish? You need a laxative!" According to TV advertisements often targeted at older adults, millions of Americans suffer from "irregularity" that can be corrected by taking various over-the-counter remedies. Are serious health problems linked to bowel habits? Can making certain dietary changes improve bowel functioning? What causes intestinal gas?

The frequency and ease of bowel movements influence the health of the large intestine. Constipation (infrequent bowel movements) often results in straining to expel feces during bowel movements. Such straining can increase pressure inside the large intestine and force small portions of tissue to form tiny sacs called colonic **diverticula** (Fig. 5.15). In most people, diverticula do not produce symptoms, but they can become painfully inflamed when bacteria and food particles are trapped within them. When this condition (*diverticulitis*) occurs, the affected person may need surgery to remove the damaged section of large intestine. Hemorrhoids are clusters of small rectal veins that become swollen, making them likely to bleed and cause discomfort and itching (Fig. 5.16). This condition commonly affects adults and may be more likely to occur when a person sits for long periods or strains during bowel movements. Although hemorrhoids are generally not a sign of a serious health problem, you should consult a physician if you experience any bleeding during bowel movements, because it may also be a sign of colorectal cancer, a major cancer site for Americans.

Your diet, particularly its fiber content, affects your bowel habits. The insoluble fiber in food attracts water and swells in the digestive tract, forming a large, soft mass that applies pressure to the inner muscular walls of the large intestine, stimulating the muscles to push the residue quickly through the tract. People who often eat foods that contain insoluble fiber have softer and more regular bowel movements, and they are less likely to strain while having bowel movements than people whose diets lack fiber. Thus, people generally do not need to rely on over-the-counter laxatives to treat constipation. Eating more fiber-rich foods is the natural way to become "regular."

Fiber and Colorectal Cancer In the United States and throughout the world, colon or *colorectal* cancer (cancer of the two lower portions of the large intestine) is one of the most common cancers.[49,50] In the early 1970s, a group of scientists noted that rural African populations who typically ate high-fiber diets rarely developed colorectal cancer. When these populations moved to urban areas and adopted relatively low-fiber Western diets, their risk of colorectal cancer increased. As a result of these observations, the scientists suggested that high-fiber diets were protective against colorectal cancer. By 2005, however, an analysis of the results of several large epidemiological studies indicated diets high in dietary fiber did not reduce the risk of colorectal cancer.[51] Other research indicates that eating *whole* grains,[52] fruits, and vegetables may help protect against the disease.[53] Nutrition experts recommend eating high-fiber foods because they provide other important health benefits, such as reducing the risk of cardiovascular disease.[54]

Fiber and Heart Health

Diets rich in fiber, particularly soluble types of fiber, can reduce the risk of cardiovascular disease by reducing blood cholesterol levels.[54] High blood levels of cholesterol are associated with increased risks of cardiovascular disease. The liver uses cholesterol to make bile, a substance that helps digest fats. The gallbladder stores bile and releases the substance into the small intestine during meals. Instead of eliminating bile along with fecal matter in bowel movements, the intestinal tract breaks it down and absorbs its components, which eventually enter the liver. The liver recycles bile components to make new bile. When you eat oat cereal, the soluble fiber in oats interferes with this recycling process, because it binds to the bile components in the intestinal tract and prevents them from being absorbed. (See Figure 6.14.) Thus, the bile components are eliminated in bowel movements. As a result, blood cholesterol levels drop as the liver removes cholesterol from the blood to make new bile. The healthful benefits of soluble fiber in oats is so important, the FDA permits manufacturers of oat cereals to use the American Heart

MY DIVERSE PLATE

Red Lentils

For thousands of years, people living in Mediterranean countries, the Middle East, India, and other countries of southeastern Asia have eaten lentils, a type of *legume*. Peas and beans are also legumes. Lentils, particularly green varieties, are an excellent source of fiber. Lentils also provide protein, iron, potassium, and folate. Red lentils soften quickly with cooking and can be used in stews, sauces, or dips.

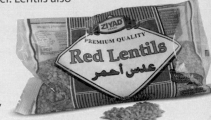

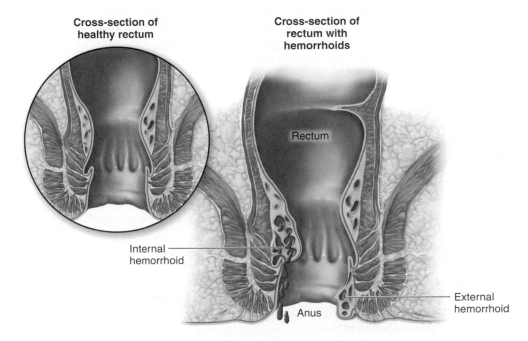

Figure 5.16 Hemorrhoids. Hemorrhoids are clusters of swollen rectal veins that can bleed, cause pain, and become itchy.

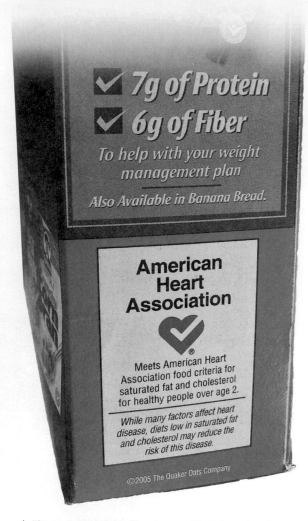

Figure 5.17 Soluble fiber in oats. The U.S. Food and Drug Administration (FDA) permits oat cereal manufacturers to include the American Heart Association's heart-healthy symbol and a special claim on the label.

Association's heart-healthy symbol (Fig. 5.17) and make the following claim on package labels: "Oatmeal helps remove cholesterol. Three grams of soluble fiber from oatmeal daily in a diet low in saturated fat and cholesterol may reduce the risk of heart disease."

Fiber and Weight Control

If you are trying to lose excess body fat, you may find it helpful to add more fiber-rich foods to your diet. High-fiber foods tend to be "filling" by increasing the volume of food eaten, which results in satiety. Additionally, a serving of a high-fiber food generally has lower energy content than the same volume of a low-fiber food.[54] As a result, energy intake usually decreases when people switch their consumption from low-fiber to high-fiber diets. The following section describes practical ways you can increase the fiber content of your snacks and meals. The Recipes for Healthy Living feature of Chapter 5 includes high-fiber waffle and oatmeal recipes.

Increasing Your Fiber Intake

The recommended Adequate Intakes (AIs) for fiber are 38 and 25 g/day for young men and women, respectively, but the typical American diet supplies only about 15 g of dietary fiber/day.[54] You can estimate your daily fiber intake by completing the Personal Dietary Analysis at the end of this chapter. The Food & Nutrition Tips box on page 148 provides tips for increasing the fiber content of your diet. No Tolerable Upper Intake Level (UL) for fiber has been determined. However, eating excessive amounts of fiber may produce severe intestinal gas and interfere with the intestinal absorption of certain minerals. In rare instances, consuming too much dietary fiber results in intestinal blockage, especially if fluid intake is low.

Intestinal bacteria produce gases when they metabolize fiber; therefore, dietitians recommend that people adjust by gradually increasing their fiber intake. Although having more intestinal gas than usual is a good sign—a sign that the diet contains more fiber—many people would rather experience a different indication of improved digestive health! To reduce the likelihood of having uncomfortable and embarrassing intestinal gas, you can add products such as Beano® to dishes that contain beans before eating them. Beano® contains natural enzymes that break down undigested complex carbohydrates before they can be fermented by intestinal bacteria. Nevertheless, athletes may choose to avoid notorious gas-forming foods, such as broccoli, cabbage, onions, and beans, 24 to 48 hours before competing. Practices that result in swallowing air, such as eating quickly; drinking carbonated beverages, especially with a straw; and chewing gum, also contribute to intestinal gas.

Concept **Checkpoint**

15. What are the signs and symptoms of type 1 and type 2 diabetes?
16. Erika wants to prevent the development of type 2 diabetes. What health-related lifestyle practices can she follow to reduce her risk of this serious metabolic disease?
17. Identify at least three signs of metabolic syndrome.
18. What is lactose intolerance?
19. List at least three ways to increase dietary fiber intake.
20. Discuss the health benefits of including soluble and insoluble fiber in diets.
21. How can a person easily determine the carbohydrate and fiber content in a serving of a packaged food?

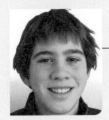

REAL *People*

REAL *Stories*

Tyler Smith

If you visit the Smith household, you'll see a wall covered with fascinating photographs—two that are especially attention grabbing. One photo shows a teenage boy holding a record-breaking 20-pound peacock bass and another photo is of the same teenager kneeling proudly next to a slain wild boar. Tyler Smith, the teenager in the photos, is only 18 years old, but he's done a lot of amazing things that most 18-year-olds don't even dream about doing. Tyler has taken two fishing trips on the Amazon River in South America. On one of those trips, he caught the huge bass. While on a hunting trip in Florida, Tyler shot the wild boar. Closer to home, Tyler enjoys hunting quail and pheasant. Aside from his enthusiasm for hunting, the young man is an Eagle Scout and serious NASCAR fan; he's often in the stands watching one of the races. Tyler has other interests. Since he was 2 years old, he has helped raise money for his local branch of the American Diabetes Association. For the past several years, the Association has honored Tyler for being the number one individual fundraiser in his area. The money that's collected by the American Diabetes Association is used to fund research efforts to find a cure for diabetes and support summer camps for children with the disorder. While attending one of those camps as a young child, Tyler learned how to give himself insulin injections. Why? Since he was 14 months old, Tyler has had type 1 diabetes.

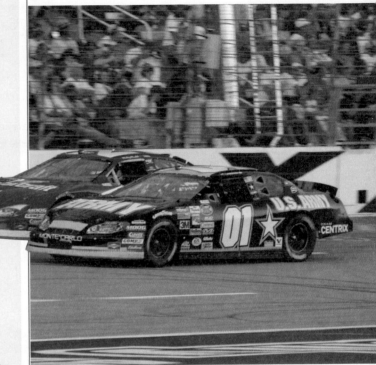

As you can tell from Tyler's busy lifestyle, he doesn't let diabetes interfere with his life. Today, he doesn't need to take insulin injections four times a day; he wears an external insulin pump on his belt that is programmed to deliver tiny amounts of the hormone into his body continuously. If Tyler needs extra insulin, he can push a button and the device provides an additional dose of the hormone. Although using an insulin pump has made Tyler's ability to manage diabetes easier, he still watches his diet. He avoids consuming foods that contain high amounts of simple sugars, such as candy bars and regular soft drinks. According to Tyler, "Sometimes, when I order a diet soft drink, the restaurant worker asks, 'Why? You don't look like you need a diet drink.'" Tyler responds by informing the person, "I have to; I'm a diabetic."

Tyler's friends don't give him any special treatment, but they're aware of the signs of hyperglycemia and hypoglycemia. According to Tyler, "My friends know when my blood sugar is too high and I need insulin because I'm really thirsty and I have to go to the bathroom [urinate] a lot. When I'm hypoglycemic, I get agitated and shaky, and I have trouble concentrating on what I'm doing. Then my friends know to get me something with sugar in it."

For now, Tyler focuses on school and his part-time job as a service consultant for a small business. As for the future, Tyler is convinced that medical research is close to finding a cure for diabetes. "If transplanting cells that produce insulin into the pancreas works, I would be willing to have the procedure," he says. Until then, Tyler knows he must continue using his insulin pump and taking care of himself. When asked to provide a message to people who do not have diabetes, he replied, "We're [diabetics] just like everyone else. We just have to do something extra for our health."

Food & Nutrition *tips*

- For healthy breakfasts or snacks, eat whole-grain, bran, or oatmeal breads and cereals. Read the ingredient label to find out if a bread or cereal product is whole grain; whole grain or bran should be the first ingredient.

- When comparing bread or cereal products, don't rely on the product's name or appearance. Check the ingredients. Terms such as "100% wheat," "multi-grain," or "stone-ground wheat" are misleading, because the product may contain little or no whole grain.

- Brown rice has more fiber and flavor than white rice. If you are concerned about convenience, instant-cooking brown rice takes less time to cook than regular brown rice.

- Substitute whole-wheat pasta for regular pasta or use half whole-wheat and half regular pasta in pasta dishes.

- Snack on pieces of fresh, frozen, or dried fruit.

- Instead of removing them, eat the edible peels, pulp, and seeds of fruits and vegetables. Eat vegetables as snacks.

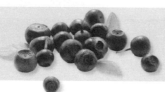

- Include more nuts, beans, and seeds in your diet.

- Spread peanut or soy butter on whole-grain crackers for a fiber-filled snack.

- Sprinkle nuts or hulled sunflower seeds on pancakes, waffles, or salads.

- Add frozen, dried, or fresh fruit such as berries, raisins, or bananas instead of sugar or honey to sweeten cereal or plain yogurt.

- Add a small amount of uncooked oatmeal and wheat germ to raw ground meats when making hamburgers or meatloaf.

- Adding bran, wheat germ, and uncooked oatmeal to pancake or waffle batter also enhances the batter's fiber content.

- Good dietary sources of fiber contain at least 2.5 g of fiber per serving.

- You can determine a serving of the food's fiber content by reading the Nutrition Facts panel on the product label.

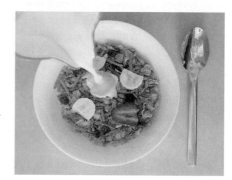

Chapter 5 Highlight

GLYCEMIC INDEX AND GLYCEMIC LOAD

In the early 1980s, researchers noted that the body digested carbohydrate-rich foods at different rates, and its insulin response to each food varied. Foods that contained large amounts of refined carbohydrates were digested rapidly, and the rapid flow of glucose into the bloodstream raised blood glucose and insulin levels sharply. Other carbohydrate-rich foods that had high fiber contents were digested slowly and did not cause such a dramatic increase in blood glucose and insulin levels. This observation led to the development of the dietary concepts *glycemic index* and *glycemic load*. Currently, the notion that a food's glycemic index could influence health has spurred the publication of popular diet books recommending avoiding foods with high glycemic indices, such as potatoes and bread. What is the glycemic index? Should you avoid foods that have high glycemic indices?

The glycemic index (GI) is a way of classifying foods by comparing the rise in blood glucose that occurs after eating a portion of a food that supplies 50 g of digestible carbohydrate to the rise that occurs after eating a standard source of carbohydrate, such as 50 g of glucose.[55] A related value, the glycemic load (GL), is the grams of carbohydrate in a serving of food multiplied by the food's GI; this figure is then divided by 100. Compared to the GI, the GL may be a more realistic way of rating foods because the value indicates the relative rise in blood glucose levels after eating a *typical* serving of a carbohydrate-containing food.

Table 5.11 lists average GIs and GLs of several commonly eaten foods. Note that sucrose and other sugary foods, as well as highly refined starchy foods such as cornflakes, baked potatoes, and white rice, have high GIs (70 or more). Honey, apples, carrots, spaghetti, milk, and peanuts have low to moderate GIs (less than 70). It is important to note that the GL of a food is usually lower than its GI. For example, the GI for 30 g of cornflakes is 81, but the GL value for cornflakes is only 21. Foods with low GLs have values below 15; high GL foods have values of more than 20.

Critics of the GI and GL think the standards have limited usefulness as a menu-planning tool because the values can vary too much. Therefore, the values shown in Table 5.11 may vary significantly, depending on where the food was grown, its degree of ripeness, or the extent of its processing. Additionally, after eating a particular carbohydrate-rich food, the resulting rise in blood glucose level varies among individuals. Furthermore, the values reflect a single food's effect on blood glucose levels. The effect may be reduced when the food is eaten as part of a meal that contains a mixture of macronutrients and fiber.

Despite the criticism directed at the indices, epidemiological studies suggest an association between high GI/GL diets and serious chronic diseases.[56] As people in developing countries abandon traditional diets and eat more high GI/GL foods, they become more likely to develop obesity and type 2 diabetes, as well as cardiovascular disease and certain cancers.[57] Low GI diets may improve blood lipid levels and reduce the risk of cardiovascular disease[58] and improve HbA1c levels.[59] People with diabetes can follow a low GI or low GL diet while monitoring their total carbohydrate intake to control their blood glucose levels.[60] More long-term research is needed before nutrition experts recommend low GI or low GL diets for the general population.

TABLE 5.11

Glycemic Index and Load: Average Values of Selected Foods

Food	GI Glycemic Index*	GL Glycemic Load
Glucose	121	–
Potato (baked)	121	26
Cornflakes cereal	81	21
Jelly beans	112	22
Gatorade	111	12
French fries	63	22
Bagel, white plain	103	25
Popcorn	103	8
White rice, boiled	78	29
Snickers candy bar	97	23
Ice cream, vanilla reduced fat	87	8
Sucrose	84	–
Coca-Cola	83	16
Banana	51	12
Orange juice	50	13
Baked beans, canned	69	7
Spaghetti (cooked)	49	20
Peach, raw	60	5
Apple, raw	36	6
Honey	46	7
Fat-free milk	46	4
Fructose	29	–
Carrots, raw	23	1
Peanuts	21	1

* Compared to white bread (GI = 100)

Source: Data from Foster-Powell K and others: International table of glycemic index and glycemic load values. *American Journal of Clinical Nutrition* 76(1):5, 2002.; Atkinson FS and others: International tables of glycemic index and glycemic load values: 2008. *Diabetes Care* 31(12):2281, 2008.

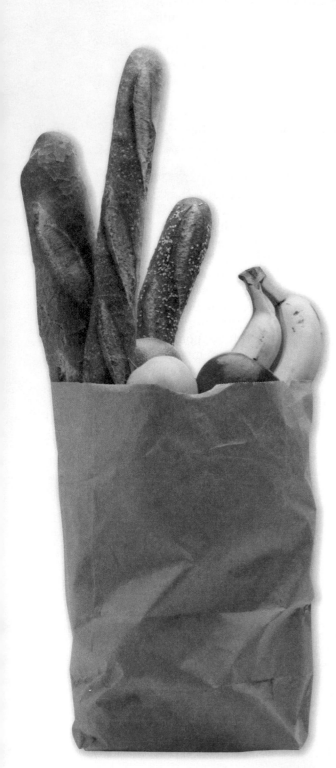

CHAPTER REFERENCES

See Appendix I.

SUMMARY

Carbohydrates are an important source of energy for the body. Plants use energy from the sun to make carbohydrates from water and carbon dioxide. Some of the energy is stored in the bonds that hold the carbon and hydrogen atoms together. Cells break down those bonds, releasing the energy that powers various forms of cellular work.

The three most important dietary monosaccharides are glucose, fructose, and galactose. Glucose is a primary fuel for muscles and other cells; nervous system and red blood cells rely on glucose for energy under normal conditions. Lactose and sucrose are major dietary disaccharides. Starch, glycogen, and most forms of dietary fiber are polysaccharides.

Glucose is the primary end product of carbohydrate digestion. Hormones, particularly insulin and glucagon, maintain normal blood glucose levels. Insulin allows glucose to enter cells, where the sugar is metabolized for energy. Additionally, insulin stimulates glycogen production. Glucagon stimulates the liver to break down glycogen into glucose molecules and release them into the bloodstream.

People in industrialized nations tend to eat less complex carbohydrates and more highly refined sugars than people living in less-developed countries. Healthy Americans should consume diets that furnish 45 to 65% of energy from carbohydrates, primarily complex carbohydrates. Refined sugar is often blamed for causing obesity, diabetes, and hyperactivity, but tooth decay is the only health problem that is clearly associated with eating carbohydrates. Many adults are lactose intolerant because they do not produce enough lactase, the intestinal enzyme needed to digest the disaccharide.

Diabetes mellitus is characterized by elevated blood glucose levels. Diabetes can result in cardiovascular disease, kidney failure, blindness, and lower limb amputations. There are two major types of diabetes mellitus, type 1 and type 2 diabetes. Type 2 diabetes is the more common form of the disease. In the United States, the prevalence of type 2 diabetes has reached epidemic proportions. People who are sedentary, are overweight, eat Western diets, and have a close relative with type 2 diabetes are at risk of developing this form of the disease.

Eating fiber-rich foods may reduce your risk of obesity, type 2 diabetes, cardiovascular disease, and certain intestinal tract disorders. High-fiber diets, especially those with ample amounts of insoluble fiber, are associated with lower risk of constipation and hemorrhoids compared to diets that contain little fiber. Additionally, foods that contain soluble fiber may improve cardiovascular health by reducing cholesterol absorption in the intestines. Plant foods generally contain both forms of fiber.

The glycemic index (GI) and glycemic load (GL) are ways of classifying certain foods by their carbohydrate contents. Results of some epidemiological studies suggest an association between high GI/GL diets and serious chronic diseases. However, more long-term research is needed before nutrition experts recommend low GI or low GL diets for the general population.

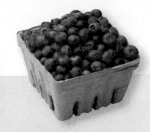

Recipes for Healthy Living

Berry-Good Hot Oatmeal Cereal

You don't have time to make or eat breakfast, especially a nutritious, hot breakfast? Think again. This single-serving recipe is a very good source of carbohydrate and provides 7 g of fiber. Furthermore, the recipe takes less than 10 minutes to make. For variety, substitute raisins, frozen or fresh strawberries, or raspberries for the blueberries. A serving of this oatmeal supplies 296 kcal, 14 g protein, 4 g fat, 51 g carbohydrate, 7 g fiber, 295 mg calcium, and 2 mg iron.

INGREDIENTS:

½ cup frozen or fresh unsweetened blueberries
½ cup quick cooking oats
¾ cup fat-free milk
1 tsp sugar
pinch of ground cinnamon (optional)

PREPARATION STEPS:

1. Place ingredients in a microwaveable bowl and stir.

2. Microwave on "high" for about 2.5 minutes.

3. Stir before eating.

Cleanup tip: After eating, soak cereal bowl in cold water before washing it.

Fiber-Power Waffles

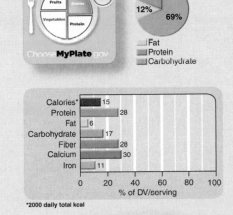

If you're tired of eating commercial toaster waffles, try this recipe for making your own high-fiber "brand." You can freeze cooked waffles in plastic storage bags; reheat individual waffles in a toaster oven. The recipe makes approximately six 6"-diameter round waffles; the batter also can be used to make high-fiber pancakes. One waffle provides about 220 kcal, 8 g protein, 7.5 g fat, 30 g carbohydrate, 5 g fiber, and 2.5 mg iron.

INGREDIENTS:

¾ cup whole-wheat commercial pancake & waffle mix
    (Do not use "Complete" mixes.)
¾ cup regular commercial pancake & waffle mix
    (Do not use "Complete" mixes.)
2 Tbsp dry roasted, unsalted, hulled sunflower seeds
2 Tbsp wheat germ
⅓ cup all-bran ready-to-eat cereal
¼ cup quick cooking dry oats
1 large egg (lightly beaten)
2 Tbsp vegetable oil
1 ½ cup fat-free fluid milk

PREPARATION STEPS:

1. Mix dry ingredients together.

2. Add egg, oil, and milk to dry ingredients and stir until moistened.

3. Pour ½ cup of the batter into the center of a heated waffle iron and close iron on batter. Follow the waffle iron manufacturer's directions for making waffles—waffles generally take 1½ to 2 minutes to cook. Top with fresh raspberries or sliced strawberries, or serve with berry sauce (see recipe).

Berry Easy Sauce

This recipe makes about ¾ cup of raspberry berry sauce. Each ¼ cup of sauce supplies about 45 kcal, 11 g carbohydrates, 1.3 g fiber, and 12 mg vitamin C. Berry sauce is a more nutritious choice than maple syrup. A ¼-cup serving of maple-flavored regular pancake and waffle syrup that contains 2% maple syrup provides about 220 kcal, 55 g carbohydrate , no fiber, and no vitamin C. You can substitute other kinds of frozen fruit, such as strawberries or blueberries, for the raspberries.

INGREDIENTS:

1 cup thawed unsweetened frozen
    raspberries
1 tsp white sugar

PREPARATION STEPS:

1. Place thawed berries in a microwave-safe dish, sprinkle sugar over berries, and cover for 30 minutes.

2. Heat berries in microwave oven for about 20 seconds.

3. Stir gently before serving. Sauce will be thick. Place unused portion in a covered container and store in the refrigerator.

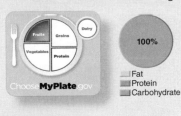
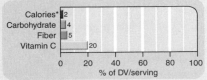

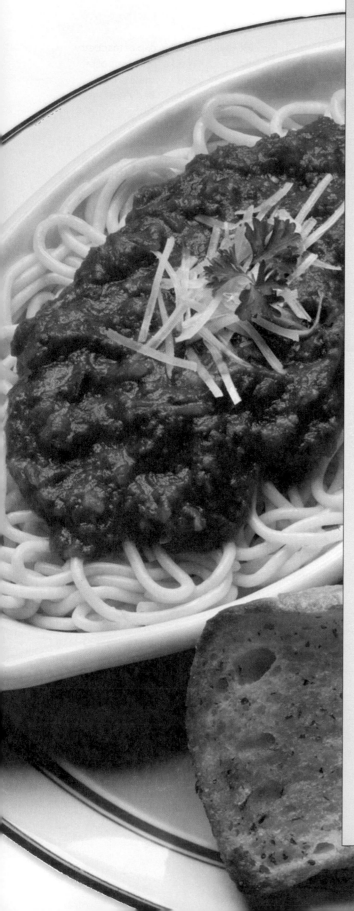

Personal *Dietary* Analysis

1. Refer to the 3-day food log from the Personal Dietary Analysis feature in Chapter 3. List the total number of kilocalories you consumed for each day of record keeping. Add the figures to obtain a total, divide the total by 3, then round the figure to the nearest whole number to obtain your average daily energy intake for the 3-day period.

Sample Calculation:

Day 1   2500 kcal   **Day 2**   3200 kcal   **Day 3**   2750 kcal
Total kcal 8450 ÷ 3 days = **2817** kcal/day
        (average kilocalorie intake, rounded to the nearest whole number)

Your Calculation:

Day 1   _____ kcal   **Day 2**   _____ kcal   **Day 3**   _____ kcal
Total kcal _____ ÷ 3 days = _____ kcal/day
        (average kilocalorie intake, rounded to the nearest whole number)

2. Add the number of grams of carbohydrate eaten each day of the period. Divide the total by 3 and round to the nearest whole number to calculate the average number of grams of carbohydrate consumed daily.

Sample Calculation:

Day 1   300 g   **Day 2**   495 g   **Day 3**   475 g   **Total =** 1270 g
Total g 1270 ÷ 3 days = **423** g/day
        (average, rounded to the nearest whole number)

Your Calculation:

Day 1   ____ g   **Day 2**   ____ g   **Day 3**   ____ g   **Total =** ____ g
Total g ____ ÷ 3 days = ____ g of carbohydrate/day
        (average, rounded to the nearest whole number)

3. Each gram of carbohydrate provides about 4 kcal; therefore, you must multiply the average number of grams of carbohydrate obtained in step 2 by 4 to obtain the number of kcal from carbohydrates.

Sample Calculation:

423 g/day × 4 kcal/g = **1692** kcal from carbohydrates

Your Calculation:

____ g/day × 4 kcal/g = ____ kcal from carbohydrates

4. To calculate the average daily percentage of kilocalories that carbohydrates contributed to your diet, divide the average kilocalories from carbohydrate obtained in step 3 by the average total daily kilocalorie intake obtained in step 1; round figure to the nearest

one-hundredth. Multiply the value by 100, drop decimal point, and add the percent symbol.

Sample Calculation:

1692 kcal ÷ 2817 kcal = 0.60

0.60 × 100 = 60%

Your Calculation:

_____ kcal ÷ _____ kcal = _____

_____ × 100 = _____ %

5. On average, did you consume *at least* the RDA of 130 g of carbohydrate? Yes _____ No _____

6. Did your average carbohydrate intake meet the recommended 45 to 65% of total energy? Yes _____ No _____

a. If your average carbohydrate intake was less than 130 g or below 45% of total calories, list five nutrient-dense, carbohydrate-rich foods you could eat that would boost your intake of carbohydrates.
Foods: _____

7. Review the log of your 3-day food intake. Calculate your average daily intake of fiber by adding the grams of fiber consumed over the 3-day period and dividing the total by three.

Your Calculation:

Day 1   _____ g

Day 2   _____ g

Day 3   _____ g

Total =   _____ g

Total g _____ ÷ 3 days = _____ g of fiber daily

a. What was your average daily fiber intake? _____ g

b. Did your average daily fiber intake meet the recommended Adequate Intakes of 38 and 25 g/day for young men and women, respectively? Yes _____ No _____

c. If your response is yes, list foods that contributed to your fiber intake.

d. If you did not meet the recommended level of fiber intake, list at least five foods that you would eat to increase your fiber intake to the recommended level.

CRITICAL THINKING

1. One of your friends thinks honey is more nutritious and safer to eat than table sugar. He wants you to avoid table sugar and use only honey as a sweetener. What would you tell this person about the nutritive value and safety of honey compared to sugar?

2. Prepare a pamphlet that describes the health benefits of dietary fiber. In addition to English, you may prepare the pamphlet in Spanish, Vietnamese, or another modern language.

3. How did you feel about drinking regular soft drinks before reading Chapter 5? Has your opinion changed? If so, explain how.

4. If you were 25 pounds overweight, explain why you would or would not follow a weight-loss diet that supplied less than 15% of calories from carbohydrate.

5. Consider the fiber content of your diet. Do you consume enough fiber each day? If your fiber intake is adequate, what foods do you eat regularly that contribute soluble and insoluble fiber to your diet? If your fiber intake is low, list foods you would consume to increase your intake of both types of fiber.

PRACTICE TEST

Select the best answer.

1. Which of the following substances is a disaccharide?

   a. fructose
   b. sucrose
   c. galactose
   d. glycogen

2. _____ is a primary fuel for muscles and other cells.

   a. Protein
   b. Cholesterol
   c. Glucose
   d. HFCS

3. Which of the following substances is a polysaccharide?

   a. glycogen
   b. glucose
   c. lactose
   d. insulin

4. Sugar contributes to

   a. browning of baked cereal products.
   b. food preservation.
   c. a food's energy value.
   d. All of the above are correct.

5. Dietary fiber

   a. supplies more energy, gram per gram, than fat.
   b. is not digested by the human intestinal tract.
   c. promotes tooth decay.
   d. is only in animal sources of food.

6. Insoluble fiber

   a. is in beef and pork.
   b. dissolves or swells in water.
   c. is in whole-grain products, including brown rice.
   d. increases the risk of heart disease.

7. _____ is the hormone that enables glucose to enter cells.

   a. Glucagon
   b. Insulin
   c. Glycerol
   d. Ketonine

8. _____ are the primary source of added sugars in the typical American diet.

   a. Candies
   b. Regular soft drinks
   c. Refined cereals
   d. Canned fruits

9. Type 2 diabetes is

   a. a disease that primarily affects young children.
   b. characterized by severe hypoglycemia.
   c. often associated with excess body weight.
   d. caused by eating refined sugars.

10. Which of the following signs is associated with metabolic syndrome?

    a. low blood pressure
    b. high fasting blood glucose
    c. low hemoglobin
    d. high fasting HDL cholesterol

11. Which of the following conditions is clearly associated with eating dietary carbohydrates, especially sticky sugars?

    a. tooth decay
    b. type 1 diabetes
    c. attention deficit hyperactivity disorder
    d. hypertension

12. Which of the following substances is an enzyme that breaks down lactose?

    a. galactose
    b. salivary amylase
    c. lactase
    d. lactic acid

13. Which of the following foods is the best source of soluble fiber?

    a. raw fruit
    b. whole-grain oat cereal
    c. sports drinks
    d. cooked meat

14. Which of the following foods has a high glycemic index?

    a. nonfat milk
    b. cornflakes cereal
    c. salted peanuts
    d. raw carrots

Answers to Chapter 5 Quiz *Yourself*

1. Compared to table sugar, honey is a natural and far more nutritious sweetener. **False.** (p. 125)

2. Ounce per ounce, sugar provides more energy than starch. **False.** (pp. 126, 129)

3. Eating a high-fiber diet can improve the functioning of your large intestine and reduce your blood cholesterol levels. **True.** (pp. 144, 145)

4. The average American consumes 80% of his or her energy intake as refined sugars. **False.** (p. 135)

5. The results of clinical studies indicate that eating too much sugar makes children hyperactive. **False.** (p. 144)

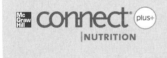

Additional resources related to the features of this book are available on ConnectPlus® Nutrition. Ask your instructor how to get access.

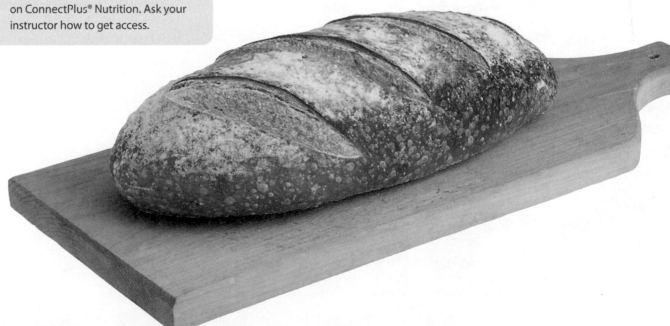

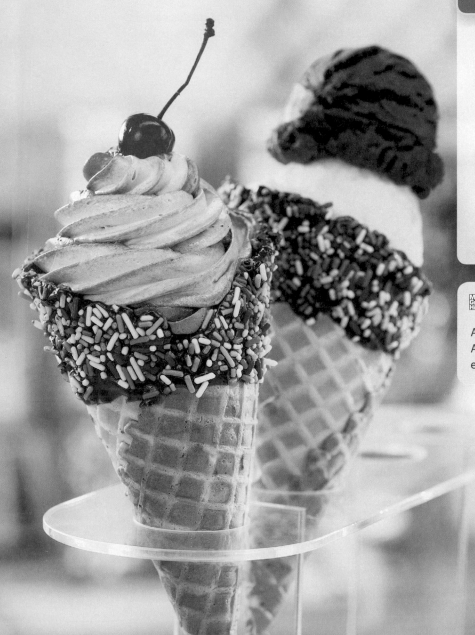

CHAPTER 6

Fats and Other Lipids

Chapter Learning Outcomes

After reading Chapter 6, you should be able to

1. Distinguish various lipids and identify at least one physiological role of each type of lipid.

2. Identify major food sources of lipids, including trans fatty acids.

3. Explain the process of atherosclerosis and list at least six risk factors of cardiovascular disease.

4. Distinguish HDL cholesterol from LDL cholesterol.

5. Identify major dietary sources of omega-3 fatty acids.

6. List dietary and other lifestyle actions that can reduce the risk of cardiovascular disease.

7. Discuss alcohol's effects on health.

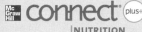

|NUTRITION   **www.mcgrawhillconnect.com**

A wealth of proven resources are available on ConnectPlus® Nutrition! Ask your instructor about ConnectPlus, which includes an interactive eBook, an adaptive learning program and much, much more!

WHAT DO YOU think when you hear the word *fat* or *cholesterol?* Does "bad," "heart attack," or "deadly" enter your mind? If your answer is "yes," are you concerned about the amounts and types of fat in your diet? Do you avoid eating eggs because of their cholesterol content? Does your concern have anything to do with having a family history of heart disease?

Fat and cholesterol are **lipids,** a class of nutrients that generally do not dissolve in water. You probably know fat is a major source of energy and eating too much fat can result in excess weight gain, which is unhealthy. Additionally, you may know that cholesterol is associated with heart attacks. However, you may not be aware of the many important roles that fat, cholesterol, and other lipids play in the body (Table 6.1). Lipids are crucial components of the plasma membrane that surround each human cell. In fact, a person cannot claim to be "fat free," because every cell in the body contains fat as well as other lipids. The layer of fat under your skin (subcutaneous fat) stores energy, insulates you against cold temperatures, protects you against minor bruising, and contributes to your body's contours. In addition to storing energy, the fat deposits in your abdominal region cushion your vital organs from jarring movements and damaging blows.

In food, lipids enhance intestinal absorption of fat-soluble vitamins and phytochemicals. Dietary lipids also provide nonnutritional benefits by contributing to the rich flavor, smooth texture, and appetizing aroma of foods. Whether fat is naturally in food or added to it, the nutrient often makes foods taste more appetizing. For example, if you are used to consuming whole milk that is about 3.25% fat by volume, you will recognize the difference fat makes to "mouth feel" when you drink fat-free milk that contains less than 0.5% fat.

It is not surprising that many Americans are confused about the roles of fat and cholesterol in health. The results from numerous studies conducted over the past 60 years indicate that consuming high amounts of certain lipids may increase the risk of serious health conditions, including obesity,[1] certain cancers,[2] and cardiovascular disease (CVD), which includes heart disease and stroke.[3, 4] On the other hand, some fat is essential to good health. By reading Chapter 6, you will learn about the roles of lipids in your foods and body as well as their major food sources. Additionally, you will learn how certain lipids may influence your health.

Quiz *Yourself*

What are trans and omega-3 fats, and which foods contain these fats? How much dietary fat is recommended? Should you avoid eating eggs because they contain cholesterol? Test your knowledge of fat and other lipids by taking the following quiz. The answers are found on page 199.

1. To lose weight, use regular, stick margarine instead of butter because it has 25% fewer calories per teaspoon.
   _____ T _____ F

2. Egg yolks are a rich source of cholesterol. _____ T _____ F

3. Taking too many fish oil supplements may be harmful to health.
   _____ T _____ F

4. On average, Americans consume 60% of their calories from fat.
   _____ I _____ F

5. Increasing your intake of trans fats will reduce your risk of heart disease. _____ T _____ F

TABLE 6.1
Major Functions of Lipids in the Body

Fats and certain other lipids are important for:

- Providing and storing energy (fat)
- Maintaining cell membranes
- Producing certain hormones
- Insulating the body against cold temperatures
- Cushioning the body against bumps and blows
- Contributing to body contours
- Absorbing fat-soluble vitamins and phytochemicals
- Enhancing the flavor, texture, and aroma of foods

lipids class of nutrients that do not dissolve in water

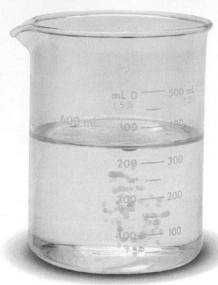

| Oil and water do not mix.

6.1 Understanding Lipids

Lipids include fatty acids, triglycerides (*try-glis'-er-eyeds*), phospholipids (*fos-foe-lip'-ids*), and cholesterol. In general, lipids are insoluble in water. Consider what happens when you mix vinegar and olive oil to make a vinaigrette salad dressing. Vinegar is 95% water; oil is 100% lipid. Therefore, the oil does not dissolve in water to make a solution. Additionally, oil is less dense than water, so it rises to the top of the vinegar in small globules when added to vinegar. The globules join others to form an oily layer that floats on the vinegar until you shake the mixture. Shaking the ingredients mixes them temporarily. When left undisturbed, the oil and vinegar soon separate; hence the saying, "Oil and water don't mix." The following sections take a closer look at each major type of lipid.

Fatty Acids

Most lipids have fatty acids in their chemical structures. Fatty acids provide energy for muscles and most other types of cells. As Figure 6.1 illustrates, a fatty acid is comprised of a **hydrocarbon chain,** a chain of carbon atoms bonded to each other and to hydrogen atoms. The first carbon in the molecule has three hydrogen atoms attached to it. Chemists call this part of the molecule *omega* or the *methyl end*. The last carbon in the fatty acid molecule forms an *acid group*.

In nature, common fatty acids have even numbers of carbon atoms. *Short-chain* fatty acids have 2 to 4 carbons; *medium-chain* fatty acids have 6 to 12 carbons; and *long-chain* fatty acids have 14 to 24 carbons. The molecules shown in Figure 6.1 contain 18 carbons; thus, they are long-chain fatty acids. Chemists identify a fatty acid by its number of carbon atoms and type of bond between carbon atoms in the hydrocarbon chain. Additionally, these factors influence how various fatty acids can affect your health.

Saturation

Fatty acids can be saturated or unsaturated. The carbons in the fatty acid chain shown in Figure 6.1a have single bonds between them. Note that each carbon in the chain has two

hydrocarbon chain chain of carbon atoms bonded to each other and to hydrogen atoms

saturated fatty acid fatty acid that has each carbon atom within the chain filled with hydrogen atoms

Figure 6.1 Fatty acids.
A fatty acid is comprised of a hydrocarbon chain. The methyl end (*omega*) contains the first carbon in the molecule; the last carbon in the molecule forms an acid group. Note that each of these fatty acids has 18 carbon atoms, but they differ in the number and location of double bonds. (*a*) A saturated fatty acid has single bonds between the carbon atoms in the hydrocarbon chain. (*b*) An unsaturated fatty acid has two neighboring carbons within the chain that are missing two hydrogen atoms, and a double bond holds those particular carbons together. (*c*) A polyunsaturated fatty acid has two or more double bonds between carbons in the hydrocarbon chain.

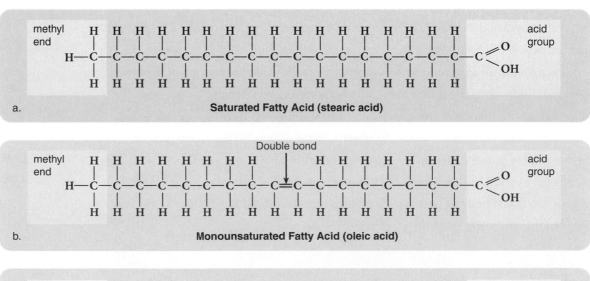

hydrogen atoms attached to it. This is a **saturated fatty acid** because each carbon within the chain is saturated, that is, completely filled with hydrogen atoms.

An **unsaturated fatty acid** has two neighboring carbons within the chain that are missing two hydrogen atoms, and a double bond holds those particular carbons together (Fig. 6.1b). Unsaturated fatty acids can be either monounsaturated or polyunsaturated. The fatty acid illustrated in Figure 6.1b has only one double bond linking two carbon atoms; therefore, it is referred to as a *monounsaturated fatty acid*. The fatty acid shown in Figure 6.1c is also unsaturated, but it has three double bonds within its hydrocarbon chain. A fatty acid that has two or more double bonds between carbons is a *poly*unsaturated **fatty acid** (PUFA).

What is the difference between fats and oils? Although both substances contain fatty acids, fats are solid and oils are liquid at room temperature. Compared to foods that contain high amounts of unsaturated fatty acids, foods that are rich sources of long-chain saturated fatty acids tend to be more solid at room temperature. A pat of butter, for example, contains more long-chain saturated fatty acids than a pat of margarine. Thus, butter keeps its shape better than margarine when it is not refrigerated. The "Lipids and Health: Cardiovascular Disease" section of Chapter 6 discusses the health effects of eating diets that are rich in saturated or unsaturated fats.

Essential Fatty Acids

The body cannot synthesize two polyunsaturated fatty acids, **alpha-linolenic** (*al'-fah lin'-o-len'-ik*) **acid** and **linoleic** (*lin'-o-lay'-ik*) **acid**. These lipids are **essential fatty acids** because they must be supplied by the diet. Alpha-linolenic acid is an **omega-3 fatty acid**. The "3" refers to the position of the first double bond that appears in the fatty acid's carbon chain, when you start counting carbons at the omega end of the molecule. Cells use alpha-linolenic acid to synthesize two other omega-3 fatty acids, eicosapentaenoic (*eye'-ko-seh-pen'-tah-e-no'-ik*) acid (EPA) and docosahexaenoic (*doe'-ko-seh-hek'-seh-e'-no'-ik*) acid (DHA). Linoleic acid is an *omega-6 fatty acid*. Cells can convert linoleic acid to arachidonic (*a'-ra-keh'-don-ik*) acid (AA). The body uses EPA, DHA, and AA to make several compounds that have hormonelike functions, including *prostaglandins*. Prostaglandins produce a variety of important effects on the body, such as stimulating uterine contractions, regulating blood pressure, and promoting the immune system's inflammatory response. Figure 6.2 shows relationships among the essential fatty acids.

Essential fatty acids are necessary in small amounts for good health. Infants require DHA and EPA for nervous system development, and babies do not grow properly when their diets lack essential fatty acids. Other signs of essential fatty acid deficiency include scaly skin, hair loss, and poor wound healing. The Adequate Intake (AI) for alpha-linolenic acid is 1.6 g/day for men and 1.1 g/day for women. The AI for linoleic acid is 17 g/day for men and 12 g/day for women who are 19 through 50 years of age.[5] These amounts can be met by eating 2 to 3 tablespoons of vegetable fat daily, especially products made with canola and soybean oils, and meals that contain fatty fish, such as salmon and tuna, at least twice a week.

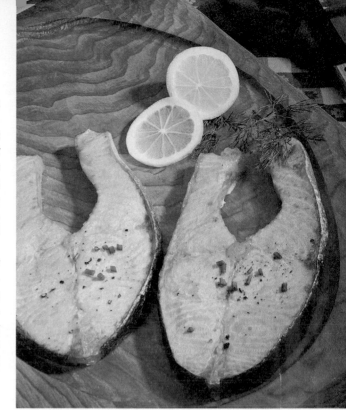

To obtain omega-3 fatty acids, consider including fatty fish such as salmon in your meals at least twice a week.

unsaturated fatty acid fatty acid that is missing hydrogen atoms and has one or more double bonds within the carbon chain

monounsaturated fatty acid fatty acid that has one double bond within the carbon chain

polyunsaturated fatty acid fatty acid that has two or more double bonds within the carbon chain

alpha-linolenic acid an essential fatty acid

linoleic acid an essential fatty acid

essential fatty acids lipids that must be supplied by the diet

omega-3 fatty acid type of polyunsaturated fatty acid

Figure 6.2 Essential fatty acids. Alpha-linolenic acid and linoleic acid are not synthesized by the body; they must be supplied in the diet. The body uses these essential fatty acids to make DHA, EPA, and arachidonic acid.

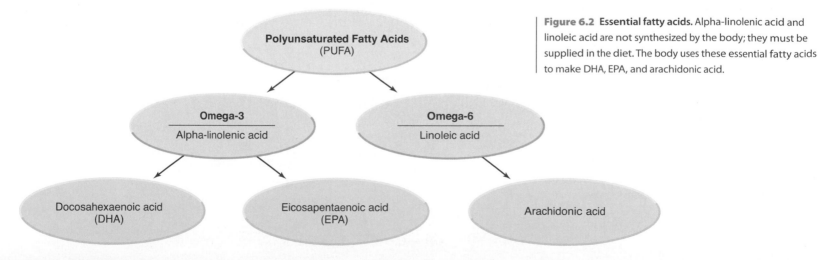

trans fats unsaturated fatty acids that have a *trans* double bond

hydrogenation food manufacturing process that adds hydrogen atoms to liquid vegetable oil, forming trans fats

triglyceride lipid that has three fatty acids attached to a three-carbon compound called glycerol

In the United States, essential fatty acid deficiency is uncommon because most Americans eat plenty of fat, especially linoleic acid. This omega-6 fatty acid is in vegetable oils often used for frying foods and making margarines and salad dressings. Additionally, whole-grain products contain linoleic acid. Certain fish are rich sources of omega-3 fatty acids, including DHA and EPA. Many Americans eat relatively small amounts of omega-3 fatty acids. The "Lipids and Health: Cardiovascular Disease (CVD)" section of Chapter 6 presents more information about essential fatty acids and their health effects.

Trans Fats

Trans fats are unsaturated fatty acids that have at least one *trans* double bond in their chemical structure rather than the more common *cis* configuration. The trans double bond enables the hydrocarbon chain to be relatively straight. The cis double bond, however, forms a kink in the hydrocarbon chain (Fig. 6.3).

Whole milk and whole milk products, butter, and meat naturally contain small amounts of trans fats. However, processed foods and margarines contribute the largest share of trans fat in the American diet. Most of the trans fat in processed food results from the **hydrogenation** process. *Partial hydrogenation* is a food manufacturing process that adds hydrogen atoms to some unsaturated fatty acids in liquid vegetable oil. The hydrogenation process also converts many of the oil's naturally occurring cis fatty acids into trans fatty acids. Structurally, a trans fatty acid resembles a saturated fatty acid and provides properties of long-chain saturated fatty acids to foods that contain them. Thus, fats that contain a high proportion of trans fatty acids are more solid at room temperature than those with a high proportion of cis fatty acids. As a result of the partial hydrogenation process, vegetable oil can be made into shortening or shaped into sticks of margarine. Shortening is often used to prepare deep-fat fried foods and cakes, pastries, and frostings.

Foods made with partially hydrogenated fat can be stored for longer periods of time than foods that contain cis fatty acids. Why? Trans fatty acids are less likely to undergo *oxidation*, a chemical process that alters the compound's structure. When oxidized, the fat in food becomes rancid and develops an unappetizing odor and taste. Unsaturated fatty acids that have the cis double-bond arrangement, especially polyunsaturated fatty acids, are very susceptible to oxidation. Instead of relying on trans fats to extend the shelf life of products, manufacturers can preserve fat and other ingredients in foods by adding antioxidants to them. Certain food additives, vitamins, and plant pigments function as antioxidants (see Chapter 8).

Although the body can use trans fatty acids for energy, these lipids are not essential, and medical researchers have not discovered any positive health effects from consuming them.[6] In the body, trans fats function like certain saturated fats, raising blood cholesterol levels, which may increase the risk of heart disease.[7] According to the American Heart Association, people should limit their trans fat intake to less than 1% of daily caloric intake.[8]

Did You Know?

Cooks often use shortening to make pie crust because the partially hydrogenated fat results in a flaky, tender crust. When making pie dough, oil can be substituted for shortening, but it produces a crumbly texture that may be undesirable.

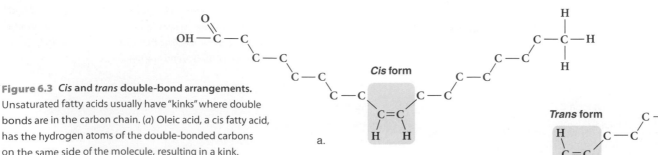

Figure 6.3 *Cis* and *trans* **double-bond arrangements.** Unsaturated fatty acids usually have "kinks" where double bonds are in the carbon chain. (*a*) Oleic acid, a cis fatty acid, has the hydrogen atoms of the double-bonded carbons on the same side of the molecule, resulting in a kink. (*b*) Elaidic acid, a trans fatty acid, has the hydrogen atoms of the double-bonded carbons on opposite sides, resulting in a straighter arrangement of the fatty acid chain. For simplicity, most of the hydrogen atoms in these molecules are not shown.

As American consumers have become more aware of the potential health problems associated with trans fat consumption, many food manufacturers have removed ingredients that contain trans fats from their products. However, the trans fat may have been replaced with other unhealthy types of fat. By 2010, several cities and the state of California banned the use of trans fats in the preparation of food sold in restaurants. In response to consumer concerns, some fast-food chains voluntarily stopped using rich sources of trans fat during food preparation.

The use of a synthetic lipid, *interesterified* (*in'-ter-eh-stear'-ih-fide'*) oil, to replace trans fats in processed foods may also have undesirable health effects. Results of a short-term study involving 30 adults found that consuming interesterified oils not only lowered the beneficial form of cholesterol in blood but also raised blood glucose levels.[9] More research is needed to determine the long-term safety of consuming foods that contain interesterified oil. Processed foods that include "fully hydrogenated" or "interesterified" oil in their ingredient lists are sources of interesterified fat.

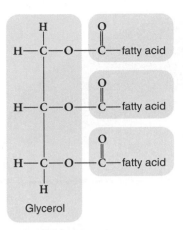

Triglyceride

Figure 6.4 Triglycerides. A triglyceride has three fatty acids attached to a glycerol "backbone."

Triglycerides

A **triglyceride** has three fatty acids attached to glycerol (*glis'-er-ol*), a three-carbon compound that is often referred to as the "backbone" of the triglyceride (Fig. 6.4). Triglycerides comprise about 95% of lipids in your body and food. Triglycerides are often referred to as fats and oils. The body stores energy as triglycerides (fat).

Most triglycerides contain mixtures of unsaturated and saturated fatty acids. In a particular food, such as olives or cheese, the unsaturated and saturated fats occur in different proportions, but one type of fatty acid (saturated, monounsaturated, or polyunsaturated) often predominates. Figure 6.5 compares the percentages of saturated,

Figure 6.5 Fats and oils. This figure shows approximate percentages of the three major types of fatty acids in common fats and oils.

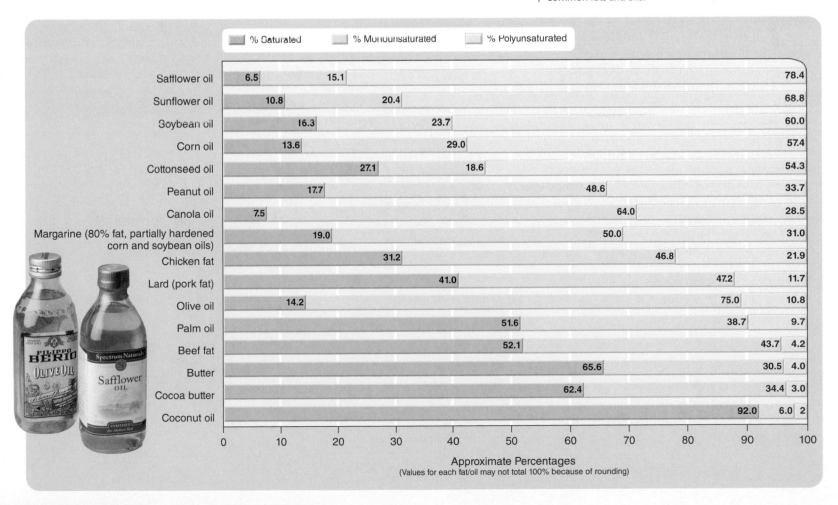

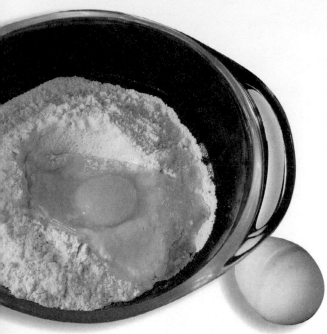

Whole eggs or egg yolks are often included in recipes that involve mixing oily and watery ingredients to form emulsions. Cake batter, for example, is an emulsion.

Did You Know?

Lard is pork fat. In some parts of the United States, lard is used to make biscuits, pie dough, and refried beans. Lard is high in saturated fat (41%), but it is not as highly saturated as butter (66%).

monounsaturated, and polyunsaturated fatty acids in commonly eaten fats. Note that the fat in beef and dairy products contains more saturated than unsaturated fatty acids; olive oil is a rich source of monounsaturated fatty acids; and liquid corn oil contains a greater proportion of unsaturated than saturated fatty acids. Certain animal foods, especially beef and dairy foods such as cheese, cream, and butter, contain higher percentages of saturated fatty acids than most plant fats. Important exceptions are tropical oils such as coconut and palm oils. Tropical oils contain more saturated than unsaturated fatty acids. Fats and oils that contain high amounts of saturated or unsaturated fatty acids are commonly called saturated fats or unsaturated fats.

Why is it important to understand the differences between saturated, unsaturated, and trans fats, and identify foods that contain high amounts of these fats? Populations that consume diets rich in saturated fat and trans fat have higher risk of cardiovascular disease than populations whose diets contain more unsaturated than saturated fat.[10] For more information about this topic, see the "Lipids and Health: Cardiovascular Disease (CVD)" section of Chapter 6.

Phospholipids

A **phospholipid** is chemically similar to a triglyceride, except that one of the fatty acids is replaced by chemical groups that contain phosphorus and, often, nitrogen (Fig. 6.6a). Phospholipids are naturally found in plant and animal foods. *Lecithin* (*less'-eh-thin*) is the major phospholipid in food; egg yolks, liver, wheat germ, peanut butter, and soybeans are rich sources of lecithin.

Unlike triglycerides, phospholipids are partially water soluble because the phosphorus-containing portion of the molecule is **hydrophilic** (*hydro* = water; *philic* = loving); that is, it attracts water (Fig. 6.6b). A phospholipid molecule also has a **hydrophobic** (*phobic* = fearing) portion that avoids watery substances and attracts oily ones. By having both hydrophilic and hydrophobic regions, a phospholipid can serve as an **emulsifier**, a substance that keeps water-soluble and water-insoluble compounds

Figure 6.6 Phospholipids. A phospholipid such as lecithin has a chemical structure that is similar to that of a triglyceride molecule. (*a*) The chemical structure of lecithin has a glycerol backbone, a phosphorus (P)–containing phosphate group, and a nitrogen (N)–containing compound called choline. (*b*) Phospholipids have hydrophilic and hydrophobic portions. As a result, a phospholipid can serve as an emulsifier, a substance that keeps water-soluble and water-insoluble compounds mixed together.

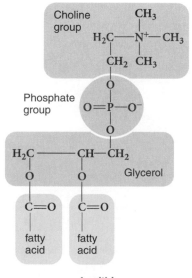

Lecithin
(phospholipid molecule)

a.

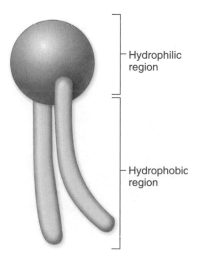

b.

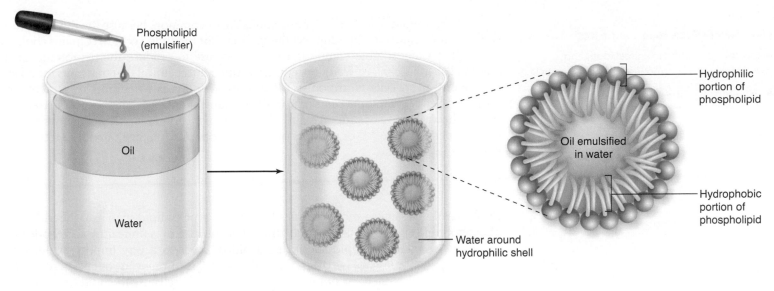

Figure 6.7 Emulsification. Emulsification enhances lipid digestion and absorption by keeping lipids dispersed in small particles, increasing their surface area. As a result, lipases gain greater access to the lipid molecules and can digest them more readily.

mixed together (Fig. 6.7). Manufacturers may add emulsifiers to foods to keep oily and watery ingredients from separating during storage. Processed foods, such as cheese food, salad dressing, and ice cream, often have phospholipids added as emulsifying agents. Egg yolk, for example, naturally contains phospholipids and is used to emulsify oil and vinegar when making mayonnaise or mixing oil and milk in cake batters.

In the body, phospholipids are major structural components of cell membranes. Cell membranes are comprised of a double layer that is mostly phospholipids (Figure 6.8). The chemical structure of the phospholipids enables the membrane to be flexible and function properly. Phospholipids are also needed for normal functioning of nerve cells, including those in the brain.

phospholipid type of lipid needed to make cell membranes and for proper functioning of nerve cells

hydrophilic part of molecule that attracts water

hydrophobic part of molecule that avoids water and attracts lipids

emulsifier substance that helps water-soluble and water-insoluble compounds mix with each other

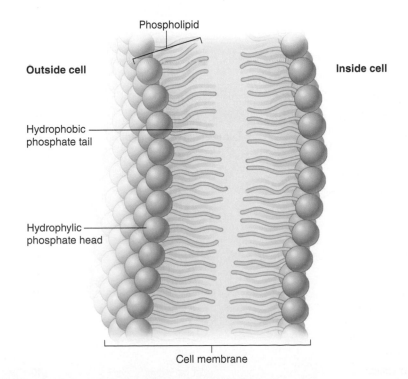

Figure 6.8 Phospholipids in cell membranes. In the human body, cell membranes are comprised of a double layer of phospholipids. Cholesterol and proteins are embedded in the membrane (not shown).

choline water-soluble compound in lecithin

cholesterol lipid found in animal foods and precursor for steroid hormones, bile, and vitamin D

bile emulsifier that aids lipid digestion

Phospholipid deficiencies among adults are uncommon, because the lipids are in a variety of foods and healthy adults synthesize these compounds. Lecithin contains **choline** (*co'-leen*), a water-soluble compound that nerves use to produce the neurotransmitter *acetylcholine* (*ah-see'-till-co'-leen*). A neurotransmitter is a chemical that transmits messages between the nerve cells. Nutritionists often classify choline as a vitamin-like nutrient, because deficiency symptoms can occur under certain conditions.[11] The results of scientific studies, however, do not support claims that lecithin or choline supplements improve the physical performance[12, 13] or memory of healthy people.[14] Chapter 8 provides more information about choline.

Cholesterol

Cholesterol is a *sterol*, a more chemically complex type of lipid than a triglyceride or a phospholipid (Fig. 6.9). Many people think that cholesterol is unhealthy and foods that contain the lipid should be avoided, but it is a very important nutrient. Cholesterol is a component of every cell membrane in your body. Although cholesterol is not metabolized for energy, cells use the lipid to synthesize a variety of substances, including vitamin D, and steroid hormones such as estrogen and testosterone. The liver uses cholesterol to make **bile**, an emulsifier that facilitates lipid digestion. The gallbladder stores bile until it is needed for digesting lipids.

Although triglycerides are widespread in foods, cholesterol is found only in animal foods. Egg yolk, liver, meat, poultry, whole milk, cheese, and ice cream are rich sources of cholesterol (Table 6.2). Even if you do not eat animal foods, your body produces cholesterol, primarily in the liver. If your body makes too much cholesterol, the excess can increase your risk of CVD.

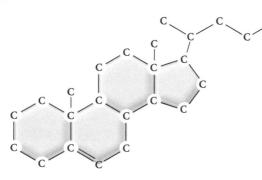

Figure 6.9 Cholesterol. Cholesterol is a complex organic molecule. For simplicity, this illustration shows only the molecule's carbon atoms.

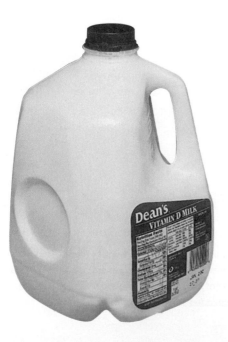

TABLE 6.2 *Approximate Cholesterol Content of Some Foods/Serving*

Food	Serving Size	Cholesterol (mg)
Liver	3 oz	234
Egg	1 large	212
Egg yolk	1	212
Sardines	3 oz	121
Single-patty cheeseburger	1	111
Beef	3 oz	88
Turkey, ground	3 oz	84
Danish fruit-filled pastry	2½ oz	81
Shrimp	6 large, breaded and fried	80
Ham	3 oz	80
Ice cream, soft-serve	½ cup	78
Ground beef, lean (15% fat)	3 oz	77
Salmon	3 oz	75
Turkey, dark meat	3 oz	71
Egg noodles	1 cup	53
Chicken breast	3 oz	49
Hot dog	1	44
Chocolate milkshake	16 oz	43
Whole milk	1 cup	34
Cottage cheese	1 cup	32
Cheddar cheese	1 oz	30

Concept **Checkpoint**

1. What are the major lipids in food and the body?
2. What is the difference between a saturated and an unsaturated fatty acid? What is the difference between a monounsaturated and a polyunsaturated fatty acid?
3. Identify at least one food that is a rich source of saturated fat, monounsaturated fat, and polyunsaturated fat.
4. Identify the two essential fatty acids.
5. What structural characteristic distinguishes a trans fatty acid from a cis fatty acid? Identify at least two foods that are rich sources of trans fat.
6. What is an omega-3 fatty acid?
7. A recipe mixes ¼ cup of oil with ¾ cup of milk. What common food could you add to keep the oil and milk emulsified?
8. Which foods contain cholesterol? List at least three functions of cholesterol in the body.

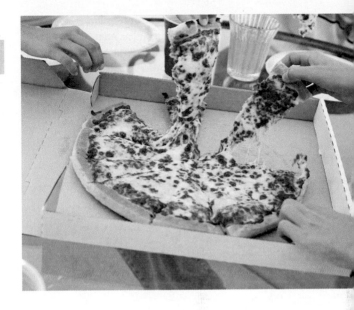

 ## 6.2 What Happens to Lipids in Your Body?

Digesting lipids is a more complicated process than digesting carbohydrates, because the majority of the lipids in food are not water soluble and the digestion process involves considerable amounts of water. Triglycerides and phospholipids need to be broken down by special enzymes called **lipases** before they can be absorbed. When you eat a cheeseburger and French fries, an inactive lipase in saliva mixes with the food. As the food enters the stomach, the organ's acid environment activates the lipase, enabling some lipid breakdown to occur. The small intestine, however, is the primary site of lipid digestion.

As the fatty chyme leaves the stomach and enters your small intestine, it stimulates certain intestinal cells to release the hormone **cholecystokinin** (*kol'-e-sis'-toe-kye'-nin*) **(CCK)**. CCK signals the pancreas to secrete digestive enzymes, including *pancreatic lipase*, into the duodenum of the small intestine. **Pancreatic lipase** digests triglycerides by removing two fatty acids from each triglyceride molecule. This action converts most triglycerides into *monoglycerides* (Fig. 6.10). A **monoglyceride** has a single fatty acid attached to the glycerol backbone of the molecule. Some triglycerides are completely broken down into glycerol and fatty acid molecules.

The process of digesting phospholipids is similar to that of digesting triglycerides. The enzyme *phospholipase* removes two fatty acids from a phospholipid molecule. The remaining structure contains the lipid's phosphate group (see Fig. 6.6). Cholesterol does not undergo digestion; small intestinal cells can absorb cholesterol directly from your food. Glycerol, fatty acids, monoglycerides, cholesterol, and phospholipid fragments are the end products of lipid digestion.

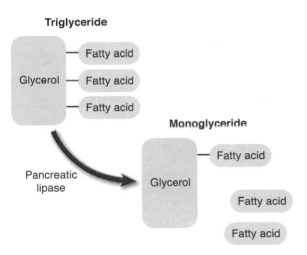

Figure 6.10 Triglyceride digestion. Pancreatic lipase digests triglycerides by removing two fatty acids from each triglyceride molecule. This process converts most triglycerides into monoglycerides.

Did You Know?

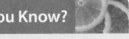

Monoglycerides and diglycerides may be listed as ingredients on food labels. These lipids result from the breakdown of triglycerides, and they may be added to foods during processing to improve the product's texture.

Bile

Another function of the hormone CCK is stimulating the gallbladder to contract. This action forces some *bile* into the duodenum, where it mixes with chyme. Bile contains *bile salts,* compounds that enhance digestion and absorption by keeping lipids dispersed in small particles,

lipases enzymes that break down lipids

cholecystokinin (CCK) hormone that stimulates the gallbladder to release bile and pancreas to secrete digestive enzymes

pancreatic lipase digestive enzyme that removes two fatty acids from each triglyceride molecule

monoglyceride single fatty acid attached to a glycerol backbone

Figure 6.11 Lipid digestion and absorption. Pancreatic lipase and bile facilitate lipid digestion. After lipids enter absorptive cells of the small intestine, triglycerides are re-formed. Triglycerides and other lipids are coated with a layer of protein, phospholipids, and cholesterol to form chylomicrons.

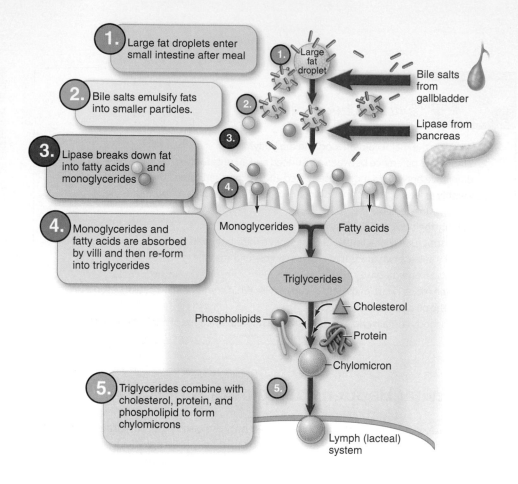

1. Large fat droplets enter small intestine after meal

1. Large fat droplet

Bile salts from gallbladder

2. Bile salts emulsify fats into smaller particles.

Lipase from pancreas

3. Lipase breaks down fat into fatty acids and monoglycerides

4. Monoglycerides and fatty acids are absorbed by villi and then re-form into triglycerides

Monoglycerides   Fatty acids

Triglycerides

Phospholipids

Cholesterol

Protein

Chylomicron

5. Triglycerides combine with cholesterol, protein, and phospholipid to form chylomicrons

Lymph (lacteal) system

---

lipoprotein water-soluble structure that transports lipids through the bloodstream

lipoprotein lipase enzyme in capillary walls that breaks down triglycerides

enterohepatic circulation process that recycles cholesterol (bile salts) in the body

---

increasing their surface area (Fig. 6.11). As a result, pancreatic lipase gains greater access to the lipid molecules and digests them more readily. If bile is not secreted into the duodenum, lipids clump together in large fatty globules, making lipid digestion less efficient.

What Are Lipoproteins?

Under normal conditions, the small intestine digests and absorbs nearly all of the triglycerides and phospholipids in food, but only about 50% of the dietary cholesterol is absorbed. After being absorbed, short- and medium-chain fatty acids can enter the bloodstream directly. Most fatty acids, glycerol, monoglycerides, and phospholipid fragments are reassembled into triglycerides and phospholipids within the absorptive cells of the small intestine. Cholesterol and the reassembled triglycerides are coated with a thin layer of protein, phospholipids, and cholesterol to form chylomicrons (see Fig. 6.11). A *chylomicron* (ky′-low-my′-kron) is a type of *lipoprotein*. **Lipoproteins** are water-soluble structures that transport lipids through the bloodstream. Chylomicrons are too large to be absorbed directly into the bloodstream. These lipoproteins must pass through the larger openings of *lacteals* (lak′-te-als), lymphatic system vessels in each villus (see Fig. 4.29).

The lymphatic system transports chylomicrons to the thoracic duct, where they enter the bloodstream through the left subclavian vein in the chest (Fig. 6.12). As chylomicrons circulate through the body, **lipoprotein lipase,** an enzyme in the walls of capillaries, breaks down their load of triglycerides into fatty acids and glycerol. Nearby cells can pick up the fatty acids and glycerol molecules to use for energy. Ten to 12 hours after a meal, most chylomicrons have been reduced to small cholesterol-rich remnants. The liver clears these remnants from the bloodstream and uses their contents to synthesize new lipids and other lipoproteins that are released into the general circulation. Figure 6.13 provides a summary of lipid digestion and absorption.

Certain lipoproteins carry lipids from the liver to cells. Other lipoproteins convey lipids from cells to the liver, where they may be converted into new compounds. The

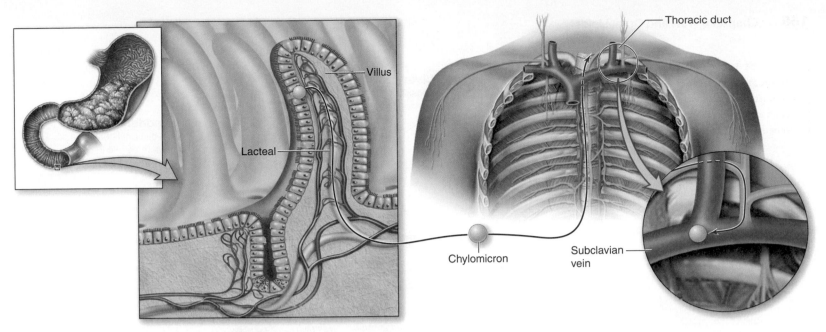

"Lipids and Health: Cardiovascular Disease (CVD)" section of Chapter 6 provides more information about lipoproteins and their effects on cardiovascular health.

Recycling Bile Salts

Most bile salts are absorbed in the ileum, where the compounds enter the bloodstream and travel to the liver. The liver uses the bile salts to make new bile. The process of recycling bile from the intestinal tract is called **enterohepatic** (*ent'-eh-roe-hih-pah'-tik*) **circulation**

Figure 6.12 **Journey into the general circulation.** Chylomicrons are too large to be absorbed directly into the bloodstream. These lipoproteins must pass through the larger openings of lacteals, lymphatic system vessels in each villus. The lymphatic system transports chylomicrons to the thoracic duct, where they enter the bloodstream through the left subclavian vein in the chest.

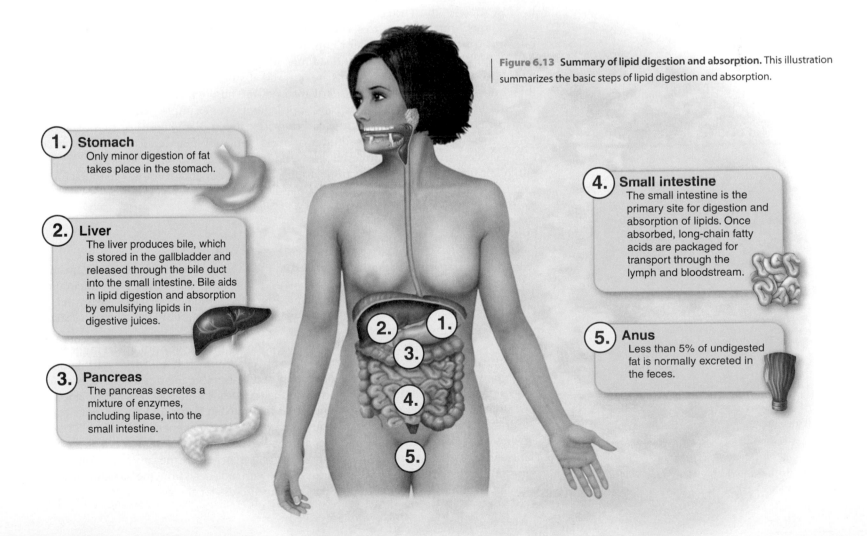

Figure 6.13 **Summary of lipid digestion and absorption.** This illustration summarizes the basic steps of lipid digestion and absorption.

1. Stomach
Only minor digestion of fat takes place in the stomach.

2. Liver
The liver produces bile, which is stored in the gallbladder and released through the bile duct into the small intestine. Bile aids in lipid digestion and absorption by emulsifying lipids in digestive juices.

3. Pancreas
The pancreas secretes a mixture of enzymes, including lipase, into the small intestine.

4. Small intestine
The small intestine is the primary site for digestion and absorption of lipids. Once absorbed, long-chain fatty acids are packaged for transport through the lymph and bloodstream.

5. Anus
Less than 5% of undigested fat is normally excreted in the feces.

Figure 6.14 Enterohepatic circulation. Enterohepatic circulation is the process of recycling bile salts. As a result of this process, the liver conserves cholesterol. Soluble fiber, however, interferes with bile salt absorption. When the intestine absorbs less bile salts, the liver needs to use cholesterol to form new bile salts.

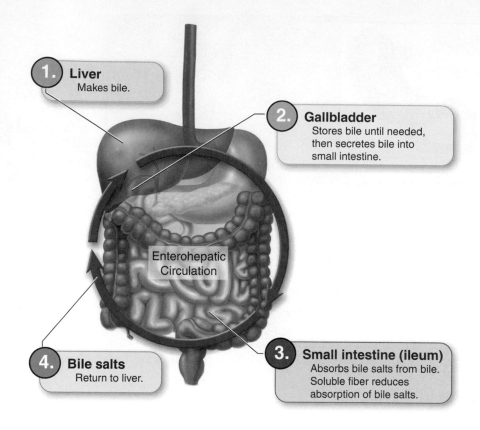

1. **Liver** Makes bile.

2. **Gallbladder** Stores bile until needed, then secretes bile into small intestine.

Enterohepatic Circulation

4. **Bile salts** Return to liver.

3. **Small intestine (ileum)** Absorbs bile salts from bile. Soluble fiber reduces absorption of bile salts.

sterols/stanols types of lipids made by plants

adipose cells fat cells

(Fig. 6.14). Interfering with enterohepatic circulation can reduce blood cholesterol levels, because the liver must use cholesterol to make new bile salts.

Plants contain substances, such as soluble fiber, that interfere with cholesterol and bile absorption (see Table 5.6 for common food sources of soluble fiber). Plants also make small amounts of **sterols** and **stanols**, lipids that are chemically related to cholesterol. Although plant sterols/stanols are not well absorbed by the human intestinal tract, these substances can reduce cholesterol absorption. Thus, plant sterols/stanols are added to certain foods, beverages, and dietary supplements. For example, synthetic margarine-like spreads such as Benecol® and TakeControl® contain plant sterols or plant stanols. Eating these products instead of butter or stick margarine may reduce mildly elevated blood cholesterol levels.[15] Cholesterol-lowering margarines and other products that contain plant sterols/stanols are functional foods, because they are specifically manufactured to provide beneficial health effects (see Chapter 3).

Using Triglycerides for Energy

Most cells can metabolize fatty acids for energy. Fat is more energy dense than carbohydrate or protein: a gram of fat supplies 9 kcal, whereas a gram of carbohydrate or protein provides only 4 kcal. Thus, a high-fat food is a more concentrated source of energy than a high-carbohydrate food. For example, you would need to eat 2½ tablespoons of sugar to obtain the amount of energy in 1 tablespoon of oil.

In many instances, your body does not need the energy from the fat in the food you have just eaten. **Adipose** (*ad'-eh-pose*) **cells,** commonly called fat cells, remove fatty acids and glycerol from circulation and reassemble them into triglycerides for storage. Most cells in your body contain triglycerides, but adipose cells are designed to store large amounts of fat (triglycerides). As illustrated in Figure 6.15, a fat droplet comprises most of an adipose cell's volume. When your body needs energy, adipose cells break down some stored triglycerides into fatty acid and glycerol molecules and release these substances into your bloodstream. Muscle and other cells then remove the fatty acids from circulation and metabolize them. The liver clears the glycerol molecules from the bloodstream and converts them into glucose molecules that cells can also use for energy.

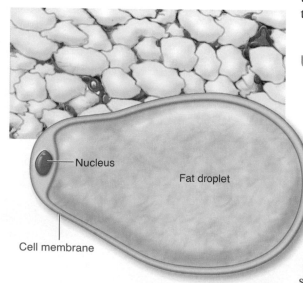

Nucleus

Fat droplet

Cell membrane

Figure 6.15 Adipose cells. A primary function of an adipose cell is storing a fat droplet.

Eating too much fat contributes to unwanted weight gain, but consuming too much energy from protein and carbohydrates also increases body fat. Why? The body can convert excess glucose and certain amino acids into fatty acids that are used to make triglycerides. Additionally, the nonnutrient alcohol stimulates triglyceride synthesis, and excess body fat can accumulate as a result of alcohol consumption. Alcohol has many other effects on the body, some of which are beneficial to cardiovascular health. To learn more about alcohol and assess your use of the substance, read the Chapter 6 Highlight, "Drink to Your Health?" on page 184. For more information about energy metabolism, see Appendix D.

Concept **Checkpoint**

9. Describe what happens to the fat in a piece of fried chicken as it undergoes digestion and absorption in your intestinal tract. In your description, include the roles of bile, CCK, pancreatic lipase, villi, and chylomicrons.

6.3 Lipid Consumption Patterns

On average, Americans ate about 54 pounds of fat per year in 1987–1988.[16] Twenty years later, the typical American consumed 63 pounds of fat per year, which is an increase of almost 17%, compared to the earlier period.[17] Fat contributes 34% of the average American's daily energy intake. Although there is no RDA or AI for total fat (for people over 1 year of age), the Acceptable Macronutrient Distribution Range (AMDR) for the macronutrient is 20 to 35% of total calories.[5] According to the American Heart Association, people should limit their fat intake to less than 25 to 35% of total calories and emphasize foods that are rich sources of polyunsaturated and monounsaturated fatty acids, such as fish, nuts, and vegetable oils.[8] To meet this recommendation, you do not need to eat only low-fat foods. By balancing your intake of low-fat and high-fat foods, your daily fat intake can average less than 35% of total energy.

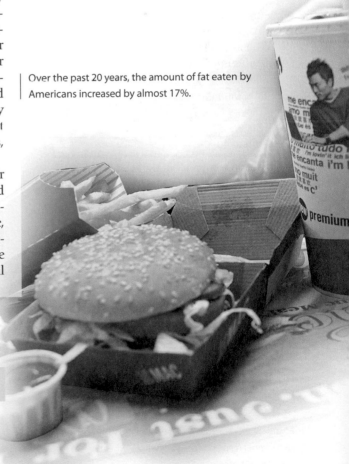

Over the past 20 years, the amount of fat eaten by Americans increased by almost 17%.

According to the Dietary Guidelines, adults should consume less than 10% of their total calories from saturated fatty acids, keep their trans fat intake as low as possible, and limit their cholesterol intake to 300 mg/day.[18] In 2007–2008, the average American consumed about 11% of his or her total daily energy intake from saturated fat.[17] On average, trans fats contributed about 2% of a person's daily energy intake.[18] In 2007–2008, cholesterol intake for Americans was about 280 mg/day. To estimate your average percentage of total energy from fat as well as your cholesterol intake per day, complete the "Personal Dietary Analysis" activity at the end of Chapter 6.

Concept **Checkpoint**

10. Fat contributes what percentage of total energy in the typical American's diet?
11. What is the AMDR for fat?
12. Describe *Dietary Guidelines for Americans 2010* recommendations concerning saturated fat, cholesterol, and trans fat intakes for adults.

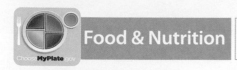

Food & Nutrition *tip*

To lower the fat content of their products, manufacturers of "lite" spreads may have water as the first ingredient. Therefore, replacing the margarine, butter, oil, or shortening in a recipe with a reduced-fat spread could alter the product's taste, texture, and appearance. It is a good idea to read the reduced-fat spread's label to determine whether the product is suitable to use in recipes.

Nutrition Facts

Serving Size 1 slice (38 g)
Servings Per Container 18

Amount Per Serving

Calories 100

Calories from Fat 20

	% Daily Value*
Total Fat 2g	3%
Saturated Fat 0g	0%
Trans Fat 0g	
Polyunsaturated Fat 1g	
Monounsaturated Fat 0g	
Cholesterol 0mg	0%
Sodium 160mg	7%
Total Carbohydrate 17g	6%
Dietary Fiber 2g	8%
Sugars 3g	
Protein 4g	

Vitamin A	10%
Vitamin C	0%
Calcium	10%
Iron	8%

* Percent Daily Values are based on a 2,000 calorie diet. Your daily values may be higher or lower, depending on your calorie needs:

		Calories	2,000	2,500
Total Fat	Less than		65g	80g
Sat Fat	Less than		20g	25g
Cholesterol	Less than		300mg	300mg
Sodium	Less than		2,400mg	2,400mg
Total Carbohydrate			300g	375g
Dietary Fiber			25g	30g

INGREDIENTS: Whole-wheat flour, Water, Brown sugar, Wheat gluten, Cracked wheat, Wheat bran, Yeast, Salt, Molasses, Soybean oil, Calcium propionate (preservative), Mono–and diglycerides, Lecithin, Reduced fat milk

Figure 6.16 Nutrition Facts panel (2011). This Nutrition Facts panel from a package of whole-wheat bread displays the amount of total fat as well as the amounts of saturated, unsaturated, trans fat, and cholesterol in one serving.

6.4 Understanding Nutritional Labeling: Lipids

You can determine how much total fat, saturated fat, trans fat, and cholesterol are in most packaged food products by reading the Nutrition Facts panel. As you can see in Figure 6.16, grams of total fat in one serving of bread (a slice) are shown, and under it, the number of grams of the different fats that comprise the total amount. The panel indicates that there are 2 g of total fat in each slice, and of that amount, 1 g is polyunsaturated fat. According to the panel, there are 0 g of saturated, trans, and monounsaturated fats in a slice of the bread. You may be asking yourself, why do the amounts of the various types of fat not add up to 2 g? What happened to the other 1 g of fat? If a food has less than 0.5 g of a specific type of fat, the amount can be reported as *0 g*. When the fractions of fat are added together, however, the total amount, in this example, is 2 g. In 2012, the FDA may introduce a new format for the Nutrition Facts panel that indicates more specific amounts of fat in products.

You can use information from the Nutrition Facts panel to determine the percentage of calories that are from fat in a product. In Figure 6.16, the panel indicates that a slice of whole-wheat bread provides 100 kcal, 20 of which are from fat. To calculate the percentage of energy from fat, divide the number of kilocalories from fat (20 kcal) by the total number of kilocalories (100 kcal) in the serving. Move the decimal point two places to the right, and then replace the decimal point with a percentage sign (e.g., 20 kcal ÷ 100 kcal = .20; .20 ⟶ 20%). In a serving of this type of bread, fat contributes 20% of the energy. By reading the list of ingredients shown at the bottom of the panel, you will note that soybean oil is the main source of fat in this bread.

The Nutrition Facts panel also provides information about the cholesterol content of a food. In the panel, the amount of cholesterol in a serving is shown below that of total fat. According to information listed on the Nutrition Facts panel shown in Figure 6.16, a slice of whole-grain bread provides 0 mg of cholesterol.

Concept **Checkpoint**

13. According to the Nutrition Facts panel, a serving of potato chips supplies 150 kcal, and fat contributes 100 of the total kcal in the serving of chips. Calculate the percentage of energy from fat in these chips.

6.5 Lipids and Health: Cardiovascular Disease (CVD)

Cardiovascular disease (CVD) includes diseases of the heart and blood vessels. According to estimates, more than one in three adult Americans has one or more forms of CVD.[19] Heart disease (**coronary artery disease,** or **CAD**) and stroke, the most common forms of CVD, are among the top four leading causes of death in the United States. In 2009, heart disease and strokes were responsible for about 30% of deaths in the United States.[20] CVD does not affect just elderly people: in 2006, one-third of Americans who died of CVD were younger than 75 years of age.

From Atherosclerosis to Cardiovascular Disease

Most cases of heart disease and stroke result from **atherosclerosis** (*athero* = lipid containing; *sclerosis* [*skleh-ro'-sis*] = hardening), a chronic process that negatively affects the functioning of arteries. Normal arteries have a smooth lining (Fig. 6.17.1). When

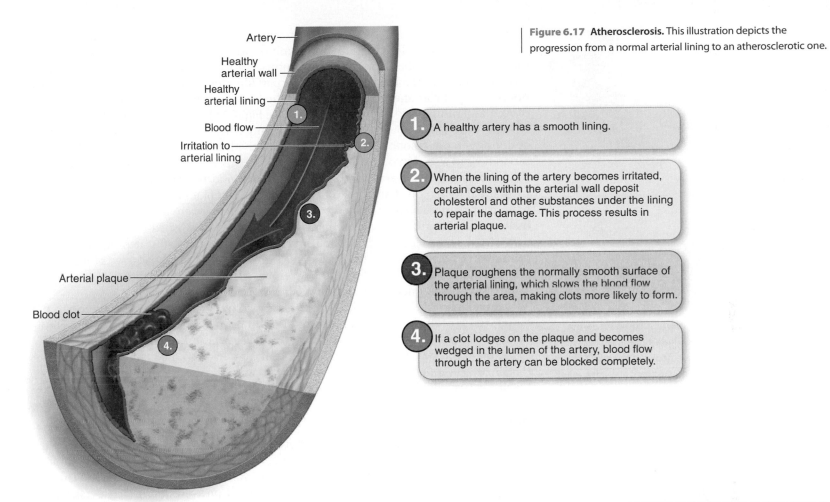

Artery

Healthy arterial wall

Healthy arterial lining

Blood flow

Irritation to arterial lining

Arterial plaque

Blood clot

1. A healthy artery has a smooth lining.

2. When the lining of the artery becomes irritated, certain cells within the arterial wall deposit cholesterol and other substances under the lining to repair the damage. This process results in arterial plaque.

3. Plaque roughens the normally smooth surface of the arterial lining, which slows the blood flow through the area, making clots more likely to form.

4. If a clot lodges on the plaque and becomes wedged in the lumen of the artery, blood flow through the artery can be blocked completely.

Figure 6.17 Atherosclerosis. This illustration depicts the progression from a normal arterial lining to an atherosclerotic one.

something in the bloodstream, such as excess cholesterol or glucose, compounds from cigarette smoke, or certain bacteria, irritates the lining of an artery, a cascade of events begins that results in atherosclerosis (Fig. 6.17.2). The body's immune system responds to the irritation by producing inflammation within the artery. Inflammation can stimulate healing, but the process can also trigger certain cells within the arterial wall to deposit cholesterol and other substances under the artery's lining. As a result, arterial plaque forms (Fig. 6.17.3). Plaque interferes with circulation in the affected area of the artery, because it narrows and may even block the opening through which blood flows (*lumen*). Furthermore, plaque roughens the normally smooth surface that lines the artery. The rough lining slows blood flow in the area and makes clots more likely to form (Fig. 6.17.4). If a plaque *ruptures* (tears open), repairing the damage also involves clot formation, and such blood clots can be life threatening. Figure 6.18 shows cross sections of a healthy artery and one that is almost completely blocked by plaque.

cardiovascular disease (CVD) group of diseases that affect the heart and blood vessels

coronary artery disease (CAD) a major form of CVD

atherosclerosis long-term disease process in which plaque build up inside arterial walls

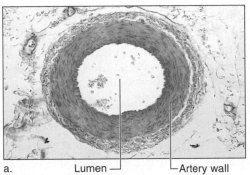

a. Lumen of the artery — Artery wall

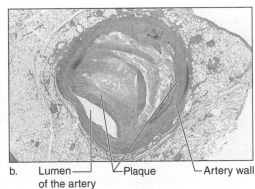

b. Lumen of the artery — Plaque — Artery wall

Figure 6.18 Healthy and atherosclerotic arteries. Note the differences between the cross section of a healthy artery (*a*) and that of an artery nearly completely blocked as a result of atherosclerosis (*b*).

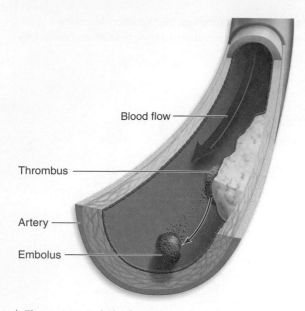

Figure 6.19 Embolus formation. A thrombus or part of a plaque that breaks free from where it formed and travels through the bloodstream is an embolus. If an embolus lodges in an artery, the material can create the same serious consequences as a stationary bunch of clots (thrombus).

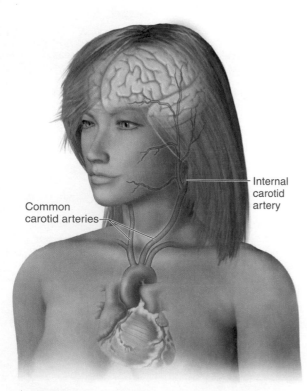

Figure 6.20 Carotid arteries. The carotid arteries convey blood to the brain. Atherosclerosis in these arteries can result in reduced blood flow to the brain and increase the risk of stroke.

Blood must be able to clot, especially when blood vessels have been injured; otherwise, a person could bleed to death from a minor bruise. In some instances, however, clots form too readily at the injury site. A **thrombus** is a fixed bunch of clots that remains in place and disrupts blood flow. If a thrombus partially closes off the lumen of an artery that nourishes the heart, the affected section of the heart muscle is unable to receive enough oxygen and nutrients to function properly (see Fig. 6.18). As a result, the affected person typically experiences bouts of chest pain, especially when his or her heart beats faster, such as during intense emotional states or physical activities. If a thrombus completely blocks blood flow to a section of the heart muscle, the muscle dies and a **myocardial infarction** (*my'-oh-card-e-al in-farc'-shun*) (heart attack) occurs. Sudden death can result from a severe myocardial infarction. A stroke can happen when a clot blocks an artery in the brain and brain cells that are nourished by the vessel die. When an artery to a limb is blocked, the tissue in the extremity dies, causing gangrene to occur. If the affected area is large, amputation of the gangrenous limb is often necessary to prevent life-threatening infection. A thrombus or part of a plaque that breaks free from where it formed and travels through the bloodstream is an **embolus** (Fig. 6.19). An embolus that lodges in an artery can create the same serious consequences as a stationary thrombus.

Certain arteries are more likely to be damaged by atherosclerosis; in addition to the blood vessels of the heart and brain, the blood supply in the kidneys, eyes, and legs is vulnerable. When atherosclerosis occurs in the *common carotid arteries* in the neck, blood flow to the brain can be decreased and clots can form that travel to the brain, causing a stroke (Fig. 6.20). Although atherosclerosis can begin during adolescence and young adulthood, the disease usually does not produce signs or symptoms of CVD until decades later.

Arteriosclerosis

In addition to interfering with blood flow, plaques reduce the flexibility of arteries, causing **arteriosclerosis** (*arterio* = artery), a condition commonly called "hardening of the arteries." Arteriosclerosis contributes to the development of **hypertension,** a chronic condition characterized by abnormally high blood pressure levels that persist even when the person is relaxed. Hypertension is a major risk factor for atherosclerosis and heart disease. The heart of a person with hypertension must work harder to circulate blood through abnormally stiff arteries. Furthermore, elevated blood pressure can cause hardened arteries to tear or burst, causing serious bleeding problems and even sudden death, depending on the artery's size and location.

Risk Factors for Atherosclerosis

The National Heart Lung and Blood Institute has identified risk factors for atherosclerosis.[21] The more risk factors a person has, the greater his or her likelihood of developing CVD. Table 6.3 lists major risk factors and indicates which ones are nonmodifiable or modifiable. Increasing age, male sex, race/ethnic background, and family history are nonmodifiable risk factors. The risk of atherosclerosis increases as people grow older, and men are more likely to have heart attacks than women. Although a woman's risk of heart attack increases after menopause, her risk is still less than that of a man of the same age. Americans with African, Mexican, or Native American ancestry are more likely to have heart disease than people with other racial or ethnic backgrounds. Another trait people cannot change is their family history. For example, if your father had his first heart attack when he was 42 years old, you have a greater risk of developing heart disease at a relatively young age than someone whose father had his first heart attack at 75 years of age. Characteristics such as age, male sex, ancestry, and family history of CVD cannot be modified, but controlling other risk factors, such as smoking and hypertension, can reduce the risk of atherosclerosis.[21]

Sleep apnea, a common disorder among overweight and obese people, may be a risk factor for atherosclerosis.[21] While asleep, a person with sleep apnea stops breathing intermittently or does not breathe deeply. As a result, the person wakes up several times and does not feel refreshed after sleeping. Sleep apnea can be treated; untreated sleep apnea can contribute to hypertension, heart attack, and stroke.

TABLE 6.3 *Atherosclerosis: Major Risk Factors*

Nonmodifiable Risk Factors
Family history of CVD (especially before 60 years of age)
Increasing age
Race/ethnic background
Male sex

Modifiable Risk Factors
Hypertension
Diabetes mellitus
Elevated blood cholesterol (especially LDL cholesterol)
Excess body fat
Physical inactivity
Tobacco use or exposure to tobacco smoke

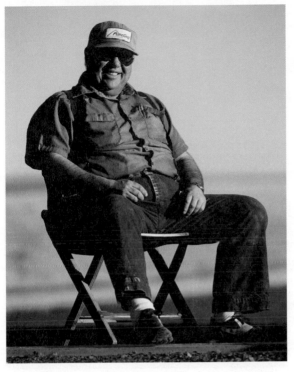

Major risk factors for CVD include male sex, increasing age, excess body fat, and physical inactivity.

Genetics and CVD

Genetics (family history) is a major risk factor for atherosclerosis and CVD that cannot be modified. A person's genes, for example, may code for various physical conditions that increase risk of heart disease, such as hypertension and diabetes. Additionally, genes may influence the way in which the circulatory and immune systems respond to diet. Thus, some people may be protected against the development of atherosclerosis, whereas other persons with similar diets develop serious arterial plaques early in life and die prematurely of CVD as a result.

Until recently, much of the research examining the role of diet in the development of atherosclerosis focused on the association between lipids and CVD. Nevertheless, some people with no apparent CVD risk factors still had heart attacks, strokes, and related blood vessel diseases. In many cases, affected individuals were under 40 years of age. This puzzling observation led to the discovery that the amino acid **homocysteine** (*ho'-mo-sis-teen*) may be associated with CVD. Amino acids are the chemical units that comprise proteins. Although homocysteine is an amino acid, the substance is not found in human proteins, and higher-than-normal blood levels of homocysteine can be toxic. High blood levels of homocysteine may injure arterial walls and contribute to atherosclerosis.[22] A few people have a rare genetic abnormality that causes the amino acid to accumulate in their bloodstream. These individuals have a higher risk of premature CVD than persons who do not have the genetic defect. Cells use two vitamins, B-6 and folate, to convert homocysteine into safer compounds. Deficiencies of certain B vitamins can also cause homocysteine levels to become elevated. Some medical experts think an elevated blood homocysteine level may be a "marker" in blood that indicates a person has CVD. Nevertheless, more studies are needed to determine whether elevated blood homocysteine plays a role in the development of CVD among the general population.

Modifiable Risk Factors

Several major risk factors for atherosclerosis involve lifestyle choices that can be modified. Hypertension, diabetes, excess body fat, and elevated blood cholesterol are modifiable risk factors that can be influenced by diet and exercise. Many people, for example, can reduce their chances of developing atherosclerosis by avoiding tobacco use, limiting their intake of saturated fat, exercising regularly, and maintaining a healthy body weight.

Nearly one in three adult Americans has hypertension, chronically elevated blood pressure.[19] Hypertension is often referred to as a "silent disease," because people with the condition frequently feel healthy and do not have obvious symptoms that indicate trouble within their circulatory system. The condition, however, is quite serious because it damages arterial walls and increases the risk of stroke, heart failure, and kidney disease.

thrombus fixed bunch of clots that remains in place

myocardial infarction heart attack

embolus thrombus or part of a plaque that breaks free and travels through the bloodstream

arteriosclerosis condition that results from atherosclerosis and is characterized by loss of arterial flexibility

hypertension abnormally high blood pressure levels that persist

homocysteine amino acid that may play a role in the development of atherosclerosis

Chapter 9 presents information about hypertension, including healthy blood pressure values (see Tables 9.8 and 9.9). Chapter 9 also discusses ways to reduce the likelihood of developing the condition.

Diabetes is another modifiable risk factor for atherosclerosis. Adults who have diabetes are two to four times more likely to die of heart disease or stroke than adults without diabetes.[23] Chapter 5 discusses diabetes in detail. Excess body fat, especially in the abdominal region, increases the risk of type 2 diabetes and hypertension; Chapter 10 focuses on sensible ways to lose body fat. Physical inactivity also contributes to excess body fat. Chapter 11 (Nutrition for Physically Active Lifestyles) provides suggestions for becoming more physically active. Elevated blood lipids, particularly certain lipoproteins, are a risk factor for atherosclerosis. The "Reducing Your Risk of Atherosclerosis: Dietary Changes" section of Chapter 6 presents ways people can modify their diets to reduce their chances of developing atherosclerosis.

Tobacco use is another major risk factor for atherosclerosis that is modifiable. Compared to nonsmokers, smokers have two to four times the likelihood of developing heart disease and having a stroke.[24] Smokers expose other people in their environment to *secondhand smoke*, which is a combination of the smoke from the burning end of cigarette and exhaled air of the person who is smoking. Exposure to secondhand smoke is a risk factor for heart disease.[25] If you smoke, simply improving your diet is unlikely to reduce your risk of atherosclerosis; therefore, if you smoke, make every effort to quit using tobacco products. If you do not smoke, avoid breathing secondhand smoke.

Emotional stress, particularly anger, also plays a role in the development of atherosclerosis.[21] Although individuals respond to stress differently, chronic stress generally causes physical changes in the body that can damage arteries and contribute to atherosclerosis. Furthermore, people who are "stressed out" may make unhealthy food choices, drink too much alcohol, and get inadequate exercise.

It is important to understand that a risk factor is not the same as a *cause* of disease. AIDS, for example, is caused by human immunodeficiency virus (HIV); a person cannot develop AIDS without being infected with HIV. Atherosclerosis, however, is an extremely complex disease process. In most cases, no single cause for the condition can be identified. Instead, having one or more risk factors increases a person's chances of developing the condition.

Lipoproteins and Atherosclerosis   Because lipoproteins transport lipids, including cholesterol, in the bloodstream, these structures play major roles in the development of atherosclerosis. In addition to chylomicrons, the body makes three major types of lipoprotein. Each type of lipoprotein carries different proportions of protein, cholesterol, triglycerides, and phospholipids (Fig. 6.21). **High-density lipoprotein (HDL)** carries more protein than cholesterol. HDL conveys lipids away from tissues and to the liver, where they can be processed and eliminated. Thus, the cholesterol carried by

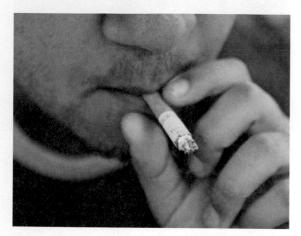

Smoking is a major risk factor for atherosclerosis. Furthermore, smoking exposes nonsmokers to cigarette smoke, which is also a risk factor for heart disease. If you smoke, simply improving your diet is unlikely to reduce your risk of heart disease; therefore, make every effort to quit using tobacco products.

Figure 6.21 Major lipoproteins. Lipoproteins contain different percentages of lipid and protein. Low-density lipoprotein (LDL) carries more cholesterol in the bloodstream than do the other lipoproteins.

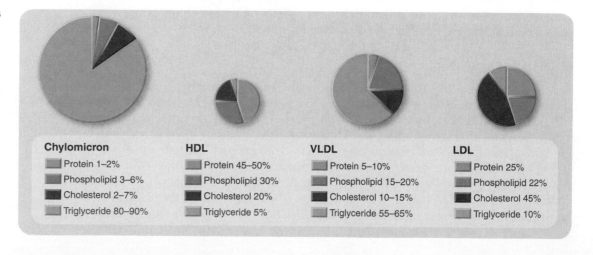

Chylomicron
Protein 1–2%
Phospholipid 3–6%
Cholesterol 2–7%
Triglyceride 80–90%

HDL
Protein 45–50%
Phospholipid 30%
Cholesterol 20%
Triglyceride 5%

VLDL
Protein 5–10%
Phospholipid 15–20%
Cholesterol 10–15%
Triglyceride 55–65%

LDL
Protein 25%
Phospholipid 22%
Cholesterol 45%
Triglyceride 10%

HDL (*HDL cholesterol*) is often called "good" cholesterol because it does not contribute to plaque formation.

Low-density lipoprotein (LDL) transports more cholesterol than HDL in the bloodstream. The cholesterol carried by LDL (*LDL cholesterol*) is often referred to as "bad" cholesterol, because LDL conveys the lipid to tissues, including cells in the arterial walls that make atherosclerotic plaques. However, there are different types of LDL, and not all forms of the lipoprotein are unhealthy. LDL is needed to transport lipids to tissues, where the nutrients are used to make cell structures and vital compounds.

Some LDLs are smaller and denser than others. People with high levels of small dense LDLs are more likely to develop atherosclerosis than people with low levels of these LDLs.[26] Additionally, chemically unstable substances (radicals) can damage LDL, forming *oxidized LDL*. This particular type of LDL is not beneficial because it is taken up by arterial cells, and over time, the cholesterol that was in the LDL contributes to atherosclerosis. Cigarette smoking is one lifestyle behavior that increases the oxidation of LDL.[27] Figure 6.22 illustrates the roles of HDL, LDL, and oxidized LDL.

A third major class of lipoproteins, **very-low-density lipoprotein (VLDL),** may also contribute to atherosclerosis. This particular lipoprotein contains only about 15% of the cholesterol in the bloodstream; VLDL carries a larger share of triglycerides than cholesterol. As blood triglyceride levels increase, concentrations of HDL cholesterol tend to decrease. Some medical researchers think elevated triglyceride levels contribute to the development of CVD, but the mechanisms are unclear at this point.

Assessing Your Risk of Atherosclerosis

You may not be able to prevent having a heart attack or stroke some day, but there is plenty of scientific evidence that suggests you can forestall CVD and live a longer, more satisfying life by reducing or eliminating modifiable risk factors for atherosclerosis. Diet, for example, influences the likelihood of atherosclerosis and is highly modifiable.

To determine your risk of atherosclerosis, it is a good idea to have regular medical checkups in which a physician checks your blood pressure and listens to blood flow in your carotid arteries to assess whether the arteries are becoming blocked. The physician

high-density lipoprotein (HDL) lipoprotein that transports cholesterol away from tissues and to the liver, where it can be eliminated

low-density lipoprotein (LDL) lipoprotein that carries cholesterol into tissues

very-low-density lipoprotein (VLDL) lipoprotein that carries much of the triglycerides in the bloodstream

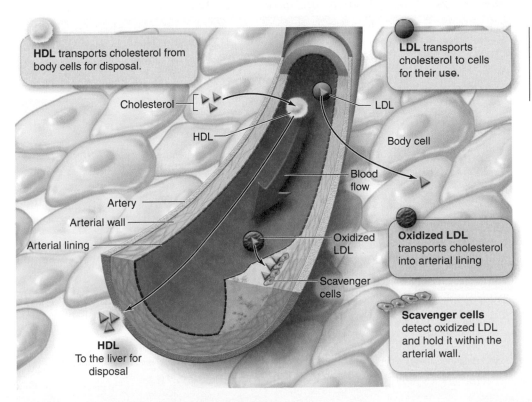

Figure 6.22 HDL, LDL, and oxidized LDL. The body makes HDL and LDL. A particular form of LDL, oxidized LDL, is harmful. Oxidized LDL is taken up by certain arterial cells, and over time, the cholesterol that was in the LDL builds up and contributes to atherosclerosis.

HDL transports cholesterol from body cells for disposal.

LDL transports cholesterol to cells for their use.

Cholesterol

HDL

LDL

Body cell

Blood flow

Artery

Arterial wall

Arterial lining

Oxidized LDL

Oxidized LDL transports cholesterol into arterial lining

Scavenger cells

Scavenger cells detect oxidized LDL and hold it within the arterial wall.

HDL To the liver for disposal

high-sensitivity C-reactive protein (hs-CRP)
protein produced primarily by the liver in response to inflammation; a marker for CVD

may request a lipoprotein profile to assess your total serum cholesterol level as well as serum HDL cholesterol, LDL cholesterol, and triglyceride levels. Although this textbook generally refers to "blood cholesterol" or "blood lipids," the amount of lipids in serum or plasma rather than whole blood is usually measured. Serum is the liquid portion of blood; plasma is similar to serum except that it contains clotting factors.

Table 6.4 presents classifications for healthy and unhealthy blood lipid levels. The desirable range for total cholesterol is less than 200 mg/dl. In 2005–2008, the average American had a total blood cholesterol level of 198 mg/dl.[28] Do you know what your blood cholesterol level is? Even if it is below 200 mg/dl, you may still have a high risk of atherosclerosis. Why? Although knowing the concentration of cholesterol carried by all lipoproteins is important, the amounts of certain lipoproteins in your blood, particularly LDL and HDL, are more critical risk factors. As mentioned earlier, LDL carries cholesterol to cells and HDL transports cholesterol away from cells.

The LDL cholesterol component of your total blood cholesterol level should be less than 100 mg/dl and the HDL cholesterol component should be 40 mg/dl or more (see Table 6.4). People with a high ratio of total cholesterol to HDL cholesterol usually have too much LDL cholesterol in their blood and an increased risk of heart disease and stroke. For example, a young man has a total blood cholesterol level of 180 mg/dl. Of that amount, only 30 mg/dl are carried by high-density lipoprotein. A healthy ratio of total cholesterol to HDL cholesterol is 4:1 or lower[29], whereas this man's ratio of total cholesterol to HDL cholesterol is 6:1 (180 mg /30 mg). If this person felt his risk of atherosclerosis and CVD was low because his cholesterol level was less than 200 mg/dl, he could be mistaken.

The ratio of LDL to HDL cholesterol in blood may also predict the risk of CVD.[30] Simply put, it is healthier to have higher levels of HDL cholesterol than to have higher levels of LDL cholesterol. To calculate your risk of having a heart attack during the next 10 years, use the risk assessment tool at http://hp2010.nhlbihin.net/atpiii/calculator .asp?usertype=pub.

Someday, scientists may be able to locate genes that are involved in the process of atherosclerosis and develop a blood test that identifies biological markers produced by the abnormal genes. Thus, young people could undergo testing to determine their risk of atherosclerosis well before the signs and symptoms of the condition appeared. Until

TABLE 6.4 *Classification of Blood Lipid Levels*

Total Cholesterol (mg/dl)	Classification
< 200	Desirable
200 to 239	Borderline high
≥ 240	High
LDL Cholesterol (mg/dl)	**Classification**
< 100	Optimal
100 to 129	Near optimal/Above optimal
130 to 159	Borderline high
160 to 189	High
≥ 190	Very high
HDL Cholesterol (mg/dl)	**Classification**
< 40 (for men); < 50 (for women)	Low
≥ 60	High
Triglycerides (mg/dl)	**Classification**
< 150	Normal
150 to 199	Borderline high
≥ 200	High

Source of data: American Heart Association, 2009. http://www.americanheart.org/presenter.jhtml?identifer=4500.

then, it is wise to have regular health checkups that include blood pressure and lipid measurements (*lipoprotein profile*). Ask your physician for a copy of the laboratory results, and keep them along with others in your personal "medical file" for future reference.

C-reactive Protein

Chronic inflammation is involved in the development of CVD. The liver responds to certain kinds of inflammation by producing and releasing **high-sensitivity C-reactive protein (hs-CRP)** into the bloodstream. People with high levels of hs-CRP are more likely to develop CVD.[31] Thus, elevated hs-CRP may be a marker for atherosclerosis, like homocysteine. If you have a family history of premature CVD, consider having your homocysteine and hs-CRP levels measured.

Coronary Calcium

Cigarette smoking and elevated total cholesterol level in early adulthood are significantly associated with the formation of *coronary calcium*, calcium deposits in arteries of the heart later in life.[27] High amounts of coronary calcium are associated with increased risk of atherosclerosis. *Computerized tomography* (*CT*) scans, special computerized images that show the body's internal structures, can detect coronary calcium deposits. A CT scan, however, involves exposure to ionizing radiation, so physicians generally reserve its use for other diagnostic purposes.

Reducing Your Risk of Atherosclerosis: Dietary Changes

Specific recommendations for consumption of various types of fat are primarily based on the results of epidemiological studies that examined the effects of dietary lipids on blood lipids and risk of CVD. Populations that consume diets rich in saturated fats generally have higher rates of heart disease than populations that eat less saturated fat. Saturated fat alters the structure of liver cell membranes so they no longer function properly. As a result, the liver removes less cholesterol from the bloodstream.[32] Most saturated fatty acids increase blood cholesterol levels, by raising concentrations of both LDL and HDL cholesterol. Trans fats also raise blood cholesterol levels.[33] However, trans fats raise LDL cholesterol while reducing beneficial HDL cholesterol levels.[32] High intakes of cholesterol can also raise LDL cholesterol levels.

Monounsaturated fatty acids generally lower LDL cholesterol without reducing HDL cholesterol levels. Foods rich in monounsaturated fat include peanuts and peanut oil, canola oil, olives and olive oil, almonds, and avocados. The "Recipes for Healthy Living" feature of Chapter 6 includes an easy-to-prepare snack made with almonds and cashews, nuts that are rich sources of monounsaturated fat.

Diets containing high amounts of polyunsaturated fatty acids may reduce blood levels of total cholesterol and LDL cholesterol. In some individuals, however, polyunsaturated fat also reduces beneficial HDL cholesterol. Nevertheless, polyunsaturated fatty acids tend to be beneficial because they do not promote atherosclerosis. Foods rich in polyunsaturated fat include safflower, corn, soybean, and cottonseed oils, as well as some types of sunflower seed oil (see Fig. 6.5).

To reduce the population's risk of CVD, *U.S. Dietary Guidelines 2010* recommend limiting saturated fat intake to less than 10% of total energy intake by replacing foods that are rich sources of saturated fat with foods that contain high amounts of unsaturated fat.[18] People should limit their trans fat intake as much as possible. You can reduce your trans fat intake by eating fewer solid fats, especially foods made with partially hydrogenated oils, such as stick margarine.

What About Omega-3 and Omega-6 Fats? The typical American eats far more omega-6 foods than foods that contain omega-3 fatty acids.[34] The primary omega-6 fatty acid, linoleic acid, increases inflammation and blood clotting. Some inflammation is necessary because it attracts immune system cells to disease-causing microorganisms that have entered

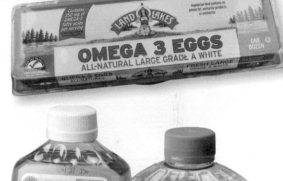

Did You Know?

Chicken eggs normally contain very low amounts of omega-3 fatty acids. By feeding hens ground flaxseed, farmers can increase the amount of omega-3 fatty acids in eggs. In supermarkets, such omega-3 enriched eggs are often sold beside cartons of regular eggs. Expect to pay more for the enriched eggs.

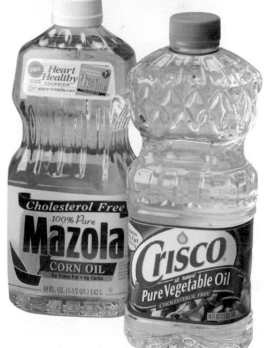

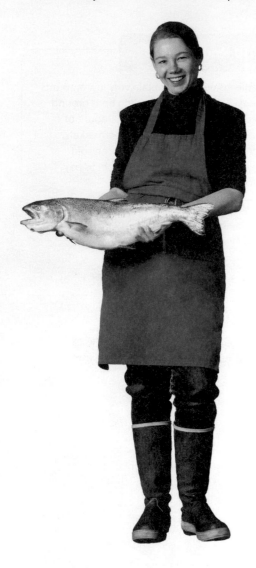

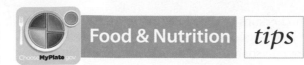

Food & Nutrition *tips*

- Eat seafood, especially fatty cold-water fish, two times a week. Before cooking, marinate fresh fish in olive or canola oil that has been seasoned with a small amount of garlic, pepper, and lemon juice. The light coating of oil on fish can help keep the food from drying out during cooking.

- Bake, grill, or broil fish.

- Add water-packed tuna to salads, or mix tuna with a little olive oil and spread on toast.

- If you don't want the flavor of olive oil in a food, use canola oil, soybean oil, or soft margarines made from these oils for frying or sautéing.

- Sprinkle chopped walnuts on salads, yogurt, or cereal, or simply eat the nuts as a snack.

the body. Inflammation, however, can also damage the inside of arteries. Clotting is also an important function of blood, but excess blood clotting can increase the risk of strokes, heart attacks, and other serious blood vessel disorders. In 2009, experts with the American Heart Association issued an advisory statement indicating that consuming 5 to 10% of energy in the form of omega-6 fatty acids *reduces* the risk of heart disease.[35] The role of omega-6 fats in preventing this major cause of death among Americans is controversial among medical experts. Thus, more research is needed to clarify the pros and cons of following diets that contain high amounts of these particular fatty acids.

Eating foods that supply omega-3 fatty acids reduces the risk of heart disease to a greater extent than does eating foods with omega-6 fatty acids.[34] The body incorporates omega-3 fatty acids into cell membranes and uses these lipids to make compounds that can reduce inflammation, serum triglycerides, and blood clotting. Table 6.5 lists foods that are rich sources of omega-3 fatty acids, including several species of fish. Certain fatty fish are rich sources of DHA and EPA, long-chain omega-3 fatty acids.

Alpha-linolenic acid is an omega-3 fatty acid that the body can convert to DHA and EPA (see Figure 6.2). Flaxseeds, soybeans, and walnuts are good sources of alpha-linolenic acid. However, the body can only make small amounts of DHA and EPA from alpha-linolenic acid. Therefore, it is important to include other sources of these long-chain fatty acids in your diet.

To obtain beneficial long-chain omega-3 fatty acids such as DHA, the Dietary Guidelines recommend that Americans eat 8 ounces of cold-water fatty fish, such as sardines, salmon, and tuna, a week.[18] Because large species of fish can contain high amounts of the toxic compound *methyl mercury*, young children, pregnant and breastfeeding women, and women who are likely to become pregnant should not eat shark, king mackerel, tilefish, and swordfish.[18] Shrimp, canned light tuna, salmon, pollock, and catfish are low in methyl mercury. According to the Dietary Guidelines, women who are pregnant or breastfeeding can safely consume up to 12 ounces of low-mercury fish and shellfish weekly. The "Recipes for Healthy Living" feature of Chapter 6 includes an easy recipe made with salmon.

What if you do not like to eat fish? Are fish oil supplements safe? Fish oil supplements can reduce elevated triglyceride levels, but doses higher than 3 g/day may interfere with blood clotting and increase the risk of strokes. Therefore, check with your physician before you embark on a campaign to increase the omega-3 fatty acid content of your diet by taking fish oil supplements. The "Food & Nutrition Tips" on this page provides some ideas for increasing your intake of omega-3 fatty acids from dietary sources.

Should You Avoid Eggs?   Eggs are a relatively economical source of protein and many micronutrients. However, egg yolks are the most concentrated source of cholesterol in the typical American's diet. One yolk contains 5 grams of fat and about 210 mg of cholesterol, which is about two-thirds of the limit recommended by the Dietary Guidelines.[18] To

TABLE 6.5   *Rich Food Sources of Omega-3 Fats*

Fish/Shellfish
Herring, salmon, sablefish, anchovies, tuna, bluefish, sardines, catfish, striped bass, mackerel, trout, shark, swordfish, halibut, pollock, flounder, shrimp, mussels, crab
Oils
Flaxseed, walnut, canola, soybean
Nuts and Seeds
Walnuts, flaxseeds
Other
Seaweed

reduce their cholesterol consumption, many Americans eat fewer fresh eggs than in the past. Whole eggs, however, are often hidden in commonly eaten foods such as salad dressings, noodles, frozen custards, sauces, and baked goods.

Does eating egg yolks and other cholesterol-rich animal foods raise the risk of atherosclerosis? Studies designed to determine the effects of dietary cholesterol on blood cholesterol levels have provided mixed results.[36] In general, the cholesterol in food does not have as much effect on blood cholesterol levels as the saturated fat does. Why? In a healthy person, the liver produces less cholesterol when large amounts of cholesterol are eaten. On the other hand, eating large amounts of saturated fat increases the liver's cholesterol production. Because foods that are high in cholesterol are often rich sources of saturated fat, dietary cholesterol was blamed for raising blood cholesterol levels.

Egg whites have no fat or cholesterol. For those who must limit their cholesterol intake, egg whites can often be used in recipes that call for whole eggs. Products that substitute for whole eggs are available in supermarkets.

Is It Safe to Eat Butter? Many Americans have replaced butter with partially hardened vegetable oil margarines because of concern over butter's cholesterol and saturated fat content. In the late 1990s, however, news reports alerted Americans that eating trans fat in margarine was more harmful than consuming the natural lipids in butter. If you use margarine, should you be concerned about its trans fat content, and switch to using butter?

Compared to butter, a serving of margarine provides more unsaturated fat, less saturated fat, and cholesterol. However, margarine made from partially hardened vegetable oil contains considerable amounts of unhealthy trans fat.[37] The amount of saturated and trans fat in soft margarines is less than the amount in hard "stick" margarines or butter. You can reduce your intake of trans fats by using soft (tub) or liquid margarines, or trans fat-free spreads that resemble margarine, instead of stick margarine or butter. However, if you enjoy butter, occasionally having some is unlikely to clog your arteries. The "Food & Nutrition Tips" feature below suggests ways to reduce your trans fat intake.

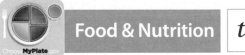

Food & Nutrition *tips*

- Read the Nutrition Facts panel and the ingredient list on the label when choosing processed foods, especially margarine. Compare margarines to find the product with 0 g of trans fat. Margarines that have "liquid" vegetable oil as the first ingredient generally have less trans fat than stick margarines.

- Avoid products that include "interesterified" (fully hydrogenated) oil, partially hydrogenated fat, or shortening in the ingredient list.

- Eat fewer commercially prepared baked goods, snack foods, and fried fast-food items.

- Purchase brands of microwave popcorn that have little added fat or no trans fats. Buy plain popcorn, and to pop the kernels use a small amount of hot oil in a covered saucepan or use a hot-air machine.

- Commercial frostings that are made with vegetable shortenings are likely to be high in hydrogenated oils. Remove most of the frosting from a serving of cake before eating it. (Frosting is primarily sugar and fat—empty calories.) You can make your own frosting by mixing soft margarine or smooth peanut butter with a little milk, powdered sugar, and vanilla flavoring.

- Pastry dough may be made with shortening. Replace shortening with oil or soft margarine to make your own pastry dough "from scratch."

MY DIVERSE PLATE

Ghee (Indian Clarified Butter)

Ghee is a solid fat that is used for cooking, primarily in India. Traditionally, ghee was made from the milk of a type of buffalo that was native to India and Pakistan, but milk from other animals can be used. To make ghee, butter is heated until its water content evaporates completely and the solids (primarily lactose and some proteins) brown and sink to the bottom. After heating, the fat is strained to remove the solids. Ghee, the product that remains, is pure fat.

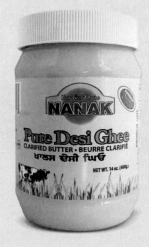

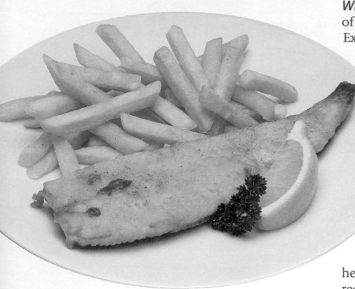

When foods such as chicken or fish are breaded and fried, the breading soaks up fat, greatly increasing the food's energy value.

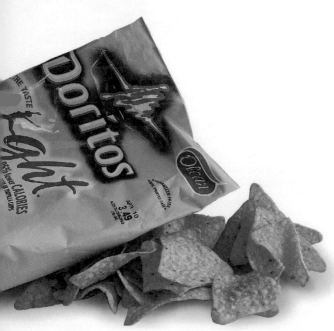

Some food products contain synthetic fat replacers such as Olean (olestra) to substitute for some or all of the fat in them.

Will Weight Loss and Exercise Help?   Having a healthy body weight can reduce the risk of CVD, and low-fat diets are often recommended for preventing weight gain and CVD. Excess body fat, especially around the midsection of the body, is associated with unhealthy LDL cholesterol and triglyceride levels. Physical inactivity and excess energy consumption contribute to unwanted weight gain. Performing moderate-intensity physical activity nearly every day and balancing energy intake with energy expenditure each day can help people achieve and maintain healthy body weights. Taking such steps can also reduce elevated LDL cholesterol and triglyceride levels.

Food Selection and Preparation

You can change your food selection and preparation practices to reduce the amount of fat and calories in your diet. Fatty meats such as rib steaks are often more tender and expensive than leaner cuts such as chuck roasts. Certain cooking methods, however, can increase the tenderness of lean cuts of meat. Moist cooking methods, such as pot roasting or tightly covering the baking dish with foil, help tenderize meats without adding fat. In addition to using a moist cooking method, reduce the oven temperature from 350°F to less than 325°F. The meat will take longer to cook, but it is less likely to toughen and dry out. After cooking, avoid eating the visible fat that remains. For example, trim away much of the fat from the meat and do not use pan drippings to make sauces or gravies. Steaming meats and vegetables is a cooking method that does not require adding fat during preparation. Stir-frying pieces of raw vegetables, meat, fish, shellfish, and poultry in small amounts of hot vegetable oil cooks them quickly and preserves micronutrients. Additionally, when you brown ground beef in a pan, drain much of the fat before you add other ingredients to the meat. Dipping raw foods in batter and deep-fat frying them adds considerable amounts of fat to your diet, because breading serves as a sponge that soaks up oil. If you prepare breaded fried foods, place the items on paper towels after cooking them to soak up as much excess fat as possible. Some people think the breading is the "best part" of a fried food, but removing some or all of the breading before eating the item can reduce your overall fat intake. Although it is easy to peel greasy breading from fried fish, much of the fat that you eat is hidden in foods and beverages. For example, do you drink 2% milk? Fat comprises only 2% of the milk's volume, but the lipid contributes 37% of the beverage's calories. Fat-free milk actually contains less than 0.5% fat by volume, and fat contributes essentially no energy to the beverage.

What about the fat content of the cream cheese, margarine, or butter that you spread on a piece of toast? About 90% of the calories in cream cheese and about 100% of the calories in butter and margarine are from fat. Vegetable oils are almost 100% fat, so fat contributes all the energy in most salad dressings. Fried foods, chips, and salad dressings are high in fat; bacon, sausage, hot dogs, luncheon meats, and hard cheeses are also fatty foods. Nuts, including peanuts and almonds, have high fat contents, but they generally contain high amounts of healthy monounsaturated fats.

Instead of striving to eliminate all fatty foods from your diet, try reducing your intake of them, especially solid fats. For example, if you drink 2% or whole milk, switch to 1% or fat-free milk. Nearly all the lipids in fat-free milk have been removed; that is why it tastes watery to people who are not accustomed to drinking it. Except for energy and lipid content, the nutritional value of fat-free milk is basically the same as that of whole and 2% milks. Rather than eat a large order of French-fried potatoes, have a baked potato topped with a teaspoon of soft margarine. By eating the baked potato instead of French fries, you will consume about 300 fewer kilocalories and 21 fewer grams of fat. The "Food & Nutrition Tips" feature on the next page provides more practical suggestions for reducing your fat and cholesterol intake.

Fat Replacers   In response to consumer demand for more fat-reduced and fat-free foods, manufacturers can use several synthetic fat replacers to substitute for some or all

Food & Nutrition *tips*

- Reduce your intake of fried foods, including French-fried potatoes.

- Purchase lean meats and trim visible fat from meat before cooking. Before eating cooked meat, trim and discard any remaining visible fat.

- Try replacing some fatty foods with reduced-fat or fat-free alternatives. For example, substitute plain, fat-free yogurt in recipes that call for sour cream. Place a spoonful of the yogurt, instead of butter or sour cream, on a baked potato.

- Because most nuts are rich sources of healthy unsaturated fats, replace foods that contain saturated fat with nuts. For example, use peanut or soy nut butters instead of cheese or luncheon meat in sandwiches. Some nut butters contain trans fats and added sugars, so read the Nutrition Facts panel and ingredients list before selecting these products.

- Replace some or all of the solid fat in recipes for baked goods with unsweetened applesauce. In general, 1 cup of applesauce can replace 1 cup of fat.

- Pretzels, air-popped popcorn, and most fruits and vegetables are low fat and generally more nutrient dense than chips, cookies, pastries, and candy bars.

- Patronize fast-food restaurants that offer low-saturated fat menu items such as salads without added cheese and meat, baked or broiled chicken and fish, low-fat yogurt, and bean burritos.

- Use less salad dressing on salads. When in restaurants, order salad dressings "on the side" so you can control the amount that is added.

- Replace butter in recipes with trans fat-free margarines (60% oil). Use olive or canola oils in recipes that call for "vegetable oil."

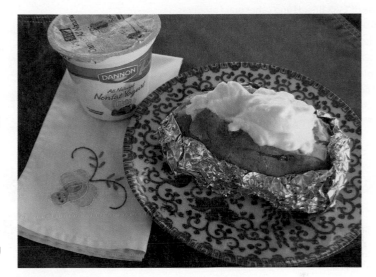

| Plain yogurt is a low-fat substitute for sour cream.

of the fat in their products. Oatrim, Simplesse, and Olean are brands of fat replacers used in a variety of processed foods. The ideal synthetic fat is safe, provides little or no energy, mimics natural fat's contribution to the taste and texture of food, and withstands typical cooking temperatures. Olean, for example, is used to make snack foods such as potato chips. This particular fat replacer contains *olestra*, a chemical that has fatty acids arranged in an unnatural configuration and is not digested. As a result, olestra passes through the intestinal tract unchanged and unabsorbed. Some people, however, report experiencing diarrhea when they eat large amounts of food made with olestra. Additionally, olestra can attract fat-soluble vitamins and interfere with their absorption; therefore, products containing olestra are fortified with these vitamins.

People who are concerned about their energy intake should recognize that fat-reduced and fat-free foods are not "calorie-free." Moreover, food manufacturers often increase the amounts of added sugars in these products to improve taste and compensate for reduced fat content. Nevertheless, fat replacers can help people reduce their total fat intake.[39]

Other Dietary Modifications

In addition to modifying your fat intake, you can reduce your risk of CVD by making other dietary changes. Eating foods that are rich sources of fiber, particularly soluble

Did You Know?

Garlic, onions, and chives are sources of sulfur-containing compounds, such as allicin, that have antioxidant properties. Fresh garlic and garlic supplements have been promoted to lower blood cholesterol levels. However, studies do not provide strong scientific support for consuming fresh garlic or garlic supplements to reduce elevated blood lipids.[38] As is often the case, more research is needed to determine whether eating garlic or taking garlic supplements helps prevent CVD.

Figure 6.23 Mediterranean Diet Pyramid. Nutrition experts often promote the traditional Mediterranean diet for healthy eating as well as reducing elevated blood lipid levels and the risk of CVD. Breads and other grain products, legumes, nuts, fruits, and vegetables form the foundation of this food guide pyramid. Note that fish and poultry are emphasized instead of red meats, fat is primarily from olive oil, a daily glass of wine may be consumed, and regular physical activity is recommended. *Source: Oldways Preservation & Exchange Trust, 2009.*

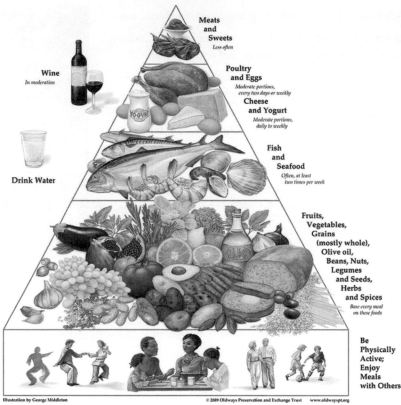

Did You Know?

Eggs with brown shells are not more nutritious than eggs with white shells; the color of an eggshell is determined by the breed of hen that laid it. Also, grading does not reflect the nutritional content of an egg. When cracked open and placed on a plate, the membrane of a "AA" grade egg tends to hold the yolk and white together better than membranes of lower-grade eggs.

fiber (see Chapter 5), can reduce LDL cholesterol levels without lowering beneficial HDL cholesterol levels. If your triglyceride level is too high (> 150 mg/dl), consider cutting back on your intake of refined carbohydrates by eating less candy and pastries and drinking fewer sugar-sweetened soft drinks. Furthermore, consuming less alcohol and losing excess body fat can help reduce elevated triglyceride levels.

Drinking small amounts of alcohol (1 to 2 drinks/day) can raise beneficial HDL cholesterol levels. Consuming too much alcohol, however, contributes to hypertension and damages every organ of the body. Furthermore, excess alcohol consumption has devastating effects on society as well as on personal safety and relationships. If you consume several alcoholic beverages regularly, consider reducing your intake to no more than one serving per day. The Chapter 6 "Highlight" discusses alcohol.

Dietitians and other nutrition experts often promote the traditional Mediterranean diet for healthy eating as well as reducing elevated blood lipid levels and the risk of CVD. The Mediterranean diet (Fig. 6.23) recommends eating more fish and seafood and smaller amounts of red meat; using heart-healthy unsaturated fatty acids; engaging in regular physical activity; and drinking a glass of wine daily. This diet also emphasizes phytochemical-rich fruits, vegetables, beans, and nuts. Table 6.6 summarizes ways certain actions, such as dietary manipulations and other therapeutic lifestyle changes, may alter a person's blood lipid levels.

What If Lifestyle Changes Do Not Work?

Some people are unable to lower their risk of CVD significantly by making dietary changes, exercising regularly, and losing excess body fat. If your blood lipids are too high and the levels have remained elevated even after you have made these lifestyle

TABLE 6.6 *Ways to Lower Your Risk of CVD*

Action	Potential Benefits
Increase physical activity level.	Raises HDL levels
Lose excess body fat.	Lowers elevated triglycerides, blood pressure, and risk of type 2 diabetes May increase HDL
Quit smoking.	May raise HDL and lower LDL levels
Make specific dietary changes:	
Reduce intake of saturated fats and avoid trans fats.	Raises HDL and lowers LDL
Replace saturated fats with polyunsaturated and monounsaturated fats.	Lowers LDL
Include some omega-3 and omega-6 fats. (Discuss the need for fish oil supplements with your physician.)	Reduces triglycerides; may raise HDL and reduce blood pressure
Replace margarine or butter with spread made from plant sterols/stanols.	Reduces LDL
Eat more whole-grain, fiber-rich foods, especially those containing soluble fiber.	Reduces total cholesterol and LDL without altering HDL
Consume foods that contain antioxidant nutrients and certain phyto-chemicals, such as red grapes and red wine (see Table 1.3). Dietary supplements of these compounds are not recommended.[3]	Reduces risk of heart disease, but the mechanism is unclear
Reduce alcohol and sugar intake.	Lowers triglyceride levels

modifications, it is important to discuss additional treatment options with your physician. Millions of Americans take a class of prescription drugs called *statins* to reduce their elevated blood lipid levels. Statins interfere with the liver's metabolism of cholesterol, effectively reducing LDL cholesterol and triglyceride levels as a result. Statins are relatively safe when taken as directed. Zetia® is a drug that works differently from a statin. Zetia inhibits intestinal absorption of cholesterol and, as a result, lowers LDL cholesterol levels. However, questions have been raised about the safety of this medication, particularly when it is taken with other cholesterol-lowering medications.[40]

Concept **Checkpoint**

14. Define atherosclerosis, arteriosclerosis, arterial plaque, thrombus, and embolus. Discuss the series of physiological changes that occur in arteries and contribute to the development of CVD.
15. What is the American Heart Association's recommendation concerning the percentage of daily total calories that are from fat? What is the recommended percentage of total calories from trans fat per day?
16. List at least three major risk factors for atherosclerosis that are nonmodifiable, and at least five that are modifiable.
17. Bernard's total blood cholesterol level is 195 mg/ml, and his HDL cholesterol level is 62 mg/dl. Based on this information, does Bernard have a high risk or low risk of CVD? Explain your answer.
18. What is "hs-CRP"? What can you learn about your risk of heart disease and stroke from having a lipoprotein profile performed on your blood?
19. Suggest at least four ways people can reduce their intakes of saturated and trans fats and increase their intakes of unsaturated fats.
20. Identify foods that are rich sources of omega-3 fatty acids and foods that are rich sources of omega-6 fatty acids.
21. What role does homocysteine play in the development of heart disease?
22. What is a statin?

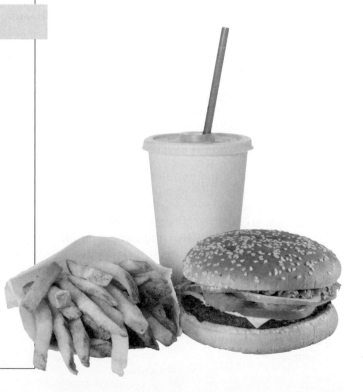

Chapter 6 Highlight

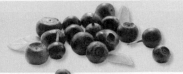

DRINK TO YOUR HEALTH?

What do beer, wine, vodka, whiskey, sake (*sak'-e*), koumiss (*koo'-mis*), and kefir (*keh-feer'*) have in common? These beverages contain *ethanol*, a two-carbon compound that chemists classify as an alcohol. Alcohols such as ethanol, glycerol, and cholesterol are organic molecules that have one or more *hydroxyl* (*OH*) groups in their chemical structures (Fig. 6.24). This textbook refers to ethanol simply as "alcohol."

Offering wine in religious ceremonies, toasting the bride and groom with champagne at a wedding, or barhopping with friends on their twenty-first birthdays—for many Americans, alcohol consumption is a part of celebrating religious rites and life's milestones. When consumed in moderation, alcoholic beverages can make social situations more enjoyable. Many people, however, experience serious problems as a result of their drinking habits. The Chapter 6 "Highlight" focuses on alcohol metabolism as well as the chemical's effects on the body.

Alcohol Production

Throughout the world, people have been producing and drinking alcoholic beverages for thousands of years. The chemical process that results in alcohol is not complicated and occurs naturally. The process requires certain microbes, warm conditions, and a source of simple sugars. Although some types of bacteria produce alcohol, commercial alcoholic beverage production relies on *yeast*, one-celled fungi (*fun'-ji*) that break down (*ferment*) simple sugars in the absence of oxygen to obtain energy and the metabolic waste product, alcohol. Grains, fruit, and potatoes—just about anything that contains simple sugars—will ferment under the proper conditions. Yeast will even ferment lactose in milk. In arid parts of southeastern Europe, Central Asia, and the Middle East, the climate and land are generally not suitable for growing grains, fruit, or other fermentable plant foods. The nomadic populations who live in these regions drink fermented mare's milk (koumiss) or camel's milk (kefir).

Alcohol is soluble in water, and alcoholic beverages generally contain a considerable amount of water. Beers are typically 3 to 6% alcohol, wines contain about 8 to 14% alcohol, and wine coolers are about 10% alcohol by volume. Alcohol is poisonous (*toxic*), and yeast die when the concentration of alcohol in the fermenting solution reaches 14 to 16%. The distilling process increases the alcohol concentration of an alcoholic beverage.

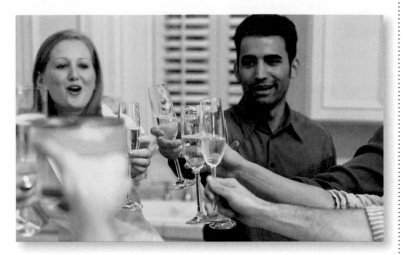

Distilled spirits (hard liquors) such as whiskey, bourbon, and vodka are generally 40 to 50% alcohol. You can determine the percentage of alcohol in hard liquor by dividing the "proof" declaration on the label by two. Tequila, for example, is "80 proof," or 40% alcohol.

Although each gram of alcohol provides 7 kcal, alcohol is not a nutrient; it is a mind-altering drug that is often classified as a food. Beer and wine contain simple carbohydrates and small amounts of certain minerals and B vitamins. Distilled spirits have essentially no nutritional value other than water. Mixing distilled spirits with juices, cocktail mixes, or other flavorings increases the alcoholic beverage's energy content and may add some nutrients, particularly simple sugars, depending on the ingredients in the mixer. Table 6.7 indicates the grams of alcohol and carbohydrates

TABLE 6.7

Approximate Alcohol, Carbohydrate, and Energy Contents of Alcoholic Beverages*

Beverage	Amount (fl oz)	Kcal	Alcohol (g)	Carbohydrates (g)
Beer				
Regular	12.0	139	13	11
Lite	12.0	103	11	5
Table Wines	5.0	114	14	5
Distilled Spirits	1.5	96	14	0
Gin, rum, vodka, whiskey				

* Protein and fat contribute little or nothing to the caloric content.

Source: U.S. Department of Agriculture.

Figure 6.24 Ethanol. Alcohol (ethanol) is a simple two-carbon compound.

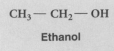

$$CH_3 — CH_2 — OH$$

Ethanol

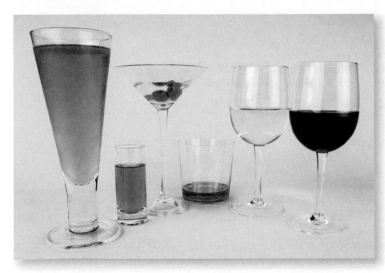

Figure 6.25 What's a standard drink? A standard drink is approximately 12 ounces of beer or wine cooler, 1½ ounces of liquor, or 5 ounces of wine. Each standard drink contains 13 to 14 grams of alcohol.

in certain alcoholic drinks as well as their caloric content. A standard drink (approximately 12 ounces of beer or wine cooler, 5 ounces of wine, or 1½ ounces of liquor) contains 13 to 14 grams of alcohol (Fig. 6.25).

How the Body Processes Alcohol

Alcohol requires no digestion and readily passes through the tissues lining the inside of the mouth, esophagus, stomach, and small intestine. When alcohol is consumed with meals, food delays its absorption from the stomach and slows the rate in which the drug enters the bloodstream. To reduce alcohol's harmful effects, the body detoxifies the simple chemical by converting it into less damaging compounds. Detoxification begins in the stomach, where the enzyme gastric alcohol dehydrogenase metabolizes up to 20% of the alcohol. Most of the remaining alcohol passes through the small intestinal wall and circulates to the liver, the primary site for metabolizing alcohol. Since alcohol is a poison, the liver shifts its metabolic focus from macronutrient metabolism to alcohol detoxification when the compound enters its tissues.

The liver relies on two biochemical pathways to metabolize alcohol. When relatively low doses are consumed, the enzyme alcohol dehydrogenase converts most of the alcohol to acetaldehyde, a substance that is more toxic than alcohol. Another enzyme, acetaldehyde dehydrogenase, reacts with acetaldehyde to form

Figure 6.26 Alcohol metabolism: Major metabolic steps. This diagram simplifies the major chemical steps involved in the metabolism of low doses of alcohol to less toxic compounds. Acetyl-CoA is an important by-product of ethanol metabolism, because the molecule can be further metabolized to carbon dioxide (CO_2) and water (H_2O), or used to form fatty acids. Thus, people who drink alcohol can experience an increase in body fat.

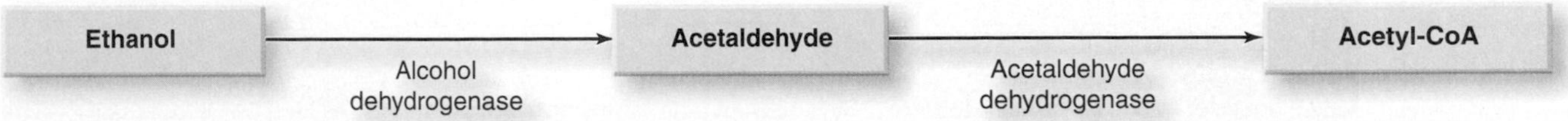

acetyl-CoA, an important molecule in energy metabolism. Acetyl-CoA may be further metabolized to carbon dioxide (CO_2) and water (H_2O), or the molecule can be used to synthesize fatty acids (Fig. 6.26).

If a person consumes excessive amounts of alcohol such as during a drinking binge, the alcohol overwhelms the liver's ability to metabolize the drug using the dehydrogenase pathway. When this occurs, the second method of processing alcohol, the microsomal ethanol oxidizing system (MEOS), takes over. Unlike the alcohol dehydrogenase pathway, MEOS wastes energy in the form of body heat that dissipates into the environment. Thus, alcoholics typically gain little weight from their energy intake when alcohol supplies most of their energy.

Factors That Influence Alcohol Metabolism You may have noticed that a few of your friends who drink can "hold their liquor" better than others. Why are some people able to drink more alcohol at one time than others? Several factors account for the variability. In addition to the amount and timing of alcohol consumption, personal characteristics such as sex, body size and composition, age, and prior drinking history affect the body's detoxification rate. For example, a healthy person who weighs 154 pounds (70 kg) metabolizes about 1 alcoholic drink per hour. Drinking caffeinated beverages, exercising, or taking vitamins does not increase this rate. To sober up, the drinker must stop consuming alcohol and give his or her liver time to metabolize the drug.

Alcohol is not stored in the body. Until the liver can detoxify the toxic chemical, it circulates in the bloodstream and diffuses into the watery fluids within and surrounding cells. The lungs and perspiration eliminate some of the alcohol; that's why you can smell alcohol when you're around someone who's been drinking. The kidneys also filter some of the drug from the bloodstream and eliminate it in urine. To determine whether someone is legally intoxicated as a result of drinking alcohol, law enforcement officials use special devices to analyze the alcohol in blood, urine, or expired air to estimate the person's blood alcohol concentration (BAC). BAC is reported as a percentage that indicates the amount of alcohol in the blood. In the United States, a BAC of 0.08% is the legal limit for intoxication for automobile operators who are 21 years of age or older.

Men and women have different physical responses to alcohol. Women tend to become more impaired than men do after drinking the same amount of alcohol, even when differences in body weight are taken into account. The reasons for these sexual differences are unclear, but they probably involve physiological factors including body size and composition. The average man is larger than the average woman, and larger people can often drink more alcohol without showing ill effects than smaller individuals, because they have bigger livers that detoxify more alcohol at a time. Additionally, a healthy 150-pound man typically has more body water than a healthy 150-pound woman. After the man drinks a

Ethanol → **Acetaldehyde** → **Acetyl-CoA**

Alcohol dehydrogenase Acetaldehyde dehydrogenase

beer, the alcohol diffuses out of his bloodstream and into the water compartments of his body. Since the woman's body has less water, more alcohol remains in her bloodstream after she drinks a beer. As a result, her BAC rises faster and she becomes more intoxicated after drinking the same amount of alcohol as her male counterpart (Fig. 6.27). Compared to men who drink heavily, women have a higher risk of serious health problems, especially damage to their liver, brain, and heart, when they abuse the same amounts of alcohol.[41]

Prior alcohol exposure also influences the rate of alcohol metabolism. People who drink regularly develop tolerance. Tolerance occurs as the levels of liver enzymes needed to metabolize alcohol increase, and as a result, the rate of alcohol metabolism increases. Consequently, the regular drinker needs to consume more alcohol at a time to achieve the same mind-altering effects as a person who drinks infrequently. Tolerance can lead to alcohol dependence (alcoholism).

Classifying Drinkers

In 2009, slightly more than 50% of Americans who were 12 years of age or older reported being current alcohol drinkers during the 30 days prior to the survey.[42] Almost one-quarter of the current drinkers engaged in binge drinking at least once, and nearly 7% of current drinkers drank heavily during this period.

What is "moderate drinking" or "binge drinking"? Although there is no universally accepted definition for "light," "moderate," or "heavy" drinking, medical practitioners and alcohol researchers often follow the classification guidelines listed in Table 6.8. Binge drinking is a form of heavy drinking, but the definition of binge drinking often differs according to sex. According

TABLE 6.8

Classifying Drinkers

Level	Amount of Alcohol Consumed (Standard Drinks)
Abstainer	None or fewer than 12 drinks/year
Light	1 to 13 drinks/month
Moderate	4 to 14 drinks/week
Heavy	3 or more drinks/day
Binge drinker	5 or more drinks/occasion (males)
Binge drinker	4 or more drinks/occasion (females)

Source: Modified from: Dufour MC: What is moderate drinking? Defining "drinks" and drinking levels. *Alcohol Research & Health*, 23(1): 5, 1999.

to the Centers for Disease Control and Prevention, binge drinking is defined as having four or more drinks during an occasion for females and five or more drinks during an occasion for males.[43] Regardless of their backgrounds, binge drinking is a common practice among Americans.

As a college student, you may have observed binge drinking or engaged in the practice. In 2009, Americans who were 18 to 24 years of age were more likely to binge drink than Americans in other age groups.[44] Youthful binge drinking is a serious public health concern because the behavior is often associated with driving while drunk. Furthermore, the practice may increase a person's later risk of alcoholism and can result in death.

Binge drinking has become an expected "rite of passage" for American youth celebrating their twenty-first birthday. The practice of trying to consume 21 drinks quickly while celebrating "power hour" ("21 for 21") can have deadly consequences. On March 15, 2004, Jason Reinhardt was living in a fraternity house

Figure 6.27 Alcohol consumption and BAC. This table shows the relationship between the number of alcoholic drinks consumed within the same period and BACs for healthy men and women. For example, a 170-pound man will have his BAC reach 0.05% after he has three drinks, whereas a 137-pound woman will have her BAC reach 0.05% after drinking only two drinks. However, alcohol's effects on individuals can vary. In the United States and Canada, a person is legally intoxicated when his/her BAC is 0.08% or higher.

at Minnesota State University, Moorhead. While celebrating his twenty-first birthday with friends in a bar, Jason rapidly drank 16 shots of alcohol. Although he managed to return to the fraternity house and go to bed, his lifeless body was discovered a few hours later. The young man's blood alcohol concentration was 0.361, well within the deadly range. Jason's death was not an isolated incident; cases in other states have also been reported. What makes binge drinking so dangerous?

Binge drinking increases a person's BAC rapidly and to a point at which signs of alcohol poisoning occur. An individual suffering from alcohol poisoning is confused, "passes out" and cannot be aroused (*comatose*), breathes slowly and irregularly, and has pale or bluish skin. Alcohol poisoning can cause the heartbeat to slow down and the lungs to stop functioning, resulting in death. Additionally, if a comatose person vomits, his or her stomach contents can enter the lungs, causing the person to choke to death. Jason died in his sleep from alcohol poisoning. His breathing rate slowed, his heartbeat became irregular, and his organs gradually shut down while he slept. Thus, it is important to recognize that alcohol poisoning is a life-threatening condition. If you suspect someone has consumed a deadly amount of alcohol, don't waste time trying to estimate how many drinks that person has drunk; call 911 immediately.

Alcohol Dependence and Abuse

A person who is *dependent* on alcohol (an alcoholic) has an uncontrollable need to drink; is unable to limit his or her alcohol consumption; suffers withdrawal symptoms, such as shakiness

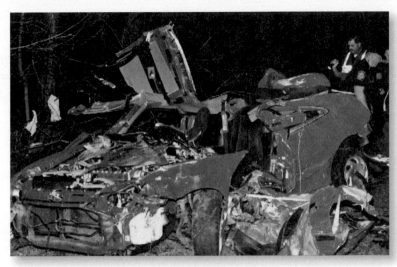

The three teenagers who died in this automobile had consumed alcohol before the accident.

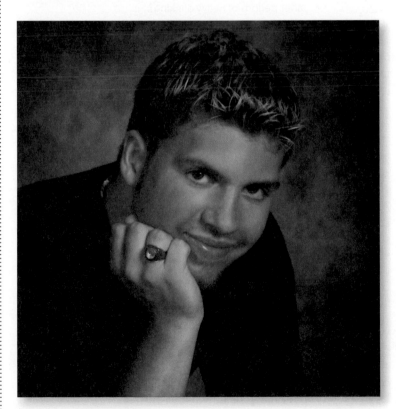

Jason Reinhardt tragically died after binge drinking with friends in celebration of his twenty-first birthday.

and anxiety, when alcohol is unavailable after a period of heavy drinking; and experiences *tolerance* to the drug. Tolerance develops over time as the drinker's body becomes better able to metabolize the alcohol. As a result, the alcohol-dependent person needs to consume more of the drug to obtain the same effects that he or she experienced prior to becoming dependent. About 17% of men and about 8% of women become dependent on alcohol at some point in their lives.[45] Table 6.9 is a self-assessment you can take to indicate whether you are at risk of alcoholism.

The alcohol abuser experiences problems at home, work, and school that are associated with his or her drinking habits. Both abusers and alcoholics engage in behaviors that place themselves and others in danger, such as drinking and driving. Table 6.10 lists signs of alcohol abuse, which often lead to alcoholism. If your drinking behaviors correspond to any of those listed in this table, you may be abusing alcohol. Some individuals should avoid alcohol completely because of their health status or responses to the drug.

Alcohol and Health

Alcohol is a central nervous system depressant. Mild alcohol intoxication often produces pleasant sensations and relaxed inhibitions. Consuming large amounts, however, depresses normal motor functioning, including breathing, and death can result. Excessive alcohol use is the third leading lifestyle-related cause of death in the United States.[43] The drug is often involved in motor vehicle accidents, falls, and drownings, as well as acts of violence and abuse. An estimated 79,000 Americans died each year as a result of excessive alcohol use.[43] Thousands of other people suffer physical injuries and have damaged interpersonal relationships related to excess alcohol consumption.

The potentially harmful physiological effects of abusing the drug vary from person to person, primarily because of differences in overall health, drinking habits, and genetic background. Alcohol affects every cell in the body, and when consumed in excess, the drug damages every system in the body, particularly the

TABLE 6.9

What Are the Signs of Alcoholism?

Here is a self-test to help you review the role alcohol plays in your life. These questions incorporate many common symptoms of alcoholism. This test is intended to help you determine if you or someone you know needs to find out more about alcoholism; it is not intended to be used to establish the diagnosis of alcoholism.

YES	NO		YES	NO	
❏	❏	1. Do you ever drink heavily when you are disappointed, under pressure or have had a quarrel with someone?	❏	❏	14. Have you sometimes failed to keep promises you made to yourself about controlling or cutting down on your drinking?
❏	❏	2. Can you handle more alcohol now than when you first started to drink?	❏	❏	15. Have you ever had a DWI (driving while intoxicated) or DUI (driving under the influence of alcohol) violation, or any other legal problem related to your drinking?
❏	❏	3. Have you ever been unable to remember part of the previous evening, even though your friends said that you did not pass out?	❏	❏	16. Do you try to avoid family or close friends while you are drinking?
❏	❏	4. When drinking with other people, do you try to have a few extra drinks when others won't know about them?	❏	❏	17. Are you having more financial, work, school and/or family problems as a result of your drinking?
❏	❏	5. Do you sometimes feel uncomfortable if alcohol is not available?	❏	❏	18. Has your physician ever advised you to cut down on your drinking?
❏	❏	6. Do you sometimes feel a little guilty about your drinking?	❏	❏	19. Do you eat very little or irregularly during the periods when you are drinking?
❏	❏	7. Are you in more of a hurry to get your first drink of the day than you used to be?	❏	❏	20. Do you sometimes have the "shakes" in the morning and find that it helps to have a "little" drink, tranquilizer, or medication of some kind?
❏	❏	8. Has a family member or close friend ever expressed concern or complained about your drinking?	❏	❏	21. Have you recently noticed that you can't drink as much as you used to?
❏	❏	9. Have you been having more memory blackouts recently?	❏	❏	22. Do you sometimes stay drunk for several days at a time?
❏	❏	10. Do you often want to continue drinking after your friends say they've had enough?	❏	❏	23. After periods of drinking do you sometimes see or hear things that aren't there?
❏	❏	11. Do you usually have a reason for the occasions when you drink heavily?	❏	❏	24. Have you ever gone to anyone for help about your drinking?
❏	❏	12. When you're sober, do you sometimes regret things you did or said while drinking?	❏	❏	25. Do you ever feel depressed or anxious before, during or after periods of heavy drinking?
❏	❏	13. Have you tried switching brands or drinks, or following different plans to control your drinking?	❏	❏	26. Have any of your blood relatives ever had a problem with alcohol?

Any "yes" answer indicates that you may be at greater risk for alcoholism. More than one "yes" answer may indicate the presence of an alcohol-related problem or alcoholism and the need for consultation with an alcoholism professional. To find out more, contact the National Council on Alcoholism and Drug Dependence in your area.

Source: National Council on Alcoholism and Drug Dependence, Inc.

TABLE 6.10

Signs of Alcohol Abuse

Not everyone who drinks alcohol regularly abuses the drug, but you might be abusing alcohol if you:

Drink to relax, forget your worries, or improve mood

Lose interest in food as a result of your drinking habits

Consume drinks in a few quick gulps or binge drink

Lie about your drinking habits or try to hide them

Drink alone more often than you did in the past

Hurt yourself or someone else while drinking

Were drunk more than three or four times last year

Need to drink more alcohol than you used to drink to get "high"

Feel irritable and resentful when you are not drinking

Have medical, social, or financial problems caused by drinking habits

Have been cited for driving while intoxicated (DWI) or driving under the

influence of alcohol (DUI)

Source: National Institute of Alcohol Abuse and Alcoholism. www.niaaa.nih.gov/publications/agepage.htm

gastrointestinal, nervous, and cardiovascular systems. Figure 6.28 summarizes major damaging physiological effects of alcohol.

Alcohol and the Gastrointestinal Tract   If you have consumed distilled spirits without adding mixers, you probably felt a burning sensation as the alcohol entered your throat and stomach. This sensation is an indication of alcohol's irritating effects on the lining of your gastrointestinal tract. Not surprisingly, chronic drinking contributes to intestinal ulcer formation, particularly in the esophagus and stomach. An ulcer is a sore. Intestinal ulcers can cause chronic bleeding and may penetrate through the intestinal wall. When this occurs, intestinal contents leak into the abdominal cavity, causing serious and often deadly infections. Although the reasons are unclear, chronic alcohol consumption increases the risk of *alcoholic pancreatitis*, a painful and sometimes fatal condition characterized by inflammation and destruction of the pancreas.

People who consume alcohol have an increased risk of mouth, throat, voicebox, esophagus, liver, colorectal, and pancreatic

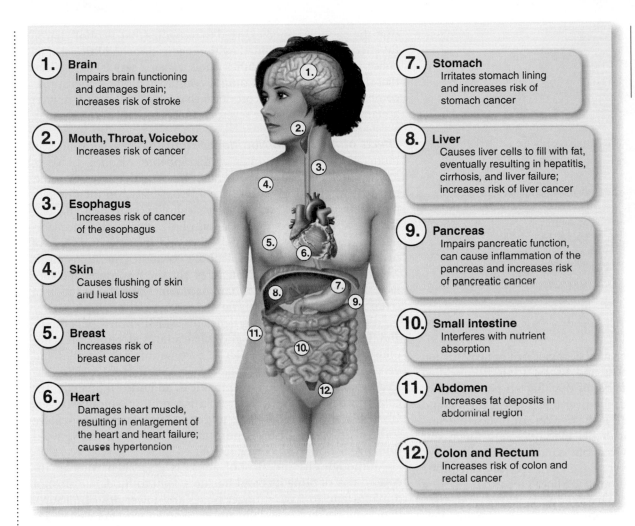

Figure 6.28 Some of alcohol's effects on the body. Chronic alcohol abuse seriously damages various organs and increases the risk of various cancers.

1. Brain
Impairs brain functioning and damages brain; increases risk of stroke

2. Mouth, Throat, Voicebox
Increases risk of cancer

3. Esophagus
Increases risk of cancer of the esophagus

4. Skin
Causes flushing of skin and heat loss

5. Breast
Increases risk of breast cancer

6. Heart
Damages heart muscle, resulting in enlargement of the heart and heart failure; causes hypertension

7. Stomach
Irritates stomach lining and increases risk of stomach cancer

8. Liver
Causes liver cells to fill with fat, eventually resulting in hepatitis, cirrhosis, and liver failure; increases risk of liver cancer

9. Pancreas
Impairs pancreatic function, can cause inflammation of the pancreas and increases risk of pancreatic cancer

10. Small intestine
Interferes with nutrient absorption

11. Abdomen
Increases fat deposits in abdominal region

12. Colon and Rectum
Increases risk of colon and rectal cancer

cancers.[46] Women who drink alcohol are more likely to develop breast cancer than women who abstain from alcohol.

Alcohol and the Brain Alcohol's effects on the central nervous system, especially the brain, appear within a few minutes of having a drink. Alcohol acts as a depressant, slowing the transmission of messages between nerve cells. At low BACs (< 0.06%), the drinker is relaxed and less inhibited socially as regions of the brain that control decision making and reasoning ability are depressed. If the person continues to drink and his or her BAC increases to between 0.08 and 0.15%, the person loses control over voluntary muscles, particularly muscles that move the lips, eyes, and limbs. As a result, the drinker's speech is slurred, his or her eyes have difficulty focusing on objects, and the person's ability to drive or operate any heavy equipment is seriously compromised. When the drinker's BAC reaches 0.20 to 0.30%, his or her brain is unable to process information. Higher BACs (0.30 to 0.50%) usually result in loss of consciousness ("passing out"). Moreover, coma and even death can occur as the brain loses control over lung and heart functioning. Table 6.11 lists BAC levels and typical nervous system effects at each level.

Alcohol can kill nerve cells (neurons) in the brain, and the organ is unable to replace many types of neurons. The brain of a chronic alcoholic has lost so many neurons that major regions shrink and the organ develops other structural abnormalities. Confusion and memory loss are common signs of the extensive brain damage that occurs in a chronic heavy drinker.

Alcohol and the Liver In addition to harming the brain, alcohol can damage the liver. Some acetyl-CoA that forms when alcohol is metabolized enters the complex series of biochemical pathways that eventually produce carbon dioxide, water, and ATP, the primary energy storage molecule for cells. The liver, however, also uses acetyl-CoA to make fatty acids for synthesizing

TABLE 6.11

Typical Effects of Alcohol at Various BAC Levels (Adults)

BAC	Typical Effects*
0.02 to 0.06	Positive mood; less inhibited; relaxed
0.06 to 0.08	Slight speech and vision impairment; elevated mood; impaired decision making
0.08 to 0.15	Reduction in motor skills; loss of emotional control; rapid eye movements; slurred speech; aggressive behavior in some individuals
0.20 to 0.30	Loss of motor and cognitive skills; decreased level of consciousness
0.30 to 0.35	Severe intoxication; barely aware of environment
> 0.35	Loss of consciousness; death

*Effects vary among adults.

Sources: Doty CI, Shah BR: Toxicity, ethanol. Last Updated: March 30, 2006. www.emedicine.com/PED/topic2715.htm.

Miller WR: *Characteristic effects of various BAC levels: Alcohol and its effects on behavior.* Center on Alcoholism, Substance Abuse, and Addictions. Last modified: July 25, 2005.

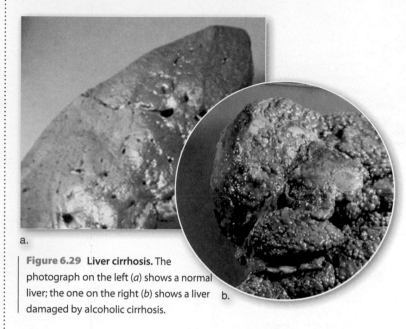

a.

b.

Figure 6.29 Liver cirrhosis. The photograph on the left (a) shows a normal liver; the one on the right (b) shows a liver damaged by alcoholic cirrhosis.

triglycerides (see Fig. 6.26). Even after a single bout of heavy drinking, fat accumulates in liver cells and causes a condition called "fatty liver." Fatty liver is reversible; if the affected person avoids alcohol for an extended period, the liver metabolizes the fat, and the organ eventually heals itself. If the person continues to drink, the buildup of fat destroys his or her liver cells, and tough scar tissue replaces them. This irreversible condition is called liver cirrhosis or hardening of the liver (Fig. 6.29). Alcoholics are prone to develop hepatitis, inflammation of the liver. Hepatitis can cause cirrhosis and increases the risk of liver cancer.

The scarred regions of an alcoholic's liver have no function other than holding the organ together. Under normal conditions, a healthy liver can regenerate sections of itself, but when destruction of liver cells is extensive, the organ begins to fail. In this situation, the affected person will die unless he or she undergoes liver transplantation. Chronic alcohol abuse is a major cause of liver failure among adult Americans.

Alcohol and the Cardiovascular System

When consumed in low to moderate intakes (1 to 2 drinks/day), alcohol reduces the risk of heart disease. Excess consumption, however, can damage heart muscle and elevate blood pressure to dangerous levels. As a result, chronic alcoholics often have enlarged but weakened hearts and suffer strokes.

Alcohol and Cancer

Compared to people who do not consume alcohol, chronic drinkers are more likely to develop certain cancers. Alcohol causes changes to cells that increase the drinker's risk of oral cavity, esophageal, stomach, liver, pancreatic, and colorectal cancer. Women who consume two or more drinks daily have a higher risk of breast cancer than women who abstain from alcohol or drink less than two drinks per day. Heavy drinkers who smoke tobacco products have a much greater risk of developing cancers of the oral cavity and esophagus than people who drink less and do not smoke.

Alcohol and Drug Interactions

People who drink alcohol while taking other drugs, including prescription medications and over-the-counter remedies, need to recognize that alcohol's harmful effects may be amplified by the medications. Additionally, alcohol may interact with other drugs, causing serious side effects that do not occur when a drug is consumed alone. For example, combining alcohol with products that contain the pain-reliever acetaminophen can cause severe liver damage and even death.

Effects of Alcohol on Nutritional Status

When consumed in moderation, alcohol stimulates the appetite. Alcohol, however, lowers blood glucose levels and raises blood triglycerides. Chronic, excessive alcohol intake can have adverse effects on the drinker's nutritional intake and status. Many alcoholics consume a considerable portion of their energy as alcohol, which often displaces nutrient-dense foods from their diets and increases their risk of malnutrition. Even when an alcoholic consumes nutritious meals while drinking, the alcohol interferes with the absorption, metabolism, and storage of various vitamins and increases the excretion of certain nutrients, particularly fat and the mineral magnesium.

Poor diets contribute to deficiencies of vitamin A, vitamin C, and the B vitamins thiamin and folate among alcoholics. It is not unusual for chronic alcoholics to become thiamin deficient and develop *Wernicke-Korsakoff syndrome*, a brain disorder characterized by mental confusion, memory loss, and uncoordinated muscular movements. The person with this condition typically staggers when trying to walk. Taking thiamin supplements can resolve some of the signs of the syndrome, but the person must avoid drinking alcohol while being treated.

Although chronic alcohol abuse is associated with an increased risk of bone loss and fractures, light to moderate alcohol drinkers tend to have stronger bones and lower risk of fractures than nondrinkers, especially among women who are past childbearing age. More research, however, is needed to determine the effects of alcohol on bone health.

Alcohol and Body Water

Billboard and commercial advertisements for alcoholic beverages often show sweaty, physically active young adults gulping down beer or liquor to relieve their thirst. These ads are misleading. Alcohol is not a good "thirst quencher" because it's a diuretic that suppresses the production of antidiuretic hormone (ADH) by the pituitary gland. Without ADH's action, the kidneys produce more urine, and the body loses water and certain vitamins and minerals along with it. If a dehydrated drinker consumes even more alcohol to relieve thirst, this response only increases his or her water losses. Drinking water and other non-alcoholic drinks is the best way to keep the body well hydrated.

Fetal Alcohol Spectrum Disorders

When a pregnant woman drinks alcohol, her embryo/fetus also "drinks" alcohol, because the drug passes freely from the mother's bloodstream into the embryo/fetus's bloodstream. Alcohol is most devastating when it affects an embryo, because organs develop during the first 2 months after conception. Unfortunately, many women are not aware that they are pregnant during this early stage of their child's prenatal (before birth) development, and they may drink socially or binge drink. Alcohol is toxic to cells, including rapidly dividing embryonic cells. An infant born with a *fetal alcohol spectrum disorder* (FASD) has some degree of developmental abnormalities as a result of its mother's

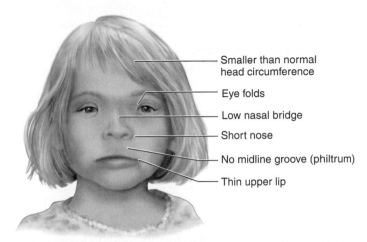

- Smaller than normal head circumference
- Eye folds
- Low nasal bridge
- Short nose
- No midline groove (philtrum)
- Thin upper lip

Figure 6.30 Fetal alcohol syndrome. Physical deformities and developmental delays are characteristics of fetal alcohol syndrome (FAS), a type of fetal alcohol spectrum disorder.

consumption of alcohol during pregnancy. *Fetal alcohol syndrome* (*FAS*) is a devastating form of FASD. A child with FAS is born with certain facial and heart defects as well as extensive, irreversible damage to its nervous system that causes intellectual disability (Fig. 6.30). Children with FAS also experience delayed and abnormal physical development.

The amount of alcohol that can be safely consumed by a pregnant woman has not been determined. Therefore, if you or someone you know is trying to conceive or is pregnant, you or that person should "play it safe" and avoid alcohol. The risks are too high to justify even one drink. Table 6.12 identifies people, including pregnant women, who should not drink alcohol.

Health Benefits of Alcohol

Consuming light to moderate amounts of alcohol raises HDL cholesterol levels; reduces blood levels of fibrinogen, an important blood-clotting factor; and decreases platelet stickiness. Platelets are cell fragments involved in the blood-clotting process. Reducing the likelihood of blood clot formation lowers the risk of heart attack and certain types of strokes.

Some medical researchers think drinking beer and red wine is healthier than consuming white wines or spirits. Although the

TABLE 6.12

Who Should Avoid Alcohol?

Women who suspect they are pregnant, know they are pregnant, or are trying to become pregnant

People who plan to drive or use heavy machinery

People taking certain over-the-counter or prescription medications

People with medical conditions that alcohol can aggravate

Recovering alcoholics

People younger than 21 years of age

Source: Adapted from National Institute on Alcohol Abuse and Alcoholism. *FAQs for the general public*. www.niaaa.nih.gov/FAQs/General-English/default.htm#safe-level Accessed: December 1, 2009.

alcohol in beer is the same as that in wine and distilled spirits, red wine and beer have higher levels of certain antioxidants and B vitamins than other alcoholic beverages, which may explain their health benefits. Other researchers point to studies that suggest all alcoholic beverages confer the same heart-healthy benefits, when adults consume moderate amounts of alcohol.[47] (Moderate alcohol consumption was defined as no more than 2 drinks/day for men and no more than 1 drink/day for women.) Purple grape juice, which is used to make red wine, contains the same antioxidants as the wine and appears to protect against heart disease as well.[48] The role of moderate alcohol consumption in coronary artery disease prevention is controversial. Drinking small amounts of alcohol seems to reduce the risk of heart disease, but consuming moderate to excessive amounts of alcohol is associated with increased risks of addiction, hypertension, heart failure, cancer, liver cirrhosis, and motor vehicle accidents. More research is needed to determine if alcohol alone or other compounds present in certain alcoholic beverages provide beneficial effects on health when consumed in moderation.

Alcohol and Physical Performance

Although some athletes may think consuming a small amount of alcohol before a competitive event might help relieve anxiety, alcohol reduces eye-hand coordination and slows reaction times even when BACs are relatively low (0.02 to 0.05%). Studies indicate conflicting findings concerning the effects of low to moderate amounts of alcohol on strength and endurance. In some instances, low to moderate intakes of alcohol reduce endurance and have negative effects on strength, but in other cases, this level of alcohol consumption produces no detrimental effects on strength and endurance. Alcohol can contribute to dehydration, which impairs muscular performance and causes heat injuries such as heat exhaustion and heat stroke. Chronic alcohol abuse causes muscular wasting that affects skeletal as well as heart muscle. Obviously, such effects will have negative effects on muscular mass, strength, and endurance.

According to the American College of Sports Medicine, athletes should learn about alcohol's effects on health, and avoid consuming excess alcohol during the 48 hours before an event. After exercise, and until his or her body recovers its normal fluid status, the athlete should focus on consuming nonalcoholic beverages.

Where to Get Help for Alcohol Abuse or Dependence

If you think you are abusing alcohol or are dependent on the drug, seek help from your personal physician. For information about alcohol abuse, you can contact the National Drug and Alcohol Treatment Referral Routing Service at 1-800-662-HELP. You can also visit the websites of Alcoholics Anonymous (www.aa.org/), the National Clearinghouse for Alcohol and Drug Information (http://ncadi.samhsa.gov/), or Al-Anon/Alateen (www.al-anon.alateen.org/).

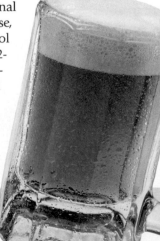

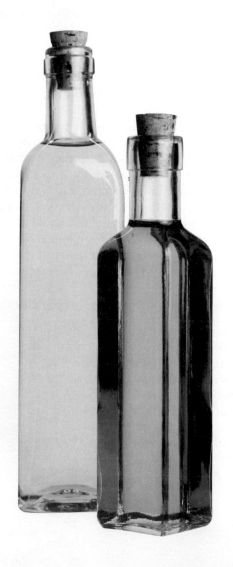

CHAPTER REFERENCES

See Appendix I.

SUMMARY

Lipids are needed for energy, proper growth and development, nerve functioning, maintenance of healthy skin and hair, and the production of bile and several hormones. Major lipids are triglycerides, phospholipids, and sterols. In addition to being a source of fuel, body fat contributes to body contours, insulates the body against cold temperatures, and protects against damaging blows.

Triglycerides, an important fuel for the body, comprise most of the lipid content of your food and body. Lipids can be sources of the essential fatty acids. Furthermore, the fat in food enhances absorption of fat-soluble vitamins and phytochemicals. Dietary lipids also contribute to the appealing flavor, texture, and aroma of foods. Although consuming some lipids is essential for health, high amounts may increase your risk of serious health conditions, including obesity, certain cancers, and CVD.

Most lipids have fatty acids in their chemical structures. Fatty acids can be saturated or unsaturated, and unsaturated fatty acids can be either monounsaturated or polyunsaturated. The body cannot synthesize the omega-6 fatty acid linoleic acid or the omega-3 fatty acid alpha-linolenic acid; these essential fatty acids must be supplied by the diet. The typical American eats more omega-6 fat than omega-3 fat. Fatty cold-water fish, canola and soybean oils, walnuts, and flaxseed are rich sources of the omega-3 fats.

Trans fatty acid molecules have a different configuration than cis fatty acid molecules. This difference enables fats that contain a high proportion of trans fatty acids to be more solid at room temperature than fats with a high proportion of cis fatty acids. Most of the trans fat in food results from the hydrogenation process. Partial hydrogenation partially hardens the oil so that it can be made into shortening or shaped into sticks of margarine. Diets that contain high amounts of trans fats are associated with an increased risk of heart disease and stroke.

A triglyceride has three fatty acids attached to glycerol. Triglycerides comprise about 95% of lipids in the body and in food. Triglycerides usually contain mixtures of unsaturated and saturated fatty acids, but one type of fatty acid (saturated, monounsaturated, or polyunsaturated) tends to predominate. In general, animal fats contain higher percentages of saturated fatty acids than plant fats. Important exceptions are the highly saturated coconut, palm, and palm kernel oils.

Phospholipids have both hydrophilic and hydrophobic regions, and as a result, they are partially soluble in water and can serve as emulsifiers. Phospholipids are the major structural component of cell membranes and are needed for proper functioning of nerve cells, including those in the brain. Lecithin is the major phospholipid in food; egg yolks, liver, wheat germ, peanut butter, and soybeans are rich sources of this compound.

The sterol cholesterol is a component of every cell membrane. Cells use cholesterol to make a variety of substances, including vitamin D, bile, and steroid hormones such as estrogen and testosterone. Cholesterol is found only in animal foods. Plants synthesize sterols and stanols that are not well absorbed by humans. Plant sterols and stanols, however, may be beneficial to health because they interfere with cholesterol absorption.

The triglycerides and phospholipids in food undergo digestion primarily in the upper part of the small intestine. Cholesterol is not broken down and is absorbed through the intestinal wall. Before leaving the small intestine, triglycerides, cholesterol, and other lipids are coated with a layer that contains protein to form chylomicrons. Chylomicrons enter the lymphatic system of the small intestine and eventually reach the bloodstream. The liver uses lipids from chylomicrons to make various lipoproteins, substances that transport lipids in the bloodstream. Enterohepatic circulation enables the liver to recycle bile salts to make new bile.

Triglycerides and carbohydrates are major sources of cellular energy. If energy is not needed, adipose cells remove fatty acids and glycerol from circulation and use them to synthesize triglycerides for storage. When energy is needed, adipose cells break down some stored triglycerides and release glycerol and fatty acids into the bloodstream.

Fat contributes about 34% of the average American's daily energy intake. Recommended diets for healthy people generally limit fat to 25 to 35% of total energy intake; the AMDR for fat is 20 to 35% of total calories. Consumers can use nutrient labels to determine how much fat, saturated fat, trans fat, and cholesterol are in packaged food.

CVD affects the heart and blood vessels. In the United States, heart disease is the leading cause of death; stroke is the fourth leading cause of death. Atherosclerosis is a long-term process that can result in CVD. Numerous risk factors are associated with atherosclerosis; some risk factors are inherited and difficult to modify, but many are related to lifestyle practices that can be altered. Smoking cigarettes, eating certain fats, and being physically inactive are lifestyle practices that increase a person's risk of atherosclerosis and CVD.

Your blood lipid levels can have a major influence on your risk of atherosclerosis. Lipoproteins transport much of the lipid content of the blood. Having high blood levels of HDL cholesterol is healthier than having high LDL cholesterol levels, because elevated LDL cholesterol contributes to atherosclerosis, whereas elevated HDL cholesterol reduces the risk of this condition.

Exercising and replacing saturated and trans fats with unsaturated fats may reduce LDL levels and increase HDL levels. On the other hand, physical inactivity and eating high amounts of saturated fat can raise LDL and blood triglyceride levels, increasing one's risk of atherosclerosis. Many people, however, do not experience an increase in their blood cholesterol levels when they eat cholesterol in foods.

Although oils, fatty spreads, and salad dressings are obvious sources of dietary fat, much of the fat we eat is not visible. Saturated fat contributes much of the calories in fatty meats, luncheon meats, sausage, hot dogs, hard cheeses, and whole milk. If people make dietary modifications, lose excess weight, and exercise regularly, and their blood lipid levels still remain elevated, they should discuss additional treatment options with their physicians. Millions of Americans take prescription statin medications to reduce their elevated blood lipid levels.

Alcohol (ethanol) is a water-soluble, two-carbon compound that is toxic to cells. Beers are typically 3 to 6% alcohol, wines contain about 8 to 14% alcohol, and wine coolers are about 10% alcohol by volume. Each gram of alcohol provides 7 kcal, but alcohol is not a nutrient; it is a mind-altering drug. A standard drink (approximately 12 ounces of beer or wine cooler, 5 ounces of wine, or 1½ ounces of liquor) contains 13 to 14 grams of alcohol.

Alcohol requires no digestion and readily passes through the tissues lining the inside of the mouth, esophagus, stomach, and small intestine. The body detoxifies alcohol by converting the chemical into less damaging compounds. Until the liver has had enough time to metabolize all the alcohol that has been consumed, the amount of the drug that remains circulates in the bloodstream. In the United States, a blood alcohol concentration of 0.08% is the legal limit for intoxication for automobile operators who are 21 years of age or older. Binge drinking is a major public health problem in the United States.

Although drinking light to moderate amounts of alcohol raises HDL, excessive amounts of the drug damages every system in the body, particularly the gastrointestinal, nervous, and cardiovascular systems. Alcohol has especially devastating effects on an embryo. Infants born with fetal alcohol syndrome (FAS) have certain facial and heart defects as well as extensive, irreversible damage to their nervous systems that causes intellectual disability. Therefore, pregnant women should not drink alcohol.

Recipes for Healthy Living

Nutty Stuff

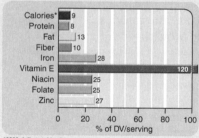

Looking for a snack that's more nutritious and tasty than chips? It's easy to make your own heart-healthy, high-fiber portable snack. The basic recipe is provided, and you can use it as the foundation for your own combinations of nuts and dried fruit. For example, you can replace the dried cranberries with raisins, chopped dates, or dried apricots; and you can use walnuts or peanuts instead of cashews. Adding some dark chocolate chips to the mixture is another option. This particular recipe makes about four ½-cup servings. Although the fats in most nuts are healthy fats, you may want to limit your serving size to less than ½ cup because of the caloric load—unless you have higher-than-average energy needs. Each ½-cup serving of this snack supplies 185 kcal, 3.8 g protein, 8.5 g fat, 2.5 g fiber, 5 mg iron, 145 mg potassium, 4 mg zinc, 100 mcg folate (a vitamin), 5 mg niacin (a vitamin), and 36 mg vitamin E.

INGREDIENTS:

¼ cup unsalted almonds
¼ cup unsalted cashews
½ cup dried cranberries
1 cup multigrain
   ready-to-eat oat cereal

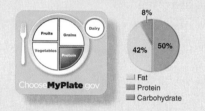

ChooseMyPlate.gov

8%
42% 50%
☐ Fat
■ Protein
☐ Carbohydrate

	% of DV/serving
Calories*	9
Protein	8
Fat	13
Fiber	10
Iron	28
Vitamin E	120
Niacin	25
Folate	25
Zinc	27

*2000 daily total kcal

PREPARATION STEPS:

1. Mix nuts, cereal, and dried fruit together.

2. Measure ½-cup servings, place in plastic sandwich bags, and seal the bags.

3. Store in a dry place. Mixture tastes best if eaten fresh or within a day or two.

Salmon Salad Sandwiches

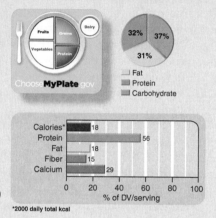

Are you tired of eating burgers? Try something different that's easy to prepare and a rich source of omega-3 fatty acids—salmon salad sandwiches. You can use canned salmon or leftover baked salmon to make the salad. This recipe makes enough salad for two sandwiches. Each sandwich provides approximately 350 kcal, 12 g fat, 28 g protein, 3.7 g fiber, and 290 mg calcium.

INGREDIENTS:

1 cup canned
  or cooked
  salmon
2 Tbsp pickle
  relish
2 Tbsp minced
  (finely chopped)
  sweet onion
1½ Tbsp lite mayonnaise
4 slices whole-wheat bread
1 slice fresh tomato (optional)
1 piece leaf lettuce (optional)

ChooseMyPlate.gov

32% 37%
31%
☐ Fat
■ Protein
☐ Carbohydrate

	% of DV/serving
Calories*	18
Protein	56
Fat	18
Fiber	15
Calcium	29

*2000 daily total kcal

PREPARATION STEPS:

1. If using canned salmon, drain fluid from salmon. In a bowl, break up salmon with a fork, including the small bones. Add other ingredients to the salmon and mix until well blended.

2. Toast slices of whole-wheat bread.

3. Spread ½ cup of salad on one slice of the toasted bread. Add a fresh tomato slice or piece of leaf lettuce, if desired.

Personal *Dietary* Analysis

1. Refer to the 3-day food log from the "Personal Dietary Analysis" feature in Chapter 3. List the total number of kilocalories you consumed for each day of record keeping. Add the figures to obtain a total, divide the total by 3, then round the figure to the nearest whole number to obtain your average daily energy intake for the 3-day period.

Sample Calculation:

Day 1   <u>2000</u>   kcal

Day 2   <u>1700</u>   kcal

Day 3   <u>2350</u>   kcal

Total kcal <u>6050</u> ÷ 3 days = <u>2017</u> kcal/day

      (average kilocalorie intake, rounded to the nearest whole number)

Your Calculation:

Day 1   _____   kcal

Day 2   _____   kcal

Day 3   _____   kcal

Total kcal _____ ÷ 3 days = _____ kcal/day

      (average kilocalorie intake, rounded to the nearest whole number)

2. Add the number of grams of fat eaten each day of the period. Divide the total by 3 and round to the nearest whole number to calculate the average number of grams of fat consumed daily.

Sample Calculation:

Day 1   <u>50</u> g

Day 2   <u>57</u> g

Day 3   <u>42</u> g

Total =   149 g

Total grams   <u>149</u> ÷ 3 days = 50g/day (average)

Your Calculation:

Day 1   _____ g

Day 2   _____ g

Day 3   _____ g

Total =   _____ g

Total grams   _____ ÷ 3 days = _____ g of fat/day

      (average, rounded to the nearest whole number)

(continued)

3. Each gram of fat provides about 9 kcal; therefore, you must multiply the average number of grams of fat that you ate daily (step 2) by 9 to obtain the average number of kilocalories from fat.

Sample Calculation:

<u>50</u> g/day × 9 kcal/g = <u>450</u> kcal from fat

Your Calculation

_____ g/day × 9 kcal/g = _____ kcal from fat

4. To calculate the average percentage of calories that fat contributed to your diet, divide the average number of calories from fat obtained in step 3 by the average total daily calorie intake obtained in step 1, and round to the nearest one-hundredth. Multiply the value by 100, drop the decimal point, and add the percent symbol.

Sample Calculation:

<u>450</u> kcal ÷ <u>2017</u> kcal = 0.22

0.22 × 100 = <u>22</u> %

Your Calculation

_____ kcal ÷ _____ kcal = _____

_____ × 100 = _____ %

5. Did your average daily fat intake meet the American Heart Association's recommended 25 to 35% of total energy?
Yes _____ No _____

6. If your average fat intake was more than 35% of your total energy intake, which foods contributed to your intake of fats?
Foods: _____

7. Review the log of your 3-day food intake. Calculate your average daily intake of cholesterol by adding the milligrams of cholesterol consumed over the 3-day period and dividing the total by 3.

Your Calculation:

Day 1 _____ mg

Day 2 _____ mg

Day 3 _____ mg

Total = _____ mg

Total g _____ ÷ 3 days = _____ mg of cholesterol daily

a. What was your average daily cholesterol intake? _____ grams

b. Was your average daily cholesterol intake less than the Dietary Guideline's recommended limit for an adult (300 mg)?

c. If your average cholesterol intake was greater than 300 mg, list foods that contributed to your cholesterol intake.

Using Nutrient Labels: Fats and Cholesterol

1. Remove the labels from two different packaged foods that contain fat. Using information from each of the product's Nutrition Facts panel, answer the following questions.

   a. Name of product #1 _____

      Name of product #2 _____

   b. How many kcal are in one serving of each food?

      Product 1 _____ kcal
      Product 2 _____ kcal

   c. How many grams of fat, saturated fat, trans fat, and cholesterol are in a serving?

      Product 1

      _____ grams of fat

      _____ grams of saturated fat

      _____ grams of trans fat

      _____ milligrams of cholesterol

      Product 2

      _____ grams of fat

      _____ grams of saturated fat

      _____ grams of trans fat

      _____ milligrams of cholesterol

   d. Calculate the percentage of total kcal/serving that are from saturated fat. First, multiply the number of grams of saturated fat by 9 (number of kcal per gram of fat). Then, divide the number of kcal contributed by saturated fat by the total number of kcal per serving. (The Nutrition Label uses the term "Calories" for kcal.) To obtain the percentage, move the decimal point two places to the right, remove the decimal point, and insert % symbol.

      Product 1 _____ grams of saturated fat $\times$ 9 kcal = _____ kcal of saturated fat/serving

      _____ % total kcal/serving contributed by saturated fat

      Product 2 _____ grams of saturated fat $\times$ 9 kcal = _____ kcal of saturated fat/serving

      _____ % total kcal/serving contributed by saturated fat

   e. Read the list of ingredients for each product. If the food contains saturated fat and cholesterol, identify ingredients that contributed saturated fat or cholesterol to the product.

      Saturated fat ingredients in Product 1 _____

      Cholesterol ingredients in Product 1 _____

      Saturated fat ingredients in Product 2 _____

      Cholesterol ingredients in Product 2 _____

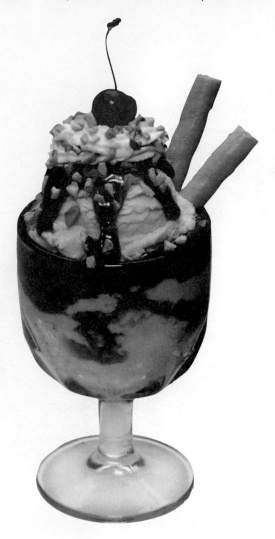

Assessment: Evaluating Your Solid Fat Intake

Do you consume:	Rarely or Never	1 to 2 Times/ Week	3 to 5 Times/ Week	Daily
1. Bacon, hot dogs, sausage, salami, bologna, or other fatty luncheon meat?	0	1	2	3
2. Whole milk?	0	1	2	3
3. 2% milk?	0	1	2	3
4. Ice cream or milkshakes?	0	1	2	3
5. Sour cream or cream cheese?	0	1	2	3
6. Fatty cuts of pork or beef?	0	1	2	3
7. Hard cheeses, such as cheddar or Swiss?	0	1	2	3
8. Butter?	0	1	2	3
9. Stick margarine?	0	1	2	3
10. Gravy, cheese sauce, or cream-based sauce?	0	1	2	3
11. Buttered popcorn or "rinds"?	0	1	2	3
12. Biscuits, croissants, doughnuts, Danish pastries, pies, cakes, or cookies?	0	1	2	3
13. Products made with lard?	0	1	2	3
14. Cream in your coffee or tea?	0	1	2	3
15. Pizza?	0	1	2	3
16. Creamed soups such as cream of potato soup or New England clam chowder?	0	1	2	3
TOTAL	_____	_____	_____	_____

Scoring: Add points in each column and then add those figures together. (The higher the total points, the higher your solid fat intake.)

My "Solid Fat Score" is _____

If your score is 30 or more: Your solid fat intake is probably too high. Note which of these fatty foods you eat more than three times per week. Consider reducing your intake of these items and replacing them with foods that do not contain solid fat.

CRITICAL THINKING

1. Calculate your risk of having a heart attack by completing the American Heart Association's risk calculator at https://www.heart.org/gglRisk/locale/en_US/index.html?gtype=health. Based on your results, should you be concerned about your risk of CVD? If you are concerned, discuss steps you can take to reduce your risk of atherosclerosis and CVD.

2. Do you avoid fried foods and look for "lite" and "fat-reduced" foods when shopping for groceries? If your answer is "no," explain why.

3. Plan a meal that supplies 25% to 35% of energy from fat. The meal should include foods from the major food groups and provide 700 to 900 kcal.

4. Prepare a pamphlet that provides information about risk factors for CVD. In addition to English, you may prepare the pamphlet in Spanish, French, Vietnamese, or another modern language.

5. Develop a lesson for middle-school-aged children that describes atherosclerosis and the role that personal choices (lifestyles) play in the development of the disease.

6. If you drink alcohol, use Table 6.9 to assess your alcohol consumption habits. After taking this assessment, ask yourself if you are abusing alcohol. If your answer is "yes," what aspects of your behavior make you an alcohol abuser? What can you do to obtain help?

PRACTICE TEST

Select the best answer.

1. Fats in foods

   a. add taste and contribute to "mouth feel."
   b. are digested and absorbed in the stomach.
   c. carry water-soluble nutrients.
   d. need to be eliminated to have a healthful diet.

2. Solid fats generally have a high proportion of _____ fatty acids.

   a. unsaturated
   b. saturated
   c. polyunsaturated
   d. monounsaturated

3. A saturated fatty acid has

   a. one double bond within the hydrocarbon chain.
   b. two double bonds within the hydrocarbon chain.
   c. no double bonds within the hydrocarbon chain.
   d. None of the above is correct.

4. Which of the following statements is true?

   a. Certain fish are rich sources of omega-3 fatty acids.
   b. Omega-3 fatty acids increase the risk of cardiovascular disease.
   c. Trans fats are rich sources of omega-3 fatty acids.
   d. The human body converts dietary fiber into omega-3 fatty acids.

5. Trans fatty acids are

   a. naturally in many foods.
   b. a by-product of the hydrogenation process.
   c. essential to good health.
   d. All of the above are correct.

6. Phospholipids

   a. do not have fatty acids in their chemical structures.
   b. lack glycerol in their chemical structures.
   c. do not occur naturally.
   d. are partially water soluble.

7. Cholesterol is

   a. metabolized for energy.
   b. found only in animal foods.
   c. not made by the human body.
   d. harmful to health.

8. The primary site of triglyceride digestion and absorption is the

   a. stomach.
   b. liver.
   c. small intestine.
   d. gallbladder.

9. Lipoproteins

   a. are water insoluble.
   b. transport lipids in the bloodstream.
   c. contain glucose.
   d. are toxic to cells.

Answers to Chapter 6 Quiz *Yourself*

1. To lose weight, use regular, stick margarine instead of butter because it has 25% fewer calories per teaspoon. **False.** (p. 179)

2. Egg yolks are a rich source of cholesterol. **True.** (p. 178)

3. Taking too many fish oil supplements may be harmful to health. **True.** (p. 178)

4. On average, Americans consume 60% of their energy from fat. **False.** (p. 169)

5. Increasing your intake of trans fats will reduce your risk of heart disease. **False.** (p. 160)

10. Modifiable risk factors for atherosclerosis include

    a. family history.
    b. age.
    c. tobacco use.
    d. All of the above are correct.

11. Homocysteine is a(n)

    a. form of folate.
    b. lipid that lowers blood pressure.
    c. possible marker for cardiovascular disease.
    d. essential amino acid.

12. Alcohol metabolism is not influenced by a person's

    a. sex.
    b. level of caffeine consumption.
    c. prior history of alcohol use.
    d. body size and composition.

13. After her college graduation party, Jade's BAC was 0.16%. This level is ___ times the legal limit.

    a. 5
    b. 4
    c. 3
    d. 2

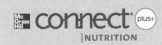

Additional resources related to the features of this book are available on ConnectPlus® Nutrition. Ask your instructor how to get access.

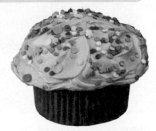

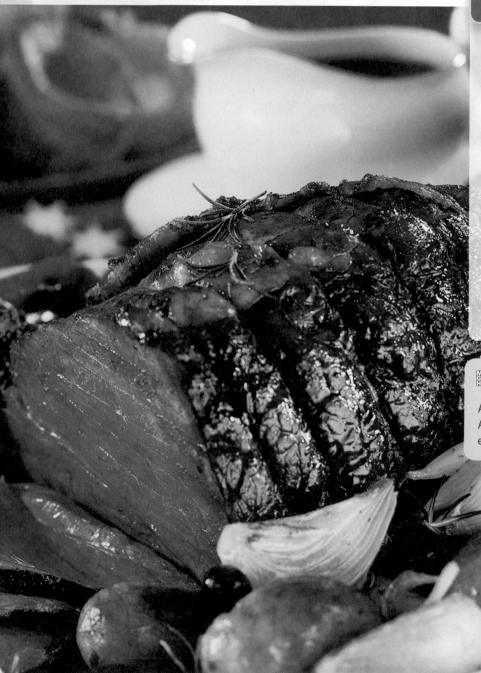

CHAPTER 7

Proteins

Chapter Learning Outcomes

After reading Chapter 7, you should be able to

1. List the primary functions of proteins in the body.

2. Identify the basic structural unit of proteins.

3. Distinguish between essential and nonessential amino acids.

4. Explain the basic steps of protein synthesis and digestion.

5. Discuss conditions that contribute to positive nitrogen balance, negative nitrogen balance, and nitrogen balance.

6. Identify food sources of protein and foods that provide high- and low-quality proteins.

7. Plan meals and snacks that reduce animal protein intakes.

8. Discuss the pros and cons of vegetarian diets.

9. Describe how protein-energy malnutrition (PEM) can affect the body.

10. List practical ways to save money on food.

connect plus+
NUTRITION **www.mcgrawhillconnect.com**

A wealth of proven resources are available on ConnectPlus® Nutrition! Ask your instructor about ConnectPlus, which includes an interactive eBook, an adaptive learning program and much, much more!

SINCE ANCIENT TIMES, many people have believed that eating animal foods, particularly meat, was necessary for good health and optimal physical performance. Milo of Croton, an ancient Greek Olympian wrestler with extraordinary strength, reportedly consumed about 20 pounds of meat daily. Although accounts of Milo's superhuman capacity for eating meat are unreliable, modern athletes often make protein-rich foods and protein supplements the foundation of their diets. Furthermore, it is not unusual for nonathletes to associate meat with protein and a lack of protein with poor muscular development and weak muscular strength.

Many Americans think a meal is not adequate unless it contains large portions of meat. Although it is true that meat is a rich source of protein, other foods, including those from plants, are often overlooked as sources of protein. The beef patty of a cheeseburger provides protein, as well as the melted cheese that tops the burger and the bun that makes the sandwich convenient to eat.

Protein is an important class of nutrients, but it is not more valuable to your health than other nutrients. Nutrients work together in your body like members of a well-trained basketball team on the playing court. Making one player the star while neglecting to develop the other athletes' skills can have disastrous effects on the team's success. Similarly, overemphasizing one class of nutrients in your diet, such as protein, while ignoring other nutrients, can lead to nutritional imbalances that result in serious health problems. By reading Chapter 7, you will learn about the roles of proteins in your body and their major food sources. You will also learn how proteins influence your health.

Quiz *Yourself*

How much protein is recommended for optimal health? Can people obtain enough protein by eating only plant foods? What happens if you eat more protein than your body needs? After reading Chapter 7, you will learn to identify good food sources of protein and understand the nutrient's roles in the body. You will also learn how the amount and quality of the protein in your diet can affect your health. Before reading Chapter 7, take the following quiz to test your knowledge of protein. The answers are on page 239.

1. Animal foods such as meat and eggs are almost 100% protein. ____T ____F

2. Foods made from processed soybeans can be sources of high-quality protein. ____T ____F

3. Americans typically consume more protein from animal sources than from plant foods. ____T ____F

4. Registered dietitians generally recommend that healthy people take amino acid supplements to increase their protein intake. ____T ____F

5. People can nourish their hair by using shampoo that contains protein. ____T ____F

proteins large, complex organic molecules made up of amino acids

hormones chemical messengers that regulate body processes and responses

7.1 What Are Proteins?

Proteins are complex organic molecules that are chemically similar to lipids and carbohydrates because they contain carbon, hydrogen, and oxygen atoms. Proteins, however, contain nitrogen, the element cells need to make a wide array of important biological compounds. Plants, animals, bacteria, and even viruses contain hundreds of proteins.

Proteins are necessary for muscle development and maintenance, but the more than 200,000 different proteins in your body have a wide variety of functions, including those shown in Table 7.1.[1] Skin, blood, nerve, bone—all cells in your body—contain proteins. Structural proteins such as *collagen* are in your cartilage, ligament, and bone tissue. *Keratin* is another structural protein; it is in your hair, nails, and skin. Contractile proteins in your muscles enable you to move, and the pigment protein *melanin* determines the color of your eyes, hair, and skin. Proteins are also necessary for your blood to clot properly.

Certain hormones, such as insulin and glucagon, are proteins. **Hormones** are chemical messengers that regulate body processes and responses, such as growth,

TABLE 7.1 *Proteins in the Body*

The body uses proteins to make or function as:
New cells and many components of cells
Structures such as hair and nails
Enzymes
Lubricants
Clotting compounds
Antibodies
Compounds that help maintain fluid and pH balance
Certain hormones and neurotransmitters
Energy source (minor, under usual conditions)

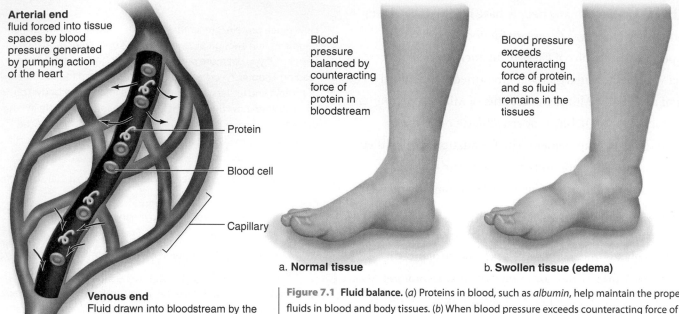

Arterial end
fluid forced into tissue spaces by blood pressure generated by pumping action of the heart

Protein

Blood cell

Capillary

Venous end
Fluid drawn into bloodstream by the proteins as blood pressure declines in the capillaries

Blood pressure balanced by counteracting force of protein in bloodstream

Blood pressure exceeds counteracting force of protein, and so fluid remains in the tissues

a. **Normal tissue**

b. **Swollen tissue (edema)**

Figure 7.1 Fluid balance. (*a*) Proteins in blood, such as *albumin*, help maintain the proper distribution of fluids in blood and body tissues. (*b*) When blood pressure exceeds counteracting force of blood proteins, fluid remains in tissues, causing edema.

enzymes compounds that speed up chemical reactions

antibodies infection-fighting proteins

edema accumulation of fluid in tissues

acid-base balance maintaining the proper pH of body fluids

buffer substance that can protect the pH of a solution

metabolism, and hunger. Nearly all **enzymes** are proteins. Enzymes speed up the rate of (*catalyze*) chemical reactions without becoming a part of the products (see Fig. 4.8). Additionally, infection-fighting **antibodies** are proteins. Although cells can use proteins for energy, normally they metabolize very little for energy, conserving the nutrient for other important functions that carbohydrates and lipids are unable to perform.

In the bloodstream, proteins transport nutrients and oxygen. Proteins in blood, such as *albumin*, also help maintain the proper distribution of fluids in blood and body tissues (Fig. 7.1). The force of blood pressure moves watery fluid out of the bloodstream and into tissues. Blood proteins help counteract the effects of blood pressure by attracting the fluid, returning it to the bloodstream. During starvation, the level of protein in blood decreases, and as a result, some water leaks out of the bloodstream and enters spaces between cells. The resulting accumulation of fluid in tissues is called **edema** (*eh-dee′mah*).

Proteins also help maintain **acid-base balance,** the proper pH of body fluids. To function properly, blood and tissue fluids need to maintain a pH of 7.35 to 7.45, which is slightly basic.[1] (To review the concept of pH, see Chapter 4.) Metabolic processes can produce acidic or basic by-products. If a particular body fluid becomes too acidic or too basic, cells can have difficulty functioning and may die. A **buffer** can protect the pH of a solution. Proteins can act as buffers, because they have acidic and basic components. For example, if cells form an excess of hydrogen ions (H^+), the pH of tissues decreases. To help restore the pH level to within the normal range, the basic portions of protein molecules bind to the excess H^+, neutralizing the excess ions and raising the pH.

Amino Acids

Proteins are comprised of smaller chemical units called **amino acids.** The human body contains proteins made from 20 different amino acids (see Appendix E). To understand how the body uses amino acids, it is necessary to learn some basic chemistry that relates to these compounds.

Each amino acid has a carbon atom that anchors a hydrogen atom and three different groups of atoms: the **amino** or **nitrogen-containing group,** the **R group** (sometimes called the **side chain**), and the **acid group.** The chemical structure of the amino acid *alanine* shown in Figure 7.2 indicates these three groups. Note that the nitrogen atom is in the amino group. The R group identifies the molecule as a particular amino acid, such as

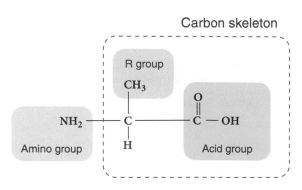

Carbon skeleton

R group

CH_3

NH_2 — C — C — OH

H

Amino group

Acid group

Alanine molecule

Figure 7.2 Amino acid: Basic chemical structure. Alanine has the typical chemical features of an amino acid—the nitrogen-containing or amino group, R group, and acid group. When the nitrogen-containing component is removed from an amino acid, the "carbon skeleton" remains.

TABLE 7.2 *Amino Acids*

Essential		Nonessential	
Histidine	Threonine	Alanine	Cysteine*
Isoleucine	Tryptophan	Aspartic acid	Glutamine*
Leucine	Valine	Asparagine	Glycine*
Lysine		Glutamic acid	Proline*
Methionine		Serine	Tyrosine*
Phenylalanine		Arginine*	

*Under certain conditions, this amino acid can become essential.

serine or *lysine*. When the nitrogen-containing group is removed, the R group, acid group, and anchoring carbon atom form the "carbon skeleton" of an amino acid (see Fig. 7.2). The carbon skeleton is an important component of an amino acid, because the body can convert the carbon skeletons of certain amino acids to glucose and use the simple sugar for energy.

Classifying Amino Acids

Traditionally, nutritionists classify amino acids as either nonessential or essential according to the body's ability to make them. A healthy human body can make 11 of the 20 amino acids. These compounds are the **nonessential amino acids.** The remaining nine amino acids are **essential amino acids** that must be supplied by foods, because the body cannot synthesize them or make enough to meet its needs. Sometimes, nonessential and essential amino acids are referred to as "dispensable" and "indispensable" amino acids, respectively. Table 7.2 lists amino acids according to their classification as essential and nonessential.

Several nonessential amino acids are "conditionally essential," which means they become essential in certain situations. For example, cells can make cysteine from methionine and serine. If a person's methionine and serine intake is inadequate, his or her body cannot make enough cysteine to meet its needs and dietary sources of the amino acid are necessary.

amino acids nitrogen-containing chemical units that comprise proteins

amino or nitrogen-containing group portion of an amino acid that contains nitrogen

R group (side chain) part of amino acid that determines the molecule's physical and chemical properties

acid group acid portion of a compound

nonessential amino acids group of amino acids that the body can make

essential amino acids amino acids the body cannot make or make enough to meet its needs

Concept **Checkpoint**

1. What is the chemical unit that makes up a protein?
2. List at least four different functions of proteins in the body.
3. Identify the three groups of atoms that make up a typical amino acid.
4. What is the "carbon skeleton" of an amino acid?
5. How many different kinds of amino acids are needed to make human proteins? How many of these amino acids are essential?

7.2 Proteins in Foods

People often associate animal foods with protein, but beans, nuts, seeds, grains, and certain vegetables are good sources of protein too. In fact, nearly all foods contain protein, but no naturally occurring food is 100% protein. Protein comprises only about 20 to 30% of the weight of a piece of beef; 25% of the weight of drained, water-packed tuna fish; and only 12% of an egg's weight. Nevertheless, animal foods generally provide higher amounts

legumes plants that produce pods with a single row of seeds

high-quality (complete) protein protein that contains all essential amino acids in amounts that support the deposition of protein in tissues and the growth of a young person

low-quality (incomplete) protein protein that lacks or has inadequate amounts of one or more of the essential amino acids

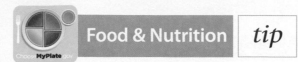

Food & Nutrition *tip*

Commercially canned beans often have considerable amounts of salt added to them. Consider purchasing canned or frozen beans that have little or no added salt. Dried beans do not have salt added to them, but they take a long time to cook, unless you soak them for several hours before cooking. The soaking process softens the beans, reducing cooking time and making them more digestible and less likely to contribute to intestinal gas. (See the Recipes for Healthy Living on page 235 for a black bean recipe.)

of protein than similar quantities of plant foods. A 3-ounce serving of broiled lean ground beef supplies 23 g of protein; a 3-ounce serving of steamed broccoli or cooked carrots provides only about 1 g of protein. In general, most plant foods provide less than 3 g of protein per ounce. Table 7.3 lists some commonly eaten foods and their approximate protein content per serving.

Certain parts of plants contain more protein than other parts. Seeds, tree nuts, and legumes supply more protein per serving than servings of fruit or the edible leaves, roots,

TABLE 7.3 *Approximate Protein Content of Some Commonly Eaten Foods/Portion*

Food	Serving Size	Protein g/serving
Chicken, breast, roasted, meat only	4 oz	40
Hamburger, 80% lean, broiled	4 oz	34
Tuna, canned, water-packed, drained	4 oz	34
Ham, lean, cooked	4 oz	30
Pepperoni pizza, regular crust, 14" pie	2 slices (200 g)	25
Miso (soybean product)	½ cup	16
Lasagna with meat sauce	8 oz	15
Cottage cheese, 2% low-fat	4 oz	16
Milk, fat-free	1 cup	8
Peanut butter	2 Tbsp	8
Tofu, regular	½ cup	8
Bagel, plain	1 (3½" diam)	7
American processed cheese	1 oz	7
Baked beans, vegetarian	½ cup	6
Egg, hard cooked	1	6
Vanilla ice cream	1 cup	4
White rice	1 cup	4
Peas, green	½ cup	4
Banana	1	1

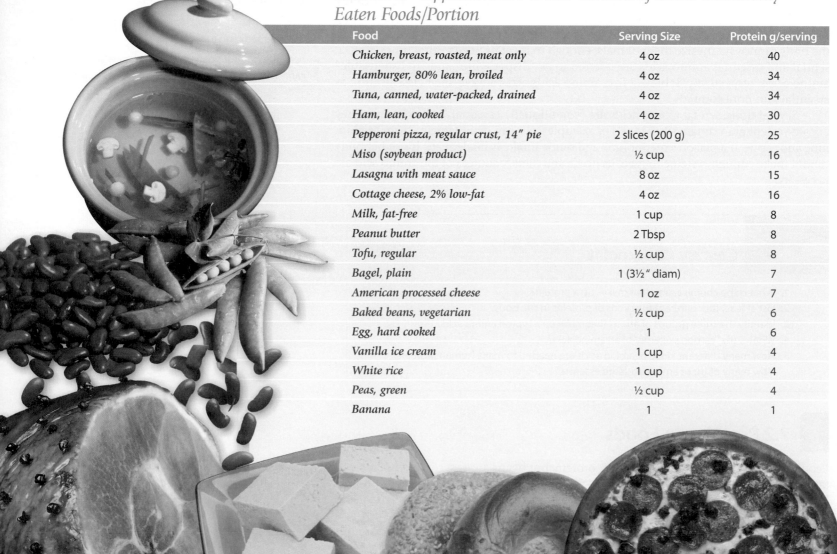

flowers, and stems of vegetables. Tree nuts include walnuts, cashews, and almonds; **legumes** are plants that produce pods that have a single row of seeds, such as soybeans, peas, peanuts, lentils, and beans (Fig. 7.3). A 3-ounce serving of almonds, dry-roasted peanuts, or sunflower seed kernels supplies about 20 g of protein. Many seeds and nuts, however, pack a lot of calories from fat. Snack on just 3 ounces of almonds, dry-roasted peanuts, or sunflower seed kernels, and you will add almost 500 kcal to your diet!

Peas, lentils, and most kinds of beans contain more protein and complex carbohydrate than fat. Eating a 3-ounce serving of vegetarian baked beans, for example, adds about 4 g of protein, 14 g of carbohydrate, and less than 1 g of fat to your diet. Although soybeans contain more fat than carbohydrate, soy fat is high in unsaturated fatty acids. The health benefits of unsaturated fatty acids are discussed in Chapter 6.

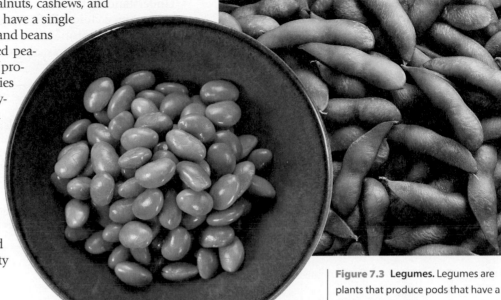

Figure 7.3 Legumes. Legumes are plants that produce pods that have a single row of seeds.

Protein Quality

Foods differ not only in the amount of protein they contain but also in their protein quality. A **high-quality** or **complete protein** contains all essential amino acids in amounts that support protein deposition in muscles and other tissues, as well as a young child's growth.[2] High-quality proteins are well digested and absorbed by the body. Meat, fish, poultry, eggs, and milk and milk products contain high-quality proteins. Egg protein generally rates very high for protein quality because it is easy to digest and has a pattern of essential amino acids that closely resembles that needed by humans.

A **low-quality** or **incomplete protein** lacks or contains inadequate amounts of one or more of the essential amino acids. Furthermore, the human digestive tract does not digest low-quality protein sources as efficiently as foods containing high-quality protein. The essential amino acids that are in relatively low amounts are referred to as *limiting* amino acids, because they reduce the protein's ability to support growth, repair, and maintenance of tissues. In most instances, tryptophan, threonine, lysine, and the sulfur-containing amino acids methionine and cysteine are the limiting amino acids in foods.[3]

Most plant foods are not sources of high-quality proteins. *Quinoa (keen'-wa)* and soy protein are exceptions. Quinoa is botanically related to sugar beets and spinach, but the quality and amount of protein in quinoa seeds are superior to those of many cereal grains.[4] Cooked quinoa is often used as a cereal (see "Recipes for Healthy Living" at the end of Chapter 7). After being processed, the quality of soy protein is comparable to that of most animal proteins.[5] Processed soybeans are used to make a variety of nutritious foods, including soy milk, infant formula, and meat substitutes. Furthermore, eating foods made from soybeans may reduce the risk of osteoporosis, cardiovascular disease, and certain cancers.[6] More research, however, is needed to determine the long-term health benefits of eating diets that contain soy products.

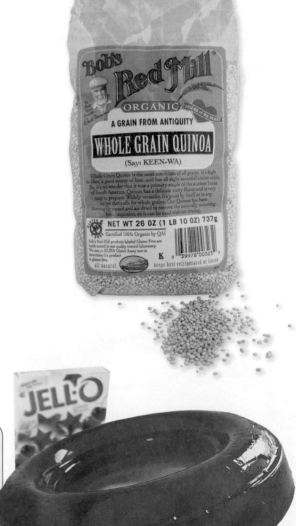

Did You Know?

Gelatin is made from *collagen*, a protein derived from the connective tissue of animals, but it is not a complete source of protein. Furthermore, eating gelatin will not make your fingernails stronger. Fingernails are composed of *keratin*, a protein that is different from collagen.

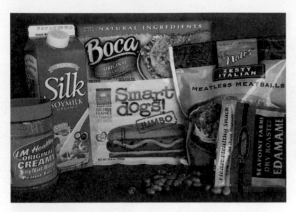

After being processed, the quality of soy protein is comparable to that of most animal proteins.

Understanding the concept of protein quality is important. Regardless of how much protein is eaten, a child will fail to grow properly if his or her diet lacks essential amino acids. The "Vegetarianism" section of Chapter 7 explains how you can obtain these and other essential nutrients by eating only plant foods.

Concept **Checkpoint**

6. Explain the difference between a high-quality protein and a low-quality protein.
7. Identify at least three dietary sources of high-quality protein and three dietary sources of low-quality protein.
8. List at least three essential amino acids that are most likely to be limiting amino acids.

DNA hereditary material that provides instructions for making proteins

peptide bond chemical attraction that connects two amino acids together

peptides small chains of amino acids

polypeptides proteins comprised of 50 or more amino acids

gene portion of DNA

7.3 What Happens to Proteins in Your Body?

In a television crime series, police in a major city are investigating what could be a homicide. A man has been reported missing by his parents, who suspect foul play and their daughter-in-law's involvement in their son's disappearance. While knocking on the door of the missing man's house, police notice some dried blood on the front porch. The man's wife, who lives in the house, tells police that the blood is from her injured dog. How can police know she is telling the truth? The blood holds important clues. Every organism synthesizes proteins—including those in blood—that are unique. Samples of the blood can be analyzed to determine whether it contains proteins from a dog or another animal, such as a human. We will leave it to your imagination to finish this story, but we will examine a real-life story—how human cells make proteins.

How Your Body Synthesizes Proteins

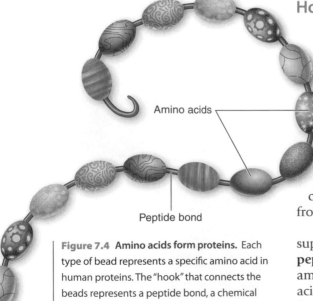

Amino acids

Peptide bond

Figure 7.4 Amino acids form proteins. Each type of bead represents a specific amino acid in human proteins. The "hook" that connects the beads represents a peptide bond, a chemical attraction between the acid group of one amino acid and the amino group of another amino acid.

Your body makes proteins by following information coded in your **DNA,** or deoxyribonucleic (*de-ox'-e-rye'-bow-new-klay'-ik*) acid, the hereditary material in a cell's nucleus. To make proteins, cells assemble the 20 amino acids in specific sequences according to the information provided by DNA. To understand this process, imagine proteins as various chains made from 20 different amino acid "beads." Figure 7.4 illustrates some of these beads and how they can be assembled into chains. Note that each bead has two metal wires that are used to link it with another bead. To make a copy of a particular beaded chain, you would follow directions for connecting the beads in a specific order and length by hooking the metal wires of each bead together. Consider the vast variety of beaded chains comprised of different bead sequences and chain lengths that you could make from just 20 different beads.

In living things, the beaded chains are proteins that contain amino acids. DNA supplies the directions for synthesizing each protein and the "hook" on each bead is a **peptide bond,** a chemical attraction between the acid group of one amino acid and the amino group of another amino acid (Fig. 7.5). A dipeptide forms when two amino acids bond and a molecule of water is released in the process. **Peptides** usually contain fewer than 15 amino acids. Most naturally occurring proteins are **polypeptides** (*poly* = many; *peptides* = amino acids) comprised of 50 or more amino acids.

Figure 7.6 summarizes the basic steps of protein synthesis. Protein synthesis begins with DNA in the cell's nucleus. DNA is a twisted, two-stranded molecule referred to as a double helix. To begin the process, a section of the DNA double helix unwinds, exposing a gene. A **gene** is a portion of DNA that contains information concerning the order of amino acids that comprise a specific protein. *Messenger ribonucleic acid (mRNA)*, a compound that is chemically similar to DNA, "reads" or transcribes the gene. The actual production of a protein occurs in the cytoplasm, so mRNA leaves the nucleus and moves to ribosomes—protein-manufacturing sites in the cytoplasm. Ribosomes translate the gene's coded instructions for adding amino acids to the polypeptide chain. During this translation process, *transfer ribonucleic acid (tRNA)* conveys specific amino acids, one at a time, to the ribosomes. At the ribosomes, the amino acid from tRNA is added to the last amino acid, causing the peptide chain to grow longer. After the mRNA is read completely, the ribosome releases the polypeptide, and then the new protein generally undergoes further processing at other sites within the cytoplasm.

Diets that contain low-quality protein can result in poor growth, slowed recovery from illness, and even death. These situations occur because protein synthesis in cells cannot proceed when the supply or "pool" of amino acids does not have one or more of the essential amino acids needed for constructing the polypeptide chain. When this happens, production of the protein stops. The partially made polypeptide chain is dismantled, and its amino acids are returned to the pool.

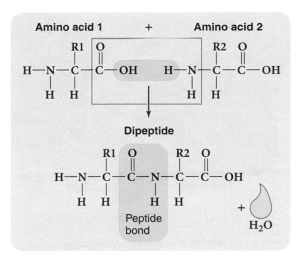

Figure 7.5 Peptide bond. A peptide bond is a chemical attraction between the acid group of one amino acid and the amino group of another amino acid. A dipeptide forms when two amino acids bond and a molecule of water is released in the process.

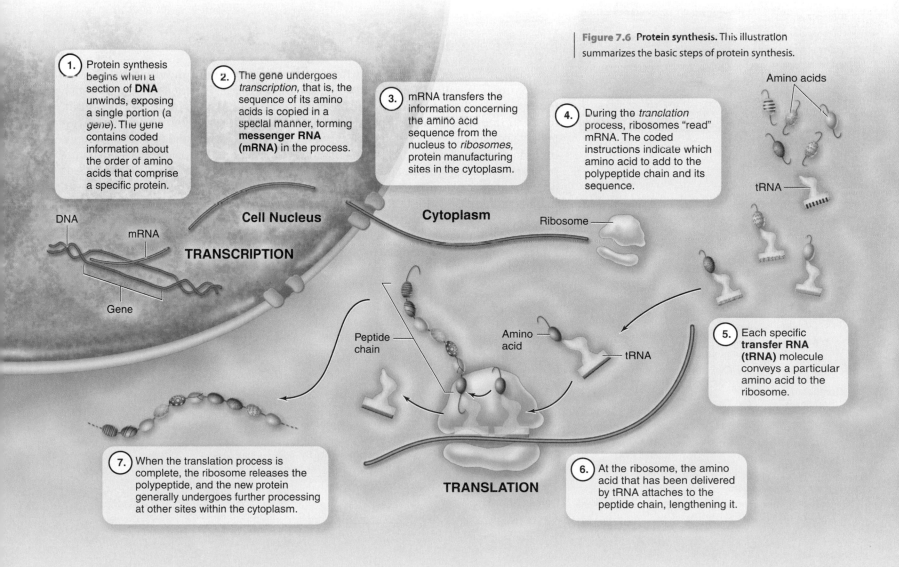

Figure 7.6 Protein synthesis. This illustration summarizes the basic steps of protein synthesis.

1. Protein synthesis begins when a section of **DNA** unwinds, exposing a single portion (a *gene*). The gene contains coded information about the order of amino acids that comprise a specific protein.

2. The gene undergoes *transcription*, that is, the sequence of its amino acids is copied in a special manner, forming **messenger RNA (mRNA)** in the process.

3. mRNA transfers the information concerning the amino acid sequence from the nucleus to *ribosomes*, protein manufacturing sites in the cytoplasm.

4. During the *translation* process, ribosomes "read" mRNA. The coded instructions indicate which amino acid to add to the polypeptide chain and its sequence.

5. Each specific **transfer RNA (tRNA)** molecule conveys a particular amino acid to the ribosome.

6. At the ribosome, the amino acid that has been delivered by tRNA attaches to the peptide chain, lengthening it.

7. When the translation process is complete, the ribosome releases the polypeptide, and the new protein generally undergoes further processing at other sites within the cytoplasm.

DNA

mRNA

Cell Nucleus

TRANSCRIPTION

Gene

Cytoplasm

Ribosome

Amino acids

tRNA

Peptide chain

Amino acid

tRNA

TRANSLATION

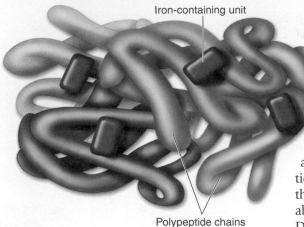

Iron-containing unit

Polypeptide chains

Figure 7.7 Shaping of a protein. A polypeptide chain can fold and coil into characteristic three-dimensional shapes, such as the four polypeptide chains of a hemoglobin molecule. In a hemoglobin molecule, each chain is associated with an iron-containing unit.

Figure 7.8 Sickle cell anemia. This microscopic view of red blood cells shows (*a*) normal disk-shaped cells and (*b*) a sickle cell that contains abnormal hemoglobin.

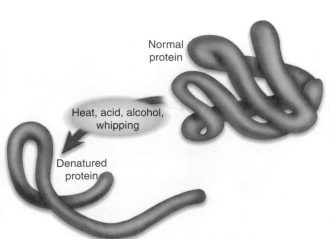

When assembly of the new protein has been completed, the polypeptide acid chain coils and folds into a three-dimensional shape that is characteristic of that particular protein. In some instances, more than one polypeptide chain curl around each other to form large protein complexes. For example, *hemoglobin*, a protein in red blood cells, is comprised of four polypeptide chains coiled together (Fig. 7.7). The shape of a protein is important because it influences the compound's activity in the body.

Occasionally, the wrong amino acid is introduced into the amino acid chain during the protein synthesis process. Cells usually check for such errors and replace the amino acid with the correct one. If the DNA code is faulty, however, the wrong amino acid will be inserted into the chain consistently, forming an abnormal polypeptide. Such errors often cause genetic defects that have devastating, even deadly, effects on the organism. *Sickle cell anemia*, for example, is an inherited condition characterized by abnormal hemoglobin. Cells in red bone marrow synthesize hemoglobin by following DNA instructions concerning proper amino acid sequencing. If the DNA codes for the insertion of the wrong amino acid in two of hemoglobin's four polypeptide chains, the resulting protein is defective and does not function correctly. Figure 7.8a shows a red blood cell that contains normal hemoglobin; the red blood cell shown in Figure 7.8b has the defective hemoglobin associated with sickle cell anemia. Crescent-shaped red blood cells cannot transport oxygen efficiently. As a result, the abnormal cells can clog small blood vessels, causing pain, organ damage, and premature death. Sickle cell anemia is a common genetic disorder that generally affects people with African, Caribbean, or Mediterranean ancestry.

Protein Denaturation

A protein undergoes **denaturation** when it is exposed to various conditions that alter the macronutrient's natural folded and coiled shape (Fig. 7.9). We often cook protein-rich foods to make them more digestible and safe to eat, but heat also causes the proteins in foods to unfold. The protein in raw egg white, for example, is almost clear and has a jellylike consistency. When you cook egg white, it becomes white and firm as its proteins become denatured. Other treatments often used during food preparation also denature proteins, including whipping or exposing them to alcohol or acid. Wine, for example, is often used in marinades, because the alcohol it contains denatures proteins in meat, helping tenderize it. Adding acidic lemon juice to milk denatures ("curdles") the proteins in milk. In your stomach, hydrochloric acid denatures food proteins, making them easier to digest. Denaturation does not "kill" a protein (because proteins are not living), but the process usually permanently alters the protein's shape and functions. Once an egg white has been cooked or milk has curdled, the food cannot return to its original state.

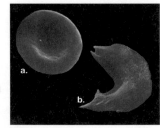

Normal protein

Heat, acid, alcohol, whipping

Denatured protein

Figure 7.9 Denaturation. A protein undergoes denaturation when exposed to various conditions that alter its natural folded shape.

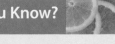

Did You Know?

Despite information provided in commercials or advertisements, you cannot "feed" your hair, nails, or skin by using shampoos, conditioners, or lotions containing proteins or other nutrients. Hair, nails, and the outermost layer of skin are not living. By eating a nutritious diet, you will provide your body with the nutrients it needs to make healthy hair, nails, and skin.

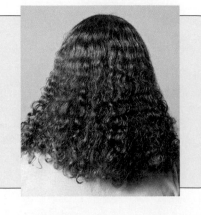

Protein Digestion and Absorption

When you eat oatmeal mixed with milk for breakfast, the large proteins in these foods must be digested before undergoing absorption. Protein digestion begins in the stomach, where hydrochloric acid denatures food proteins and **pepsin**, an enzyme, digests proteins into smaller polypeptides. Soon after the polypeptides enter the small intestine, the pancreas secretes protein-splitting enzymes, including trypsin (*trip'-sin*) and chymotrypsin (*ki'-mo-trip'-sin*). *Trypsin* and *chymotrypsin* break down polypeptides into shorter peptides and amino acids. Enzymes released by the absorptive cells of the small intestine break down most of the shortened peptides into dipeptides, tripeptides, and individual amino acids. Dipeptides and tripeptides are compounds that consist of two and three amino acids, respectively. Within the absorptive cells, di- and tripeptides are broken down into amino acids. Thus, amino acids are the end products of protein digestion. After being absorbed, the amino acids enter the portal vein and travel to the liver, where they may enter the general circulation. Protein digestion and absorption is very efficient: very little dietary protein escapes digestion and is eliminated in feces. Figure 7.10 summarizes protein digestion and absorption.

denaturation altering a protein's natural shape and function by exposing it to conditions such as heat, acids, and physical agitation

pepsin gastric enzyme that breaks down proteins into smaller polypeptides

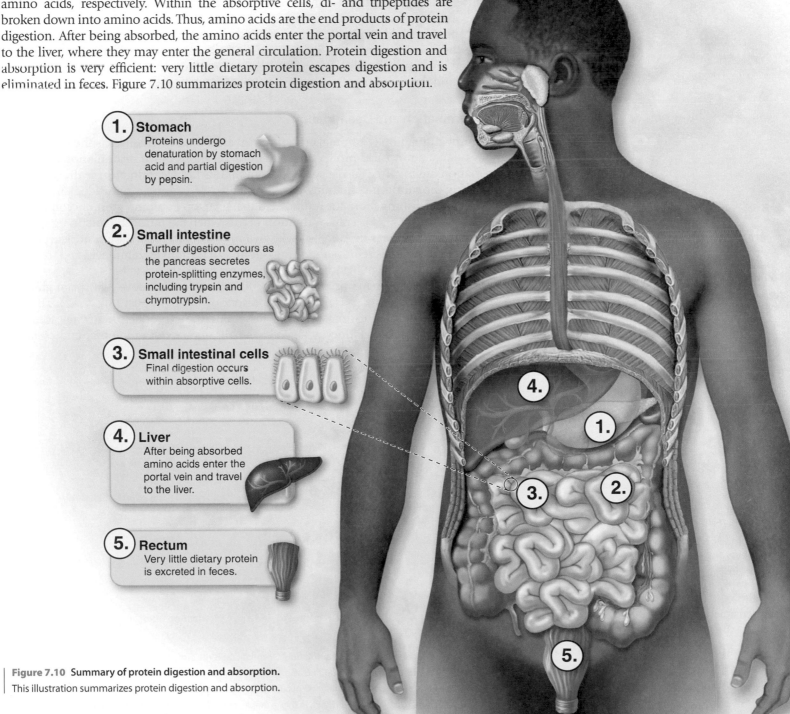

1. Stomach Proteins undergo denaturation by stomach acid and partial digestion by pepsin.

2. Small intestine Further digestion occurs as the pancreas secretes protein-splitting enzymes, including trypsin and chymotrypsin.

3. Small intestinal cells Final digestion occurs within absorptive cells.

4. Liver After being absorbed amino acids enter the portal vein and travel to the liver.

5. Rectum Very little dietary protein is excreted in feces.

Figure 7.10 Summary of protein digestion and absorption. This illustration summarizes protein digestion and absorption.

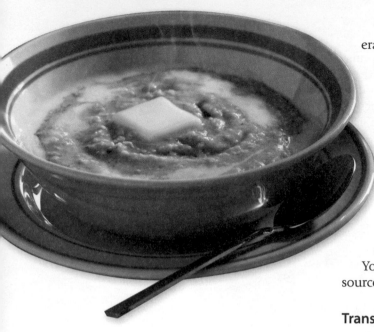

The liver keeps some amino acids for its needs and releases the rest into the general circulation. By the time cells obtain amino acids from blood, they cannot distinguish the ones that were originally in oat proteins from those that were in milk proteins. The cells, however, now have all the amino acids they need to make *your* body's proteins.

Protein Turnover

Not all protein must be supplied by the diet. **Protein turnover,** the process of breaking down old or unneeded proteins into their component amino acids and recycling them to make new proteins, occurs constantly within cells. Amino acids that are not incorporated into proteins become part of a small amino acid pool, a readily available supply of amino acids that cells can use for future protein synthesis. The amino acid pool is an *endogenous*, or internal, source of nitrogen. Your body obtains about two-thirds of its amino acid supply from endogenous sources and the remainder from *exogenous* (dietary) sources.

Transamination and Deamination

A healthy human body can make 11 of the 20 amino acids. The liver is the main site of nonessential amino acid production. Chemical reactions called deamination and transamination are involved in the synthesis of amino acids. **Deamination** is the process of removing the nitrogen-containing group (usually NH_2) from an unneeded amino acid. As a result of deamination, the amino acid that gives up its amino group becomes a carbon skeleton (Fig. 7.11). **Transamination** occurs when the nitrogen-containing group is transferred to another substance to make an amino acid. To make the amino acid alanine, for example, liver cells remove the amino group (NH_2) from glutamic acid and transfer it to pyruvic acid (see Fig. 7.11). Transamination reactions are reversible.

Deamination occurs primarily in the liver. Liver cells remove NH_2 from glutamic acid, forming ammonia (NH_3), a highly poisonous waste product (Fig. 7.12). The liver can use the ammonia to make **urea,** a metabolic waste product that is released into your bloodstream. The kidneys filter urea, small amounts of ammonia, and *creatinine*

protein turnover cellular process of breaking down proteins and recycling their amino acids

deamination removal of the nitrogen-containing group from an amino acid

transamination transfer of the nitrogen-containing group from an unneeded amino acid to a carbon skeleton to form an amino acid

urea waste product of amino acid metabolism

nitrogen balance (equilibrium) balancing nitrogen intake with nitrogen losses

positive nitrogen balance state in which the body retains more nitrogen than it loses

negative nitrogen balance state in which the body loses more nitrogen than it retains

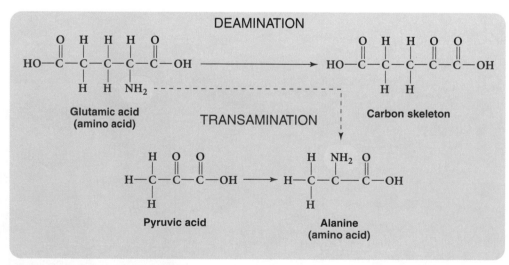

Figure 7.11 Deamination and transamination. Deamination is the process of removing the nitrogen-containing group from an unneeded amino acid. In this example, glutamic acid loses its amino group and becomes a carbon skeleton. Transamination occurs when the nitrogen-containing group is transferred to another substance to make an amino acid. In this example, pyruvic acid receives the amino group from glutamic acid, forming alanine, a nonessential amino acid.

(a nitrogen-containing waste produced by muscles) from blood and eliminate the compounds in urine. After an amino acid undergoes deamination, the carbon skeleton that remains can be used for energy or converted to other compounds, such as glucose. Muscle cells can deaminate certain amino acids and use their carbon skeletons for energy.

If you consume more protein than you need, what happens to the extra amino acids? The body does not store excess amino acids in muscle or other tissues. The unnecessary amino acids undergo deamination, and cells convert the carbon skeletons into glucose or fat, or metabolize them for energy.

Nitrogen Balance

Although your body conserves nitrogen by recycling amino acids, each day you lose some protein and nitrogen from your body. Urinary elimination of urea and creatinine accounts for most of the lost nitrogen.[7] Daily nitrogen losses also occur as your nails and hair grow, and when you shed the outermost layer of your skin and cells from your intestinal tract. Your body uses amino acids from foods to replace the lost nitrogen.

Normally, an adult's body maintains its protein content by maintaining **nitrogen balance** or **nitrogen equilibrium**, that is, balancing nitrogen intake and protein turnover with losses. During certain stages of life or physical conditions, however, nitrogen intake and retention do not equal nitrogen losses. When the body is in a state of **positive nitrogen balance,** it retains more nitrogen than it loses as proteins are added to various tissues. In this case, a person must eat more protein to satisfy the increased need for the nutrient. Positive balance occurs during periods of rapid growth such as pregnancy, infancy, and puberty, and when people are recovering from illness or injury. Hormones such as insulin, growth hormone, and testosterone stimulate positive nitrogen balance. Performing weight (resistance) training also leads to nitrogen retention.[8] When the body is in a state of **negative nitrogen balance,** the body loses more nitrogen than it retains and protein intake is less than what the body needs. Negative balance occurs during starvation, serious illnesses, and severe injuries. Recovery from the illness or injury and refeeding protein results in positive nitrogen balance until nitrogen equilibrium is restored. Figure 7.13

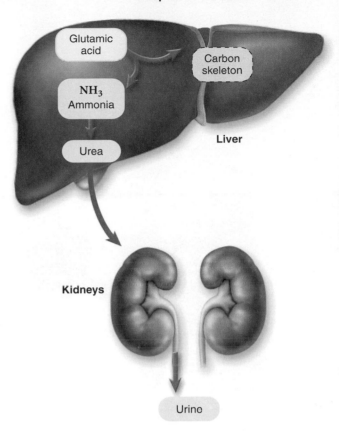

Figure 7.12 Deamination. The process of deamination results in the production of the highly toxic compound ammonia in the liver. The liver converts ammonia to urea and releases it into the blood. Kidneys pick up urea and other nitrogen-containing wastes and eliminate them in urine.

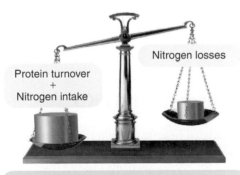

Positive Nitrogen Balance

- Growth
- Pregnancy
- Recovery from illness/injury
- Increased levels of the hormones insulin, testosterone, and growth hormone
- Resistance exercise

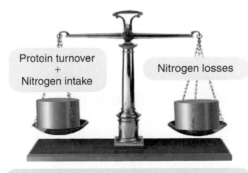

Nitrogen Equilibrium

- Healthy adult meets protein and energy needs

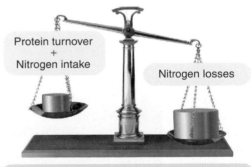

Negative Nitrogen Balance

- Inadequate protein intake or digestive tract diseases that interfere with protein absorption
- Increased protein losses resulting from certain kidney diseases or blood loss
- Bed rest
- Fever, injuries, or burns
- Increased secretion of thyroid hormone or cortisol (a "stress hormone")

Figure 7.13 Nitrogen balance. This diagram illustrates the concept of nitrogen balance and lists conditions that result in positive and negative nitrogen balance. Note that nitrogen balance occurs when nitrogen intake plus turnover equals nitrogen losses.

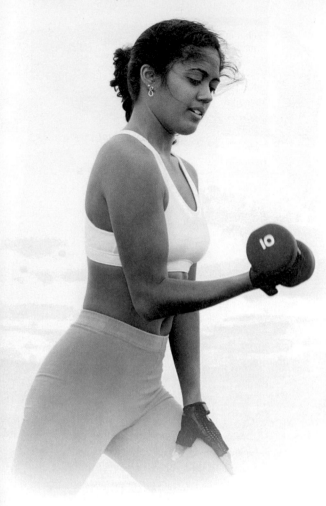

illustrates the concept of nitrogen balance and lists conditions that result in positive and negative nitrogen balance.

How Much Protein Do You Need?

The Estimated Average Requirement (EAR) for protein is 0.66 g of protein/kg of body weight.[3] The EAR for protein increases during pregnancy, breastfeeding, periods of rapid growth, and recovery from serious illnesses, blood losses, and burns. Recall from Chapter 3 that scientists use EARs to establish Recommended Dietary Allowances (RDAs). A healthy adult's RDA for protein is 0.8 g/kg of body weight.[3] By reviewing DRI tables (inside back cover of this book), you will note that the RDAs for protein vary during certain ages and conditions.

To determine your RDA for protein, multiply your weight in kilograms by 0.8 grams. If you are underweight or overweight, use a healthy weight for your height when making this calculation (see the body mass index chart in Chapter 10). For example, a healthy man who is 5'10" tall and weighs 75 kilograms (his weight in pounds divided by 2.2) should consume 60 grams of protein daily (75 kg × 0.8 g) to meet his RDA for the nutrient. The "Personal Dietary Analysis" at the end of Chapter 7 can help you estimate your daily protein intake.

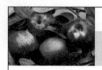

Concept **Checkpoint**

9. Explain the basic steps involved in protein synthesis.
10. Define denaturation, deamination, and transamination.
11. Describe conditions that can cause the body to be in negative nitrogen balance. Describe conditions in which the body is in positive nitrogen balance.
12. A healthy young woman weighs 143 pounds. Calculate her RDA for protein.
13. Explain what happens to proteins in beans as they undergo digestion and absorption in the human digestive tract.

 ## 7.4 Food Allergies, Celiac Disease, and PKU

There is no question that cells need amino acids to function properly. In some instances, however, certain amino acids or proteins cause havoc in the body, resulting in serious health problems and even death. The following sections take a closer look at three protein-related conditions that affect the lives of millions of Americans. By following special diets, people with these conditions can live normal and productive lives.

What Is a Food Allergy?

Have you ever experienced an allergic reaction after eating certain foods or drinks? A food allergy is an inflammatory response that results when the body's immune system reacts inappropriately to one or more harmless substances (*allergens*) in the food. In most instances, the allergen is a protein. For reasons that are unclear, some protein in a

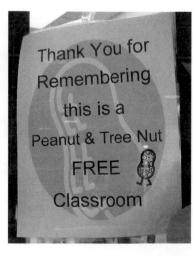

This sign on the door of an elementary school classroom lets people know to avoid bringing anything containing peanuts and tree nuts into the room.

food that is eaten does not undergo digestion, and the small intestine absorbs the whole molecule. Immune system cells in the small intestine recognize the food protein as a foreign substance and try to protect the body by mounting a defensive response. As a result of the immune response, the person who is allergic to that food experiences typical signs and symptoms. Common signs and symptoms of food allergies include *hives*, red raised bumps that usually appear on the skin; swollen or itchy lips; skin flushing; a scaly skin rash (eczema); difficulty swallowing; wheezing and difficulty breathing; and abdominal pain, vomiting, and diarrhea. Allergic reactions generally occur within a few minutes to a couple of hours after eating the offending food. In severe cases, sensitive people who are exposed to food allergens can develop *anaphylactic shock*, a serious drop in blood pressure that affects the whole body. Anaphylaxis (*an-a-pha-lax'-is*) can be fatal, unless emergency treatment is provided. Genetics play a major role in the risk of food allergies; people who have family histories of allergies to foods or other environmental triggers are more likely to develop these conditions.

Although any food protein has the potential to cause an allergic reaction in a susceptible person, the most allergenic proteins are in cow's milk, eggs, peanuts and other nuts, wheat, soybeans, fish, and shellfish. Allergic responses to nonprotein food dyes or other food additives such as *sulfites* can also occur. Sulfites are a group of sulfur-containing compounds that result from the metabolism of certain amino acids. Sulfites can be found naturally in foods, but the compounds are often added to wines, potatoes, and shrimp as a preservative.[9] People who suffer from asthma often develop breathing difficulties after consuming food treated with sulfites. Other sulfite-sensitive people report skin flushing (redness and warmth), hives, difficulty swallowing, vomiting, diarrhea, and dizziness after consuming foods that contain the compounds.

In the United States, approximately 6% of young children suffer from food allergies.[10] Since 1997, the prevalence of food allergies among children under 18 years of age has been increasing in the United States. Children with food allergies are more likely than other children to experience other allergies and asthma. Most youngsters outgrow their food allergies by the time they are 5 years old. Allergies to nuts, seafood, and wheat, however, usually are not outgrown. According to the American Academy of Allergy, Asthma, and Immunology, 3 to 4% of adults in the United States have one or more food allergies.[10]

Accurate diagnosis of a food allergy should be undertaken by an immunologist, a physician who specializes in the diagnosis and treatment of allergies. Skin testing is a reliable way to identify allergens. Although hair analysis, cytotoxic or electrodermal testing, and kinesiology are promoted by alternative medical practitioners to diagnose allergies, these are unproven diagnostic methods.[11]

Treatment of food allergies involves strict avoidance of the offending foods. Parents or caregivers of young children with food allergies should read food labels carefully to check for allergens listed among ingredients. Additionally, they should educate teachers and other adults who associate with the allergic child about the importance of not exposing the youngster to specific foods. In 2004, the U.S. Congress passed the Food Allergen Labeling and Consumer Protection Act, which required food manufacturers to

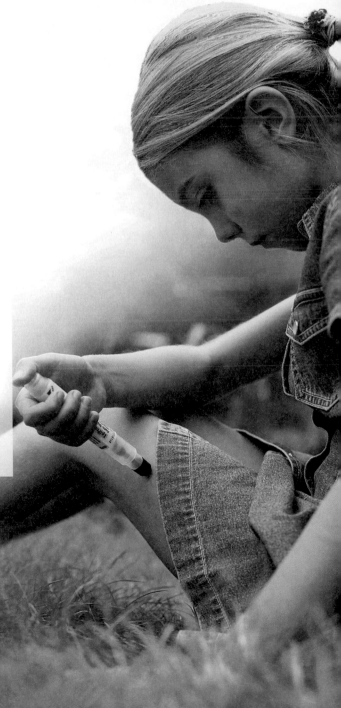

Emergency treatment for anaphylaxis often involves injecting a medication that prevents or blunts the allergic response. This child is using an *autoinjector pen,* a special syringe, to inject herself with a dose of the medication.

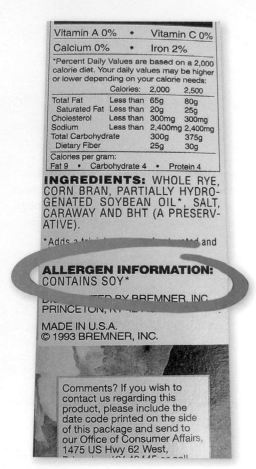

	Calories:	2,000	2,500
Vitamin A 0%	•	Vitamin C 0%	
Calcium 0%	•	Iron 2%	

*Percent Daily Values are based on a 2,000 calorie diet. Your daily values may be higher or lower depending on your calorie needs:

		2,000	2,500
Total Fat	Less than	65g	80g
Saturated Fat	Less than	20g	25g
Cholesterol	Less than	300mg	300mg
Sodium	Less than	2,400mg	2,400mg
Total Carbohydrate		300g	375g
Dietary Fiber		25g	30g

Calories per gram:
Fat 9 • Carbohydrate 4 • Protein 4

INGREDIENTS: WHOLE RYE, CORN BRAN, PARTIALLY HYDRO-GENATED SOYBEAN OIL*, SALT, CARAWAY AND BHT (A PRESERV-ATIVE).

*Adds a trivial ... and

ALLERGEN INFORMATION: CONTAINS SOY*

DISTRIBUTED BY BREMNER, INC. PRINCETON, KY ...

MADE IN U.S.A.
© 1993 BREMNER, INC.

Comments? If you wish to contact us regarding this product, please include the date code printed on the side of this package and send to our Office of Consumer Affairs, 1475 US Hwy 62 West, ...

Figure 7.14 Allergen labeling. According to the Food Allergen Labeling and Consumer Protection Act, food manufacturers must identify potentially allergenic ingredients, such as soy, milk, and peanuts, on product labels.

identify potentially allergenic ingredients, such as soy, milk, and peanuts, on product labels (Fig. 7.14).[12]

What Is Celiac Disease?

Celiac (see'-lee-ak) disease is a common inherited condition that results in poor absorption of nutrients (malabsorption) from the small intestine. People with the disease cannot tolerate foods that contain gluten, a group of related proteins in wheat, barley, and rye. Gluten provides the chewy texture and stiff structure of breads and other baked products made from wheat, barley, and rye. After a person with celiac disease eats foods or is exposed to substances that contain gluten, the protein stimulates the body to mount an immune response in the small intestine that inflames or destroys villi. (Villi are the tiny, fingerlike projections of small intestine that absorb nutrients [see Figure 4.26].) Even though the affected person's food intake may be nutritionally adequate, malnutrition results because his or her intestinal tract lacks healthy villi. Celiac disease is also known as nontropical sprue and gluten-induced or gluten-sensitive enteropathy (*ent-er-op'-a-thee*).

The signs and symptoms of celiac disease vary from person to person but usually include abdominal bloating, chronic diarrhea, and weight loss. Children with this condition also experience poor growth due to nutrient malabsorption and protein malnutrition. Some people have no obvious signs or symptoms of the disease, despite the damage occurring to their small intestines. Serious health problems such as anemia (a blood disorder), osteoporosis (weak bones), infertility, liver disease, and intestinal cancer can result from untreated celiac disease.

In the United States, about 1 in 133 people has celiac disease.[13] Although the tendency to develop the disease is probably inherited, environmental factors often play a role by triggering the condition. A serious viral infection or severe emotional stress, for example, may activate the disorder in a genetically susceptible person. Infants who consume formula may be more likely to develop the condition than breastfed babies.[13] Also, infants who are fed gluten-containing foods when they are too young (3 months of age, for example) may have a higher risk of developing celiac disease than infants who are not introduced to such foods until they are older.

No single medical test is effective in determining whether a person has celiac disease. However, blood testing and intestinal biopsies are often used to diagnose the condition. The biopsy involves removing tiny pieces of tissue from the small intestine. The tissue samples undergo microscopic examination to evaluate the condition of the villi. The presence of damaged villi can help confirm the diagnosis of celiac disease.

There is no cure for celiac disease, but persons with the condition can achieve and maintain good health by following a special gluten-free diet very carefully. Many supermarkets carry a variety of gluten-free foods (Figure 7.15). Table 7.4 lists foods that must be avoided by people with celiac disease as well as those that are safe for them to consume. Although people with the condition can eat corn, rice, and soy products, these foods may be contaminated with gluten if they are processed in factories that also manufacture wheat products. Because gluten may be used to make medications, dietary supplements, and lipsticks, people with celiac disease should read ingredient lists to determine whether such "hidden" sources of gluten are present. At the time of this writing, the U.S. Food and Drug Administration (FDA) was preparing rules for the use of the claim "gluten-free" on product labels.

Katie Adams was diagnosed with celiac disease when she was in college. The "Real People, Real Stories" feature on page 215 introduces Katie and describes how she manages her diet to avoid signs, symptoms, and complications of celiac disease.

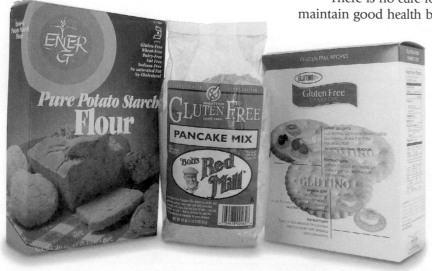

Figure 7.15 Gluten-free foods. Gluten-free foods are often available in supermarkets.

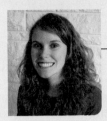

REAL *People*
REAL *Stories*

Katie Adams

When Katie Adams was an American college student, she had the opportunity to attend England's renowned Cambridge University during her junior year. Being at Cambridge was a wonderful educational opportunity for the young woman, but being thousands of miles away from her family made her homesick. Within a few months after Katie began her studies in England, she began to experience frequent bouts of abdominal pain not long after eating. Making matters even worse, she suffered from nearly constant diarrhea. Although her weight was at a healthy level when she first went to England, she began to lose pounds despite eating adequate amounts of food. Unaware that she could have a serious intestinal disorder, Katie attributed her weight loss and abdominal discomfort to emotional stress and irritable bowel syndrome (see Chapter 4's "Highlight").

Eventually, Katie reached the point at which she could no longer ignore her health problems. While at Cambridge, she was examined by a physician who thought her signs and symptoms were the result of celiac disease. Although Katie was unfamiliar with the disease, she decided to forego being tested for the condition until she returned to the United States.

After coming home from England, Katie underwent specialized testing by a gastroenterologist, a physician who diagnoses and treats conditions affecting the intestinal tract. The tests included determining whether certain antibodies, proteins produced by the immune system in response to foreign substances, were present in her blood. This testing detected the presence of antibodies to proteins in gluten. She also underwent an endoscopic examination of her upper gastrointestinal tract. This exam enabled the gastroenterologist to see the condition of her small intestine and remove a small part of the damaged tissue to view under a microscope. As a result of these definitive tests, Katie was diagnosed with celiac disease. The only treatment for celiac disease is complete avoidance of gluten-containing foods.

At first, Katie cried when she learned her diagnosis. However, she soon realized that her health would improve dramatically when she took strict control of her food choices. For a person with celiac disease, eating foods that contain gluten poses serious consequences, so Katie learned how to shop for and prepare gluten-free foods. After a couple of weeks on a gluten-free diet, she began to feel better.

Eating out is especially difficult for people with celiac disease, because of restaurants' widespread inclusion of breads, rolls, pasta, and desserts made from wheat flour in menus. Katie learned how to locate the few restaurants in her community that cater to people with celiac disease by having kitchens that are dedicated to gluten-free food preparation. People with the condition can patronize these eating establishments without worrying about eating any gluten-containing or contaminated foods.

Today, Katie maintains her good health by continuing to avoid gluten. Although her diet is very restrictive, she knows from experience that if she "cheats" by eating even a small amount of food that contains gluten, she'll get sick again. After such occasions, she returns to following a gluten-free diet, and within several days, her intestinal tract heals itself.

According to Katie, people who are unfamiliar with celiac disease should take the condition seriously and accommodate the special dietary needs of people who have the disease. For example, if you invite someone with celiac disease to share a meal or snack with you, wash your hands after you prepare foods that contain gluten and don't offer those foods to the person. Additionally, prepare some gluten-free foods for your guest who has celiac disease to eat safely. She says, "It's discouraging when people think I'm simply a 'picky eater' and just making life hard for them. The more people who understand celiac disease, the easier my life becomes!"

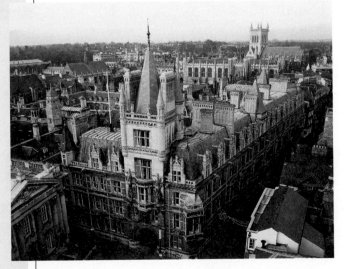

TABLE 7.4 *Gluten-Free Diet*

People with celiac disease should avoid foods that contain:
wheat, including wheat, enriched, durum, graham, and semolina flours; farina, wheat bran, wheat germ, cracked wheat, and wheat protein
barley
rye
triticale
Unless contaminated with any of the above foods, products that contain the following ingredients are generally safe to eat for people with celiac disease:
arrowroot, buckwheat, cassava, corn, flax, oats (small amounts), millet, nuts, quinoa, rice, sorghum, soy, and tapioca

What Is PKU?

Phenylketunuria (*fen-ul-key-toe-nur'-e-ah*) or PKU is a rare genetic metabolic disorder that affects about 1 in 10,000 to 1 in 15,000 infants in the United States.[14] PKU usually occurs when cells are unable to produce an enzyme that converts the essential amino acid phenylalanine (*fen-ul-al'-ah-neen*) to other compounds. As a result, phenylalanine or its toxic by-products build up in tissues and damage cells, including nerve cells in the brain. If PKU is not diagnosed and treated within a few weeks of birth, the affected infant can develop intellectual disability within the first year of life.[14]

To diagnose PKU, physicians generally rely on a simple blood test that is conducted on infants within 48 hours after their birth. In the United States, more than 98% of newborns undergo testing for PKU and several other treatable inherited diseases.[15] Infants who have PKU are generally given special formulas that lack phenylalanine. Phenylalanine is essential for growth and development; therefore, young children can consume a small amount of the amino acid. As the children grow and mature, fruits, vegetables, and special low-protein foods can be added to their formula diet. However, children and adults with the disorder need to avoid foods that are rich sources of phenylalanine, such as nuts, milk products, eggs, meats, and other animal foods. Additionally, people with PKU should not consume diet soft drinks and other foods and beverages containing the alternative sweetener aspartame, because the sweetener is a source of phenylalanine (see Chapter 5 for information about aspartame).

Throughout their lives, individuals with PKU should follow the restrictive diet.[14] Discontinuing the phenylalanine-restricted diet can lead to behavioral problems and brain damage. Furthermore, people with the disorder need to undergo frequent blood tests to make sure they are maintaining a healthy concentration of phenylalanine in their bodies. Monitoring blood phenylalanine is especially important during pregnancy. An expectant woman who has PKU must carefully control her phenylalanine level to avoid exposing her embryo/fetus to excessive amounts of the amino acid. If she fails to control the concentration of phenylalanine in her blood, she can give birth to a baby with severe birth defects, including a smaller-than-normal brain. The "Real People, Real Stories" on page 217 features Dallas Clasen, a teenager who has PKU.

Concept **Checkpoint**

14. List three common signs or symptoms of food allergy and celiac disease.
15. Discuss what parents of infants with PKU can do to help their children grow and develop normally.

 ## 7.5 Protein Consumption Patterns

In 2007–2008, protein comprised about 15% of the typical adult American's total energy intake for a day.[16] For healthy adults, this level of consumption is within the Acceptable Macronutrient Distribution Range (AMDR), which is 10 to 35% of energy from protein.[3] In 2005–2006, Americans generally ate about the same percentage of total daily calories

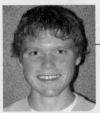

REAL *People*
REAL *Stories*

Dallas Clasen

Dallas Clasen is an energetic teenager who loves mountain bike and road bike racing, downhill skiing, wrestling, and playing football. Not only is he athletic, he is also smart—his grades place him at the top of his class. According to his proud parents, Dallas is the perfect son—"a nice boy." Dallas *is* a special young man, but he also needs a special diet. Dallas was born with phenylketonuria (PKU).

A few days after birth, Dallas underwent standard newborn blood testing. The results of the test indicated that the level of phenylalanine in his blood was about 40 times higher than the normal amount, a sign of the inherited disorder PKU. To avoid developing severe brain damage and other physiological effects of PKU, the infant needed to receive the care of a physician who specializes in treating children with the disorder. The primary treatment for PKU is a low-phenylalanine diet.

Most foods that are rich sources of protein, especially high-quality animal proteins, contain more phenylalanine than people with PKU can tolerate. Thus, from the time Dallas was a week old, he has consumed a formula that does not contain the amino acid. In addition to the formula, Dallas eats special foods that resemble "regular" foods but are not available in supermarkets. To obtain low-phenylalanine foods, his parents order them from companies that manufacture such products. Dallas can eat limited amounts of grain products and most fruits and vegetables. To determine whether the diet is working, Dallas must have the level of phenylalanine in his blood checked weekly.

Dallas's parents and his two younger sisters do not have PKU. At home, he eats the low-phenylalanine foods, while the other members of his family consume regular foods. Foods that are eaten away from home can present problems for people with PKU. In Dallas's case, his mother provides his school with a supply of low-phenylalanine foods for the teen's lunches. When the family visits restaurants, Dallas usually orders French fries, which are allowed in his diet. Dallas is so accustomed to his special diet, he thinks meat looks "gross."

In the past, children with PKU were often allowed to eat regular foods after they were about 6 years of age. However, the importance of continuing the low-phenylalanine diet became evident when many of the children experienced learning and behavioral problems as they matured. Dallas is aware of the consequences that can occur if he does not limit his phenylalanine intake, and he accepts the need to follow the special diet for the rest of his life. According to Dallas, "Being on a strict diet has not only made me disciplined, it has taught me to do whatever is needed to always take good care of myself. I have learned that we are all different, anyway. So, accept who you are!"

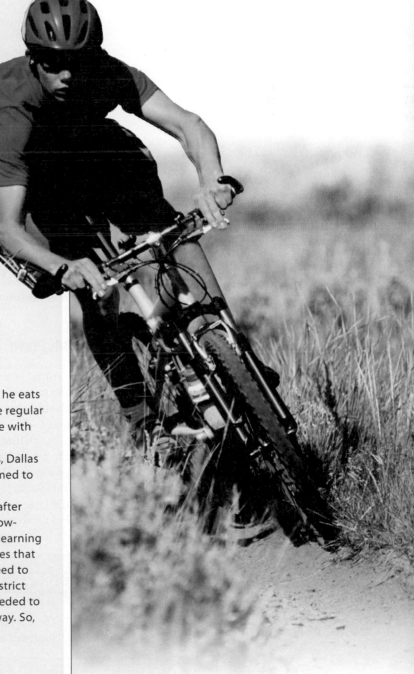

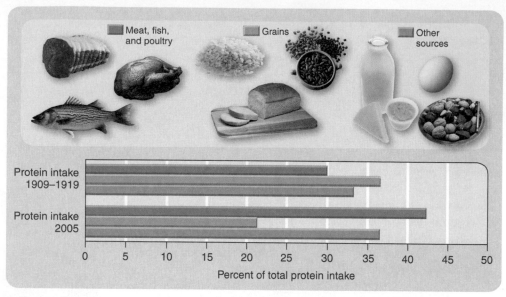

Figure 7.16 **Protein consumption patterns.** In 2005, Americans ate almost 20% more protein than they did in the early 1900s. Much of this increase reflects the population's greater consumption of protein from fish, milk products, and poultry.

Ham, bacon, sausage, frankfurters, and deli meats, such as salami and bologna, generally contain high amounts of fat and sodium.

from protein as they did in the early 1900s.[17] Americans, however, consumed more protein from meat, fish, and poultry than from plant foods (Fig. 7.16). During the years from 1909 to 1919, grain products contributed approximately 37% of the typical American's protein intake. At that time, meat, fish, and poultry accounted for 30% of the protein in the typical American's diet. By 2005–2006, grain products supplied only 21% of the average American's protein intake, whereas meat, fish, and poultry provided most of the protein (about 42%) in the diet.[17]

MyPlate: Recommendations for Protein Intake

Animal sources of protein are often rich sources of saturated fat and cholesterol. According to guidelines of the U.S. Department of Agriculture's MyPlate food plan, Americans should choose lean or low-fat meat and poultry.[18] The leanest cuts of beef include round, and top round, loin, and top sirloin steaks, as well as chuck and arm roasts.

Before cooking a piece of beef, you can reduce its fat content by trimming the visible fat away from the meat. When buying ground beef, consider choosing "extra lean" products. The label on a package of extra lean ground beef should state that the meat is at least 90% lean. When cooked, extra lean ground beef can taste "dry." You can improve the taste of the beef by adding a small amount of "heart healthy" olive oil to the raw meat before shaping it into hamburger patties. The leanest cuts of pork include pork loin, tenderloin, and center loin.

Did You Know?

There is nothing inherently "bad" about eating small portions of red meat. Red meat is a good source of zinc and iron, minerals that are often less bioavailable from plant foods.

You can choose lean turkey, roast beef, or low-fat luncheon meats for sandwiches, instead of processed meat products. Processed meat products, such as ham, bacon, sausage, frankfurters, and bologna and salami, generally contain a lot of fat, and they also have high amounts of added sodium. Excessive sodium intakes are associated with increased risk of hypertension. If you decide to purchase processed meats, check the Nutrition Facts panels on products' labels to compare fat as well as sodium contents.

The MyPlate plan also recommends varying your protein choices. For example, consider eating fish that are rich sources of beneficial omega-3 fatty acids, such as salmon, trout, and herring. You can also replace main menu items that contain meat with dishes made with dry beans, peas, or foods made from soybeans. Additionally, consider snacking on nuts, such as peanuts, almonds, cashews, walnuts, and pecans, instead of pieces of meat or cheese.

Concept **Checkpoint**

16. What is the AMDR for adult protein intake?
17. Describe how Americans' food sources of protein have changed since the early 1900s.
18. Consider your usual food choices. Using the recommendations of the MyPlate food guide, discuss ways you can reduce your intake of protein from animal foods.

7.6 Understanding Nutritional Labeling

You can determine how much protein is in a packaged food product by reading the Nutrition Facts panel on the label. As you can see in Figure 7.17, one serving of whole-wheat bread contains 4 g of protein. The panel does not provide information about a product's protein quality, but you can judge from the list of ingredients. This particular brand of bread, for example, contains proteins from various cereal grains and some seeds, but its ingredients do not include sources of high-quality proteins such as eggs, milk, or processed soybeans. Although this bread is not a source of complete protein, its protein quality is improved if the bread is eaten with foods that contain high-quality proteins; it could be eaten with a glass of milk, folded over a slice of cooked chicken, or spread with soy nut butter. The "Eating Well for Less" section of Chapter 7 explains how you can use plant proteins to obtain high-quality protein.

Concept **Checkpoint**

19. Discuss how you can use information on a food product's label to determine whether the food is a source of high-quality protein.

Figure 7.17 Nutrition Facts panel (2011). The Nutrition Facts panel provides information about a product's protein content.

Nutrition Facts

Serving Size 1 slice (38 g)
Servings Per Container 18

Amount Per Serving

Calories 100
Calories from Fat 20

	% Daily Value*
Total Fat 2g	3%
Saturated Fat 0g	0%
Trans Fat 0g	
Polyunsaturated Fat 1g	
Monounsaturated Fat 0g	
Cholesterol 0mg	0%
Sodium 160mg	7%
Total Carbohydrate 17g	6%
Dietary Fiber 2g	8%
Sugars 3g	
Protein 4g	

Vitamin A	10%
Vitamin C	0%
Calcium	10%
Iron	8%

* Percent Daily Values are based on a 2,000 calorie diet. Your daily values may be higher or lower, depending on your calorie needs:

		Calories	2,000	2,500
Total Fat		Less than	65g	80g
Sat Fat		Less than	20g	25g
Cholesterol		Less than	300mg	300mg
Sodium		Less than	2,400mg	2,400mg
Total Carbohydrate			300g	375g
Dietary Fiber			25g	30g

INGREDIENTS: Whole-wheat flour, Water, Brown sugar, Wheat gluten, Cracked wheat, Wheat bran, Yeast, Salt, Molasses, Soybean oil, Calcium propionate (preservative), Mono–and diglycerides, Lecithin

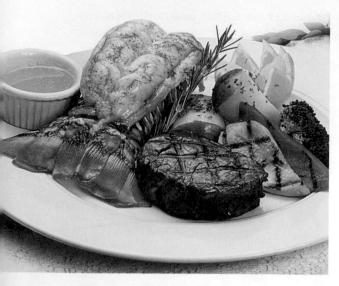

Animal foods contribute the largest share of the protein in the typical American's diet. Some of these foods, however, are among the most expensive items on our grocery lists.

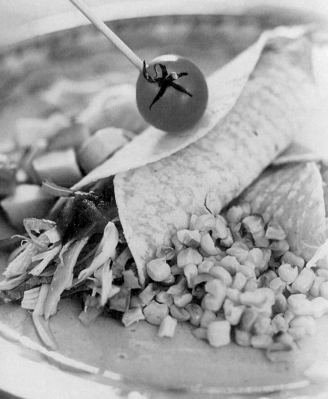

A taco or burrito combines a relatively large amount of a grain product with smaller amounts of lysine-rich meat, seafood, chicken, or cheese. The proteins in the animal foods enhance the quality of the wheat or corn proteins.

7.7 Eating Well for Less

Does your favorite breakfast include some slices of ham, two fried eggs, a slice of toast, and a glass of milk? For lunch, would you enjoy eating a submarine sandwich made with three different types of cold cuts and two kinds of cheese? Perhaps your mouth waters at the thought of a dinner eating "surf and turf"—lobster tail accompanied by a steak. If you are a typical American, animal foods contribute the largest share of the protein in your diet. In fact, animal foods, including eggs and milk products, supply almost two-thirds of the protein in the American diet.[17] Some of these foods, however, are among the most expensive items on our grocery lists, and you may be able to reduce your food costs if you eat less of them. Furthermore, you may reap substantial health benefits by reducing your animal protein intake and increasing your consumption of plant foods.

Animal foods are among the best dietary sources of essential amino acids, so is it safe to eat less animal protein? Yes! One way you can lower your intake is to include only one animal source of protein in a meal and reduce its serving size. For example, if your breakfast is a 6-ounce slice of ham with two large fried eggs, you are obtaining over 500 kcal and almost 60 g of high-quality protein. That is enough protein in one meal to meet the RDA for a person who weighs 132 pounds. Instead of eating such a large serving of ham with the fried eggs, have 3 ounces of ham without the eggs, or skip the ham and eat just the eggs. Two fried eggs supply 12.5 g of high-quality protein and only 180 kcal.

An easy way to reduce your meat consumption is to replace meat with other high-quality protein sources. Eggs, milk, cheese, and yogurt are animal sources of high-quality protein that you can substitute for meat, fish, or poultry items in your diet. For example, simply have a cheese sandwich instead of eating a submarine sandwich made with various luncheon meats and cheeses. If you are interested in eating less fat, a serving of low-fat cottage cheese or low-fat yogurt makes a protein-rich substitute for the "sub" or cheese sandwich.

Another way to reduce the amount of animal food in your diet and your food costs is to make meals that contain less animal protein and more plant protein. Many commonly eaten menu items provide the proper amounts and mixtures of essential amino acids without relying heavily on animal products. Throughout the world, people with limited access to meat and other animal foods rely heavily on recipes that combine small amounts of animal protein with larger portions of certain plant proteins. Proteins in animal foods contain enough essential amino acids to extend or "beef up" the lower quality plant proteins in peas, beans, cereals, and other grain products. Pasta made from white flour, for example, contains cereal (wheat) proteins that have limiting amounts of lysine. By mixing large amounts of cooked pasta with smaller amounts of lysine-rich meat, seafood, chicken, or cheese, the proteins in the animal foods enhance the quality of the wheat proteins. As a result, the body can use the amino acids in pasta for growth, repair, and maintenance of tissues.

Pancakes, waffles, crepes, and cornflakes with milk are examples of breakfast foods that extend egg and milk proteins with large amounts of cereal proteins. Many popular Asian dishes mix small amounts of chicken, beef, or seafood with large portions of rice; Italian dishes often combine pasta with small amounts of cheese or meat sauce. Serving meals that extend the high-quality protein in animal foods is an economical way to feed

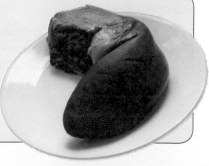

large numbers of people. For example, you can use 1 pound of ground meat to make a single hamburger for each of your four friends. However, you will have enough chili con carne to feed six or more friends if you combine that pound of ground meat with three cans of kidney beans and a couple of large cans of tomatoes. The ground meat has plenty of cysteine and methionine, the essential amino acids that are low in kidney beans. By mixing plant and animal sources of protein together in chili con carne, the beef protein extends the quality of the protein in the kidney beans. Although the chili recipe calls for adding tomatoes to the meat and beans, tomatoes are botanically classified as fruit, so they add very little protein to the dish. (Imagine eating chili con carne without tomatoes!) If you want to extend the chili even more, add cooked macaroni to the mixture. Macaroni is made from wheat, so it contains cereal proteins that are enhanced by the proteins in the meat and beans. For more practical ways to "stretch" your food dollars without sacrificing the nutritional quality of your diet, read the "Highlight" at the end of this chapter.

Combining Complementary Proteins

Although research findings indicate that it is not necessary to consume all essential amino acids during a meal for the body to utilize them for growth, certain plant-based recipes ensure that these compounds are consumed at one time. **Complementary combinations** are mixtures of certain plant foods that provide all essential amino acids without adding animal proteins. However, to make dishes that contain complementary amino acid combinations, you must know which plant foods are good protein sources and which essential amino acids are limiting or low in those plant foods. Most plant foods are poor sources of one or more essential amino acids, particularly tryptophan, threonine, lysine, and methionine. Green peas, for example, are good sources of lysine, but they contain low amounts of tryptophan and methionine. Cereal grains such as wheat, rice, and corn are good sources of tryptophan and methionine, but they tend to be low in lysine. Wheat germ, however, is a rich source of lysine. Legumes are low in methionine. Seeds such as sesame and sunflower seeds are generally low in lysine. Walnuts, cashews, almonds, and other tree nuts also contain low amounts of lysine. Although most fruits and some kinds of vegetables are poor sources of protein, they add appealing colors and textures as well as vitamins, minerals, and phytochemicals to plant-based meals.

Many cultures have traditional foods that combine complementary plant proteins. For example, a peanut butter sandwich combines two foods that supply complementary plant proteins. Peanuts are a fair source of lysine. Bread contains some methionine, but the grain product is very low in lysine. Serving the two foods together as a peanut butter sandwich provides adequate amounts of these essential amino acids. Table 7.5 lists some other foods that are examples of complementary protein combinations. When menu planning, you can combine a variety of legumes, grains, tree nuts, and seeds with

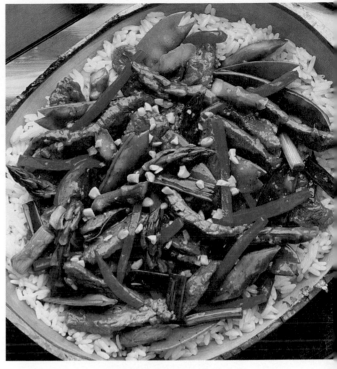

Traditional Asian dishes, such as beef stir-fry, combine small amounts of animal protein with larger amounts of cereal and vegetable proteins.

complementary combinations mixing certain plant foods to provide all essential amino acids without adding animal protein

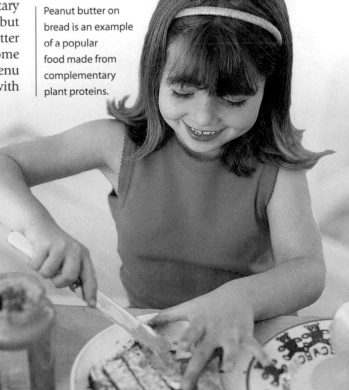

Peanut butter on bread is an example of a popular food made from complementary plant proteins.

TABLE 7.5 *Complementary Protein Dishes*

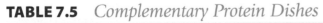

Red beans and rice

Peanut or soy nut butter on bagel, sprinkled with wheat germ

Hummus (mashed chickpeas/garbanzo beans) with sesame seeds*

Hummus on whole-grain pita bread

Black beans and cornmeal tortilla*

Split pea soup with toasted whole-wheat bread

Meatless kidney bean chili with macaroni

Cornmeal tortilla with black bean salsa

Peanut butter on whole-grain crackers, sprinkled with wheat germ

Green beans with brown rice and cashews

* See the "Recipes for Healthy Living" feature for a black bean recipe.

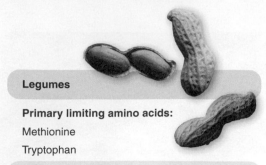

Legumes

Primary limiting amino acids:

Methionine

Tryptophan

Peas

Peanuts and peanut butter

Soy beans, soy products, and other beans

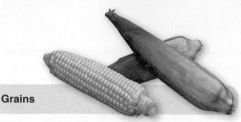

Grains

Primary limiting amino acid:

Lysine

Wheat and products made from wheat flour

Rice, oats, millet, barley, bulgur

Corn and products made from corn

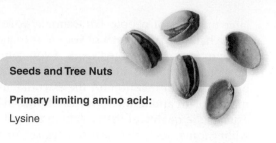

Seeds and Tree Nuts

Primary limiting amino acid:

Lysine

Sesame seeds, sunflower seed kernels, pumpkin seeds

Cashews, pistachios, walnuts, pine nuts, almonds

Figure 7.18 Complementary combinations. Combining certain plant foods can result in complementary combinations of essential amino acids. To ensure an adequate mix of proteins, combine one or more foods from at least two of the plant food groups shown in the above illustration (legumes, grains, and seeds and tree nuts).

vegetables to prepare dishes that provide adequate mixtures of the essential amino acids. Figure 7.18 shows three categories of plant proteins (legumes, grains, and tree nuts and seeds) that make complementary combinations when one or more foods from at least two different groups are mixed together.

Not every mixture of plant foods creates a complementary combination. For example, making a fruit salad by combining apples, grapes, and oranges will not provide a complementary mixture of essential amino acids. Fruits are nutritious foods, but they are generally poor sources of protein. Combining Boston, iceberg, and romaine varieties of lettuce with carrots and onions makes a tasty salad, but simply mixing leafy greens with

 Food & Nutrition *tips*

The following information describes popular soybean foods and tips for how to use them in menu planning.

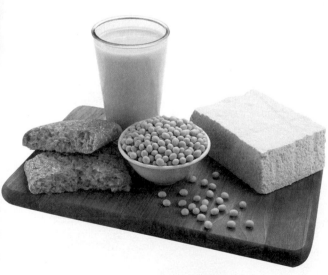

- Tofu is made from pureed soybeans and has the consistency of thick jelly. Plain tofu has little flavor, so it can be added to a variety of foods, including stir-fried vegetables and scrambled eggs.

- Tempeh is a fermented soybean and grain mixture that can substitute for meat in sandwiches and casseroles.

- Miso is also made from fermented soybeans. Miso can be used to boost the protein content and add flavor to other foods, but it is high in sodium and should be used sparingly.

- Soy nuts are roasted soybeans that are often eaten as a snack. Ground soy nuts form a spread that is used like peanut butter.

- Soy milk is made from crushed soybeans. Soy milk is usually fortified with calcium and vitamins A, D, B-12, and riboflavin. Read the Nutrition Facts panel for information about the percentage of calcium and vitamin D in the milk. Regular soy milk can substitute for cow's milk as a beverage or in recipes. Soy milk cheeses and yogurt are also available.

- Texturized soy protein (TSP) is made from soybean flour. TSP is often processed to imitate the texture, taste, and appearance of meat or poultry. A TSP product that resembles ground beef can be used to replace half or all of the ground beef in meatloaf, meatball, chili, taco, or meat sauce recipes.

- Soy protein concentrate is a high-protein, high-fiber refined soybean product that is used to boost the protein content of foods.

other vegetables does not make a complementary combination, because vegetables have small amounts of protein that tend to contain low amounts of essential amino acids. However, adding sunflower seed kernels, kidney or black beans, cashews, and bread cubes to the salad boosts the amount of protein and provides a complete mix of amino acids. To increase the essential amino acid content of the salad even further, you can add a small amount of hard-cooked egg, shredded cheese, or bits of *tofu*, a soybean product, to it. Processed soybean foods are good sources of essential amino acids. If you are interested in trying foods made from soybeans, the "Food & Nutrition Tips" feature on page 222 provides information about some of the more popular foods made from soybeans.

Concept **Checkpoint**

20. Explain the difference between substituting high-quality proteins and extending high-quality proteins. Give examples of common foods that are high-quality substitutes for meat and foods that extend a source of high-quality protein.
21. Does a recipe that combines apples and oranges with peanuts provide a complementary mixture of proteins? Explain why or why not.
22. A recipe mixes cereals made from wheat, rice, and corn. What plant foods could you add to this combination of cereals to make the recipe a source of high-quality protein?

vegetarians people who eat plant-based diets

lactovegetarian vegetarian who consumes milk and milk products for animal protein

ovovegetarian vegetarian who eats eggs for animal protein

lactoovovegetarian vegetarian who consumes milk products and eggs for animal protein

vegan vegetarian who eats only plant foods

7.8 Vegetarianism

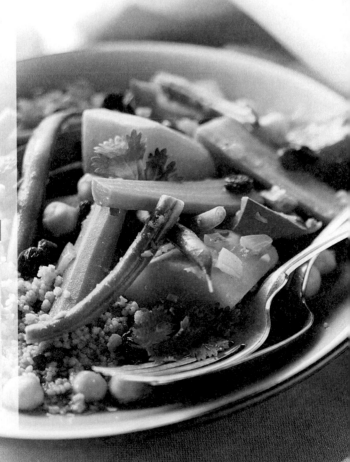

A vegan, or total vegetarian, might enjoy this dish: couscous with vegetables and chickpeas. Couscous is a grain product.

Are you or is anyone you know vegetarian? If you are vegetarian, do you eat any animal foods? **Vegetarians** rely heavily on plant foods and may or may not include some animal foods in their diets. About 2.3% of American adults do not eat meat, fish, or poultry; about 1.4% of adults avoid eating any foods from animal sources.[19]

There are many different types of vegetarian diets, including some that contain animal foods. A semivegetarian, for example, avoids red meat but consumes other animal foods, including fish, poultry, eggs, and dairy products. Other vegetarians have more restrictive diets, particularly when choosing whether to eat animal foods. A **lactovegetarian** (*lacto* = milk) consumes milk and milk products, including yogurt, cheese, and ice cream, to obtain animal protein. An **ovovegetarian** (*ovo* = egg) eats eggs, and a **lactoovovegetarian** consumes milk products and eggs. A **vegan,** or total vegetarian, eats only plant foods. Table 7.6 lists common types of vegetarian diets.

TABLE 7.6 *Common Types of Vegetarian Diets*

Type of Vegetarian Diet	Animal Foods Included
Semivegetarian	All except red meats
Lactovegetarian	Milk and milk products No animal flesh or eggs
Ovovegetarian	Eggs but no other animal foods
Lactoovovegetarian	Milk and milk products and eggs but no other animal foods
Vegan *Fruitarian*	No animal foods Fruits, nuts, and seeds only
*Macrobiotic**	Organically grown whole grains, fruits and vegetables, and soups made with vegetables, seaweed, grains, beans, and miso

*For more details about macrobiotic diets, visit http://www.cancer.org/Treatment/TreatmentsandSideEffects/ComplementaryandAlternativeMedicine/DietandNutrition/macrobiotic-diet?sitearea=ETO .

Vegetarians have various reasons for eating few or no animal products. Many vegetarians have religious, ethical, and other philosophical beliefs that do not support the practice of killing and eating animals. For others, vegetarianism is a matter of concern for the environment and economics; plant foods are generally less expensive than animal foods. Some vegetarians believe that humans are not physically able to digest animal foods. This is not true. The omnivore's intestinal tract is able to obtain nutrients from both plants and animals, and humans are omnivores. Nevertheless, eating more plant than animal sources of protein may provide important health benefits.

Is Vegetarianism a Healthy Lifestyle?

Vegetarian diets are often lower in fat and energy than "Western diets" that contain animal foods, particularly plenty of red meat. Compared to people who eat meat, vegetarians tend to have a lower risk of obesity, type 2 diabetes, hypertension, and certain cancers.[20] Furthermore, vegans tend to be leaner than nonvegans.[21] It is difficult, however, to pinpoint diet as responsible for vegetarians' health status. Why? Vegetarians often adopt other healthy lifestyle practices, such as exercising regularly; practicing relaxation activities, such as meditation; and avoiding tobacco products and excess alcohol.

Compared to the typical American diet, vegetarian diets provide more fiber, phytochemicals, folic acid (a B vitamin), vitamins E and C, and the minerals potassium and magnesium.[21] Furthermore, vegetarian diets often supply less saturated fat and cholesterol than diets that include animal foods.

In general, plant foods have low energy density: they add bulk to the diet without adding a lot of calories. Thus, vegetarians may feel "full" soon after eating a meal of plant foods, and they may not consume as much energy and nutrients as they need. Poorly planned plant-based diets may not contain enough energy; high-quality protein; omega-3 fatty acids; vitamins B-12, D, and riboflavin; and minerals zinc, iron, and calcium to meet a person's nutritional needs.[20,21] Humans digest animal proteins to a greater extent than plant proteins.[22] Therefore, vegetarians may need to increase their protein intakes by about 10%. Total vegetarians, including vegan athletes, can obtain adequate amounts of the essential amino acids by eating processed soybean products and foods that combine complementary plant proteins.

Vegetarians who do not consume fish may need to obtain DHA and EPA (omega-3 fatty acids) by taking fish oil supplements or eating certain algae. Plant foods contain little or no vitamin B-12,[23] and there are few dietary sources of vitamin D other than fortified cow's milk. Furthermore, mineral nutrients such as calcium and iron are more available from animal than from plant foods. Plants often contain phytochemicals that interfere with the body's absorption of minerals, particularly iron, zinc, and calcium. Vegans have lower calcium intakes and higher risk of bone fractures than vegetarians who include milk and milk products in their diets.[20]

Vegans can obtain vitamin B-12, vitamin D, iron, zinc, and many other micronutrients by consuming fortified foods such as soy and rice beverages, "Red Star" vegetarian nutritional yeast, and breakfast cereals. Vegetarians can also take a multiple vitamin/mineral supplement to provide dietary "insurance." Table 7.7 summarizes the nutritional advantages and possible nutritional disadvantages of vegetarian diets.

Children have higher protein and energy needs per pound of body weight than an adult. Since plant foods add bulk to the diet, vegan children are likely to eat far less food than adult vegans because they become full sooner during meals. Thus, very young vegans may be unable to eat enough plant foods to meet their protein and energy needs. Therefore, it is very important for parents or other caretakers to plan nutritionally adequate diets for vegetarian children and monitor the youngsters' growth rates.

Vegan women who breastfeed their infants may produce milk that is deficient in vitamin B-12, particularly if the mothers' diets lack the vitamin. These infants of vegan mothers have a high risk of developing severe developmental delays associated with neurological damage, especially when breast milk is their only source of vitamin B-12.[24]

MY DIVERSE PLATE

Miso

Miso, a seasoning paste made from fermented soybeans, is a staple of traditional Japanese diets. Miso is added to soup (misoshiru) and vegetables. Two tablespoons of miso supply about 70 kcal, 4 g protein, 2 g fat, and 1280 mg sodium. Although miso adds flavor to foods, the paste is very salty; therefore, it should be used in small amounts.

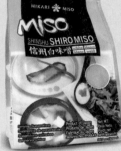

TABLE 7.7 *Vegetarian Diets: Nutritional Aspects*

Advantages	Possible Disadvantages
High: Vitamins C , E, and folic acid	**Low:** Vitamins B-12, D, and riboflavin
Phytochemicals	Zinc, iron, and calcium
Fiber	Omega-3 fatty acids
Magnesium and potassium	Certain essential amino acids
Low: Fat (saturated) Cholesterol	Energy

Pregnant vegan women should consult with their physicians about the need to take a vitamin B-12 supplement to reduce the likelihood of having a baby who is deficient in this nutrient. Additionally, vegan mothers who breastfeed their infants may need to provide the babies with a source of vitamin B-12 as well.

Many American teenagers and young adults are adopting vegetarian diets. Switching from the typical Western diet to vegetarianism can be a healthy practice for teens; vegetarian youth often eat more fruits and vegetables and less fat than their nonvegetarian peers.[20] On the other hand, vegetarian teenagers may have a higher risk of unhealthy weight control practices and eating disorders, such as *anorexia nervosa*, than young people who eat meat. Anorexia nervosa ("anorexia") is a serious psychological disorder that can result in starvation and suicide. The Chapter 10 "Highlight" provides more information about anorexia nervosa and other eating disorders.

Meatless Menu Planning

Many common menu items can be converted into vegetarian foods by removing the meat, fish, or poultry. For example, pizza and lasagna can be prepared without meat and still provide plenty of protein from the cheese as well as the crust or pasta. Stir-fried foods can also be a reliable source of protein without adding meat, fish, or poultry. To stir-fry, heat a small amount of peanut or canola oil in a frying pan and add cooked rice and pieces of raw vegetables. While the mixture is heating, add a beaten egg to it and stir so the egg cooks thoroughly. Before serving the dish, sprinkle cashews or sunflower seed kernels over the hot rice and vegetable mixture. Table 7.8 presents more meatless menu suggestions.

Commercially prepared vegetarian foods that substitute for meat, fish, and poultry items are often available in the frozen food section of supermarkets. These vegetarian products can look and taste like their nonvegetarian counterparts, but they generally do not contain cholesterol and may be lower in saturated fat. Such foods include soy-based sausage patties or links, soy hot dogs, "veggie" burgers, and soy "crumbles" that look like bits of cooked ground beef. Asian restaurants usually offer vegetarian dishes. Some "Western-style" restaurants offer vegetarian menu items, or their cooks can modify menu items by substituting meatless sauces, omitting meat from stir-fries, and adding vegetables or pasta in place of meat.

TABLE 7.8 *Meatless Menu Ideas*

- Cooked pasta with marinara sauce and grated Parmesan or part-skim mozzarella cheese
- Vegetable lasagna with layers of thinly sliced zucchini, mushrooms, and bell peppers
- Vegetable stir-fry with bits of tofu and cheese
- Grilled vegetable kabobs served over cooked rice and black beans
- Black or red bean burritos
- Bean and corn tacos

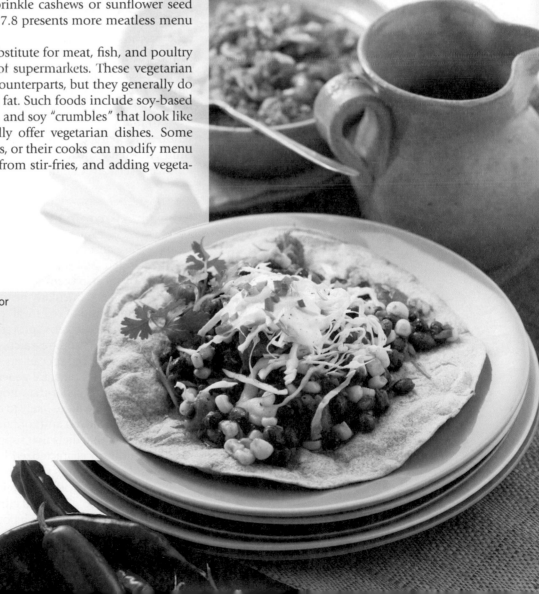

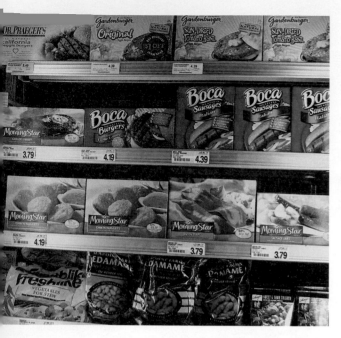

Commercially prepared vegetarian foods are often available in the frozen food section of supermarkets.

With careful planning, vegetarians can overcome the nutritional limitations of a plant-based diet and consume adequate diets.[19] If you are interested in learning more specific details about vegetarian cookery and menu planning, contact a registered dietitian (R.D.) or University Extension nutritionist in your area. The MyPlate website also offers suggestions for planning nutritionally adequate meatless meals. For more information, visit http://www.choosemyplate.gov/tipsresources/vegetarian_diets.html.

Concept **Checkpoint**

23. Describe how the diets of semivegetarians differ from other vegetarian diets.
24. Identify nutrients that are most likely lacking in a vegan's diet.
25. Explain why vegans must be careful when planning vegan meals for children.

7.9 Protein Adequacy

If some protein is necessary for proper growth and good health, can eating extra amounts of the nutrient make you *extra* healthy or physically fit? Intuitively, the idea of eating more protein to improve your health seems logical, but protein is no different from the other nutrients. If your diet contains adequate amounts of protein, then eating "more is not better."

In many parts of the world, the lack of foods containing high-quality proteins is a serious problem, particularly for young children. Protein deficiency interferes with a child's normal growth and development, and contributes to many childhood deaths. The following sections examine protein malnutrition.

Excessive Protein Intake

Heart disease and cancer are the leading causes of death in developed countries, including the United States. In these nations, the typical Western diet that contains high amounts of meat protein and saturated fat is associated with increased risk of certain chronic diseases, particularly heart disease, colorectal cancer,[25] and possibly prostate cancer.[26] Consumption of red meat, pork, and processed meats is associated with increased risk of pancreatic cancer;[27] processed, smoked, and/or salted meats increase the risk of stomach cancer.[28] More research, however, is needed to clarify the role of high-protein diets in the risk of certain cancers.

High-protein diets are generally not recommended for healthy individuals. Such diets may lead to higher-than-normal urinary losses of the mineral nutrient calcium.[29] Such losses may be more likely to occur when people, particularly women, consume diets that are low in calcium and contain more animal than vegetable proteins. Some nutrition experts suspect that diets that supply a lot of animal protein are associated with osteoporosis, a condition characterized by thin bones that fracture easily. Chapter 9 discusses dietary and other factors that contribute to osteoporosis.

Excess amino acid or protein intake can lead to dehydration, because the kidneys need more water to dilute and eliminate the toxic waste products of amino acid metabolism in urine. Dehydration is a potentially life-threatening condition in which the body's water level is too low. People with liver or kidney diseases may need to avoid protein-rich diets and amino acid supplements because metabolizing the excess amino acids is a burden to their bodies.

What About High-Protein Weight-Loss Diets?

Certain popular weight-loss diets, such as the Atkins, Protein Power, and Sugar Busters! diets, promote high intakes of protein. While following high-protein diets to lose weight, people often report decreased feelings of hunger and increased sense of fullness (satiety) after meals.[30] This response is probably because protein contributes to satiety to a greater extent than fat or carbohydrate.[8] Chapter 10 provides information about the safety and effectiveness of various popular weight-loss diets.

Protein Deficiency

Although food insecurity exists in the United States, protein deficiency is uncommon. (See the Chapter 1 "Highlight" for information about food insecurity.) People suffering from alcoholism, anorexia nervosa, or certain intestinal tract disorders are at risk of protein undernutrition. People with low incomes, especially those who are elderly, are also at risk of protein deficiency. Many elderly Americans have limited incomes and must make difficult choices concerning their expenses. If you were old, chronically ill, and on a low fixed income, what would you think was more important—purchasing nutritious foods or costly prescription medications that control your serious health problems?

As discussed in the Chapter 1 "Highlight," undernutrition, the lack of food, is often widespread in poor nations in which populations endure frequent famine resulting from crop failures, political unrest, or civil wars. In these countries, protein-energy malnutrition (PEM) affects people whose diets lack sufficient protein as well as energy. The failure to consume nourishing food also results in vitamin and mineral deficiencies.

When food is limited, it is often more difficult for children to obtain nutritionally adequate diets than for adults to do so. Why? Adults may be able to consume enough plant proteins to meet their protein and energy needs, but children have smaller stomachs and higher energy and protein needs per pound of body weight than adults. They are unable to eat enough plant foods to meet their relatively high protein and other nutrient requirements.

In children, underweight is often a sign of (PEM). According to the World Health Organization (WHO), 18% of children are underweight.[31] Impoverished children in Asia and Africa are most likely to be underweight, and the effects of undernutrition are especially devastating for the very young. Children whose diets lack sufficient protein and energy do not grow and are very weak, irritable, and vulnerable to dehydration and infections, such as measles, that can kill them. If these children survive, their growth may be permanently stunted and their intelligence may be lower than normal because undernutrition during early childhood can cause permanent brain damage.

Protein-Energy Malnutrition

At one time, nutrition experts thought there were only two types of PEM, **kwashiorkor** and **marasmus.** The distinctions between these conditions, however, are often blurred, because protein deficiency is unlikely when a person's energy intake is adequate. Nevertheless, dietitians generally consider *kwashiorkor, marasmic kwashiorkor,* and *marasmus* as forms of PEM.

Kwashiorkor (*qwash'-e-or'-kor*) primarily occurs in developing countries where mothers commonly breastfeed their infants until they give birth to another child. The older youngster, who is usually a toddler, is fairly healthy until abruptly weaned from

kwashiorkor form of undernutrition that results from consuming adequate energy and insufficient high-quality protein

marasmus starvation

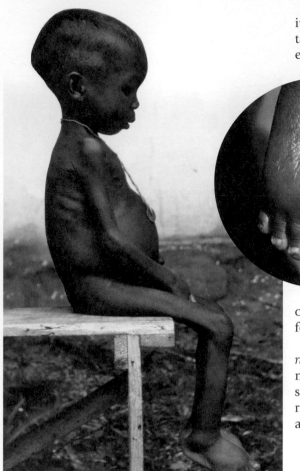

its mother's milk to make way for the younger sibling. Although the toddler may obtain adequate energy by consuming a traditional diet of cereal grains, the diet lacks enough complete protein to meet the youngster's high needs, and he or she soon develops signs of protein deficiency. Children affected by kwashiorkor have stunted growth (see Fig. 1.13); unnaturally blond, sparse, and brittle hair; and patches of skin that have lost their normal coloration. Children with kwashiorkor have some subcutaneous (under the skin) fat and swollen cheeks, arms, legs, and bellies that make them look well fed, but their appearance is misleading. An important function of certain proteins in blood is to maintain proper fluid balance within cells and blood vessels, as well as between cells. During starvation, levels of these proteins decline, resulting in edema, which can make the protein-deficient child look plump and overfed instead of thin and undernourished. In many cases, the child suffering from kwashiorkor does not obtain enough energy and eventually develops marasmic kwashiorkor, a condition characterized by edema and wasting (Fig. 7.19). Wasting is the loss of organ and muscle proteins as the body tears down these tissues to obtain amino acids for energy metabolism.

Severe PEM causes extreme weight loss and a condition called marasmus (*mah-raz'-mus*), which is commonly referred to as starvation (Fig. 7.20). Obvious signs of marasmus are weakness and wasting. The body of a starving person loses most of its subcutaneous fat and deeper fat stores. The marasmic person is so thin that his or her ribs, hips, and spine are visible through the skin. People suffering from marasmus avoid physical activity to conserve energy, and they are often irritable.

Figure 7.19 Mild to moderate protein-energy malnutrition. This Nigerian child is suffering from marasmic kwashiorkor. Note the edema in the child's abdomen, lower legs, and feet. The inset photo shows "pitting" edema—swollen tissues that become deformed when pressed with a finger. These photos were taken during the Nigerian civil war that occurred in the late 1960s.

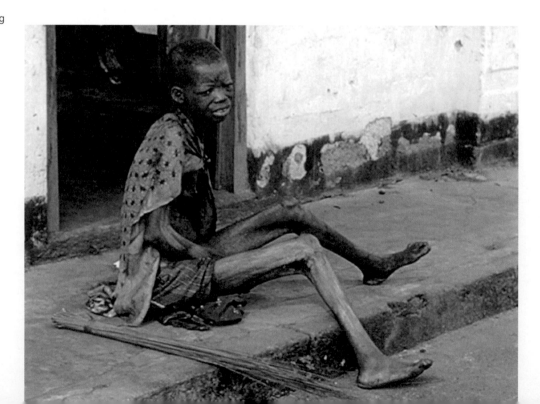

Figure 7.20 Severe protein-energy malnutrition. This photo of a Nigerian person suffering from marasmus was taken during the civil war that occurred in the late 1960s.

Concept **Checkpoint**

26. In the United States, which groups of people are most likely to suffer from protein-energy malnutrition?

27. Why is protein-energy malnutrition a devastating condition for young children?

28. Police bring a 2-year-old child into a clinic; the child has a swollen belly and feet, but the arms and upper legs are so thin, the skin hangs from them. The police report indicates the child was severely neglected by the parents. According to this information, is this child suffering from PKU, severe protein-energy malnutrition, sickle cell anemia, or anorexia nervosa? Choose one of these conditions and explain why you selected it.

7.10 Proteins: General Advice for Athletes

It is not surprising that people often associate protein with muscle. Approximately 43% of the protein in an average person's body is in his or her skeletal muscle mass. Athletes and other people interested in building their muscle mass often rely on eating large portions of animal foods as well as taking amino acid and protein supplements to boost their protein intakes. This practice, however, does not build bigger, stronger muscles.[32] The only effective way to increase muscle mass safely is to combine a nutritionally adequate diet with a program of muscle-strengthening exercises, particularly resistance exercise, such as weight lifting. During resistance exercise, proteins in working muscles break down, but protein synthesis occurs during the recovery period that follows and lasts about 24 to 48 hours.[33] As a result, muscles grow larger and stronger. Over time, resistance training induces a state of positive nitrogen balance. It should be noted, however, that 70% of muscle tissue is water and only about 22% is protein.[33] Thus, resistance training adds a considerable amount of water to muscle tissue.

An athlete's diet should supply enough calories from carbohydrate and fat to support energy needs for increased physical activity and spare the use of protein for growth, repair, and maintenance of muscle tissue. Therefore, athletes should not overly focus on their protein intake. Eating a snack that supplies both protein and carbohydrate before or after exercise is recommended. Nutritious choices include a bowl of cereal and fat-free milk, low-fat cottage cheese and a whole-wheat bagel, or a sandwich made with lean meat or poultry. If you do not have time to prepare these foods, energy drinks and bars are convenient ways to obtain carbohydrate and protein.

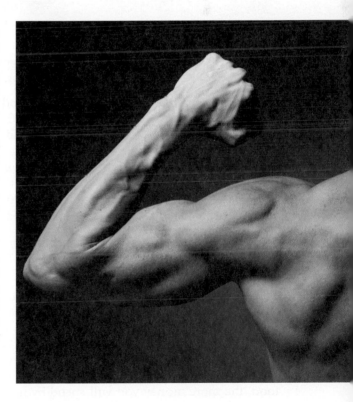

What About Protein Supplements?

Healthy people may adapt to protein intakes that are higher than the AMDR for the macronutrient and not experience health problems as a result. However, taking protein supplements is not recommended for healthy persons, especially if the products supply individual amino acids. Why? The human digestive system is designed to digest large protein molecules from the mixture of proteins that naturally occurs in foods. Consuming supplements that supply large amounts of individual amino acids can upset intestinal cells' ability to absorb other amino acids. Moreover, excessive intakes of certain amino acids, particularly methionine and tyrosine, can be toxic.

The results of studies indicate that injecting various amino acids into the bloodstream can stimulate the pituitary gland in the brain to release human growth hormone (HGH). Although HGH fosters muscle tissue growth, the results of studies examining the effects of consuming individual amino acids on HGH release do not support the use of these nutrients for stimulating muscle growth. Nevertheless, supplements that contain the amino acids arginine, lysine, and ornithine are popular among resistance athletes.

For thousands of years, humans have obtained amino acids directly by eating plants and animals. The use of amino acid and protein supplements as sources of the nutrient is a relatively recent development, and little is known about the long-term safety of using these products. Chapter 11 provides more information about nutrition for physically active people and examines the evidence concerning the value and safety of using certain foods and dietary supplements to enhance physical performance.

Concept **Checkpoint**

29. Explain why athletes should avoid taking amino acid supplements.

Chapter 7 Highlight

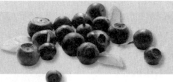

STRETCHING YOUR FOOD DOLLARS

Are you concerned about the high cost of food? If you are, how can you lower your food costs without sacrificing proper nutrition? You can trim food costs, and preserve and even improve the nutritional quality of your diet, by analyzing your food buying practices and making a few changes. This "Highlight" focuses on ways you can eat well for less. Please note that the pricing of products reflects food costs during the summer of 2011 in a major Midwestern city, but you should find them useful for comparing current prices where you live.

Where and What You Buy

Where you buy foods and beverages and what you decide to purchase are major factors in determining your overall food expenditures. If you frequently purchase meals and snacks from vending machines, convenience stores, fast-food outlets, and other restaurants, you may be spending too much on such "convenience" foods. In general, the less time you spend preparing food, the more money you will spend by having someone at a commercial outlet prepare the food for you. Even if a fast-food restaurant hamburger seems like a bargain because it is "only $1.00," you are likely paying a premium for the French fries and soft drink that you purchase to accompany the sandwich. From a nutrition standpoint, fast foods are often energy-dense—high in fat and sugar—and low in micronutrients (except sodium), fiber, and phytochemicals.

You probably already know that supermarkets have the same snack foods and staple items (bread and milk) as convenience stores and usually offer these foods at lower prices. Furthermore, supermarkets have a much larger selection of foods, particularly more nutrient-dense raw or less processed foods, than convenience stores. It may be easier to run into a convenience store and load up on foods while you load up on gas than to shop in a supermarket. However, you pay extra for the convenience and your diet may suffer as a result of poor food choices.

A good way to save money is to buy foods in large quantities at "bulk" food stores or at smaller, "no frills," cash-only grocery stores. Although shopping at these places can reduce your food costs, food choices are usually more limited than the selection in supermarkets. It is important to recognize that buying food in bulk is a bargain only if you can use the item before it spoils.

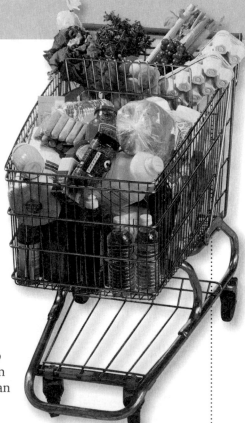

How to Shop Wisely in Supermarkets

To lower your food costs, plan your meals and snacks before you shop for food. Prepare a shopping list to help avoid needless or impulse purchases and having to return to the store to buy forgotten items. Keep the grocery list in a convenient place, such as on the refrigerator, and jot down items as they become depleted.

When shopping for groceries, you will need to compare *unit costs* of similar food products. A "unit" of a packaged food item is usually indicated in ounces or pounds. Food packages and containers are available in different sizes and hold different amounts of food, which can make comparing costs of similar foods difficult. Using a small calculator to compare prices can be helpful. For

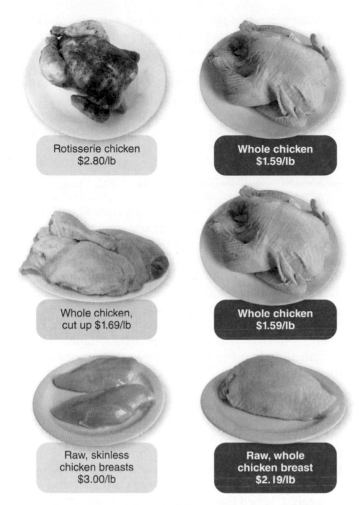

Figure 7.21 Convenience—Is it worth it? You can save money by purchasing a raw whole chicken and cutting it into parts, or a whole chicken breast and removing the skin and bones.

salt, fat, or sugar. To save money and improve your diet, rely less on prepared foods and more on "slow foods"—foods that require some of your time and effort to prepare. Figure 7.21 uses various forms of chicken to illustrate this point. A 2.5–lb rotisserie-cooked chicken costs $2.80/lb, but you can save over a dollar per pound by purchasing a whole chicken ($1.59/lb) and roasting it yourself. Instead of buying raw, skinless, boneless chicken breasts ($3.00/lb), buy raw split chicken breasts that have the bones and skin ($2.19/lb). Remove the skin and bones after the chicken breasts are cooked. You can use the cooked chicken immediately, freeze the meat in containers for a future meal, or chill the meat before chopping it to make chicken salad.

Eating more fruits and vegetables is the natural way to add micronutrients, fiber, and phytochemicals to your diet. Many supermarkets offer fresh fruit and vegetables that have been trimmed, cut up, and packed into containers. Before you reach for one of these items, compare its price with that of its raw counterpart. For example, a 2.2–oz, "single-serving" package of sliced apples sells for $1.25, and a pound of raw apples is priced at $1.99. In this case, buying the raw apples and slicing them yourself is a money-saving practice. To make this determination, you will need to calculate the unit price of each product (Fig. 7.22). An ounce of the packaged apples costs about 57 cents ($1.25 divided by 2.2 oz/package). A pound of apples equals 16 ounces, so an ounce of these apples costs about 12 cents ($1.99 divided by 16). Thus, the prepackaged sliced apples cost almost five times more than the bulk raw apples.

example, a box of one brand of shredded wheat cereal contains 15.0 ounces of cereal and costs $3.49; a box of a different brand of shredded wheat that contains 11.5 ounces of cereal costs $3.29. Which box of cereal is lower in cost? To answer this question, determine the unit price of the cereal in each box by dividing the cost of the entire package by the number of units of food it contains.

Box #1

$3.49 entire box ÷ 15.0 ounces = approximately $.23/ounce

Box #2

$3.29 entire box ÷ 11.5 ounces = approximately $.29/ounce

In this situation, the larger box of cereal is a better buy, even though it costs more than the smaller box. Some supermarkets indicate unit prices on shelf tags, but the tags may be difficult to read or confusing.

Supermarkets offer a wide variety of prepared foods, including deli items, frozen entrées, fresh cut-up fruit packaged in single serving plastic bags or bins, and rotisserie chicken. Although these "fast foods" are convenient, food processing and packaging add to the cost of food. Such foods may contain unhealthy amounts of

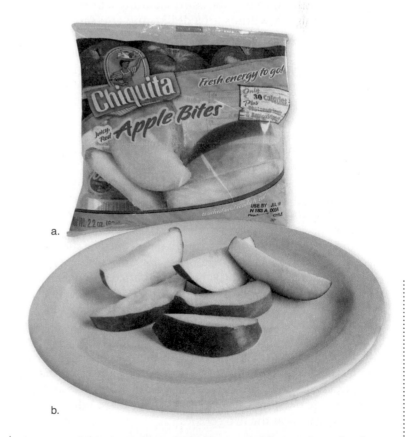

Figure 7.22 Comparing apples to apples. The cost of a 2.2–oz. package of apple slices (*a*) is almost five times the cost of the same amount of fresh, sliced raw apples (*b*).

Produce that is grown in the United States is usually less expensive when it is in season and more plentiful. For example, berries are plentiful in the spring and early summer, tomatoes and melons in late summer, and apples in the fall. "Fresh" produce that is shipped long distances to supermarket suppliers is often picked before its peak ripeness. As a result, the fruits and vegetables may not taste as good or be as nutritious as locally grown produce. Produce loses some of its vitamin C content when it is bruised or becomes wilted. Therefore, consider buying fresh produce directly from local farmers, if possible. Although you still need to compare prices of farmers' market items with those of fresh produce sold in supermarkets, you may be able to find reasonably priced produce that is grown within 100 miles of your home at farmers' markets. Buying produce from local farmers helps support your community's economy, too.

An alternative to buying produce directly from growers is to purchase frozen or canned fruits and vegetables. These products are often less expensive than their fresh counterparts. Furthermore, produce that is destined to be frozen is generally harvested when ripe and frozen immediately, maximizing much of its vitamin content and fresh flavor.

While shopping for foods in supermarkets, you can save money if you

- Use unit pricing to compare costs of similar packaged products.
- Are wary of appealing offers that are not bargains. For example, items marked "3 for $1.00" or "10 for $10.00" can be confusing to consumers. It is important to understand that you do not need to buy the entire quantity. For example, if a store offers 3 kiwifruits for a dollar, and you cannot use 3 of them, buy one for 34 cents. That price is still a bargain compared to buying kiwifruits that are "2 for $1.00." Also, beware of offers such as "10 oranges for $10." Paying $1 for an orange is not a bargain! The same store may be selling a bag of 10 oranges for $5. At that price, each orange costs only 50 cents.
- Package sizes can be misleading, so ignore the size of a package and compare net weights of package contents to determine the best value.
- Compare the unit price of organic foods and similar conventionally produced items. If an organic food item is more expensive, consider purchasing the conventional product instead.
- Compare unit prices of preportioned snack foods such as chips or cookies in 100-Calorie packages with prices of the typical, larger package size products. Such preportioned snacks may be convenient and helpful if you are trying to control your calorie intake, but they are usually more costly per ounce than the same foods purchased in larger packages. Furthermore, people may eat more of the preportioned snack foods, because they think they are lower in calories than the same items packed in larger containers. Make your own preproportioned snacks. For example, buy a large package of oatmeal cookies and place two-cookie portions into reusable storage bags. When you want a snack, eat the two cookies.

- Use coupons when purchasing brand-name items. However, be aware that many stores offer similar products, often referred to as "store brands," that are less expensive than the brand-name items. Although store brand items do not have name recognition, these products are usually just as nutritious as their corresponding brand-name items.
- Limit your carbonated soft drink, commercially prepared coffee, and bottled water purchases. When you are thirsty, locate the nearest water fountain and have a drink for free!
- Check "sell by," "best if used by," or "use by" dates on packages of perishable foods such as eggs and dairy products. Compared to canned and frozen foods, perishable foods lose their appealing sensory qualities, such as fresh taste and appearance, more rapidly during storage. The "sell by" date informs store employees about the length of time the product should be displayed for sale. Obviously, it is best to buy foods before the sell by date. The "best if used by" or "use by" dates indicate the last day to use the product before it loses its best flavor and other appealing sensory qualities. The date does not indicate the last day to purchase the food because of safety concerns.[34] Also, read food product labels for storage information. Many products must be refrigerated after opening to delay spoilage. Chapter 12 provides more information about proper food storage practices.
- Have at least one vegetarian meal a week.
- Use more chicken, turkey, and fish. Red meats are among the most expensive protein sources.
- Have a meal with canned, baked, broiled, or grilled fish as the primary source of animal protein at least once a week.
- Incorporate canned fish, such as tuna, salmon, and sardines, in meals. Canned fish can be a less expensive choice than fresh fish, because there is less waste (skin and large bones).
- Remember that any food product is not a good buy if the item spoils before you can use it.

For more ways to save money on food, read the "Food & Nutrition Tips" on page 233.

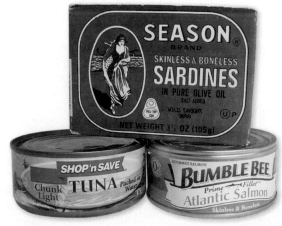

Canned fish, such as tuna, salmon, and sardines, can be a less expensive choice than meat or fresh fish.

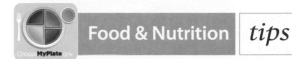 Food & Nutrition *tips*

- Prepare a shopping list to help avoid needless or impulse purchases and having to return to the store to buy forgotten items. Keep the grocery list in a convenient place, such as on the refrigerator, and jot down items as they become depleted.

- Empty-calorie foods often look more appealing when your stomach is empty. To reduce the likelihood of buying such foods on impulse, avoid shopping for groceries when you are hungry.

- Be wary of buying food items that are displayed near or along checkout aisles. They are usually energy-dense foods and are not nutrient dense, such as candy bars and baked goods.

- Many perishable foods, such as margarine, shredded cheese, and fluid fat-free milk, can be frozen.

- If you drink coffee, buy a small coffeemaker, a can of ground coffee, and coffee filters to make the beverage. Consider carrying a small thermos of coffee in your backpack. It is much less expensive to make a cup of your own coffee than to buy one from a coffeehouse.

- Canned beans are often sold in large cans that may be cheaper per ounce than beans in smaller cans. If the larger-sized product is less expensive, buy it. After opening the large can of beans, remove the amount needed for the meal, and freeze the remainder in an air-tight container for a future meal.

- For fresh seasoning, grow your own herbs. Basil, oregano, parsley, cilantro, and thyme grow well in flower pots placed in a sunny area. Snip as many leaves as needed for recipes, while keeping the rest of the plants intact.

- Share potluck dinners with friends. Plan the menu and ask your friends to bring certain items, such as vegetable or fruit salads and whole-grain rolls or breads. Inexpensive entrees (the main food items on the menu) include spaghetti and meat sauce, chicken burritos, vegetarian chili, tuna and noodle casserole, and tacos made with tuna fish.

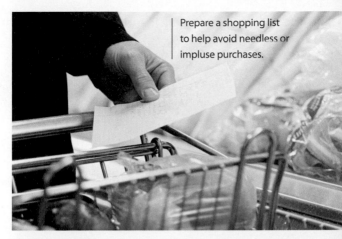
Prepare a shopping list to help avoid needless or impulse purchases.

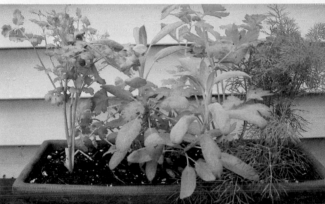
For fresh seasonings, grow your own herbs such as basil, oregano, parsley, and thyme.

 ## CHAPTER REFERENCES

See Appendix I.

 ## SUMMARY

Proteins are organic compounds that contain nitrogen, the element cells need to make a wide array of important biological compounds with structural or metabolic functions in the body. Proteins, for example, participate in muscular movement, catalyze chemical reactions, transport nutrients, and help maintain proper fluid and acid-base balance. Additionally, a relatively small amount of protein contributes to the body's energy needs. Numerous vital functions as well as physical growth and development would not be possible without specific proteins.

The typical amino acid has nitrogen-containing or amino, acid, and "R" groups. The diet must supply nine of the amino acids, because the body cannot make them or make enough of them to meet its needs. Under normal conditions, cells can synthesize the remaining amino acids if the raw materials are available.

Human proteins are comprised of 20 different amino acids arranged in various combinations. Cells produce proteins by linking amino acids together in specific sequences that are dictated by instructions coded in DNA. Faulty DNA results in the wrong amino acids being inserted into peptide chains, causing genetic defects. If an essential amino

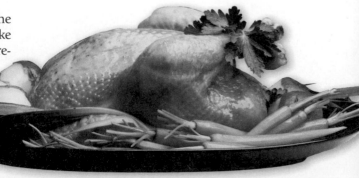

acid is not available when protein synthesis occurs, proteins in muscles and organs can provide the essential amino acids. Otherwise, protein synthesis halts, and the amino acids in the unfinished peptide are removed and returned to the amino acid pool. Excess amino acids are metabolized for energy or converted into body fat.

Protein turnover is the process of breaking down old or unneeded proteins into their component amino acids and recycling them to make new proteins. The body conserves nitrogen by recycling amino acids, but each day, it loses some protein and nitrogen, primarily in urine, nails, hair, feces, and skin. Amino acids from food replace the lost nitrogen. An adult's body maintains its protein content by carefully balancing nitrogen intake and losses. In positive nitrogen balance, the body retains more nitrogen than it loses; in negative nitrogen balance, the body loses more nitrogen than it retains.

A healthy adult requires only about 0.5 g of protein/kg of body weight daily. The protein requirement increases during pregnancy, breastfeeding, periods of growth, and recovery from serious illnesses, blood losses, and burns. The adult RDA for protein is 0.8 g/kg of body weight daily.

Protein digestion begins in the stomach, where hydrochloric acid denatures food proteins and pepsin breaks proteins into polypeptides. In the small intestine, enzymes secreted by the pancreas and absorptive cells digest polypeptides primarily into di- and tripeptides. The absorptive cells pick up these compounds and convert the peptides into amino acids. The end-products of protein digestion, amino acids, travel to the liver. The liver uses the amino acids or releases them into the general circulation.

The AMDR for adults is 10 to 35% of energy intake from protein. Although total protein consumption as a percentage of daily calories has remained about the same since the early twentieth century, Americans now eat less red meat and more poultry, fish, nuts, and legumes. People can reduce their intake of animal protein without sacrificing the protein quality of their diets.

The average American consumes more protein than the RDA for the nutrient. Protein-rich diets that contain animal products generally contain high amounts of saturated fat and cholesterol, and such diets are associated with increased risk of certain chronic diseases, particularly heart disease and certain cancers. High-protein diets may result in amino acid imbalances, high urinary losses of calcium, and dehydration.

Animal foods generally provide more protein than similar quantities of plant foods. High-quality, or complete, protein is well digested and contains all essential amino acids in amounts that will support protein deposition and a young child's growth. Low-quality, or incomplete, protein is low in one or more of the essential amino acids and often is poorly digested. In general, meat, fish, poultry, eggs, milk, and milk products contain high-quality proteins. When compared to animal foods, most plant foods provide low-quality protein. Quinoa and foods made from processed soybeans are good plant sources of essential amino acids.

Vegetarian diets are based on plant foods and limit animal foods to some extent. Although vegetarians are generally healthier than people who eat Western diets, it is difficult to pinpoint diet as responsible for vegetarians' better health. If not properly planned, plant-based diets may not contain enough energy, high-quality protein, omega-3 fatty acids, vitamins B-12 and D, and zinc, iron, and calcium to meet a person's nutritional needs, especially children's needs.

PEM affects people whose diets lack sufficient protein as well as energy; children are more likely to be affected by PEM than adults. In impoverished developing countries, PEM is a major cause of childhood deaths. Severely undernourished children do not grow and are very weak, irritable, and vulnerable to dehydration and life-threatening infections. Undernutrition during early childhood can cause permanent brain damage.

Eating large portions of animal foods as well as taking amino acid and protein supplements does not build bigger, stronger muscles. The only effective way to increase muscle mass safely is to combine a nutritionally adequate diet with a program of muscle-strengthening exercises. Seventy percent of muscle tissue is water and only about 22% is protein. Thus, resistance training adds a considerable amount of water to muscle tissue. An athlete's diet should supply enough calories from carbohydrate and fat to support energy needs for increased physical activity and spare the use of protein for growth, repair, and maintenance of muscle tissue.

Although "fast foods" are convenient, food processing and packaging add to the cost of food. In general, the less time a person spends preparing food, the more money he or she will spend by having someone else prepare the food. Convenience foods are often energy dense—high in fat and sugar—and low in other micronutrients (except sodium), fiber, and phytochemicals. Supermarkets generally offer the same products as convenience stores but often at lower prices. Supermarkets also have a much larger selection of foods, particularly more nutrient-dense foods, than convenience stores. A good way to save money is to buy foods in large quantities at "bulk" food stores, but buying food in bulk is a bargain only if the items can be used before they spoil.

Recipes for Healthy Living

Trendy Black Beans

You've probably eaten ordinary canned baked beans as an accompaniment to hot dogs and hamburgers. If you are interested in eating a more trendy kind of bean then baked beans, try this recipe for black beans. Although canned black beans are more convenient to use in recipes than dried black beans, the canned products generally contain a lot of salt. Consider purchasing canned beans that contain less salt.

This black bean recipe makes about four ½-cup servings. Each serving supplies approximately 120 kcal, 8 g protein, less than 1 g fat, 7.5 g fiber, 2 mg iron, 70 mg sodium, and 130 mcg folate (a B vitamin). To make the beans a complementary protein source, serve them wrapped in a soft burrito or on cooked rice.

INGREDIENTS:

1 cup dried black beans (or 2 cups canned, low-salt beans)
¼ cup coarsely chopped green pepper
¼ cup peeled, chopped yellow onion
1 large clove garlic, peeled and minced
⅛ tsp ground black pepper
⅛ tsp salt (don't add if using canned beans)
3–5 drops hot pepper sauce (optional)

Pie chart: Fat 3%, Protein 27%, Carbohydrate 70%

Bar chart (% of DV/serving):
Calories* 6
Protein 16
Fiber 30
Iron 11
Folate 33
*2000 daily total kcal

PREPARATION STEPS:

1. If using dried beans, rinse beans in cold water, draining excess water. If using canned beans, skip steps 1 through 4 and place beans in a saucepan.

2. Place the beans in a saucepan and add 1¾ cups of water.

3. Heat beans and water on high heat until mixture boils. Boil for 2 minutes, then turn off heat, and remove saucepan from the burner. Cover saucepan and allow beans to remain in the hot water for 1 hour.

4. Do not drain water from beans. Simmer beans on low heat, in the covered saucepan, for 45 minutes. Stir occasionally.

5. Add green pepper, onion, garlic, black pepper, and salt to beans. Stir and simmer for 15 minutes.

6. Serve hot. Cooked beans can be frozen.

Apricot Quinoa

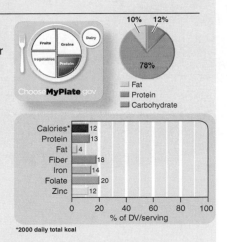

The ancient Incas of South America cultivated quinoa and relied on the protein-rich vegetable as a dietary staple. Today, cooked quinoa is often added to vegetable salads. This recipe is easy to make, and the quinoa can be served as a breakfast item or an accompaniment to chicken or pork.

This quinoa recipe makes about two ½-cup servings. Each serving provides about 230 kcal, 8 g protein, 2.5 g fat, 4.5 g fiber, 2.6 mg iron, 2 mg zinc, and 80 mcg folate.

INGREDIENTS:

1⅓ cups water
½ cup quinoa
⅓ cup dried apricots, chopped
¼ tsp ground cinnamon
1 Tbsp maple syrup

Pie chart: Fat 10%, Protein 12%, Carbohydrate 78%

Bar chart (% of DV/serving):
Calories* 12
Protein 13
Fat 4
Fiber 18
Iron 14
Folate 20
Zinc 12
*2000 daily total kcal

PREPARATION STEPS:

1. Add water to a small saucepan and bring to a boil. Add quinoa to boiling water.

2. Cover saucepan and cook quinoa over medium heat until all the water is absorbed (about 12–15 minutes).

3. Remove from heat; fluff quinoa with fork; and stir chopped apricots into the quinoa.

4. Place quinoa into a bowl; drizzle with maple syrup; and sprinkle cinnamon on the quinoa.

5. If desired, garnish with fresh fruit. Serve warm.

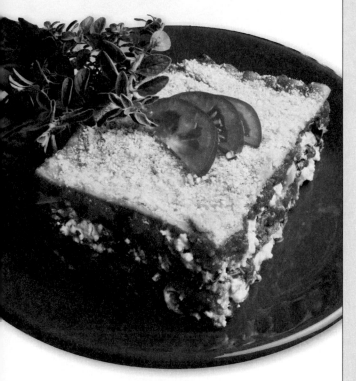

Personal *Dietary* Analysis

1. Refer to the 3-day food log from the "Personal Dietary Analysis" feature in Chapter 3. Calculate your average protein intake by adding the grams of protein eaten each day, dividing the total by 3, and rounding the figure to the nearest whole number.

Sample Calculation:

Day 1	<u>76</u> g
Day 2	<u>55</u> g
Day 3	<u>103</u> g
Total grams	<u>234</u> g ÷ 3 days = **<u>78</u>** g of protein/day

Your Calculation:

Day 1	_____ g
Day 2	_____ g
Day 3	_____ g
Total grams	_____ ÷ 3 days = _____ g/day

My average daily protein intake was _____ g.

2. The RDA for protein is based on body weight. Using the RDA of 0.8 g of protein/kg of body weight, calculate the amount of protein that you need to consume daily to meet the recommendation. To determine your body weight in kilograms, divide your weight (pounds) by 2.2, then multiply this number by 0.8 to obtain your RDA for protein. Then round the figure to the nearest whole number.

   My weight in pounds _____ ÷ 2.2 = _____ kg

   My weight in kg _____ × 0.8 = _____ g

   My RDA for protein = _____ g

   a. Did your average intake of protein meet or exceed your RDA level that was calculated in step 1? _____ yes _____ no

   b. If your answer to 2a is "yes," which foods contributed the most to your protein intake?

3. Review the log of your 3-day food intake. Calculate the average number of kilocalories that protein contributed to your diet each day during the 3-day period.

   a. Each gram of protein provides about 4 kcal; therefore, you must multiply the average number of grams of protein obtained in step 1 by 4 kcal to obtain the average number of kcal from protein.

Sample Calculation:

78 g/day × 4 kcal/g = 312 kcal from protein

Your Calculation:

_____ g/day × 4 kcal/g = _____ average number of kcal from protein

4. Determine your average energy intake over the 3-day period by adding the kilocalories for each day and dividing the sum by 3, and round to the nearest whole number.

Sample Calculation:

Day 1	<u>2500</u> kcal
Day 2	<u>3200</u> kcal
Day 3	<u>2750</u> kcal
Total kcal	<u>8450</u> ÷ 3 days = <u>2817</u> kcal/day (average caloric intake)

Your Calculation:

Day 1	_____ kcal
Day 2	_____ kcal
Day 3	_____ kcal
Total kcal	_____ ÷ 3 days = _____ kcal/day (average)

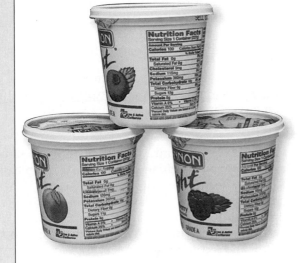

5. Determine the average percentage of energy that protein contributed to your diet by dividing the average kilocalories from protein obtained in step 3 by the average total daily energy intake obtained in step 4. Then round this figure to the nearest one-hundredth. Multiply this value by 100, move the decimal point two places to the right, drop the decimal point, and add a percent symbol.

Sample Calculation:

<u>312</u> kcal from protein ÷ <u>2817</u> kcal intake = <u>0.11</u> (rounded)

0.11 × 100 = 11%

Your Calculation:

_____ kcal from protein ÷ _____ kcal intake = _____

_____ × 100 = _____ %

6. Did your average intake of protein meet the recommendation of 10 to 35% of total calories? If your average protein intake was below 10%, list at least five foods you could eat that would boost your intake.

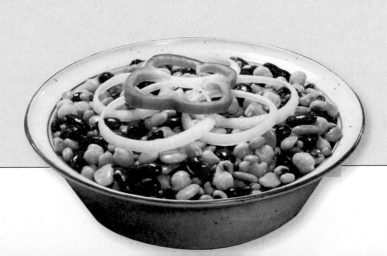

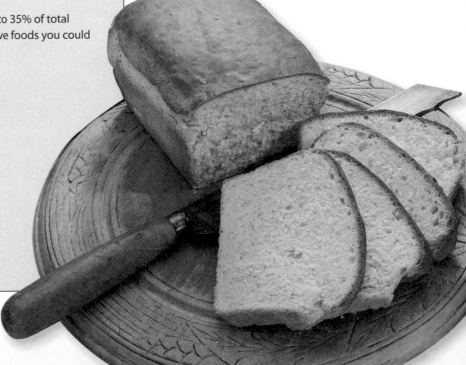

CRITICAL THINKING

1. Have you used or are you currently using protein or amino acid supplements?

_____ yes _____ no

If you answered "yes," explain why you use these supplements.

2. Are you a vegetarian? If so, describe your dietary practices (e.g., vegan or semivegetarian) and explain why you decided to become vegetarian. If you are not a vegetarian, explain why you would or would not consider this lifestyle.

3. Plan a day's meals and snacks for a healthy 132-pound (60 kg) adult lactoovovegetarian female who is not pregnant or breastfeeding. The menu should contain all essential amino acids but contain no animal foods other than eggs and foods from the dairy group. Your meal plan can range from 1800 to 2200 kcal, and it should include foods from the major food groups and follow the recommendations of the U.S. Department of Agriculture's MyPlate food guide.

4. Using only plant foods, plan a day's meals and snacks for a healthy 154-pound (70 kg) adult vegan male. The menu should supply at least 2200 kcal, follow the recommendations of the MyPlate food plan, and include foods from the major food groups (except for the dairy group, unless calcium-fortified soy milk is used).

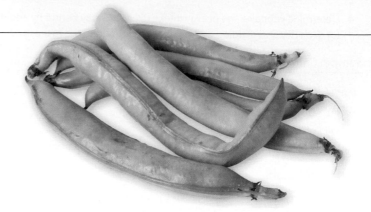

5. A recipe for bean salad has the following main ingredients:

1 cup kidney beans
1 cup green beans
1 cup butter beans
1 cup black beans
1½ cups wine vinegar
⅓ cup canola oil
¼ cup chopped onion

Explain why this recipe is not a complementary mixture of plant proteins. What plant foods could you add to the recipe to make it a complementary mixture?

 PRACTICE TEST

Select the best answer.

1. A protein
   a. is comprised of glucose molecules.
   b. has nitrogen in its chemical structure.
   c. provides more energy per gram than carbohydrate.
   d. is a complex inorganic molecule.

2. Which of the following statements is false?
   a. Certain hormones are proteins.
   b. Nearly all enzymes are proteins.
   c. Proteins are part of triglycerides.
   d. The body uses amino acids to make antibodies.

3. Which of the following foods generally provides the least amount of protein per serving?
   a. fruits
   b. milk
   c. nuts
   d. seeds

4. Which of the following foods is not a source of complete protein?
   a. peanut butter
   b. cheese
   c. fish
   d. eggs

5. In cells, _____ controls the assembly of amino acids into proteins.
   a. PEU
   b. DNA
   c. IOM
   d. ATP

6. _____ is the process of removing nitrogen from an amino acid.
   a. Transamination
   b. Denaturation
   c. Hydrogenation
   d. Deamination

7. Which of the following physical states is (are) characterized by positive nitrogen balance?

a. starvation
b. illness
c. puberty
d. All of the above are correct.

8. What is the RDA for protein of a healthy adult woman who weighs 62 kg?

a. 49.6 g
b. 59.6 g
c. 69.6 g
d. 79.6 g

9. Which of the following foods is not a source of complementary protein?

a. red beans and rice
b. hummus on pita bread
c. soynut butter on a bagel
d. whole-wheat bread with fruit spread

10. A person following a vegan diet would eat

a. eggs.
b. cheese.
c. nuts.
d. fish.

11. By eating more protein than needed, a person can

a. build bigger muscles.
b. lose weight.
c. absorb more calcium.
d. become dehydrated.

12. People with celiac disease should

a. take amino acid supplements.
b. limit their protein intake to 20 g per day.
c. avoid foods that contain gluten.
d. eliminate protein from plant sources.

13. Which of the following tips is a recommended way to reduce food costs?

a. buying food in bulk, if it can be used before spoiling
b. purchasing preportioned, packaged foods
c. shopping at convenience stores, if the stores are within 5 miles of your home
d. eating at fast-food outlets at least three times a week

Answers to Chapter 7 Quiz *Yourself*

1. Animal foods such as meat and eggs are almost 100% protein. **False.** (p. 203)

2. Foods made from processed soybeans can be sources of high-quality protein. **True.** (p. 205)

3. Americans typically consume more protein from animal sources than from plant foods. **True.** (p. 218)

4. Registered dietitians generally recommend that healthy people take amino acid supplements to increase their protein intake. **False.** (p. 229)

5. People can nourish their hair by using shampoo that contains protein. **False.** (p. 208)

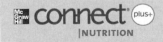

Additional resources related to the features of this book are available on ConnectPlus® Nutrition. Ask your instructor how to get access.

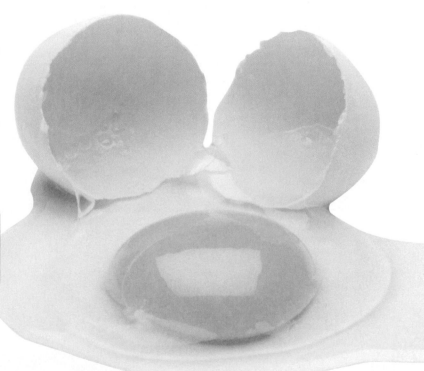

Vitamins

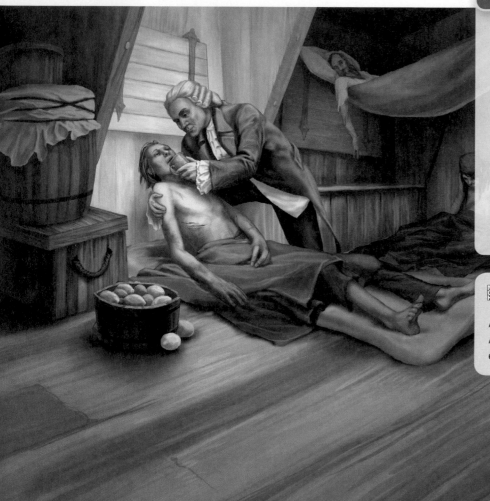

Chapter Learning Outcomes

After reading Chapter 8, you should be able to

1. Classify vitamins according to whether they are fat soluble or water soluble.

2. List major functions and food sources for each vitamin.

3. Describe deficiency and/or toxicity signs and symptoms for certain vitamins, including A, D, thiamin, B-6, niacin, and C.

4. Discuss ways to conserve the vitamin content of foods.

5. Evaluate the use of vitamin supplements with respect to their potential health benefits and hazards.

6. Identify lifestyle practices associated with increased risk of certain cancers.

McGraw Hill **connect** plus+
|NUTRITION   **www.mcgrawhillconnect.com**

A wealth of proven resources are available on ConnectPlus® Nutrition! Ask your instructor about ConnectPlus, which includes an interactive eBook, an adaptive learning program and much, much more!

FOR CENTURIES, taking lengthy ocean voyages was a dangerous venture, not just because of the threat of severe storms and pillaging pirates but also because of a terrifying and deadly disease called **scurvy.** The first signs and symptoms of scurvy—fatigue and *petechiae* (*peh-tee'-key-eye*), pinpoint hemorrhages in skin—occurred about 20 to 40 days after setting sail. As the disease progressed, the affected person's skin bruised easily; gums swelled, became spongy, and bled after being barely touched; teeth loosened and fell out. Not surprisingly, the person suffering from scurvy also became irritable and depressed. A particularly devastating sign of the disease was the opening up of old scars, exposing wounds that could become infected. Scurvy victims eventually died, generally from infections, brain hemorrhages, or heart complications.

In 1753, British physician James Lind published an article describing an experiment he had performed on 12 sailors suffering from scurvy. Lind divided the sick sailors into 6 pairs, and each pair received a different treatment. The six treatments were cider, vinegar, sulfuric acid, seawater, nutmeg, or oranges and lemons. Lind observed that the pair of sailors given the citrus fruit were the only ones to recover from scurvy. By today's standards, Lind's experiment was primitive, but as a result of his testing, Lind found the cure for scurvy—eating oranges and lemons. Eventually, food rations for British sailors included lemon juice to prevent the disease. The sailors earned the nickname "limeys" because at that time, people often referred to citrus fruits collectively as "limes."

Today, we know that scurvy results from a deficiency of vitamin C and that citrus fruits are among the richest dietary sources of the vitamin. Although Lind is often credited with having discovered the cure for scurvy, he did not suspect the disease resulted from the lack of something in the typical seafarer's diet. At that time, scientists were unaware that food contained vitamins. Lind thought scurvy was a digestive system disorder that could be treated with substances associated with warm climates.[1] In his experiment, Lind happened to administer citrus fruits to a pair of the sailors with scurvy because these fruits were associated with such climates.

In 1911, Polish chemist Casimir Funk discovered a substance in an extract made from rice bran that he thought would cure the disease beriberi. Funk called the compound a "vitamine" (*vita* = necessary for life; *amine* = a type of nitrogen-containing substance) because of its chemical structure. The term *vitamine* was later modified to *vitamin*, when scientists determined that there were several kinds of these substances in

(continued)

scurvy vitamin C–deficiency disease

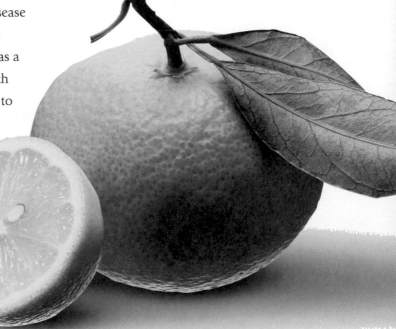

foods and not all were amines. By the end of the twentieth century, scientists had added riboflavin, niacin, biotin, B-6, B-12, pantothenic acid, folate, ascorbic acid, A, D, E, and K to the list of vitamins. Humans also require *choline*, especially during *prenatal* (before birth) development. Like vitamin D, the body can make choline, but under certain conditions, the body does not synthesize enough to meet its needs.[2] Choline is considered to be a *vitamin-like* essential nutrient.

It is unlikely that any vitamins still need to be discovered. Why? Babies grow and thrive on infant formulas, synthetic liquid diets containing vitamins and other nutrients known to be essential for health. Additionally, very ill people who cannot eat solid food can be kept alive for years on liquid synthetic feedings that contain all known nutrients, including vitamins. If a vitamin remained undiscovered, infants and people who are unable to consume solid foods would not be able to survive on formula diets.

Chapter 8 presents information about the 13 vitamins and choline, including physiological roles and major food sources. By reading Chapter 8, you will learn what can happen to the body when consumption of certain vitamins is too small or too great. Many Americans take vitamin supplements to prevent disease; the "Vitamins as Medicines" section of Chapter 8 examines current scientific evidence concerning the usefulness of taking megadoses of certain vitamins. In general, a megadose is at least 10 times the recommended amount of the micronutrient.[3]

 ## 8.1 Vitamins: Basic Concepts

> **vitamin** complex organic molecule that regulates certain metabolic processes
>
> **fat-soluble vitamins** vitamins A, D, E, and K
>
> **water-soluble vitamins** thiamin, riboflavin, niacin, vitamin B-6, pantothenic acid, folate, biotin, vitamin B-12, and vitamin C

What is a vitamin? A **vitamin** is a complex organic compound that regulates certain metabolic processes in the body. A vitamin meets the following criteria:

- the body cannot synthesize the compound or make enough to maintain good health;

- the compound naturally occurs in commonly eaten foods;

- signs and symptoms of a health problem (*deficiency disorder*) eventually occur when the substance is missing from the diet; and

- good health is restored, if the deficiency disorder is treated early by supplying the missing substance.

Although vitamins are organic molecules in foods, they are distinctly different from carbohydrates, fats, and proteins. Foods generally contain much smaller amounts of vitamins than of macronutrients. A slice of whole-wheat bread, for example, weighs 28 grams. Of that weight, only about 0.005% (1.48 mg) is comprised of vitamins; carbohydrate, water, protein, fat, and minerals make up the remaining weight of the bread. Furthermore, the body requires vitamins in milligram or microgram amounts, but it needs grams of macronutrients.

To estimate the vitamin contents of packaged foods, you can check the Nutrition Facts panels on food labels. Food manufacturers are required to indicate amounts of vitamins A and C in a serving of food as percentages of these micronutrients' Daily Values (%DVs). Daily Values have been established for most vitamins (see Appendix C).

In the past, amounts of most vitamins in foods, particularly fat-soluble vitamins, were often expressed in *International Units* (*IUs*). Today, IUs have largely been replaced by more precise milligram or microgram measures. One microgram of vitamin D, for example, equals 40 IUs of the vitamin. Food composition tables and the information panels on food and supplement labels often still list IU values for fat-soluble vitamins.

Classifying Vitamins

Vitamins A, D, E, and K are **fat-soluble vitamins.** These vitamins are in the lipid portions of foods and tend to associate with lipids in the body. Thiamin, riboflavin, niacin, vitamin B-6, pantothenic acid, folate, biotin, vitamin B-12 (collectively known as the B vitamins), and vitamin C are **water-soluble vitamins.** Water-soluble vitamins dissolve in the watery components of food and the body. (Choline is also water soluble.) Table 8.1 presents the vitamins and provides some other names that may be used to identify them.

Why is it important to know the difference between fat- and water-soluble vitamins? The body generally has more difficulty eliminating *excess* fat-soluble vitamins because these nutrients do not dissolve in watery substances such as urine. As a result, the body stores extra fat-soluble vitamins, primarily in the liver and in body fat. Over time, these vitamins can accumulate and cause toxicity. On the other hand, the body stores only limited amounts of most water-soluble vitamins—vitamin B-12 is an exception. Furthermore, kidneys can filter excesses of water-soluble vitamins from the bloodstream and eliminate them in urine. Thus, water-soluble vitamins are generally not as toxic as fat-soluble vitamins.

Roles of Vitamins

Vitamins play numerous roles in the body, and each of these micronutrients generally has more than one function (Fig. 8.1). Some vitamins, such as vitamin D, act as hormones; other vitamins, such as vitamin C and thiamin, participate in chemical reactions by accepting or donating electrons. In general, vitamins regulate a variety of body processes, including those involved in cell division and development as well as the growth and maintenance of tissues.

Advertisements for vitamins often promote the notion that the micronutrients can "give" you energy. Vitamins, however, are not a source of energy, because cells do not metabolize them for energy. Although the body does not use vitamins directly for energy, many vitamins participate in the chemical reactions that release energy from glucose, fatty acids, and amino acids. The diagram in Appendix F presents a simplified view of energy metabolism and indicates vitamins that are involved in the various steps of the process.

Most vitamins have more than one chemical form that functions in the body. For example, *retinol*, *retinal*, and *retinoic acid* are chemically related types of vitamin A that have roles in the body. Additionally, some vitamins have precursors (*provitamins*) that do not function as vitamins until the body converts them into active forms. For example, the plant pigment beta-carotene is a provitamin for vitamin A, and the amino acid tryptophan is a precursor for the B-vitamin niacin.

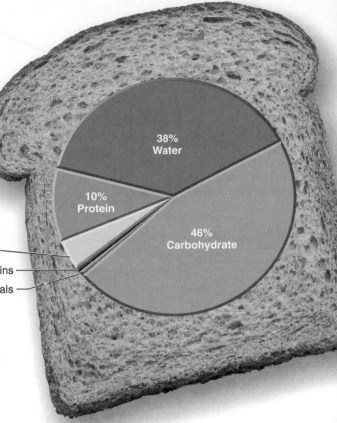

38% Water

10% Protein

46% Carbohydrate

4% Fat

<1% Vitamins

<1% Minerals

A slice of bread weighs about 1 ounce (28 g). Vitamins comprise only about 0.005% (1.48 mg) of the weight of the bread.

TABLE 8.1 *Classifying Vitamins*

Fat-Soluble Vitamins
A (retinol)
D
E (alpha-tocopherol, other tocopherols)
K
Water-Soluble Vitamins
Thiamin (thiamine, B-1)
Riboflavin (B-2)
Niacin (B-3, nicotinamide, nicotinic acid)
B-6 (pyridoxine)
B-12 (cobalamin, cobalamine)
Biotin (H)
Pantothenic acid (B-5)
Folate (folic acid, folacin)
C (ascorbic acid)
Vitamin-like
Choline

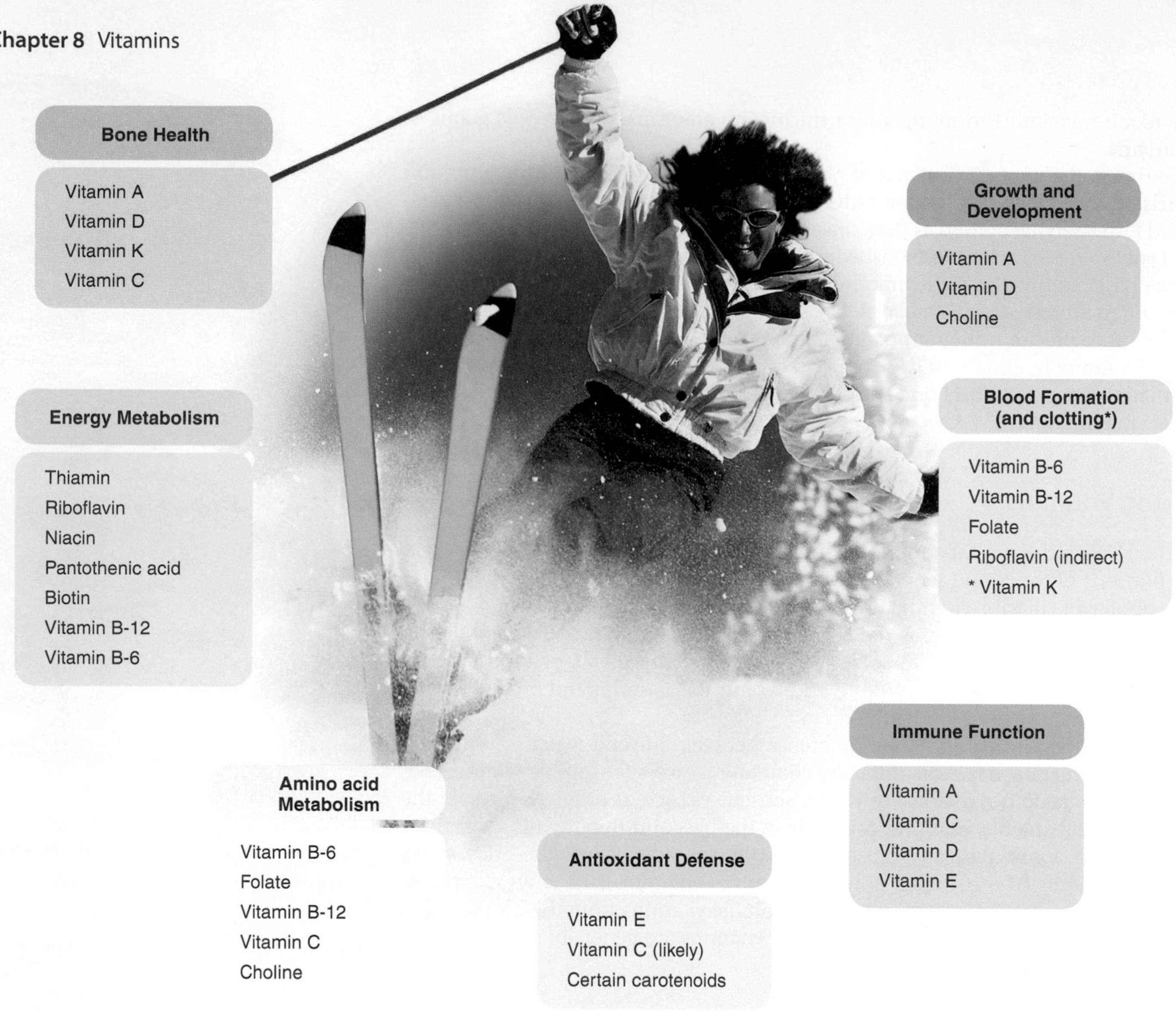

Bone Health

Vitamin A
Vitamin D
Vitamin K
Vitamin C

Growth and Development

Vitamin A
Vitamin D
Choline

Energy Metabolism

Thiamin
Riboflavin
Niacin
Pantothenic acid
Biotin
Vitamin B-12
Vitamin B-6

Blood Formation (and clotting*)

Vitamin B-6
Vitamin B-12
Folate
Riboflavin (indirect)
* Vitamin K

Amino acid Metabolism

Vitamin B-6
Folate
Vitamin B-12
Vitamin C
Choline

Immune Function

Vitamin A
Vitamin C
Vitamin D
Vitamin E

Antioxidant Defense

Vitamin E
Vitamin C (likely)
Certain carotenoids

Figure 8.1 Functions of vitamins and related compounds. Groups of vitamins and related compounds (e.g., choline and certain carotenoids) work together to maintain good health.

Did You Know?

Rancidity results when fat in food, particularly the unsaturated fat, undergoes oxidation. Rancid fat makes the food smell and taste bad, and people usually refuse to eat it. To inhibit oxidation of fatty acids and increase a food's "shelf life," manufacturers add antioxidants such as BHT and BHA to the food during production.

What Is an Antioxidant?

When many biochemical reactions take place, the compounds participating in the reactions lose or gain electrons. When an atom or molecule gains one or more electrons, it has been *reduced*. When an atom or molecule loses one or more electrons, it has been *oxidized*. An **oxidizing agent** or **oxidant** is a substance that removes electrons from atoms or molecules. An oxidation reaction can form a **radical** (commonly referred to as a "free radical"), a substance with an unpaired electron. Radicals are highly reactive (chemically unstable), and they remove electrons from more stable molecules, such as proteins, fatty acids, and DNA (Fig. 8.2). As a result, radicals can damage or destroy these molecules. If the loss of electrons is uncontrolled, a chain reaction can occur in which excessive oxidation takes place and affects many cells. Many medical researchers suspect excess oxidation is responsible for promoting chemical changes in cells that ultimately lead to heart attack, stroke, cancer, Alzheimer's disease, and even the aging process.

Some radical formation in the body is necessary and provides some benefits.[4] Radicals, for example, stimulate normal cell growth and division. Additionally, white blood cells generate radicals as part of their activities that destroy infectious agents. Under normal conditions, cells regulate oxidation reactions by using antioxidants such as vitamin E. **Antioxidants** protect cells by giving up electrons to radicals. When a chemically unstable substance accepts an electron, it can form a more stable structure that does not pull electrons away from other compounds. By sacrificing electrons, antioxidants protect molecules such as polyunsaturated fatty acids in the membrane or DNA in the nucleus from being oxidized (Fig. 8.3).

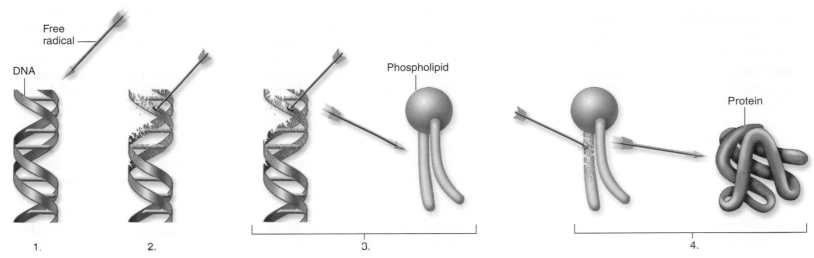

Sources of Vitamins

Plants, animals, fungi, and even bacteria supply natural forms of vitamins in our diets. In addition to foods, vitamin supplements are another source of these micronutrients. Although chemists can synthesize vitamins, certain types of bacteria and algae produce vitamins. These organisms can be grown in laboratory settings for the purpose of "harvesting" their vitamins to use in supplement production.[5]

Regardless of whether a particular vitamin is naturally in foods or synthesized in a laboratory, it generally has the same chemical structure and works equally well in the body—but there are exceptions. The natural form of vitamin E has more **biological activity**, that is, it produces more effects in the body, than synthetic vitamin E. On the other hand, *synthetic folic acid*, the type of folate that is added to flour and many ready-to-eat and cooked cereals, has almost twice the biological activity as the natural form of the vitamin.

Many adult Americans take multivitamin supplements that contain two or more vitamins and may also supply one or more minerals (*multivitamin-multimineral supplement*).[6] According to data collected in the Third National Health and Examination Survey in 1999–2000, 35% of adults reported regular use of a multivitamin-multimineral supplement that contained at least three vitamins.[7] Such products are often marketed as "one-a-days" or for a particular target audience, such as men, people with diabetes, athletes, or older adults.

Figure 8.2 What is a radical? A radical is a highly reactive substance because it has an unpaired electron. Radicals remove electrons from more stable molecules, such as DNA in the cell's nucleus. A radical acts as an "arrow" by hitting a vulnerable molecule (1, 2). The damaged molecule becomes the source of another radical that "strikes" another vulnerable molecule, in this case, a phospholipid (3). The reaction repeats itself as another radical forms and attacks another vulnerable molecule, such as a protein (4).

oxidizing agent or **oxidant** substance that removes electrons from atoms or molecules

radical substance with an unpaired electron

antioxidant substance that gives up electrons to radicals to protect cells

biological activity describes vitamin's degree of potency or effects in the body

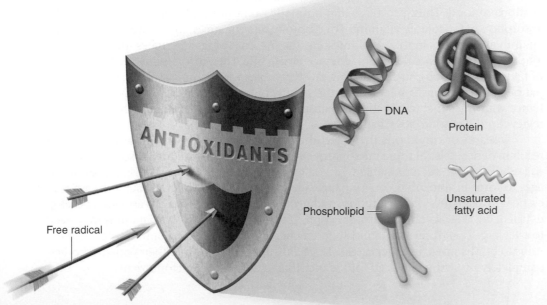

Figure 8.3 Antioxidant action. Antioxidants can protect the cell's plasma membrane and DNA from radicals. By sacrificing electrons, antioxidants protect molecules such as polyunsaturated fatty acids in the plasma membrane or DNA in the nucleus from being oxidized.

enrichment addition of specific amounts of thiamin, riboflavin, niacin, folic acid, and iron to refined flour and cereals

fortification addition of one or more nutrients to foods during their manufacturing process

It is not necessary to consume 100% of every vitamin each day. If you are healthy and usually follow a nutritionally adequate diet, your cells should contain a supply of vitamins that can last for several days and possibly even years, depending on the vitamin. Furthermore, bacteria that reside in your lower intestinal tract produce certain vitamins, particularly biotin and vitamin K, and you can absorb these micronutrients to some extent. Additionally, your body can synthesize vitamin D and niacin under certain conditions.

Vitamin Enrichment and Fortification

Cereal grains such as wheat, rice, and corn lose considerable amounts of their natural vitamin contents during milling (refinement). The federally regulated **enrichment** program specifies amounts of four B vitamins (thiamin, riboflavin, niacin, and folic acid) and the mineral iron that manufacturers must add to their refined flour and other milled grain products. At present, health experts are considering whether vitamin B-12 should be included as an enrichment nutrient. Enrichment helps protect Americans from developing the deficiency diseases associated with the lack of these nutrients. However, enrichment does not replace the vitamin E, vitamin B-6, potassium, magnesium, several other micronutrients, and fiber that were naturally in the unrefined grains. This is the major reason dietitians and other nutrition experts promote regular consumption of whole-grain products, such as whole-wheat bread and brown rice.

Fortification involves the addition during manufacturing of one or more vitamins (and/or other nutrients) to a wide array of commonly eaten foods. The vitamins that are added may or may not be in the food naturally. For example, milk is often fortified with vitamins A and D, and many ready-to-eat cereals are sprayed with additional vitamins before packaging.[8] In the United States, fortification and enrichment of foods have improved vitamin intakes of Americans. However, some food manufacturers add vitamins to foods and beverages, particularly flavored drinks, that would otherwise be considered "empty-calorie" items. Many nutrition experts are concerned that by substituting such human-made products for more natural foods and beverages, Americans may consume excessive amounts of a few vitamins while reducing their intake of others.

Vitamin Absorption

The small intestine is the primary site of vitamin absorption. However, the intestine does not absorb 100% of the vitamins in food. Vitamin absorption tends to increase when the body's needs for the micronutrients are also higher than usual. The body's requirements for vitamins generally increase during periods of growth, such as infancy and adolescence, and during pregnancy and breastfeeding.

Fat-soluble vitamins are chemically similar to lipids, and the vitamins are in fatty portions of food. Thus, processes that normally occur during fat digestion facilitate the absorption of fat-soluble vitamins. For example, bile enhances lipid as well as fat-soluble vitamin absorption. In the small intestine, the presence of fat stimulates the secretion of a hormone that causes the gallbladder to release bile. Therefore, adding a small amount of fat to low-fat foods, such as tossing raw vegetables with some salad dressing, adding a pat of soft margarine to steamed carrots, or stir-frying green beans in peanut oil, can enhance your intestinal tract's ability to absorb the fat-soluble vitamins in these foods. To review lipid digestion, see Chapter 6.

Diseases or conditions that affect the GI tract can reduce vitamin absorption and result in deficiencies of these micronutrients. People with the inherited disease *cystic fibrosis (sis'-tik fie-broe'-sis)* are unable to digest fat properly, because the disease causes blockages to form in ducts that convey pancreatic enzymes to the small intestine. As a result, cystic fibrosis reduces fat absorption, and people suffering from the disease often develop deficiencies of fat-soluble vitamins. People who are unable to absorb vitamins may need to take large oral doses of vitamin supplements just to enable small amounts of the vitamins to be absorbed. In other cases, physicians inject vitamins into their patients' bodies, completely bypassing the need for the intestine to absorb the micronutrients.

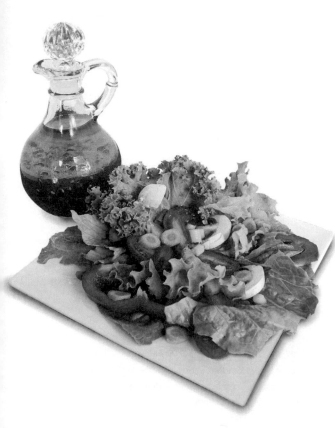

Vitamin Deficiency and Toxicity Disorders

A diet that contains adequate amounts of a wide variety of foods, including minimally processed fruits, vegetables, and whole-grain breads and cereals, can help supply the vitamin needs of most healthy people. Vitamin deficiency disorders generally result from inadequate diets or conditions that increase the body's requirements for vitamins, such as reduced intestinal absorption or higher-than-normal excretion of the micronutrients. Today, severe vitamin deficiencies are uncommon in the United States, thanks in part to modern food preservation practices, food enrichment and fortification, and the year-round, widespread availability of fresh fruits and vegetables from other countries. Many Americans, however, consume considerably less than recommended amounts of certain vitamins, particularly E, D, and the vitamin-like compound choline.[9]

A few segments of the population have a high risk of vitamin deficiencies. These vulnerable people include alcoholics, older adults, and patients who are hospitalized for lengthy periods. Additionally, people who suffer from anorexia nervosa, have intestinal conditions that interfere with vitamin absorption, or have rare metabolic defects that increase their vitamin requirements are more likely to develop vitamin deficiency disorders than people who do not have these conditions.

If your usual diet is nutritionally adequate but you occasionally have low intakes of vitamins, you are unlikely to develop vitamin deficiency diseases, because your cells store these micronutrients to some extent. The likelihood of developing a deficiency disease increases when a person's diet consistently lacks the vitamin. When this happens, the person's body stores or tissue levels of the vitamin become depleted, and the signs and symptoms of the nutrient's deficiency disease begin to occur. A person, for example, can become vitamin C–deficient after about a month of consuming a diet that lacks the vitamin.[10]

If you are considering taking vitamin supplements or are taking them already, you need to recognize that "more" is not necessarily better. When cells are saturated with a vitamin, they contain all they need and cannot accept additional amounts of the micronutrient. When this situation occurs, continuing to take the vitamin can produce a toxicity disorder, because exposure to the excess micronutrient or its by-products can damage cells.

Do you need to be concerned about developing a vitamin toxicity disorder? Probably not, unless you are taking excessive amounts (megadoses) of vitamin supplements or consuming large amounts of vitamin-fortified foods regularly. In their natural states, most commonly eaten foods do not contain toxic levels of vitamins. Taking a "one-a-day" type of multivitamin supplement regularly is unlikely to cause toxic effects in adults, because these products usually contain less than two times the Daily Values of each micronutrient component.

Preserving the Vitamin Content of Foods

Regardless of whether you pick fruits and vegetables from your own garden or buy them from a farmer's market or supermarket, many kinds of produce, especially berries and leafy vegetables, are highly perishable. Therefore, these foods should be eaten as soon as they are harvested or purchased to ensure maximum vitamin retention. In many instances, unpackaged ("bulk") fresh fruits or vegetables that are sold in supermarkets do not have dates indicating when they should be used, and consumers have no way of knowing when the produce was harvested.

Fresh fruits and vegetables can lose substantial amounts of vitamins as a result of improper handling

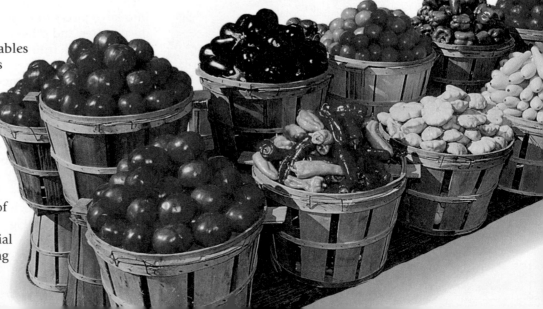

A farmer's market can be a source of locally grown fresh produce during the growing season.

or lengthy storage conditions. Therefore, select fresh produce carefully when buying it in grocery stores. Avoid produce that is bruised, wilted, or shriveled, or shows signs of decay such as mold. If you are uncertain how to choose ripe fruits and vegetables, ask the person who manages the produce section of the store for advice.

Some vitamins, such as niacin and D, resist destruction by usual food storage conditions or preparation methods. Other vitamins—particularly vitamin C, thiamin, and folate—are easily destroyed or lost by improper food storage and cooking methods. Fresh produce is more likely to retain its natural vitamin content when stored at temperatures near freezing, in high humidity, and away from air. Therefore, you should keep most fresh fruits and vegetables in plastic packaging and chilled until you are ready to use them. Tomatoes, bananas, and garlic should be stored at room temperature. Although precut, packaged salad greens and other vegetables may be convenient to use, they are highly perishable and should be used soon after purchasing.

Exposure to excessive heat, alkaline substances, light, and air can destroy certain vitamins, especially vitamin C. To reduce such losses, trim, peel, and cut raw fruits and vegetables just before eating or serving them. The darker leaves of vegetable greens generally contain more vitamins than the inner, paler color leaves or stems. Therefore, lightly trim away the outer leaves of lettuce and cabbage, and keep edible peels intact—just remove rotten or shriveled parts.

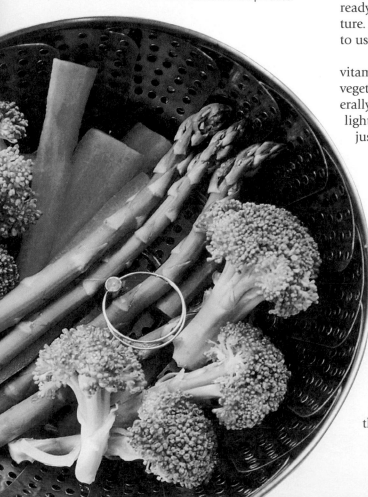

Figure 8.4 Conserving vitamins. Steaming vegetables can conserve much of the vitamin content of the produce.

Water-soluble vitamins can leach out of food and dissolve in the cooking water, which is often discarded. By cooking vegetables in small amounts of water and reusing that water for soups or sauces, you are likely to consume those water-soluble nutrients. When preparing produce for cooking, cut the food into large pieces to reduce the amount of surface area that will be exposed to heat, water, and other conditions that can increase vitamin losses. Whenever possible, cook fruits and vegetables in their skins, and if the skins are edible, eat them too.

Quick cooking methods that involve little contact between produce and water, such as microwaving, steaming, and stir-frying, can conserve much of the vitamin content of the food. According to the Food and Drug Administration (FDA), microwave cooking does not reduce the nutrient content of foods any more than do conventional cooking methods.[11] Microwave cooking may help conserve more vitamins in food because the method cooks quickly and without the need to add much water.

To steam vegetables, place them in a steamer basket that fits inside a pot, add enough water to touch the bottom of the basket, cover the pot, and then heat the water until it boils (Fig. 8.4). As the steam gently cooks the vegetables, add more water, if necessary. To stir-fry vegetables, heat a small amount of oil in a wok or pan that has deep sides, add small pieces of fresh vegetables, and stir the mixture, lightly coating the vegetables with oil (Fig. 8.5). Stir-fried vegetables should be cooked until they are barely tender to retain their nutrients as well as appealing textures, flavors, and colors. The "Recipe for Healthy Living" feature of Chapter 8 has a recipe for stir-fried vegetables.

Are fresh fruits and raw vegetables better sources of vitamins than canned or frozen versions? Sometimes they are. During the canning process, the heating of food can cause the destruction of certain vitamins. However, produce that is frozen immediately after being harvested and then properly stored can be just as nutritious as fresh produce. Frozen fruits and vegetables are often economical alternatives to fresh produce, but they need to be cooked without thawing to conserve much of their vitamin content. The thawing process causes some of the water that was naturally in the produce to drip out, taking water-soluble vitamins with it. If this water is discarded, vitamins in the fluid are lost. The following "Food & Nutrition Tips" box provides practical ways to preserve the vitamin content of food.

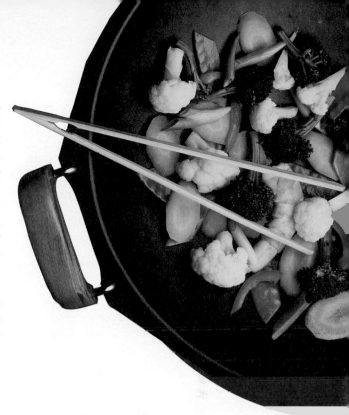

Figure 8.5 Conserving vitamins. Stir-frying conserves vitamins by cooking vegetables quickly without adding water.

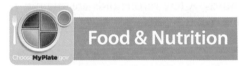

Food & Nutrition *tips*

- Eat fresh fruits and vegetables along with their edible peels or skins whenever possible.

- Cook fresh vegetables by microwaving, steaming, or stir-frying. Vegetables generally have high water content; therefore, add no water or just a small amount when microwaving vegetables.

- Do not overcook vegetables and minimize reheating, because prolonged heating reduces vitamin content.

- Do not add margarine or butter to vegetables during cooking, because fat-soluble vitamins and phytochemicals may enter the fat and be discarded when the fat is drained before serving. Fat in foods can enhance the body's absorption of fat-soluble vitamins; therefore, you can add some fat, such as olive oil or soft margarine, to vegetables after they are cooked.

- Store canned foods in a cool place. Canned foods can vary in the amount of nutrients they contain, largely because of differences in storage times and temperatures. If the can has been on the shelf for an extended period of time, the food's vitamin content may have deteriorated and its taste and texture may be less than desirable. To get maximal nutritive value from canned vegetables, drain the liquid that is packed with the food and use it as a base for soups, sauces, or gravies. If the liquid is too salty, discard it.

Concept **Checkpoint**

1. List at least three criteria used to designate a substance as a vitamin.
2. List three factors that distinguish vitamins from macronutrients.
3. Define the following terms: provitamin, antioxidant, and radical.
4. Explain the difference between enrichment and fortification.
5. Discuss at least five ways to preserve the vitamin content of fruits and vegetables during food preparation and storage.

> **retinol (preformed vitamin A)** most active form of vitamin A in the body
>
> **carotenoids** yellow-orange pigments in fruits and vegetables
>
> **epithelial cells** cells that form protective tissues that line the body

8.2 Fat-Soluble Vitamins

This section of Chapter 8 focuses on fat-soluble vitamins. Table 8.2 presents a summary of general information about all fat-soluble vitamins. Unless otherwise noted, RDA/AI values are for adults 19 to 50 years of age, excluding pregnant or breastfeeding women. Figure 8.6 indicates food groups of MyPlate that are good sources of fat-soluble vitamins.

Vitamin A

Do you associate vitamin A with eating carrots and good vision? It is true that vitamin A is involved in the visual process and carrots contain vitamin A precursors. However, vitamin A can multitask: it has numerous functions in the body. Furthermore, carrots are not the only source of vitamin A precursors; many fruits and vegetables are rich sources of these compounds.

Vitamin A is actually a family of compounds that includes retinol. **Retinol (preformed vitamin A)** is the most active form of the vitamin in the body. Although retinol and the other forms of vitamin A are only in animal foods, plants contain hundreds of yellow-orange pigments called **carotenoids.** A few carotenoids are vitamin A precursors, because the body can use them to make some retinol.

TABLE 8.2 *Summary of Fat-Soluble Vitamins*

Vitamin	Major Functions in the Body	Adult RDA/AI (adult RDA = bold)	Major Dietary Sources	Major Deficiency Signs and Symptoms	Major Toxicity Signs and Symptoms
Vitamin A (preformed and provitamin A)	Normal vision and reproduction, cellular growth, and immune system function	**700–900 mcg RAE**	Preformed: liver, milk, fortified cereals Provitamin: yellow-orange and dark green fruits and vegetables	Night blindness, xerophthalmia, poor growth, dry skin, reduced immune system functioning	**Adult Upper Limit (UL) = 3,000 mcg/day** Nausea and vomiting, headaches, bone pain and fractures, hair loss, liver damage, interference with vitamin K absorption
Vitamin D	Absorption of calcium and phosphorus, maintenance of normal blood calcium, calcification of bone, maintenance of immune function	**15–20 mcg**	Vitamin D–fortified milk, fortified cereals, fish oils, fatty fish	Rickets in children, osteomalacia in adults: soft bones, depressed growth, and reduced immune system functioning	**Adult UL = 100 mcg/day** Poor growth, calcium deposits in soft tissues
Vitamin E	Antioxidant	**15 mg** (alpha-tocopherol)	Vegetable oils and products made from these oils, certain fruits and vegetables, nuts and seeds, fortified cereals	Loss of muscular coordination, hemolysis of red blood cells resulting in anemia	**Adult UL = 1000 mg/day** Excessive bleeding as a result of interfering with vitamin K metabolism
Vitamin K	Production of active blood-clotting factors	90–120 mcg	Green leafy vegetables, canola and soybean oils, and products made from these oils	Excessive bleeding	**Adult UL = undetermined** Unknown

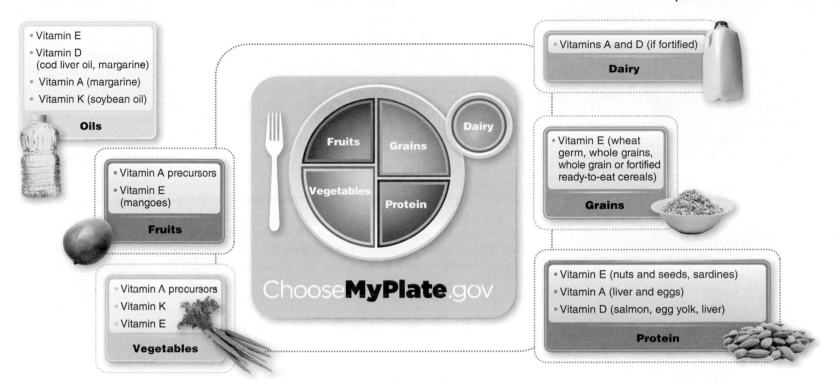

- Vitamin E
- Vitamin D
  (cod liver oil, margarine)
- Vitamin A (margarine)
- Vitamin K (soybean oil)

Oils

- Vitamin A precursors
- Vitamin E
  (mangoes)

Fruits

- Vitamin A precursors
- Vitamin K
- Vitamin E

Vegetables

- Vitamins A and D (if fortified)

Dairy

- Vitamin E (wheat germ, whole grains, whole grain or fortified ready-to-eat cereals)

Grains

- Vitamin E (nuts and seeds, sardines)
- Vitamin A (liver and eggs)
- Vitamin D (salmon, egg yolk, liver)

Protein

ChooseMyPlate.gov

Figure 8.6 MyPlate and fat-soluble vitamins. This illustration highlights MyPlate food groups that are generally good sources of fat-soluble vitamins.

All cells in the body need vitamin A to develop and function properly. Vitamin A participates in the processes of cell production, growth and development, function, and maintenance. For example, the vitamin is necessary for the production and maintenance of **epithelial cells,** cells that form protective tissues that line the body, including skin and linings of the digestive, respiratory, and reproductive tracts (Fig. 8.7). Certain epithelial cells secrete *mucus,* a sticky fluid that keeps the tissue moist and forms a barrier against many environmental pollutants and infectious agents. When the mucus-secreting epithelial cells do not have vitamin A, they deteriorate and no longer produce mucus. A lack of vitamin A can also reduce fertility, because the vitamin is required for maintaining the epithelial cells that line the reproductive tracts of men and women.

Certain white blood cells produce antibodies, which are proteins that participate in the body's immune response. Antibodies help destroy infectious agents such as bacteria. Vitamin A plays a role in regulating the activity of the immune system. Thus, vitamin A–deficient people are at greater risk of infections than those with adequate levels of the vitamin in their bodies.

Normal bone growth and development also require vitamin A. Although your bones do not appear to change their shape, they are constantly remodeled by processes that involve tearing down and rebuilding the tissues to meet the physical demands that you place on them each day. Vitamin A participates with other vitamins and minerals in the bone remodeling process.

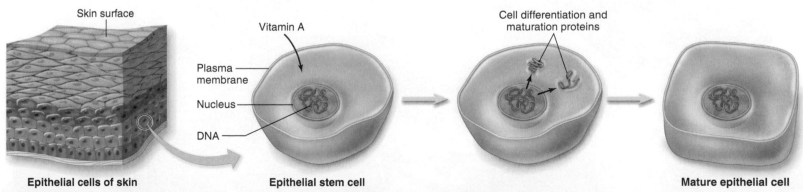

Figure 8.7 Vitamin A and epithelial cells. Vitamin A is necessary for epithelial *stem cells* to differentiate and mature properly.

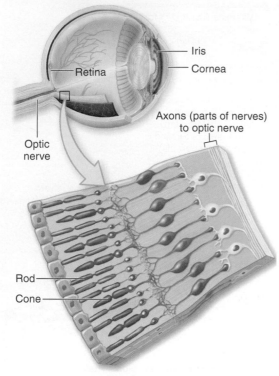

Figure 8.8 Vitamin A and vision. The retina, the light-sensitive area inside each eye, contains *rods* and *cones*, specialized nerve cells that are essential for vision. Rods and cones need vitamin A to function properly.

What Is Night Blindness?   Have you ever walked from a brightly lit theatre lobby into the darkened movie auditorium and felt blinded for a few seconds? This is a normal visual response to the sudden and dramatic reduction in light intensity. The *retina*, the light-sensitive area inside each eye, contains *rods* and *cones*, specialized nerve cells that are essential for vision (Fig. 8.8). Rods enable you to adapt to poorly lit environments and see objects as shades of black. Cones are responsible for color vision and function in well-lit environments. Rods and cones need vitamin A, particularly retinol, to function properly.

Figure 8.9 illustrates the *visual cycle* involving rods. Rods remove retinol from the bloodstream and convert it to retinal. In dark conditions, retinal binds to a protein called *opsin* to form **rhodopsin** (*visual purple*). Rhodopsin is necessary for vision in dim light. When you are in a dark environment and exposed to a small amount of light, such as moonlight, the light strikes your rods, activating rhodopsin. Activation alters the shape of the retinal portion of rhodopsin and bleaches the compound. This process causes retinal to split away, reforming opsin. The transformation of rhodopsin to opsin stimulates the rod to send a nervous impulse to the brain that signals the visual processing areas to interpret what is seen. After splitting away from opsin, retinal can bind to the protein, forming rhodopsin again.

As a result of the visual process shown in Figure 8.9, some retinal is destroyed. To replace the retinal, rods remove some retinol (vitamin A) from the bloodstream and convert it to retinal. *Night blindness*, the inability to see in dim light, occurs if retinol is unavailable. Night blindness is an early sign of vitamin A deficiency. Although cone cells also need vitamin A to function, the inability to see certain colors (color blindness) is not the result of a vitamin A deficiency.

Food & Nutrition   *tip*

When preparing salads or meals, do not discard the edible dark green leaves of lettuce, cabbage, or broccoli. These darkly pigmented parts of the plants contribute more provitamin A carotenoids to your diet than the lighter-colored parts. Use them in salads or on sandwiches. In addition to carotenoids, many fruits and vegetables contain hundreds of other phytochemicals that may benefit your health. To obtain a variety of these compounds, include colorful vegetables and fruits in your meals and snacks.

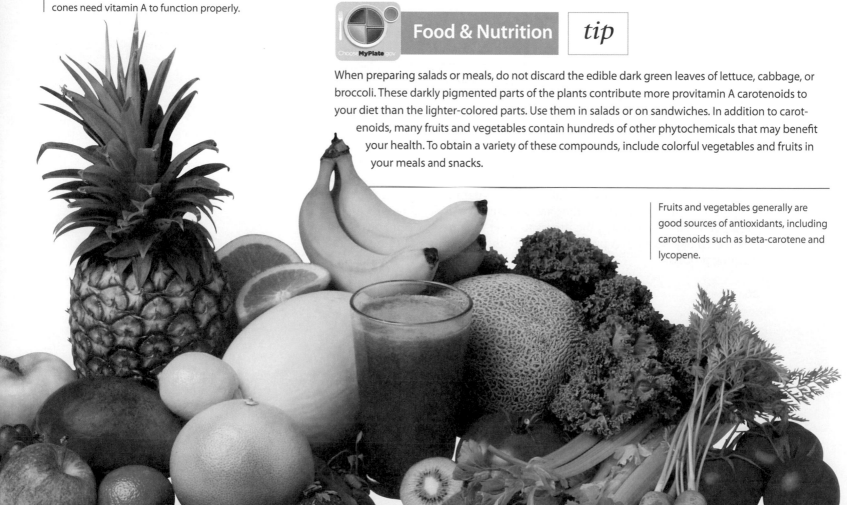

Fruits and vegetables generally are good sources of antioxidants, including carotenoids such as beta-carotene and lycopene.

Figure 8.9 Vitamin A and the visual cycle. Rod cells in the retina need retinol, a form of vitamin A, to function properly. Steps 1–6 illustrate the visual cycle.

Disc

Retinol (vitamin A)

Bloodstream

Opsin

Retinal (vitamin A)

Outside of disk membrane

Nucleus

Disc membrane

Rod

1. In dark conditions retinal is attached inside opsin to make rhodopsin.

Dark

Rhodopsin — Opsin / Retinal

6. Retinal attaches to opsin to form rhodopsin. (Return to step 1.)

2. Light activates rhodopsin by causing retinal to change shape, which causes opsin to change shape.

Low light

Retinal

Energy

5. Energy is required to bring retinal back to its original form.

Low light

Retinal

4. Following rhodopsin activation, retinal detaches from opsin.

Vision

3. Activated rhodopsin stimulates rod cell changes that result in vision.

Food Sources of Vitamin A

Animal foods such as liver, butter, fish, fish oils, and eggs are good sources of preformed vitamin A. Some foods are fortified with the vitamin during processing. Vitamin A–fortified milk, yogurt, margarine, and cereals are important sources of the nutrient for Americans. Carrots, spinach and other leafy greens, pumpkin, sweet potatoes, broccoli, mangoes, and cantaloupe are rich sources of **beta-carotene,** a carotenoid that the body can convert to vitamin A. However, the body obtains only 1 mcg of retinol from every 12 mcg of beta-carotene in a food. Furthermore, vitamin A precursors in plant foods are not as well absorbed as retinol in animal foods.[12]

In addition to beta-carotene, common carotenoids include lutein (*loo'-tee-en*), zeaxanthin (*zee-ah-zan'-thin*), and lycopene (*lie'-ko-peen*). Green, leafy vegetables, such as spinach and kale, have high concentrations of lutein and zeaxanthin. Tomato juice and other tomato products, including pizza sauce, contain considerable amounts of lycopene. Although lutein, zeaxanthin, and lycopene are carotenoids, the body does not convert them to vitamin A. Nevertheless, these plant pigments may function as beneficial antioxidants in the human body.

rhodopsin vitamin A–containing protein that is needed for vision in dim light

beta-carotene carotenoid that the body can convert to vitamin A

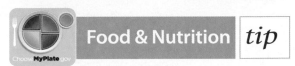

Food & Nutrition *tip*

Be wary of claims that taking vitamin A supplements will improve your vision so you will not need to wear eyeglasses or contact lenses. Vitamin A deficiency does not cause the kinds of visual defects that are correctable with glasses or contacts. Furthermore, large doses of vitamin A are toxic.

Did You Know?

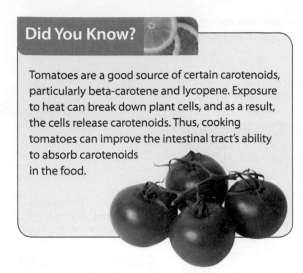

Tomatoes are a good source of certain carotenoids, particularly beta-carotene and lycopene. Exposure to heat can break down plant cells, and as a result, the cells release carotenoids. Thus, cooking tomatoes can improve the intestinal tract's ability to absorb carotenoids in the food.

Darkly pigmented fruits and vegetables usually contain more beta-carotene and other provitamin A carotenoids than lightly colored produce. For example, carrots, sweet potatoes, mangoes, and peaches contain more beta-carotene than celery, white potatoes, apples, and bananas. Dark green fruits and vegetables also contain carotenoids, but their green pigment *chlorophyll* contents hide the yellow-orange pigments.

Table 8.3 lists some foods that are sources of vitamin A and its precursors. Amounts of vitamin A in food are often reported as micrograms of retinol activity equivalents (RAE). One RAE is approximately 1 mcg of retinol.

Dietary Adequacy

For adults, the RDA for vitamin A is 700 to 900 mcg RAE. Deficiencies of the vitamin are rare in the United States.[12] Preschool children who do not eat enough vegetables, urban poor, older adults, and people with severe alcoholism, fat malabsorption, or liver diseases are at risk for vitamin A deficiency.

Vitamin A Deficiency Epithelial cells are among the first to become affected by a deficiency of vitamin A. In skin, vitamin A–deficient epithelial cells produce too much **keratin,** a tough protein found in hair, nails, and the outermost layers of skin. Keratin accumulates within the skin and makes the tissue rough and bumpy. Keratin also forms in tissues that do not normally contain the protein, such as the *cornea,* the clear covering over the iris of the eye (see Fig. 8.8). The cornea enables light to enter the eye. The epithelial cells that line the inner eyelids secrete mucus that helps keep the cornea moist

TABLE 8.3 *Vitamin A Content of Selected Foods*

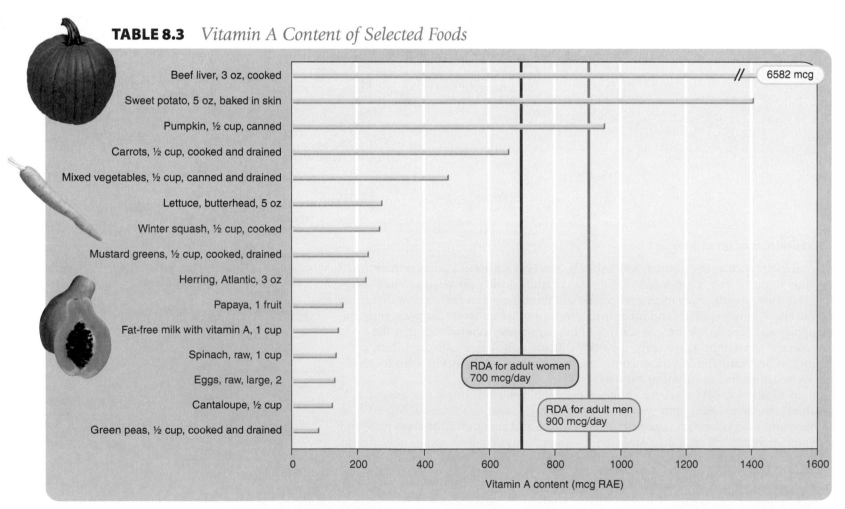

Source: Data from U.S. Department of Agriculture, Agricultural Research Service, USDA Nutrient Data Laboratory: Vitamin A, RAE (µg) content of selected foods by common measure, sorted by nutrient content. *USDA national nutrient database for standard reference, release 18. 2004.*

and clean. In a person suffering from chronic vitamin A deficiency, these cells accumulate keratin, and the white of the eye develops "foamy" areas (Fig. 8.10). Eventually, the epithelial cells harden and stop producing mucus. This condition is called **xerophthalmia** (*zir-op-thal'-me-a*) or "dry eye." Corneas affected by xerophthalmia can be damaged easily by dirt and bacteria. Unless a person with xerophthalmia receives vitamin A, the condition eventually leads to blindness.

Each year, thousands of children in developing nations, especially in Africa and Southeast Asia, become blind because of severe vitamin A deficiency.[13] Vitamin deficiency also reduces the effectiveness of the immune system, and many children suffering from vitamin A deficiency die from infections such as measles. In countries where vitamin A deficiency is widespread, public health efforts are being taken to reduce the prevalence of the condition. Such efforts include educating people about the need to eat regionally grown foods that are rich in beta-carotene and giving vitamin A injections periodically to vulnerable populations. In some countries, governments encourage food manufacturers to fortify commonly eaten foods, such as sugar and margarine, with vitamin A.

The results of animal studies suggest that women who are vitamin A deficient during pregnancy may give birth to infants with circulatory, urinary, skeletal, and nervous system defects.[14] However, pregnant women should not take vitamin A supplements to prevent birth defects without consulting with their physicians. When taken during pregnancy, excess vitamin A is a **teratogen,** an agent that causes birth defects.

Vitamin A Toxicity   The UL for vitamin A intake is 3000 mcg/day for adults. Excessive consumption of vitamin A can damage the liver, because the organ is the main site for vitamin A storage. Toxicity signs and symptoms include headache, nausea, vomiting, visual disturbances, hair loss, bone pain, and bone fractures.

Miscarriage and birth defects may result when excessive amounts of vitamin A are taken early in pregnancy. Women of childbearing age should limit their overall intake of vitamin A to about 100% of the Daily Value (5000 IU). In addition, women who may become pregnant or who are pregnant should restrict their intake of rich food sources of vitamin A, such as liver and fish liver oils.

Carotenemia (*kar'-et-eh-ne'-me-ah*), a condition characterized by yellowing of the skin, can result from eating too much beta-carotene-rich produce or taking too many beta-carotene supplements. This condition occasionally develops in infants who eat a lot of baby foods that contain carrots, apricots, winter squash, or green beans.[15] In most instances, carotenemia is harmless. The skin's natural color eventually returns to normal when the carotenoid-rich foods are no longer eaten.

keratin tough protein found in hair, nails, and the outermost layers of skin

xerophthalmia condition affecting the eyes that results from vitamin A deficiency

teratogen an agent that causes birth defects

carotenemia yellowing of the skin that results from excess beta-carotene in the body

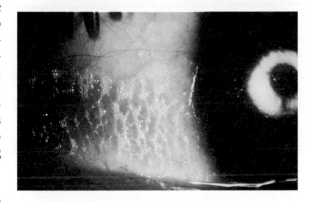

Figure 8.10 Early sign of xerophthalmia. Vitamin A deficiency can cause drying of the surface of the eye. The white foamy areas are signs of such dryness. If untreated, this condition can lead to blindness.

Did You Know?

In the early 1900s, teams of explorers raced to discover and explore the North and South Poles. Starvation was a major risk of embarking on such expeditions. Some explorers learned survival techniques from the Inuits, an Eskimo population who inhabit the Arctic region of North America. The Inuits warned the explorers to avoid eating polar bear and seal livers because severe illness and death could result. Unfortunately, many Western explorers did not know that their sled dogs were also not safe for human consumption.

From 1911 to 1913, Douglas Mawson and Xavier Mertz were on an ill-fated expedition to explore an area near the South Pole. As the two men struggled to return to their winter base camp, they had to eat their sled dogs, particularly the animals' livers, to avoid starvation. Both men suffered terribly from the diet; Mertz did not survive. Over 50 years later, scientists determined that sled dogs can accumulate large amounts of vitamin A in their livers without showing ill effects. However, eating just a few ounces of sled dog liver can be toxic for humans.

Physicians may prescribe medications derived from vitamin A, such as isotretinoin (Retin-A), to treat severe acne and other skin disorders. Although these medications are less toxic than natural vitamin A, ingesting excessive amounts can produce harmful symptoms. Furthermore, vitamin A derivatives can cause miscarriage or severe birth defects in the offspring of women who use them during pregnancy. Therefore, women of childbearing age should avoid pregnancy while using these medications.

Vitamin D

By the 1700s, some people in parts of northern Europe had learned that exposing children to sunlight or giving the youngsters fish liver oil could prevent or treat **rickets.** Children with rickets have bones that are soft and can become misshapen. Leg bones, for example, bow under the weight of carrying the upper part of the body (Fig. 8.11). Additionally, the affected child's joints, rib cage, and hips (pelvis) become deformed, and the child may complain of muscle pain. In 1922, scientists discovered a fat-soluble factor in cod liver oil that was needed for proper bone health and preventing rickets. The scientists thought the factor that cured rickets was a vitamin, and they named the substance *vitamin D.* The fat-soluble factor in cod liver oil is still considered a vitamin, because rickets can be prevented and treated by taking vitamin D supplements or eating vitamin D–rich foods. However, vitamin D is actually a hormone.

The body can make vitamin D when skin cells are exposed to the sun's ultraviolet radiation (*UVB*, in particular), which explains why the nutrient is often called the "sunshine vitamin." The radiation converts a substance in skin that is derived from cholesterol into a prohormone (*vitamin D_3*). Vitamin D_3 circulates to the liver where the substance is converted to the inactive compound *25-OH vitamin D*. Eventually, the kidneys convert *25-OH vitamin D* into the active hormone we call "vitamin D" (Fig. 8.12).

Why Is Vitamin D Necessary?

Vitamin D is necessary for the metabolism of the minerals calcium and phosphorus, and the production and maintenance of healthy bones. Vitamin D also stimulates small intestinal cells to absorb calcium and phosphorus from food. When vitamin D is lacking, the

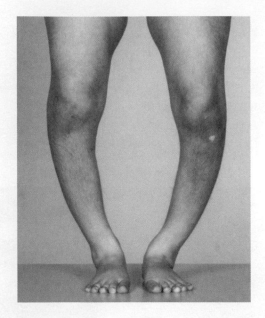

Figure 8.11 Rickets. A child suffering from rickets has soft bones that do not grow properly. The youngster's leg bones bow under the weight of carrying the upper part of the body, and his or her joints, rib cage, and hips (pelvis) also become deformed.

rickets vitamin D deficiency disorder in children

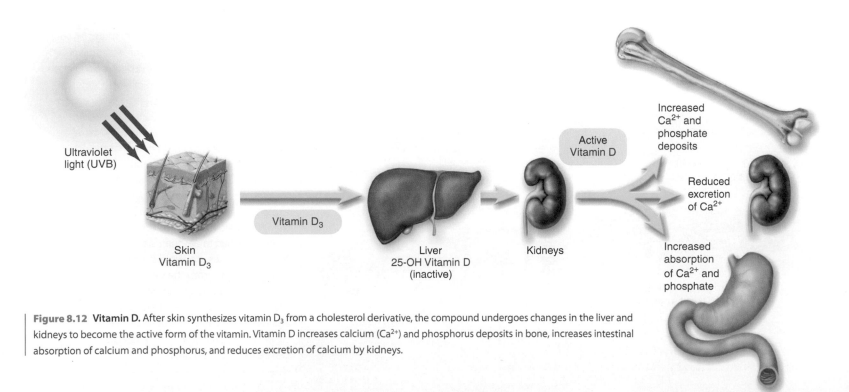

Figure 8.12 Vitamin D. After skin synthesizes vitamin D_3 from a cholesterol derivative, the compound undergoes changes in the liver and kidneys to become the active form of the vitamin. Vitamin D increases calcium (Ca^{2+}) and phosphorus deposits in bone, increases intestinal absorption of calcium and phosphorus, and reduces excretion of calcium by kidneys.

intestine absorbs only 10 to 15% of the calcium in foods; with the vitamin, intestinal absorption of dietary calcium increases to 30 to 80%.[16] Vitamin D also stimulates bone cells to form *calcium phosphate*, the major mineral compound in bone. Without adequate vitamin D, bone cells cannot deposit enough calcium and phosphorus to produce strong bones (see Fig. 8.12).

When blood calcium levels drop, vitamin D works with *parathyroid hormone* (*PTH*) to signal bones to release calcium. PTH also stimulates the kidneys to increase vitamin D production and decrease the elimination of calcium in urine. These actions help raise the level of calcium in blood to normal (Fig. 8.13). Removing too much calcium from bones can weaken them, but calcium is essential for normal heartbeat and other muscle contractions. If bones did not supply calcium for such vital functions, a person could experience serious, even fatal consequences.

Vitamin D has other roles in the body, including regulating neuromuscular and immune function and reducing inflammation.[17] Vitamin D is also involved in controlling cell growth, and as a result, the micronutrient may reduce the risk of certain cancers. However, more research is needed to clarify the vitamin's role in immune function and disease prevention.

Sources of Vitamin D

Fish liver oils and fatty fish, especially salmon, herring, and catfish, are among the few foods that naturally contain vitamin D. Milk is routinely fortified with vitamin D, and some brands of ready-to-eat cereals, orange juice, and margarine have the vitamin added to them as well. Table 8.4 lists some food sources of vitamin D. Food composition tables often list the vitamin D content of foods in International Units; 1 mcg of vitamin D equals 40 IU.

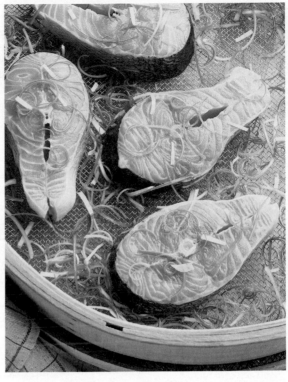

Salmon is a good source of vitamin D.

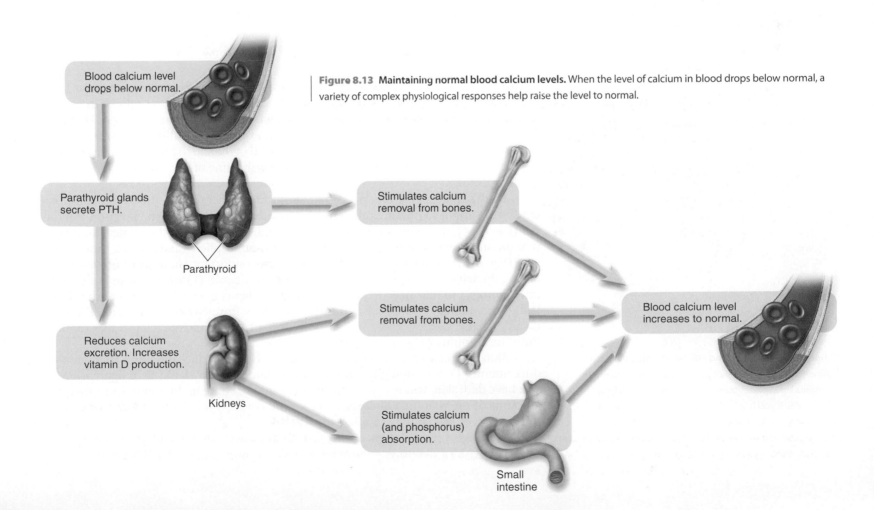

Figure 8.13 Maintaining normal blood calcium levels. When the level of calcium in blood drops below normal, a variety of complex physiological responses help raise the level to normal.

Blood calcium level drops below normal.

Parathyroid glands secrete PTH.

Parathyroid

Reduces calcium excretion. Increases vitamin D production.

Kidneys

Stimulates calcium removal from bones.

Stimulates calcium removal from bones.

Stimulates calcium (and phosphorus) absorption.

Small intestine

Blood calcium level increases to normal.

TABLE 8.4 *Vitamin D Content of Selected Foods*

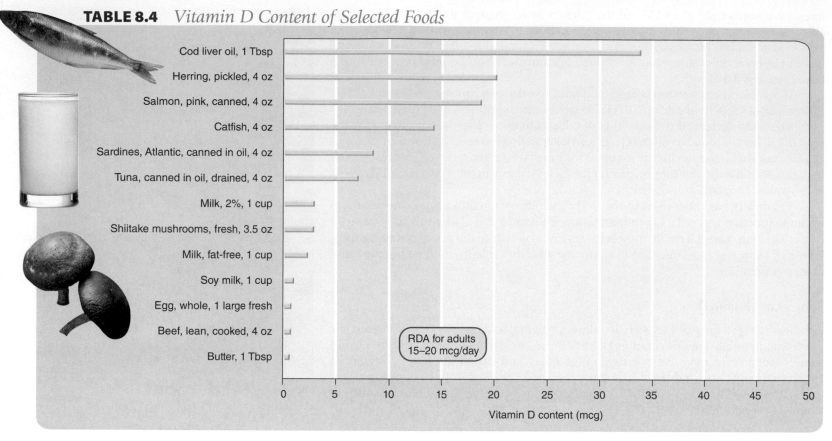

Food	Vitamin D content (mcg)

Cod liver oil, 1 Tbsp
Herring, pickled, 4 oz
Salmon, pink, canned, 4 oz
Catfish, 4 oz
Sardines, Atlantic, canned in oil, 4 oz
Tuna, canned in oil, drained, 4 oz
Milk, 2%, 1 cup
Shiitake mushrooms, fresh, 3.5 oz
Milk, fat-free, 1 cup
Soy milk, 1 cup
Egg, whole, 1 large fresh
Beef, lean, cooked, 4 oz
Butter, 1 Tbsp

RDA for adults
15–20 mcg/day

Vitamin D content (mcg)

Source: Data from U.S. Department of Agriculture, Human Nutrition Information Service: *Provisional table on the vitamin D content of foods.* HNIS/PT-108, 1991, Revised 1999.

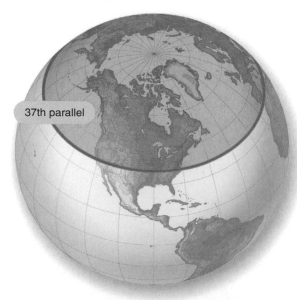

37th parallel

Figure 8.14 Latitude and vitamin D status. In North America, the 37th parallel extends from about southern Virginia through southern Missouri to San Francisco, California. If you live in North America south of the 37th parallel and are outdoors when sunlight is most intense during the day, you are likely to obtain enough sun exposure to synthesize vitamin D most of the year.

Vitamin D and Sunlight   Vitamin D is not widespread in food; therefore, your body depends on sun exposure to synthesize the vitamin. If you live south of the 37th parallel and are outdoors for about 5 to 30 minutes when sunlight is most intense (between 10 A.M. and 3 P.M.), you may obtain enough sun exposure to synthesize vitamin D most of the year.[17] The amount of time you need to spend in the sun to form adequate amounts of vitamin D depends primarily on your location, the time of day and year, and your age and skin color.

Earth's atmosphere blocks UV radiation. In North America, the 37th parallel extends from about southern Virginia through southern Missouri to San Francisco, California (Fig. 8.14). If you live north of the 37th parallel, the angle of the winter sun is such that the sun's rays must pass through more of the atmosphere than at other times of the year (Fig. 8.15). As a result, your skin cannot make sufficient amounts of provitamin D during the winter, and you may not have adequate vitamin D stored in your body to last until spring. You may need to take a supplement that contains 100% of the adult Daily Value for vitamin D (400 IU or 10 mcg), especially from November through February. Clouds, shade, window glass, and air pollution are environmental factors that can also limit the amount of UV radiation that reaches your skin.

Skin contains *melanin*, the brown pigment that can reduce the skin's ability to produce vitamin D from sunlight. Darker skin contains more melanin than lighter skin. If you have dark skin, you may need to spend even more time in the sun to form adequate amounts of the vitamin. Otherwise, you should consider consuming foods that contain the vitamin or a vitamin D supplement regularly.

Although you may think tanned skin is attractive, tanning and severe sunburn increase the risk of developing wrinkles and skin cancer. Ultraviolet (UV) radiation is a

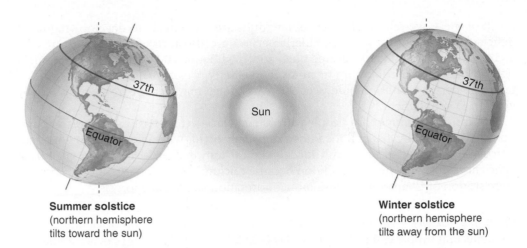

Summer solstice
(northern hemisphere
tilts toward the sun)

Sun

Winter solstice
(northern hemisphere
tilts away from the sun)

Figure 8.15 Seasonal variations in sunlight intensity. If you live north of the 37th parallel, the angle of the winter sun is such that the sun's rays must pass through more of the atmosphere than at other times of the year. As a result, skin tends to form less prohormone vitamin D in the winter.

major risk factor for skin cancer, including melanoma, the most deadly form of skin cancer. Dermatologists often advise people to apply sunscreens consistently before going outdoors. Using a sunscreen, however, limits skin's ability to synthesize prohormone vitamin D₃. When properly applied, a sunscreen with a *sun protection factor* (*SPF*) of 8 or more blocks sunlight that is needed to form the prohormone.[17] To allow your body to synthesize some vitamin D, you can expose your skin to the sun for about 15 minutes *before* applying a commercial sunscreen. Concerns about the risk of skin cancer have made it difficult for scientists to develop guidelines for the amount of sunlight exposure that is necessary to optimize vitamin D synthesis.

Did You Know?

Information provided by tanning parlors may include claims that the tanning process is safe. Nevertheless, the ultraviolet radiation emitted by tanning beds increases the risk of wrinkles and skin cancer. Therefore, the use of tanning beds should be avoided.

Dietary Adequacy

For adults under 70 years of age, the RDA for vitamin D is 15 mcg/day. Many Americans do not consume enough vitamin D to meet the RDA.[9] Nevertheless, blood levels of vitamin D were, on average, within the adequate range, according to findings of a nationwide survey conducted in 2005–2006.[17] Younger people generally have higher blood levels of the vitamin than older adults.

In the United States, a national effort to fortify milk with vitamin D began in the 1930s, and as a result, rickets became rare in this country. Although severe rickets is uncommon, public health officials are concerned about the recent increase in the number of cases reported among infants and toddlers. Breast milk contains insufficient amounts of vitamin D to prevent rickets. Infants who are most likely to develop rickets are breastfed, and they have dark skin, minimal sunlight exposure, and little or no vitamin D intake.[17] Exposing breastfed babies to sunlight reduces their risk of the disease, but as mentioned earlier, medical experts do not know how much sun exposure is necessary. Thus, breastfed infants should consume a supplement containing 10 mcg (400 IU) of vitamin D per day soon after birth. The adult form of rickets is called **osteomalacia** (*ahs'-tee-o-mah-lay'-she-a*). The bones of people with osteomalacia have normal amounts of *collagen*, the protein that provides structure for the skeleton, but they contain less-than-normal amounts of calcium. The bones are soft and weak, and break easily as a result. Muscle weakness is also a symptom of osteomalacia.

Adults who are confined indoors or almost fully covered during the day, such as for religious reasons, are at risk for osteomalacia (Fig. 8.16).[17] Osteomalacia is a risk for adults who have kidney, liver, or intestinal diseases, because these conditions may reduce both vitamin D production and calcium absorption. Exposing skin to sunlight, eating vitamin D–rich foods, or taking vitamin D supplements can help adults avoid vitamin D deficiency and osteomalacia.

As a person ages, production of prohormone vitamin D₃ in skin declines and conversion of the prohormone to active vitamin D in kidneys also decreases. As a

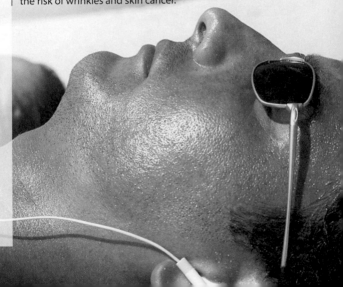

Exposure to ultraviolet radiation from the sun can increase the risk of wrinkles and skin cancer.

result of these age-related changes, older adults are more likely to develop vitamin D deficiency than younger persons. Elderly persons are also at risk for bone fractures. An analysis of several studies indicated older adults who took 700 to 800 IUs of vitamin D per day had a lower risk of hip fractures than elderly persons who took 400 IUs of vitamin D per day. Thus, people over 50 years of age may benefit from using a daily vitamin D supplement.[18]

It is not uncommon for people with osteomalacia to also have *osteoporosis*, a condition characterized by loss of bone mass that usually occurs with aging.[19] Although osteoporosis is usually associated with inadequate calcium intakes, a long-term vitamin D deficiency contributes to the condition because calcium absorption is reduced.[17] The calcium section of Chapter 9 provides more information about osteoporosis.

Vitamin D Toxicity   The body stores vitamin D. Long-term ingestion of vitamin D supplements that supply 250 to 1250 mcg/day (10,000 to 50,000 IU/day) can accumulate in the body and produce toxicity.[17] When excess vitamin D is consumed, the small intestine absorbs too much calcium from foods and the mineral is deposited in soft tissues, including the kidneys, heart, and blood vessels. The calcium deposits can interfere with cells' ability to function and cause cellular death. Other signs and symptoms of vitamin D toxicity include muscular weakness, loss of appetite, diarrhea, vomiting, and mental confusion. You do not have to be concerned about your body making toxic levels of vitamin D when exposed to sunlight, because skin limits its production of prohormone vitamin D$_3$. The Upper Limit (UL) for vitamin D is 100 mcg/day (4000 IU/day).

Vitamin E

Vitamin E has several forms, but only the *alpha-tocopherol* (*al'-fah toe-koff'-e-roll*) form is maintained in plasma and used by the body.[20] **Alpha-tocopherol** (*vitamin E*) protects polyunsaturated fatty acids in cell membranes from being damaged by radicals (Fig. 8.17). Such oxidative damage may be associated with the development of atherosclerosis, the process that occurs within arteries and contributes to heart attack and stroke; cancer; and premature cellular aging and death. Other roles for vitamin E include maintaining nervous tissue and immune system function.

Food Sources of Vitamin E

Rich food sources of vitamin E include sunflower seeds, almonds, and plant oils, especially sunflower, safflower, canola, and olive oils. Products made from vitamin E–rich plant oils—margarine and salad dressings—also supply the micronutrient. Other important dietary sources of the vitamin include fish, whole grains, nuts, seeds, and certain vegetables. Meats, processed grain products, and dairy products generally do not contain much vitamin E. Table 8.5 lists some common foods that are sources of the micronutrient.

Harvesting, processing, storage, and cooking methods influence the amount of vitamin E retained in food. During the milling process, most of the vitamin E that is in whole grains is lost, and it is not restored by enrichment. Furthermore, vitamin E is highly susceptible to destruction by exposure to oxygen, metals, and light, as well as high temperatures that occur when heating oil for deep-fat frying.

Dietary Adequacy

For adults, the RDA for vitamin E is 15 mg/day of alpha-tocopherol. Although many American adults do not consume recommended amounts of vitamin E, vitamin E deficiency is rare.[20] A healthy body stores the vitamin in body fat, skeletal muscle, and the liver.

Amounts of vitamin E may be reported as a number of IUs. One mg of alpha-tocopherol is about 1.5 IU of the natural form of the vitamin. Synthetic vitamin E is used to fortify foods and produce supplements that contain the vitamin. One mg of vitamin E is equal to 2.22 IU of the synthetic form of the vitamin.[20]

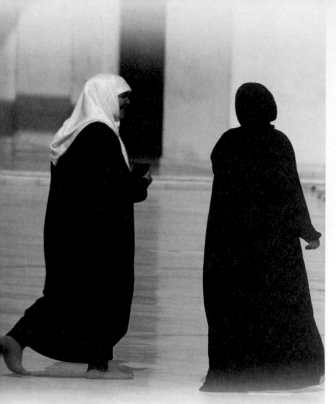

Figure 8.16 Clothing and vitamin D status. Adults who are almost fully covered during the day, such as for religious reasons, are at risk for osteomalacia.

osteomalacia adult rickets; condition characterized by poorly mineralized (soft) bones

alpha-tocopherol vitamin E

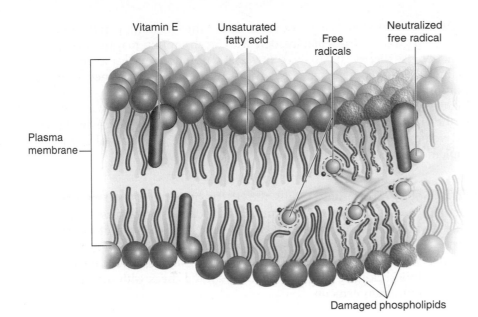

Vitamin E   Unsaturated fatty acid   Free radicals   Neutralized free radical

Plasma membrane

Damaged phospholipids

Figure 8.17 Vitamin E and the cell membrane. Vitamin E protects unsaturated fatty acids in cell membranes from being damaged by radicals.

Vitamin E Deficiency A vitamin E deficiency can result in red blood cell (RBC) membranes that are vulnerable to damage by oxidizing agents. When damaged, RBC membranes break easily, and the cells undergo **hemolysis** (*hemo* = blood; *lysis* = disintegrate), that is, they break apart and die. Hemolysis can cause **anemia,** a disorder characterized by

TABLE 8.5 *Vitamin E Content of Selected Foods*

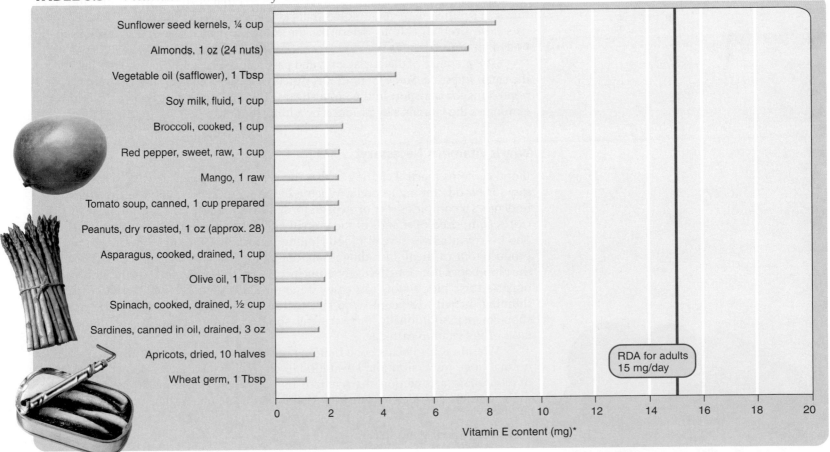

Sunflower seed kernels, ¼ cup
Almonds, 1 oz (24 nuts)
Vegetable oil (safflower), 1 Tbsp
Soy milk, fluid, 1 cup
Broccoli, cooked, 1 cup
Red pepper, sweet, raw, 1 cup
Mango, 1 raw
Tomato soup, canned, 1 cup prepared
Peanuts, dry roasted, 1 oz (approx. 28)
Asparagus, cooked, drained, 1 cup
Olive oil, 1 Tbsp
Spinach, cooked, drained, ½ cup
Sardines, canned in oil, drained, 3 oz
Apricots, dried, 10 halves
Wheat germ, 1 Tbsp

RDA for adults 15 mg/day

Vitamin E content (mg)*

*As alpha-tocopherol.
Source: Data from U.S. Department of Agriculture, Agricultural Research Service, USDA Nutrient Data Laboratory: Vitamin E (alpha-tocopherol) (mg) content of selected foods by common measure, sorted by nutrient content. *USDA national nutrient database for standard reference, release 18.* 2004.

hemolysis disintegration of red blood cells

anemia disorder characterized by too few red blood cells

too few RBCs. Vitamin E deficiency can also reduce the functioning of the immune system. People who have diseases that interfere with fat absorption may become deficient in vitamin E, because dietary fat enhances intestinal absorption of the micronutrient. Long-term vitamin E deficiency damages the nervous system and results in nerve damage, loss of neuromuscular control, and blindness.[20]

Infants who are born too early (premature infants) may have low vitamin E stores, because the vitamin is transferred from mother to fetus late in pregnancy. If premature infants develop signs of vitamin E deficiency, they can be given special infant formulas and supplements that provide the vitamin.

Vitamin E Toxicity For healthy adults, the UL for vitamin E is 1000 mg/day of alpha-tocopherol. Consuming amounts of vitamin E in foods has not been associated with any negative effects on health.[20] However, taking dietary supplements that supply excessive amounts of the vitamin may interfere with vitamin K's role in blood clotting and lead to uncontrolled bleeding (hemorrhage). Therefore, people who are taking medications that interfere with blood clotting ("blood thinners") should check with their physicians before using vitamin E supplements.

Vitamin K

In the early 1930s, Danish researcher Henrick Dam discovered a factor in alfalfa that played a role in blood clotting (coagulation). Dam named the factor vitamin "K" after *koagulation*, the Danish spelling of coagulation. Vitamin K is a family of compounds that includes *phylloquinone* (fill-o-kwin'-own) from plants and *menaquinones* (men-eh-kwin'-owns) in fish oils and meat. Bacteria that normally live in the large intestine also synthesize menaquinones that can be absorbed by the body. However, scientists have been unable to determine the extent to which bacteria contribute to the body's vitamin K supply.[21]

The presence of dietary fat, bile, and pancreatic juice help vitamin K be absorbed in the small intestine. Some vitamin K is stored in the liver and some is incorporated in lipoproteins for transport in the bloodstream. The liver also breaks down vitamin K and eliminates the vitamin's by-products by adding them to bile.

Why Is Vitamin K Necessary?

Blood contains inactive clotting factors and cell fragments called *platelets* that are necessary for blood clotting to occur. When a blood vessel is cut, blood in the injured area undergoes a complex series of steps to form a clot that stops the bleeding (Fig. 8.18). A clot is comprised of strands of the protein *fibrin* that traps blood cells, forming a mesh. The liver synthesizes several blood-clotting factors, and the organ needs vitamin K to produce four of them, including *prothrombin*, properly. When vitamin K is unavailable, the blood does not clot effectively. Some people take the prescribed medication warfarin because their blood clots too easily. Vitamin K can interfere with warfarin's "blood-thinning" activity, so people who take the medication should not consume vitamin K supplements. Additionally, these patients should try to maintain consistent dietary intakes of the vitamin each day.

Vitamin K also helps bone-building cells produce *osteocalcin*, a protein needed for normal bone mineralization. Low blood levels of vitamin K are associated with the risk of *osteoporosis*, a condition characterized by bones with low mineral density. However, more research is needed to clarify the vitamin's role in bone health.

Food Sources of Vitamin K

Major food sources of vitamin K are green leafy vegetables such as kale, turnip greens, salad greens, cabbage, and spinach; broccoli; and green beans. Other reliable sources of

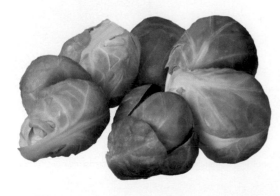

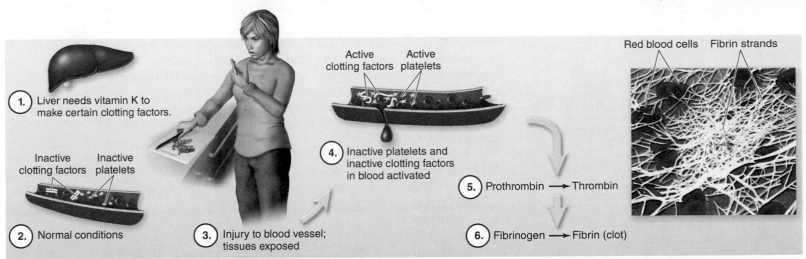

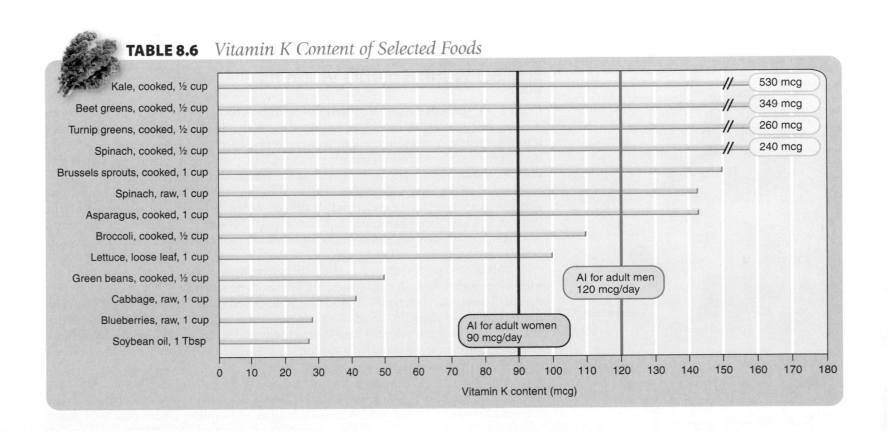

Figure 8.18 Vitamin K and blood clotting. When a blood vessel is cut, blood in the injured area undergoes a series of steps to form a clot that stops the bleeding. The liver needs vitamin K to make prothrombin and three other blood-clotting factors.

the vitamin are soybean and canola oils, and products made from these oils, such as margarine and salad dressing. Table 8.6 lists some foods that are sources of the vitamin. The chemical structure of vitamin K is very stable and resists being destroyed by usual cooking methods.

Dietary Adequacy

No RDAs for vitamin K have been established, but AIs for the vitamin are 120 mcg/day for men and 90 mcg/day for women. The AIs can be met easily be eating a salad that contains 1 cup of leafy vegetables and 2 tablespoons of salad dressing made with soybean oil.

TABLE 8.6 *Vitamin K Content of Selected Foods*

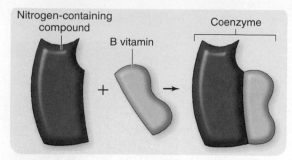

Figure 8.19 Coenzyme. To synthesize a coenzyme, cells combine a B vitamin with a nitrogen-containing, nonprotein compound.

coenzyme ion or small molecule that interacts with enzymes, enabling the enzymes to function

Figure 8.20 Coenzyme action. Many enzymes need coenzymes to function. This illustration shows a coenzyme activating an enzyme, which enables it to split a substrate into two parts.

Vitamin K: Deficiency and Toxicity Although the body stores very little vitamin K, deficiencies among adults rarely occur.[21] Vitamin K deficiency, however, can develop in people who have liver diseases or conditions that impair fat absorption, such as cystic fibrosis. Additionally, long-term antibiotic therapy can reduce the number of bacteria in the colon that synthesize vitamin K and, as a result, contribute to a deficiency of the nutrient. The most reliable sign of vitamin K deficiency is an increase in the time it takes for blood to clot.

Babies are generally born with low vitamin K stores, and a deficiency of the vitamin can occur soon after birth. Vitamin K–deficient infants are at risk of serious bleeding because their bodies are unable to make certain blood-clotting factors. To prevent vitamin K deficiency from developing during infancy, newborns generally receive a single injection of vitamin K.

Ingesting amounts of vitamin K that exceed the AIs has not been reported to be harmful to humans. Therefore, members of the Food and Nutrition Board did not set a UL for the micronutrient.

Concept **Checkpoint**

6. Prepare a table for fat-soluble vitamins. For each vitamin, indicate its major function in the body, major food sources, deficiency disorder (if it has a specific name), and major signs and symptoms of the deficiency disorder. If the vitamin is known to be toxic, also indicate major toxicity signs and symptoms. Check your table against the information provided in Table 8.2.

8.3 Water-Soluble Vitamins

In the body, most water-soluble vitamins function as components of specific coenzymes. A **coenzyme** is a *cofactor*, an ion or small molecule that interacts with enzymes and, as a result, regulates a chemical reaction. To synthesize a coenzyme, cells combine one of the B vitamins with a nitrogen-containing, nonprotein compound (Fig. 8.19). When activated by the coenzyme, the enzyme enables the reaction to occur (Fig. 8.20).

Many of the chemical reactions involved in the metabolism of carbohydrates, fats, and amino acids involve coenzymes that contain B vitamins. Thiamin, riboflavin, niacin, vitamin B-6, and pantothenic acid function as part of coenzymes involved in energy metabolism. Coenzymes containing these vitamins are also necessary for synthesizing glucose, amino acids, and certain lipids.

Foods contain B vitamins in their coenzyme forms. Health-food stores often sell supplements that contain coenzymes, but buying these products is a waste of money. In the small intestine, coenzymes in food or supplements are not absorbed intact. The compounds undergo digestion to release their B vitamin components. The small intestine absorbs many of the B vitamins that were in foods and supplements, and the micronutrients eventually enter the general circulation. Cells then remove the free vitamins from the bloodstream and use them to rebuild coenzymes.

This section of Chapter 8 focuses on seven water-soluble vitamins: thiamin, riboflavin, niacin, B-6, folate, B-12, and C. Table 8.7 provides a summary of general information about all the water-soluble vitamins and choline. Unless otherwise noted,

TABLE 8.7 *Summary of Water-Soluble Vitamins and Choline*

Vitamin	Major Functions in the Body	Adult RDA/AI (adult RDA = bold)	Major Dietary Sources	Major Deficiency Signs and Symptoms	Major Toxicity Signs and Symptoms
Thiamin	Part of coenzyme needed for carbohydrate metabolism and the metabolism of certain amino acids; may help produce neurotransmitters	**1.1–1.2 mg**	Pork, wheat germ, enriched breads and cereals, brewer's yeast	Beriberi and Wernicke-Korsakoff syndrome: Weakness, abnormal nervous system functioning	None (Upper limit [UL] not determined)
Riboflavin	Part of coenzymes needed for carbohydrate, amino acid, and lipid metabolism	**1.1–1.3 mg**	Milk, yogurt, and other milk products; enriched breads and cereals; liver	Inflammation of the mouth and tongue, eye disorders	None (UL not determined)
Niacin	Part of coenzymes needed for energy metabolism	**14–16 mg**	Enriched breads and cereals, beef, liver, tuna, salmon, poultry, pork, mushrooms	Pellagra: • Diarrhea • Dermatitis • Dementia • Death	**Adult UL = 35 mg/ day** Flushing of facial skin, itchy skin, nausea and vomiting, liver damage
Pantothenic acid	Part of the coenzyme that is needed for synthesizing fat and releasing energy from macronutrients	5 mg	Beef and chicken liver, sunflower seeds, mushrooms, yogurt, soy milk, fortified cereals	Rarely occurs	Unknown (UL not determined)
Biotin	Cofactor needed for synthesizing glucose and fatty acids	30 mcg	Liver, eggs, peanuts, salmon, pork, mushrooms, sunflower seeds	Rarely occurs: Skin rash, hair loss, convulsions, and other neurological disorders; developmental delays in infants	Unknown (UL not determined)
Vitamin B-6	Part of coenzyme needed for amino acid metabolism, involved in neurotransmitter and hemoglobin synthesis	**1.3–1.7 mg**	Meat, fish, and poultry; potatoes, bananas, spinach, sweet red peppers, broccoli	Dermatitis, anemia, depression, confusion, and neurological disorders such as convulsions	**Adult UL = 100 mg/ day** Nerve destruction
Folate	Part of coenzyme needed for DNA synthesis and conversion of cysteine to methionine, preventing homocysteine accumulation	**400 mcg DFE**	Dark green, leafy vegetables, liver, legumes, asparagus, broccoli, orange juice, enriched breads and cereals (folic acid)	Megaloblastic anemia, diarrhea, neural tube defects in embryos	**Adult UL = 1000 mcg/day** May stimulate cancer cell growth
Vitamin B-12	Part of coenzymes needed for various cellular processes, including folate metabolism; maintenance of myelin sheaths	**2.4 mcg**	Animal foods, fortified cereals, fortified soy milk	Pernicious anemia: megaloblastic anemia and nerve damage resulting in paralysis and death	None (UL not determined)
Ascorbic acid (vitamin C)	Connective tissue synthesis and maintenance; antioxidant; synthesis of neurotransmitters and certain hormones; immune system functioning	**75–90 mg** (nonsmokers)	Peppers, citrus fruits, papaya, broccoli, cabbage, berries	Scurvy: Poor wound healing, pinpoint hemorrhages, bleeding gums, bruises, depression	**Adult UL = 2000 mg/ day** Diarrhea and GI tract discomfort
Choline	Neurotransmitter and phospholipid synthesis; methionine metabolism	425–550 mg	Widely distributed in foods and human biosynthesis	Liver damage	Fishy body odor and reduced blood pressure

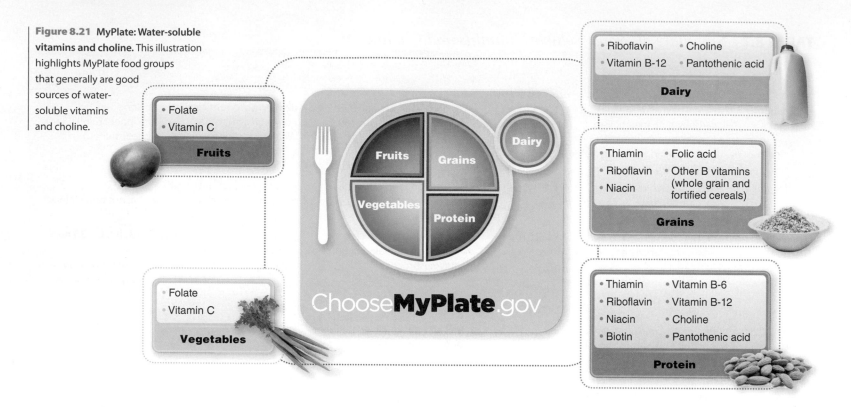

Figure 8.21 MyPlate: Water-soluble vitamins and choline. This illustration highlights MyPlate food groups that generally are good sources of water-soluble vitamins and choline.

beriberi thiamin deficiency disease

RDA/AI values are for adults 19 to 50 years of age, excluding pregnant or breastfeeding women. Figure 8.21 indicates food groups that are good sources of water-soluble vitamins.

Thiamin

In the body, thiamin is used to make a coenzyme that participates in chemical reactions involved in the release of energy from carbohydrates. Additionally, the thiamin-containing coenzyme plays a role in the metabolism of certain amino acids, and the coenzyme may be necessary for the synthesis of neurotransmitters. A neurotransmitter is a chemical produced by a nerve cell that enables the cell to communicate to other nerve cells.

Food Sources of Thiamin

Foods that contribute thiamin to American diets include whole-grain and enriched breads and cereals, pork, legumes, and orange juice. Brewer's yeast is a rich source of thiamin, but most Americans do not eat the product. Table 8.8 lists some common foods that are good sources of thiamin. Overcooking and cooking food in alkaline solutions can destroy thiamin.

Dietary Adequacy

The adult RDA for thiamin is 1.2 mg/day and 1.1 mg/day for men and women, respectively. There are no reports of toxicity from consuming high amounts of thiamin from food or supplements,[22] probably because the excess vitamin is readily excreted in urine. Thus, no UL has been established for thiamin.

The thiamin deficiency disease is called **beriberi.** People suffering from beriberi are very weak and have poor muscular coordination (Fig. 8.22). The severe lack of thiamin also negatively affects the functioning of the cardiovascular, digestive, and nervous systems.

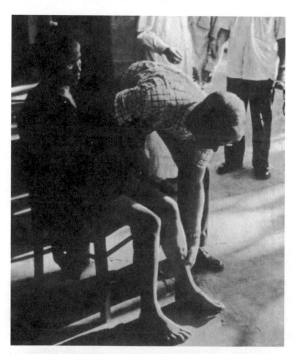

Figure 8.22 Beriberi. The woman sitting in the chair has a form of beriberi called "wet beriberi." In addition to suffering from fatigue and nervous system disorders, she has cardiovascular abnormalities that result in severe "pitting" edema in her lower legs.

TABLE 8.8 *Thiamin Content of Selected Foods*

Food	Thiamin content (mg)
Canned lean ham, 3 oz	0.9
Pork chops, 4 oz	0.6
Wheat germ, ¼ cup	0.5
Canadian bacon, 2 oz	0.5
Soy milk, 1 cup	0.4
Flour tortilla, 1	0.4
Fresh orange juice, 1 cup	0.2
Cooked green peas, ½ cup	0.2
Baked beans, ½ cup	0.2
Corn, ½ cup	0.2
White bread, enriched, 1 slice	0.1
Whole-wheat bread, enriched, 1 slice	0.1

RDA for adult women 1.1 mg/day

RDA for adult men 1.2 mg/day

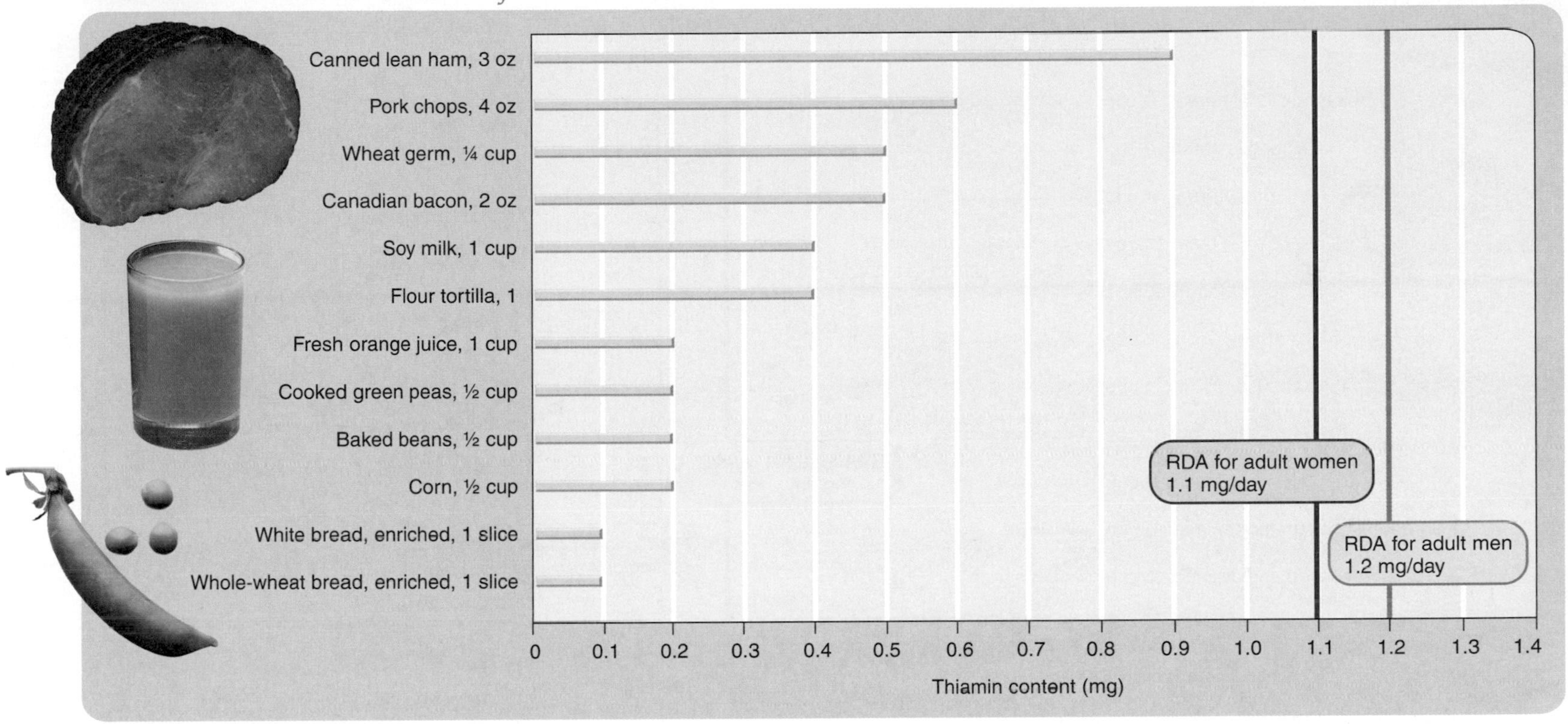

Source: Data from U.S. Department of Agriculture, Agricultural Research Service, USDA Nutrient Data Laboratory: Thiamin (mg) content of selected foods by common measure, sorted by nutrient content. *USDA national nutrient database for standard reference, release 18.* 2004.

In the United States, the degenerative brain disorder associated with thiamin deficiency is called **Wernicke-Korsakoff syndrome** (*vear'-nih-key kor'-sah-koff*). Most cases of Wernicke-Korsakoff syndrome occur in alcoholics, because alcohol reduces thiamin absorption and increases the vitamin's excretion. People with alcoholism also tend to have poor eating habits that contribute to deficiencies of thiamin and other vitamins. Signs of Wernicke-Korsakoff syndrome include abnormal eye movements, staggering gait, and distorted thought processes. Treatment involves avoiding alcohol and obtaining thiamin injections. Without prompt treatment, people with Wernicke-Korsakoff syndrome can become disabled permanently or die.

Wernicke-Korsakoff syndrome degenerative brain disorder resulting from thiamin deficiency that occurs primarily among alcoholics

Riboflavin

Riboflavin is a component of two coenzymes that play key roles in metabolism of carbohydrates, lipids, and amino acids. Milk, yogurt, and other milk products; enriched cereals; and liver are among the best sources of riboflavin. Mushrooms, broccoli, asparagus, and spinach and other green leafy vegetables also contain substantial amounts of the vitamin. Table 8.9 lists these and other food sources of riboflavin. Riboflavin's chemical structure is fairly stable, but exposure to light causes the vitamin to break down rapidly. Therefore, riboflavin-rich foods, such as milk and milk products, should not be packaged or stored in clear glass containers.

Dietary Adequacy

The RDA for riboflavin is 1.1 mg/day for women and 1.3 mg/day for men. The typical riboflavin intake of North Americans is about 1.5 mg/day for women and 2.1 mg/day for men.[22] In the United States, riboflavin deficiency rarely occurs, because many commonly

Did You Know?

Riboflavin is naturally yellow. If you take a dietary supplement that contains high amounts of riboflavin, your kidneys will excrete the excess, and you may notice the bright yellow color of your urine.

TABLE 8.9 *Riboflavin Content of Selected Foods*

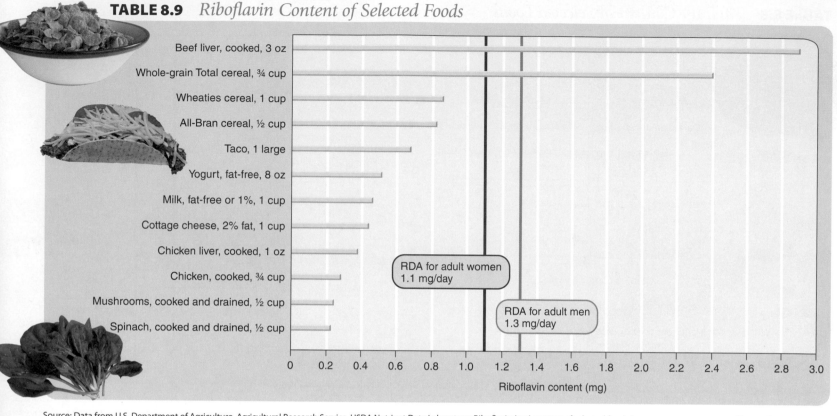

Source: Data from U.S. Department of Agriculture, Agricultural Research Service, USDA Nutrient Data Laboratory: Riboflavin (mg) content of selected foods by common measure, sorted by nutrient content. *USDA national nutrient database for standard reference, release 18*. 2004.

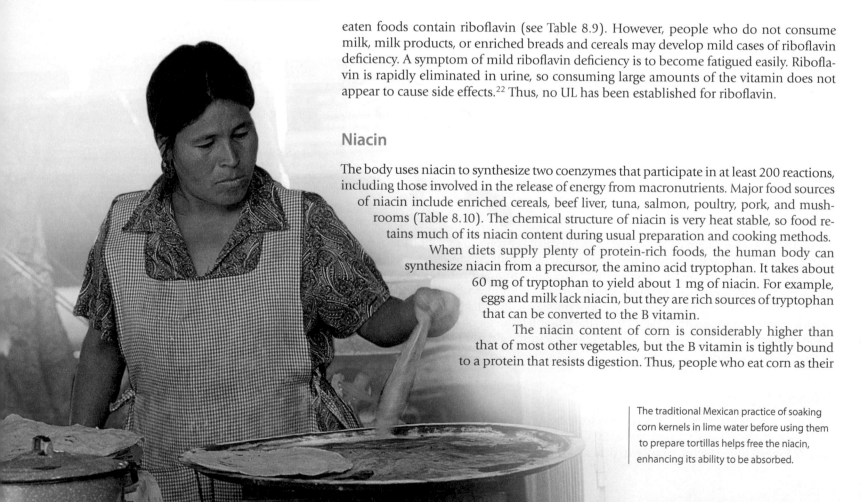

eaten foods contain riboflavin (see Table 8.9). However, people who do not consume milk, milk products, or enriched breads and cereals may develop mild cases of riboflavin deficiency. A symptom of mild riboflavin deficiency is to become fatigued easily. Riboflavin is rapidly eliminated in urine, so consuming large amounts of the vitamin does not appear to cause side effects.[22] Thus, no UL has been established for riboflavin.

Niacin

The body uses niacin to synthesize two coenzymes that participate in at least 200 reactions, including those involved in the release of energy from macronutrients. Major food sources of niacin include enriched cereals, beef liver, tuna, salmon, poultry, pork, and mushrooms (Table 8.10). The chemical structure of niacin is very heat stable, so food retains much of its niacin content during usual preparation and cooking methods.

When diets supply plenty of protein-rich foods, the human body can synthesize niacin from a precursor, the amino acid tryptophan. It takes about 60 mg of tryptophan to yield about 1 mg of niacin. For example, eggs and milk lack niacin, but they are rich sources of tryptophan that can be converted to the B vitamin.

The niacin content of corn is considerably higher than that of most other vegetables, but the B vitamin is tightly bound to a protein that resists digestion. Thus, people who eat corn as their

The traditional Mexican practice of soaking corn kernels in lime water before using them to prepare tortillas helps free the niacin, enhancing its ability to be absorbed.

TABLE 8.10 *Niacin Content of Selected Foods*

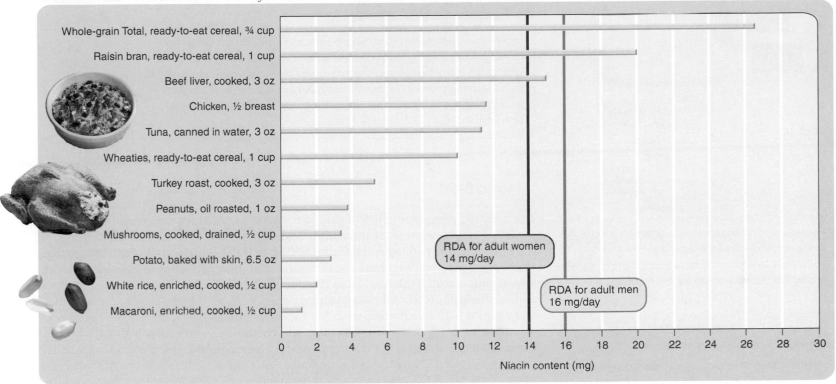

Source: Data from U.S. Department of Agriculture, Agricultural Research Service, USDA Nutrient Data Laboratory: Niacin (mg) content of selected foods by common measure, sorted by nutrient content. *USDA national nutrient database for standard reference, release 18.* 2004.

staple food are prone to develop pellagra. The traditional Mexican diet is corn based, but pellagra was not a widespread disease in Mexico when it was a major health concern in other parts of the world. Why? The Mexican practice of soaking corn kernels in lime water before using them to prepare tortillas helps free the niacin, enhancing its ability to be absorbed. In the United States, corn products such as hominy and grits are sources of niacin because they have been treated with lime before cooking.

Dietary Adequacy

The adult RDA for niacin is 14 to 16 mg/day. In the United States, people with alcoholism and those with rare disorders that disrupt tryptophan metabolism are generally the only groups at risk of niacin deficiency. Early signs and symptoms of mild niacin deficiency include poor appetite, weight loss, and weakness. If the affected person continues to consume a niacin-deficient diet, the condition worsens and **pellagra** (*peh-lah'-gra* or *peh-lay'-gra*) develops. The classic signs and symptoms of pellagra are dermatitis, diarrhea, dementia, and death—the "4 Ds of pellagra" (Fig. 8.23). In the early twentieth century, pellagra was widespread in the southeastern United States (see the introduction to Chapter 2). Today, the disease is rare in Western societies, but it still occurs among impoverished populations in developing countries, particularly in regions of Africa, India, and China.

The adult UL for niacin (nicotinic acid) is 35 mg/day. There have been no reports indicating that the niacin naturally in foods can cause toxicity.[22] Physicians may prescribe megadoses of nicotinic acid supplements to treat elevated blood cholesterol levels. However, patients taking such high doses of the vitamin may experience side effects such as facial flushing and even liver damage. The "Vitamins as Medicines" section of Chapter 8 discusses the use of niacin supplements to reduce cholesterol levels.

pellagra niacin deficiency disease

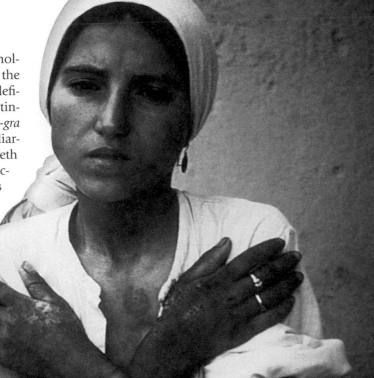

Figure 8.23 Pellagra. This person with pellagra shows one of the classic signs of the niacin deficiency disease—dermatitis, particularly on parts of the body exposed to sun.

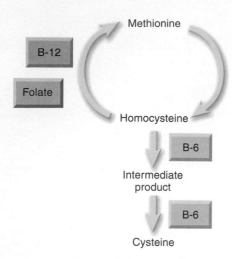

Homocysteine can be converted to cysteine, a nonessential amino acid, in reactions that depend on B-6-containing coenzymes. Methionine can be recycled from homocysteine in reactions that involve vitamins B-12 and folate.

homocysteine amino acid that is a toxic by-product of methionine metabolism

hemoglobin iron-containing protein in red blood cells that transports oxygen

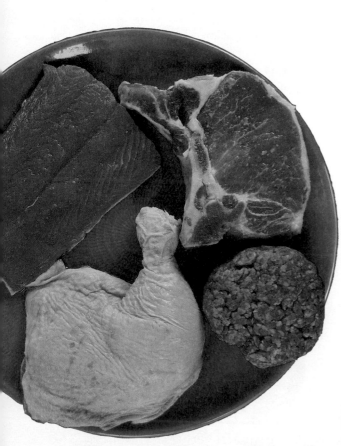

Meat, fish, and poultry are among the best dietary sources of vitamin B-6.

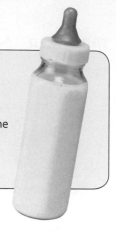

Did You Know?

In the early 1950s, some infants became unusually irritable and developed convulsions after being fed a commercial formula. It was determined that the vitamin B-6 in the formula had been destroyed by excessive heating during the manufacturing process. The convulsions may have resulted from a lack of neurotransmitters in the infants' brains. The babies were effectively treated with vitamin B-6.

Vitamin B-6

The body requires vitamin B-6 to make a coenzyme needed for amino acid metabolism, including the conversion of the amino acid tryptophan to niacin and transamination reactions that form nonessential amino acids (see Fig. 7.11). The coenzyme that contains vitamin B-6 also helps convert a toxic amino acid, **homocysteine,** to cysteine, a nonessential amino acid. If the body lacks vitamin B-6, homocysteine can accumulate in blood and may contribute to cardiovascular disease in some individuals (see Chapter 6). Folate and vitamin B-12 also participate in homocysteine metabolism.

During red blood cell production, the coenzyme participates in the synthesis of heme. Heme is the iron-containing portion of **hemoglobin,** the protein in RBCs that transports oxygen. If vitamin B-6 is unavailable for heme synthesis, a type of anemia develops. Vitamin B-6 is also involved in the synthesis of *neurotransmitters*, chemicals that nerves produce to transmit messages.

Food Sources of Vitamin B-6

Liver, meat, fish, and poultry are among the best dietary sources of vitamin B-6. Additionally, potatoes, bananas, spinach, sweet red peppers, and broccoli are good sources of vitamin B-6. During the refining process, the vitamin B-6 that is naturally in grains is lost, and the nutrient is not added back to the grain products during enrichment. However, many ready-to-eat and cooked cereals have been fortified with the vitamin. Table 8.11 lists some foods that are major sources of vitamin B-6. During cooking, excessive heat can cause major losses of the vitamin.

Dietary Adequacy

The adult RDAs for vitamin B-6 range from 1.3 to 1.7 mg/day. In the United States, the average adult consumes more than the RDA of the vitamin. Therefore, cases of vitamin B-6 deficiency are rare, but they can result from alcoholism or genetic conditions that affect vitamin B-6 metabolism. Signs and symptoms of vitamin B-6 deficiency include dermatitis, anemia, convulsions, depression, and confusion.

The adult UL for vitamin B-6 is 100 mg/day. Unlike most B vitamins, megadoses of vitamin B-6 are toxic.[23] The "Vitamins as Medicines" section of Chapter 8 provides information about vitamin B-6 toxicity.

Folate

"Folate" is the name for a group of related compounds that includes **folic acid** and **folacin.** Folic acid refers specifically to the synthetic form of the vitamin found in supplements and added to fortify foods. In the body, cells convert all forms of folate to a group of folate-containing coenzymes collectively called **tetrahydrofolic** (*the'-tra-hi-drow-foe-lik*) **acid** or simply **THFA.** THFA accepts a single-carbon group, such as CH_3, from one compound and transfers it to another substance. As a result, THFA participates in many

TABLE 8.11 *Vitamin B-6 Content of Selected Foods*

Food	Vitamin B-6 content (mg)
All-Bran, ready-to-eat cereal, ½ cup	(bar to ~3.6)
Tuna, yellowfin, cooked, 3 oz	~0.9
Beef liver, cooked, 3 oz	~0.9
Potato, baked, flesh and skin, 6.5 oz	~0.7
Chicken, cooked, ½ breast	~0.6
Beef, broiled, 3 oz	~0.5
Pork, cooked, 3 oz	~0.4
Salmon, sockeye, cooked, 5 oz	~0.3
Broccoli, cooked, 1 cup	~0.3
Banana, raw, ½ cup	~0.2
Sweet potato, canned, ½ cup	~0.2
Pinto beans, cooked, ½ cup	~0.2

RDA for adults 1.3 mg/day

RDA for adult women over 50 1.5 mg/day

RDA for adult men over 50 1.7 mg/day

Scale: 0, 0.5, 1.0, 1.5, 2.0, 2.5, 3.0, 3.5, 4.0

Source: Data from U.S. Department of Agriculture, Agricultural Research Service, USDA Nutrient Data Laboratory: Vitamin B-6 (mg) content of selected foods by common measure, sorted by nutrient content. *USDA national nutrient database for standard reference, release 18.* 2004.

chemical reactions involved in DNA synthesis and amino acid metabolism. As cells prepare to divide, they need THFA to make DNA.

Certain roles of folate and vitamin B-12 are interrelated. THFA can transfer a CH_3 group to vitamin B-12, which, in turn, transfers the CH_3 group to homocysteine, forming methionine (Fig. 8.24). This process recycles methionine. When vitamin B-12 is unavailable, folate cannot be used, and a deficiency of the vitamin occurs, even though dietary intakes of folate are adequate.

folic acid and **folacin** forms of folate

tetrahydrofolic acid (THFA) folate coenzyme

Food Sources of Folate

Leafy vegetables, liver, legumes, asparagus, broccoli, and orange juice are good sources of naturally occurring folate. The synthetic folic acid that is used to fortify or enrich food is better absorbed than naturally occurring forms of folate. Thus, enriched grain products and fortified cereals are among the richest sources of folate in the American diet. Enriched grain products currently supply U.S. adults with about 200 mcg folic acid/day—half the RDA.[9]

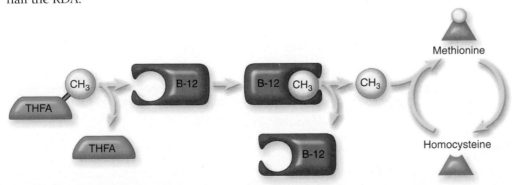

Figure 8.24 Folate and vitamin B-12: Working together.
This diagram shows how folate (THFA) works with vitamin B-12 to transfer a methyl group (CH_3).

The folate content of foods may be reported as micrograms of *dietary folate equivalents* (*DFEs*). DFE units account for differences in the body's ability to absorb folic acid and natural forms of folate. Table 8.12 lists the folate content of selected foods in micrograms of DFE.

Folate is extremely susceptible to destruction by heat, oxidation, and ultraviolet light. Food processing and preparation can destroy 50 to 90% of the folate in food. By eating fresh fruits and raw or lightly cooked vegetables, you are likely to obtain most of the foods' folate content.

Dietary Adequacy

The adult RDA for folate is 400 mcg (DFE)/day. In the United States, the prevalence of low blood levels of folate among people 4 years of age and older has declined significantly since 1988–1994.[24] Less than 1% of this population is deficient in folate. The risk of folate deficiency increases during periods of rapid growth, such as pregnancy, infancy, and childhood.[25]

Folate deficiency usually results from nutritionally inadequate diets, but excess alcohol consumption and use of certain medications can negatively affect the body's ability to absorb and use folate, resulting in deficiencies of the vitamin. Initially, folate deficiency affects cells that rapidly divide, such as red blood cells. Mature RBCs do not have nuclei, and they live for only about 4 months. Thus, the body must replace old or worn-out RBCs constantly. To keep up with their rapid rate of cell division, the precursor cells that mature into RBCs must actively synthesize DNA. Without folate, RBC precursor cells that reside in bone marrow enlarge, but they cannot divide normally, because they are unable to form new DNA. Bone marrow releases some of the abnormal RBCs into the bloodstream before they mature (Fig. 8.25). This condition, called megaloblastic (*mega =*

TABLE 8.12 *Folate Content of Selected Foods*

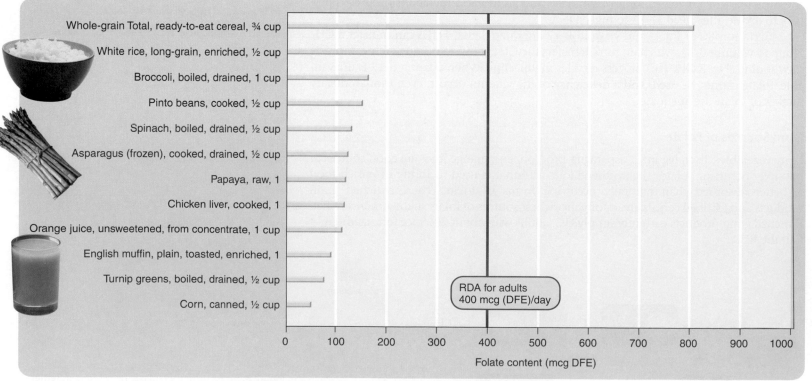

Source: Data from U.S. Department of Agriculture, Agricultural Research Service, USDA Nutrient Data Laboratory: Folate, DFE (µg) content of selected foods by common measure, sorted by nutrient content. *USDA national nutrient database for standard reference, release 18.* 2004.

large; *blast* = immature cell) anemia, is characterized by large, immature RBCs (*megalo-blasts*) that still have nuclei and do not carry normal amounts of oxygen.

Because many of folate's metabolic roles are related to those of vitamin B-12, diets that lack either vitamin produce a number of identical deficiency signs and symptoms. For example, being deficient in folate or vitamin B-12 can cause megaloblastic anemia. Therefore, a person with this type of anemia needs further analysis of his or her blood to determine which vitamin is lacking.

Although the folate naturally in foods does not appear to be toxic, the UL for the synthetic form of the vitamin (folic acid) is 1000 mcg/day. The UL was established because taking folic acid supplements can cure not only the anemia that occurs in folate deficiency but also the anemia that is a sign of vitamin B-12 deficiency. Folic acid supplementation, however, does not prevent the serious nervous system damage that accompanies the B-12 deficiency. Furthermore, some medical experts are concerned that taking folic acid supplements and consuming foods that contain the micronutrient may cause excess folic acid to accumulate in blood and produce negative health effects as a result.[76] Thus, more research is needed to determine whether ingesting too much folic acid poses health risks.

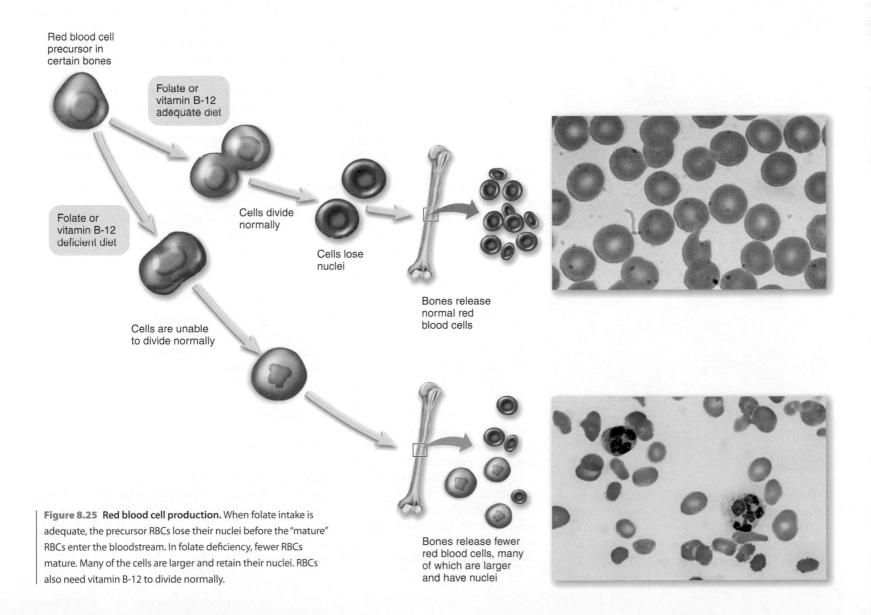

Red blood cell precursor in certain bones

Folate or vitamin B-12 adequate diet

Folate or vitamin B-12 deficient diet

Cells divide normally

Cells lose nuclei

Cells are unable to divide normally

Bones release normal red blood cells

Bones release fewer red blood cells, many of which are larger and have nuclei

Figure 8.25 Red blood cell production. When folate intake is adequate, the precursor RBCs lose their nuclei before the "mature" RBCs enter the bloodstream. In folate deficiency, fewer RBCs mature. Many of the cells are larger and retain their nuclei. RBCs also need vitamin B-12 to divide normally.

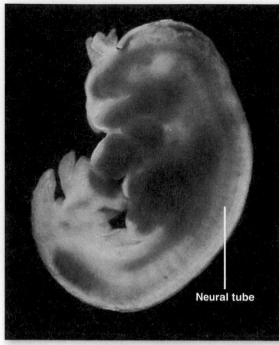

Neural tube

a.

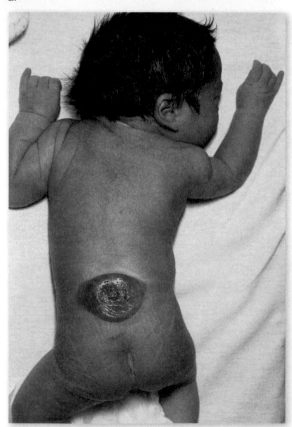

b.

Figure 8.26 **Neural tube defect.** (*a*) During the first few weeks after conception, the neural tube forms in the human embryo. (*b*) Infants born with severe spina bifida have a section of their spinal cord or a sac containing some spinal fluid bulging through their backs.

Neural Tube Defects   A woman's diet before and during pregnancy provides the raw materials for her developing offspring's needs as well as her body's needs. Not surprisingly, recommendations for intakes of many nutrients increase during pregnancy. A pregnant woman has an increased requirement for folate, because DNA synthesis and cell division take place at a rapid pace during embryonic development.

During the first few weeks after conception, the **neural tube** forms in the human embryo (Fig. 8.26a). This tube eventually develops into the brain and spinal cord. Pregnant women who suffer from folate deficiency have high risk of giving birth to infants with neural tube defects. The two most common neural tube defects are **spina bifida** (*spy'-na bif'-eh-dah*) and **anencephaly** (*an-en-sef'-ah-lee*). Spina bifida occurs when the embryo's spine does not form properly, and the bones fail to enclose the spinal cord. As you can see in Figure 8.26b, infants with severe spina bifida have a section of their spinal cord or a sac containing some spinal fluid bulging through an opening in their backs. Often, people with spina bifida are unable to use muscles in the lower part of their bodies, and as a result, they cannot walk independently. Infants born with anencephaly have much of their brain malformed or missing, and they usually die shortly after birth.

In 1992, officials with the U.S. Public Health Service (USPHS) recommended that all women capable of becoming pregnant consume 400 mcg of folic acid daily to prevent neural tube defects. In January 1998, the Food and Drug Administration required the addition of folic acid to enriched flour and cereals. According to medical experts, adequate folic acid intake can prevent most cases of spina bifida.[27] For pregnant women, adequate folate status is critical early in pregnancy, because the neural tube begins to form about 21 days after conception. This developmental milestone occurs when many women are not even aware they are pregnant.

Each year, 1 in every 5,000 babies is born with anencephaly[28] and about 1500 babies are born with spina bifida in the United States.[29] However, the prevalence of these neural tube defects has declined by about 30% since enrichment of foods with folic acid began.

Because women of childbearing age may become pregnant at some point, they need to be aware of the association between the lack of folate and neural tube defects. In addition to including folate-rich foods in their diets, young women can prepare for pregnancy by taking a daily multivitamin supplement that contains 400 mcg of synthetic folic acid.[27] Although folic acid intakes have increased among Americans since the United States began enriching grain products with the vitamin, only 30% of women who are 18 to 24 years of age take a daily folic acid supplement that supplies at least 400 mcg.[30]

Vitamin B-12

Cells require vitamin B-12 to make coenzymes that participate in a variety of cellular processes, including the transfer of CH_3 groups in the metabolism of folate. Vitamin B-12 is also needed to convert folate to coenzyme forms that are needed for metabolic reactions, including DNA synthesis. Vitamin B-12 also participates in homocysteine metabolism.

There is one vital function of vitamin B-12 that does not involve folate— maintaining the *myelin sheaths* that wrap around parts of certain nerve cells, insulating them. Myelin enables the nerves to communicate effectively. Without vitamin B-12, segments of myelin sheath gradually undergo destruction that can lead to paralysis. If a person who is vitamin B-12 deficient does not obtain treatment with the vitamin, he or she can die as a result of the deficiency.

Absorbing the vitamin B-12 that is naturally in food requires a complex series of steps that are unique for a vitamin (Fig. 8.27). Natural vitamin B-12 is bound to animal protein that prevents its absorption. When the food enters the stomach, the vitamin is released from the protein, primarily by the actions of hydrochloric acid (HCl) in gastric juice. Synthetic vitamin B-12 in dietary supplements or fortified foods is not bound to food protein, so it does not need stomach acid to release the protein.

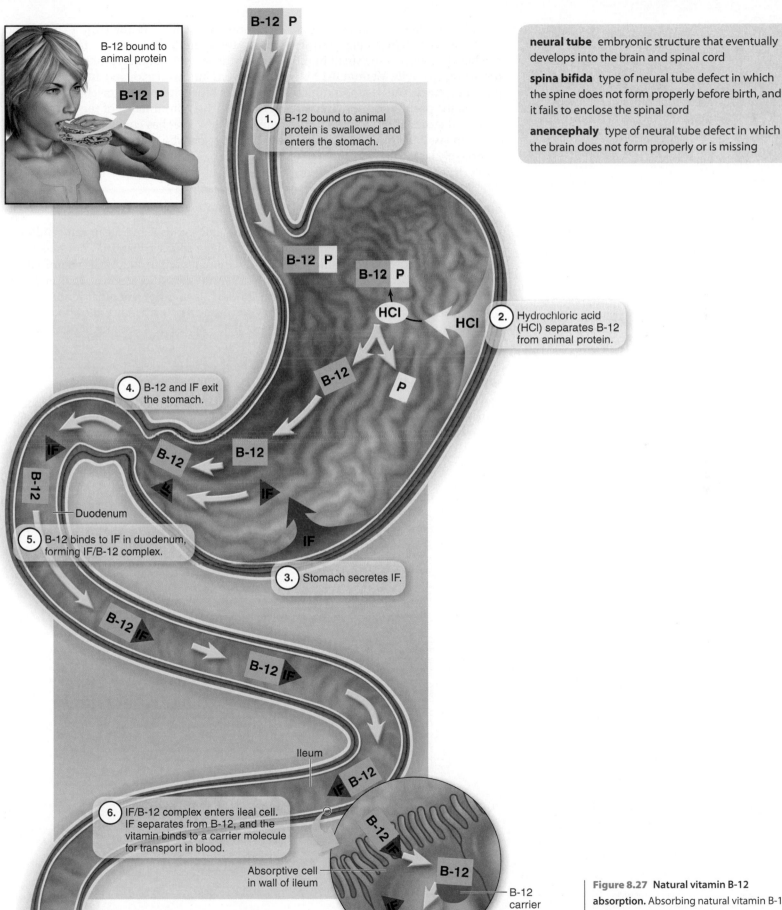

B-12 bound to animal protein

B-12 P

1. B-12 bound to animal protein is swallowed and enters the stomach.

2. Hydrochloric acid (HCl) separates B-12 from animal protein.

4. B-12 and IF exit the stomach.

Duodenum

5. B-12 binds to IF in duodenum, forming IF/B-12 complex.

3. Stomach secretes IF.

Ileum

6. IF/B-12 complex enters ileal cell. IF separates from B-12, and the vitamin binds to a carrier molecule for transport in blood.

Absorptive cell in wall of ileum

B-12 carrier molecule

To blood-stream

neural tube embryonic structure that eventually develops into the brain and spinal cord

spina bifida type of neural tube defect in which the spine does not form properly before birth, and it fails to enclose the spinal cord

anencephaly type of neural tube defect in which the brain does not form properly or is missing

Figure 8.27 Natural vitamin B-12 absorption. Absorbing natural vitamin B-12 from food requires a complex series of steps.

intrinsic factor (IF) substance produced in the stomach that facilitates intestinal absorption of vitamin B-12

pernicious anemia condition caused by the lack of intrinsic factor and characterized by vitamin B-12 deficiency, nerve damage, and megaloblastic RBCs

ascorbic acid vitamin C

In the small intestine, vitamin B-12 binds to **intrinsic factor (IF)**, a compound produced by certain stomach cells. Eventually, the vitamin B-12/intrinsic factor complex reaches the ileum of the small intestine, where the vitamin complex is absorbed. Within the absorptive cells, vitamin B-12 is separated from intrinsic factor and attached to transport molecules. The transport molecules enter the bloodstream and travel to the liver via the hepatic portal vein. The liver removes vitamin B-12 from many of the carrier molecules and stores about 50% of the vitamin. A healthy liver has enough vitamin B-12 reserves to last 5 to 10 years.[31] Therefore, a healthy person who decides to follow a diet that completely lacks vitamin B-12 is not likely to experience signs and symptoms of the vitamin's deficiency disorder for as long as 10 years.

Food Sources of Vitamin B-12

Only bacteria, fungi (for example, mushrooms and molds), and algae can synthesize vitamin B-12. Animals obtain the vitamin from these sources. Plants do not make vitamin B-12; therefore, we rely almost entirely on animal foods to supply the vitamin naturally. Major sources of vitamin B-12 in the typical American's diet are meat, milk and milk products, poultry, fish, shellfish, and eggs. Although liver is not a popular food, it is one of the richest sources of vitamin B-12. Many soy products, such as soy milk, and ready-to-eat cereals are fortified with synthetic vitamin B-12. Table 8.13 lists some foods that provide vitamin B-12.

Dietary Adequacy

The adult RDA for vitamin B-12 is 2.4 mcg/day. Most Americans who eat animal products consume more than the RDA.[32] No UL has been established for vitamin B-12, because no adverse effects have been observed with excess intake from food or dietary supplements.

TABLE 8.13 *Vitamin B-12 Content of Selected Foods*

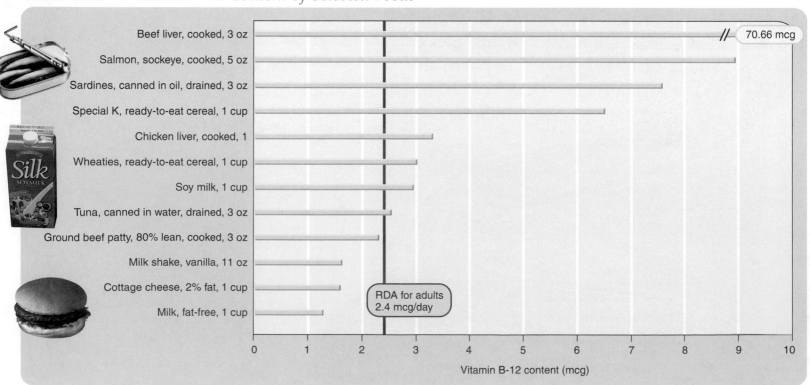

Source: Data from U.S. Department of Agriculture, Agricultural Research Service, USDA Nutrient Data Laboratory: Vitamin B-12 (µg) content of selected foods by common measure, sorted by nutrient content. *USDA national nutrient database for standard reference, release 18.* 2004.

Vitamin B-12 Deficiency Vitamin B-12 deficiency is characterized by nerve damage and megaloblastic RBCs. Other common signs and symptoms of the deficiency include muscle weakness, sore mouth, smooth and shiny tongue, memory loss, confusion, difficulty walking and maintaining balance, and numbness and tingling sensations, particularly in the lower extremities. Most cases of vitamin B-12 deficiency result from problems that interfere with intestinal absorption of the vitamin (cobalamin) in foods (*food-cobalamin malabsorption*) and not from inadequate intakes.[31]

Vitamin B-12 deficiency is common among older adults. As people age, HCl production in their stomachs declines. Thus, many older adults have *food-cobalamin malabsorption* because they are unable to release vitamin B-12 from animal protein.[33] People with this condition develop vitamin B-12 deficiency disorder despite consuming diets that contain the vitamin. In addition to advanced age, chronic alcoholism, gastric bypass surgeries for weight reduction, and certain medications, particularly those that reduce stomach acid secretion, can contribute to food-cobalamin malabsorption. People with this form of malabsorption produce intrinsic factor, so they can absorb synthetic forms of the vitamin in dietary supplements that contain B-12.

About 1 to 2% of older adults have an autoimmune disorder that causes inflammation and destruction of the cells in the stomach that produce intrinsic factor.[33] (An autoimmune disorder results when a person's immune system attacks his or her own cells.) In these cases, diets may supply adequate amounts of vitamin B-12, but the lack of intrinsic factor prevents most of the micronutrient from being absorbed. Eventually, people who lack intrinsic factor develop a disease called **pernicious** ("deadly") **anemia.** As its name implies, pernicious anemia can lead to vitamin B-12 deficiency and death. Treatment involves bypassing the need for intrinsic factor and intestinal absorption, usually by providing routine vitamin B-12 injections. Furthermore, taking large doses of vitamin B-12 floods the intestinal tract with the vitamin and enables a small amount to be absorbed without the need for intrinsic factor.

In addition to advanced age, family history is a risk factor for pernicious anemia. Therefore, it is a good idea to have your blood tested for signs of vitamin B-12 deficiency as you grow older, and especially if you have a close relative with pernicious anemia.

Vegans ("total" vegetarians) avoid eating animal products. Plant foods supply little vitamin B-12, so vegans need to be concerned about their intakes of the nutrient (see the "Vegetarianism" section of Chapter 7). People who eat few or no animal products should consume foods that have been fortified with vitamin B-12, such as fortified soy milk and cereals, or take supplements that supply the vitamin. Vegan women who breastfeed their babies need to be aware that their breast milk may contain inadequate amounts of vitamin B-12. Babies who consume only vitamin B-12–deficient breast milk are likely to develop megaloblastic anemia and serious nervous system problems, including diminished brain growth and spinal cord damage. The signs and symptoms of the deficiency are likely to occur during the first few months of life, particularly when the infants' mothers did not supplement their diets with vitamin B-12 during pregnancy. Providing vitamin B-12 to the deficient babies effectively treats the anemia, but some of the damage to the children's nervous systems may be permanent.[34]

Vitamin C

Most animals do not need dietary sources of vitamin C **(ascorbic acid)** because they can synthesize all the vitamin they need. Humans and guinea pigs are among the few species that are unable to make vitamin C, and for these animals, the micronutrient is essential.

Vitamin C absorption occurs in the small intestine. As intakes of the vitamin increase, the amount absorbed decreases. The intestine, for example, absorbs 50% or less of the vitamin when intakes are 1 g or more/day. Additionally, the kidneys increase their excretion of the vitamin in response to high intakes. Therefore, taking megadoses of vitamin C may be wasteful, because such high amounts of the vitamin are not well absorbed and excesses are eliminated in urine.

MY DIVERSE PLATE

Guava

Guava is a tropical fruit that is available in many varieties. Although guavas can be eaten fresh, the fruit is often used to make sauces, jellies, and juices. Guavas are an excellent source of fiber and vitamin C. The white or pink flesh of a guava contains more vitamin C than an orange.

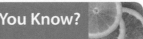

Did You Know?

Vitamin C plays a role in the absorption of the mineral iron (Fe). Plants are major sources of *nonheme* iron (Fe^{+++}). The small intestine, however, absorbs Fe^{++} more readily than Fe^{+++}. Vitamin C promotes iron absorption by donating an electron to Fe^{+++}, forming Fe^{++} as a result. The vitamin may also form a complex with iron that enhances the body's ability to absorb the mineral. Therefore, adding citrus fruits, broccoli, peppers, or other vitamin C–rich foods to meals can increase absorption of nonheme iron.

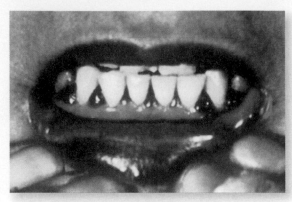

| Swollen gums that bleed easily are a sign of scurvy.

collagen fibrous protein that gives strength to connective tissue

prooxidant substance that promotes free radical production

Functions of Vitamin C

Vitamin C does not function as part of a coenzyme as do B vitamins, but the vitamin serves as a nutrient cofactor that facilitates certain chemical reactions. Vitamin C performs a variety of important cellular functions, primarily by donating electrons to other compounds. In the body, vitamin C has widespread physiological roles; the following sections describe some of the micronutrient's most well-understood functions.

Collagen Synthesis   Vitamin C participates in reactions that form and maintain collagen. **Collagen** is a fibrous protein that gives strength to *connective tissue*. Connective tissues, such as bone, cartilage, and tendons, connect and support other structures in the body. During collagen formation, vitamin C helps create numerous cross-connections between the amino acids in collagen that greatly strengthen the connective tissue (Fig. 8.28). If vitamin C is unavailable, the body forms weak connective tissue and is unable to maintain existing collagen. Some of the more obvious signs of scurvy, such as swollen gums that bleed easily, teeth that loosen and fall out of their sockets, skin that bruises easily, and old scars that open, are primarily the result of poorly formed and maintained collagen.

Antioxidant Activity   Results of some experiments indicate that vitamin C can act as an antioxidant by donating electrons to radicals. Vitamin C also may donate electrons to another antioxidant—vitamin E. Thus, vitamin C recycles vitamin E so it can regain its antioxidant function. Scientists, however, do not know the extent of vitamin C's antioxidant abilities in the human body. Taking excessive amounts of vitamin C may be harmful, because in high doses, the vitamin has **prooxidant** effects. A prooxidant promotes radical production.

Other Roles of Vitamin C in the Body   Vitamin C plays a role in the body's immune function, and the vitamin is necessary for the synthesis of bile and certain neurotransmitters. Vitamin C is also involved in the production of various hormones, including the "stress hormone" cortisol; adolsterone, a hormone involved in blood pressure regulation; and thyroxin, the thyroid hormone that regulates energy metabolism.

Food Sources of Vitamin C

Plant foods are the best dietary sources of vitamin C. Peppers, citrus fruit, papaya, broccoli, cabbage, and berries contain relatively high amounts of the micronutrient

Figure 8.28 Vitamin C and collagen formation. The action of vitamin C results in the formation of numerous cross-connections between the amino acids in collagen, greatly strengthening the connective tissue.

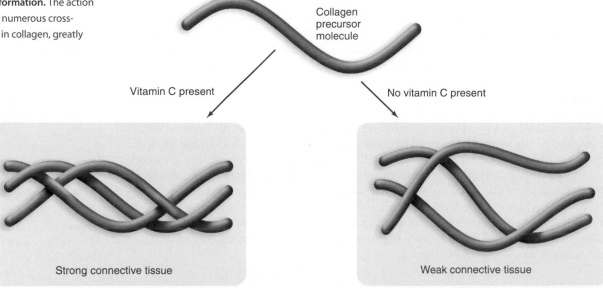

TABLE 8.14 *Vitamin C Content of Selected Foods*

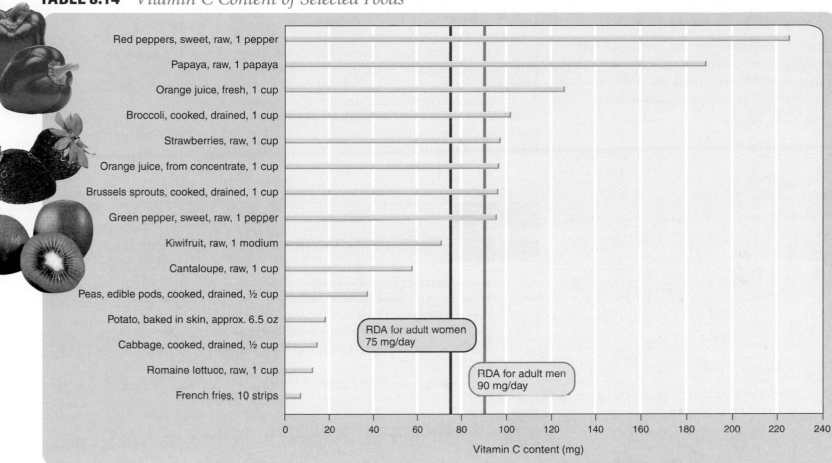

Red peppers, sweet, raw, 1 pepper
Papaya, raw, 1 papaya
Orange juice, fresh, 1 cup
Broccoli, cooked, drained, 1 cup
Strawberries, raw, 1 cup
Orange juice, from concentrate, 1 cup
Brussels sprouts, cooked, drained, 1 cup
Green pepper, sweet, raw, 1 pepper
Kiwifruit, raw, 1 modium
Cantaloupe, raw, 1 cup
Peas, edible pods, cooked, drained, ½ cup
Potato, baked in skin, approx. 6.5 oz
Cabbage, cooked, drained, ½ cup
Romaine lettuce, raw, 1 cup
French fries, 10 strips

RDA for adult women
75 mg/day

RDA for adult men
90 mg/day

Vitamin C content (mg)

Source: Data from U.S. Department of Agriculture, Agricultural Research Service, USDA Nutrient Data Laboratory: Vitamin C, total ascorbic acid (mg) content of selected foods by common measure, sorted by nutrient content. *USDA national nutrient database for standard reference, release 18.* 2004.

(Table 8.14). Potatoes and vitamin C–fortified fruit drinks and ready-to-eat cereals also supply vitamin C. Most animal foods are not sources of the micronutrient.

Vitamin C is very unstable in the presence of heat, oxygen, light, alkaline conditions, and the minerals iron and copper. Storing vitamin C–rich foods in cool conditions, such as in the refrigerator, will help preserve the micronutrient. Because vitamin C is easily lost during cooking, eat raw fruits and vegetables whenever possible.

Dietary Adequacy

The adult RDA for vitamin C is 75 to 90 mg/day for women and men, respectively. Cigarette smokers need to add an extra 35 mg/day to their RDA, because exposure to cigarette smoke increases radical formation in their lungs.[4] By including vitamin C–rich fruits and vegetables in their diets, healthy people can obtain adequate amounts of vitamin C.

The adult UL for vitamin C is 2000 mg/day. When people exceed this amount of the vitamin, gastrointestinal upsets, including diarrhea, often occur.[4] Taking megadoses of vitamin C supplements is wasteful, because the small intestine reduces absorption of the micronutrient when intakes of the vitamin exceed 200 mg/day. Furthermore, when cells are saturated with vitamin C, the excess vitamin and *oxalate*, a by-product of breaking down vitamin C, circulate in the bloodstream. The kidneys filter and eliminate these unnecessary substances in urine. Excess oxalate excretion raises the risk of kidney stones.[35] Therefore, people who are susceptible to develop such stones should avoid consuming

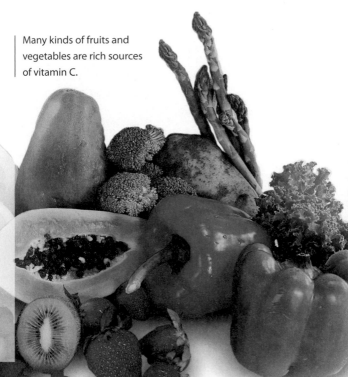

Many kinds of fruits and vegetables are rich sources of vitamin C.

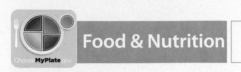

vitamin C supplements. The "Vitamins as Medicines" section of Chapter 8 provides more information about the value of taking megadoses of vitamin C to prevent or treat colds and other disorders.

Even if you do not regularly eat foods that naturally contain the vitamin or take a vitamin C supplement, you are unlikely to develop a vitamin C deficiency, because most people require less than 10 mg of the vitamin daily to prevent scurvy. A 6-ounce serving of fresh orange juice provides about 60 mg of vitamin C—well beyond the requirement. Additionally, Americans rarely develop scurvy because vitamin C is added to many processed foods, including fruit and sports drinks, ready-to-eat cereals, and nutrition or power bars. If you would still like to take a vitamin C supplement daily, consider choosing a product that provides 50 to 100 mg of the vitamin in each tablet.

Concept **Checkpoint**

7. Prepare a table for water-soluble vitamins and choline. For each of these micronutrients, indicate its major function in the body, major food sources, deficiency disorder (if it has a specific name), and major signs and symptoms of the deficiency disorder. If the micronutrient is known to be toxic, also indicate major toxicity signs and symptoms. Check your table against the information provided in Table 8.7.

8.4 Vitamins as Medicines

Are you among the millions of Americans who take vitamin supplements? If your answer is "yes," why do you use them? Many people take multiple vitamin/mineral supplements as an "insurance policy" in case their diets are not nutritionally adequate. Other people use specific vitamin supplements because they think the practice will result in optimal health. Vitamin supplements are effective for treating people with specific vitamin deficiency diseases, metabolic defects that increase vitamin requirements, and a few other medical conditions. However, scientific evidence generally does not support claims that megadoses of vitamins can prevent or treat everything from gray hair to lung cancer.

How did vitamins earn the reputation of being cure-alls? The fact that a very small amount of a vitamin can prevent or cure the vitamin's deficiency disease provides the foundation for beliefs that these micronutrients are useful for preventing or treating serious chronic diseases. Furthermore, many people think that vitamins are helpful and safe in any amount. When ingested in high doses, however, vitamins and related compounds such as carotenoids often have druglike effects in the body. In some cases, these physiological responses are beneficial, but in other instances, vitamin excesses cause unpleasant and even dangerous side effects. Therefore, people should be just as cautious about using megadoses of vitamins as they need to be when taking medications. This section of Chapter 8 focuses on some current scientific evidence regarding the usefulness and safety of using large doses of vitamins and related compounds as medications.

Niacin as Medicine?

In Chapter 6, we discussed the association between elevated blood levels of LDL cholesterol and increased risk of cardiovascular disease (CVD), the number one killer of Americans. Heart disease and stroke are the major forms of CVD. Megadoses of dietary supplements containing *nicotinic acid*, a form of niacin, can reduce elevated LDL cholesterol levels and increase beneficial HDL cholesterol levels in blood. However, such therapy may have side effects, including flushing of the skin, usually on the face and chest; itchy skin; and GI tract upsets, such as nausea and vomiting. High doses of nicotinic acid can also cause liver damage. Some people experience these side effects while taking only 50 mg/day. (The adult RDA for niacin ranges from 14 to 16 mg.) Therefore, a physician should supervise the use of niacin megadoses to treat elevated LDL cholesterol levels.

Vitamin B-6 as Medicine?

Popular sources of nutrition information often recommend large doses of vitamin B-6 to treat *premenstrual syndrome* (*PMS*), a condition that many women experience a few days before their menstrual period begins, and *carpal tunnel syndrome,* a painful nerve disorder that affects the wrist. However, studies investigating the value of vitamin B-6 supplementation for relieving PMS and carpal tunnel syndrome do not provide evidence that supports the use of the micronutrient to treat these disorders.[23]

Unlike most other B vitamins, vitamin B-6 is toxic in high doses, causing severe sensory nerve damage when taken in doses that exceed the UL for extended periods. Signs and symptoms of vitamin B-6 toxicity include walking difficulties and numbness of the hands and feet. The nerve damage resolves when affected people stop ingesting megadoses of vitamin B-6.

Folic Acid, B-6, and B-12 as Medicine?

Deficiencies of folic acid, vitamin B-6, and vitamin B-12 are associated with elevated blood levels of homocysteine. High homocysteine levels may be a biochemical marker (an indicator in the body) or a risk factor for cardiovascular disease. However, results of research do not provide evidence that lowering homocysteine levels by taking these B vitamins reduces the risk of heart disease.[23] More research is needed to determine whether healthy people can reduce their risk of heart disease and other forms of CVD by using folic acid, B-6, and B-12 supplements for long periods.

Elevated blood homocysteine levels may also be a marker or risk factor for Alzheimer's disease (AD). Alzheimer's disease is characterized by a gradual progressive decline in cognitive functioning, including memory and decision-making skills. There is no cure or effective treatment for the disease. The results of one study suggested a relationship between mild cognitive impairment (an early sign of AD) and both folate deficiency and high blood levels of homocysteine.[36] In another study, low intakes of folate, vitamin B-12, and vitamin B-6 were associated with high blood levels of homocysteine and reduced cognitive functioning in aging men.[37] Although taking megadoses of these B vitamins can reduce homocysteine levels, such treatment does not improve cognitive functioning.[23] As is often the case, more research is needed to determine whether using supplements that contain these micronutrients can reduce the risk of cognitive decline or slow the progression of AD.

Vitamin C as Medicine?

In 1970, Nobel Prize–winning American chemist Dr. Linus Pauling (1901–1994) published *Vitamin C and the Common Cold*. This bestselling book established the popular belief that megadoses of vitamin C could prevent colds. As a result of Pauling's claim, many Americans take megadoses of the micronutrient when they notice the first cold symptoms.

In the years that followed the publication of *Vitamin C and the Common Cold*, Pauling became more convinced of vitamin C's health benefits. He claimed large doses of vitamin C could battle a variety of diseases, including influenza, cancer, and CVD. He even believed the vitamin could slow the aging process. Despite Pauling's impressive credentials in chemistry, conventional nutrition scientists have approached his ideas about vitamin C's health benefits with caution and skepticism.

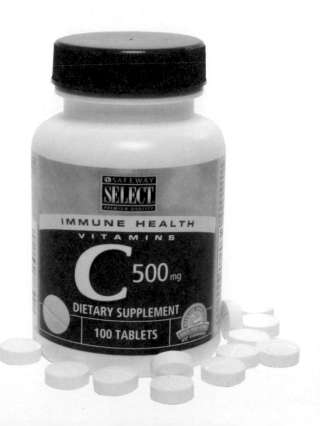

Can taking vitamin C protect you against infection by cold viruses? The evidence collected from several scientific studies indicates that routine vitamin C supplementation (200 mg or more of the vitamin daily) does not prevent colds in the general population.[38] However, taking such large doses of the vitamin may reduce the duration of cold symptoms by a day or so. Additionally, vitamin C may reduce the severity of cold symptoms because the micronutrient acts like an antihistamine when taken in very large doses.[4]

Beyond the Common Cold

When LDL cholesterol is oxidized, it is more likely to contribute to atherosclerosis than nonoxidized LDL cholesterol (see Chapter 6). As an antioxidant, vitamin C may reduce the oxidation of LDL cholesterol, lowering the risk of CVD. Studies to determine whether vitamin C can help prevent CVD have not provided consistent evidence that the micronutrient reduces the risk of CVD or dying from the condition.[39] Atherosclerosis takes years and probably decades to result in heart attack, strokes, and other forms of CVD. Thus, more research is needed to determine whether long-term vitamin C supplementation can reduce the risk of this leading killer of Americans.

Results of some observational studies suggest that high intake of vitamin C–rich foods may reduce the risk of Alzheimer's disease.[40] Several studies have examined the benefits of using combinations of antioxidant vitamin supplements, particularly vitamins C and E, to lower the risk of this dreaded disease. In general, the results of these studies were mixed: some findings indicated the antioxidant supplements were useful in reducing the risk of AD, while findings from other studies were not as encouraging.[41]

According to findings of epidemiological studies, people who consume diets containing high amounts of vitamin C–rich fruits and vegetables have lower risk of cancer than people who do not eat much of these foods. However, taking megadoses of vitamin C can damage DNA, which may actually increase the likelihood of cancer.[42]

Although there is some encouraging scientific evidence that vitamin C may be useful in treating cancer,[43] the vitamin may interfere with certain cancer-fighting medications, lowering their effectiveness.[44] The Chapter 8 "Highlight" provides more information concerning the role of diet in cancer development and prevention.

It is important to note that complex chronic diseases such as CVD, Alzheimer's disease, and cancer generally do not have simple causes. Inherited factors as well as lifestyle practices other than diet—smoking, obesity, and lack of physical activity—contribute to the development of these diseases. Therefore, it is unlikely that people will be able to prevent or treat cancer simply by taking vitamin C (or any other supplement).

Vitamin E as Medicine?

In the early 1980s, epidemiological reports indicated that populations who ate vitamin E–rich diets had lower risk of heart disease than groups who ate diets that did not contain high amounts of the micronutrient. Additionally, results of other studies suggested that vitamin E might reduce the risk of cancer, particularly lung cancer in smokers. Soon more good news about vitamin E appeared in the medical literature. Some researchers promoted the use of vitamin E megadoses to slow the decline in mental functioning that is associated with Alzheimer's disease. Not surprisingly, sales of vitamin E supplements increased dramatically between 1987 and 2000.[45]

Over the past few years, the scientific community's enthusiasm for using high doses of vitamin E supplements to prevent or treat chronic diseases, including CVD and cancer, has subsided considerably. Major long-term trials failed to show that high intakes of vitamin E consistently reduce the risk of these chronic diseases.[20] Furthermore, use of vitamin E supplements has been associated with an increased risk of hemorrhagic stroke.

Studies generally do not provide evidence that vitamin E helps people with signs of *mild cognitive impairment,* a condition characterized by declining thought-processing abilities that can progress to Alzheimer's disease.[20, 41] Furthermore, taking vitamin E supplements does not reduce the likelihood of developing age-related forms of cognitive decline.[20, 41]

More clinical research is needed to determine whether combinations of vitamin E and other antioxidant nutrients can delay or prevent the cognitive decline that often accompanies the aging process.

Did scientists *prove* vitamin E supplements are useless or "bad"? No. Vitamin E has several forms, and it is possible that the alpha-tocopherol form of vitamin E that is typically in supplements does not have any beneficial druglike effects on the body. The dosage of vitamin E and the length of time the supplements are administered during clinical tests may provide other reasons why research findings do not always support epidemiological observations. To detect positive effects on health, scientists may need to test higher doses of the vitamin than have been studied in the past. Additionally, studies that last longer may be necessary; the health benefits of vitamin E supplementation may take several years to become evident.

Vitamin A and Carotenoids as Medicine?

Findings of observational studies suggest an association between eating diets rich in fruits and vegetables and lower risk of certain cancers, heart disease, and *age-related macular degeneration (AMD)*, a leading cause of blindness in the United States (see the section on "Carotenoid Supplements and AMD" in Chapter 8). Such diets provide plenty of beta-carotene and other antioxidant carotenoids. Scientists have conducted numerous large-scale studies to determine whether carotenoid supplements provide health benefits. The following sections summarize research findings regarding the health effects of taking these supplements.

CVD and Cancer

Results of clinical studies have not provided support for taking vitamin A or beta-carotene supplements to reduce the risk of CVD.[39] Furthermore, the use of beta-carotene supplements does not reduce the risk of cancer.[12] In two major studies, smokers who took beta-carotene supplements were *more* likely to die of lung cancer than smokers who took placebos.[12] Nevertheless, more research is needed to determine whether other carotenoids, such as lycopene and *beta-cryptoxanthin* (*bay'-ta krip-teh-zan'-thin*), protect against CVD and cancer.

Carotenoid Supplements and AMD

In developed countries, age-related macular degeneration (AMD) is one of the leading causes of blindness among older adults.[46] The disease is associated with changes in the *macula*, the region within the eye that provides the most detailed central vision (Fig. 8.29). When the macula is damaged, objects appear to be distorted as in the grid shown in Figure 8.30 (right side). Major risk factors for

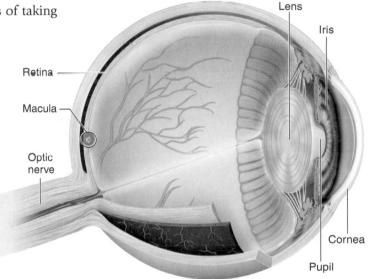

Figure 8.29 **The macula.** The macula is the region within the eye that provides the most detailed central vision.

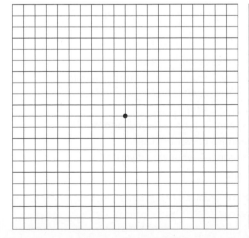 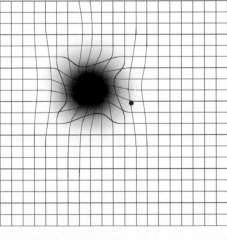

Figure 8.30 **Visual effect of macular degeneration.** When shown a grid comprised of straight lines, people with normal vision see the grid on the left. However, people with age-related macular degeneration (AMD) would see distorted gridlines, as shown in the right illustration.

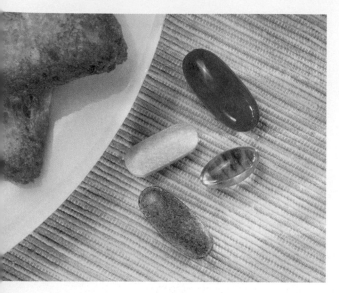

AMD are genetics, smoking, and advanced age, but diet also plays a role in the development of the condition.

The macula contains the carotenoids lutein and zeaxanthin. In the Age-Related Eye Disease Study (AREDS), patients who already had advanced AMD took dietary supplements that contained relatively high amounts of vitamins C and E, beta-carotene, and the mineral zinc.[47] The combination of these substances slowed the progression of vision loss associated with macular degeneration. However, there was no clear scientific evidence that taking antioxidant supplements *prevents* healthy people from developing AMD. Additionally, the long-term use of these supplements could be harmful.

Some Final Thoughts

According to a report issued by the U.S. Preventive Services Task Force, people do not need to be discouraged from taking vitamin supplements unless there is strong evidence to indicate the practice is harmful, as in the case of smokers who use beta-carotene supplements.[48] Nevertheless, the Task Force report states, ". . . taking vitamins does not replace the need to eat a healthy diet." Although the health benefits of vitamin supplementation are often uncertain, there is more consistent evidence that a diet high in fruits, vegetables, and legumes has important benefits. It is possible that other constituents besides vitamins may account for the benefits of such diets.

Consuming a wide variety of vitamins, antioxidants, and phytochemicals in their natural states and concentrations (in foods) may be the most effective way to lower your risk of CVD, cancer, and many other serious chronic diseases. Why? These substances probably work together to enhance health, and isolating them from their natural sources or synthesizing and concentrating them into supplements may reduce their usefulness and increase their risks.[49] Therefore, dietitians recommend that adults eat a variety of fruits and vegetables each day rather than take antioxidant or phytochemical supplements.

Nutrition experts tend to emphasize the importance of combining a nutritious diet with regular exercise for achieving and maintaining good health. However, an overwhelming amount of scientific evidence links tobacco use to several forms of cancer, heart disease, AMD, and other serious chronic conditions. If you smoke tobacco, quitting may have a greater beneficial impact on your long-term health than improving your diet or increasing your physical activity level while still continuing tobacco use.

Concept **Checkpoint**

8. Explain why people should be careful about taking megadoses of vitamin supplements.
9. List three side effects from taking megadoses of nicotinic acid.
10. Explain why people should avoid taking high doses of vitamin B-6.
11. A friend of yours takes 1000 mg of vitamin C daily, because she thinks the vitamin prevents colds, heart attacks, and Alzheimer's disease. After reading section 8.4, what would you tell your friend about her vitamin C use?
12. Dorothy is 85 years of age. She has excellent vision, but she takes megadoses of vitamins C and E, because she thinks these vitamins prevent macular degeneration. Based on the information in section 8.4, what would you tell Dorothy about her vitamin C and vitamin E use?

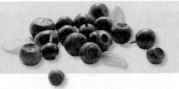

Chapter 8 Highlight

DIET AND CANCER

For many people, no diagnosis evokes more fear than *cancer*. Although modern medical technologies have enabled physicians to make great progress in treating many types of cancer successfully, the disease is still the second-leading cause of death in the United States. According to the American Cancer Society, one in four Americans dies as a result of cancer.[50]

In 2011, the three leading sites of new cancer cases (excluding common types of skin cancer) for American men were prostate, lung, and colon and rectal (colorectal) cancers. The three leading sites of new cancer cases in American women were breast, lung, and colorectal cancers. As shown in Figure 8.31, lung cancer is responsible for more cancer deaths than prostate (males), breast (females), and colorectal cancers. There is good news: The majority of cancer deaths are preventable.

This "Highlight" focuses on the roles of diet and exercise in the development, progression, and possible prevention of certain cancers. For more information about cancer, including specific forms of cancer, visit the American Cancer Society's website at www.cancer.org or the National Cancer Institute's website at www.cancer.gov.

What Is Cancer?

Cancer is the term for a group of chronic diseases characterized by cells that have undergone damage to certain genes (*mutations*). Genes are portions of DNA that code for the production of specific proteins (see Chapter 7). DNA dictates cellular growth, division, and eventual death. The rate at which healthy cells develop, grow, divide, and die occurs in a controlled fashion. As a normal body cell develops and matures, it acquires specialized functions. Examples include the ability of muscle cells to contract and that of certain stomach cells to secrete hydrochloric acid.

Cancerous (*malignant*) cells are literally "out of control"—they divide repeatedly and frequently, and they do not die. If genes that regulate cellular growth, division, and death mutate, abnormal cell development, rapid cell growth, and unchecked cell division can result. When a cell becomes malignant, it does not perform the specialized functions of the cells from which it was derived. A cancerous liver cell, for example, does not remove toxins from the bloodstream or store nutrients properly.

As a result of their rapid growth rate, many types of cancer cells form masses, called *malignant tumors*. Malignant cells often break away from the tumor. These cells can move to and invade other parts of the body. When cancer spreads to other tissues, the disease has *metastasized* (*meh-tass'-tah-sized*).

Some cells multiply excessively and form *benign* (*bih-nine'*) masses or tumors as a result. A benign tumor is not cancerous, because the tumor's cells do not destroy nearby tissues or metastasize. Benign tumors are usually harmless. In some cases, however, a benign tumor grows large enough to interfere with the functioning of healthy structures, such as a blood vessel or brain tissue. When this occurs, the tumor needs to be treated to reduce its size or remove it.

A *carcinogen* (*car-sin'-o-jin*) is an environmental factor, such as radiation, tobacco smoke, or a virus, that triggers cancer. Carcinogens can irritate tissues, causing an inflammatory response by the body. Over time, the inflammation may result in cancer development. Some carcinogens damage DNA, causing mutations to genes that control certain cell behaviors. Over time, repeated exposures to various carcinogens take their toll on cells, making malignant cells more likely to develop. In fact, it is not unusual for cancerous cells to develop during a person's lifetime. However, a healthy immune system identifies the malignant cells and destroys them before

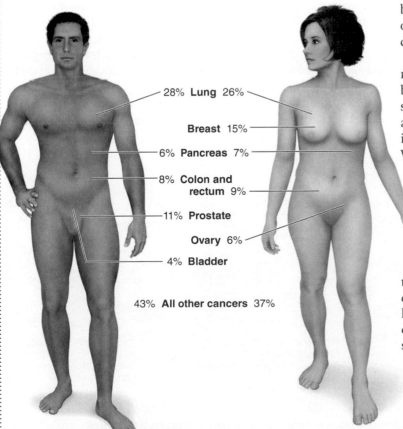

28% **Lung** 26%

Breast 15%

6% **Pancreas** 7%

8% **Colon and rectum** 9%

11% **Prostate**

Ovary 6%

4% **Bladder**

43% **All other cancers** 37%

Figure 8.31 Leading cancer sites and deaths. This figure indicates leading sites of cancer deaths and percentages of cancer deaths according to 2011 estimates. *Source: American Cancer Society: Cancer Facts & Figures 2011. www.cancer.org. Accessed: July 27, 2011.*

they multiply uncontrollably. Nutrient deficiencies, the aging process, and environmental insults, such as exposure to radiation and certain chemicals, reduce the effectiveness of the immune system. As a result, cancer cells are able to divide unchecked and eventually metastasize. Figure 8.32 illustrates major steps in the development and behavior of most cancerous cells.

Because of their rapid growth and frequent cell divisions, malignant cells require more nutrients than normal cells. To supply enough nutrients to meet their needs, cancerous tumors stimulate the body to form blood vessels that divert blood away from healthy cells and into the tumor (see Fig. 8.32). Much of the severe body wasting that usually accompanies advanced cases of cancer happens because healthy tissues are unable to obtain adequate supplies of nutrients, and they die.

Regular health checkups and various screening methods can detect cancer in its early stages, when many forms can be effectively treated. Screening methods include testing blood for the level of *prostate specific antigen* (*PSA*) to detect prostate (a male reproductive organ) cancer and using a special scope to view the inside of the lower gastrointestinal tract to detect colorectal cancer (*colonoscopy*). Conventional medical treatments for cancer typically involve surgical removal of cancerous tissue; chemotherapy, medications that are toxic to cancer cells or limit their growth; and radiation that kills cancer cells. Early diagnosis of cancer is very important. Once cancer metastasizes, it is far more difficult to treat.

What Causes Cells to Become Cancerous?

Why do many smokers develop lung cancer and some not develop it? Why do some women have breast cancer and others remain free of the disease? Medical researchers have discovered several risk factors for many forms of the disease, including the following:

- Aging (most cancers occur in people over 65 years of age)
- Having a family history of cancer
- Using tobacco
- Being exposed to some forms of radiation

- Being exposed to certain environmental substances, such as irritants
- Having certain viral and bacterial infections
- Having elevated levels of certain hormones
- Consuming alcohol and certain foods
- Being physically inactive and having excess body fat[51]

People can lower their risk of cancer by avoiding known carcinogens, especially tobacco smoke. Approximately one of every three cancer deaths is associated with smoking tobacco, and nearly 90% of lung cancer deaths are caused by exposure to tobacco smoke.[50] In 2011, experts with the American Cancer Society predicted that nearly 157,000 Americans would die from lung cancer. Mouth, larynx ("voicebox"), esophageal, stomach, pancreatic, kidney, and bladder cancers are also associated with tobacco use.

Cancer causation is a complex process. Therefore, it may be impossible to pinpoint a single cause of a patient's cancer. Individuals differ widely in their genetic makeups, lifestyle practices, environmental exposures, and nutritional states. Some forms of the disease are likely to be inherited, but lifestyle factors, including diet, contribute to most cases of cancer.[52] The following sections examine relationships between dietary factors and the risk of cancer.

The Role of Diet in Cancer Development

Rates of specific cancers vary widely among different populations. Men and women living in Asian countries, for example, have lower risks of prostate and breast cancer, respectively, than men and women living in Western countries. After Asian men and women migrate to Western countries, their risks of prostate and breast cancer increase and eventually become similar to the risks of their adopted country's native population. Such findings provide epidemiological evidence of associations between cancer and certain lifestyle choices.

According to results of observational and experimental studies, certain substances in foods and beverages promote cancer

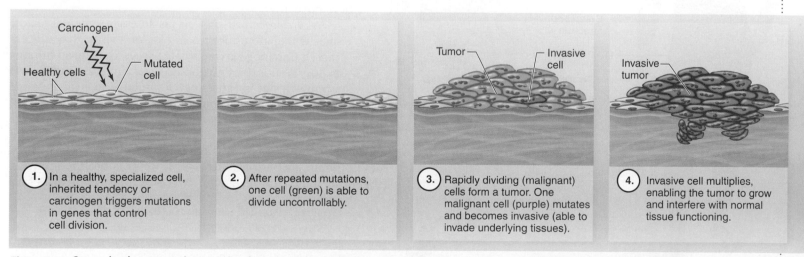

Figure 8.32 Cancer development and progression. Several steps are involved as a normal cell progresses into a cancerous one that multiplies out of control.

development. Alcohol, for example, is a carcinogen. People who consume two or more alcoholic drinks daily have higher risks of cancers of the mouth, throat, esophagus, larynx, liver, and breast.[50] The risk rises as the amount of alcohol consumed increases and when cigarette smoking is combined with drinking. To reduce your risk of cancer, avoid alcoholic beverages or drink in moderation—no more than one standard drink per day for women and no more than two standard drinks per day for men. (A *standard* alcoholic drink is 1.5 oz of liquor, 12 oz of regular beer, and 5 oz of wine.)

Certain molds that can grow on nuts or grains produce a chemical called *aflatoxin* (*ah'-fla-tox-in*). Consuming foods that are contaminated with these molds increases the risk of liver cancer. Although liver cancer is not common among Americans, populations that consume peanuts and grains that have been stored improperly have high rates of this type of cancer. Chapter 12 discusses toxic molds and ways to protect the food supply from them and other food-borne health threats.

High red meat and dairy intakes may contribute to prostate cancer.[53] Diets that contain large amounts of processed and/or red meat (defined as beef, pork, and lamb) are associated with increased risk of colon cancer.[53] Processed meat ("deli" meat) has sodium nitrate and sodium nitrite added to it during production. Under certain conditions, these chemicals form *nitrosamines* (*nitros'-ah-menes*), which are carcinogens. Eating high amounts of smoked or salt-preserved (*pickled*) foods, such as salted fish, may increase the risk of stomach cancer.

According to findings of some studies, the risk of colorectal cancer is greater in populations that consume a lot of fried, grilled, or broiled meats.[54] The high temperatures used to cook the meat may cause the formation of a group of carcinogens in the food called *heterocyclic* (*het'-eh-ro-si'-klic*) amines. Therefore, you may be able to reduce your risk of certain cancers by limiting your intake of grilled meats and avoiding charred parts of charcoal-grilled meats. Also, covering the grate with aluminum foil, poking a few holes in the foil, and placing the meat on top of it will reduce charring of the meat.

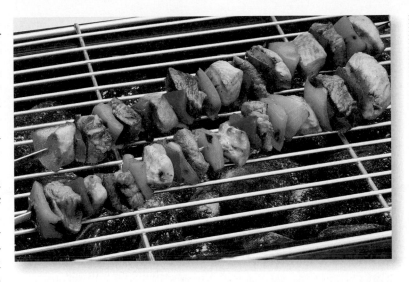

Excess Body Fat Diets that provide a surplus of calories result in a person becoming overweight or obese, conditions characterized by excess body fat (see Chapter 10). Obese people have higher risks of cancers of the colon, breast (in postmenopausal women), uterus, kidney, and esophagus than people who have healthy amounts of body fat.[55] Hodgkin's lymphoma (cancer of the immune system) and cancers of the pancreas, gallbladder, prostate, thyroid, cervix, and ovaries are also associated with obesity.

The reasons for the relationship between excess body fat and cancer development are unclear. However, overweight and obese people often have elevated insulin, estrogen, and testosterone levels. Excesses of these and possibly other hormones may stimulate the production of cell factors that promote malignant cell development and growth. In some cases, cancer triggers are easier to identify. For example, overweight and obesity are associated with the increased risk of esophageal cancer. Excess abdominal fat contributes to the reflux of stomach acid into the esophagus by restricting the ability of the stomach to expand during meals. As a result, the gastroesophageal sphincter is unable to keep the stomach's contents from moving into the esophagus. (See the Chapter 4 "Highlight.") Chronic exposure to stomach acid irritates

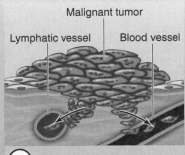

5. Malignant cells break away from the tumor, and enter circulatory or lymphatic systems (metastasize).

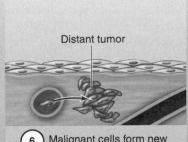

6. Malignant cells form new tumors in other parts of the body.

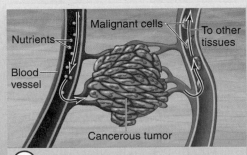

7. Tumor stimulates development of its own blood supply, depriving the rest of the body of nourishment.

TABLE 8.15

Possible Diet-Related Carcinogens

Possibly Carcinogenic	Common Dietary Sources	Possible or Known Action
Aflatoxin	Moldy nuts and grains	Can cause liver damage
Arsenic	Natural contaminant in drinking water	May increase risk of bladder cancer
Alcohol	Alcoholic beverages	Unclear, but may increase certain hormone levels or the body's breakdown of alcohol may result in carcinogens
Bisphenol A	Food or beverages stored in plastic containers made with BPA	Unclear whether the substance is carcinogenic, but it may disrupt the hormone estrogen
Excess calorie intake	All macronutrients	Excess calorie intake is linked to obesity
Heterocyclic amines	Foods exposed to high temperature, especially grilled meat that has charred areas	Formation of heterocyclic amines that alter DNA of colon cells
High glycemic diet	High-carbohydrate foods such as those listed in Table 5.11	Unclear, but may increase risk of breast cancer
Sodium nitrate and nitrite	Cured meats, such as deli meats, hot dogs, and bacon	Formation of nitrosamines
Trans fat	Partially hydrogenated fats used to make shortening, "stick" margarines, and baked goods	Unclear whether trans fats are carcinogenic, but they may alter the normal balance of fatty acids in the colorectum

the lining of the esophagus, making cancerous cells more likely to develop in the affected area.

Table 8.15 indicates dietary factors that may be associated with increased risk of various cancers. Currently, there is no scientific evidence that consuming artificial sweeteners, such as aspartame; coffee; fluoridated water; or foods preserved by radiation (*irradiated foods*) causes cancer.[54] However, some dietary practices may *reduce* the risk of cancer.

Diet: Cancer Prevention

Consuming a nutritious diet that contains adequate fluids and a variety of foods, especially plant foods, may prevent or delay the development of certain cancers. Drinking enough water and other nonalcoholic fluids may reduce the risk of bladder cancer, because water dilutes carcinogens that may be present in urine.[53] Adequate fluid intake also encourages frequent urination, which reduces the time that carcinogens remain in contact with the walls of the bladder.

High intakes of fruits and vegetables reduce the risk of cancer, especially lung, mouth, throat, esophageal, stomach, pancreatic, and colorectal cancers.[53] Fruits and vegetables are rich sources of vitamin C as well as carotenoids and other phytochemicals that

may have antioxidant activity in the body. Antioxidants protect DNA from free radical damage, preventing potentially cancer-causing mutations from occurring. Although research is ongoing, results of scientific studies generally do not provide evidence that taking dietary supplements that contain antioxidants reduces the risk of cancer.[56] Some medical experts are concerned that taking antioxidant supplements may *increase* the risk of lung and prostate cancers, especially among smokers and men with family histories of prostate cancer.[57]

Many plant foods naturally contain chemicals that reduce carcinogens' ability to damage DNA. Other phytochemicals inhibit tumor growth by being toxic to cancer cells, interfering with their ability to form supportive blood vessels, or creating conditions that make it difficult for cancer cells to flourish. For example, broccoli; cabbage; Brussels sprouts, and other *cruciferous* (*crew-siff'-er-us*) vegetables; and *turmeric* (*tur'-mur-ik*), a spice found in curry powder, contain substances that are toxic to cancer cells. Table 8.16 lists these and some other foods, beverages, and spices that may have anticancer activity. Medical researchers do not know whether taking supplements that contain phytochemicals from these dietary sources offers the same benefits as consuming the chemicals in their natural forms. Currently, much of the evidence about the cancer-protective benefits of specific plant-based chemicals is from laboratory experiments on animals or cell cultures. Testing the chemicals in clinical settings is necessary to determine whether the results observed in laboratories also occur in people. Thus, more research is needed to support the use of phytochemicals to prevent or treat cancer.

Reducing the Risk Although medical researchers are studying the cancer-fighting potential of various chemicals naturally in

TABLE 8.16

Foods, Beverages, and Spices: Possible Cancer Prevention

Although more research is necessary, consuming one or more of these foods each day **may reduce your risk of cancer:**

Cruciferous vegetables (Brussels sprouts, broccoli, cauliflower, cabbage)

Garlic, onions

Spinach

Soy and other legumes

Tomato products

Blueberries, raspberries, blackberries, cranberries

Grapes

Dark chocolate (70% cocoa)

Citrus fruit

Green tea

Red wine (in moderation)

Turmeric, curry powder

Black pepper

Whole grains

Water and other fluids

Sources: Béliveau R and Gingras D: Role of nutrition in preventing cancer. Canadian Family Physician 53:1905, 2007; American Cancer Society: The Complete Guide—Nutrition and Physical Activity: Nutrition and physical activity guidelines for cancer prevention: Revised 2008. http://www.cancer.org/docroot/PED/content/PED_3_2X_Diet_and_Activity_Factors_That_Affect_Risks.asp?siteare.

food, no major breakthroughs have occurred. At this point, the best course of action is to take steps to prevent cancer. According to the American Cancer Society, people can reduce their risk of cancer by

- Avoiding exposure to tobacco smoke
- Achieving and maintaining a healthy weight
- Adopting a physically active lifestyle
- Eating a healthy diet that limits intakes of red and processed meats and emphasizes intakes of plant foods, including fruits, vegetables, and whole grains.[53]

Avoiding obesity by establishing healthy eating and physical activity habits, especially early in life, may reduce the risk of cancer. According to results of epidemiological studies, people who exercise regularly have lower risks of certain cancers, including colon and breast cancer. Regular physical activity may reduce the risk by helping to control weight, improving immune system functioning, and enhancing the body's regulation of various hormones. Following the American Cancer Society's recommendations does not guarantee zero risk of cancer. As mentioned earlier in this "Highlight," an individual's cancer risk is ultimately determined by the complex interaction of numerous factors, not just diet and physical activity. However, people may be able to reduce their risk of many types of cancer significantly by improving their dietary choices and increasing their physical activity.

CHAPTER REFERENCES

See Appendix I.

SUMMARY

Vitamins are organic compounds that the body cannot synthesize or make enough of to maintain good health; that naturally occur in commonly eaten foods; that cause deficiency disease when they are missing from diets; and that restore good health when added back to the diet. Foods generally contain much smaller amounts of vitamins than of macronutrients.

Vitamins play numerous roles in the body, and each vitamin generally has more than one function. In general, vitamins regulate a variety of body processes, including those involved in cell division and development as well as the growth and maintenance of tissues. Vitamins, however, are not a source of energy, because cells do not metabolize them for energy. Most vitamins have more than one chemical form that functions in the body. Additionally, some vitamins have precursors (provitamins), that do not function as vitamins until the body converts them into active forms.

An oxidation reaction can form a radical, a substance with an unpaired electron. Radicals are highly reactive, and they damage or destroy molecules by removing electrons from them. Many medical researchers suspect excess oxidation is responsible for promoting chemical changes in cells that ultimately lead to heart attack, stroke, cancer, Alzheimer's disease, and even the aging process. Cells normally regulate oxidation reactions by using antioxidants such as vitamin E.

Vitamins A, D, E, and K are fat-soluble vitamins; thiamin, riboflavin, niacin, vitamin B-6, pantothenic acid, folate, biotin, vitamin B-12, and vitamin C are water-soluble vitamins. (The vitamin-like compound called choline is water soluble.) The body generally has more difficulty eliminating excess fat-soluble vitamins than doing so with water-soluble vitamins. As a result, the body stores extra fat-soluble vitamins. Over time, these vitamins can accumulate and cause toxicity. Water-soluble vitamins are generally not as toxic as fat-soluble vitamins.

The enrichment program specifies amounts of thiamin, riboflavin, niacin, and folic acid and the mineral iron that manufacturers must add to their refined flour and other milled grain products. However, enrichment does not replace the vitamin E, vitamin B-6, potassium, magnesium, several other micronutrients, and fiber that were naturally in the unrefined grains. Fortification involves the addition of one or more vitamins (and/or other nutrients) to a wide array of commonly eaten foods during manufacturing. The vitamins that are added may or may not be in the food naturally.

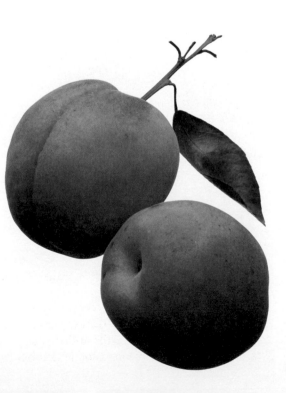

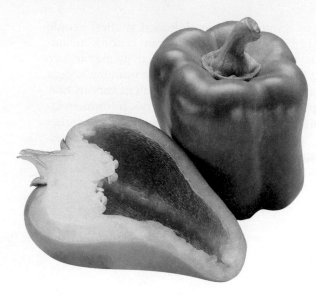

Vitamin deficiency disorders generally result from inadequate diets or conditions that increase the body's requirements for vitamins, such as reduced intestinal absorption or higher-than-normal excretion of the micronutrients. Although severe vitamin deficiencies are uncommon in the United States, certain segments of the population, particularly alcoholics, elderly persons, and patients who are hospitalized for lengthy periods, are at risk of vitamin deficiencies. The chances of developing a vitamin deficiency disease increase when the diet consistently lacks the micronutrient and levels of the nutrient in the body become depleted.

Most commonly eaten foods do not contain toxic levels of vitamins. Vitamin toxicity is most likely to occur in people who take megadoses of vitamin supplements or consume large amounts of vitamin-fortified foods regularly. A diet that contains adequate amounts of a wide variety of foods, including minimally processed fruits, vegetables, and whole-grain breads and cereals, can help supply the vitamin needs of healthy people.

Vitamin A is involved in vision, immune function, and cell development. The vitamin A precursor, beta-carotene, functions as an antioxidant. Dietary sources of preformed vitamin A include liver, fish, and fish oils; provitamin A carotenoids are especially plentiful in dark green and orange fruits and vegetables. Excess vitamin A can be quite toxic and cause birth defects when taken during pregnancy.

Vitamin D is both a hormone and a vitamin. Exposure to sunlight enables human skin to synthesize a precursor of the vitamin from a cholesterol-like substance. The body can convert this substance to the active form of the vitamin. A few foods, including fatty fish and fortified milk, are dietary sources of the vitamin. Vitamin D helps regulate the level of blood calcium by increasing calcium absorption from the intestine. Infants and children who do not obtain enough vitamin D may develop rickets, and adults with inadequate amounts of the vitamin in their bodies may develop osteomalacia. Older people and breastfed infants often need a supplemental source of the vitamin. Excess intakes of vitamin D can cause the body to deposit calcium in soft tissues.

Vitamin E functions primarily as an antioxidant. By donating electrons to electron-seeking compounds, vitamin E neutralizes them. This effect shields cell membranes and red blood cells from breakdown. Plant oils and products made from these oils are generally rich sources of vitamin E.

Thiamin, riboflavin, and niacin play key roles as part of coenzymes in energy-yielding reactions. These water-soluble vitamins help cells metabolize carbohydrates, fats, and proteins. Enriched grain products are common sources of all three of the vitamins. Beriberi is the severe thiamin deficiency disease; pellagra results from a severe lack of niacin. Excess intakes of niacin can cause toxicity.

Vitamin B-6 is involved in protein metabolism, especially in synthesizing nonessential amino acids. The vitamin also participates in the synthesis of neurotransmitters and the metabolism of homocysteine. Healthy people can obtain enough vitamin B-6 by eating a varied diet that contains animal foods and rich plant sources of the micronutrient. High doses of vitamin B-6 should be avoided because the vitamin can cause nervous system damage.

Folate plays important roles in DNA synthesis and homocysteine metabolism. Rich food sources of folate are leafy vegetables, organ meats, and orange juice. Signs of folate deficiency include megaloblastic anemia. Pregnancy increases the body's needs for folate; a deficiency during the first month of pregnancy can result in neural tube defects in offspring. Women of childbearing age can meet the RDA for the vitamin by taking dietary supplements that contain synthetic folic acid. Excess folate in the diet can mask a vitamin B-12 deficiency.

The body needs vitamin B-12 to metabolize folate and homocysteine, and maintain the insulation surrounding nerves. Although vitamin B-12 does not occur naturally in plant foods, the vitamin is in animal foods and products that have been fortified with the micronutrient. Vitamin B-12 deficiency is more common in older adults. As people age, they produce less HCl, which can result in B-12 deficiency even though adequate amounts of the micronutrient are consumed in foods. Loss of intrinsic factor production in the stomach also causes vitamin B-12 deficiency and a condition called pernicious anemia.

The body uses vitamin C to synthesize and maintain collagen, a major protein in connective tissue. Vitamin C also functions as an antioxidant. Fresh fruits and vegetables, especially citrus fruits, are generally good sources of the micronutrient. Because vitamin C is readily lost in cooking, diets should emphasize fresh or lightly cooked fruits and vegetables. Smoking increases the body's requirement for vitamin C. Scurvy is the vitamin C deficiency disease. Excess vitamin C may cause diarrhea and increase the risk of kidney stones in some people.

Although the health benefits of vitamin supplementation remain uncertain, there is consistent epidemiological evidence that a diet high in fruits, vegetables, and legumes may lower the risk of CVD, cancer, and other serious chronic disease. Consuming a wide variety of vitamins, antioxidants, and phytochemicals in their natural states and concentrations (in foods) may be the most effective way to achieve good health. Therefore, people should consume a variety of fruits and vegetables daily rather than take vitamin or antioxidant supplements. Combining a nutritious diet with regular exercise is essential for achieving and maintaining good health. Furthermore, smokers need to recognize that quitting tobacco use is more likely to benefit their long-term health than simply improving their diets or increasing their physical activity levels.

Cancer occurs when genes that regulate cellular growth, division, and death mutate, resulting in abnormal cell development, rapid cell growth, and unchecked cell division. Maintaining a healthy body weight, exercising regularly, consuming diets that supply plenty of fruits and vegetables, limiting intakes of red and/or processed meats, and avoiding tobacco smoke and excess alcohol may reduce the risk of cancer.

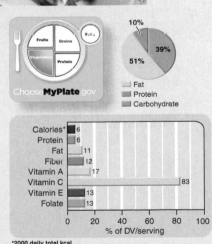

Recipe for Healthy Living

Stir-Fried Vegetable Medley

"Eat your vegetables!" Does this order bring back some not-so-fond dinnertime memories? If you are like many Americans, cooked vegetables were not high on your list of favorite foods when you were a child. Corn on the cob was fun to eat, but you may have picked at your peas and carrots, and refused to eat broccoli unless it was smothered in a gooey cheese sauce. You probably drew a "line in the sand" when offered Brussels sprouts. Now that you have read Chapter 8, you should appreciate the nutritional contribution that a wide variety of colorful vegetables can make to your diet. Your parents told the truth when they said, "Vegetables are good for you."

This vegetable medley can be the foundation of a vegetarian meal or a colorful accompaniment to main dishes. You don't need to use all the vegetables in the recipe—feel free to improvise, especially when certain fresh vegetables are in season and plentiful. If you use fresh vegetables, wash them in cool water and drain on paper towels before cutting them into bite-size pieces. If you use frozen vegetables, add them directly to the hot oil, without thawing them first. Be careful because ice from the vegetables can cause hot oil to spatter.

Your goal is to heat the vegetables in a small amount of hot oil only until they are still colorful and crisp—about 4 to 8 minutes. Add the quicker-cooking vegetables (for example, mushrooms) last, so they don't overcook. Use a slotted spoon to drain oil from vegetables and serve immediately.

This recipe (without rice or noodles) makes about four ½-cup servings. Each serving supplies approximately 123 kcal, 3 g protein, 7 g fat, 3 g fiber, 50 mg vitamin C, 53 mcg folate, 173 RAE vitamin A, and 4 mg vitamin E.

INGREDIENTS:

1 Tbsp low-sodium soy sauce
2 Tbsp water
1 Tbsp brown sugar
⅛ tsp ground black pepper
2 Tbsp vegetable oil
1 large garlic clove, minced
½ cup onions, sliced
1 cup asparagus, cut into 2"- long pieces
½ cup broccoli, small pieces
½ cup carrots, sliced into "coins"
½ medium green pepper, cut in
   2" strips, about ¼" wide
½ medium sweet red pepper, cut in
   2" strips, about ¼" wide
6 button mushrooms, crosscut into
   quarters

PREPARATION STEPS:

1. In a small dish, prepare mixture of soy sauce, water, and brown sugar. Set aside.

2. Heat oil in a wok or large deep frying pan over medium-high heat. Add garlic and onions. Stir.

3. When onions and garlic are translucent, add asparagus, broccoli, carrots, peppers, and mushrooms. Stir mixture constantly to coat vegetables with oil.

4. Add soy sauce, water, and brown sugar mixture.

5. Add zucchini. Sprinkle black pepper over vegetables.

6. Do not overcook. If the mixture seems too dry, add another tablespoon of water.

7. Serve immediately over cooked rice or noodles.

Personal *Dietary* Analysis

Using the DRIs

1. Refer to your 1- or 3-day food log from the "Personal Dietary Analysis" feature in Chapter 3.

  a. Find the RDA/AI values for vitamins under your life stage/gender group category in the DRI tables (see the inside back cover of this book). Write those values under the "My RDA/AI" column in the table on the following page.

  b. Review your personal dietary assessment. Find your 3-day average intakes of vitamins A, E, C, D, folate, B-12, thiamin, riboflavin, and niacin. Write those values under the "My Average Intake" column of the table.

  c. Calculate the percentage of the RDA/AI you consumed for each vitamin by dividing your intake by the RDA/AI amount and multiplying the figure you obtain by 100. For example, if your average intake of vitamin C were 100 mg/day, and your RDA for the vitamin were 75 mg/day, you would divide 100 mg by 75 mg to obtain 1.25. To multiply this figure by 100, simply move the decimal point two places to the right, and replace the decimal point with a percentage sign (125%). Thus, your average daily intake of vitamin C was 125% of the RDA. Place the percentages for each vitamin under the "% of My RDA/AI" column.

  d. Under the "> , < , =" column, indicate whether your average daily intake was greater than (>), less than (<), or equal to (=) the RDA/AI.

2. Use the information you calculated in the first part of this activity to answer the following questions:

  a. Which of your average vitamin intakes equaled or exceeded the RDA/AI value?

  b. Which of your average vitamin intakes was below the RDA/AI value?

  c. What foods would you eat to increase your intake of the vitamins that were less than the RDA/AI levels? (Review sources of certain vitamins in Chapter 8.)

  d. Turn in your completed table and answers to your instructor.

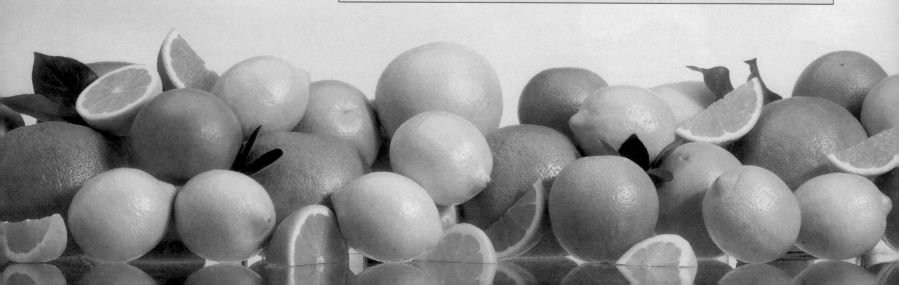

Personal Dietary Analysis: Vitamins

Vitamin	My RDA/AI	My Average Intake	% of My RDA/AI	>, <, or =
A				
E				
C				
D				
Folate				
B-12				
Thiamin				
Riboflavin				
Niacin				

 CRITICAL THINKING

1. Choose a vitamin and type the nutrient's name in the search box of an Internet browser. Locate three sites that sell products containing the vitamin. Review the pages of each site, making notes about claims, prices, and the kinds of links provided. Then write a three- to five-page report that describes and compares the information you found at the sites. In your paper, discuss any claims made on behalf of these products that you consider false or misleading. Include the URLs for the sites in your report.

2. Choose three different websites that sell vitamin supplements. Choose three different products and compare prices for the same product at the different websites. Then compare prices of the vitamins from these sites with the prices you would pay at a local supermarket, discount department store, or drugstore. Make sure to compare products with the same chemical composition (single vitamin, for example) and that have the same amount of the vitamin or vitamin-like compound in each dose. Write a one-page report about your findings.

3. While watching an infomercial on TV, you hear a so-called nutrition expert make claims for a substance that he or she claims to be a vitamin. What questions would you ask the expert to ascertain whether the substance truly is a vitamin?

4. One of your friends takes megadoses of vitamin A, C, B-6, and E because she thinks they help her stay healthy. What would you tell her about taking such large doses of these vitamins?

5. According to MyPlate, a person who needs 2000 kcal/day should consume 2 cups of fruit and 2.5 cups of vegetables daily. Plan a day's meals and snacks that provide these amounts of fruits and vegetables. In your plan, incorporate foods you like to eat. For information concerning how much of a certain form of fruit or type of vegetable equals 1 cup of fruit, visit www.choosemyplate.gov and click on the "Fruits" and then the "Vegetables" sections of the plate.

PRACTICE TEST

Select the best answer.

1. Megadoses of vitamins are
   a. safe to take, if the vitamins are water soluble.
   b. useful for preventing chronic diseases.
   c. available naturally from a wide variety of foods.
   d. None of the above is correct.

2. Vitamins
   a. are metabolized to yield energy.
   b. occur in gram amounts in foods.
   c. are organic molecules.
   d. are macronutrients.

3. People who are unable to absorb fat are likely to develop a _____ deficiency.
   a. vitamin A
   b. folate
   c. vitamin B-12
   d. riboflavin

4. Enriched grain products have specific amounts of _____ added during processing.
   a. vitamin C
   b. vitamin A
   c. vitamin B-12
   d. thiamin

5. The vitamin content of a plant can be affected by
   a. soil composition.
   b. the plant's maturity when harvested.
   c. sunlight exposure.
   d. All of the above are correct.

6. Which of the following foods is not a rich source of provitamin A?
   a. beef
   b. carrots
   c. squash
   d. sweet potato

7. Children who lack vitamin D can develop
   a. pellagra.
   b. rickets.
   c. beriberi.
   d. scurvy.

8. During pregnancy, excess _____ intake is known to be teratogenic.
   a. vitamin A
   b. biotin
   c. vitamin K
   d. folate

9. Lack of vitamin _____ causes scurvy.
   a. A
   b. C
   c. D
   d. K

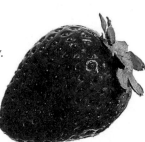

10. Vitamin K can be produced by
    a. skin exposure to ultraviolet radiation.
    b. hydrolysis of seawater.
    c. intestinal bacteria.
    d. conversion of lactic acid into lactate.

11. Diets that lack niacin can lead to
    a. rickets.
    b. beriberi.
    c. pellagra.
    d. pernicious anemia.

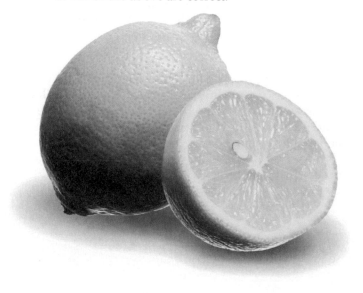

12. To reduce the likelihood of giving birth to babies with neural tube defects, women of childbearing age should obtain adequate
    a. folate.
    b. biotin.
    c. cellulose.
    d. niacin.

13. Major food sources of vitamin B-12 include
    a. enriched grain products.
    b. meat and milk products.
    c. fruit and vegetables.
    d. nuts and seeds.

14. Which of the following statements is false?
    a. Intrinsic factor is needed for vitamin B-12 absorption.
    b. Vitamin B-12 deficiency is common among elderly persons.
    c. Patients with pernicious anemia are treated with high doses of folic acid.
    d. If untreated, pernicious anemia can be deadly.

15. Which of the following foods is a rich source of vitamin C?
    a. whole milk
    b. egg white
    c. hamburger patty
    d. green pepper

16. Which of the following practices may reduce your risk of cancer?
    a. eating fruits and vegetables
    b. eating grilled meats regularly
    c. smoking no more than 10 cigarettes daily
    d. consuming two to three standard alcoholic drinks daily

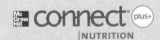

Additional resources related to the features of this book are available on ConnectPlus® Nutrition. Ask your instructor how to get access.

Answers to Chapter 8 Quiz *Yourself*

1. Natural vitamins are better for you because they have more biological activity than synthetic vitamins. **False.** (p. 245)

2. Certain vitamins are toxic. **True.** (p. 243)

3. Vitamin E is an antioxidant. **True.** (p. 244)

4. Vitamins are a source of "quick" energy. **False.** (p. 243)

5. According to scientific research, taking large doses of vitamin C daily prevents the common cold. **False.** (p. 282)

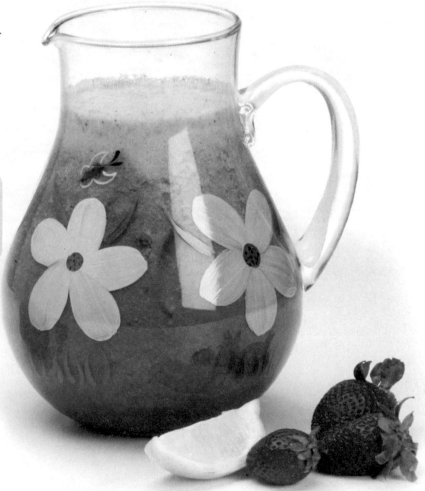

9

Water and Minerals

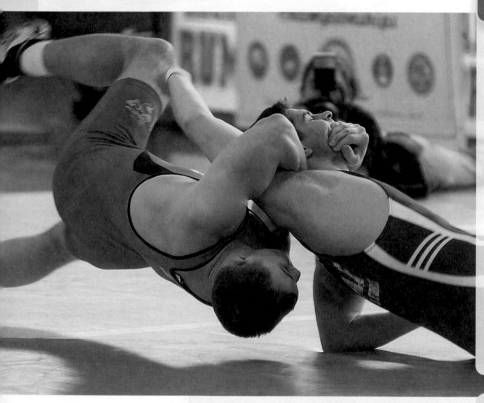

Chapter Learning Outcomes

After reading Chapter 9, you should be able to

1. Discuss the functions of water in the body as well as typical sources of intake and loss.

2. Discuss how the body maintains its water balance.

3. List major signs and symptoms of heat-related illnesses.

4. Classify mineral nutrients as major, trace, or possible essential minerals.

5. Describe factors that can affect the absorption, retention, and availability of mineral nutrients.

6. List key functions and major food sources of mineral nutrients.

7. Identify signs and symptoms associated with deficiencies as well as excesses of mineral nutrients.

8. Describe roles of minerals in achieving and maintaining good health.

9. Identify major risk factors for hypertension and osteoporosis.

10. Discuss the pros and cons of drinking bottled water.

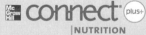 **www.mcgrawhillconnect.com**

A wealth of proven resources are available on ConnectPlus® Nutrition! Ask your instructor about ConnectPlus, which includes an interactive eBook, an adaptive learning program and much, much more!

IN LATE AUGUST 1997, a 19-year-old student wrestler who weighed 233 pounds attended a university in North Carolina. The young man was anxious to lose enough weight to qualify for the 195-pound weight class when the collegiate wrestling season began later that semester. By November 6, the wrestler had lost 23 pounds, but the first tournament was to be held in two days and he was still 15 pounds too heavy. To lose ("cut") the extra weight, he engaged in an intense, almost nonstop training session. In a 12-hour period that spanned November 6 and 7, the wrestler restricted his water and food intake severely. Additionally, he wore a special suit made from a rubberized material that was *vapor impermeable*, and he even covered it with a cotton warm up outfit. By wearing this combination of clothing, the young man perspired profusely. Sweating can cause the body to lose a significant amount of "water weight"; however, sweating can also cause **dehydration** (body water depletion), especially when a person restricts his or her fluid intake. Severe dehydration is a life-threatening condition that requires urgent medical care.

At 3 P.M. on November 6, the college wrestler began exercising vigorously in a hot environment. By 11:30 P.M. that night, he had lost 9 pounds. After resting for about 2 hours, the young man resumed his exercise regimen in a desperate effort to lose the remaining 6 pounds. Around 2:45 A.M. on November 7, he had to discontinue exercising—he was extremely fatigued and unable to communicate. An hour later, he stopped breathing and his heart ceased beating. Attempts to revive him were unsuccessful.[1]

During the 33 days that followed this young man's death, two more young male wrestlers died under similar circumstances at two other universities. As in the first wrestler's case, the two student athletes were trying to lose approximately 15% of their pre–wrestling season body weights in a relatively short period of time. At the time of their deaths, all three wrestlers suffered from dehydration. Furthermore, the young men presented signs of **hyperthermia** (very high body temperature) that may have contributed to their deaths.[1]

The rapid weight-loss practices that resulted in the deaths of these young wrestlers were prohibited by National Collegiate Athletic Association (NCAA) regulations. However, the NCAA's guidelines concerning weight management practices for wrestlers were often ignored by the athletes. Why? At that time, many wrestlers were determined to lose enough weight prior to a meet so they could compete in weight categories that were lower than their preseason weights. By competing in a lower weight class, the wrestlers hoped to increase their competitive edge over opponents. After weighing in for an event, the dehydrated athletes counted on having enough time to restore their body's normal water status before the start of the match.

(continued)

dehydration body water depletion

hyperthermia very high body temperature

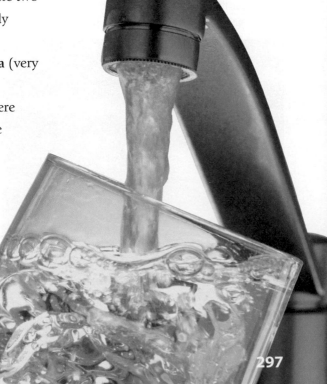

After the deaths of these athletes, the NCAA instituted sweeping changes establishing new guidelines concerning weight certification, weight classification, and weighing-in procedures for college wrestlers. NCAA rules prohibit the athletes from losing weight rapidly by restricting food and fluid intakes excessively; staying in hot boxes, saunas, or other rooms designed to produce sweating; wearing vapor-impermeable suits to cause sweating; and using laxatives, self-induced vomiting, or medications that increase urine production. Failure to follow the NCAA's wrestling guidelines can result in suspension from competition. Since these rules were established, no dehydration-related deaths among college wrestlers have been reported.

The tragic and preventable deaths of the three young wrestlers emphasize the importance of water and the consequences of dehydration. Many of water's functions involve certain minerals. The mineral nutrients are key components of body structures and play vital roles in metabolism, water balance, muscle movement, and various physiological processes. Mineral deficiencies can cause serious health problems and, in severe cases, death. In Chapter 9, we will focus on water first and then discuss some of the essential minerals that are of major concern for public health officials in the United States and other parts of the world.

Perspiring helps maintain normal body temperature because water can hold a lot of heat. As sweat evaporates from skin, it takes some heat along with it, cooling the body.

 ## 9.1 Water

Compared to other nutrients, water is so unusual, it is in a class by itself. Water is a simple compound; a molecule of water is comprised of two hydrogen atoms and one oxygen atom (H_2O). Water does not need to be digested, and it is easily absorbed by the intestinal tract.

Depending on a person's age, sex, and body composition, 50 to 75% of his or her body is water weight (see Fig. 1.2). Lean muscle tissue contains more water (about 73%) than fat tissue (about 20%). On average, young adult men have more lean tissue than young women. Approximately 55 to 60% of an average young man's body weight is water; the average young adult woman's body has more fat and, therefore, slightly less water than an average young man's body. A person's percentage of body weight that is water declines from birth to old age. Water may comprise only 45% of a typical older adult's weight.[2]

Water is a major solvent; many substances, including glucose, dissolve in water. Water often participates directly in chemical reactions, such as those involved in digesting food. Water's other physiological roles include transporting substances, removing waste products, lubricating tissues, and regulating body temperature and acid-base balance (proper blood pH). Furthermore, water is a major component of blood, saliva, sweat, tears, mucus, and the fluid in joints. Table 9.1 lists roles of water in the body.

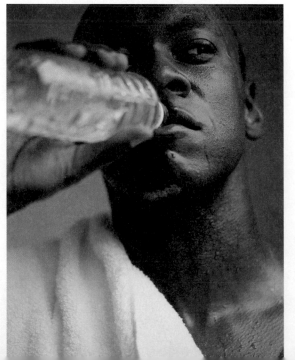

Although water has numerous functions in the body, this unique nutrient does not provide energy.

We often take water for granted, but this simple molecule is highly essential. You can survive for weeks, even months, if your diet lacks carbohydrates, lipids, proteins, and vitamins. But if you do not have any water, your life will end within a week or two. Fortunately, your body obtains water from beverages and foods, especially fruits, vegetables, and meats. The body also makes some water as a result of its metabolism.

Did You Know?

The layer of fat that is under the skin (*subcutaneous fat*) interferes with the transfer of heat to the skin. This explains why overweight people who are in warm conditions are more uncomfortable and perspire more than slender people.

Membrane Transport

One reason why water is such a vital nutrient is its role in helping cells obtain materials from their environment and eliminate wastes. To understand some of water's functions in the body, it is necessary to understand how water-soluble substances can become distributed when they are in water. In some instances, the molecules move by **simple diffusion**; that is, the molecules move from where they are highly concentrated to where they are less concentrated (Fig. 9.1). For example, simple diffusion occurs when a sugar cube is dropped into a cup of hot tea. As the cube dissolves, the concentration of sugar molecules around the cube becomes higher than the concentration of sugar molecules near the surface of the tea. However, the sugar molecules spontaneously diffuse throughout the tea, and eventually, the concentration of sugar molecules and water molecules becomes evenly distributed within the beverage.

Simple diffusion also occurs when there is a greater concentration of molecules on one side of a *selectively permeable membrane* than on the other. A **selectively permeable membrane** is a barrier that allows the passage of certain substances and prevents the movement of other substances through it. **Osmosis** is the diffusion of *water* through a selectively permeable membrane, such as the plasma membrane of a human cell. The concentration of substances dissolved in the water, such as sodium ions or glucose, influences osmosis. Water moves from a region that has

TABLE 9.1 *Functions of Water in the Body*

Water
is a solvent
is a major component of blood, saliva, sweat, tears, mucus, joint fluid
removes wastes
helps transport substances
lubricates tissues
regulates body temperature
helps digest foods
participates in many chemical reactions
helps maintain proper blood pH

simple diffusion molecular movement from a region of higher to lower concentration

selectively permeable membrane barrier that allows the passage of certain substances and prevents the movement of other substances

osmosis movement of water through a selectively permeable membrane

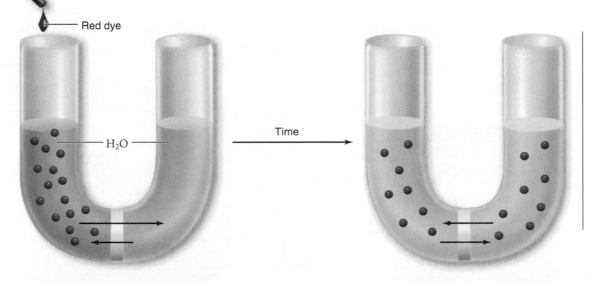

Red dye

H_2O

Time

Figure 9.1 Simple diffusion. Simple diffusion can occur when there is a greater concentration of a substance in one region than in another. In this example, the dye is more concentrated on the left side of the container than on the right side. Eventually, the dye molecules diffuse (move) from where they are more concentrated to where they are less concentrated. The diffusion stops when the concentrations of dye molecules are equally distributed throughout the container.

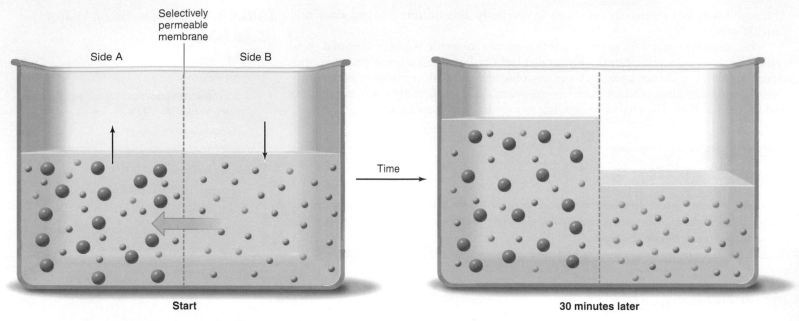

Figure 9.2 Osmosis. Osmosis is the diffusion of water through a selectively permeable membrane. Water moves from a compartment that is less concentrated to a compartment that has more material dissolved in it.

less material dissolved in it (dilute) to a region that has more material dissolved in it (Fig. 9.2). The diffusion stops when the concentrations of the material on either side of the plasma membrane are equal.

To survive, a human cell carefully controls the passage of substances through its plasma membrane. Some materials, such as oxygen and carbon dioxide, easily pass through the cell's plasma membrane by simple diffusion. Large molecules, such as proteins, may be unable to pass through the cell's membrane, or they may need special carrier molecules to enter the cell. Chapter 4 discussed other ways cells can obtain substances from their environment.

Body Water Distribution

The body has two major fluid compartments—intracellular water and extracellular water (Fig. 9.3). **Intracellular water** is inside cells. **Extracellular water** surrounds cells (tissue

Figure 9.3 Fluid compartments in the body. Intracellular water is inside cells; extracellular water surrounds cells (tissue fluid) or is the fluid in blood (*plasma*). Water is exchanged between plasma and tissue fluid (large arrows) as well as between tissue and intracellular fluids (small arrows).

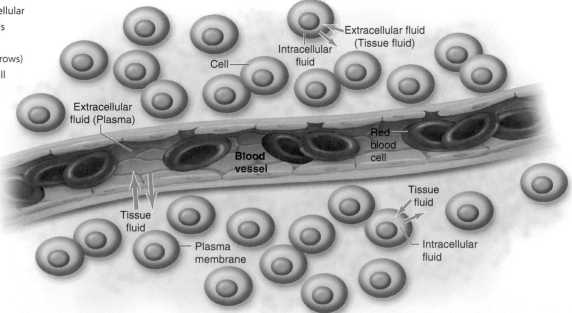

fluid) or is the fluid portion of blood (*plasma*). About two-thirds of the body's water is in the intracellular compartment.

The body maintains the balance of compartmental fluids and proper **hydration,** adequate water status, primarily by controlling concentrations of ions in each compartment. Ions are elements or small molecules that have electrical charges (electrolytes). Water is attracted to ions, such as sodium, potassium, phosphate, and chloride ions. Overall, where ions go, water follows.

Maintenance of intracellular water volume depends to a large extent on the intracellular concentration of potassium and phosphate ions. On the other hand, maintenance of extracellular water volume depends primarily on the extracellular concentration of sodium and chloride ions. Changes in the normal concentrations of these ions can cause water to shift out of one compartment and move into the other. For example, if extracellular fluid has fewer-than-normal sodium ions, water moves from the extracellular compartment into cells. When this occurs, the cells swell and can burst (Fig. 9.4a). On the other hand, if extracellular fluid has an excess of sodium ions, water moves out of cells. As a result, the cells shrink and die because they lack enough intracellular fluid to function (Fig. 9.4b). Recall from Chapter 7 that edema (*eh-dee'-mah*) occurs when an excessive amount of water moves into the space surrounding cells (see Fig. 7.1). To function normally, the body must maintain intracellular and extracellular water volumes within certain limits.

Sources of Water

How much water is necessary to drink for good health? Contrary to popular belief, there is no "rule of thumb" recommendation that specifies how many glasses of water to consume each day.[3] Factors such as environmental temperatures, health conditions, physical activities, and dietary choices influence individual water requirements. Thus, total water intakes vary widely. **Total water intake** refers to water ingested by consuming beverages and foods.

intracellular water water that is inside cells

extracellular water water that surrounds cells or is in blood

hydration water status

total water intake water in beverages and foods

Figure 9.4 Maintaining proper hydration. Cells, such as red blood cells, need to maintain their fluid balance. Changes in the normal concentrations of ions can cause water to shift out of one compartment and move into the other. The cell in beaker *(a)* is placed in a solution that contains few sodium ions (Na$^+$) in relation to the concentration of Na$^+$ in the cell. As a result, water moves from the solution and into the red blood cell. The cell can swell and burst. The solution in beaker *(b)* has an excess of sodium ions (Na$^+$) compared to the concentration of Na$^+$ inside the cell. Water moves out of the red blood cell placed in beaker *(b)*. As a result, the cell shrinks, and can die.

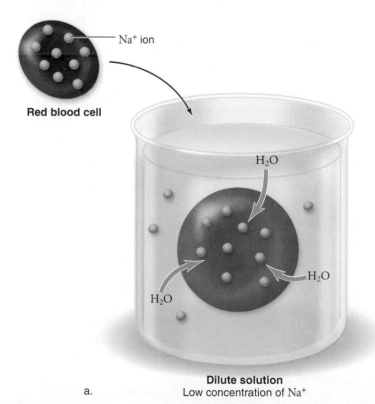

a.   **Dilute solution**
Low concentration of Na$^+$

b.   **Concentrated solution**
High concentration of Na$^+$

Na$^+$ ion

Red blood cell

H$_2$O

metabolic water water formed by cells as a metabolic by-product

antidiuretic hormone (ADH) hormone that participates in water conservation

aldosterone hormone that participates in sodium and water conservation

The Adequate Intake (AI) for *total* water intake is approximately 11 cups (2.7 L) for young women and approximately 15.5 cups (3.7 L) for young men.[4] These amounts do not need to be consumed in the form of water. Other sources of water include fruit juice, milk, soup, coffee, tea, soft drinks, and flavored bottled water. Most solid foods also contain some water. Fruits and vegetables appear to be solid, but they generally contain 60 to 95% water weight. Table 9.2 lists some commonly consumed foods and their water content by weight. About 80% of our total water intake is from water and other beverages; food supplies the remaining amount of our water intake.[4]

In addition to the water in beverages and foods, a considerable amount of water enters the digestive tract daily through secretions from the mouth, stomach, intestine, pancreas, and gallbladder. The intestinal tract absorbs most of this water too. Each day, only about 0.4 to 0.8 cup (100 to 200 ml) of the water that enters the digestive tract is not absorbed. The body eventually eliminates the unabsorbed water in feces.

Cells also form some water as a by-product of metabolism. Physically inactive people typically form about 1 to 1.5 cups (250 to 350 ml) of water per day; very active people can produce about 2 to 2.5 cups (500 ml to 600 ml) of water daily.[4] **Metabolic water** also contributes to the body's fluid balance.

The Essential Balancing Act

An average healthy adult consumes and produces approximately 2.5 quarts (2500 ml) of water daily (Fig. 9.5).[2] The body eliminates about 2.5 quarts of water in urine, exhaled air, feces, and perspiration (see Fig. 9.5). Thus, a healthy person's average daily water input equals his or her average daily losses (output).

Various factors influence a person's fluid input and output. Environmental factors such as temperature, humidity, and altitude can affect body water losses. Physiological conditions, especially fever, vomiting, and diarrhea, as well as lifestyle practices, such as exercise habits and sodium and alcohol intakes, can also alter the body's fluid balance.

Perspiration is body water that is secreted by sweat glands in skin. When perspiration reaches the skin's surface, it evaporates into the air. This process helps cool the body and maintain its normal temperature. *Insensible perspiration* is body water that

TABLE 9.2 *How Much Water Is in That Food or Beverage?*

Food	Water % by Weight
Lettuce	95
Tomato	95
Watermelon	91
Milk, 1% fat	90
Apple, with skin	86
Avocado	79
Potato, white, baked with skin	75
Banana	75
Chicken, white meat, roasted	65
Ground beef, 80% lean	56
Bread, whole wheat	38
Margarine, stick	16
Crackers, saltines	5
Vegetable oil	0

Source: Data from U.S. Department of Agriculture, Agricultural Research Service, USDA Nutrient Data Laboratory: *USDA national nutrient database for standard reference, release 19.* 2006.

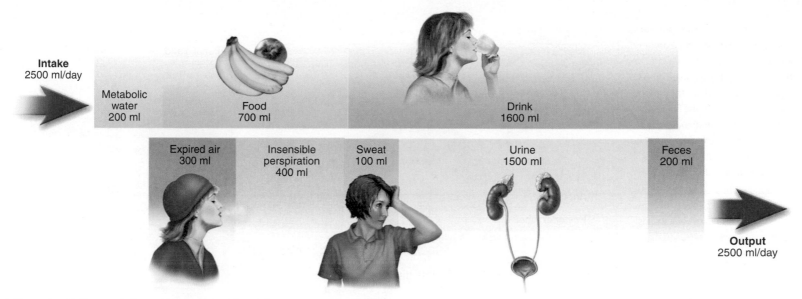

Intake
2500 ml/day

Metabolic
water
200 ml

Food
700 ml

Drink
1600 ml

Expired air
300 ml

Insensible
perspiration
400 ml

Sweat
100 ml

Urine
1500 ml

Feces
200 ml

Output
2500 ml/day

Figure 9.5 Daily water balance. An average healthy adult consumes and produces approximately 2500 ml of water and eliminates about 2500 ml of water daily. A healthy person's average daily water input equals his or her average daily losses.

diffuses through the layers of skin or is exhaled from the lungs instead of being secreted by sweat glands.[3] People are usually unaware that their bodies are constantly losing water in this manner—hence, the term "insensible" perspiration.

Kidneys and Hydration

The kidneys are the major regulator of the body's water content and ion concentrations. In a healthy person, the kidneys maintain proper hydration by filtering excess ions from blood as it flows through the kidney's tissues. When the kidneys remove ions such as sodium, water follows and becomes the main component of urine. If you drink more watery fluids than your body needs, your kidneys excrete the excess water in urine.

Kidneys also remove drugs and metabolic waste products, such as urea, from the bloodstream. Sometimes, minerals and waste products settle out of urine and collect into crystals. If the crystals enlarge and form a hard mass, the object is called a kidney stone (Fig. 9.6). Kidney stones often contain the mineral calcium.[2] As a kidney stone moves out of the kidney and enters the tube leading to the bladder, it may cause considerable pain and bloody urine until it passes out of the body. Dehydration increases the likelihood of forming kidney stones.

The amount of urine a person produces is determined primarily by his or her total water intake. A healthy person produces about 1 to 2 quarts (1 to 2 L) of urine per day. Healthy kidneys can form more urine, but they become less efficient at urine production when fluid intakes are less than about 2 cups (500 ml) per day.

Water Conservation

As mentioned in the opener of this chapter, body water depletion is called dehydration. Dehydration can be a life-threatening condition. When you are hot and perspiring heavily, your kidneys try to conserve as much water as possible to avoid dehydration. **Antidiuretic hormone (ADH)** and **aldosterone** (*al-dahs'-te-rown*) are two hormones that participate in the body's efforts to maintain fluid balance. In response to dehydration, the posterior pituitary gland in the brain releases antidiuretic hormone. Antidiuretic hormone stimulates the kidneys to conserve water. Additionally, the adrenal glands secrete aldosterone. Aldosterone signals kidneys to reduce the elimination of sodium in urine and, as a result, the kidneys return the mineral to the general circulation. Because water follows sodium, it is conserved as well. The diagram

Figure 9.6 Kidney stones. Some people form kidney stones. Although small enough to fit on a fingertip, such stones can be quite painful when they move from the kidneys and are eliminated in urine.

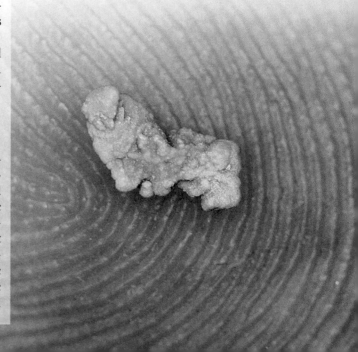

Figure 9.7 Effects of antidiuretic hormone and adolsterone on kidneys. In response to dehydration, the posterior pituitary gland in the brain secretes antidiuretic hormone (ADH), which signals the kidneys to conserve water. Additionally, the adrenal glands secrete the hormone aldosterone. Aldosterone reduces urinary excretion of sodium. When the kidneys retain sodium, they return the mineral to the general circulation. Because water follows sodium, it is conserved as well.

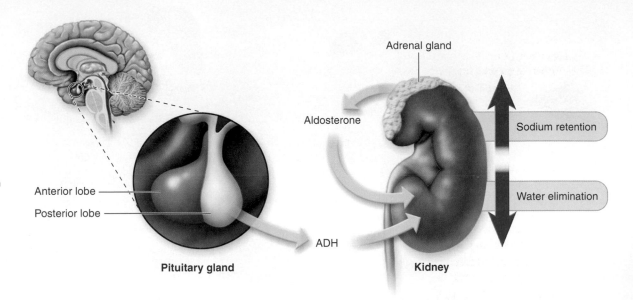

in Figure 9.7 summarizes the effects of antidiuretic hormone and aldosterone on the kidneys.

The simplest way to determine if you are consuming enough water is to observe the volume of your urine. When your fluid intake is adequate, your kidneys will produce enough urine to maintain fluid balance. If you consume more fluid than needed, your kidneys will eliminate the excess, and you will produce plenty of urine. On the other hand, if you limit your fluid intake or have high fluid losses such as in sweat, you will produce small amounts of urine.

In addition to urine volume, the color of urine may be a useful indicator of hydration status. Straw-colored (light yellow) urine can indicate adequate hydration, whereas dark-colored urine may be a sign of dehydration. However, the color of urine is not always a reliable guide for judging a person's hydration status.[5] It is important to recognize that having urinary tract infections or ingesting certain medications, foods, and dietary supplements, especially those containing the B-vitamin riboflavin, can alter urine's color.

What Is a Diuretic? Caffeine is a **diuretic,** a substance that increases urine production. Coffee, tea, energy drinks, and soft drinks often contain caffeine or caffeine-related compounds. However, the water consumed in caffeinated beverages is not completely lost in urine, so drinking these fluids may still contribute to meeting your water needs.[4]

diuretic substance that increases urine production

Did You Know?

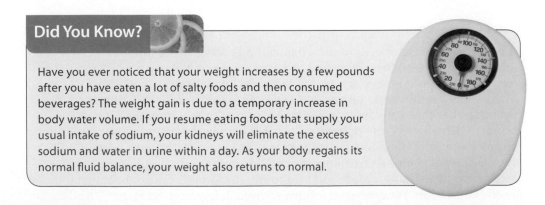

Have you ever noticed that your weight increases by a few pounds after you have eaten a lot of salty foods and then consumed beverages? The weight gain is due to a temporary increase in body water volume. If you resume eating foods that supply your usual intake of sodium, your kidneys will eliminate the excess sodium and water in urine within a day. As your body regains its normal fluid balance, your weight also returns to normal.

Alcohol is also a diuretic. Normally, antidiuretic hormone signals the kidneys to conserve water. Alcohol, however, inhibits ADH secretion from the pituitary gland in the brain, enabling the kidneys to eliminate more urine than normal. Alcohol consumption actually results in urinary water losses that are greater than the volume of fluid consumed. Therefore, alcohol contributes to dehydration.

Scientists do not know what causes a "hangover," the headache and overall discomfort that occurs a few hours after drinking too much alcohol. Dehydration, the body's immune response, and *congeners* may be responsible for the unpleasant, delayed side effects of excess alcohol consumption.[6] Congeners are substances in alcoholic drinks that contribute to the taste and color of the beverages. (Beer and vodka have lower congener contents than red wine and whiskey.) Alcoholic drinks with high congener contents tend to produce more severe hangovers than drinks with lower contents of these substances.

Dehydration

Despite the body's mechanisms to balance its water content, some fluid is constantly being lost, primarily via the skin and lungs. If a person does not consume enough fluids to replace that water, dehydration can occur. Rapid weight loss is a sign of dehydration. Every 16 ounces (about 0.5 L) of water that the body loses represents a pound of body weight. If you lose 1 to 2% of your usual body weight in fluids, you will feel fatigued and thirsty. If you weigh 150 pounds, for example, and your weight drops 3 pounds after exercising in hot conditions, you have lost 2% of your body weight, primarily as water weight.

As the loss of body water approaches 4% of body weight, muscles lose considerable amounts of strength and endurance. By the time body weight is reduced by 7 to 10% as a result of body fluid losses, severe weakness results. At a 20% reduction of body weight, coma and death are likely.

Thirst is the primary regulator of fluid intake.[2] The thirst response alerts you to the need to replenish water that was lost by sweating and other means. The majority of healthy people meet their AI for water by letting thirst be their guide.[4] Thirst stimulates people to drink fluids *before* severe dehydration occurs. However, people who are dehydrated and older than 60 years of age do not sense thirst as accurately as younger adults.[7] Furthermore, older adults may be more susceptible to develop dehydration than younger persons, because as kidneys age, they become less able to conserve water when fluid intakes are low. Therefore, it may be necessary to remind older adults to drink more watery fluids, especially when they are physically active or in warm conditions. Nevertheless, healthy elderly persons who live independently are generally able to maintain adequate hydration.[7]

People who are sick, especially children with fever, vomiting, diarrhea, and increased perspiration, may need to be given special solutions of water and electrolytes to prevent dehydration. Athletes and other people who work or exercise outdoors, especially in hot conditions, also need to stay properly hydrated to avoid dehydration and heat-related illnesses such as heat exhaustion. Chapter 11 provides information about heat-related illnesses.

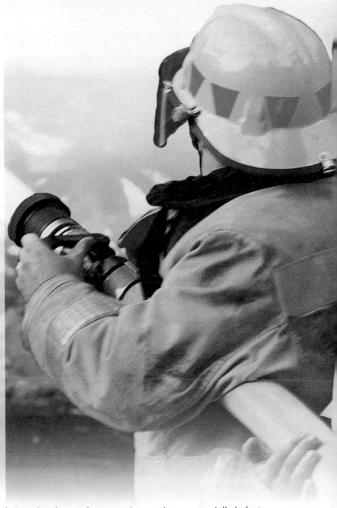

People who work or exercise outdoors, especially in hot conditions, need to stay hydrated to avoid dehydration and heat-related illnesses.

During the aftermath of the January 12, 2010, earthquake, members of the U.S. military provided safe bottled water to desperate Haitian citizens.

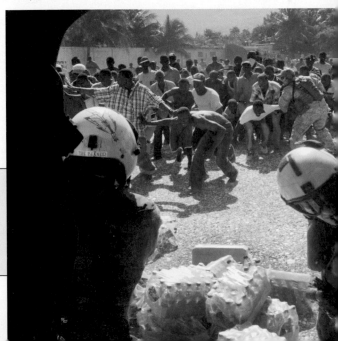

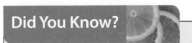

Did You Know?

A massive earthquake struck the island nation of Haiti on January 12, 2010, devastating a region that included the island's highly populated major city, Port-au-Prince. As a result of the earthquake, many Haitians had no access to drinkable water. People can survive for a few days in such conditions before dehydration contributes to their deaths.

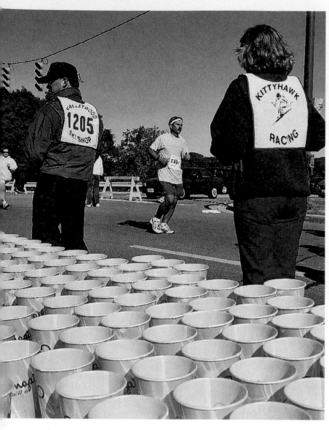

Marathon runners who consume large amounts of plain water in an effort to keep hydrated during competition may be at risk of water intoxication.

Cheese is a good source of calcium, phosphorus, and sodium.

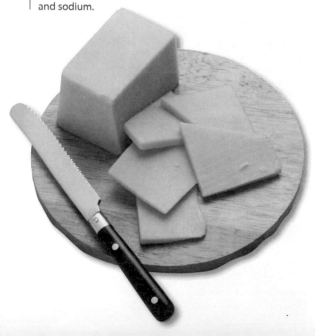

Can Too Much Water Be Toxic?

There is no Upper Limit (UL) for water. **Water intoxication,** however, can occur when an excessive amount of water is consumed in a short time period or the kidneys have difficulty filtering water from blood. The excess water dilutes the sodium concentration of blood, disrupting water balance. As a result of the imbalance, too much water moves into cells, including brain cells. Signs and symptoms of water intoxication may include dizziness, headache, confusion, inability to coordinate muscular movements, bizarre behavior, and seizures.[8] If the condition is not detected early and treated effectively, coma and death can result.

Healthy people rarely drink enough water to become intoxicated. However, water intoxication can develop in people with disorders that interfere with the kidney's ability to excrete water normally. Marathon runners who consume large amounts of plain water in an effort to keep hydrated during competition may be at risk of water intoxication. Chapter 11 discusses the importance of proper hydration for athletes.

Concept **Checkpoint**

1. List at least five different functions of water in the body.
2. Define osmosis.
3. Which ions are found primarily in extracellular water? Which ions are found primarily in intracellular water?
4. Discuss ways the body obtains and loses water.
5. What can happen to cells if the body is unable to regulate its water balance?
6. How do antidiuretic hormone and aldosterone help maintain fluid balance in the body?
7. How much water do healthy young men and women need to consume daily (AI values)?
8. What is a diuretic? Identify two diuretics commonly consumed by Americans.
9. List at least three signs and symptoms of dehydration.
10. List at least three signs and symptoms of water intoxication.

9.2 Minerals: Basic Concepts

Minerals, such as iron and calcium, are a group of elements in Earth's rocks, soils, and natural water sources. Plants, animals, and other living things cannot synthesize minerals. Plants obtain the minerals they need from soil or fertilizer; animals generally

TABLE 9.3 *Minerals with Known or Possible Roles in the Body**

Major Mineral	Trace Mineral	Possible Essential Mineral
Calcium (Ca)	Chromium (Cr)	Arsenic (As)
Chloride (Cl)	Fluoride (F)**	Boron (B)
Magnesium (Mg)	Copper (Cu)	Lithium (Li)
Phosphorus (P)	Iodine (I)	Nickel (Ni)
Potassium (K)	Iron (Fe)	Silicon (Si)
Sodium (Na)	Manganese (Mn)	Vanadium (V)
Sulfur (S)	Molybdenum (Mo)	
	Selenium (Se)	
	Zinc (Zn)	

*Chemical symbol is shown in parentheses next to mineral's name.
**Although fluoride is not essential, the mineral plays an important role in strengthening teeth and bones.

obtain minerals when they consume plants and other animals or substances that contain these elements.

About 15 mineral elements have known functions in the body and are necessary for human health. The body requires these particular micronutrients in milligram or microgram amounts. The essential minerals are classified into two groups—**major minerals** and **trace minerals** (Table 9.3). If we require 100 mg or more of a mineral per day, the mineral is classified as a major mineral; otherwise, the micronutrient is a trace mineral. The body also contains very small amounts of other minerals, such as nickel and arsenic. The essential nature of this particular group of minerals has not been fully determined.

Several minerals, including lead and mercury, are often found in the human body, but they are environmental contaminants that have no known functions. The body can eliminate most minerals in urine. However, exposure to excessive amounts of minerals can cause toxicity.

Unlike vitamins, minerals are indestructible. Because minerals cannot be destroyed, heating a food or exposing it to most other environmental conditions will not affect the food's mineral content. However, minerals are water soluble, and they can leach out of a food and into cooking water. By using the cooking water to make soups or sauces, you can obtain minerals from the food that would otherwise be discarded.

Why Are Minerals Necessary?

Essential minerals have diverse roles in the body (Fig. 9.8). Some minerals form inorganic structural components of tissues, such as calcium and phosphorus in bones and teeth. Minerals may also function as inorganic ions, substances that have negative or positive charges (see Chapter 4). For example, calcium ions (Ca^{++}) participate in blood clotting and sodium ions (Na^+) help maintain fluid balance. Sodium, potassium, and chloride ions are among the ions that participate in acid-base balance. Some ions, such

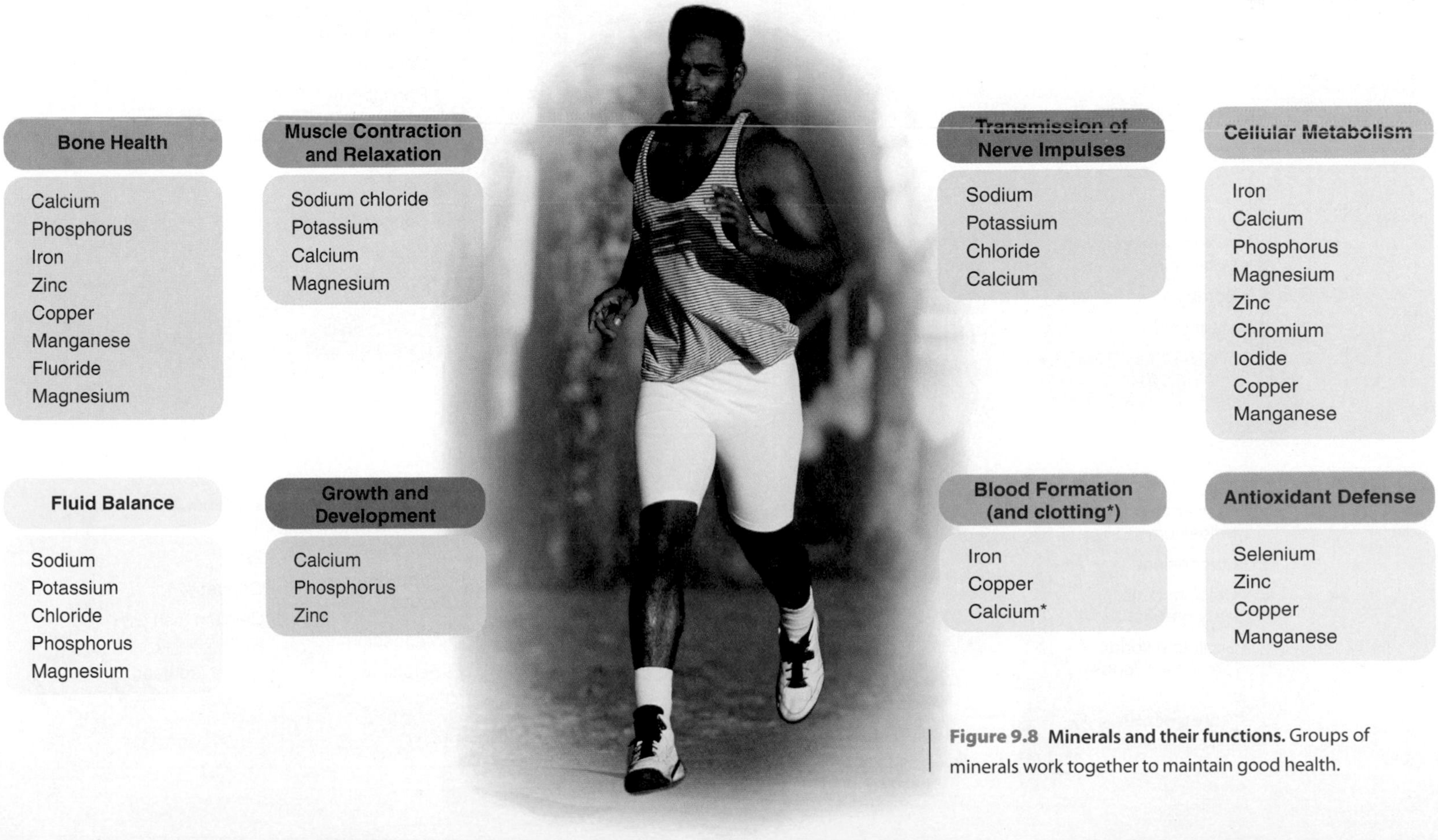

water intoxication condition that occurs when too much water is consumed in a short time period or the kidneys have difficulty filtering water from blood

major minerals essential mineral elements required in amounts of 100 mg or more per day

trace minerals essential mineral elements required in amounts that are less than 100 mg per day

Bone Health

Calcium
Phosphorus
Iron
Zinc
Copper
Manganese
Fluoride
Magnesium

Muscle Contraction and Relaxation

Sodium chloride
Potassium
Calcium
Magnesium

Transmission of Nerve Impulses

Sodium
Potassium
Chloride
Calcium

Cellular Metabolism

Iron
Calcium
Phosphorus
Magnesium
Zinc
Chromium
Iodide
Copper
Manganese

Fluid Balance

Sodium
Potassium
Chloride
Phosphorus
Magnesium

Growth and Development

Calcium
Phosphorus
Zinc

Blood Formation (and clotting*)

Iron
Copper
Calcium*

Antioxidant Defense

Selenium
Zinc
Copper
Manganese

Figure 9.8 Minerals and their functions. Groups of minerals work together to maintain good health.

cofactor ion or molecule that catalyzes chemical reactions

as magnesium (Mg⁺⁺) and copper (Cu⁺⁺), are cofactors. A **cofactor** is an ion or molecule that catalyzes chemical reactions. Many minerals are components of various enzymes, hormones, or other organic molecules, such as cobalt in vitamin B-12, iron in hemoglobin, and sulfur in the amino acids methionine and cysteine. Although cells cannot metabolize minerals for energy, certain minerals are involved in chemical reactions that release energy from macronutrients.

In some instances, the digestive tract absorbs more minerals than the body needs, but the excess is excreted, primarily in urine or feces. In other instances, the body stores the extra minerals in the liver, bones, or other tissues. Toxicity signs and symptoms occur when minerals accumulate in the body to such an extent that they interfere with the functioning of cells. Under normal conditions, the human body does not store large quantities of most minerals, and it loses small amounts of these essential elements every day. Therefore, people should choose their diets carefully so their bodies can maintain an adequate supply of minerals.

Sources of Minerals

Although most foods contain small amounts of minerals, Figure 9.9 indicates food groups from MyPlate that are generally rich sources of various minerals. The digestive tract, however, does not absorb 100% of the minerals in foods or dietary supplements. The body's ability to absorb and use minerals (*bioavailability*) depends on many factors. A major factor is the body's need for the mineral. In general, requirements increase during periods of growth, such as infancy and puberty, and during pregnancy and breastfeeding. During these critical life stages, the bioavailability of minerals also tends to increase to help meet the body's demand.

Figure 9.9 MyPlate: Food sources of minerals. Each MyPlate food group contributes minerals to the diet.

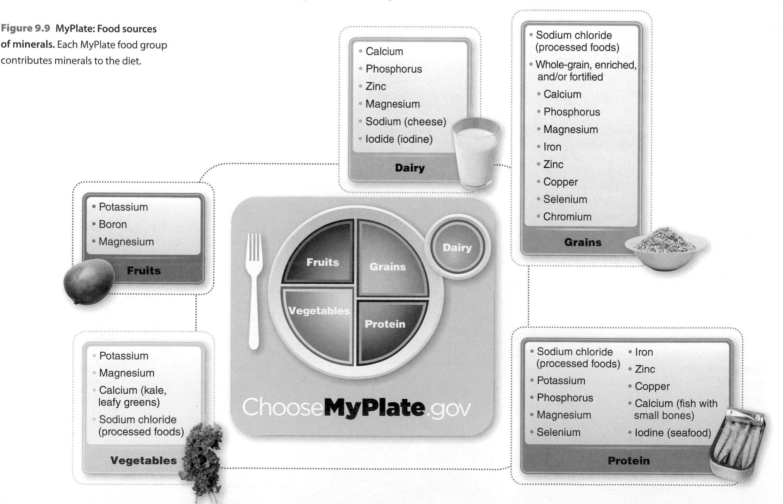

Compared to plant foods, animal foods tend to be more reliable sources of minerals, such as iron and calcium. Why? Animal products often have higher concentrations of these minerals. Additionally, plant foods can contain substances that reduce the bioavailability of minerals, particularly calcium, zinc, and iron. On the other hand, plants supply more magnesium and manganese than animal foods.

In general, the more processing a plant food undergoes, the lower its natural mineral content. Cereal grains, for example, naturally contain selenium, zinc, copper, and some other minerals, but these micronutrients are lost during refinement. Iron is the only mineral added to grains during enrichment. To obtain a variety of minerals, include some whole-grain products in your diet each day. By following the recommendations of MyPlate.gov (see Chapter 3) and eating a variety of plant and animal foods, you are likely to obtain adequate amounts of all essential minerals.

To estimate the mineral contents of packaged foods, you can check the panels on food labels. Food manufacturers are required to indicate amounts of iron and calcium in a serving of food as percentages of these micronutrients' Daily Values (%DVs). Daily Values have been established for several mineral nutrients (see Appendix C).

Other Sources of Minerals

The tap water in your community may be a source of minerals that you may have overlooked. "Hard" water naturally contains a variety of minerals, including calcium, magnesium, sulfur, iron, and zinc. Water with high mineral content often tastes and smells unpleasant. Many people drink bottled water as a substitute for tap water because they think bottled water tastes better and it is safer. To learn more about bottled water, read the Chapter 9 "Highlight."

Fluoride is often added to public water supplies. Although fluoride is not essential for life, the mineral strengthens bones and teeth when consumed in adequate amounts. In 2008, over 195 million people, or about 72% of the United States population served by public water supplies, drank water that contained optimal fluoride levels.[9]

Dietary supplements are another source of minerals. A daily multiple vitamin and mineral supplement is generally safe for healthy people, because a dose of this type of supplement does not provide high amounts of minerals. However, people need to be careful when taking dietary supplements that contain individual minerals, such as iron or selenium. Many minerals have a narrow range of safe intake; therefore, it is easy to consume a toxic amount, especially by taking supplements that contain only a particular mineral (Fig. 9.10). Additionally, an excess of one mineral can interfere with the absorption or metabolism of other minerals. For example, the presence of a large amount of zinc in the intestinal tract decreases copper absorption. Single-mineral supplements are usually unnecessary unless they are prescribed to treat a specific medical condition, such as iron deficiency.

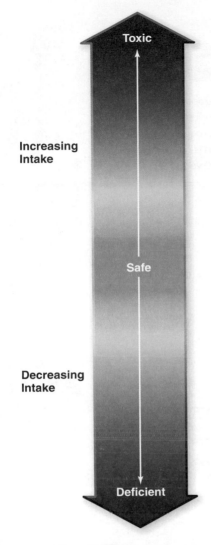

Figure 9.10 Mineral intake. Many minerals have a narrow range of safe intake. As a result, it is relatively easy to consume a toxic amount, especially by taking supplements that only contain a particular mineral.

Concept **Checkpoint**

11. List at least three different functions of minerals in the body, and provide an example of a mineral that performs each function.
12. What is the primary difference between a major mineral and a trace mineral? List three major minerals and three trace minerals.
13. Explain how foods that are naturally good sources of minerals can become poor sources of those minerals by the time you eat them.
14. Discuss factors that influence mineral absorption in the digestive tract.
15. In the United States, which mineral is required to be added to grain products as part of the enrichment program?

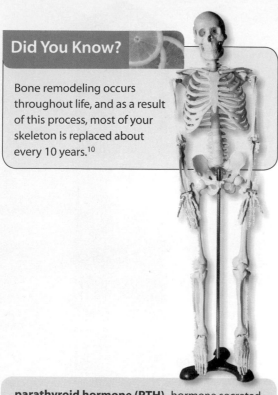

9.3 Major Minerals

Table 9.4 summarizes nutrition-related information about the major minerals. This section focuses on calcium, sodium, potassium, and magnesium because Americans tend to consume too much or too little of them. Unless otherwise noted, RDA/AI values are for adults, excluding pregnant or breastfeeding women. For more information about Dietary Reference Intake values for minerals, see the inside back cover of this textbook.

Calcium (Ca)

Calcium is the most plentiful mineral element in the human body. All cells need calcium, but more than 99% of the body's calcium is in an inorganic compound that forms the structural component of bones and teeth. The remaining calcium is in muscle tissue and extracellular fluid.

Why Is Calcium Necessary?

Although the body needs calcium to form bones and teeth, the mineral is vital to all cells. Calcium is involved in muscle contraction, blood clot formation, nerve impulse transmission, and cell metabolism. Additionally, calcium may play important roles in maintaining healthy blood pressure and functioning of the immune system.

parathyroid hormone (PTH) hormone secreted by parathyroid glands when blood calcium levels are too low

osteoclasts bone cells that tear down bone tissue

Maintaining Normal Blood Calcium Levels   The body has complex hormonal systems to maintain calcium homeostasis. The thyroid and parathyroid glands help regulate blood calcium levels (Fig. 9.11). In response to falling blood calcium levels, the parathyroid glands secrete **parathyroid hormone (PTH),** which signals special bone cells called **osteoclasts** to tear down bone tissue. This process releases calcium from bones so the

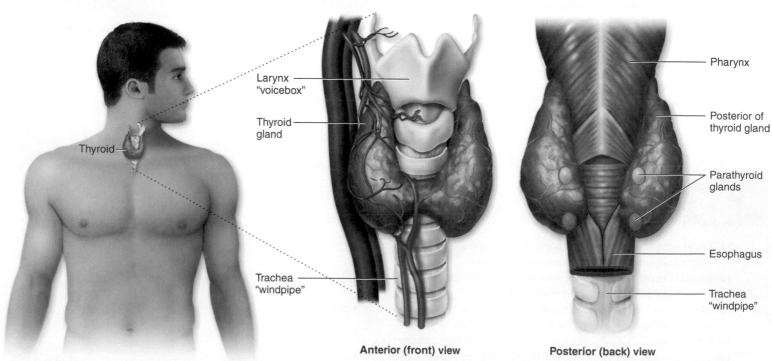

Larynx "voicebox"

Thyroid gland

Thyroid

Trachea "windpipe"

Pharynx

Posterior of thyroid gland

Parathyroid glands

Esophagus

Trachea "windpipe"

Anterior (front) view   **Posterior (back) view**

Figure 9.11 Thyroid and parathyroid glands. The thyroid gland has the four parathyroid glands imbedded in the back (posterior) of the organ. Hormones secreted by the thyroid and parathyroid glands help regulate blood calcium levels.

TABLE 9.4 *Summary of Major Minerals*

Mineral	Major Functions in the Body	Adult RDA/AI* (adult RDA = bold)	Major Dietary Sources	Major Deficiency Signs and Symptoms	Major Toxicity Signs and Symptoms
Calcium (Ca)	• Structural component of bones and teeth • Blood clotting • Transmission of nerve impulses • Muscle contraction • Regulation of metabolism	**1000–1200** mg	Milk and milk products, canned fish, tofu made with calcium sulfate, leafy vegetables, calcium-fortified foods such as orange juice	• Increased risk of osteoporosis • May increase risk of hypertension	UL = 2.0 to 2.5 g/day • Intakes > 2.5 g/day may cause kidney stones and interfere with absorption of other minerals.
Sodium (Na)	• Maintenance of proper fluid balance • Transmission of nerve impulses • Muscle contraction • Transport of certain substances into cells	1500 mg (19–50 years of age)	Table salt; luncheon meats; processed foods; pretzels, chips, and other snack foods; condiments; sauces	• Muscle cramps	UL = 2300 mg/day • Contributes to hypertension in susceptible individuals • Increases urinary calcium losses
Potassium (K)	• Maintenance of proper fluid balance • Transmission of nerve impulses • Maintenance of acid-base balance	4700 mg	Fruits, vegetables, milk, meat, legumes, whole grains	• Irregular heartbeat • Muscle cramps	No UL has been determined. • Slowing of heart rate that can result in death
Magnesium (Mg)	• Strengthens bone • Cofactor for certain enzymes • Heart and nerve functioning	Men: **400–420 mg** Women: **310–320 mg**	Wheat bran, green vegetables, nuts, chocolate, legumes	• Muscle weakness and pain • Poor heart function	UL = 350 mg/day • Diarrhea
Phosphorus (P)	• Structural component of bones and teeth • Maintenance of acid-base balance • Component of DNA, phospholipids, and other organic compounds	**700 mg**	Dairy products, processed foods, soft drinks, fish, baked goods, meat	• None reported	UL = 4 g/day • Poor bone mineralization
Chloride (Cl)	• Maintenance of proper fluid balance • Production of stomach acid • Transmission of nerve impulses • Maintenance of acid-base balance	2300 mg (19–50 years of age)	Processed foods, salty snacks, table salt	• Convulsions (observed in infants)	UL = 3600 mg/day • Hypertension (because of the association with sodium in sodium chloride [table salt])
Sulfur (S)	• Component of organic compounds such as certain amino acids and vitamins	None	Protein-rich foods	• None reported	• Unlikely from dietary sources

*Component of organic compounds such as certain amino acids and vitamins

Figure 9.12 **Bone tissue.** Normal spine tissue is on the left; the spine tissue on the right is from a person with osteoporosis.

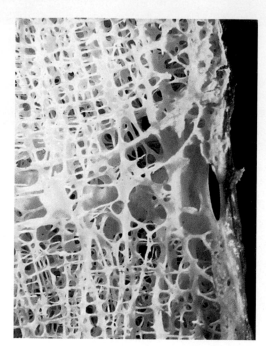
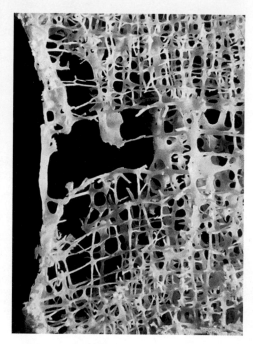

Certain leafy vegetables, such as bok choy and collard greens, contain calcium that is bioavailable.

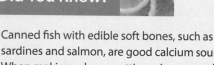

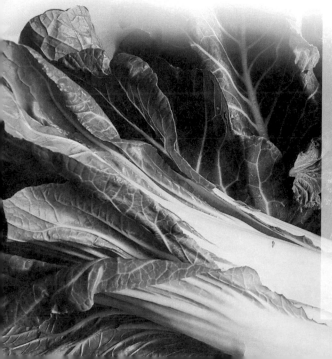

mineral can enter the bloodstream. PTH also works with vitamin D to increase intestinal calcium absorption and reduce calcium excretion in urine (see Fig. 8.12).

When the level of calcium in blood is too high, the thyroid gland secretes the hormone **calcitonin** (*cal'-sih-toe-nin*). Calcitonin signals another type of bone cell (**osteoblasts**) to remove excess calcium from blood and build bone tissue. All these physiological responses help maintain your blood calcium level within the normal range.

Bone Development and Maintenance Although your bones do not appear to change shape, they are being remodeled continually in response to the physical stresses placed on them. The remodeling process involves breaking down bone where there is little stress and building bone where there is more stress. For example, if you begin to play tennis regularly and hold the racket in your right hand, osteoblasts in the bones of your right arm build bone tissue where it is needed to help support the muscular activity. As a result, the bones in that arm become denser than the bones in your left arm. Bones that are denser have greater bone mass. As a result, they are stronger and less likely to fracture than less dense bones. Figure 9.12 shows x-rays of bone tissue. By just looking at the photos, can you tell which bone is denser and has greater mass?

Sources of Calcium

Table 9.5 includes some foods that are among the richest sources of calcium. Milk products, such as fluid milk, yogurt, and cheese, provide about 75% of the calcium in American diets.[11] Moreover, the calcium in milk products is well absorbed and used by the body. Not all products made from milk are rich sources of calcium. Cottage cheese, for example, does not supply as much calcium as the milk from which it is made, because the milk loses about half of its calcium content when it is processed to make cottage cheese (see Table 9.5). Although butter, sour cream, and cream cheese are made from whole milk, people generally do not eat enough of these high-fat foods to contribute much calcium to their diets.

Certain foods from plants contain calcium, but the foods also contain *phytic* (*fite'-ik*) *acid* or *oxalic* (*awk-sal'-ik*) *acid,* naturally occurring substances that interfere with calcium absorption. Phytic acid is a compound in whole grains and in certain seeds and beans. Spinach, collard greens, and sweet potatoes have high amounts of oxalic acid. In fact, rhubarb leaves are toxic because they contain such high amounts of the chemical.

TABLE 9.5 *Calcium Content of Selected Foods*

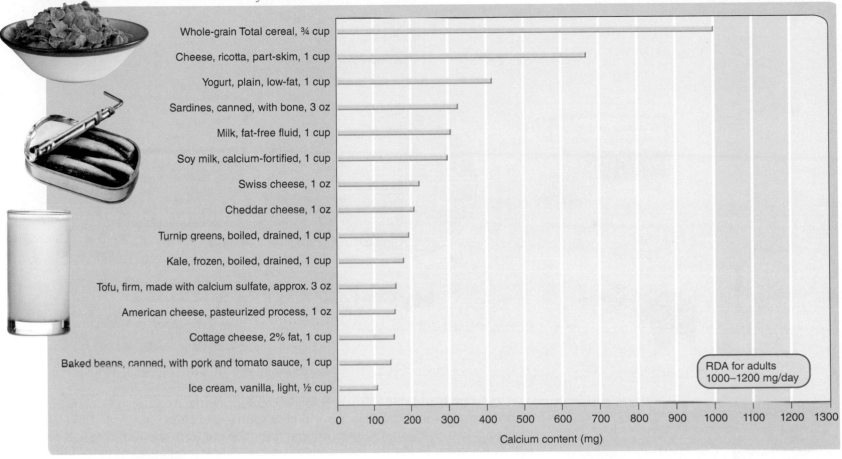

Whole-grain Total cereal, ¾ cup
Cheese, ricotta, part-skim, 1 cup
Yogurt, plain, low-fat, 1 cup
Sardines, canned, with bone, 3 oz
Milk, fat-free fluid, 1 cup
Soy milk, calcium-fortified, 1 cup
Swiss cheese, 1 oz
Cheddar cheese, 1 oz
Turnip greens, boiled, drained, 1 cup
Kale, frozen, boiled, drained, 1 cup
Tofu, firm, made with calcium sulfate, approx. 3 oz
American cheese, pasteurized process, 1 oz
Cottage cheese, 2% fat, 1 cup
Baked beans, canned, with pork and tomato sauce, 1 cup
Ice cream, vanilla, light, ½ cup

RDA for adults
1000–1200 mg/day

Calcium content (mg)
0 100 200 300 400 500 600 700 800 900 1000 1100 1200 1300

Good plant sources of calcium include broccoli and leafy greens, especially kale, collard, turnip, bok choy, and mustard greens. Nevertheless, the calcium in plant foods is generally not as bioavailable as the calcium in milk and milk products. For example, 1 cup of fat-free milk supplies almost 300 mg of calcium, and about 30% of the calcium in milk is bioavailable.[12] A cup of raw spinach supplies 30 mg of calcium, but only about 13% of that amount is bioavailable. Figure 9.13 shows how much spinach, broccoli, and kale a person would need to eat to obtain about the same amount of calcium that is in 1 cup of fat-free milk.

calcitonin hormone secreted by the thyroid gland when blood calcium levels are too high

osteoblasts bone cells that add bone to where the tissue is needed

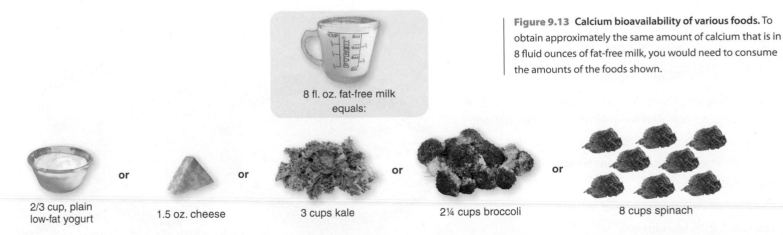

8 fl. oz. fat-free milk equals:

Figure 9.13 Calcium bioavailability of various foods. To obtain approximately the same amount of calcium that is in 8 fluid ounces of fat-free milk, you would need to consume the amounts of the foods shown.

2/3 cup, plain low-fat yogurt — or — 1.5 oz. cheese — or — 3 cups kale — or — 2¼ cups broccoli — or — 8 cups spinach

Figure 9.14 MyPlate: Food sources of calcium. The foods listed in these MyPlate groups are good food sources of calcium.

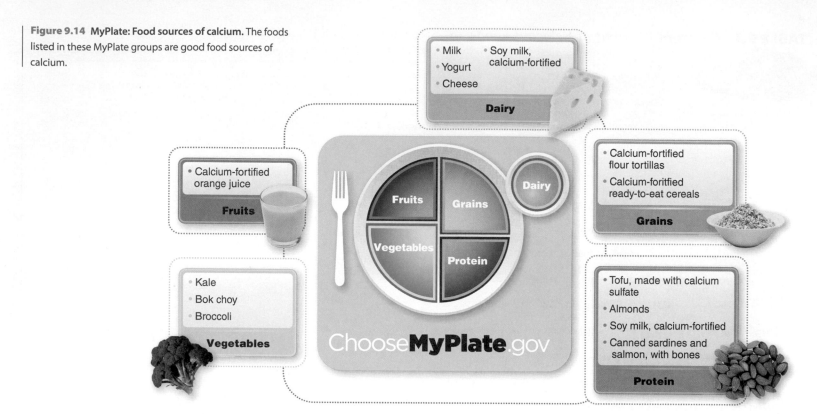

hypercalcemia condition characterized by higher-than-normal concentration of calcium in blood

osteoporosis chronic disease characterized by bones with low mass and reduced structure

Calcium is added to a variety of foods, including fortified orange juice, margarine, soy milk, cereals, and breakfast bars. Another source of calcium is soybean curd (tofu) that is made with calcium sulfate. You can read labels to learn about the calcium content of packaged foods; the information is a mandatory component of the Nutrition Facts panel. Figure 9.14 indicates food groups from MyPlate that are good sources of calcium.

Calcium Supplements Many adults find it difficult to consume enough milk products and other calcium-rich foods to achieve adequate intakes of the mineral. Thus, taking calcium supplements or antacids that contain calcium has become a common practice, especially among older adults. Dietary supplements containing calcium carbonate are the most commonly used type of calcium supplement. Supplements made with calcium citrate are also available. The body absorbs both forms of calcium to about the same extent. If you choose to take a calcium supplement, consider products that include vitamin D, because the vitamin enhances calcium absorption. Taking only 500 mg of calcium at a

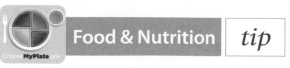 **Food & Nutrition** *tip*

Each of the following foods contains about the same amount of calcium that is in 1 cup of fat-free milk (approximately 300 mg):

2 cups low-fat (2% milk) cottage cheese

2.3 oz processed cheese (American cheese)

⅔ cup plain, low-fat yogurt

1.5 oz natural cheese (e.g., cheddar or Swiss)

1 cup calcium-fortified soy milk

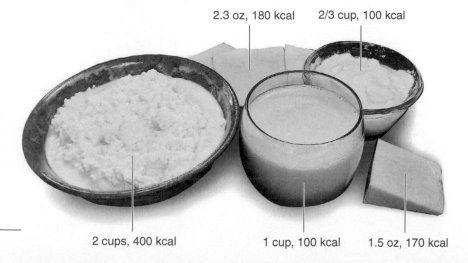

2.3 oz, 180 kcal   2/3 cup, 100 kcal

2 cups, 400 kcal   1 cup, 100 kcal   1.5 oz, 170 kcal

time and ingesting the supplement with meals will also improve the mineral's absorption. Some calcium supplements contain lead, a nonnutrient mineral that is highly toxic. Therefore, it is important to avoid supplements made from dolomite, oyster shell, or bonemeal, because they are most likely to contain lead.[13]

Dietary Adequacy

The adult RDA for calcium ranges from 1000 to 1200 mg/day. For children and adolescents between the ages of 9 and 18, the RDA is higher (1300 mg/day) to allow for increases in bone mass during growth and development. In the United States, average calcium intakes were approximately 1040 mg/day for men and 833 mg/day for women in 2007–2008.[14] Thus, women consumed less than the RDA for calcium, whereas most men had intakes that were roughly equivalent to the RDA. Total vegetarians (vegans) and people who are lactose intolerant are at risk of calcium deficiency, because they often avoid consuming milk and milk products, the most reliable dietary sources of calcium.

Healthy adults absorb about 30% of the calcium in foods, but this percentage varies, depending on the type of food.[15] During stages of life when the body needs extra calcium—such as infancy and pregnancy—absorption can be as high as 60%. Vitamin D enhances calcium absorption.

Older people, especially aging women, do not absorb calcium as well as younger people. Thus, recommendations for calcium intakes are higher for people over 50 years of age than for younger adults. In addition to advanced age, other factors that reduce calcium absorption include vitamin D deficiency and diarrhea.

Calcium Toxicity The Upper Level (UL) for calcium is 2000 to 2500 mg/day. Normally, the small intestine prevents too much calcium from being absorbed. However, taking too many calcium-containing antacids or supplements, or drinking too much vitamin D–fortified milk can result in excessive calcium absorption and hypercalcemia. **Hypercalcemia** (*hyper* = excess; *calcemia* = calcium in the blood) is a condition characterized by a higher-than-normal concentration of calcium in blood. Signs and symptoms of hypercalcemia include kidney stones, bone pain, muscle weakness, fatigue, and hypertension.[16] Treatment for hypercalcemia may include avoiding vitamin D and calcium supplements to reduce calcium absorption.

What Is Osteoporosis?

Osteoporosis is a chronic disease characterized by low bone mass and reduced bone structure (see Fig. 9.12). People with osteoporosis have weak bones that are susceptible to fractures. In the United States, osteoporosis is a major public health problem. More than 10 million Americans have osteoporosis, and another 34 million are at risk of the disease because they have low bone mass.[15] Most people with osteoporosis are older adult women.

Each year, an estimated 1.5 million Americans experience an osteoporosis-related fracture. Half of women and one-fourth of men who are over 50 years of age will have such a fracture at some point.[16] Many people do not realize their bones are becoming weaker and they have osteoporosis until they experience a fracture. People with osteoporosis may break a bone by falling, or they may experience spontaneous fractures, in which the fragile bone shatters for no apparent reason. Osteoporosis-related fractures often involve the spine, hip, wrist, or ankle bones. In severe cases, bones in the upper spine fracture and then heal in an abnormally curved position, giving the obvious "widow's hump" appearance associated with osteoporosis (Fig. 9.15).

Fractures, especially hip fractures, can be devastating events for the elderly. Only about 15% of older people who break their hip can walk without assistance six months after the fracture occurred.[16] Moreover, about 25% of older Americans who experience a broken hip die within one year of the injury.

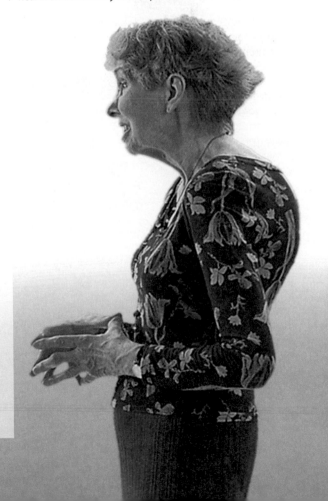

Figure 9.15 Osteoporosis. In many people with severe osteoporosis, bones in the upper spine fracture and then heal in an abnormally curved position.

estrogen hormone needed for normal bone development and maintenance

What Causes Osteoporosis? Several factors contribute to bone loss and osteoporosis. Consuming a high-protein diet may increase urinary calcium excretion, particularly when calcium intake is low. Additionally, family history of osteoporosis, cigarette smoking, and excessive alcohol consumption are also associated with increased risk of the disease. Other factors that contribute to low bone mass include small body frame size, irregular or absent menstrual cycles, prolonged bed rest, and use of certain medications. Table 9.6 lists these and other risk factors for osteoporosis. Note that some of these factors cannot be modified, but other factors can be changed to prevent or delay the development of the disease.

By 20 years of age, healthy young men and women have acquired 85 to 90% of their adult bone mass.[16] Regardless of one's sex, loss of bone tissue begins in mid-adulthood. In men, bone loss is slow and steady beginning around age 30. In women, however, the rate of bone loss increases significantly after *menopause*, that is, after menstrual cycles have ceased. At this time of life, women have the highest risk of osteoporosis. Why? The hormone **estrogen** is needed for normal bone development and maintenance. In women of childbearing age, ovaries are the primary source of estrogen. After menopause, a woman's ovaries no longer produce estrogen, and as a result, her rate of bone loss exceeds the rate of bone replacement. Because estrogen is so important to maintaining strong bones, young adult women should see a physician if they have signs of estrogen deficiency, such as irregular menstrual cycles.

A simple way to monitor bone mass is by tracking height. Losing an inch or more of adult height may be the first sign that a person has experienced fractures of the spine due to osteoporosis.[17] If osteoporosis is suspected, a person can undergo special painless x-ray testing to determine the extent of bone loss. Individuals with a family history of osteoporosis, men who have low testosterone levels, and women who are postmenopausal should ask their physician if testing to determine bone mineral density is necessary. People who are at high risk for or who already have osteoporosis may require medication to reduce their rate of bone loss. For postmenopausal women, taking calcium and vitamin D supplements may not reduce the risk of hip fractures.[18] In this life stage, it may be too late to benefit from simply taking dietary supplements to prevent osteoporosis.

Reducing the Risk of Osteoporosis Efforts to reduce the risk of osteoporosis should begin early in life. Proper diet and regular exercise are especially important from early childhood through late adolescence, because the body actively builds bone during these

MY DIVERSE PLATE

Bok Choy (Pak Choi or Chinese Cabbage)

Bok choy is a cruciferous vegetable that is typically used in Asian cookery. Cruciferous vegetables contain phytochemicals that may have cancer-fighting activity. The leaves and stalks are steamed or sautéed with other vegetables. Bok choy is a good source of minerals, especially iron, calcium, and potassium; the vegetable also contains high amounts of vitamin C.

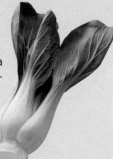

TABLE 9.6 *Risk Factors for Osteoporosis*

Factors You Can Not Change:
Being a woman
Growing older
Having white or Asian ancestry
Having a family history of osteoporosis
Having a small body frame
Factors You Can Change:
Having low estrogen levels in women, low testosterone levels in men
Following diets that contain inadequate amounts of calcium and vitamin D
Using medications such as steroids or some types of anticonvulsants
Being physically inactive
Smoking cigarettes
Consuming excessive alcohol
Consuming excess protein, sodium, and caffeine, especially when calcium intake is low

Modified from: Bennett B: The low-down on osteoporosis: What we know and what we don't. *Word on health: Consumer health information based on research from the National Institutes of Health.* 2003. www.nih.gov/news/WordonHealth/dec2003/osteo.htm Accessed: June 11, 2006.

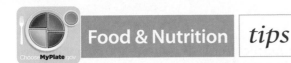

Food & Nutrition *tips*

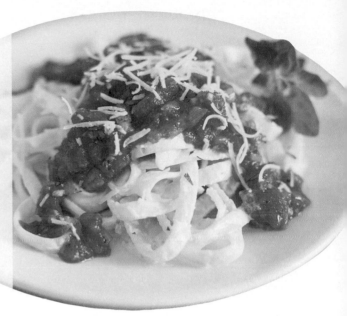

The following suggestions can add more calcium to your diet:

- Sprinkle grated low-fat cheeses on top of salads, bean or pasta dishes, and cooked vegetables.

- If you do not like the taste of plain fat-free milk, try adding a small amount of flavored syrup to the beverage. Two teaspoons of "lite" chocolate syrup add 50 kcal and some trace minerals to the milk.

- For a snack, melt a slice of low-fat cheese on half a whole-wheat bagel, whole-wheat crackers, or a slice of rye bread.

- If a recipe calls for water, substitute fat-free milk for water, if it is appropriate. For example, use fat-free milk when making cooked oatmeal or pancake batter.

- Add ¼ cup nonfat milk powder to 1 pound of raw ground meat when preparing hamburgers, meatballs, or meatloaf.

- Make homemade smoothies by blending plain low-fat yogurt with fresh or frozen fruit and fat-reduced ice cream or sherbet (see "Recipe for Healthy Living" at the end of Chapter 9).

life stages. By following the recommendations of MyPlate, most people can obtain adequate amounts of calcium from foods. Exposing skin to sunlight can stimulate the body's ability to form vitamin D, but some people will need to take calcium and vitamin D supplements.

Exercise training, especially performing weight-bearing activities, increases bone mass, because contracting muscles keep tension (physical stress) on bones.[19] Table 9.7 lists examples of weight-bearing and non-weight-bearing activities. Regardless of one's age, regular physical activity that includes weight-bearing muscular movements provides numerous benefits to health, such as improving balance and reducing the likelihood of falling.

Everyone needs to be concerned about his or her risk of osteoporosis and focus on maximizing bone mass while he or she is young. The interactive osteoporosis risk test at the International Osteoporosis Foundation's website (www.iofbonehealth.org/patients-public/risk test.html) can help you determine whether you or someone you know is at risk for the disease.

Regular weight-bearing activities provide numerous benefits to health, including strengthening bones. These older adults are performing tai chi, an activity that can improve balance and may reduce the likelihood of falling.

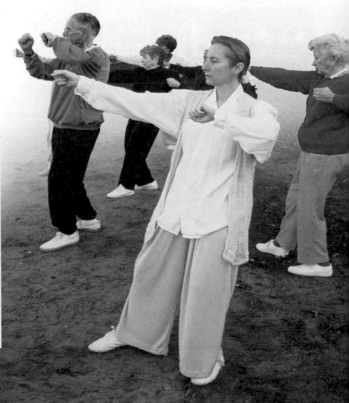

TABLE 9.7 *Examples of Weight-Bearing and Non-Weight-Bearing Activities*

Weight-bearing	Non-weight-bearing
Low-impact aerobics	Lying in bed
Basketball	Swimming
Running or jogging	Water aerobics
Walking	Cycling
Jumping rope	Traveling in reduced-gravity situations (e.g., space flight)
Dancing	
Hiking	
Stair climbing	
Strength training with weights	
Tennis and other racket sports	

Sodium (Na)

Salt is the primary source of sodium in American diets. The chemical commonly called "table salt" or simply "salt" is actually *sodium chloride*, a compound comprised of two minerals, sodium and chloride. A teaspoon of table salt supplies 2325 mg of sodium. (Unless otherwise noted, we will refer to sodium chloride simply as "salt" or "table salt.") The human digestive tract absorbs almost all of the sodium that is in foods and beverages.

Why Is Sodium Necessary?

As mentioned in the "Water" section of this chapter, sodium plays a major role in maintaining normal fluid balance. The mineral is also necessary for the transmission of impulses by nerves, for transporting small substances such as glucose and amino acids into cells, and for functioning of muscles.

Sources of Sodium

Most uncooked vegetables, raw meats, and grain products are naturally low in sodium. Thus, most of the sodium Americans consume is from the salt that is added to food during processing, during preparation, or at the table. As a food additive, salt enhances flavors and can prevent the growth of microorganisms responsible for food spoilage. Other food additives that contain sodium include sodium nitrate, sodium citrate, and *monosodium glutamate* (MSG), a seasoning that is often added to foods served in Chinese restaurants.

TABLE 9.8 *Sodium Content of Selected Foods/Food Additives*

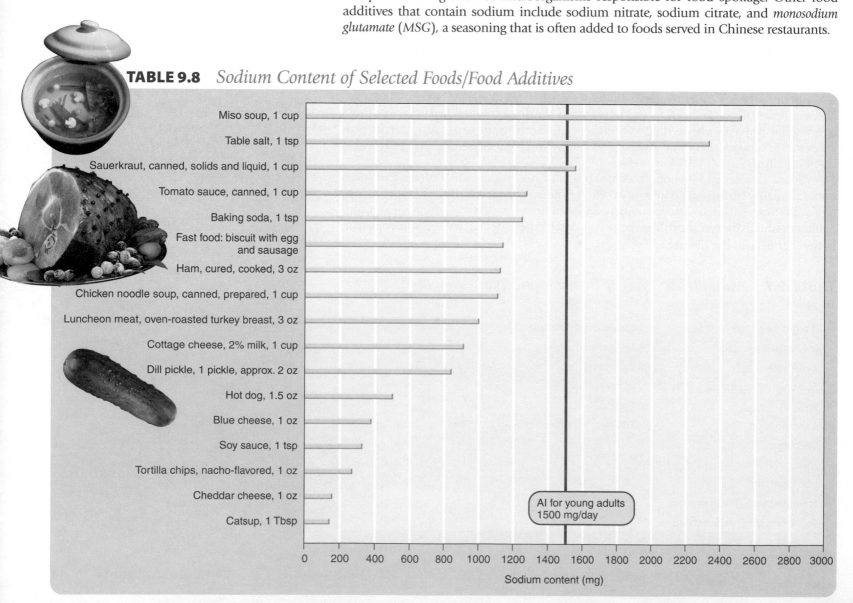

Miso soup, 1 cup
Table salt, 1 tsp
Sauerkraut, canned, solids and liquid, 1 cup
Tomato sauce, canned, 1 cup
Baking soda, 1 tsp
Fast food: biscuit with egg and sausage
Ham, cured, cooked, 3 oz
Chicken noodle soup, canned, prepared, 1 cup
Luncheon meat, oven-roasted turkey breast, 3 oz
Cottage cheese, 2% milk, 1 cup
Dill pickle, 1 pickle, approx. 2 oz
Hot dog, 1.5 oz
Blue cheese, 1 oz
Soy sauce, 1 tsp
Tortilla chips, nacho-flavored, 1 oz
Cheddar cheese, 1 oz
Catsup, 1 Tbsp

AI for young adults 1500 mg/day

0   200   400   600   800   1000   1200   1400   1600   1800   2000   2200   2400   2600   2800   3000

Sodium content (mg)

Salted snack foods, French fries, canned and dried soups, sauces and gravies, hot dogs and "deli" meats, cheeses, and pickled foods are high in sodium (Table 9.8). If you frequently eat these foods, your sodium intake is probably higher than recommended. Although sodium is an essential mineral, diets that contain high amounts of sodium are associated with increased risk of hypertension. The American Medical Association has encouraged efforts to reduce the sodium content of processed foods, fast foods, and restaurant meals by at least 50% and urged the Food and Drug Administration (FDA) to develop warnings or markers on labels to indicate foods that are high in sodium.[20]

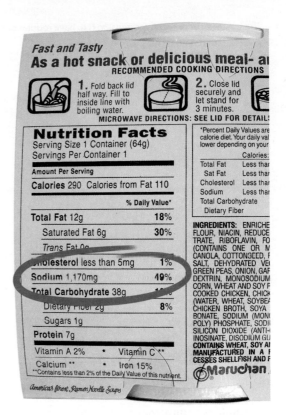

Dietary Adequacy

Humans require only about 180 mg of sodium per day, but the AI for adults under 51 years of age is 1500 mg/day. The AI for sodium does not apply for people who perspire heavily, such as marathon runners, or people who work in extremely hot conditions.[4] Sweat contains small amounts of sodium, chloride, and some other minerals. People who perspire extensively can lose large amounts of these minerals in their sweat.

Sodium Deficiency   The typical North American's diet supplies far more sodium than the AI amount, and as a result, the average person is unlikely to become sodium deficient. A healthy body is able to regulate its sodium concentration effectively, but sodium depletion can occur in certain situations. A person who loses more than 2 to 3% of body weight as a result of excessive sweating is at risk of sodium depletion. In most cases, drinking fluids and simply eating some salty foods or adding salt to foods is usually effective for restoring the body's sodium content. However, endurance athletes may need to consume sports drinks during competition to avoid dehydration and sodium depletion. Salt tablets are generally not recommended for sodium replacement. Sodium depletion also can result from diarrhea or vomiting, especially in infants. In these cases, it is necessary to obtain medical care promptly to replace the lost fluids and electrolytes, because infants can develop dehydration rapidly.

Sodium Toxicity   The adult UL for sodium is 2300 mg/day. On average, Americans consumed more than 3300 mg of sodium per day in 2007–2008.[14] According to the results of numerous studies, high sodium intakes are associated with increased risk of hypertension.[21] Thus, health experts generally recommend that Americans limit their sodium consumption. To evaluate your sodium intake, take the "Sodium Intake Assessment."

Sodium Intake Assessment ✔

For each question, place a check in the column that best describes your sodium intake habits.

How Often Do You...	Rarely	Occasionally	Often	Daily
1. Eat cured or processed meats ("deli" meats), such as bacon, sausage, hot dogs, ham, and other luncheon meats?				
2. Eat canned or frozen vegetables with sauce?				
3. Eat commercially prepared meals, main dishes, or canned or dehydrated soups?				
4. Eat processed cheeses, such as cheese spreads?				
5. Eat salted nuts, popcorn, pretzels, corn chips, or potato chips?				
6. Add salt to cooking water for vegetables, rice, or pasta?				
7. Add salt, seasoning mixes, salad dressings, or condiments—such as soy sauce, steak sauce, pickles, and catsup—to foods during preparation or at the table?				
8. Salt your food before tasting it?				
9. Ignore reading the Nutrition Facts panel for sodium content when buying foods?				
10. Choose menu items that are salty or with sauces when dining out?				

Scoring: The more checks you put in the "often" or "daily" columns, the higher your dietary sodium intake is. To reduce your sodium intake, choose low-sodium foods from each food group more often and balance high-sodium food choices with high-potassium ones.

Adapted from: USDA: *Home and Garden Bulletin*, No. 232–6, April 1986.

The best way to detect hypertension is to have regular blood pressure screenings.

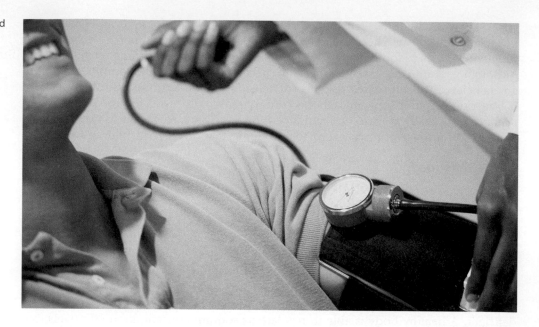

hypertension condition characterized by persistently elevated blood pressure

systolic pressure maximum blood pressure within an artery that occurs when the ventricles contract

diastolic pressure pressure in an artery that occurs when the ventricles relax between contractions

prehypertension persistent systolic blood pressure readings of 120 mm Hg to 139 mm Hg and diastolic readings of 80 mm Hg to 89 mm Hg

Did You Know?

Some homeowners install water-softening machines, because "hard water" interferes with the cleansing ability of soap and laundry detergent. Water softeners usually replace calcium and magnesium ions with sodium ions. Therefore, drinking softened water or using the treated water for preparing foods is not recommended because of its high sodium content.

Sodium and Hypertension **Hypertension,** a condition characterized by persistently elevated blood pressure, is a serious public health problem in the United States. Compared to people with normal blood pressure, hypertensive individuals have greater risk of cardiovascular disease (CVD), especially heart disease and stroke, as well as kidney failure and damage to other organs. Approximately 30% of adult Americans have hypertension.[22] Children can also develop hypertension. A study of ethnically diverse 14-year-old children in Texas, California, and North Carolina indicated that nearly one-fourth of the adolescents had hypertension.[23] Hypertension is often called the "silent killer," because high blood pressure generally does not cause symptoms until the affected person's organs and blood vessels have been damaged.

The best way to detect hypertension is to have regular blood pressure screenings. When you have your blood pressure determined, two measurements are actually taken. The first measurement is the **systolic pressure,** which is the maximum blood pressure within an artery. This value occurs when the ventricles, the heart's pumping chambers, contract. The second measurement is the **diastolic pressure,** which measures the pressure in an artery when the ventricles relax between contractions. The systolic value is always higher than the diastolic value. For adults, healthy blood pressure readings are less than 120/80 millimeters of mercury (mm Hg). After having your blood pressure measured, ask the clinician for your systolic and diastolic readings and keep a record of the values.

A person who is under physical or emotional stress can expect his or her blood pressure to rise temporarily. However, persistent systolic blood pressure readings of 120 mm Hg to 139 mm Hg and diastolic readings of 80 mm Hg to 89 mm Hg are signs of **prehypertension.**[24] People with prehypertension are more likely to develop hypertension than people with normal blood pressure. If a person's blood pressure persists at systolic values that are greater than or equal to (≥) 140 mm Hg and diastolic values that are ≥ 90 mm Hg, he or she has hypertension. Table 9.9 presents categories for blood pressure levels in adults.

What Causes Hypertension? Most cases of hypertension do not have simple causes, but advanced age, African-American ancestry, obesity, physical inactivity, smoking cigarettes, and excess alcohol and sodium intakes are among the major risk factors for the condition (Table 9.10). Blood pressure usually increases as a person ages, probably in part because plaque builds up in arteries (atherosclerosis) and interferes with the normal functioning of the blood vessels. Healthy arteries are flexible tubes that expand with each heartbeat and recoil in between beats. Atherosclerotic arteries are less flexible and cannot expand

TABLE 9.9 *Categories for Blood Pressure Levels in Adults (Ages 18 Years and Older)*

Category*	Blood Pressure Level (mm Hg)	
	Systolic	**Diastolic**
Normal	< 120 and	< 80
Prehypertension	120 to 139 or	80 to 89
Hypertension	≥ 140 or	≥ 90

*When systolic and diastolic blood pressures fall into different categories, the higher category should be used to classify blood pressure level. For example, a person with a blood pressure of 160/80 mm Hg would be classified as having hypertension. In people who are older than 50 years, elevated systolic values are a more significant risk factor for heart disease and stroke than elevated diastolic readings.
Source: National Heart, Lung, and Blood Institute: *Your guide to lowering high blood pressure: Categories for blood pressure levels in adults.* ND. http://www.nhlbi.nih.gov/hbp/detect/categ.htm. Accessed: July 28, 2011.

TABLE 9.10 *Major Risk Factors for Hypertension*

Family history
Advanced age
African-American ancestry
Obesity
Physical inactivity
Consuming excess sodium
Cigarette smoking
Consuming excess alcohol
Type 2 diabetes

as much as healthy arteries. As a result, the heart must work harder to pump blood through the stiff arteries and blood pressure becomes chronically elevated.

For reasons that are unclear, non-Hispanic African-Americans are more likely than non-Hispanic white Americans to develop hypertension, especially early in life. Diets that limit sodium but contain adequate amounts of calcium, potassium, and magnesium may decrease high blood pressure, especially among African-Americans.[21]

Obesity, a condition characterized by excessive amounts of body fat, is a major risk factor for hypertension. Physical inactivity is another leading risk factor related to hypertension. Obesity and physical inactivity are modifiable risk factors. By exercising and losing some excess fat, obese people who have hypertension often experience reductions in their blood pressure.[21]

Excessive alcohol intake increases the risk of hypertension. To reduce their chances of developing high blood pressure, people should avoid alcohol or limit their consumption to two or fewer drinks/day (men) and only one drink/day (women and older adults). Other important risk factors for hypertension include having diabetes and using tobacco.

Finally, a high-sodium diet is associated with increased risk of hypertension, and in some cases, such diets can be a cause of hypertension.[25] Many medical researchers think some people are genetically "sodium sensitive." A person who is sodium sensitive is more likely to develop hypertension as a result of consuming a high-sodium diet than an individual who lacks this sensitivity. The kidneys of a sodium-sensitive person may be unable to eliminate excess sodium as effectively as the kidneys of a healthy person. The excess sodium causes the body to retain water, and blood volume and pressure increase as a result.

Dietary Guidelines for Americans 2010 recommends less than 2300 mg of sodium daily.[26] That amount of sodium is in 6 g (about 1 teaspoon) of table salt. Members of high-risk populations, African-Americans, for example, should limit their sodium intake to no more than 1500 mg per day. People who are being treated for hypertension should check with their physician for advice concerning an acceptable sodium intake.

If you want to lower your sodium intake, try gradually reducing your use of salt and consumption of salty foods. By doing so, you will eventually become accustomed to the taste of less salty food. To replace salt as a seasoning, try using garlic, citrus juice, and herbs and spices to enhance the taste of foods. Furthermore, avoid buying seasonings with added salt, such as "garlic salt" or "onion salt," and check the ingredient list to purchase seasonings without added salt (garlic *powder* or onion *powder*) instead.

Information about a packaged food's sodium content is a mandatory component of the Nutrition Facts panel. If you take the time to read labels, you can find foods that have little or no salt added to them during processing. For example, an ounce of salted peanuts provides 230 mg of sodium; the same amount of unsalted peanuts has only 2 mg of sodium. The "Food & Nutrition Tips" feature on page 322 provides some suggestions for reducing your salt (sodium) intake.

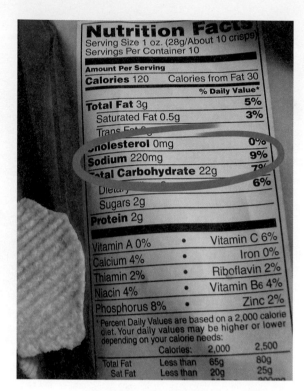

By reading the label, you can find foods that have high amounts of added sodium. A serving of these chips provides about 10% of the maximum recommended amount of sodium for a day.

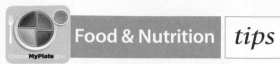

Food & Nutrition *tips*

To reduce your sodium intake, consider taking these actions:

- Prepare homemade meals and snacks as much as possible so you have control over your salt intake.
- Do not add salt while preparing foods, even though instructions tell you to "add salt."
- Taste your food *before* salting it. Adjust to eating foods with less salt in them.
- Do not keep a salt shaker on your table.
- Read the Nutrition Facts panels before purchasing packaged foods to determine sodium contents of the items.
- When ordering items in restaurants, request that no salt be added to your food while it is being prepared.

Even if your blood pressure is normal now, it is important to have regular blood pressure checks as you grow older, because the risk of hypertension increases with age. In the United States, approximately 70% of people who are 65 years of age and older have hypertension.[22] Children and young adults, however, are not immune to hypertension. Justin Steinbruegge, the college student featured in "Real People, Real Stories" on page 323, was 18 when he found out he had hypertension. When was the last time you had your blood pressure measured? What were the systolic and diastolic values?

Treatment for hypertension usually includes taking certain medications, following dietary modifications, and making some other lifestyle changes (Table 9.11). The *Dietary Approaches to Stop Hypertension* (*DASH*) diet is low in sodium, total fat, saturated fat, and cholesterol, and high in fruits, vegetables, and low-fat dairy products. Research indicates that people can lower their blood pressure and reduce their risk of CVD by following the DASH diet, losing excess body fat, and increasing their physical activity level.[26] To obtain more information about this diet and some low-sodium recipes, visit the National Heart, Lung, and Blood Institute's website: www.nhlbi.nih.gov/health/public/heart/hbp/dash/new_dash.pdf.

TABLE 9.11 *Practical Steps to Reduce Your Risk of Hypertension*

1. Follow the dietary recommendations of MyPlate concerning fruit, vegetable, and low-fat milk intakes. Furthermore, consider using fresh fruit to replace some empty calories in your daily meals and snacks. (See Chapter 3 for more information about empty calories.)
2. Reduce your consumption of salty foods and have your blood pressure checked regularly.
3. Attain and maintain a healthy body weight.
4. Incorporate more physical activity into your daily schedule. For example, walk more often and use steps instead of elevators or escalators.
5. If you drink alcohol, consume alcoholic beverages in moderation—no more than two drinks/day for men and one drink/day for women and older adults.
6. Avoid using tobacco products.

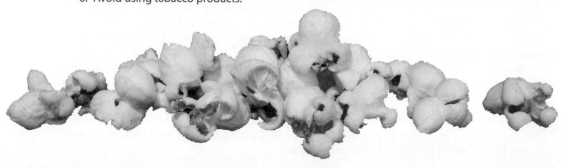

Potassium (K)

Potassium is the primary positively charged ion in the intracellular fluid. In fact, most of the body's potassium is in cells. All cells need potassium, but nerve and muscle cells contain high amounts of the mineral.

Why Is Potassium Necessary?

Like sodium, potassium plays a key role in maintaining proper fluid balance. Unlike sodium, potassium is associated with lower, rather than higher, blood pressure values. Potassium is also necessary for transmitting nerve impulses, contracting muscles, and maintaining normal kidney function. Potassium-rich diets, such as the DASH diet, may lower blood pressure, reduce the risk of developing kidney stones, and possibly decrease bone loss.[28] A natural way to counteract high sodium intakes is to consume foods naturally rich in potassium and low in sodium, such as fruits.

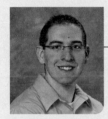

REAL *People*

REAL *Stories*

Justin Steinbruegge

If you were to meet 23-year-old Justin Steinbruegge, your first impression would be that he is the "picture" of good health. At 6'1," Justin weighs 170 pounds and appears to be in great physical condition. Justin enjoys bicycling; he also runs 3 to 5 miles a day and weight trains 3 days a week to maintain his muscle mass. In addition to being very physically active, Justin has other healthy habits—he doesn't smoke or consume caffeine or alcohol, and he keeps his salt intake low.

In the spring of his senior year of high school, Justin decided to join the Air Force after graduation. As part of military enlistment activities, Justin underwent thorough physical screening. Much to his surprise, his blood pressure was elevated to such an extent that the Air Force denied his entrance into the service. "It was a huge shock," said Justin. "I had no signs or symptoms of hypertension. I didn't even know what 'hypertension' was."

After being evaluated by his family doctor, Justin was eventually accepted into the Air Force, but he had to see a cardiologist, a physician who specializes in diseases of the heart and blood vessels. To treat his condition, Justin was given medication. He also learned to avoid salty foods and monitor his blood pressure at least three times daily.

It is unusual for physically active young adults who have healthy lifestyles and body weights to develop chronic high blood pressure. However, Justin now realizes that he was at risk for hypertension because of his family history of the disease. His mother, mother's sister, and maternal grandmother have the condition.

Although Justin decided not to enter the Air Force, he still has impressive professional goals. After completing certification training at a police academy, Justin hopes to find a position as a state police trooper. Justin has some excellent advice for college students: "As a young person, you may think you are invincible. But even if you don't think there's anything wrong with you, have your blood pressure tested. I thought I was the healthiest person ever! For people who are struggling with hypertension like me, be sure to exercise regularly, watch your diet, and remember to take your medication. We may not be able to cure hypertension, but we can do our best to control it. For those individuals fortunate enough to be healthier than I am, go to the doctor anyway and get your blood pressure checked a couple times per year. You may be surprised to discover you're hypertensive, just as I was. They don't call it 'the silent killer' for nothing."

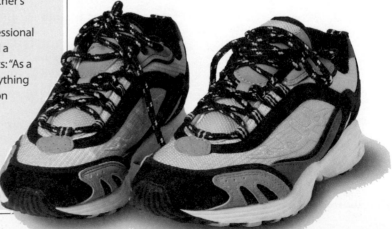

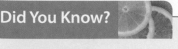

Did You Know?

Salt substitutes often contain a type of salt called potassium chloride. People who have severe kidney diseases may accumulate toxic levels of potassium in their blood. Therefore, kidney disease patients should consult their physicians before using salt substitutes made with potassium chloride. Fruits and vegetables are recommended sources of potassium instead of potassium chloride.[27]

Sources of Potassium

Overall, fresh fruits, fruit juice, and vegetables are good dietary sources of potassium. Milk, whole grains, dried beans, and meats are also major contributors of potassium to American diets. Table 9.12 lists foods that are among the richest sources of this mineral. Figure 9.16 indicates food groups that are naturally good sources of potassium.

Dietary Adequacy

The adult AI for potassium is 4700 mg per day. On average, Americans consume only about 2500 mg of potassium per day.[14] People can raise their potassium intakes by increasing their consumption of fruits, vegetables, whole-grain breads and cereals, and low-fat and fat-free milk and milk products. This eating pattern is similar to the DASH diet.

TABLE 9.12 *Potassium Content of Selected Foods*

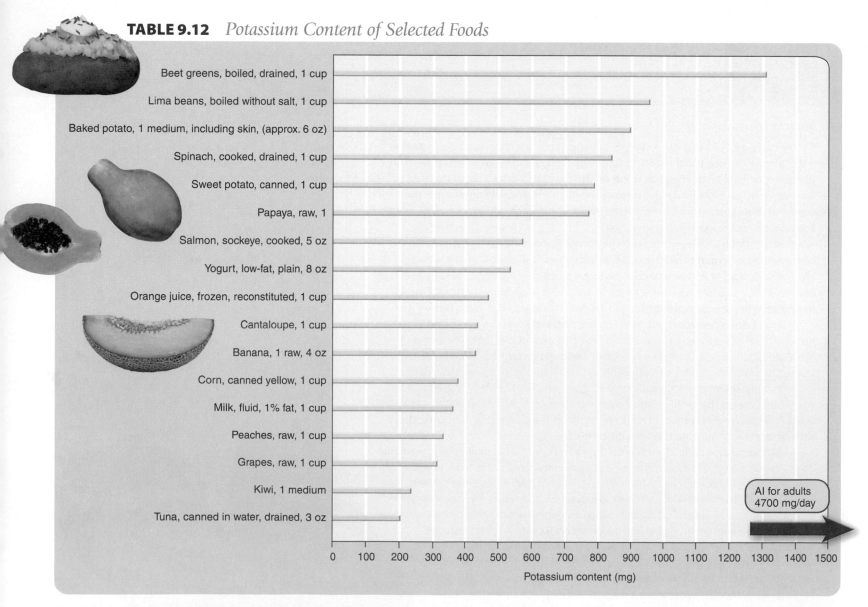

Source: Data from U.S. Department of Agriculture, Agricultural Research Service, USDA Nutrient Data Laboratory: Potassium K (mg) content of selected foods per common measure, sorted by nutrient content. *USDA national nutrient database for standard reference, release 19.* 2006.

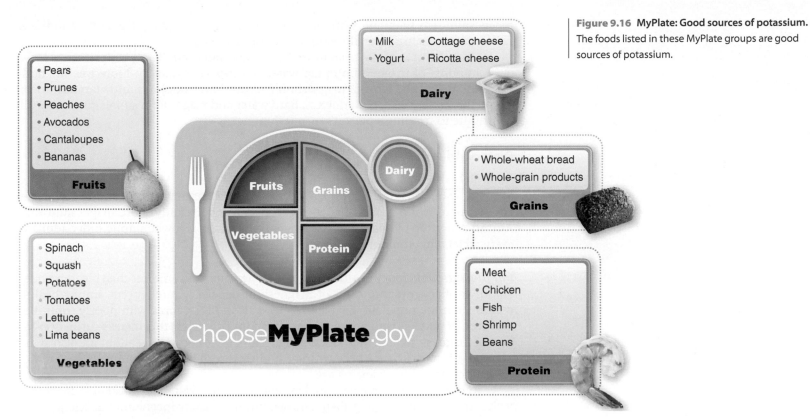

The body is unable to conserve potassium as well as sodium; therefore, the risk of potassium deficiency is greater than that of sodium deficiency. Individuals suffering from excessive sweating, vomiting, diarrhea, or kidney diseases that increase potassium excretion are at risk for potassium depletion. Symptoms of the condition generally include loss of appetite, muscle cramps, confusion, constipation, and increased urinary calcium excretion.

Although there is no UL for potassium, taking potassium supplements can upset the GI tract. Moreover, if a person's kidneys are not able to eliminate the excess potassium, the mineral accumulates in the blood and can cause the heart to stop beating. To avoid toxicity, do not take potassium supplements unless you are under a physician's care.

Magnesium (Mg)

Magnesium participates in more than 300 chemical reactions in the body.[29] The essential mineral also helps regulate normal muscle and nerve function as well as blood pressure and blood glucose levels. Additionally, the body needs magnesium to maintain strong bones and a healthy immune system. Magnesium may help prevent diabetes, hypertension, and CVD. However, more research is needed to clarify the mineral's role in these diseases.

Normally, humans absorb about 40 to 60% of the magnesium in their diets, but as much as 80% of the magnesium in food may be absorbed when the body lacks the mineral. The kidneys regulate blood concentrations of magnesium and can reduce urinary losses of the mineral when the body's level of magnesium is low.

Sources of Magnesium

Magnesium is in chlorophyll, the green pigment in plants. Therefore, it is not surprising that plant foods, such as spinach, green leafy vegetables, whole grains, beans, nuts, seeds, and chocolate, are the richest sources of magnesium. Animal products, such as milk and meats, also supply some magnesium. Table 9.13 lists some commonly eaten foods that supply magnesium. Refined grains are generally low in magnesium, because the magnesium-rich bran and germ are removed during processing. Figure 9.17 indicates food groups that are naturally good sources of magnesium.

Other sources of magnesium are "hard" tap water and dietary supplements. However, amounts of magnesium in tap water can vary considerably. Moreover, the body does not absorb the form of magnesium (magnesium oxide) in multivitamin/mineral supplements very well. Nevertheless, hard water and magnesium supplements can still contribute to meeting a person's magnesium needs.

Dietary Adequacy

Adult RDAs for magnesium range from 310 to 420 mg/day. Many people in the United States do not consume recommended amounts of magnesium.[14] Among adult men and women, white Americans tend to consume significantly more magnesium than African-Americans.[29] Nevertheless, magnesium intake is lower among older adults in every racial and ethnic group.

Magnesium Deficiency Although many Americans consume less than recommended amounts of magnesium, cases of magnesium deficiency rarely occur among healthy members of the population.[29] Nevertheless, alcoholics, people with poorly controlled diabetes, or persons who use certain medications (diuretics) that increase urinary excretion of magnesium have high risk of magnesium deficiency. Older adults are also at risk of magnesium deficiency because their bodies absorb less of the mineral and urinary losses increase with advancing age.

In humans, mild magnesium deficiency can cause irritability, weakness, loss of appetite, and muscle twitching. Signs and symptoms of severe magnesium deficiency often

TABLE 9.13 *Magnesium Content of Selected Foods*

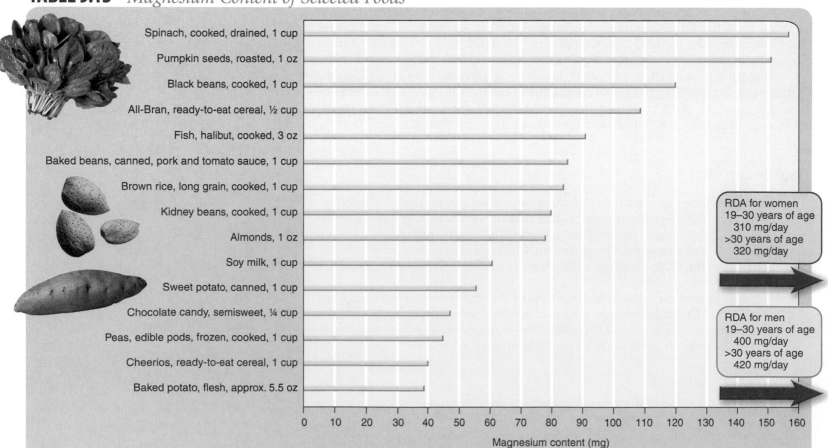

Source: Data from U.S. Department of Agriculture, Agricultural Research Service, USDA Nutrient Data Laboratory: Magnesium, Mg (mg) content of selected foods per common measure, sorted by nutrient content. *USDA national nutrient database for standard reference, release 19.* 2006.

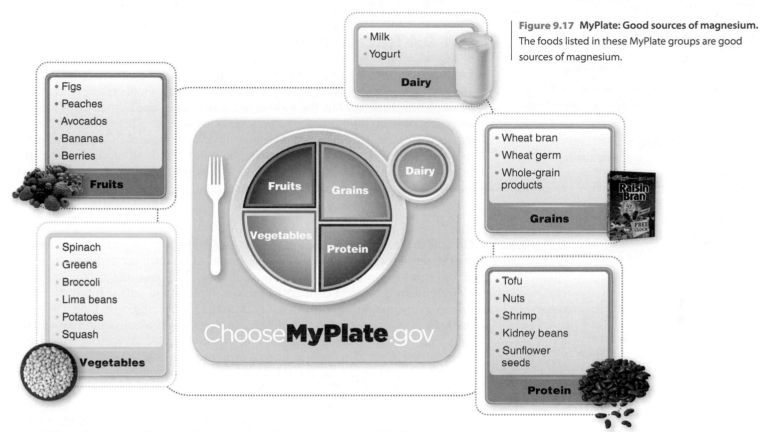

include rapid heartbeat, inability to relax muscles, disorientation, and hallucinations. Chronic magnesium deficiency may increase the risk of osteoporosis, because the deficiency lowers the level of calcium in blood.

Magnesium Toxicity Magnesium toxicity rarely occurs from eating too much magnesium-rich food.[29] Toxicity is more likely to occur from ingesting excessive magnesium from laxatives, antacids, or dietary supplements that contain the mineral. Thus, the UL for the micronutrient (350 mg/day) is for magnesium-containing medications and not food sources. A person who consumes too much magnesium often develops diarrhea.

Patients suffering from kidney failure and elderly persons have high risk of magnesium toxicity, because their kidneys do not excrete the mineral as effectively as the kidneys of younger, healthier individuals. In cases of kidney failure, the high concentration of magnesium in blood causes weakness, nausea, slowed breathing, coma, and death.

Concept **Checkpoint**

16. What is osteoporosis, and why is it a major public health concern in the United States?
17. Identify at least four major risk factors for osteoporosis. Which risk factors can be modified to reduce the risk of osteoporosis?
18. What is prehypertension? What is hypertension? What are major risk factors for hypertension?
19. What is the DASH diet? Aside from making dietary modifications, what other lifestyle changes can people with hypertension make to lower their blood pressure?
20. Prepare a table for the major minerals that includes information about each mineral's major roles in the body, primary food sources, and signs and symptoms of the mineral's deficiency as well as toxicity disorders. Check your table against the information provided in Table 9.4.

hemoglobin iron-containing protein in red blood cells that transports oxygen to tissues and some carbon dioxide away from tissues

myoglobin iron-containing protein in muscle cells that controls oxygen uptake from red blood cells

cytochromes group of proteins involved in the release of energy from macronutrients

heme iron form of iron in hemoglobin and myoglobin

nonheme iron form of iron in vegetables, grains, meats, and supplements

 ## 9.4 Trace Minerals

Although the body requires trace minerals in very small amounts, obtaining adequate amounts of these important nutrients can be difficult. Iron, for example, is one of Earth's most plentiful metals, but the total amount of iron in the human body is quite small, averaging only about 0.006% of a person's body weight.[2] This section of Chapter 9 discusses iron, zinc, iodine (iodide), selenium, and chromium in detail. Table 9.14 summarizes nutrition-related information about iron and other trace minerals. Unless otherwise noted, RDA/AI values are for adults, excluding pregnant or breastfeeding women.

Iron (Fe)

Do you think of "iron" when you think of "strength"? Associating iron with strength makes sense, because muscular strength and endurance are reduced when the body lacks iron. Iron is a component of hemoglobin and *myoglobin* (*my'-o-glow-bin*). **Hemoglobin** is the iron-containing protein in red blood cells that transports oxygen to tissues and some carbon dioxide away from tissues. Hemoglobin is also responsible for the red color of oxygenated blood. **Myoglobin** is the iron-containing protein in muscle cells that controls oxygen uptake from red blood cells. Oxygen is critical for energy metabolism. Cells also contain iron in **cytochromes** (*sigh'-toe-crowms*), a group of proteins that are necessary for certain chemical reactions involved in the release of energy from macronutrients. If the body does not have enough iron to make hemoglobin, myoglobin, and the cytochromes, cells cannot obtain the energy they need to perform work. Thus, fatigue is a major symptom of iron deficiency. Iron also plays roles in immune system function and brain development.

Dietary Sources

Beef, fish, and poultry ("meat") contain more iron than most plant foods. Some of the iron in meat is present as hemoglobin and myoglobin. These forms of iron are collectively referred to as **heme iron.** The remaining iron in meat, as well as all the iron in vegetables, grains, and supplements, is **nonheme iron.**

The intestinal tract absorbs more of the heme iron than nonheme iron in foods.[30] Some plant foods, such as spinach, contain nonheme iron, but oxalic acid in spinach binds to the mineral, reducing its absorption. Other naturally occurring compounds that reduce iron absorption include phytic acid in whole grains, tannins in tea, and substances that are chemically related to tannins in coffee.

Meat is the major source of iron in the typical American diet. Other important sources of iron are fortified cereals and products made from enriched flour, such as breads

Whole grains are good sources of several trace minerals.

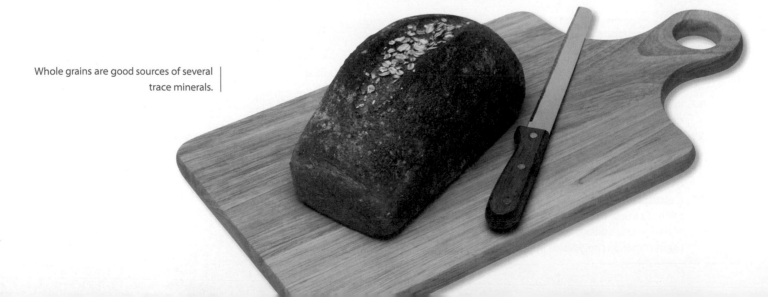

TABLE 9.14 *Summary of Trace Minerals*

Mineral	Major Functions in the Body	Adult RDA/AI* (adult RDA = bold)	Major Dietary Sources	Major Deficiency Signs and Symptoms	Major Toxicity Signs and Symptoms
Iron (Fe)	• Component of hemoglobin and myoglobin that carries oxygen • Energy generation • Immune system function	Women: **18 mg** Men: **8 mg**	Meat and other animal foods, except milk; whole-grain and enriched breads and cereals; fortified cereals	• Fatigue upon exertion • Small, pale red blood cells • Low hemoglobin levels • Poor immune system function • Growth and developmental retardation in infants	UL = 45 mg/day • Intestinal upset • Organ damage • Death
Zinc (Zn)	• Component of numerous enzymes	Women: **8 mg** Men: **11 mg**	Seafood, meat, whole grains	• Skin rash • Diarrhea • Depressed sense of taste and smell • Hair loss • Poor growth and physical development	UL = 40 mg/day • Intestinal upset • Depressed immune system function • Supplement use can reduce copper absorption.
Copper (Cu)	• Promotes iron metabolism • Component of antioxidant enzymes • Component of enzymes involved in connective tissue synthesis	**900 mcg**	Liver, cocoa, legumes, whole grains, shellfish	• Anemia • Reduced immune system function • Poor growth and development	UL = 10,000 mcg/day • Vomiting • Abnormal nervous system function • Liver damage
Selenium (Se)	• Component of an antioxidant system	**55 mcg**	Meat, eggs, fish, seafood, whole grains	• Muscle pain and weakness • Form of heart disease	UL = 400 mcg/day • Nausea • Vomiting • Hair loss • Weakness • Liver damage
Iodine (I)	• Component of thyroid hormones	**150 mcg**	Iodized salt, saltwater fish, dairy products	• Goiter • Cretinism (intellectual impairment and poor growth in infants of women who were iodine deficient during pregnancy)	UL = 1100 mcg/day • Reduced thyroid gland function
Fluoride (F)	• Increases resistance of tooth enamel to cavity formation • Stimulates bone formation	Men: 4 mg Women: 3 mg	Fluoridated water, tea, seaweed	• No true deficiency, but increased risk of tooth decay	UL = 10 mg/day • Stomach upset • Staining of teeth (mottling) during development • Bone deterioration
Chromium (Cr)	• Enhances insulin action	Men: 30–35 mcg Women: 20–25 mcg	Egg yolks, whole grains, pork, nuts, mushrooms	• Blood glucose level remains elevated after meals	• Unknown but currently under scientific investigation • May interact with certain medications
Manganese (Mn)	• Cofactor for certain enzymes, including some involved in carbohydrate metabolism	Men: 2.3 mg Women: 1.8 mg	Nuts, oats, beans, tea	• None in humans	UL = 11 mg/day • Abnormal nervous system function
Molybdenum (Mo)	• Component of certain coenzymes	**45 mcg**	Liver, peas, beans, cereal products, leafy vegetables, low-fat milk	• None in healthy humans	UL = 2000 mcg/day • Rarely occurs from usual dietary sources • Overdoses of dietary supplements containing molybdenum may cause joint pain; side, lower back, or stomach pain; swelling of feet or lower legs.

*Values are for adults, excluding pregnant or breastfeeding women.

iron deficiency condition characterized by low body stores of iron

anemia condition characterized by poor oxygen transport in blood

and rolls. Dairy products are poor sources of iron. Table 9.15 lists some foods that are among the richest sources of iron. Figure 9.18 indicates food groups that are good sources of iron.

Regulating Iron Under normal conditions, the body regulates iron absorption and conservation. The digestive tract absorbs only 5 to 15% of the iron in foods. However, the intestinal tract can absorb more iron when the body's need for the trace mineral increases. Despite iron enrichment and fortification, only about 5% of the iron added to grain products is absorbed.[30] The liver, the body's main site for iron storage, incorporates the trace mineral into the protein ferritin (*fer'-ih-tin*) until it is needed.

After red blood cells die, the body breaks them down and conserves most of the iron that was in hemoglobin. By doing so, the body can recycle the trace mineral to make hemoglobin for new red blood cells. Nonetheless, some iron is lost each day via the GI tract, urine, and skin. Any form of bleeding, including menstruation, also contributes to iron losses. Replacing the iron is essential to good health.

Dietary Adequacy

For adult men, the RDA for iron is 8 mg per day; for adult women between 19 and 50 years of age, the RDA for iron is 18 mg/day. The average daily intake for American men is about 17.5 mg, whereas the average daily intake for American women is about 13.0 mg/day.[14] Thus, women between 19 and 50 years of age are more likely than men to have inadequate iron intakes.

TABLE 9.15 *Iron Content of Selected Foods*

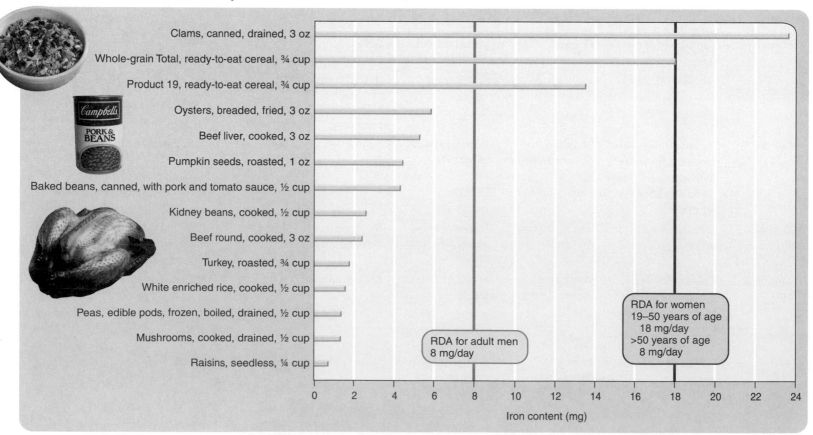

Source: Data from U.S. Department of Agriculture, Agricultural Research Service, USDA Nutrient Data Laboratory: Iron, Fe (mg) content of selected foods per common measure, sorted by nutrient content. *USDA national nutrient database for standard reference, release 19.* 2006.

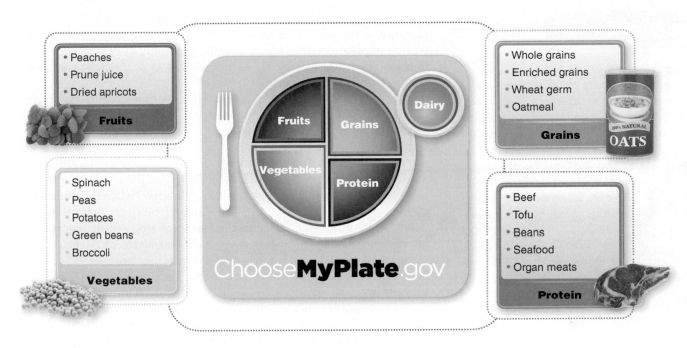

| Figure 9.18 **MyPlate: Good sources of iron.** The foods listed in these MyPlate groups are good sources of iron.

Iron Deficiency–Related Disorders Low blood iron levels usually result from losing blood, consuming diets that lack iron, or being unable to absorb dietary iron. In cases of **iron deficiency,** the body's iron stores are low but not low enough to result in severe health problems. Nevertheless, iron deficiency can still have widespread negative effects on the body, including interfering with normal growth, behavior, immune system function, cardiac function, and energy metabolism.[31] Furthermore, iron deficiency can lead to iron deficiency anemia.

Anemia occurs when oxygen transport in blood is impaired, generally because there are not enough red blood cells to carry the oxygen or the red blood cells do not contain enough hemoglobin (Fig. 9.19). If oxygen is lacking, cells cannot release considerable amounts of energy from macronutrients, so symptoms of iron deficiency anemia include lack of energy and difficulty concentrating on mental activities. Furthermore, the heart of a person suffering from anemia has to work harder to circulate oxygen-poor blood throughout the body. Over time, anemia can cause rapid or irregular heartbeat, chest pain, an enlarged heart, and even heart failure. Table 9.16 lists common signs and symptoms of iron deficiency anemia.

TABLE 9.16 *Signs and Symptoms of Iron Deficiency Anemia*

Pale skin and pale mucous membrane
Fatigue and weakness
Irritability
Shortness of breath
Brittle nails
Unusual food cravings (pica)
Decreased appetite (especially in children)
Headache

Source: U.S. Library of Medicine (Medline), National Institutes of Health: Iron deficiency anemia. *Medline plus.* www.nlm.nih.gov/medlineplus/ency/article/000584.htm. Accessed: October 12, 2011.

a. b.

Figure 9.19 **Iron-deficient red blood cells.** (*a*) Normal red blood cells. (*b*) Red blood cells in a person with iron deficiency.

There are many different kinds of anemia, but iron deficiency anemia is the most common form. According to the World Health Organization (WHO), over 30% of the world's population suffers from anemia, and many cases of the condition are due to iron deficiency.[32] In the United States, iron deficiency is the most common nutritional deficiency and the leading cause of anemia.[33]

Substantial blood loss is a common cause of iron deficiency anemia. Such losses of blood often result from serious intestinal diseases, severe physical injuries, and excessive menstrual bleeding. Diseases that reduce red blood cell formation or increase red blood cell destruction also cause anemia. It is important to note that some types of anemia are the result of genetic defects and not dietary deficiencies. Blood testing can determine which kind of anemia a person has developed, so the condition can be treated properly.

Young women are at risk for iron deficiency–related disorders because they often exclude meat and enriched bread and cereal products from their diets. Additionally, women of childbearing age generally lose some iron during menstruation. Women with heavy menstrual blood losses are especially prone to iron deficiency anemia. Although pregnant women do not have to contend with menstrual blood losses, they still need to be concerned about their iron intake. The "Food & Nutrition Tips" feature on this page suggests practical ways to increase dietary sources of iron.

During pregnancy, a woman's need for iron increases as her blood supply expands and new tissues are added to both her body and that of her fetus. Pregnant women who suffer from iron deficiency anemia have higher risk of dying during pregnancy than healthy pregnant women. Anemic pregnant women are also more likely to give birth to premature or low-birth-weight infants. Premature babies are born before the 37th week of pregnancy; normally, pregnancies last about 40 weeks from the date of the mother's last menstrual period. A low-birth-weight baby weighs less than 5½ pounds at birth. Compared to healthy newborns, premature or low-birth-weight infants are more likely to die during their first year of life.

Because of their rapid growth rates, infants and toddlers have higher needs for iron than older children. Furthermore, iron appears to be necessary for normal nervous system functioning, including brain development. Iron-deficient infants can experience delays in the development of normal motor and mental functions.[33]

Consuming too much milk may play a role in the development of iron deficiency in children. Milk is a poor source of iron. Thus, children who drink excessive amounts of milk may not have the appetite to eat foods that are more reliable iron sources. The calcium that is in milk also interferes with iron absorption when the beverage is consumed with foods that contain the mineral.[34] To reduce the risk of iron deficiency,

Food & Nutrition *tips*

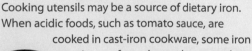

The following suggestions can add more iron to your diet:

- Eat lean meat, poultry, or fish with plant sources of iron.
- Combine soybeans with tomatoes or tomato sauce.
- Add orange segments or chopped tomatoes to spinach salads or cooked spinach.
- Add chopped onions and green peppers to peas or beans.
- Serve sweet potatoes with fresh orange segments or dried apricots.
- Add raspberries, strawberries, raisins, or dried apricots to cereal.
- Drink orange juice when eating peanut butter or soy nut butter sandwiches.
- Consume watermelon, dried plums, dried apricots, or raisins for snacks.

Iron-deficient people, particularly children and pregnant females, occasionally eat dirt or clay. Some medical researchers think they crave clay or dirt in response to being iron deficient. Other researchers think eating these nonfood items is acceptable in some cultures, and the practice *causes* iron deficiency. Why? Substances in clay and dirt can interfere with iron absorption in the digestive tract. The practice of eating nonfood items is called **pica** (*pié-kah*).

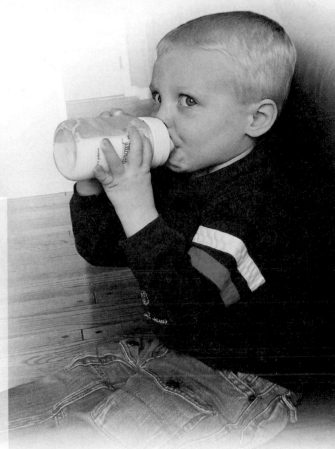

children should be encouraged to eat more iron-rich foods, such as meat, products made from soybeans, and iron-fortified cereals.

In the United States, rates of iron deficiency–related disorders in infants and preschool children have decreased over the past 30 years. The use of iron-fortified formulas and cereals in the Special Supplemental Nutrition Program for Women, Infants, and Children (the WIC program) may be responsible for improving this aspect of children's health. A summary of the WIC program is presented in Table 1.7 in the Chapter 1 "Highlight."

Total vegetarians have a higher risk of iron deficiency–related disorders than people who eat meat, because meat provides heme iron. Combining a small amount of meat with plant foods improves the bioavailability of the plant's nonheme iron. Vegetarians, however, may reject recipes that include any meat, especially red meats. Some plant foods contain high amounts of oxalic acid and phytic acid, substances that can depress iron absorption. On the other hand, vegetarian diets usually are rich in vitamin C, a factor that increases nonheme iron absorption. Thus, vegetarians should consume vitamin C–rich foods along with plant foods, especially those that contain appreciable amounts of iron, such as spinach, lentils, and soybeans. Eating iron-fortified ready-to-eat cereals can also be helpful for vegetarians, even though the form of iron used to fortify cereals is not as well absorbed as heme iron. Finally, vegetarians can take a multivitamin and mineral supplement that contains iron to ensure their iron and other mineral intakes are adequate.

Treatment for iron deficiency anemia generally includes iron supplements and the addition of iron-rich foods to the diet. It is also important to find and treat factors that may be causing the deficiency, such as intestinal bleeding.

Iron Toxicity   The UL for iron is 45 mg/day. Although not having enough iron in the body interferes with normal growth, development, and functioning, ingesting too much iron poses the risk of toxicity. Between 1988 and 1997, 29 American children under 6 years of age died as a result of accidentally taking too many iron-containing dietary supplements.[35] Early signs of acute iron poisoning include vomiting and diarrhea that may progress to coma and death.

In 1997, the FDA required a warning statement on the packaging of iron supplements to reduce the number of iron poisoning cases among young children. The agency also required unit-dose packaging of oral iron supplements that contained 30 mg of iron or more per dose. The individually wrapped supplements were designed to make it difficult for young children to ingest large quantities of the supplements at a time. After these rules were instituted, only one child died from iron poisoning between 1998 and 2002.[35] In 2003, however, a federal court ruled that the FDA did not have the legal authority to require special unit-dose packaging of iron supplements. The agency, however, could continue to require warning statements on supplement labels.

Iron Overload: Hereditary Hemochromatosis   *Iron overload* is a condition characterized by excess iron in the body. Iron overload occurs when toxic amounts of iron supplements are ingested, but the condition also results from certain genetic diseases.[36] **Hereditary hemochromatosis** (*he'-mo-crow'-ma-toe-sis*) is the most common type of iron overload disease in the United States.[37] People who have hereditary hemochromatosis (HH) absorb too much iron. The body has no way to eliminate the excess iron, so

Excess milk consumption contributes to iron deficiency in toddlers and preschool-age children.

pica   practice of eating nonfood items

 Food & Nutrition *tip*

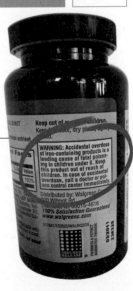

- Always treat iron and other dietary supplements as medicinal drugs and store these products in places that are inaccessible to children.

> **hereditary hemochromatosis** common inherited disorder characterized by excess iron absorption

the mineral accumulates in tissues and can cause joint pain, abnormal bronze skin color, and damage to the liver, heart, adrenal glands, and pancreas.

HH most often affects people who have northern European ancestors. In the United States, about 5 in every 1000 non-Hispanic white Americans are susceptible to developing the disease.[37] Men are more likely to be diagnosed with HH than women. Additionally, men tend to develop health problems from the excess iron at a younger age than women with the condition.

Joint pain is the most common complaint of people suffering from HH. Other common signs and symptoms of the disorder include fatigue, lack of energy, abdominal pain, loss of sex drive, and heart problems. Even though people with HH begin accumulating iron early in life, they often do not report any signs and symptoms of the disease until they are over 30 years of age. Testing is available to determine the presence of the genes that are responsible for the disease.

Many people who have HH experience vague symptoms or no symptoms at all. If the disease is not detected early and treated effectively, the organ damage resulting from the condition can be deadly. Treatment usually includes visiting a clinic periodically to have blood removed. This process stimulates the tissues that produce red blood cells to use storage iron for hemoglobin production. People with HH should avoid taking dietary supplements that contain iron.

Zinc (Zn)

In 1958, physician Ananda Prasad was working in Iran when he examined a 21-year-old man with dwarfism, intellectual disability, iron deficiency anemia, and underdeveloped sexual organs (Fig. 9.20).[38] Prasad noted that the young man ate unleavened ("flat") bread almost exclusively. After examining other patients in Iran and Egypt with similar health problems and dietary practices, Prasad hypothesized that diet was responsible for the condition. Eventually, medical researchers determined that Prasad's patients had severe zinc deficiencies. After these patients were given zinc supplements, they began to grow and develop normally. Prasad later determined that girls also experienced stunted growth and delays in sexual maturation as a result of zinc deficiency.[39]

In the regions where the men who were zinc deficient lived, the typical diet was comprised primarily of unleavened whole-wheat bread and little animal protein. Unleavened whole-wheat bread is naturally high in phytic acid and fiber, substances that decrease zinc bioavailability. In places where people use yeast to leaven (raise) bread dough, severe zinc deficiency is less likely to occur. Yeast reduces the binding effects of phytic acid and fiber, making zinc more bioavailable. Consuming zinc-rich sources of animal protein, such as meat and milk, also reduces the likelihood of zinc deficiency.

Other factors that influence the bioavailability of zinc include the body's need for the mineral and the presence of large amounts of certain other metals. During times when a healthy body needs zinc, the small intestine absorbs more. However, the presence of excess copper or iron in the small intestine interferes with zinc absorption. Thus, iron supplements should be taken between meals instead of with them.[40]

Why Is Zinc Necessary?

Zinc is a component of about a hundred enzymes.[40] Zinc is necessary for wound healing, the sense of taste and smell, DNA synthesis, and proper functioning of the immune system. Zinc is also essential for growth and development during pregnancy, childhood, and adolescence.

Sources of Zinc

Zinc is widespread in foods (Table 9.17). Red meat and poultry products supply most of the zinc in the typical American's diet. Figure 9.21 indicates MyPlate food groups that have foods that are good sources of zinc.

Figure 9.20 Zinc deficiency in young men. Zinc is necessary for normal physical growth and sexual development. This 16-year-old Egyptian boy experienced stunted growth and impaired sexual maturation as a result of a zinc-deficient diet.

TABLE 9.17 *Zinc Content of Selected Foods*

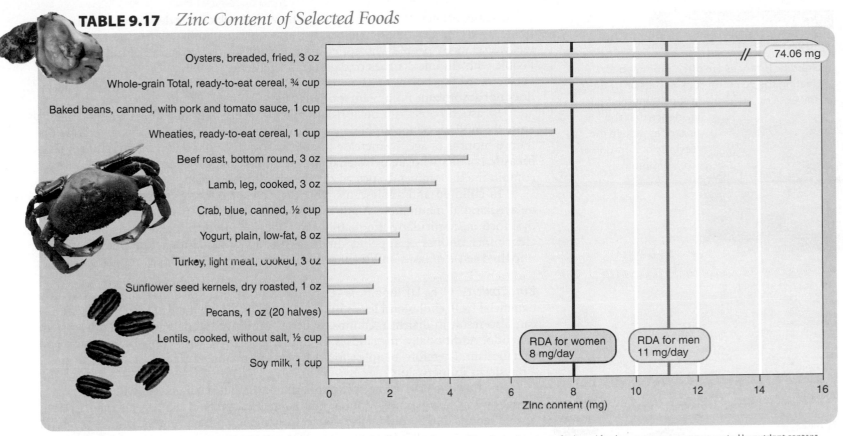

Food	Zinc content (mg)
Oysters, breaded, fried, 3 oz	74.06 mg
Whole-grain Total, ready-to-eat cereal, ¾ cup	
Baked beans, canned, with pork and tomato sauce, 1 cup	
Wheaties, ready-to-eat cereal, 1 cup	
Beef roast, bottom round, 3 oz	
Lamb, leg, cooked, 3 oz	
Crab, blue, canned, ½ cup	
Yogurt, plain, low-fat, 8 oz	
Turkey, light meat, cooked, 3 oz	
Sunflower seed kernels, dry roasted, 1 oz	
Pecans, 1 oz (20 halves)	
Lentils, cooked, without salt, ½ cup	
Soy milk, 1 cup	

RDA for women 8 mg/day

RDA for men 11 mg/day

Source: Data from U.S. Department of Agriculture, Agricultural Research Service, USDA Nutrient Data Laboratory: Zinc, Zn (mg) content of selected foods per common measure, sorted by nutrient content. *USDA national nutrient database for standard reference, release 19.* 2006.

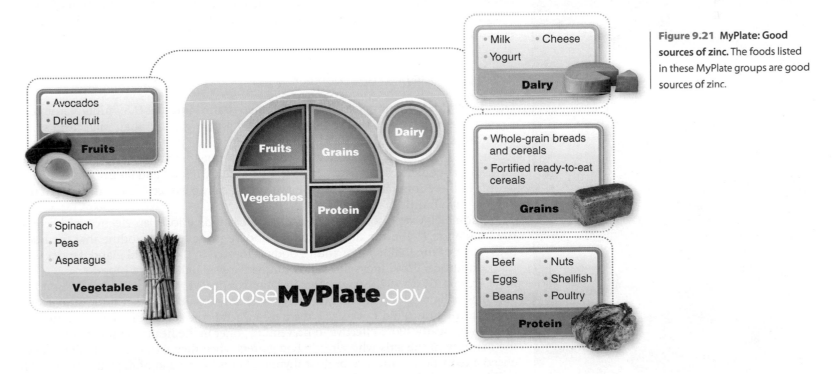

Figure 9.21 MyPlate: Good sources of zinc. The foods listed in these MyPlate groups are good sources of zinc.

- Avocados
- Dried fruit

Fruits

- Spinach
- Peas
- Asparagus

Vegetables

- Milk   • Cheese
- Yogurt

Dairy

- Whole-grain breads and cereals
- Fortified ready-to-eat cereals

Grains

- Beef   • Nuts
- Eggs   • Shellfish
- Beans   • Poultry

Protein

Dietary Adequacy

Adult RDAs for zinc range from 8 mg to 11 mg/day. In the United States, the average adult consumes adequate amounts of zinc. Thus, zinc deficiency is not a widespread problem

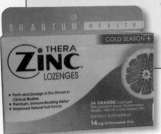
in the United States. However, alcoholics have high risk of zinc deficiency, because alcohol reduces zinc absorption and increases excretion of the mineral in urine. Making matters worse, many people who suffer from alcoholism do not consume nutritious diets. People with chronic diarrhea or digestive tract diseases can also develop zinc deficiency. Furthermore, vegetarians need more zinc than people who eat meat, because the GI tract does not absorb zinc from plant foods as well as from animal foods.[40]

Breastfed babies can be at risk of zinc deficiency. Although breast milk contains zinc, the milk does not supply enough of the trace mineral for infants who are older than 6 months of age. To increase the likelihood that their diets contain enough zinc, breastfed babies who are between 6 and 12 months of age need to consume foods that contain the trace mineral, such as zinc-fortified infant cereal.

In children and adolescents, zinc deficiency can cause growth retardation and delayed sexual maturation. Adult men who are zinc deficient may experience sexual dysfunction, particularly the inability to attain an erection. Other signs of zinc deficiency include loss of appetite, diarrhea, hair loss, dermatitis, poor wound healing, impaired sense of taste, and mental slowness.[40]

Zinc Toxicity The UL for zinc is 40 mg/day. Zinc intakes that exceed the UL can reduce beneficial HDL cholesterol levels in blood. Ingesting more than 100 mg of zinc per day can also result in diarrhea, cramps, nausea, vomiting, and depressed immune system function. Additionally, megadoses of zinc may interfere with copper absorption and metabolism. Therefore, people should avoid high intakes of zinc, unless they are under a physician's supervision.

In 2009, the FDA warned the public about using two *intranasal* ("within the nose") forms of Zicam, a nonprescription, zinc-containing product. The agency had received several reports that the alternative medical treatment for the common cold may result in loss of sense of smell.[40] In response to FDA actions, the manufacturer of Zicam voluntarily recalled the products, removing them from the marketplace. Results of studies do not provide consistent evidence that zinc helps reduce the severity or duration of colds, but more research is needed to clarify whether cold products that contain zinc may be beneficial.

Iodine (Iodide)

During World War I, physicians noted that men drafted into the U.S. military from the Great Lakes region were far more likely to have goiter (*goy'-ter*) than men from some other areas of the country. Goiter is enlargement of the thyroid gland that is not the result of cancer (Fig. 9.22). Goiters often occur among populations living in areas that have iodine-depleted soil. In general, these regions are inland and far from an ocean. If people in these communities limit their diets to locally produced foods, they might not have enough iodine in their diets.

Iodine (I_2) is poisonous, but most ingested iodine loses an electron to become the iodide ion (I^-) in the digestive tract.[30] Iodide is the form of iodine that the body uses. Most of the iodide in an adult's body is located in the thyroid gland. Under normal conditions, the kidneys filter and eliminate excess iodide from blood.

From 1917 to 1922, researchers in Ohio conducted an experiment on a group of girls in which one group of the children received doses of iodine, whereas the other group (the control group) did not receive the trace mineral. The results of the study indicated iodine was nearly 100% effective in preventing goiter in the healthy children. Moreover, the majority of the girls who already had goiters when they received the iodine experienced a reduction in the size of their thyroid glands by the end of the study.[41] In 1924, iodide was added to table salt in the United States, and as a result, cases of goiter caused by iodine deficiency rarely occur in this country. Today, use of iodized salt is the major method of preventing iodine deficiencies in developed nations, but inadequate iodine intake and goiters are still common in central Asia and central Africa.

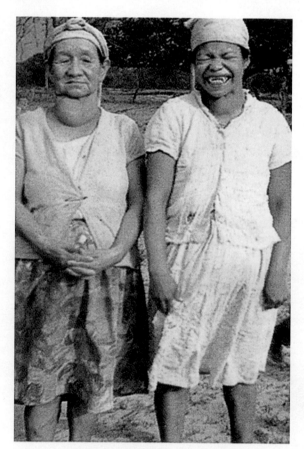

Figure 9.22 Goiter and cretinism in Bolivia, South America. The woman on the left is the mother of the woman on the right. Note that both women have goiters. Additionally, the daughter has cretinism.

Why Is Iodine Necessary?

People require iodine for normal thyroid function and for the production of thyroid hormones, collectively referred to as **thyroid hormone.** Thyroid hormone controls the rate of cell metabolism, that is, the rate at which cells obtain energy. The thyroid gland traps iodide from the bloodstream and accumulates the element for thyroid hormone synthesis. If a person's iodine intake is too low, the thyroid gland enlarges as it attempts to remove as much iodide as possible from the bloodstream. It is important to note that an enlarged thyroid gland can also be a sign of some diseases and conditions that are not related to iodine intake.

Sources of Iodine

Major sources of iodine include saltwater fish; seafood; seaweed; some plants, especially the leaves of plants grown near oceans; and iodized salt. A half teaspoon of iodine-fortified salt supplies the adult RDA for iodine. Iodide fortification of salt is voluntary in the United States, so not all salt has the trace mineral added to it. Other dietary sources of iodine include food additives that contain the mineral, such as certain dough conditioners and food dyes. Table 9.18 lists some foods that are good sources of iodine.

Dietary Adequacy

The adult RDA for iodine is 150 mcg/day. Most Americans have adequate iodine intakes.[42] As many Americans, particularly older adults, try to reduce their risk of hypertension by using less salt, iodine intakes may decline to marginal or inadequate levels.

Iodine Deficiency In cases of iodine deficiency, the thyroid gland produces insufficient amounts of thyroid hormone and goiter develops. As a result of the lack of thyroid hormone, iodine-deficient people generally have low metabolic rates and elevated blood cholesterol levels. Other signs and symptoms of iodine deficiency include fatigue,

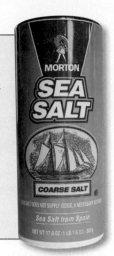

Did You Know?

The sea salt that is usually sold in supermarkets is not a good source of iodine and other minerals because it has undergone processing. Some stores sell "unrefined" or "natural" sea salt that contains much of its natural mineral content, including iodine.[42] Consumers, however, need to avoid excess sodium from all sources, including sea salt.

thyroid hormone hormone that regulates the body's metabolic rate

TABLE 9.18 *Iodine Content of Selected Foods*

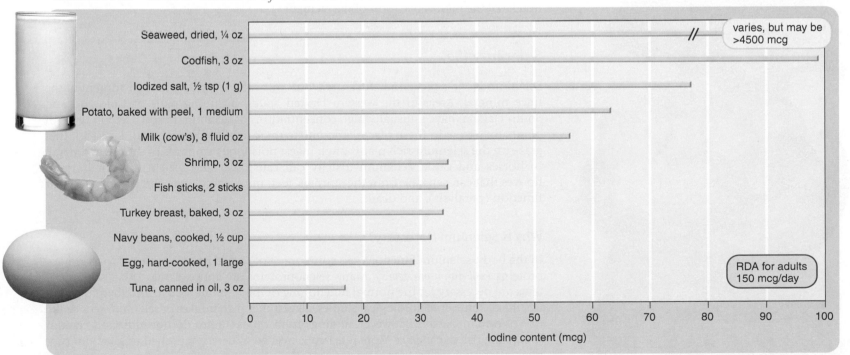

Source: Data from Higdon, J: *Iodine*. Micronutrient Information Center, Linus Pauling Institute, Oregon State University. Updated 2010. http://lpi.oregonstate.edu/infocenter/minerals/iodine/ Accessed: October 12, 2011.

cretinism condition affecting infants of women who were iodine deficient during pregnancy

goitrogens compounds that inhibit iodide metabolism by the thyroid gland

Did You Know?

Raw vegetables, particularly turnips, cabbage, brussels sprouts, cauliflower, and broccoli, contain **goitrogens.** These compounds inhibit iodide metabolism by the thyroid gland and, as a result, reduce thyroid hormone production. Unless people eat large amounts of raw vegetables that contain goitrogens or they are iodide deficient, they do not need to be concerned about eating these foods.[42] Furthermore, cooking vegetables destroys goitrogens.

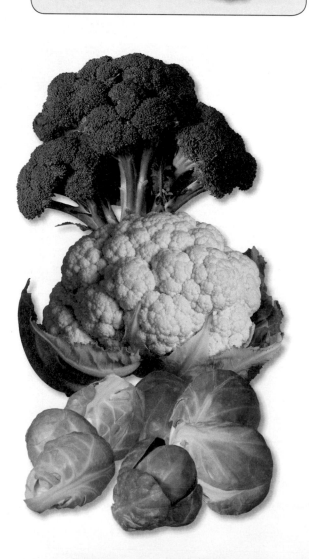

difficulty concentrating on mental tasks, weight gain, intolerance of cold temperatures, constipation, and dry skin.

Throughout the world, millions of people are at risk of iodine deficiency. Pregnant women who are iodine deficient have high risk of stillbirths (giving birth to a dead infant) or low-birth-weight babies. During fetal life, thyroid hormone is crucial for normal brain development. Thus, infants of iodine-deficient women are likely to be born with a condition called **cretinism** (*kre'-tin-ih-zim*). Babies with cretinism have permanent brain damage, reduced intellectual functioning, and growth retardation (see Fig. 9.22). Worldwide, iodine deficiency is the most common cause of preventable intellectual disability.[42] Pregnant women can reduce the risk of giving birth to infants with cretinism by consuming adequate amounts of iodine throughout pregnancy.

Iodine deficiency is a serious threat to health in places where soils are iodine deficient and commonly eaten foods are not fortified with the trace mineral, such as regions of Latin America, India, Southeast Asia, and Africa. Currently, international health organizations are engaging in efforts to eliminate iodine deficiency, primarily by promoting the use of iodized salt or iodide-fortified vegetable oils.

Iodide Toxicity   The UL for iodine is 1.1 mg/day. Over time, consuming very high amounts of iodine can cause thyroid gland enlargement and reduced production of thyroid hormone. These side effects are the same as those that occur when diets are deficient in iodine. Excess iodine is also associated with an increased risk of a form of thyroid cancer.[42]

Nuclear power plant accidents, such as the one that occurred after a major earthquake struck Japan in 2011, may release radioactive iodine (Iodine-131) into the environment. When people are exposed to radioactive iodine, the element can enter their bodies and be picked up by their thyroid glands. Exposure to a high amount of the radiation increases the risk of thyroid cancer, especially in children.[42] People who have iodine deficiency are more likely to accumulate the radioactive iodine in their thyroid glands than people who are not iodine deficient. To reduce the risk of thyroid cancer, people who are exposed to radioactive iodine can take supplements that contain 16 to 130 mg of potassium iodide, depending on their age, until the risk of extreme radiation exposure ends.[42] The thyroid gland picks up the potassium iodide, which helps block the thyroid gland's uptake of the radioactive form of the element.

Selenium (Se)

Selenium is widespread in Earth's crust, but soils can vary widely in their content of the trace mineral. Areas of the western United States, including parts of Colorado and South Dakota, have unusually high concentrations of selenium in soil. Certain types of plants that grow in these places accumulate toxic levels of the mineral. Livestock that graze on the selenium-rich plants often ingest poisonous amounts of the trace mineral. In horses and cattle, selenium toxicity can cause hair and weight loss, malformed hooves that can separate from the animals' feet, muscle weakness and loss of muscular function (paralysis), and death.

Why Is Selenium Necessary?

In the body, selenium functions as a component of several proteins referred to as selenoproteins (*sell'-in-oh-pro'-teens*). Many selenoproteins are antioxidants. Other selenoproteins are necessary for the normal functioning of the immune system and thyroid gland. Results of some epidemiological studies suggest that high intakes of selenium reduce the risk of certain cancers. However, findings from other studies do not indicate selenium lowers the risk of cancer.[43] More research is needed to determine whether selenium supplementation is useful for cancer prevention.

TABLE 9.19 *Selenium Content of Selected Foods*

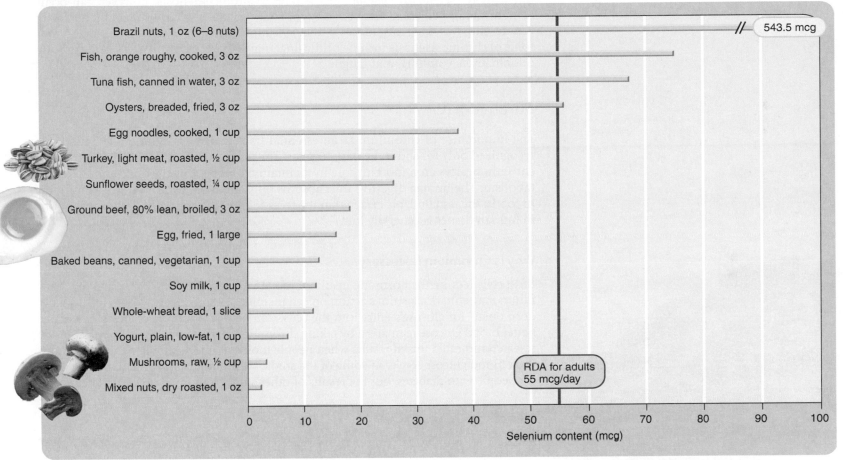

Brazil nuts, 1 oz (6–8 nuts) — 543.5 mcg
Fish, orange roughy, cooked, 3 oz
Tuna fish, canned in water, 3 oz
Oysters, breaded, fried, 3 oz
Egg noodles, cooked, 1 cup
Turkey, light meat, roasted, ½ cup
Sunflower seeds, roasted, ¼ cup
Ground beef, 80% lean, broiled, 3 oz
Egg, fried, 1 large
Baked beans, canned, vegetarian, 1 cup
Soy milk, 1 cup
Whole-wheat bread, 1 slice
Yogurt, plain, low-fat, 1 cup
Mushrooms, raw, ½ cup
Mixed nuts, dry roasted, 1 oz

RDA for adults
55 mcg/day

Selenium content (mcg)

Source: Data from U.S. Department of Agriculture, Agricultural Research Service, USDA Nutrient Data Laboratory: Selenium, Se (mcg) content of selected foods per common measure, sorted by nutrient content. *USDA national nutrient database for standard reference, release 19.* 2006.

Sources of Selenium

In most countries, plant foods are the major dietary sources of selenium.[43] Although the selenium content of foods varies, nuts, whole-grain products, seafood, and meats are generally rich sources of the trace mineral (Table 9.19). Because Brazil nuts can have very high selenium contents, people should not eat these nuts regularly.

Dietary Adequacy

Most Americans' diets meet the RDA for selenium. In the United States, selenium deficiency is uncommon, but the condition may occur in people who have serious digestive tract conditions that interfere with the mineral's absorption. Selenium deficiency reduces thyroid gland activity and can lead to goiter. The deficiency also depresses immune system function and may contribute to the development of heart disease and cancer. In parts of China where the soil lacks selenium and the population consumes locally produced foods, diets typically contain inadequate amounts of selenium. Certain types of cancer and a form of heart disease are common in these areas of China. There is not enough scientific evidence, however, to support the use of selenium supplements to prevent or treat cancer or CVD.[43]

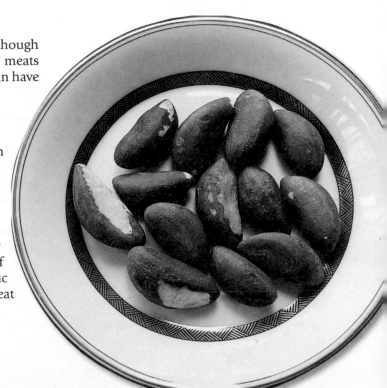

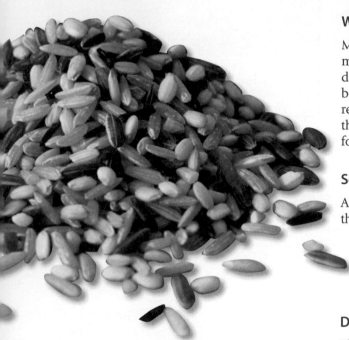

Selenium Toxicity   The UL for selenium is 400 mcg/day. In the United States, selenium toxicity (selenosis) (*sell'-in-o-sis*) is rare.[43] Chronic selenosis, however, can occur from drinking well water that naturally contains too much selenium. Selenium toxicity can develop by taking megadoses of dietary supplements. In humans, signs and symptoms of chronic selenosis include brittle fingernails, loss of hair and nails, garlicky body odor, nausea, vomiting, and fatigue.

Chromium (Cr)

The importance of chromium as an essential trace mineral in human diets has been recognized only for about the past 40 years. The results of scientific studies suggest that chromium plays an important role in maintaining proper carbohydrate and lipid metabolism. The human digestive tract absorbs only about 0.4 to 2.5% of the chromium in foods; the remainder is excreted in the feces.[44] Thus, the concentration of chromium in human tissues is generally low.

Why Is Chromium Necessary?

Most cells require the hormone insulin to obtain glucose from the bloodstream. Chromium may enhance insulin's action on cell membranes and, in a way, help to "hold the door open" for glucose's entry into the cells. Can people who have diabetes experience better blood glucose regulation by taking chromium supplements? A review of scientific research indicated mixed results when people took chromium supplements to improve their blood glucose levels. In some of the studies, chromium supplements were helpful for people with diabetes, but the results of other studies indicated no such benefits.

Sources of Chromium

Although chromium is widely distributed in foods, most foods contain less than 2 mcg of the mineral per serving.[44] Information regarding the chromium content of various foods is difficult to find, because most reliable food composition tables do not include this trace mineral. In general, meat, whole-grain products, yeast, fruits, and vegetables are good sources of chromium. Like selenium, the amount of chromium in plant foods reflects the chromium content of soils where crops are grown.

Dietary Adequacy

The adult AIs for chromium are 25 mcg/day for young women and 35 mcg/day for young men. Well-balanced diets typically contain these amounts of chromium. On average, American adults consume diets that meet or exceed their AIs for chromium.[44]

Chromium Deficiency   Signs of chromium deficiency are impaired glucose tolerance and elevated blood cholesterol and triglyceride levels. The mechanism by which chromium influences cholesterol metabolism is not known but may involve enzymes that control the body's cholesterol production. Cases of chromium deficiency have been reported in people maintained on special-formula diets that did not contain chromium, as well as in severely malnourished children.

Chromium Toxicity   The form of chromium that is naturally in foods has not been shown to produce toxicity, so no UL has been set for the trace mineral. The long-term safety of taking various chromium supplements is unknown. Data from a study using cells of mice indicated chromium picolinate may damage human DNA.[45] This finding raises concern, because damaged DNA can result in cancer. Therefore, taking supplemental chromium may be risky (see Table 11.7).

Concept **Checkpoint**

21. What is the difference between iron deficiency and iron deficiency anemia? What are the signs and symptoms of iron deficiency anemia? Which members of the population are most at risk of iron deficiency?
22. What is hemochromatosis? Identify at least three signs or symptoms of hemochromatosis. How is the condition treated?
23. Describe signs and symptoms of zinc deficiency in humans.
24. What is a goiter? What is cretinism? How can cretinism be prevented?
25. Which foods are rich sources of selenium?
26. What is the major role of chromium in the body?
27. Prepare a table for trace minerals that includes information about each trace mineral's major role or roles in the body, food sources, and signs and symptoms of the mineral's deficiency as well as toxicity disorders. Check your table against the information provided in Table 9.14.

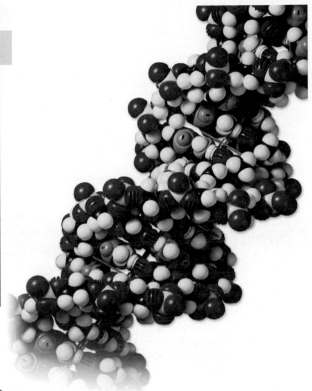

 9.5 Minerals with Possible Physiological Roles

A few minerals, including nickel, arsenic, and silicon, are found in small amounts in the body, but their roles in the body are unclear. At present, this group of minerals is not classified as essential nutrients. Table 9.20 summarizes the possible functions, suggested human intakes, and food sources of six minerals that may be essential to humans. Although there are reports of severe illness and deaths resulting from environmental exposure to high amounts of these minerals, foods generally do not contain toxic amounts of them.

TABLE 9.20 *Summary of Six Possible Essential Minerals*

Mineral	Possible Functions	Suggested Daily Human Intakes	Dietary Sources
Arsenic (As)	No clear biological function in humans, but may play a role in methionine metabolism, growth, and reproduction (animal studies)	No UL has been established; however, arsenic is highly toxic.	Fish, grains, cereals
Boron (B)	No clear biological function in humans but may be involved in steroid hormone metabolism	1–13 mg (UL: 20 mg/day)	Fruit, leafy vegetables, peanuts, beans, wine
Lithium (Li)	Reproduction Maintenance of appropriate mood	1000 mcg (No UL has been established.)	Water supply, grains, vegetables
Nickel (Ni)	Amino acid and fatty acid metabolism	25–35 mcg (UL: 1 mg/day)	Chocolate, nuts, beans, whole grains
Silicon (Si)	Connective tissue, including bone formation	25–30 mg (Insufficient data to determine UL)	Root vegetables, whole grains
Vanadium (V)	Glucose metabolism Tooth and bone mineralization	10 mcg (UL: 1.8 mg/day)	Shellfish, mushrooms, black pepper, parsley, dill

Sources: Data from Food and Nutrition Board, Institute of Medicine: *Dietary Reference Intakes for vitamin A, vitamin K, arsenic, boron, chromium, copper, iodine, iron, manganese, molybdenum, nickel, silicon, vanadium, and zinc.* Washington, DC: Standing Committee on the Scientific Evaluation of Dietary Reference Intakes. National Academy Press, 2006. Schrauzer, GN: Lithium: Occurrence, dietary intakes, nutritional essentiality. *Journal of the American College of Nutrition*, 21(1):14, 2002.

Concept **Checkpoint**

28. Identify at least four minerals that are classified as possible essential minerals.
29. Prepare a table for arsenic, boron, lithium, nickel, silicon, and vanadium that includes information about each mineral's possible function and major food sources. Check your table against the information provided in Table 9.20.

Chapter 9 Highlight

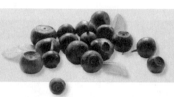

BOTTLED WATER VERSUS TAP WATER

Today, preparing for a class often involves bringing into the classroom a notebook, something to write with, and a bottle of cold water. Even many college instructors keep a bottle of water nearby as they lecture. Not long ago, most Americans got their water from a faucet ("tap water"). Now, millions of Americans are turning away from the tap and choosing to drink bottled water instead. If you prefer drinking bottled water over tap water, you are part of a growing trend. According to data provided by the Beverage Market Corporation, each American consumed 27.6 gallons of bottled water in 2009.[46] That amount of bottled water is 70% more than the amount consumed in 1999. The U.S. population drinks more bottled water than milk, juice, or any other beverage, except carbonated soft drinks. Sales revenues for bottled water were about $10.6 billion in 2009.[46]

Why do so many Americans drink bottled water when tap water is much less costly? Among adults, taste, convenience, and health concerns were major reasons they chose bottled water over other beverages. For most Americans, however, bottled water is usually unnecessary and expensive, as it is often very similar to tap water. Consumers need to be aware that the water in some bottled water products actually comes from a municipal water supply. However, when public water supplies are disrupted by hurricanes, tornadoes, or earthquakes, drinking bottled water may be a consumer's only option. What is bottled water? Is it safe to drink?

The Environmental Protection Agency (EPA) regulates the sanitation of public water supplies in the United States. Another federal agency, the Food and Drug Administration (FDA), regulates bottled water products that are marketed for interstate commerce. Neither agency "certifies" bottled water.[47]

The FDA requires bottled water producers to

• Process, bottle, hold and transport bottled water under sanitary conditions;

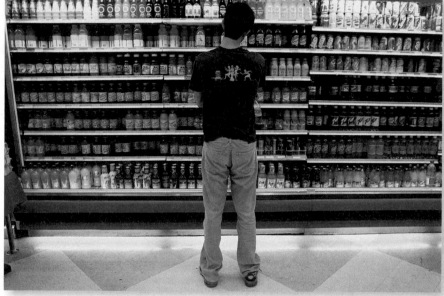

• Protect water sources from bacteria, chemicals, and other contaminants;
• Use quality control processes to ensure the bacteriological and chemical safety of the water;
• Sample and test both the source of water and the final product for contaminants.[48]

Bottled water is sealed in containers and has no added ingredients other than a substance that prevents the growth of microbes, such as bacteria. Bottled water may have fluoride added, but amounts must meet FDA guidelines. If bottled water manufacturers add flavorings or other ingredients to their products, the name of the product must indicate the added ingredients—"Bottled Water with Cherry Flavor," for example. These drinks are often called "flavored water beverages." Flavored waters may simply contain additives that make the beverage taste good, but a growing number of flavored waters also have added nutrients other than sugars, such as sodium, potassium, and amino acids. The beverage's label must identify the additives in the list of ingredients.

The FDA uses place of origin to classify some bottled waters. "Artesian well water," for example, must come from a well that taps an *aquifer*, a body of water found between porous layers of rock, sand, and earth. Table 9.21 lists common types of water used for bottling purposes and their FDA definitions.

Safety standards for bottled water are similar to those established by the EPA for tap water. According to FDA guidelines, bottled water manufacturers are responsible for producing safe products. Production procedures for bottled water must follow manufacturing regulations established and enforced by the FDA. Additionally, the FDA inspects water bottling facilities regularly.

Because of FDA regulations and oversight, consumers can be assured that their supply of bottled water is safe. Additionally, most Americans can trust the safety of their tap water because the vast majority of municipal water systems in the United States are regulated by the *Safe Drinking Water Act* (*SDWA*). As a result of this law, most tap water undergoes a thorough purification process and is constantly tested for safety. If such testing indicates the water supply may pose a threat to public health, consumers are warned through media, and a "boil order"—requirement to boil water for 10 minutes to kill harmful microorganisms—may be issued.

Although bottled water is safe to drink, the plastic used to contain it may have toxic effects on health. *Bisphenol* (*biss'-feen-ol*) *A*, which is also called *BPA*, is a chemical used to make polycarbonate plastics and epoxy resins. Polycarbonate plastics are in many consumer products that come in contact with foods and

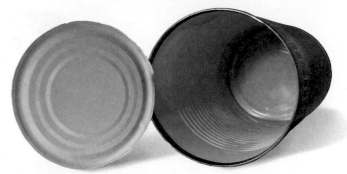

Figure 9.23 BPA and epoxy resins. The epoxy resin that is used to coat the inside of cans contains BPA.

beverages, including some water bottles and baby bottles. The epoxy resin that contains BPA is used to coat the inside of certain food cans. The coating prevents the can's metal from coming in contact with and being damaged by the food (Fig. 9.23). However, BPA can leach from polycarbonate plastic containers or epoxy resin-coated cans and enter the food or beverage stored within them.

Results of recent studies involving laboratory animals suggested that low doses of BPA were harmful. More research is needed to determine the extent to which BPA can affect human health, especially infants and children who are exposed to the chemical. Nevertheless, concern over the safety of BPA has encouraged some plastic bottle manufacturers to discontinue using the chemical in their products.[49] Plastic containers that contain BPA are marked with the symbol shown in Figure 9.24. To reduce your exposure to BPA, consider taking these actions:

- Avoid heating foods in polycarbonate plastic containers.
- Avoid plastic containers that have the symbol shown in Figure 9.24.
- Do not wash polycarbonate containers in the dishwasher or with harsh detergents.
- Reduce your intake of canned foods.
- Cook or store foods and beverages in glass, porcelain, or stainless steel containers.
- Avoid using polycarbonate dishware, cups, or eating utensils for serving foods (especially hot foods or liquids).
- Avoid baby bottles and toys that contain BPA.

TABLE 9.21 *FDA Definitions for Classifying Some Types of Water**

Water	Definition
Artesian water	Water from a well that taps a confined aquifer
Mineral water	Water containing not less than 250 ppm (parts per million) total dissolved solids and originates from a geologically and physically protected underground water source. No minerals may be added to mineral water.
Purified water	Water produced by distillation, deionization, reverse osmosis, or other suitable processes. The water must meet the definition of "purified water" in the *U.S. Pharmacopeia*.
Sparkling bottled water	Treated water that contains the same amount of carbon dioxide it had when it emerged from its source
Spring water	Water from an underground formation from which the water flows naturally to the surface of the earth at an identified location.

*For complete regulatory definitions, see 21 CFR 165.110(a)(2) at FDA's website: www.cfsan.fda.gov/~dms/botwatr.html

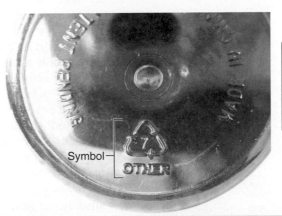

Figure 9.24 Where's the BPA? This symbol indicates that the plastic used to make this water bottle contains BPA.

Symbol

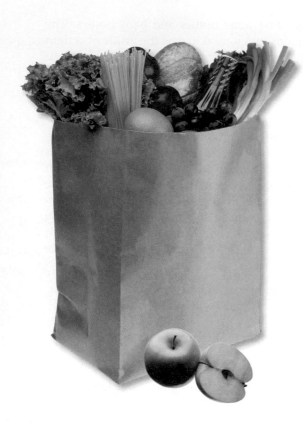

CHAPTER REFERENCES

See Appendix I.

SUMMARY

Water is a simple compound that does not undergo digestion. In the body, water is a major solvent that often participates directly in chemical reactions. Water's other physiological roles include transporting substances, removing waste products, lubricating tissues, and regulating body temperature and acid-base balance. Water does not provide energy for the body. Depending on a person's age, sex, and body composition, about 45 to 75% of his or her body is water.

The body maintains a balance between intracellular and extracellular fluids primarily by controlling concentrations of ions in each fluid compartment. Maintenance of intracellular water volume depends largely on the intracellular concentration of potassium and phosphate ions. Maintenance of extracellular water volume depends primarily on the extracellular concentration of sodium and chloride ions. If the normal concentrations of these ions change too much, water shifts out of a compartment, and cells shrink or swell as a result.

Total water intake includes water from beverages and foods. About 80% of a person's total water intake is from beverages. Most of the water that enters the digestive tract is absorbed. Metabolic water is another source of water for the body.

The body loses water in urine, perspiration, exhaled air, feces, and insensible perspiration. A healthy person's average daily total water input equals his or her average output. Environmental factors, physiological conditions, and lifestyle practices can alter the body's fluid balance.

The kidneys are the major regulator of the body's water content and ion concentrations. In a healthy person, the kidneys maintain proper hydration by filtering excess ions from blood. When the kidneys remove ions such as sodium, water follows and becomes the main component of urine. Kidneys also remove drugs and metabolic waste products from the bloodstream.

To avoid overheating, the body must dissipate the excess heat into the environment, primarily by perspiration. When water evaporates from skin, it takes some heat along with it, cooling the body.

The AI for total water intake is 2.7 L for young women and 3.7 L for young men. These amounts do not need to be consumed in the form of fluids, because most solid foods and metabolic water contribute some water to the body.

Thirst is the primary regulator of fluid intake. The majority of healthy people meet their AI for water by letting thirst be their guide. Under certain conditions, however, elderly individuals, sick persons, and people who work or exercise outdoors, especially in hot conditions, are at risk of dehydration.

Minerals are a group of elements in Earth's rocks, soils, and natural water sources. About 15 mineral elements have known functions in the body and are necessary for human health. The two primary groups of dietary minerals are major minerals and trace minerals.

Some minerals function as inorganic ions or structural components of tissues; other minerals are components of various enzymes, hormones, or other organic molecules. Cells cannot metabolize minerals for energy. The body, however, needs certain minerals to catalyze specific chemical reactions that release energy from macronutrients. Lack of energy is often a symptom of these particular mineral deficiency disorders. Excessive amounts of minerals in the body can disrupt normal cell functioning, causing toxicity.

Most foods contain small amounts of minerals. When the body's needs for minerals increase, the bioavailability of minerals generally increases to meet the demand.

Calcium is a major structural component of bones and teeth, and the mineral is necessary for blood clotting, muscle contraction, nerve transmission, and cell metabolism. Calcium absorption depends on vitamin D. Milk and milk products are rich calcium sources. Although people, especially women, are at risk of developing osteoporosis as they age, various lifestyle modifications help reduce this risk.

Sodium, the major positively charged ion found outside cells, is vital for maintaining fluid balance and transmitting nerve impulses. The typical American diet provides high amounts of sodium, primarily from processed foods and table salt. Diets high in sodium are associated with increased risk of hypertension.

Hypertensive individuals have greater risk of CVD, kidney failure, and damage to other organs than people with normal blood pressures. Advanced age, African-American ancestry, obesity, physical inactivity, cigarette smoking, and excess alcohol and sodium intakes are major risk factors for hypertension. Treatment for hypertension usually includes following dietary modifications and making some other lifestyle changes.

Potassium, the major positively charged ion found inside cells, has functions that are similar to those of sodium. Potassium-rich diets may lower blood pressure, reduce the risk of developing kidney stones, and possibly decrease bone loss. Plant foods, meat, and milk are good sources of potassium.

Magnesium is a cofactor for numerous chemical reactions and is needed for nerve and heart function. Although many Americans do not consume recommended amounts of magnesium, cases of magnesium deficiency rarely occur among healthy members of the population. Plant foods are good sources of magnesium.

Iron is a critical component of hemoglobin, myoglobin, and cytochromes. Hemoglobin in red blood cells transports oxygen from the lungs to the tissues. Iron deficiency can result in iron deficiency anemia, a condition characterized by decreased production of red blood cells. People suffering from anemia fatigue easily and lack interest in activities. In children, anemia interferes with growth and development.

Iron absorption depends on the body's need for the mineral and the form of iron in food. Heme iron is better absorbed than nonheme iron. Meat and liver are among the best sources of dietary iron. Women of childbearing age have higher needs for iron than men because of menstrual blood loss. Throughout the world, iron deficiency–related disorders are common. People who have hereditary hemochromatosis develop iron toxicity, because they absorb too much iron.

Zinc functions as a cofactor that activates many enzymes. Zinc is involved in growth and development, antioxidant activity, immune function, and taste. Zinc deficiency can result in growth failure and loss of appetite, as well as reduced intellectual and decreased immune function. Animal foods are the best dietary sources of zinc, but whole grains, peanuts, and legumes are also good sources of the trace mineral.

Iodine is needed to make thyroid hormone. When the diet lacks iodine, the thyroid gland enlarges, forming a goiter. The iodine content of the soil in which a plant is grown affects the iodine content of the plant food. Cretinism can occur in infants born to women who were iodine deficient during pregnancy. Iodine deficiency is rare in the United States because table salt is often fortified with iodide. However, the deficiency is a major health problem in parts of the world where people consume diets that lack iodine.

Selenium functions as a component of selenoproteins, many of which are antioxidants. Other selenoproteins are involved in the normal functioning of the immune system and thyroid gland. The selenium content of the soil in which a plant is grown affects the selenium content of the plant food. Meat, fish, nuts, whole grains, and seeds are good sources of selenium.

Chromium enhances the action of insulin. Chromium is found in meats and whole grains. More research is needed to determine the effects of taking chromium supplements.

A few minerals, including nickel and silicon, are found in very small amounts in the body, but their roles in the body are unclear. At present, these particular minerals are not classified as essential nutrients.

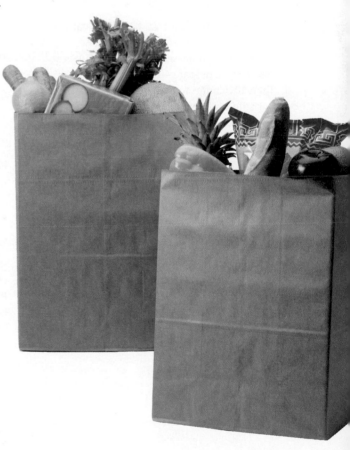

In the United States, bottled water is usually unnecessary and expensive, and it is often derived from a municipal water supply. When public water supplies are disrupted by hurricanes, tornadoes, or earthquakes, drinking bottled water may be a consumer's only option. The Environmental Protection Agency regulates the sanitation of public water supplies in the United States. The Food and Drug Administration regulates bottled water products that are marketed for interstate commerce. Bottled water may have fluoride added, but amounts must meet FDA guidelines. If bottled water manufacturers add flavorings or other ingredients to a product, the name of the product must indicate the added ingredients, and the beverage's label must identify the additives in the list of ingredients. Many public health experts are concerned about the possible effects of bisphenol A (BPA), especially to infants and children. BPA is used to make certain plastics and resins. Plastic bottles, including water bottles and baby bottles, may contain BPA. Although more research is needed to clarify the role of BPA in health, it is wise to avoid products that contain the chemical.

Recipe for Healthy Living

Easy Orange-Strawberry Smoothie

When made with fat-free milk or low-fat yogurt, smoothies are a tasty, low-fat, calcium- and potassium-rich snack. They are also easy to prepare—this recipe takes less than 10 minutes to make. For variety, substitute a banana, a mango, or raspberries for the strawberries, or use lime sherbet instead of orange sherbet. Experimenting with different fruits and flavored sherbets makes it easy to individualize smoothies, depending on your preferences and the fruit that's available. You'll need a sturdy blender to combine the ingredients.

The following recipe makes about three 8-fluid-ounce servings. Each serving supplies approximately 200 kcal, 7 g protein, 3 g fat, 343 mg calcium, 564 mg potassium, 103 mg sodium, 1 mg zinc, 5 mcg selenium, and 70 mg vitamin C.

INGREDIENTS:

¼ cup frozen orange juice concentrate, calcium fortified
1 cup orange sherbet
1½ cups low-fat, plain yogurt
1 cup fresh strawberries, washed with leafy "caps" removed (can substitute frozen strawberries)
2 ice cubes

PREPARATION STEPS:

1. Place all ingredients, except ice cubes, in blender.

2. Blend until smooth. Add ice cubes and blend again, until ice is crushed.

3. Serve.

4. Refrigerate or freeze unused portion in a covered container.
Partially thaw frozen smoothie before blending again.

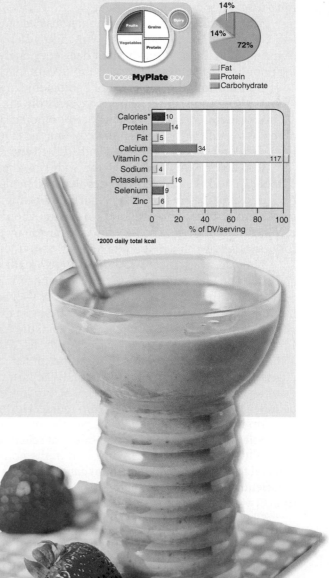

ChooseMyPlate.gov

14%
14%
72%

Fat
Protein
Carbohydrate

	% of DV/serving
Calories*	10
Protein	14
Fat	5
Calcium	34
Vitamin C	117
Sodium	4
Potassium	16
Selenium	9
Zinc	6

*2000 daily total kcal

Personal *Dietary* Analysis

Using the DRIs

1. Refer to your 3-day food log from the "Personal Dietary Analysis" feature in Chapter 3.

   a. Find the RDA/AI values for minerals under your life stage/gender group category in the DRI tables (see the inside back cover of this book). Write those values under the "My RDA/AI" column in the table below.

   b. Review your personal dietary assessment. Find your 3-day average intakes of iron, calcium, zinc, sodium, potassium, and magnesium. Write those values under the "My Average Intake" column of the table.

   c. Calculate the percentage of the RDA/AI you consumed for each mineral by dividing your intake by the RDA/AI amount and multiplying the figure you obtain by 100. For example, if your average intake of iron was 9 mg/day, and your RDA for the mineral is 18 mg/day, you would divide 18 mg by 9 mg to obtain .50. To multiply this figure by 100, simply move the decimal point two places to the right, and replace the decimal point with a percentage sign (50%). Thus, your average daily intake of iron was 50% of the RDA. Place the percentages for each mineral under the "% of My RDA/AI" column.

   d. Under the ">, <, =" column, indicate whether your average daily intake was greater than (>), less than (<), or equal to (=) the RDA/AI.

2. Use the information you calculated in the first part of this activity to answer the following questions:

   a. Which of your average mineral intakes equaled or exceeded the RDA/AI?

   b. Which of your average mineral intakes was below the RDA/AI?

   c. What foods would you eat to increase your intake of the minerals that were less than the RDA/AI levels? (Review sources of the minerals in Chapter 9.)

   d. Turn in your completed table and answers to your instructor.

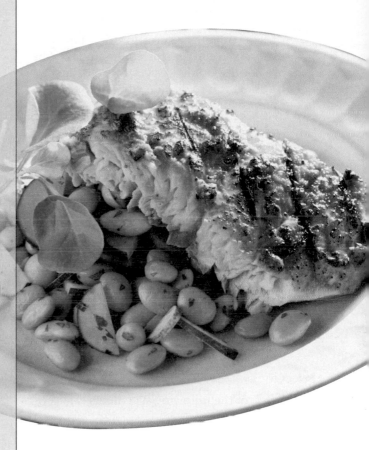

Personal Dietary Analysis: Minerals

Mineral	My RDA/AI	My Average Intake	% of My RDA/AI	>, <, or =
iron				
calcium				
zinc				
sodium				
potassium				
magnesium				

CRITICAL THINKING

1. Before the advent of refrigeration, salting meat was a common way of preventing microbes from spoiling the food. Explain why salting was effective as a means of food preservation.

2. A friend of yours refuses to drink tap water because she thinks it is contaminated. She drinks only bottled water or well water. If she asked you to explain why you drink tap water, what would you tell her?

3. A group of food manufacturers is considering fortifying some of their products with iron, chromium, boron, and iodide. Explain why you think they should or should not fortify the foods with each of these minerals.

4. What advice would you give a total vegetarian (vegan) concerning his need for calcium, iron, potassium, magnesium, and zinc?

5. Consider your family history and lifestyle to determine whether you are at risk of osteoporosis. If you are at risk, what steps can you take at this point in your life to reduce your chances of developing this disease?

6. Consider your family history and lifestyle to determine whether you are at risk of hypertension. If you are at risk, what steps can you take at this point in your life to reduce your chances of developing this disease?

7. In a televised interview, a person claiming to be a doctor recommends taking megadoses of zinc, iron, and selenium supplements to enhance muscular strength and endurance. Discuss why you would or would not follow this person's advice.

PRACTICE TEST

Select the best answer.

1. Which of the following statements is false?
   a. Lean tissue contains more water than fat tissue.
   b. Water is a major solvent.
   c. Generally, young women have more body water than young men.
   d. Water does not provide energy.

2. If the extracellular fluid has an excess of sodium ions,
   a. sodium ions move into cells.
   b. intracellular fluid moves to the outside of cells.
   c. phosphate and calcium ions are eliminated in feces.
   d. blood levels of arsenic and oxalate increase.

3. Which of the following foods has the lowest percentage of water?
   a. tomatoes
   b. oranges
   c. whole-grain bread
   d. vegetable oil

4. In the United States, table salt is often fortified with
   a. iron.
   b. selenium.
   c. potassium.
   d. iodide.

5. Which of the following foods is not a good source of calcium?
   a. butter
   b. American cheese
   c. canned sardines
   d. kale

6. Henry is concerned about his risk of osteoporosis. Which of the following characteristics is a modifiable risk factor for this chronic condition?
   a. family history
   b. racial/ethnic background
   c. physical activity level
   d. age

7. The primary source of sodium in the typical American's diet is
   a. bottled water.
   b. unprocessed food.
   c. fruit.
   d. salt.

8. Which of the following populations has the highest risk of hypertension?
   a. people with African-American ancestry
   b. young, physically active Asian men
   c. Hispanic women who do not drink alcohol
   d. young adults who consume high amounts of fruit

9. Sources of heme iron include
   a. fortified grain products.
   b. beef.
   c. spinach.
   d. cast-iron cookware.

10. Worldwide, the most common nutrient deficiency disorder is _____ deficiency.
    a. iodine
    b. cobalt
    c. iron
    d. calcium

11. Which of the following statements is false?
    a. Iodine is necessary for normal thyroid function.
    b. In the United States, milk is usually fortified with iodide.
    c. Having too much or too little iodine in the diet can cause the thyroid gland to enlarge.
    d. Saltwater fish and other seafood are sources of iodine.

12. Which of the following statements is true?
    a. Safety standards for bottled water are similar to those for tap water.
    b. Most brands of water bottled in the United States contain unsafe amounts of arsenic and lead.
    c. The EPA inspects and certifies water bottling facilities at least three times a year.
    d. The majority of Americans should drink bottled water because water from municipal systems is unsafe.

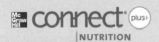

Additional resources related to the features of this book are available on ConnectPlus® Nutrition. Ask your instructor how to get access.

Answers to Chapter 9 Quiz *Yourself*

1. Your body constantly loses water through insensible perspiration, a form of water loss that is not the same as sweat. **True.** (p. 302)

2. Ounce per ounce, cottage cheese contains more calcium than plain yogurt. **False.** (p. 312)

3. Potassium, sodium, and chloride ions are involved in fluid balance. **True.** (p. 301)

4. Selenium is an essential mineral. **True.** (p. 338)

5. In general, plants are good sources of iron because the plant pigment chlorophyll contains iron. **False.** (p. 325)

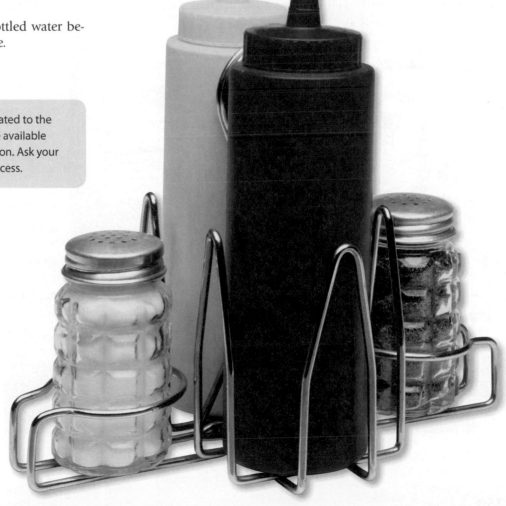

Energy Balance and Weight Control

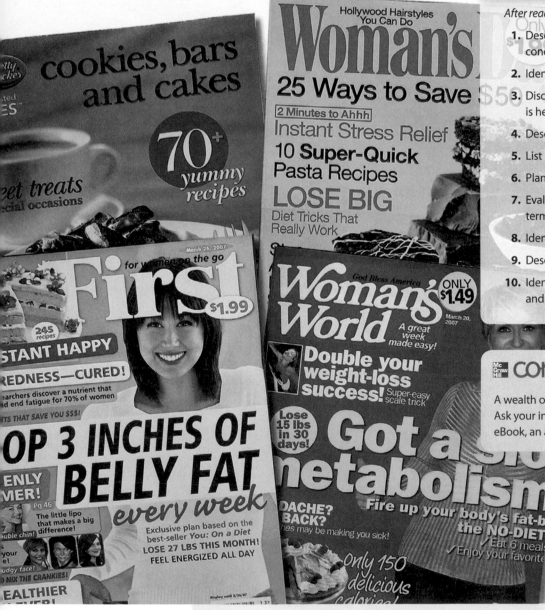

Chapter Learning Outcomes

After reading Chapter 10, you should be able to

1. Describe the uses of energy by the body and explain the concept of energy balance.

2. Identify factors that influence body weight.

3. Discuss how BMI is used to determine whether a person's weight is healthy.

4. Describe ways to measure body composition.

5. List major health risks associated with excess body fat.

6. Plan a long-term weight-loss regimen that is safe and effective.

7. Evaluate popular weight-reduction diets for safety and long-term effectiveness.

8. Identify surgical procedures for severe obesity.

9. Describe treatments for underweight.

10. Identify major kinds of eating disorders, and discuss risk factors and treatments for these conditions.

McGraw Hill **connect** plus+
| NUTRITION
www.mcgrawhillconnect.com

A wealth of proven resources are available on ConnectPlus® Nutrition! Ask your instructor about ConnectPlus, which includes an interactive eBook, an adaptive learning program and much, much more!

HAVE YOU NOTICED the array of magazines stacked next to supermarket checkout lanes? The headline on one of the popular women's magazine covers announces in large, bright pink letters: "LOSE BIG—diet tricks that really work." A photo of chocolate brownies, cookies, and fudge nearly fills the magazine's cover. The magazine next to it contains recipes for rich desserts. Another magazine cover displays a decorated cake and the statement: "Drop 3 inches of belly fat—every week." The magazine next to it suggests a way you can "Double your weight-loss success!" To ensure that the cover grabs your attention, an appealing-looking pie appears in the lower left-hand corner. Month after month, the magazines' covers and tables of contents seem to remain the same. When it comes to attracting readers, magazine covers that hype "new" weight-loss diets and recipes for rich desserts are a winning combination. The demand for weight-loss diets that promise success and recipes for high-calorie desserts indicates what is happening in our society today: many Americans are too fat, preoccupied with losing weight, and yet they want to eat whatever they want and still lose weight.

According to the National Heart Lung and Blood Institute, **overweight** refers to having extra body weight that is contributed by bone, muscle, body fat, and/or body water.[1] A professional football player, for example, may be overweight because of his muscular body build. **Obesity** is a condition characterized by excessive and unhealthy amounts of body fat. Some body fat is essential for good health, but people who have excess body fat have a greater risk of developing type 2 diabetes, hypertension, and cardiovascular disease than people who are not *overfat*.[2] To determine whether a person's weight is healthy, overweight, or obese, medical experts generally use the **body mass index (BMI).** BMI is a numerical value based on the relationship between body weight and risk of chronic health problems associated with excess body fat.

Overweight and obesity are the most common nutritional disorders in the United States.[3] According to data collected from a national survey, almost 68% of American adults 20 to 74 years of age were either overweight or obese in 2007 to 2008.[4] Slightly over one-third of these persons were overweight and slightly more than one-third of them were obese. Between 1988–1994 and 2007–2008, the percentage of overweight adults remained about the same, but the percentage of obese adults rose by almost 50%.

The maps shown in Figure 10.1 illustrate how quickly the percentage of obese adults increased in the United States between 1994 and 2010. In 1994, every state had less than 20% of its population classified as obese. By 2010, no state had less than 20% of its population who were obese.

Compared to non-Hispanic white adults, overweight and obesity are more common among non-Hispanic black and Mexican-American adults, particularly among non-Hispanic black women.[4] According to experts at the Centers for Disease Control and Prevention (CDC), cultural, behavioral, and environmental factors may be largely responsible for racial/ethnic differences in obesity rates.

Quiz *Yourself*

What is the difference between overweight and obesity? Why do most people gain body fat as they age? How can you tell whether a person is following a "fad" diet or a diet that is likely to be safe and effective? Are there any medications or dietary supplements that help people lose weight? Test your knowledge of energy balance and weight management concepts by taking the following quiz. The answers are on page 399.

1. You can determine whether you have an unhealthy amount of body fat simply by measuring your waistline. _____ T _____ F

2. The best way to lose weight and keep it off is to follow a low-carbohydrate, high-fat diet, such as the Atkins diet. _____ T _____ F

3. As people age, their muscle cells turn into fat cells. _____ T _____ F

4. When a person consumes more carbohydrates than needed, the excess is converted to fat and stored in fat cells. _____ T _____ F

5. Cellulite is a unique type of fat that can be eliminated by taking certain dietary supplements. _____ T _____ F

overweight having extra weight from bone, muscle, body fat, and/or body water

obesity condition characterized by an excessive and unhealthy amount of body fat

body mass index (BMI) numerical value of relationship between body weight and risk of chronic health problems associated with excess body fat

(continued)

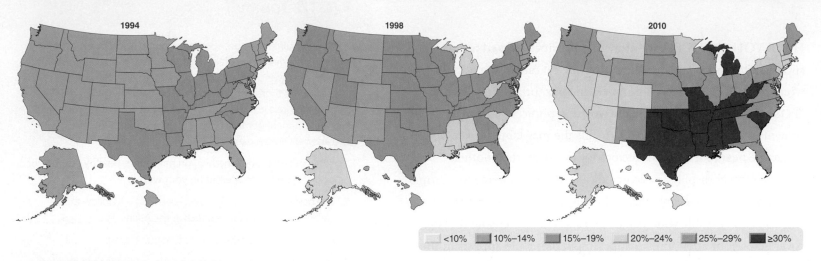

	<10%		10%–14%		15%–19%		20%–24%		25%–29%		≥30%

Figure 10.1 Obesity trends among U.S. adults: 1994 to 2010. These maps illustrate how quickly the percentage of obese adults increased in the United States between 1994 and 2010.

The prevalence of obesity among American children and adolescents has also risen sharply over the past two decades. Results of national surveys conducted from 1988 to 1994 indicated that about 11% of American children aged 6 through 11 years and 10.5% of children aged 12 through 19 years were obese.[5] By 2007–2008, almost 20% of children who were 6 through 11 years of age and slightly more than 18% of children who were 12 through 19 years of age were obese (Fig. 10.2). The percentage of overweight babies aged 6 to 23 months increased in the United States between 1988–1994 and 2003–2004. According to the CDC, 10% of babies aged 6 to 23 months were overweight in 2003–2004.[6] Public health experts are very concerned about the rising prevalence of obesity among children, because these youngsters have higher risk of maturing into obese adults than children who are not obese.

According to national target goals established in *Healthy People 2020*, the percentage of obese adults should decline to 30.6% by 2020.[7] Furthermore, the percentage of obese children aged 6 through 11 years should decline to 15.7% and the percentage of obese youth aged 12 through 19 years of age should drop to 16.1% by 2020. Based on current trends concerning rising rates of obesity within the population, these goals may be unrealistic.

Treating obesity and dealing with its consequences are costly. In 2008, the estimated medical expenses for taking care of obese patients, including economic costs (e.g., absenteeism and loss of worker productivity), was about $147 billion in the United States.[8] At that time, obesity-related costs accounted for almost 10% of spending on all forms of medical care in the nation. Unless the prevalence of obesity can be reduced, these figures are likely to continue spiraling upward, stressing the country's health care system as a result.

Although the prevalence of obesity among Americans has reached epidemic proportions, overweight and obesity rates ("globesity") are rising rapidly throughout the world. The World Health Organization (WHO) estimated that worldwide, 1 *billon* adults were overweight and 500 million adults were obese in 2008.[9] In the past, overweight and obesity were primarily problems in high-income nations, such as the United States, but the conditions are rising rapidly among populations in low- and middle-income countries. Throughout the world, overweight and obesity are responsible for more deaths than underweight.

Results of a national survey conducted in 2001 to 2002 indicated that about half of American adults had tried to lose or maintain their weight at some point during the previous year.[10] However, the likelihood that obese people can achieve and maintain healthy weights without surgery is low. According to limited data, less than 20% of overweight and obese people who intentionally lose weight can avoid regaining the weight for at least a year.[11] Overweight and obesity are chronic conditions that are difficult and expensive to treat. Therefore, preventing their development is crucial.

Regardless of whether a person wants to maintain, lose, or gain weight, the basic principles of energy balance apply. By reading Chapter 10, you will learn about energy balance, body composition, health consequences linked to having too much or too little body fat, and factors that contribute to unwanted weight gain. This chapter also provides practical tips for helping you achieve or maintain a healthy body weight through sensible eating and physical activity practices. Concern about body size can result in unhealthy eating practices. The Chapter 10 "Highlight" discusses eating disorders, including anorexia nervosa and bulimia nervosa.

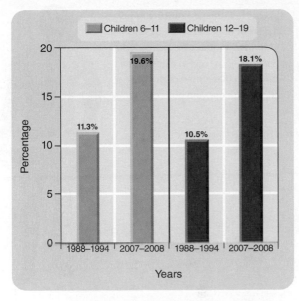

Figure 10.2 Prevalence of obesity among U.S. children. Percentages of obese children 6 through 11 years of age and 12 through 19 years of age increased considerably between 1988–1994 and 2007–2008. *Source: Ogden C, Carroll M: National Center for Health Statistics: Prevalence of obesity among children and adolescents: United States, trends 1963–1965 through 2007–2008. 2010. http://www.cdc.gov/nchs/data/hestat/obesity_child_07_08/obesity_child_07_08.htm*

10.1 Body Composition

The body is composed of two major compartments: **fat-free mass** (lean tissues) and **total body fat.** (Some scientists who study body composition divide the body into four compartments: body water, bone mineral, fat-free mass, and total body fat.)[12] Fat-free mass is comprised of body water; mineral-rich tissues such as bones and teeth; and protein-rich tissues, including muscles and organs. Total body fat includes "essential fat" and *adipose tissue*. Essential fat is in cell membranes, certain bones, and nervous tissue. Essential fat is vital for survival. Adipose tissue contains **adipose cells** that are specialized for storing energy in the form of triglycerides (fat). Overweight and obese people have excessive amounts of fat stored in their adipose tissue.

fat-free mass lean tissues

total body fat essential fat and adipose tissue

adipose cell specialized cell that stores fat

Adipose Tissue

Every cell contains some lipid, but the major function of an adult **adipose** or "fat" **cell** is to store a droplet of fat (see Fig. 6.16). When food is plentiful, adipose cells remove excess fat from the bloodstream for storage. As the amount of fat stored in adipose cells increases, the size of each cell expands, and the body gains weight. At one time, scientists thought the body could only produce fat cells during periods of rapid growth, such as childhood. However, the body can also develop more fat cells when overeating occurs in adulthood, especially in cases of extreme obesity.[13] Once fat cells form, scientists think the cells remain, unless they die or are surgically removed.

Figure 10.3 **Uneven subcutaneous fat distribution.** Subcutaneous fat is unevenly distributed. Thicker deposits occur in various regions of men's and women's bodies, especially in the abdomen, thighs, and buttocks.

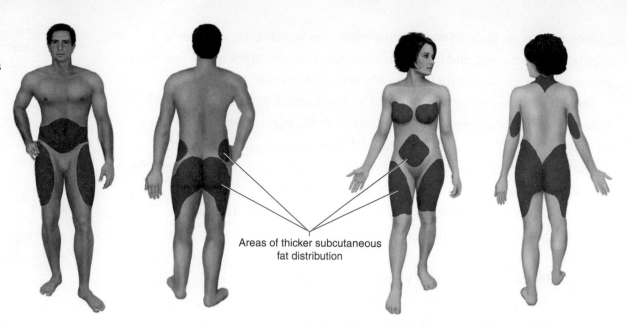

Areas of thicker subcutaneous fat distribution

Did You Know?

Cellulite, lumpy-appearing skin on thighs and buttocks of many women, is not a unique type of fat. Scientists have no clear understanding of why cellulite occurs, but it may simply be subcutaneous fat held in place by irregular bands of connective tissue. Despite claims by cosmetic manufacturers that their products eliminate cellulite, there are no effective ways to smooth the skin's dimpled appearance.[15]

When the body needs energy, adipose cells release fat for other cells to use as fuel. As each adipose cell loses some fat, it becomes smaller. If adipose cells continue to release fat, the body eventually loses weight as a result. In addition to storing and releasing fat, adipose cells secrete numerous proteins, some of which have roles in regulating food intake, glucose metabolism, and immune responses.[14]

Subcutaneous Fat and Visceral Fat

Subcutaneous (*sub* = under; cu-ta-ne-ous [*qu-tay'-nee-us*] = skin) tissue holds skin in place over underlying tissues such as muscles. Subcutaneous tissue also contains adipose cells. When subcutaneous tissue has more adipose cells than other kinds of cells, it is referred to as *subcutaneous fat*.[16] Subcutaneous fat helps insulate the body against cold temperatures and protects muscles and bones from bumps and bruises. Subcutaneous fat is unevenly distributed. This layer of fat is thicker in certain regions of men's and women's bodies, especially in the abdominal area, thighs, and buttocks (Fig. 10.3).

In addition to subcutaneous fat, the body has *visceral* (*viss'-eh-rol*) fat. Visceral fat also contains adipose cells, but this type of body fat forms a protective structure that is under the abdominal muscles and hangs over the stomach and intestines (Fig. 10.4). Although there are some racial differences, women generally have more

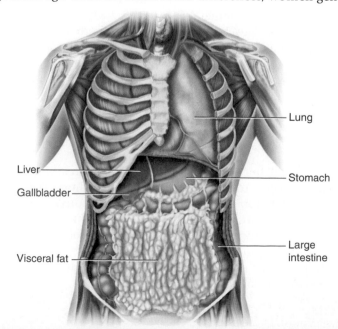

Lung

Liver

Gallbladder

Stomach

Large intestine

Visceral fat

Figure 10.4 **What is visceral fat?** Visceral fat forms a protective structure that is under abdominal muscles and hangs over the stomach and intestines.

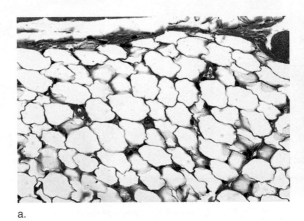

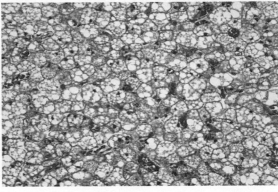

a. b.

Figure 10.5 Body fat. The majority of adipose cells are white fat (*a*). Brown fat tissue (*b*) has more mitochondria and is more richly supplied with blood than white fat tissue.

subcutaneous fat than men, whereas men tend to have more visceral fat than women.[17] Excessive amounts of visceral fat and/or subcutaneous abdominal fat result in what is commonly called a "beer belly" or the "middle-age spread."

What Is Brown Fat?

The majority of adipose cells are creamy white or yellow in appearance and may be referred to as "white fat" (Fig. 10.5a). Brown fat cells (brown adipose tissue or BAT) are specialized adipose cells that are more richly supplied with blood and contain more mitochondria, the energy-generating organelles, than white fat tissue (Fig. 10.5b). BAT uses fat for generating heat, whereas white fat tissue stores fat.

Human infants have deposits of BAT in their upper backs and abdomens. In infants, BAT may be important for maintaining normal body temperature, because the cells generate body heat without the need to shiver. Although adult humans have very small amounts of BAT, their white fat cells may have the potential to acquire brown fat cells' fat-burning ability.[18] Thus, some medical researchers think finding ways to "switch on" the development of BAT in adults may help people lose or control their weight, because brown fat cells "waste" energy as heat.

Promoters of certain dietary supplements claim their products contain ingredients that eliminate "hard-to-burn" brown fat in the thighs and abdominal area. These claims are untrue. The fat in those regions is primarily white fat. Furthermore, why would overweight or obese people want to eliminate BAT—if they had it?

Measuring Body Fat

When you weigh yourself on a scale, you cannot determine whether your weight is healthy. Why? It is healthier to have more fat-free tissue than fat tissue, but the scale does not distinguish between these two major components of your body. Information concerning your body's composition, especially its *percentage* of fat, can help you predict your risk of obesity-related diseases.

There is no direct way to measure a living person's percentage of body fat. Nevertheless, scientists can use indirect methods of measuring body fat, such as "underwater weighing," dual-energy x-ray absorptiometry, air displacement, bioelectrical impedance, and skinfold thicknesses. The following sections describe these methods of assessing body composition, including their advantages and disadvantages.

Underwater Weighing

Underwater weighing involves comparing a person's weight "on land" to his or her weight when completely submerged in a tank of water (Fig. 10.6). Lean tissue is denser than water; fat tissue is not as dense as water. Thus, a person who has more body fat will weigh less when under water than a person who has more lean tissue. The underwater weighing method can be an accurate way of assessing body composition. However, the method is not a convenient, easy, inexpensive, or practical way to estimate body fat, because it requires special testing facilities.

underwater weighing technique of estimating body composition that involves comparing weight on land to weight when completely submerged in a tank of water

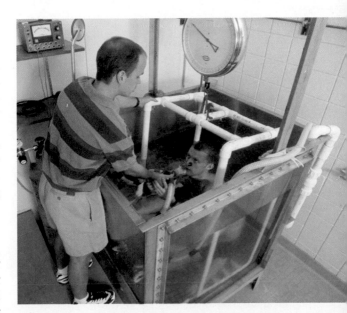

Figure 10.6 Underwater weighing. Underwater weighing involves comparing a person's weight on land to his or her weight when completely submerged in a tank of water.

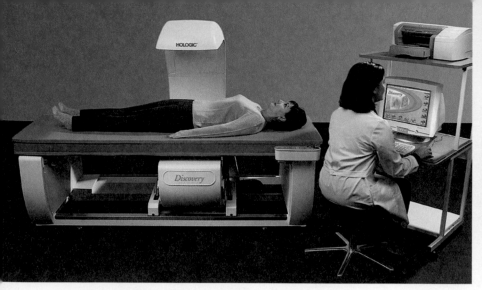

Figure 10.7 Dual-energy x-ray absorptiometry (DXA). Although DXA is a highly accurate way to estimate body fat content, the equipment is very expensive and not widely available outside of clinical settings.

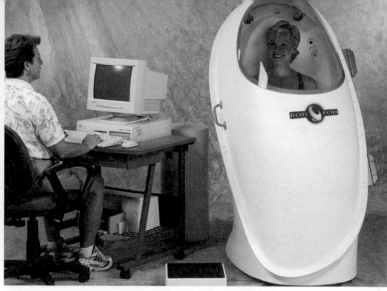

Figure 10.8 BOD POD. The BOD POD device estimates a person's body volume by measuring the space the body occupies while seated inside the chamber.

Dual-Energy X-Ray Absorptiometry (DXA)

Dual-energy x-ray absorptiometry (DXA) involves the use of multiple low-energy x-rays to scan the entire body. The method provides a detailed "picture" of internal structures, including fat deposits (Fig. 10.7). During the scanning process, the equipment emits a dose of radiation that is lower than that used for a chest x-ray. Although DXA is a highly accurate way to estimate body fat content, the equipment is very expensive and not widely available outside of clinical settings.

Air Displacement

The **air displacement** method assesses the volume of a person's body, which can be used to calculate his or her body composition. After being weighed on a very precise scale, the subject sits in the chamber of a device called the BOD POD (Fig. 10.8). This device measures the volume of air in the chamber with the person in it and compares the value with the volume of air that was in the chamber when it was unoccupied. The person's volume is the volume of air that was displaced after the subject entered the chamber. Air displacement measurements provide highly accurate estimates of body fat content, but the measuring device is expensive and not practical for most consumers to use.

Bioelectrical Impedance

Bioelectrical impedance is a quick way to estimate body fat content. This method is based on the principle that water and electrolytes conduct electricity. Body fat resists the flow of electricity, because fat tissue contains less water and electrolytes than lean tissue. The bioelectrical impedance device sends a painless, low-energy electrical current via wires connected to electrodes placed on the subject's skin (Fig. 10.9). Within a few minutes, the device converts information about the body's electrical resistance into an estimate of total body fat. The method is fairly accurate, as long as the subject's hydration status is normal. Consumers can purchase a bioelectrical impedance device that resembles a bathroom scale, but scientific data about the machine's accuracy is lacking.

Skinfold Thickness

A common technique for estimating total body fat involves taking **skinfold thickness measurements** at multiple body sites, such as over the triceps muscle of the arm (Fig. 10.10). The width of a skinfold indicates the depth of the subcutaneous fat at that site. To perform the measurements, a trained person pinches a section of the subject's skin, gently pulls it away from underlying muscle tissue, and uses special calipers to measure the thickness of the fat. After taking the measurements, the values are incorporated into a mathematical formula that provides a fairly accurate estimate of the subject's amount of body fat.

dual-energy x-ray absorptiometry (DXA) technique of estimating body composition that involves scanning the body with multiple low-energy x-rays

air displacement method of estimating body composition by determining body volume

bioelectrical impedance technique of estimating body composition in which a device measures the conduction of a weak electrical current through the body

skinfold thickness measurements technique of estimating body composition in which calipers are used to measure the width of skinfolds at multiple body sites

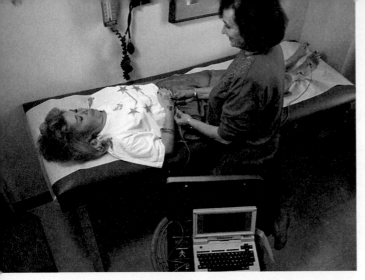

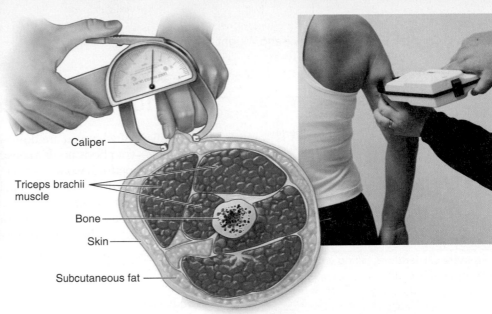

Figure 10.9 **Bioelectrical impedance.** The use of a device that measures bioelectrical impedance is a quick and painless way to estimate body fat content.

Skinfold thickness measurements are relatively easy and inexpensive to perform, but the method's accuracy largely depends on the skill of the person performing the measurements. Also, the technique may underestimate total body fat when used on overfat subjects. However, by combining data collected from skinfold, waist and hip circumference, and body frame (skeletal joint) measurements, researchers can obtain more reliable estimates of an individual's total body fat.[19]

How Much Body Fat Is Too Much?

Some body fat is essential for good health, but too much adipose tissue, especially visceral fat, can interfere with the body's ability to function normally. Percentages of body fat can be used to develop weight classifications for adults. According to one such classification system, a man is overweight when his body is 22 to 25% fat; a woman is overweight when her body is 32 to 37% fat (Table 10.1).[20] A man is obese when fat comprises 26% or more of his body; a woman is obese when fat makes up 38% or more of her body. It is important to note that the average healthy young woman has more body fat than the average healthy young man, because she needs the extra fat for hormonal and reproductive purposes.

Adults tend to gain adipose tissue as they age, but for elderly persons, some additional fat does not necessarily contribute to serious health problems. The extra fat may actually provide some health benefits, such as providing an energy reserve for a very ill person who cannot eat. Furthermore, the extra padding of fat may protect a person from being injured by falling.

Figure 10.10 **Measuring skinfold thickness.** Body fat content can be estimated by measuring skinfold thicknesses using a special device (skinfold caliper) at multiple body sites, such as the triceps muscle of the arm.

TABLE 10.1 *Adult Body Weight Classification by Percentage of Body Fat*

Classification	Body Fat (%)	
	Men	Women
Healthy	13 to 21%	23 to 31%
Overweight	22 to 25%	32 to 37%
Obese	26 to 31%	38 to 42%
Extremely obese	32% or more	43% or more

Source: Adapted from: Food and Nutrition Board: *Dietary Reference Intakes for energy, carbohydrate, fiber, fat, fatty acids, cholesterol, protein, and amino acids (macronutrients).* Table 5.5, page 126, 2005. www.nap.edu/openbook/0309085373/html/126.html
Accessed: July 30, 2011

Concept **Checkpoint**

1. Which tissues comprise total body fat and which comprise fat-free mass?
2. Discuss conditions in which fat cells can increase in size and number.
3. Why is it necessary to have some body fat?
4. List three roles for subcutaneous fat.
5. What is visceral fat?
6. What is cellulite?
7. Describe at least two differences between brown fat tissue and white fat tissue.
8. Describe three different methods of measuring body fat, including drawbacks of each method.
9. Explain why a healthy woman has more body fat than a healthy man.
10. A young man's body is 13% fat. According to information in Table 10.1, is he overweight, obese, or healthy?

10.2 Energy for Living

Regardless of what you are doing—eating, watching television, studying, exercising, even sleeping—your body needs a constant supply of energy to function. **Energy** is defined as the capacity to perform work. There are several forms of energy, but heat, mechanical, chemical, and even electrical energy occur in living things. The total amount of energy is *constant*; that is, the amount remains the same, because energy cannot be created or destroyed. Nevertheless, the various forms of energy can be stored, released, moved, or transformed from one kind to another. The following sections discuss how human cells obtain and use energy.

Energy Intake

Just as a car engine uses a mixture of gasoline, ethanol, and oxygen to run properly, your body uses a mixture of *biological fuels* and oxygen to do its work. For humans, biological fuels are foods and beverages that contain macronutrients **(energy intake).** For some individuals, nonnutrient alcohol (ethanol) also provides energy. Under normal conditions, our cells metabolize primarily glucose and fatty acids, but small amounts of amino acids are also used for energy.

Cells release the energy stored in biological fuels by breaking bonds within the compounds' molecules. The energy that is released can be captured and stored in special compounds, such as **adenosine triphosphate (ATP),** until it is needed. Cells obtain only about 40% of the energy that was in macronutrients by forming ATP. Cells release the remaining energy as heat. Figure 10.11 summarizes events that result in macronutrient storage or breakdown for energy. The diagram in Appendix D shows the complex chemical pathways that most cells use to generate ATP from the metabolism of glucose, fat, and amino acids.

Energy Output

Energy output (*energy expenditure*) refers to the energy (calories) cells use to carry out their activities. For example, muscle cells need energy to contract, liver cells use energy to convert

Figure 10.11 What happens to macronutrients?
(*a*) After being absorbed, macronutrients are used for energy or stored as glycogen or fat. (*b*) When energy is needed to fuel cells, macronutrients are released from storage and metabolized to synthesize ATP.

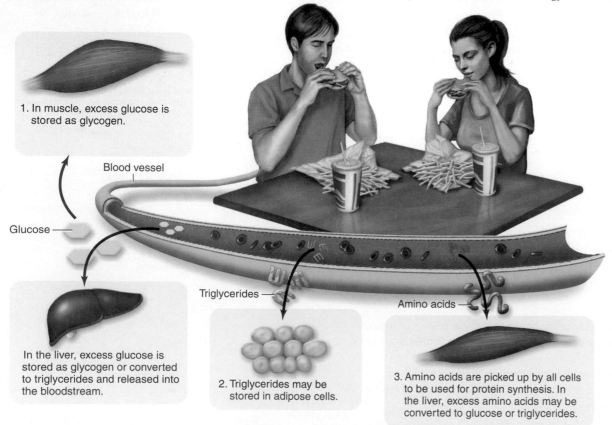

1. In muscle, excess glucose is stored as glycogen.

Blood vessel

Glucose

In the liver, excess glucose is stored as glycogen or converted to triglycerides and released into the bloodstream.

Triglycerides

2. Triglycerides may be stored in adipose cells.

Amino acids

3. Amino acids are picked up by all cells to be used for protein synthesis. In the liver, excess amino acids may be converted to glucose or triglycerides.

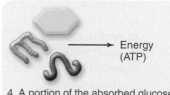

Energy (ATP)

4. A portion of the absorbed glucose, triglycerides, and amino acids are used for energy.

a.

toxic compounds to safer substances, and intestinal cells need energy to absorb certain nutrients. The following sections discuss the major ways the body uses food energy.

Basal and Resting Metabolism

Metabolism refers to all chemical changes, or reactions, that constantly occur in living cells. Anabolic reactions require energy to occur; catabolic reactions release energy. **Basal metabolism** is the minimal number of calories the body uses for vital physiological activities after fasting and resting for 12 hours. Basal metabolic processes include breathing, circulating blood, and maintaining constant liver, brain, and kidney functions. Basal metabolism does not encompass energy needed for skeletal muscle movements (physical activity), digestion of food, and absorption and processing of nutrients. For the typical active person, basal metabolism accounts for about 60 to 75% of the body's total energy use.[12]

The **resting metabolic rate (RMR)** refers to the body's rate of energy use a few hours after resting and eating. A person's RMR is slightly higher than his or her BMR (basal metabolism rate). Although there is a difference between the BMR and the RMR, researchers often use the terms interchangeably in their publications.

Thyroid hormone, secreted by the thyroid gland, regulates metabolism (see Fig. 9.11). A person who has an overactive thyroid gland produces too much thyroid hormone. As a result, this person has a higher-than-normal metabolic rate. Signs and symptoms of excess thyroid hormone production (*hyperthyroidism*) include feeling warm, sweaty, nervous, and restless; having rapid heart rate and chronic diarrhea; fatigue; and losing weight despite having an increased appetite.[21] You might think that hyperthyroidism is the key to treating unwanted weight gain, but the condition can have serious side effects, such as elevated blood pressure and heart failure. A person who suffers from *hypothyroidism* does not produce enough thyroid hormone, and as a result, he or she has a lower-than-normal metabolic rate. This individual typically complains of feeling cold, lacking energy and interest in usual activities, being constipated,

energy capacity to perform work

energy intake calories from foods and beverages that contain macronutrients and alcohol

adenosine triphosphate (ATP) biological compound that stores energy

energy output calories cells use to carry out their activities

basal metabolism minimal number of kilocalories the body uses to support vital activities after fasting and resting for 12 hours.

resting metabolic rate (RMR) body's rate of energy use a few hours after resting and eating

thyroid hormone secretion of the thyroid gland that regulates metabolism

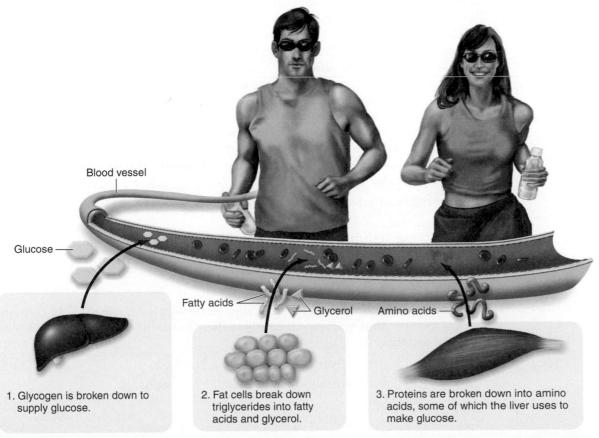

Blood vessel

Glucose

Fatty acids ← → Glycerol   Amino acids

1. Glycogen is broken down to supply glucose.

2. Fat cells break down triglycerides into fatty acids and glycerol.

3. Proteins are broken down into amino acids, some of which the liver uses to make glucose.

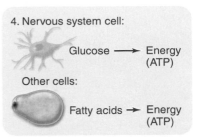

4. Nervous system cell:

Glucose → Energy (ATP)

Other cells:

Fatty acids → Energy (ATP)

b.

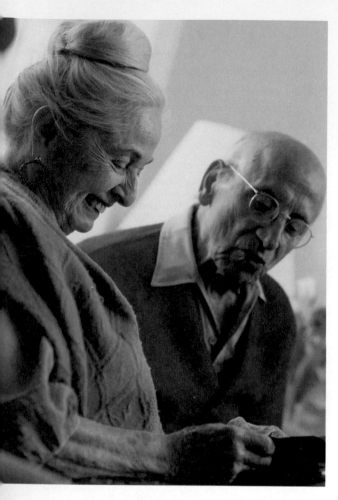

and gaining weight easily. Treatment for a hypoactive thyroid gland generally includes medication that contains a form of thyroid hormone.

Although a decline in normal thyroid hormone levels results in lower-than-normal metabolic rates, many overweight or obese people have thyroid hormone levels that are within the normal range. However, an individual who secretes slightly less thyroid hormone than other persons may be more likely to become obese.[22]

Factors That Influence the Metabolic Rate In addition to thyroid hormone, numerous factors can increase or decrease basal metabolic rates. Thus, metabolic rates vary among individuals. Factors that influence basal metabolism include these:

- *Body composition* Lean body mass is the major factor that influences the metabolic rate.[20] Muscle tissue, a component of lean body mass, is more metabolically active than fat tissue. In general, a person who has more muscle mass will have a higher metabolic rate than someone with less muscle tissue.
- *Gender* Males generally have higher metabolic rates than women because they tend to have more lean body mass.
- *Body surface area* A tall, slender person who weighs 150 pounds has a higher metabolic rate than a shorter person who also weighs 150 pounds. Why? The body constantly loses energy in the form of heat that moves to the skin's surface and then into the environment. Because the taller person's body has more surface area than the shorter person's body, the taller individual has to generate more heat energy to replace that which is lost.
- *Age* Basal metabolism declines as one grows older, primarily due to the loss of fat-free tissues such as muscle. After 20 years of age, a woman's BMR declines about 2% and a man's BMR about 3% per decade.[23] Therefore, the average adult needs about 150 fewer kilocalories per decade as he or she ages. As many adults grow older, they think their muscles have "turned into" fat. A muscle cell, however, cannot transform itself into a fat cell. During the aging process, lean tissue mass shrinks, as cells from muscle, bone, and organs die and are not replaced. Fat cells, however, can continue to develop throughout life, especially when a person overeats consistently. When adipose tissue expands in size, it can fill in spaces formerly occupied by muscle and organ tissues. Regular exercise helps build and preserve lean body mass, and to some extent, people can maintain a higher metabolic rate by being physically active as they grow older.
- *Calorie intake* Calorie intake also affects the metabolic rate. The body conserves energy use when calorie intakes are very low or lacking altogether. In one study, subjects who consumed 800 kcal/day for 10 days experienced about a 6% decline in their resting metabolic rates.[24] To enhance the rate of weight loss, an overfat person should reduce caloric intake while maintaining a normal metabolic rate. Because very-low-calorie diets reduce the metabolic rate, such diets are not generally recommended for weight loss.

The following factors increase the metabolic rate:

- *Fever*
- *Stimulant drugs* (caffeine, for example)
- *Pregnancy*
- *Milk production in a female who has given birth*
- *Recovery after exercise*

Calculating Metabolic Energy Needs Your basal metabolic rate is fairly constant from day to day.[25] Thus, you can estimate your daily metabolic rate by following a "rule of thumb" formula:

Formula for men = 1.0 kcal/kg/hr

Formula for women = 0.9 kcal/kg/hr

To estimate the number of calories you need for your basal metabolism, first convert your weight in pounds to kilograms by dividing your weight by 2.2. (A kilogram is approximately 2.2 pounds.)

_____ lb ÷ 2.2 lb = _____ kg

Then, depending on your sex, use one of the following formulas:

_____ kg × 0.9 (women) = _____ kcal/hr

_____ kg × 1.0 (men) = _____ kcal/hr

Finally, use this hourly basal metabolic rate to estimate your basal metabolic rate for an entire day by multiplying the hourly value by 24.

_____ kcal/hr × 24 hr = _____ kcal/day

These calculations only provide an estimate of your daily metabolic rate. To estimate your Estimated Energy Requirement (EER) for a 24-hour period, you need to add kilocalories used for physical and other activities to your BMR figure.

Energy for Physical Activity

Physical activity, voluntary skeletal muscle movement, increases energy expenditure above basal energy needs. The number of kilocalories expended for a particular physical activity depends largely on the type of activity, how long it is performed (duration), the degree of effort (intensity) used while performing the activity, and the weight of the person. A heavy person expends more kilocalories when performing the same activity, for the same duration, and at the same intensity than a lighter person. Why? The muscles of the heavier person must work harder to move the larger body.

To estimate your energy needs for physical activity, visit www.mypyramidtracker .gov/default.htm and click on "Assess Your Physical Activity." Table 10.2 lists various

TABLE 10.2 _Approximate Energy Expenditures of Selected Physical Activities (150-pound person)_

Physical Activity	Approximate kcal/ min.
Sitting and playing cards	1.9
Bowling	4.1
Walking (3.5 mph)	5.1
Bicycling (10 mph)	6.4
Canoeing (4 mph)	6.7
Dancing (active)	6.8
Hiking (with pack, 3 mph)	6.8
Walking (4.5 mph)	7.1
Tennis (singles, recreational)	7.5
Weight training	7.8
Touch football (vigorous)	8.3
Aerobic dancing	9.0
Swimming (vigorous breaststroke)	9.6
Running/jogging, steady pace (5.5 mph)	10.0
Bicycling (15 mph)	10.9
Karate	12.8

Source: Williams M: _Nutrition for health, fitness, and sport._ 9th edition. New York:McGraw-Hill, 2010.

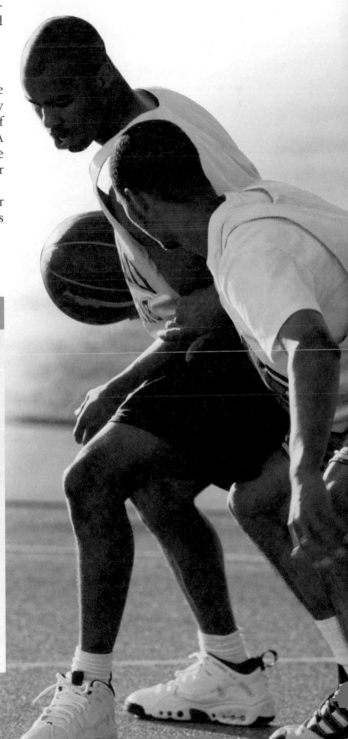

thermic effect of food (TEF) energy used to digest foods and beverages as well as absorb and further process the macronutrients

nonexercise activity thermogenesis (NEAT) involuntary skeletal muscular activities such as fidgeting

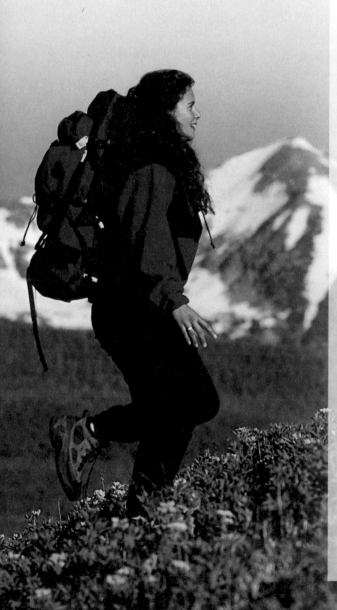

physical activities and the approximate number of kilocalories an individual who weighs 150 pounds expends while performing each activity for a minute. For example, a 150-pound person who walks for 30 minutes (3.5 mph) burns approximately 53 kcal during the walk (30 × 5.1).

The number of calories you need for physical activity can vary widely, depending on how active you are each day. Because you can control the type, intensity, and duration of your physical activities, you can manipulate your energy output to increase, decrease, or maintain your weight.

Thermic Effect of Food (TEF)

The body needs a relatively small amount of energy to digest foods and beverages as well as to absorb and further process the macronutrients. The energy used for these tasks, generally 5 to 10% of total caloric intake, is referred to as the **thermic effect of food (TEF)**. For example, if your energy intake was 3000 kcal/day, TEF would account for 150 to 300 kcal.

Nonexercise Activity Thermogenesis (NEAT)

Nonexercise activity thermogenesis (*thermo* = heat; *genesis* = production) or **NEAT** refers to *involuntary* skeletal muscle activity, that is, physical activity that a person does not consciously control. NEAT activities include shivering, fidgeting, maintaining muscle tone, and maintaining body posture when not lying down. Studies have shown that people typically expend 100 to 800 kcal daily as NEAT.[23] It is possible that some individuals resist weight gain from overeating because they have higher-than-average energy expenditures for NEAT. Nevertheless, the contribution of NEAT to overall calorie needs is fairly small for most people.

Putting It All Together

To estimate your daily energy expenditure, you could add the kilocalories you burned for basal metabolism, physical activity, TEF, and NEAT in a day. However, an easier method is to use one of the formulas published by the Food and Nutrition Board of the Institute of Medicine (FNB).[20] The following formulas are for men and women who are 19 years of age or older.

Men

$$\text{Estimated Energy Requirement (EER)} = 662 - (9.53 \times \text{AGE}) + \text{PA} \times (15.91 \times \text{WT} + 539.6 \times \text{HT})$$

Women

$$\text{Estimated Energy Requirement (EER)} = 354 - (6.91 \times \text{AGE}) + \text{PA} \times (9.36 \times \text{WT} + 726 \times \text{HT})$$

TABLE 10.3 *Physical Activity Level Estimates*

Activity Level	PA (Men)	PA (Women)
Sedentary (no exercise)	1.00	1.00
Low activity (for example, walking the equivalent of 2 miles/day at 3 to 4 mph)	1.11	1.12
Active (for example, walking the equivalent of 7 miles/day at 3 to 4 mph)	1.25	1.27
Very active (for example, walking the equivalent of 17 miles/day at 3 to 4 mph)	1.48	1.45

Source of data: Food and Nutrition Board, National Institute of Medicine: *Dietary Reference Intakes for energy, carbohydrate, fiber, fat, fatty acids, cholesterol, protein, and amino acids (macronutrients)*. Washington, DC: National Academies Press, 2005.

The variables in the formulas are:

$$AGE = \text{age in years}$$

$$PA = \text{physical activity estimate (Table 10.3)}$$

$$WT = \text{weight in kg (lb} \div 2.2)$$

$$HT = \text{height in meters (inches} \div 39.4)$$

To practice using the formula, consider a 24-year-old woman who is 5′5″ (65″) in height, weighs 145 pounds, and has a low level of physical activity. With this information, you can determine the missing values for the formula.

This young woman's age is **24** and her value for physical activity level (PA) is **1.12**. To convert her weight in pounds to kilograms, divide her weight by 2.2.

$$145 \div 2.2 = 65.9 \text{ kg}$$

To convert her height to meters, divide her height (inches) by 39.4.

$$65.0 \div 39.4 = 1.65 \text{ meters (rounded value)}$$

Now we can "plug" these values into the formula for a woman.

$$\textbf{Estimated Energy Requirement (EER)} = 354 - (6.91 \times 24) +$$
$$1.12 \times (9.36 \times 65.9 + 726 \times 1.65)$$

To solve the equation, move from left to right, but do the math in the parentheses first.

$$EER = 354 - (6.91 \times 24)$$

$$EER = 354 - 165.84$$

$$354 - 165.84 = 188.16$$

$$EER = 188.16 + 1.12 \times (9.36 \times 65.9 + 726 \times 1.65)$$

Now, do the math in the remaining parentheses on the right.
Multiply the first two numbers in the parentheses together:

$$9.36 \times 65.9 = 616.82$$

Multiply the next two numbers together:

$$726 \times 1.65 = 1197.9$$

Add the two products together:

$$616.82 + 1197.9 = 1814.72$$

Plug this value into the formula and multiply $1.12 \times 1814.72 = 2032.49$
And add the left and right sides of the formula together:

$$EER = 188.16 + 2032.49 = 2220.65$$

$$\textbf{EER = approx. 2221 kcal/day}$$

To estimate your EER, complete the "Personal Dietary Analysis" activity at the end of Chapter 10.

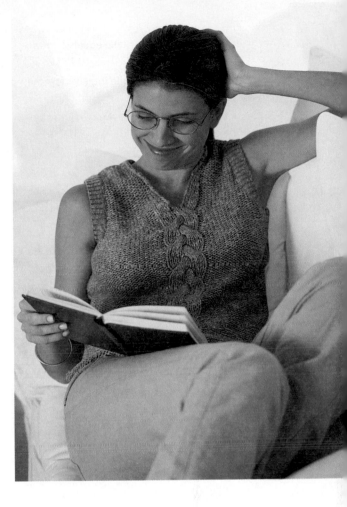

 Concept **Checkpoint**

11. Using the "rule of thumb" formula, estimate the daily basal metabolic energy needs of a woman who weighs 185 pounds.
12. List the four major ways the body uses energy (energy output).
13. For most people, which form of energy expenditure uses the most energy on a daily basis?
14. Discuss at least five factors that influence basal metabolic rate.
15. Of the four major ways the body uses energy, which one is most easily altered?
16. Explain the differences between TEF and energy needs for physical activity.
17. What is NEAT? List at least three ways the body expends energy by NEAT.

energy equilibrium calorie intake equals calorie output

negative energy balance calorie intake is less than calorie output

positive energy balance calorie intake is greater than calorie output

Did You Know?

Have you heard of the "Freshman 15," the popular belief that college students gain 15 pounds during their freshman year? Results of scientific studies confirm that freshmen are likely to gain weight, but the increase is much less than 15 pounds—only 3 pounds on average.[26] In one study, 290 college students were weighed at the beginning of their freshman year and again at the completion of their sophomore year. During their first two years in college, 70% of the students participating in the study gained weight, on average, about 9 pounds.[27]

10.3 Energy Balance

Understanding the concept of *energy balance* is critical to understanding why most people gain, lose, or maintain weight. Your body is in a state of **energy equilibrium** and "balanced" when your calorie intake from food and beverages equals your calorie output for basal metabolism, physical activity, TEF, and NEAT (Fig. 10.12). By maintaining a balanced energy state, your weight will remain relatively stable over time.

If your calorie intake is lower than your calorie output, you are in **negative energy balance.** In this state, your body needs more calories to carry out its activities than your diet is supplying. Therefore, your body metabolizes stored fat for energy. Weight loss results from being in a negative energy state. Over time, you will notice your clothes have become baggy as your adipose tissue shrinks.

If your calorie intake from macronutrients (and alcohol) is greater than your calorie output, you are in a state of **positive energy balance.** In this state, your body stores excess dietary fat in adipose cells. Additionally, the body converts surplus dietary carbohydrate, protein, and alcohol to fat and stores that fat in adipose cells. Weight gain results from being in a positive energy state, and eventually, you will notice that your clothes seem to have shrunk.

Positive energy balance is necessary for pregnant women, because extra calories are needed to add new tissues that support the pregnancy. Positive energy balance also occurs during periods of growth, such as during fetal development, infancy, childhood, and adolescence. Over time, however, even a small positive energy balance can cause anyone's weight to increase, regardless of his or her age. Maintenance of energy balance—matching calorie intake to calorie output over the long term—is critical for controlling body weight (Fig. 10.13).

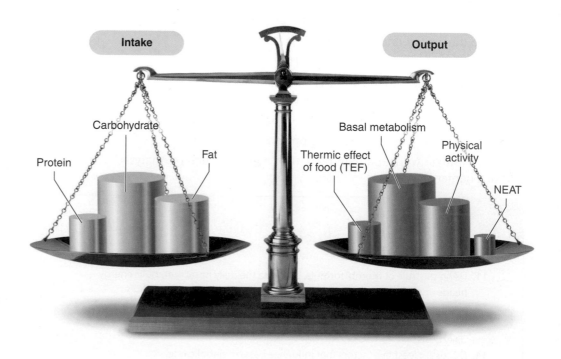

Figure 10.12 Energy balance. Your energy state is in equilibrium and "balanced" when your calorie intake from food and beverages equals your calorie output for basal metabolism, physical activity, TEF, and NEAT.

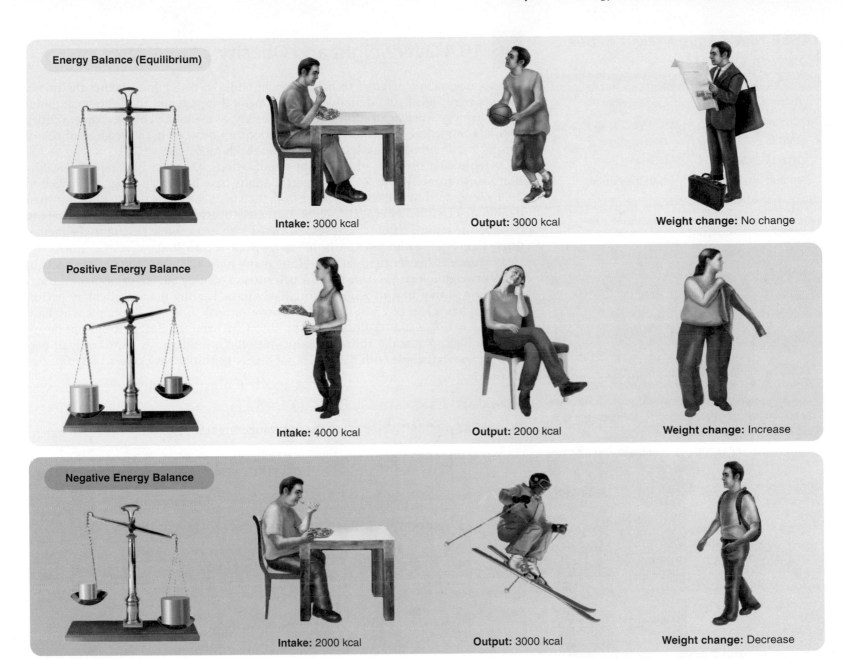

Figure 10.13 presents the following visual content:

Energy Balance (Equilibrium)
Intake: 3000 kcal Output: 3000 kcal Weight change: No change

Positive Energy Balance
Intake: 4000 kcal Output: 2000 kcal Weight change: Increase

Negative Energy Balance
Intake: 2000 kcal Output: 3000 kcal Weight change: Decrease

Figure 10.13 The body's possible energy states. This figure presents three possible energy states. In energy equilibrium, individuals consume the same amount of energy as they expend, and as a result, they experience no weight change. In a positive energy state, individuals consume more energy than they expend, and as a result, they gain weight. In a negative energy state, individuals consume less energy than they expend, and as a result, they lose weight. Maintenance of energy balance—matching calorie intake to calorie output over the long term—is critical for controlling body weight.

Concept **Checkpoint**

18. What happens to a person's body weight when he or she is in a state of positive energy balance?

19. When is it desirable for a person to be in a positive energy balance state?

20. When is a person in a negative energy balance state?

TABLE 10.4 *Adult Weight Status Categories (BMI)*

BMI	Weight Status
Below 18.5	Underweight
18.5 to 24.9	Healthy
25.0 to 29.9	Overweight
30.0 to 39.9	Obese
40 and above	Extremely obese

Source: National Heart, Lung, and Blood Institute: *The practical guide: Identification, evaluation, and treatment of overweight and obesity in adults.* NIH Publication 00-4084, 2000. www.nhlbi.nih.gov/guidelines/obesity/prctgd_c.pdf Accessed: October 17, 2011.

Extremely obese people are far more likely to develop the serious chronic diseases associated with excess body fat and die prematurely than people who have BMIs between 18.5 and 30.0.

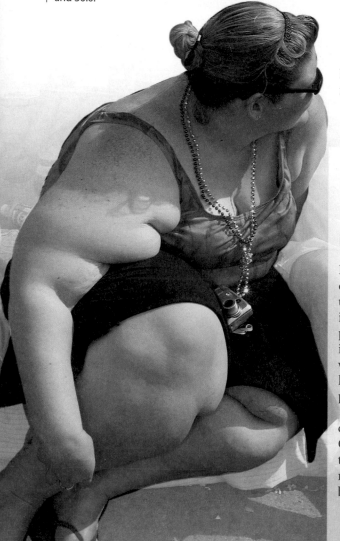

10.4 Overweight and Obesity

At one time, people referred to height/weight tables to determine whether their body weights were "ideal" or "desirable." Today, medical experts use the body mass index (BMI) to judge whether an adult's weight is healthy. As mentioned in the chapter opener, BMI is a numerical value based on the relationship between body weight and risk of chronic health problems associated with excess body fat.[20]

Table 10.4 presents adult weight classifications based on BMI ranges. Healthy BMIs range from 18.5 to 24.9. *Overweight* adults have BMIs that range from 25.0 to 29.9; *obese* adults have BMIs that range from 30.0 to 39.9. People whose BMIs are 40 or higher are classified as *extremely obese.* Extremely obese people are far more likely to develop the serious chronic diseases associated with excess body fat and to die prematurely than people who have BMIs that range from 18.5 to 30.0.

Muscle is denser than fat; therefore, many muscular people may have BMIs in the overweight range, yet have healthy percentages of body fat. For example, a muscular person with a BMI of 25.0 is more likely to be healthy than a sedentary person who also has a BMI of 25.0. The BMI may overestimate body fat in people who have lost muscle tissue as a result of aging or illness.[28] Therefore, BMIs should not be applied to highly muscular individuals, people who are elderly, or chronically ill persons. However, people with BMIs of 30 or higher generally have excess body fat.

How Can I Calculate My BMI?

To calculate your BMI, you can use the following formula:

$$\frac{\text{weight (lb)}}{[\text{height (in)}]^2 \times 703}$$

For example, a person who weighs 140 pounds and is 5′3″ (63″) has a BMI of approximately 24.8. This person's BMI is almost at the upper limit of the healthy range.

$$\text{Calculation: } [140 \div (63)^2] \times 703$$

$$(140 \div 3969) \times 703 =$$

$$0.03527 \times 703 = 24.8$$

Excess Body Fat: Effects on Health

People with BMIs greater than 25 have increased risks of CVD, hypertension, and type 2 diabetes. Many types of cancer, including cancers of the gallbladder, pancreas, cervix, uterus, breast (postmenopausal women), colon, rectum, and kidney, are more common in obese people. Furthermore, obese patients have high risk of experiencing serious complications during and after surgery. Such patients often require more anesthesia and their incisions are more likely to become infected than surgical patients whose weights are within the healthy range. Compared to people with healthy BMIs, obese people are more likely to die prematurely from all causes. According to experts, obesity contributed to approximately 112,000 preventable deaths among Americans in 2000.[29]

Overweight and obese people are more likely to develop osteoarthritis, a painful chronic condition that affects joints and interferes with the person's ability to move.[30, 31] Obese people typically have difficulty carrying out routine daily activities, especially those that require walking, carrying, kneeling, and stooping. Additionally, obese people are more likely to suffer from chronic heartburn as well as *sleep apnea*, a condition that causes breathing to stop periodically during sleep.

TABLE 10.5 *Health Problems Associated with Excess Body Fat*

Overweight and obesity increase the risk of	
Cardiovascular disease (CVD)	Chronic low back pain
Hypertension	Loss of mobility
Type 2 diabetes	Fatty liver disease (not alcohol related)
Metabolic syndrome	Erectile dysfunction in men (impotence)
Polycystic ovary syndrome	Low-grade inflammation
Infertility	Gastroesophageal reflux disorder (GERD)
Elevated blood lipid levels	Psychological depression
Gallstones	Certain cancers
Sleep apnea	Skin ulcers
Osteoarthritis	Premature death

Sources: Jackson Y and others: Summary of the 2000 Surgeon General's listening session: Toward a national action plan on overweight and obesity. *Obesity Research* 10(12):1299, 2002; Virji A, Murr MM: Caring for patients after bariatric surgery. *American Family Physician*, 73(8):1403, 2006.

Obese men and women are more likely to have fertility problems than people with healthy BMIs. *Polycystic ovary disease* often affects obese women and can reduce the women's chances of becoming pregnant. During pregnancy, obese women have high risk of *gestational diabetes* and a form of hypertension that can be deadly.[32] Additionally, obese pregnant women are at greater risk for stillbirths or giving birth to babies with birth defects than are pregnant women who have lower BMIs.

A person's mental health and self-esteem can be negatively affected by his or her "weight problem." Many Americans admire slim and muscular body builds over overfat body shapes. Thus, overfat people often suffer from poor self-images because they think their bodies are unattractive. The general public often views obesity as a condition that results from lack of willpower and the inability to "push oneself away from the table." Thus, many overfat people also deal with the negative attitude (stigma) that many people have toward them. People who are not overfat often characterize obese persons as lazy, stupid, and sloppy.[33] The stigma of obesity can result in discriminatory practices that limit an obese person's chances for career opportunities and access to adequate health care. It is not surprising that depression tends to accompany obesity. Table 10.5 lists these and other major health problems associated with excessive body fat.

Body Fat Distribution: Effects on Health

The results of medical research suggest that the distribution of excess body fat has a closer association with obesity-related diseases than does the percentage of total body fat. Some people, especially women, tend to store extra subcutaneous fat below the waist, primarily in the buttocks and thighs (Fig. 10.14a). Having this particular pattern of fat distribution (a "pear shape") adds stress to hip and knee joints that must carry the extra weight, but the pattern is not associated with increased risk of more serious chronic diseases such as type 2 diabetes.

Men and African-American women tend to store extra visceral fat in the abdominal or central region of their bodies.[34] **Central-body obesity** is characterized by a large "spare tire" that spreads beyond buttocks and thighs. A person with central-body obesity is sometimes described as having an "apple" body shape (see Fig. 10.14b). People with central-body obesity have higher risks of cardiovascular disease and type 2 diabetes ("diabesity") than people who have waists that do not extend beyond their hips.[35]

central-body obesity condition characterized by excessive abdominal fat

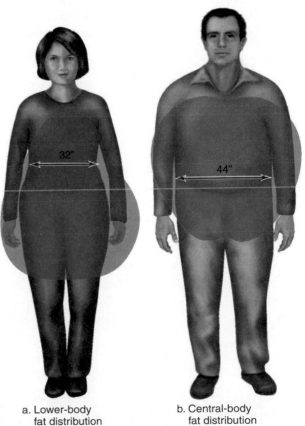

a. Lower-body fat distribution (pear shape)

b. Central-body fat distribution (apple shape)

Figure 10.14 Body fat distribution: Typical sex differences. Some people, especially women, tend to store extra subcutaneous fat below the waist, primarily in the buttocks and thighs (*a*). Men and African-American women tend to store extra visceral fat in the central region of their bodies (*b*).

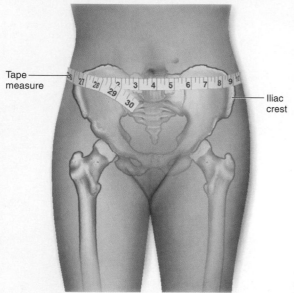

Tape measure

Iliac crest

Figure 10.15 Measuring waist circumference. A quick and easy method to determine a person's risk of obesity-related disorders is to measure the individual's waist circumference. Note the positioning of the tape at the top of the hip bones and not necessarily at the narrowest point. Additionally, the tape should be held around the waist, parallel to the floor.

Some medical researchers think central-body obesity contributes to certain chronic diseases because the surplus of visceral fat cells releases too many fatty acids into the hepatic portal vein that leads directly to the liver.[36] When flooded with fatty acids, the liver has difficulty using the lipids to make lipoproteins. When this occurs, the fatty acids circulate in blood, possibly disrupting muscle and liver glucose metabolism.[36] Furthermore, adipose cells, particularly visceral fat, make substances that cause inflammation in the body.[17] These inflammatory factors may also increase risks of type 2 diabetes and CVD.

A quick and easy method to determine your risk of obesity-related disorders is to measure your *waist circumference*. Figure 10.15 shows the recommended placement of the tape measure. Note the positioning of the tape at the top of the hip bones and not necessarily at the narrowest point.[37, 38] It is also important to use a measuring tape that does not stretch. Central-body obesity is defined by a waist circumference of greater than 40 inches in men and greater than 35 inches in women.[36]

Concept **Checkpoint**

21. A young woman's BMI is 26.2. According to this information, is this woman likely to be healthy, overweight, obese, or extremely obese?
22. List at least six different serious health problems that are associated with having too much body fat and being obese in particular.
23. What is the "stigma" of obesity?
24. Which of the two major types of body fat distribution is more likely to pose serious health risks? Which chronic diseases are more likely to develop in people who have this pattern of excess fat deposition?
25. What is a quick and easy way to determine whether a person's body fat distribution is likely to result in serious health problems, such as type 2 diabetes?

10.5 What Causes Overweight and Obesity?

Although an excess intake of calories in relation to calorie output causes weight gain, there is no simple *cause* of obesity. To lose weight, a person needs to create a negative energy state by eating fewer calories, expending more calories than the amount consumed, or taking both actions. For many people, however, it is not easy to alter calorie input and output. Physiological, environmental, behavioral, psychological, and socioeconomic forces influence a person's calorie intake and expenditure.

Physiological Factors

hunger uncomfortable feeling that drives a person to consume food

satiety sense that enough food or beverages have been consumed to satisfy hunger

ghrelin protein that stimulates eating behavior

leptin hormone that reduces hunger and inhibits fat storage in the body

From a physiological standpoint, eating behavior is complex and largely involves interactions among the nervous, endocrine, and digestive systems as well as fat tissue. *Hunger* and *satiety* are key sensations that regulate eating behavior. **Hunger** is an uncomfortable feeling that drives a person to consume food. **Satiety** is the sense that enough food or beverages have been consumed to satisfy hunger.

Physical sensations influence eating behavior. As time between meals increases, the stomach signals "it's time to eat" by contracting, causing hunger pangs. As the contractions become stronger, the person usually eats or drinks something to relieve the discomfort. The size of the stomach influences satiety. During meals, the stomach stretches as it fills. The sensation that the stomach has reached its capacity can make a person stop eating. Nevertheless, many overfat persons do not recognize the sensation of stomach fullness, and as a result, they may eat even when they should not be hungry.

An area of the *hypothalamus*, a structure in the brain, controls hunger and satiety. Scientists think this region functions as a "hunger/satiety center." The stomach, intestines, and fat tissue produce certain proteins, such as hormones and *peptide YY*, that stimulate nerve cells involved in the regulation of hunger and satiety. **Ghrelin** (*greh'-lin*), a hormone secreted mainly by the stomach, stimulates eating behavior. Some scientists think that reducing ghrelin production or activity is the key to helping people lose or maintain their weight. The small and large intestines release peptide YY, a protein that signals the stomach to reduce ghrelin secretion. The small intestine also releases *cholecystokinin (CCK)*, the hormone that stimulates the gallbladder to contract and the pancreas to release digestive enzymes (see Chapter 6). Additionally, CCK stimulates the brain and other nervous tissue, suppressing appetite as a result.

Adipose tissue helps regulate hunger and satiety. Fat cells secrete **leptin,** a hormone that reduces hunger and inhibits fat storage in the body. A person's blood leptin level is directly proportional to his or her amount of body fat.[16] The brain obtains information about the status of body fat stores by monitoring the level of leptin in blood. When researchers administer leptin to genetically engineered mice that cannot synthesize the hormone, the rodents lose weight, because the hormone reduces the animals' interest in eating and increases their rate of fat metabolism.[39] Studies involving humans, however, generally find that obese people produce high amounts of leptin, but their bodies resist the hormone's hunger-suppressing action.[40] Figure 10.16 illustrates the complex effects of ghrelin, leptin, CCK, and peptide YY on hunger and satiety.

Figure 10.16 Proteins that influence hunger. Appetite regulation involves complex factors, including the secretion of proteins by the digestive tract and fat tissue that stimulate or inhibit a region of the hypothalamus. Grehlin stimulates hunger sensations (*a*). Leptin, CCK, and PYY inhibit hunger sensations (*b*).

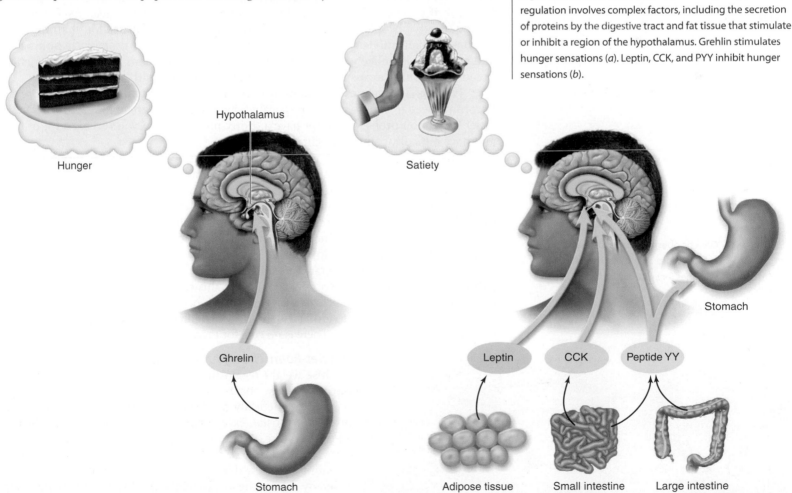

Hunger

Hypothalamus

Satiety

Ghrelin

Stomach

Leptin

CCK

Peptide YY

Stomach

Adipose tissue

Small intestine

Large intestine

a.   **Stimulating hunger**

b.   **Inhibiting hunger**

set-point theory scientific notion that body fat content is genetically predetermined

appetite desire to eat appealing food

Food Composition Factors

Dietary factors, particularly amounts of fat and certain carbohydrates in diets, can influence body fat production and appetite. Fatty foods are more energy dense than foods that contain more carbohydrate, protein, and water than fat.[41] Thus, high-fat diets are associated with excess calorie intakes and rising obesity rates.[42] Fatty foods often contain a lot of sugar. Some medical researchers think the consumption of the simple sugar fructose is associated with the current obesity epidemic. High fructose intakes may result in weight gain because the sugar decreases satiety and stimulates fat synthesis in the body.[43] For a more extensive review of the role that carbohydrates may play in weight gain, see the "Are Carbohydrates Fattening?" section of Chapter 5.

Genetic Factors

Genetics play a major role in the development of obesity. Most physical characteristics are inherited, including metabolic rate, hormone production, body frame size, and pattern of fat distribution. All of these characteristics affect body weight.

Some rats and mice are genetically predisposed to become obese because they have inherited genes for "thrifty metabolisms." Rodents with thrifty metabolisms have bodies that are more efficient at storing excess energy as fat than rodents who do not have such metabolisms. It is possible that humans who gain weight easily have genes that code for thrifty metabolisms as well. In ancient times, food was often scarce, and people had to eat as much as they could when food was available. During times when food was plentiful, individuals who had thrifty metabolisms stored more of the excess energy from food as body fat than persons who did not have such efficient metabolisms. The people who lacked thrifty metabolisms wasted the excess food energy as body heat. As a result, the energy-"thrifty" people were more likely to survive periods of starvation than the other persons. In many modern societies, however, high-calorie food is available 24 hours a day and starvation is unlikely. As a result, having thrifty metabolisms is no longer beneficial because depositing excess body fat often results in serious health problems.

If you gain weight easily, you may have inherited a thrifty metabolism. To prevent becoming overfat, you need to be physically active and make careful food choices. On the other hand, you probably do not have a thrifty metabolism if you can eat a lot of food and have difficulty gaining weight.

Medical researchers have identified several genes that contribute to human fatness. Genes also control hormones that regulate growth and metabolism, as well as grehlin and leptin production. Certain mice, for example, become obese because they lack genes for synthesizing leptin (Fig. 10.17). Researchers are interested in developing medications that regulate the influence of certain genes over metabolism and hormone production. If research indicates that such medications are safe and effective, they could help people manage their weight over the long term.

Prader-Willi syndrome is a rare genetic condition that results from the lack of genes in a particular section of a chromosome. People with this condition have skeletal deformities, delayed motor development, decreased intellectual functioning, food cravings, and insatiable appetites. If their access to food is not restricted, children with Prader-Willi syndrome eat constantly and become obese. There is no cure for Prader-Willi syndrome.

Figure 10.17 Genetic obesity in mice. Certain genetically engineered mice (the mouse on the left) become obese because they lack genes for synthesizing leptin.

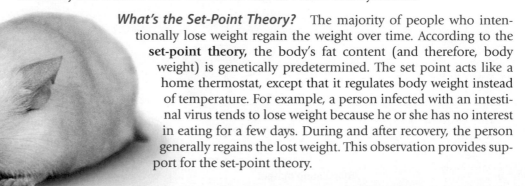

What's the Set-Point Theory? The majority of people who intentionally lose weight regain the weight over time. According to the **set-point theory**, the body's fat content (and therefore, body weight) is genetically predetermined. The set point acts like a home thermostat, except that it regulates body weight instead of temperature. For example, a person infected with an intestinal virus tends to lose weight because he or she has no interest in eating for a few days. During and after recovery, the person generally regains the lost weight. This observation provides support for the set-point theory.

Biochemical and metabolic studies also support the set-point theory. When calorie intakes are reduced, blood thyroid hormone levels decline, depressing the normal basal metabolic rate. Additionally, the caloric cost of performing weight-bearing activities decreases when a person loses weight. As a result, an activity that required 100 kcal before weight loss may burn only 80 kcal after weight loss. Furthermore, weight loss appears to make the body become more efficient at storing calories from macronutrients as fat. When a person gains weight and stays at that weight for a while, his or her body tends to establish a new and higher set point. According to the theory, all these changes protect the body from losing weight and explain why weight loss is so difficult to achieve and maintain.

Opponents of the set-point theory argue that weight does not remain constant throughout adulthood: the average person gains weight slowly, at least until old age. Thus, body weight may result more from lifestyle practices and environmental influences than predetermined biological controls such as a set point.

Environmental Influences

Consider your eating behavior during a typical holiday meal that includes a variety of attractive, tasty foods. After eating the meal, your hunger should be satisfied, but as soon as pie or cake is placed on the table, do you "find some room" in your stomach for some dessert? If you often eat when you are not hungry, then you are probably aware of the effect your environment can have on your appetite. **Appetite** is the desire to eat appealing food.

Food advertising is an aspect of the environment that has a powerful influence on your food choices. To entice you to buy their products, food manufacturers usually appeal to your senses, emphasizing the appearance and taste of food, in particular. Recently, a television ad for a fast-food chain promoted a hamburger that has three beef patties, three slices of cheese, and six bacon slices topped with mayonnaise. According to information at the fast-food company's website, this burger provides 800 kcal. The site, however, does not tell you that 800 kcal is more than one-third of a day's calorie needs for an average person! How do you respond when you see food advertisements on television? Do the ads make you hungry or eager to try a new food product?

Over the past 30 years, portion sizes of many popular foods, especially restaurant items, have become larger.[41] People may choose to purchase "supersized" portions of foods because they like the idea of getting more for their money. In many instances, however, "more" means *more* fat and calories per serving. According to some nutrition experts, the increased consumption of oversized portions of many restaurant foods contributes to the obesity epidemic in the United States.[44]

Even consuming a small amount of extra energy can result in weight gain. One pound of body fat represents about 3500 kcal. Therefore, you will gain a pound of fat if you accumulate 3500 more calories than your body needs. Consider this: If you consume only 100 extra calories and maintain the same level of physical activity each day, you will consume an extra 36,500 kcal in a year. By the end of that year, you will gain about 10 pounds (36,500 kcal ÷ 3500 kcal)!

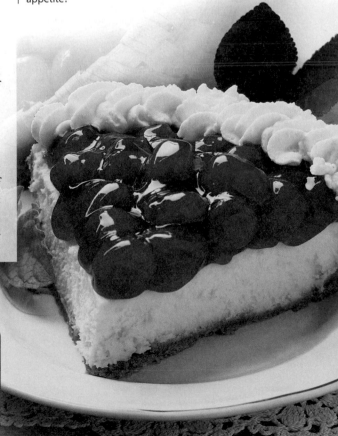

How does the presence of such appealing food affect your appetite?

Did You Know?

Regular exercise, such as walking, can shrink abdominal fat, but it is not possible to "spot-reduce" by exercising a fatty body part intensely.[12] The energy needed to fuel muscle activity comes from fatty deposits within muscle tissue and the rest of the body. Exercise, however, can improve muscle tone, so that fat tissue appears less flabby.

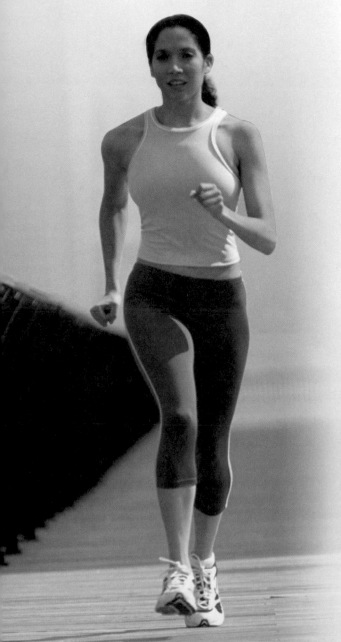

Our environment also affects whether we choose to be sedentary or physically active. In our homes, we rely on a variety of "energy-saving" devices such as dishwashing machines, TV remote controls, and garage door openers to work for us. Outside our homes, we use cars, elevators, escalators, and other motorized devices, instead of our feet, to move us from place to place. With the help of machines, our lives are considerably easier; however, we are consuming more calories than in the past.

In 2007–2008, average energy intake in one day of American men and women who were 20 to 29 years of age was 2756 kcal and 1828 kcal, respectively.[45] Overall, Americans are consuming more food energy than they consumed in the early 1970s. The increase in energy intake may help explain why the prevalence of overweight and obesity has increased among Americans over the past 40 years. According to the principles of energy balance, excess energy intake in relation to energy output results in weight gain.

By becoming more physically active, people can increase their energy output. Many Americans, however, have "desk jobs" that require little muscular movement. When we have some leisure time, we often spend it performing tasks that involve sitting—watching television, playing computer games, or chatting with people on the Internet. In a national survey conducted in 2008, approximately 25% of American adults reported that in the month before the survey, they did not engage in physical activity during their leisure time.[46] According to experts with the American College of Sports Medicine and the American Heart Association, healthy adults under 65 years of age should perform at least 30 minutes of moderate-intensity physical activity (brisk walking, for example) five days of the week.[47] Adults who include exercise in their weight-loss plan may need to engage in at least 60 minutes of moderate-intensity activity each day to achieve long-term maintenance of lower body weight.[48] Choose MyPlate.gov has information about physical activity, including examples of activities that are moderate or vigorous (http://www.choosemyplate.gov/foodgroups/physicalactivity_tips.html).

If you live on or near a university or college campus, your environment probably provides ample opportunities for engaging in exercise and sports, such as tennis courts, swimming pools, and weight-training rooms. It is relatively easy to be physically active while you are in college, *if you choose to be.* After you graduate, consider what you will do to maintain a healthy level of physical activity each day, especially if you have a sedentary job. How likely are you to use the staircase in a building when you see the elevator? Will you keep a pair of comfortable shoes at work, so you can walk for at least 20 minutes during lunch?

Genes and Environment: Interactions

It is difficult to determine the extent to which an obese person's genetic makeup or environment contributes to his or her excess body weight. Children are more likely to become overweight or obese if their mothers were overfat prior to becoming pregnant.[49, 50] This finding appears to support the hypothesis that obesity is an inherited trait. Nevertheless, genes do not control everything about our health, including our weight. Environmental and other factors can modify the expression of genes. For example, children whose mothers are obese may have inherited genes that increase risk for obesity. However, these children may avoid becoming obese if they adopt a physically active lifestyle and do not overeat. On the other hand, these children may become obese if their parents have poor eating habits and sedentary lifestyles and the youngsters follow their parents' practices.

Did You Know?

Infants born to women who smoked during pregnancy are more likely to become obese as adults than babies born to nonsmokers.[50]

Other Factors That Influence Weight

Socioeconomic factors are associated with increased likelihood of overweight and obesity among adult Americans. Level of education appears to be a stronger influence over BMI than income. In a survey of over 29,000 adults, 27.5% of the subjects who had less than a high school education were obese, whereas 17.4% of the subjects who had earned bachelor degrees were obese.[51] However, the prevalence of overweight and obesity is increasing among *all* members of the U.S. population, including people who have high incomes and are well educated.[52]

Psychological factors such as mood and self-esteem influence eating behaviors and body weight. Many people eat not because they are hungry but because they are bored, anxious, angry, or depressed. Obesity may increase the likelihood of depression, especially in American women.[53] Researchers, however, cannot easily determine whether being obese causes depression or being depressed causes obesity.

Among some segments of American society, the ideal female figure is slim but curvy and the ideal male physique is trim and muscular. As a result, societal pressures inspire many young women to idealize underweight. Consider the body shapes of many fashion models, professional ballerinas, and successful young actresses. These young women have so little subcutaneous fat that some of their bones protrude under their skin. In their relentless efforts to pursue such unrealistic body shapes, many young women adopt unhealthy and potentially life-threatening eating practices. The Chapter 10 "Highlight" focuses on eating disorders, including *anorexia nervosa*.

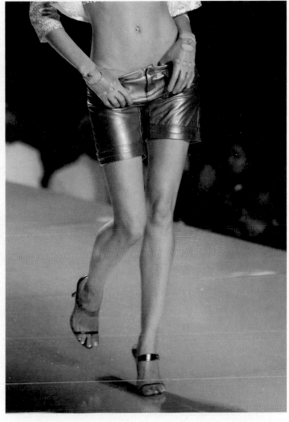

Societal pressures inspire many young women to idealize underweight people, especially thin female celebrities.

Concept **Checkpoint**

26. What is hunger? What is satiety?
27. Discuss the roles of leptin and ghrelin in regulating hunger.
28. Under what conditions would having "thrifty genes" benefit a person?
29. What is the set-point theory?
30. What is the difference between hunger and appetite?
31. Describe how the environment influences a person's food intake and physical activity level.
32. Provide at least three examples of ways that socioeconomic, psychological, and societal factors can influence eating behavior.

10.6 Weight Loss and Its Maintenance

Before you embark on an effort to lose (or gain) weight, an important first step is determining whether it is even necessary to change your weight. The need for changing your weight should be based on your overall health and family history of weight-related diseases. If you are dissatisfied with your body weight and shape, consider the following questions. Are you physically healthy at your present weight? If your BMI is within the healthy range, why do you think you need to lose or gain weight?

Using a BMI calculator (http://www.nhlbisupport.com/bmi/bmicalc.htm) or consulting a BMI table such as the one in Figure 10.18 that indicates the range of healthy

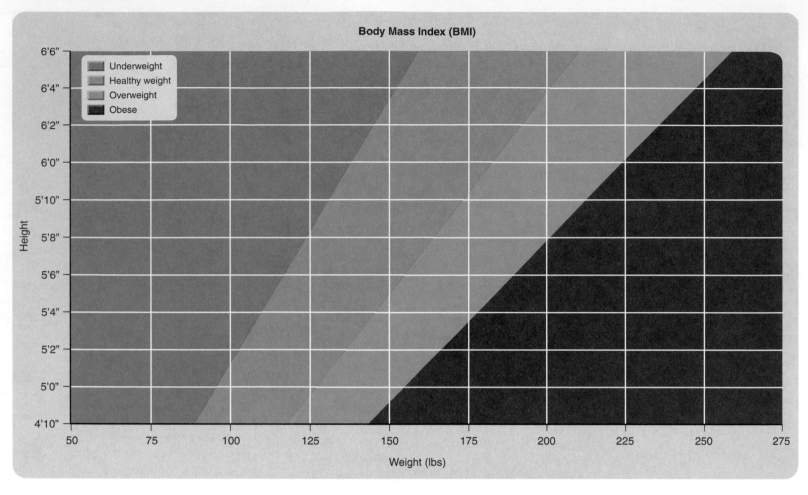

Body Mass Index (BMI)

Legend:
- Underweight
- Healthy weight
- Overweight
- Obese

Y-axis: Height (4'10" to 6'6")
X-axis: Weight (lbs) (50 to 275)

Figure 10.18 Adult BMI chart. Are you at a healthy weight?
Source of data: www.nhlbi.nih.gov/guidelines/obesity/ bmi-tbl.pdf

weights for a particular height (BMIs of 18.5 up to 24.9) can be helpful. According to this chart, an adult whose height is 5′5″ has a healthy weight range of about 111 to 149 pounds.

To determine your BMI range using the table in Figure 10.18, locate your height in the left-most column with your left index finger, then locate your weight along the bottom line of the graph with your right index finger. Read across the row with your left finger and up from the bottom with your right finger, until your fingers meet. Note the BMI range where the two fingers meet. According to this graph, is your BMI in the healthy range?

The next step, if necessary, is setting a reasonable and realistic goal weight. It is important to note that an overweight or obese person does not have to shed a lot of weight to reduce risk factors associated with CVD, stroke, and type 2 diabetes. Just losing 5 to 10% of excess body fat can increase beneficial high-density lipoprotein levels (HDL cholesterol), reduce elevated blood pressure and triglyceride levels, and improve glucose tolerance.[28]

Features of Medically Sound Weight-Loss Plans

Table 10.6 presents key features of reliable weight-loss plans. Such plans should be safe and effective, as well as flexible enough to meet the dieter's nutritional, psychological, and social needs. A medically sound weight-loss diet should emphasize a wide variety of low-calorie, readily available nutritious foods and be adaptable to the dieter's food likes and dislikes. Furthermore, reliable weight-loss plans should provide suggestions for altering environments that foster overeating and sedentary behaviors. Before beginning any weight-loss diet, overfat people need to obtain their physician's approval, especially if they have serious health conditions, such as type 2 diabetes, or they are over the age of 40 (men) or 50 (women).

Key Factors

Despite claims made in advertisements and infomercials, there are no quick cures for overweight and obesity. Successful weight loss and long-term weight maintenance involve four key elements: motivation, calorie reduction, regular physical activity, and behavior modification.

Motivation

The motivation to lose weight and keep it off requires an overfat person to recognize that there is a need to change his or her behavior and become committed to making those changes permanent. For some people, this recognition occurs when they are diagnosed with a health disorder that is associated with excess body fat. Nevertheless, many overfat people choose not to lose weight. The commitment to lose weight and enjoy better health must become far more important than the desire to overeat.

Weight-loss "triggers" often serve as motivators. For some people, seeing themselves in an unflattering photograph, being advised by their physicians to lose weight, or being unable to enjoy activities because being obese restricts their movement triggers the decision to lose weight. According to results of a large survey, adult Americans most frequently cited "medical advice" as the reason for their weight-loss efforts.[54]

Calorie Reduction

To lose a pound of weight, a person needs to create a negative energy state of 3500 kcal. A reasonable rate of weight loss is one-half to 1 pound of fat per week.[37] Overfat persons can usually accomplish this rate of loss by reducing their calorie intake or increasing their physical activity (energy output) by 300 to 500 kcal/day.[37] Overweight or obese people can lose about 1 to 2 pounds per week by cutting their calorie intakes even further—by 500 to 1000 kcal/day.[55] Although many dieters would like to shed more than 2 pounds per week, health experts recommend a slow and steady rate.

According to guidelines issued by the National Institutes of Health, reasonable calorie intakes for adults who want to lose weight range from 1000 to 1200 kcal/day for women and 1200 to 1600 kcal/day for men.[37] At these calorie intake levels, careful food choices are necessary to obtain nutritionally adequate diets. Certain diets severely limit food intake and provide fewer than 800 kcal/day. Such *very-low-calorie diets* are not recommended for most overfat persons.[55] People who follow very-low-calorie diets may lose a lot of weight rapidly, but they regain the weight quickly after they "go off" the diet and return to their former eating habits.

The healthy way to lower intake of total calories is to reduce consumption of added sugars, fats, and alcohol. People can also achieve negative energy states by reducing calorie intake *and* increasing physical activity. Nevertheless, a survey of adults who were trying to lose weight indicated that only one-third reported combining the two weight-loss strategies.[56]

Reliable weight-loss diets should follow the Acceptable Macronutrient Distribution Ranges (AMDRs): 20 to 35% of calories from fat, 45 to 65% of calories from carbohydrates, and 10 to 35% of calories from protein.[57] Increasing consumption of watery, high-fiber foods that are not energy dense, such as fruits and vegetables, may be helpful for dieters. Such foods are more likely to provide satiety sooner than energy-dense foods and, as a result, reduce the person's calorie intake.[58] No particular diet or food has a "metabolic advantage" by promoting greater calorie burning by the body. A dieter's goal should be reducing total calorie intake while obtaining all essential nutrients.

Eventually, a person who intentionally loses weight by reducing calorie intake and increasing physical activity reaches a weight *plateau*. When this occurs, the dieter is in energy balance. To continue losing weight, the person must reduce his or her calorie intake or increase physical activity beyond the present levels. For someone who is consuming

TABLE 10.6 *Key Features of Reliable Weight-Loss Plans*

A sound weight-loss plan

- Is safe and effective.
- Meets nutritional, psychological, and social needs.
- Incorporates a variety of common foods from all food groups.
- Fosters slow but steady weight loss.
- Does not require costly devices or diet books.
- Accommodates family and restaurant meals, parties and special occasions, ethnic foods, and food likes.
- Does not make the dieter feel deprived.
- Emphasizes readily available nutritious foods.
- Promotes changing habits that lead to overeating.
- Encourages regular physical activity.
- Provides suggestions for obtaining social support.
- Can be followed for a lifetime.

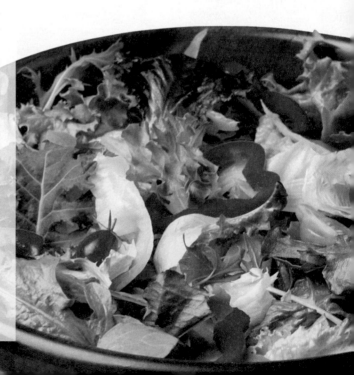

only 1000 to 1200 kcal/day, cutting calories even further can lower the metabolic rate, hindering weight loss.

Preparing nutritionally adequate but calorie-reduced meals and snacks can be easier when dietary experts have already done the calculations for consumers. For example, MyPlate (www.choosemyplate.gov/downloads/MyPyramid_Food_Intake_Patterns.pdf) provides patterns of food choices for 12 different calorie levels (1000 to 3200 kcal/day) that incorporate all food groups. Chapter 3 provides more information about MyPlate. For more general information about weight control, obesity, and nutrition, visit the Weight-control Information Network (WIN) at: http://win.niddk.nih.gov/index.htm. Other reliable sites for weight control information include www.obesity.org; and www .eatright.org.

Regular Physical Activity

It is difficult to burn much energy without being physically active. By increasing their physical activity level and burning more calories, dieters do not need to limit their food intake as excessively as they would by relying on calorie reduction alone to lose weight. You do not need to jog for 10 miles to reap the benefits of engaging in regular physical activity. Moderate-intensity activities are recommended for people who want to lose or manage their weight. Chapter 11 discusses the healthful benefits of a physically active lifestyle.

Behavior Modification

Controlling calorie intake and increasing physical activity are easier to accomplish if overfat persons analyze their faulty behaviors, identify eating *cues* and "problem" behaviors, and develop ways to change the behaviors. Eating cues are usually environmental factors that stimulate eating behavior, such as seeing an ad for a fast-food restaurant or smelling freshly baked brownies when walking past a bakery. Identifying such cues can enable people to recognize effects of the signals and avoid inappropriate ones, whenever possible. By analyzing their food-related behaviors, overfat individuals can often determine in which circumstances they tend to overeat.

Cues can also help overfat people lose weight. If, for example, you are trying to lose weight, posting an unflattering photograph of yourself on the refrigerator or pantry door can serve as a reminder to stay on course with your behavior modification plan.

Although the process may seem slow, people are more likely to change ingrained habits by focusing on changing one behavior at a time. For example, many people snack on energy-dense foods and drinks while watching television. To change this habit, a person could decide to eat only at the kitchen table and avoid all food and beverage consumption while sitting in front of a TV.

For individuals who want to lose (or gain) weight, keeping records of food intake and physical activities can be helpful for estimating daily calorie input and output. However, overfat persons often underestimate their calorie intake and overestimate their energy output.[60] Therefore, people need to record information about food choices and physical activity habits accurately.

Tips for Modifying Food- and Exercise-Related Behaviors The following suggestions may help a person lose excess weight as well as maintain a lower, healthier body weight.

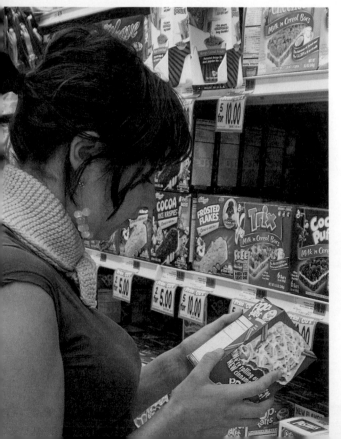

Read Nutrition Facts panels to compare calorie and fat contents of packaged foods.

- **Planning Menus**
  1. Plan meals and snacks to cover three or more days, then use the plan to prepare grocery lists.
  2. When menu planning, include sources of protein, unsaturated fat, and complex carbohydrates in meals and snacks.

3. Avoid labeling certain foods as "off limits." Depriving yourself of such items can result in bingeing on the "forbidden" food. Learning to analyze why you have difficulty controlling your intake of these foods and developing strategies to learn how to reduce your intake of them can be very helpful.

• **Grocery Shopping**

1. To reduce the likelihood of making impulsive food choices, shop for food *after* eating.
2. Shop from a grocery list. If a food is not on your list, ask yourself if you really need to buy it and if it will hinder or help your weight-loss efforts.
3. Read food labels to compare calorie and fat contents per serving.

• **Food Preparation**

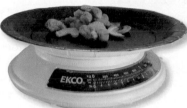

1. Reduce the use of solid fat in cooking; bake, broil, or roast meats instead of frying them.
2. Add less solid fat to foods such as cooked vegetables before serving or eating them.
3. If you sample foods while preparing them, consider the amounts you ate and at mealtimes reduce your portion sizes accordingly.
4. Prepare only enough food to provide one limited-size portion for yourself. Using measuring cups and a small scale for weighing food can be helpful.
5. Serve food on smaller plates and eat with smaller spoons.
6. Take your usual-size portion and return one-third to one-half of it to the serving dish or container.
7. Remove serving dishes from the table. Keeping foods or their containers in sight can encourage overeating.

Using a small scale for weighing food can be helpful for limiting portion sizes.

• **Eating Behavior**

1. Keep nutrient-dense, low-calorie snack foods, such as fresh fruits and vegetables, on hand.
2. Eat meals and snacks at scheduled times; do not skip meals, especially breakfast.
3. Eat all food in a "dining" area; avoid eating while engaged in other activities, such as reading a book or watching television.
4. Slow down the pace of meals by putting eating utensils down between mouthfuls and eating more slowly.
5. Leave some food on your plate.
6. Become a "defensive eater." Practice ways to refuse food graciously or request smaller portions. Be aware of people, especially relatives and friends, who *sabotage* your weight-loss efforts. Examples of such sabotage include a person who repeatedly offers calorie-dense foods to you, even though you have turned down the food and this person knows you are trying to lose weight.

• **Holidays and Parties**

1. Beforehand, think about what you will eat and drink while attending the event. Practice polite ways to decline food.
2. Consider limiting your food intake before the special occasion to avoid consuming too many calories for the day.
3. Eat a low-calorie snack about an hour before the occasion.
4. Drink fewer alcoholic beverages. Replace alcoholic beverages with ice water or diet soft drinks.

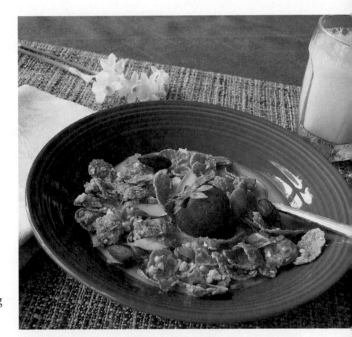

Individuals who lose excess weight and maintain the weight loss tend to eat regular meals, including breakfast.

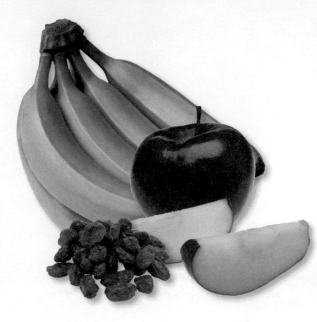

 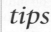

Food & Nutrition *tips*

- When you are hungry, drink some fat-free milk or eat a banana, an apple, a few whole dates, or a handful of raisins.

- Skipping meals can contribute to fatigue. Eating breakfast and small between-meal snacks can provide the carbohydrates needed to maintain blood glucose levels.

- Include foods that supply complex carbohydrate, including fiber, in each meal to provide a sense of fullness and satiety.

- **Restaurants**

   1. Avoid fried menu items or those made with butter, gravy, or cream sauce.
   2. Choose pasta with red sauce instead of white sauce.
   3. Request salad dressing "on the side" so you can control the amount.
   4. Think "small." Order an entrée and share it with another person.
   5. Do not be a member of the "clean plate club." Ask your server for a "carryout bag" when he or she brings your order to the table. Then divide the food in half, and place one-half in the container. Be sure to refrigerate the leftovers within 2 hours after the meal, and eat them for a meal the following day.
   6. If you choose a dessert item, share it with others.
   7. Avoid eating regularly at fast-food outlets.
   8. When at fast-food outlets, make substitutions, such as a salad instead of a fried fish sandwich, a regular hamburger instead of a specialty burger, or a roasted chicken sandwich instead of a breaded and fried chicken sandwich. Order a diet soft drink or water instead of a regular soft drink. If possible, order a baked potato instead of fries.

- **Physical Activity**

   1. Choose physical activities that you enjoy and can do without the need for expensive equipment.
   2. Increase the time you spend walking each day. Keep walking shoes where you can see them.
   3. Reduce the amount of time you spend sitting. For example, do more household chores yourself.
   4. Take stairs instead of elevators or escalators whenever possible.
   5. Park your car farther from your destination and walk, if you feel it is safe to do so.
   6. Perform calisthenics or lift handheld weights while watching television.
   7. Adopt moderate-intensity activities for your leisure time. For example, join a co-ed volleyball club or take a ballroom dancing class.

An easy way to monitor your daily physical activity is to use a pedometer.

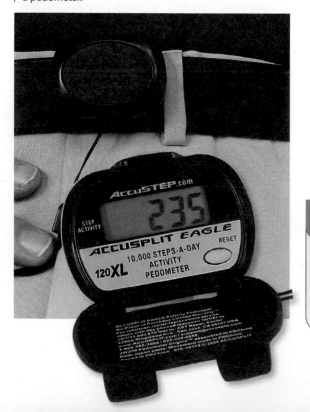

Did You Know?

A *pedometer* is a small device that records the number of steps a person takes while engaging in physical activities. According to the Shape Up America! organization (www.shapeup.org), the goal is to take at least 10,000 steps per day. If you would like to monitor your steps, you can purchase an inexpensive pedometer in sporting goods stores. The one shown in the photo clips onto socks or belts.

- **Self-Monitoring**

  1. Set reasonable weight-loss goals, for example, losing 4 pounds in 1 month. When you achieve that goal, then set another reasonable goal, and continue with this process until the goal weight is achieved.
  2. Keep a special notebook to use as a food and exercise diary where you can see it—near the kitchen table, refrigerator, or pantry, for example.
  3. In the diary, note the time and place of eating as well as the type and amount of food eaten. Also record who was present and your mood when you ate meals and snacks.
  4. Use the diary to identify your food-related problem areas, such as eating when bored or depressed.
  5. In the exercise section of the diary, record the form of moderate-intensity exercise you performed and the number of minutes you spent engaging in that activity each day. Try to achieve at least 150 minutes of moderate-intensity activities each week.
  6. Measure your waistline weekly and keep a record of the measurements.
  7. Weigh yourself at least once a week, preferably at the same time and without clothing. However, do not rely only on your weight as an indication of your progress. Regular exercise often increases muscle mass that can result in weight gain or failure to lose weight. However, adding muscle mass is healthier than maintaining too much body fat.

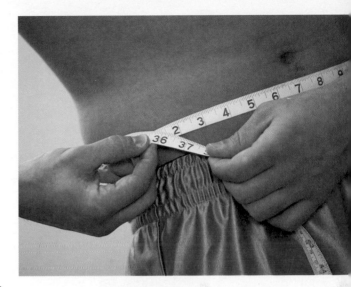

- **Rewards for New Behaviors**

  1. Plan nonfood motivators or rewards for specific behaviors. For example, "I'll buy a pair of slacks that are one size smaller than what I currently wear and hang them where I can see them," or "I'll buy that DVD I've wanted, when I lose 5 pounds."
  2. Encourage family and friends to provide praise and encouragement for your efforts to manage your weight. Let family, friends, and associates know that you are trying to lose weight and you would appreciate their help and support. Thank them when you receive their praise and support.

- **Changing Negative Thought Patterns**

  1. Do not get discouraged by occasional setbacks—relapses can be expected when changing behaviors. For example, instead of thinking, "I can't lose weight. I'm a failure," say to yourself, "OK, so I lost control and had too much to eat at the wedding. That's to be expected. I just need to get back on track. I'll pull in the reins on my eating for the next day and exercise more."
  2. Think positively about progress. "I didn't lose any weight this week, but I didn't gain any either. I must be losing fat and getting trimmer—those slacks fit better than they did 2 months ago."
  3. Counter negative thoughts with positive statements. "Next time, I'll eat two cookies instead of four. This afternoon, I'll just have to walk a little longer and harder to burn off those extra calories."

Community-Based Weight-Loss Programs

Many communities offer a variety of weight-loss programs. Registered dietitians often conduct weight-loss classes at hospitals or universities. Dietitians have extensive training in foods, nutrition, dietetics, and counseling methods to help people design safe and effective weight-loss plans. If a physician prescribes dietary counseling by a registered dietitian, the patient's health insurance may cover the cost of such treatment.

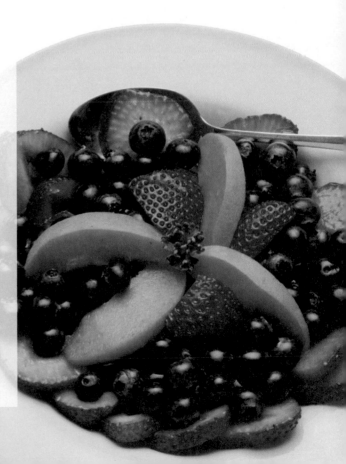

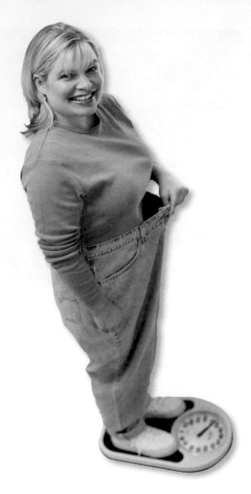

Some commercial weight-loss programs, such as *Weight Watchers,* have diet plans that have been developed by dietitians. Members who have lost weight while following the plan often conduct local meetings. Before joining any weight-loss program, consumers should obtain answers to the following questions:

- How much does the program cost? Do I pay when I attend meetings? Do I need to sign a contract? If so, for what length of time?
- Do I have to buy special foods or dietary supplements?
- Is nutrition counseling provided? Do the persons providing nutrition counseling and information have degrees in nutrition and dietetics from accredited colleges or universities? How much contact will I have with a counselor?
- Were the diet plans developed by dietitians? Does the plan emphasize the importance of making lifestyle changes, including ways to increase physical activity?
- Does the program's advertising include questionable weight-loss claims and deceptive testimonials?

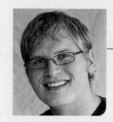

REAL *People*
REAL *Stories*

Jan Haapala

Early in 2005, 24-year-old Jan Haapala did not feel well. He slept poorly at night, and during the day, extreme fatigue seemed to be his constant companion. Frequent indigestion added to his general discomfort. Concerned about her husband's health, Jan's wife, Valerie, urged him to see a doctor and have a physical exam. That trip to the doctor's office would prove to be a major turning point in Jan's life.

During the physical exam, Jan was shocked to learn he had hypertension. The physician prescribed medication to reduce his dangerously elevated blood pressure and issued a stern warning to the young man, "If you don't change your life now, it will end sooner than expected." Why would a physician make such a frightening remark to his patient?

At the time of his doctor's appointment, Jan weighed 335 pounds and his BMI was over 45, which is in the "extremely obese" range. Obesity is a major risk factor for hypertension. If Jan could not reduce his blood pressure and maintain it at a healthy level, he was very likely to die prematurely. Taking medication can reduce elevated blood pressure and keep it under control, but losing excess fat often cures hypertension, making the medication unnecessary. The physician knew he had to say something alarming to Jan that might motivate him to lose his excess fat.

Like many overfat people, Jan was aware that his lifestyle contributed to his extreme obesity. He typically ate two doughnuts and a 20-ounce serving of a sugar-sweetened soft drink for breakfast. Lunches and dinners were "big" meals, often comprised of fast foods, especially double cheeseburgers and large portions of French fries and soft drinks. Candy bars were among his favorite snacks. "I knew those foods were unhealthy, but that didn't change what I ate once I sat down to eat." In addition to his poor food choices, Jan was physically inactive, so he didn't metabolize the excess food energy, and his body fat rapidly increased as a result.

After returning home from the doctor's office, Jan became very angry at the physician. "How could a doctor be so mean?" he thought; but after taking some time to

Successful Dieters—How Do They Manage Their Weight?

The National Weight Control Registry tracks a group of over 4000 adult Americans, mostly women, who have lost at least 30 pounds and maintained the weight loss for at least 1 year.[10] Information about members' nutrition- and exercise-related practices provides some insights into lifestyle practices that foster losing excess weight and maintaining the lower weight. Registry members tend to

- Eat low-calorie, low-fat, high-carbohydrate diets;[61] on average, a member's estimated calorie intake is 1800 kcal/day, with fat comprising about 25% of total calories.
- Maintain the same diet regimen every day of the week.
- Eat regular meals, including breakfast almost every day.
- Weigh themselves at least once a week; many registry members weigh themselves daily.
- Burn about 400 kcal by exercising at least 60 minutes daily.[62]
- Eat a limited variety of nutritious foods.[61]

think about his situation, he made up his mind to improve his health. He recalls, "I didn't want to take medicine to stay alive." Determined to lose weight, Jan heeded his wife's suggestion to join Weight Watchers, one of the oldest and most reliable commercial group weight loss programs in the country.

Although some people can lose weight on their own, others benefit from participating in group weight loss programs that offer sensible and safe nutritional guidance, including tips for controlling the size of food portions and increasing physical activity. Group membership also provides emotional support from other members, a factor that is often critical for weight loss success and maintenance.

By joining Weight Watchers, Jan acquired the information he needed to change his lifestyle to a healthier one. He also developed the motivation to follow a personalized diet and exercise plan that was very different from his past eating and physical activity patterns. In addition to choosing less fatty and sugary foods, he started a walking regimen that eventually became a running regimen. The pounds seemed to melt away from his body, and not long after he began to lose weight, he was able to discontinue taking the medication for hypertension.

When Jan joined the weight loss program, his waistline measured 46" and he wore shirts with a 21" neck size. By the time he reached his goal weight of 210 pounds, his waistline was a trim 35" and his neck size measured only 15 ½". Although it took three years, Jan had lost 125 pounds! The gradual but steady weight loss was an indication that he was making the kinds of behavioral and lifestyle changes that would be permanent.

Jan now chooses foods that support his goals of maintaining his healthy lifestyle and managing his weight. His new dietary pattern includes less processed foods, including oatmeal, whole wheat breads, fruits and vegetables, lean protein sources such as turkey and black beans, and heart-healthy fats such as almonds and olive oil.

Today, Jan is "feeling great" and running races from 5Ks to half-marathons. He has even completed his first marathon. When he was obese, he was embarrassed about exercising in public, but his self-confidence and high self-esteem helped him overcome his reluctance to work out while other people were around. His advice to overfat people who are worried about what strangers will think while they exercise: "Don't be embarrassed about doing something in public that's good for you. People won't judge you negatively for trying to become healthier." Clearly, Jan is a role model and inspiration for anyone who is overweight or obese and wants to get his or her weight (and life) under control.

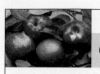

Concept **Checkpoint**

33. What are the four key elements that are necessary for weight loss and maintenance?

34. List at least six features of reliable weight-loss plans or programs.

35. What questions would it be wise for consumers to have answered before they join a weight-loss group or plan?

36. List at least three steps that members of the National Weight Control Registry often take to maintain their reduced body weights.

10.7 Medical Treatments for Obesity

Obese patients are often unsatisfied with the amount of weight they lose while following fad as well as conventional diets. The frustration of repeated dieting leads some obese persons to turn to physicians for prescription medication and surgical procedures for managing their weight.

Weight-Loss Medication

Some obese people are candidates for taking prescribed medication to aid their weight-loss efforts. Such candidates generally have BMIs of 30 or more, or they have waist circumferences that exceed 40 inches (men) or 35 inches (women). Weight-loss medications approved by the U.S. Food and Drug Administration (FDA) for long-term use are Belviq, Qsymia, and Xenical (orlistat). When orlistat is taken along with a meal, the medication reduces fat digestion by about 30%. The undigested fat is eliminated in the feces and can cause an oily, unpleasant discharge. The fat carries fat-soluble vitamins along with it, and these micronutrients are eliminated in feces as well. Therefore, patients using orlistat often need to take a multiple vitamin supplement. In 2007, the FDA approved sales of the nonprescription form of orlistat ("Alli") as a weight-loss aid for adults.

The typical patient who uses orlistat in addition to a weight loss diet for up to 2 years loses only about 7 more pounds than if he or she used the diet without the medication.[63] Overfat people need to recognize that in some instances, prescription medication can aid their weight-loss efforts but do not replace the need to reduce calorie intake and increase physical activity.

Bariatric Surgical Procedures

Bariatric (*bar-ee-a'-tric*) **medicine** is the medical specialty that focuses on the treatment of obesity. Currently, *bariatric surgery* is the only effective method of treating extreme obesity.[37, 64] Such surgical procedures drastically reduce the size of an obese person's stomach, markedly limiting his or her food intake. As a result, obese patients may lose 50% or more of their excess weight.[65] Aside from helping obese people lose considerable amounts of weight and maintain the loss, bariatric surgery can produce dramatic health benefits. Patients often achieve normal blood pressure, glucose levels, and triglyceride levels after surgery. Furthermore, overall death rates are lower for extremely obese people who lose weight after undergoing bariatric surgery. Such surgeries are relatively safe: fewer than 1% of patients die as a result of a bariatric surgical procedure.[66]

bariatric medicine medical specialty that focuses on the treatment of obesity

In the United States, the two most common surgical approaches to treating obesity are the *Roux-en-Y (ru-en-wi') gastric bypass* and *gastric banding procedures*.[66] Both of these operations can be performed *laparoscopically*, that is, by using several small incisions that allow surgeons to insert instruments and a video camera into the abdomen. Laparoscopic bariatric surgical procedures reduce recovery time and the risk of infections.

During the Roux-en-Y operation, the surgeon staples across the upper part of the stomach to create a small pouch. This procedure reduces the obese patient's stomach capacity to about 1.5 oz, which is approximately the volume of one egg. (Normally, the stomach's capacity is about 32 oz.) Additionally, the surgeon cuts the small intestine and attaches the lower end of it to the newly formed stomach pouch (see Fig. 10.19a). The "bypassed" section of the intestine does not receive food, so digestion and absorption are reduced as a result of the surgery.

Sleeve gastrectomy is another form of bariatric surgery that reduces the stomach's size. During this procedure, the surgeon staples the stomach to form a banana-shaped pouch that holds about 2 to 5 ounces of food. The surgery does not involve bypassing a section of the small intestine, so nutrient absorption is not reduced (Fig. 10.19b). People who have undergone sleeve gastrectomy can eat only small portions of solid foods, which contributes to rapid weight loss. These patients also lose weight because they are not as hungry as they were before having the surgery. Why? The portion of the stomach that secretes ghrelin is removed during surgery, and as a result, hunger sensations are reduced. Sleeve gastrectomy surgery is irreversible, because the unused portion of the stomach is removed.

Complications often associated with gastric bypass surgery include intestinal blockage and bleeding, leaks along the staple site, blood clot formation, and wound infections. After surgery, gastric bypass patients can develop micronutrient deficiencies and some bone loss. However, patients can reduce their risk of nutrient deficiencies by taking vitamin and mineral supplements.

Did You Know?

The U.S. Federal Trade Commission (FTC) can prosecute promoters making fraudulent claims about the effectiveness of their weight-loss products. Enforma Natural Products, Inc., had to pay $10 million in fines after the company used false claims in ads for its "Fat Trapper" product.

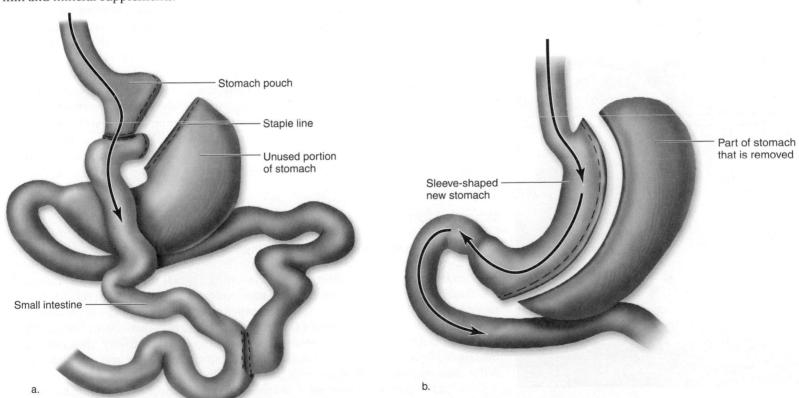

Figure 10.19 Gastric bypass surgeries. (*a*) The Roux-en-Y gastric bypass procedure reduces the obese patient's stomach capacity to about 1.5 oz. Additionally, the surgeon cuts the small intestine and attaches the lower end of it to the newly formed stomach pouch. (*b*) The sleeve gastrectomy procedure also reduces stomach volume, but the surgery does not involve an intestinal bypass. The procedure is not reversible, because the unused portion of the stomach is removed.

Figure 10.20 Adjustable gastric banding. When performing the adjustable gastric banding procedure, the surgeon creates a small stomach pouch with an adjustable band. By injecting *saline* (a weak salt water solution) into the port that lies beneath the patient's skin, the surgeon adjusts the tightness of the band and determines the size of the stomach pouch.

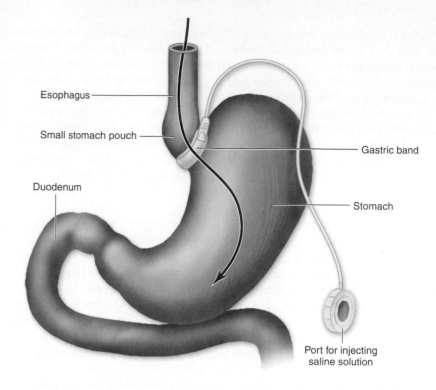

Esophagus

Small stomach pouch

Duodenum

Gastric band

Stomach

Port for injecting saline solution

liposuction surgical method of reducing the size of local fat deposits

fad trendy practice that has widespread appeal for a period, then becomes no longer fashionable

By performing the *adjustable gastric banding* procedure, the bariatric surgeon creates the small stomach pouch with an adjustable band instead of fixed surgical staples (Fig. 10.20). By adjusting the tightness of the band, the surgeon determines the size of the stomach. Laparoscopic gastric banding procedure is easier to perform and safer than the other types of bariatric surgery.[64] The procedure is also reversible. However, up to 60% of gastric bands require removal because of slippage or other complications.[66] Furthermore, obese people lose weight more slowly and they lose less weight than those who undergo gastric bypass or sleeve gastrectomy procedures.

Bariatric surgeries result in weight loss partly because the stomach pouch fills quickly with food and patients experience satiety sooner than prior to surgery. Moreover, overeating causes discomfort or vomiting. Thus, people who undergo such surgical procedures must make major lifestyle changes, such as learning to plan and consume frequent, small meals. Engaging in regular exercise and avoiding "soft calories," energy-dense high-calorie foods such as milk shakes and ice cream, are also important for maximizing weight loss and maintaining the lower body weight over time.

What Is Liposuction?

Liposuction is a surgical method of reducing the size of local subcutaneous fat deposits. Liposuction is not intended to treat obesity, but it can help a person improve the contours of his or her body. This procedure involves inserting a pencil-thin tube into an incision in the skin and suctioning the excess subcutaneous fat out of the body (Fig. 10.21). This procedure has risks, such as infection, permanent dimpling of the skin at the suctioning site, and blood clots or droplets of fat that can enter the bloodstream and be deadly. Liposuction is usually considered cosmetic rather than necessary surgery; therefore, health insurance plans are not likely to cover its costs. Despite the expense and risks, liposuction is the most common type of cosmetic surgery in the United States.

A highly promoted treatment involves injecting chemicals into subcutaneous fat tissue that supposedly "dissolve" the fat without the need for surgical suctioning. (The procedure may make you wonder what happens to the fat after it "dissolves.") At this point, there is a lack of reliable scientific evidence to support the safety and effectiveness of this method.[67]

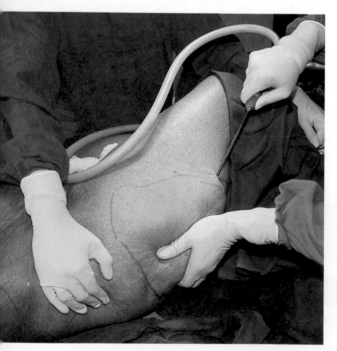

Figure 10.21 Liposuction. Liposuction is a surgical procedure that involves inserting a pencil-thin tube into an incision in the skin and suctioning the excess fat out of the body.

Concept **Checkpoint**

37. Explain how orlistat (Xenical) can aid weight-loss efforts.

38. Describe the two most common types of bariatric surgery in the United States. Why is bariatric surgery effective? Compared to gastric stapling procedures, what is a major advantage of gastric banding?

39. What is liposuction? List three risks associated with this procedure.

10.8 Unreliable Weight-Loss Methods

Each year, Americans spend about $50 billion on products and services promoted to help them lose weight.[10] Some overweight or obese people join commercial weight-loss programs that have "good track records" for encouraging successful weight loss and maintenance. Other overfat persons obtain individual dietary counseling from a registered dietitian to help them lose weight. By recognizing that it took months and probably years to gain the excess fat, individuals may be more likely to accept advice and diets that result in slow but steady weight loss. However, many overweight and obese people seek "quick fixes" to lose weight, such as *fad* diets and dietary supplements promoted to "burn" or "melt" fat fast.

Fad Diets

A **fad** is a trendy practice that has widespread appeal among a population. After a period, however, people lose interest in the practice, and it becomes no longer fashionable. Table 10.7 presents some popular fad weight-loss diets and their features.

TABLE 10.7 *Examples of Popular Fad Weight-Loss Diets*

Approach	Examples	Features	Outcomes
Restricted carbohydrates	Dr. Atkins New Diet Revolution; Calories Don't Count; The Complete Scarsdale Medical Diet; Enter the Zone; Sugar Busters!; South Beach Diet—especially initial phase; Protein Power; G.I. (*Glycemic Index*) Diet; Dr. Gott's No Flour, No Sugar Diet	Generally less than 100 g of carbohydrate daily May emphasize specific carbohydrate choices, such as eating primarily low–glycemic index foods	Ketosis due to excess burning of fat; may cause fatigue, constipation, headaches, and bad breath May improve blood lipid levels and reduce the risk of CVD for up to 1 year After 1 year, amount of weight loss is comparable to that achieved by following low-fat diets.
Low fat	The Rice Diet; Rice Diet Solution; The Macrobiotic Diet (some versions); Pritikin Diet; T-Factor Diet; Fit or Fat; The McDougall Plan; Lean Bodies; Turn Off the Fat Genes; The Pasta Diet; Eat More, Weigh Less; G-Index Diet	Generally less than 20% of calories from fat Limited or no sources of animal protein Limited nuts and seeds	Excess fiber may result in increased intestinal gas Difficult to follow for long periods because food choices are so limited Limited food choices may lead to feelings of food deprivation.
Diets with gimmicks	hCG diet; Dr. Berger's Immune Power Diet; Fit for Life; The Beverly Hills Diet; F-Plan Diet; The Princeton Diet; 3-Hour Diet; Fat Smash Diet; Ultrametabolism; Eat to Win; Cabbage Soup Diet; Grapefruit Diet; Eat Right for Your Type	Promotes certain nutrients, foods, or combinations of foods as having unique, magical, or previously unreported weight-loss-promoting properties	Undernutrition if followed for a long period Such diets generally do not encourage changing exercise and food-related habits.

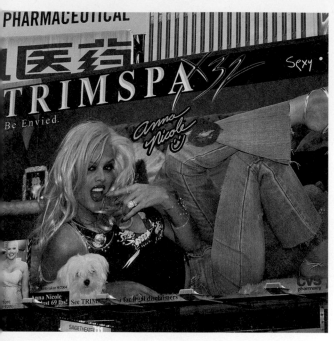

The late model Anna Nicole Smith appeared in advertisements for TrimSpa, a weight-loss supplement.

People often lose weight while following fad diets; however, they usually regain much of the weight that was lost while on the diet when they resume their prior eating and other lifestyle habits. Too often, people think of a weight-loss diet as a temporary change in their eating habits. Achieving a healthy body weight and maintaining that weight requires making lifestyle changes that a person adopts for the rest of his or her life.

Fad diets often rely on *gimmicks*. A gimmick is a novel feature that makes the diet seem to be unique and more likely to work than other diets. Some fad diets use the gimmick of emphasizing one food or food group while excluding almost all others. The cabbage soup and grapefruit diets are examples of fad diets that promote eating single foods. Dieters may lose some weight while following eating plans that restrict food variety, but the weight loss occurs because the diet is low in calories, not because cabbage, grapefruit, or other "special food" contains compounds that cause rapid weight loss. Following such diets for a few days often results in boredom and monotony. Eventually, dieters abandon such restrictive menu plans because they just cannot face another cup of cabbage soup or bowl of grapefruit. Weight regain occurs when dieters return to their former eating habits—the habits that contributed to their original overweight or obese conditions.

Fad diets will come and go. However, if you examine any diet plan carefully, you can determine whether it is probably a fad. A typical fad diet

- Offers a "quick fix"; that is, the diet promotes rapid weight loss without calorie restriction and increased physical activity.
- Limits food selections from a few food groups and dictates specific rituals, such as eating only fruit for breakfast or eating only certain food combinations.
- Requires buying a book or various gimmicks, such as expensive dietary supplements, weight-loss patches, or cellulite-reducing creams.
- Uses outlandish and unscientific claims to support its usefulness. For example, *The Beverly Hills Diet* book promoted the notion that people become fat because food "gets stuck" in their bodies, rots, and produces toxins. Another author of a fad diet book claimed people can lose weight by following diet plans based on their blood types. These notions and recommendations are not supported by scientific evidence.
- Relies on testimonials from famous people or connects the diet to trendy places such as Beverly Hills, California, and South Beach, Florida.
- Does not emphasize the need to change eating habits and physical activity patterns.

Low-Carbohydrate Approaches

Fad weight-loss diets that limit carbohydrate intakes and are high in protein and saturated fat include the Dr. Atkins' New Diet Revolution, the Scarsdale Diet, and the early phases of the South Beach Diet. A weight-reduction diet is low carbohydrate if it eliminates or severely restricts the intake of carbohydrate-rich foods such as breads, cereals, fruits, vegetables, and sweets. The lack of variety often leads to boredom with the selection of foods, and as a result, people lose weight because they tend to eat less. On the other hand, people who follow low-carbohydrate/high-protein diets tend to like the diet plan more and have less difficulty adhering to the diets than people who are on low-fat diets.[68]

Low-carbohydrate diets usually produce rapid weight loss initially, primarily because the body loses water. Why? The body produces less glycogen when carbohydrate intake is low and uses much of its stored glycogen to supply glucose for energy. Tissues maintain about 3 grams of water with each gram of glycogen, so a reduction in body glycogen content results in the need for less water to store with it. The kidneys eliminate the excess water in urine. Furthermore, a very-low-carbohydrate intake causes the liver to produce glucose, mostly from certain amino acids supplied by the body's tissue proteins. Protein tissue also contains a lot of water. When protein-rich tissues are dismantled and their amino acids used for energy, the water that was stored with the proteins also ends up in urine.

An analysis of 13 studies indicated that after 6 months, people on low-carbohydrate/high-protein diet plans lost an average of about 9 pounds more than people on low-fat/high-carbohydrate diets.[68] After 12 months, however, people on the carbohydrate-restricted diets weighed only about 2 pounds less than people following the low-fat diets. Low-carbohydrate diets resulted in more favorable high-density lipoprotein ("good cholesterol") and serum triglyceride levels. According to the authors of this review, low-carbohydrate diets may be as effective as or even more effective than low-fat diets for reducing weight and risk of cardiovascular disease (CVD) for up to 1 year. More studies, however, are needed to determine whether low-carbohydrate diets are safe and reduce the risk of CVD for longer periods.

Very-Low-Fat Approaches

Very-low-fat diets are actually very-high-carbohydrate diets. These diets supply approximately 5 to 10% of calories from fat and generally result in rapid weight loss when followed consistently. The most notable are the Pritikin Diet and Dr. Dean Ornish's "Eat More, Weigh Less" diet plans. Very-low-fat diets are not harmful for healthy adults, but they are difficult to follow for the long term. Fat contributes to the flavor and texture of foods. Extremely low-fat diets are not tasty, and they eliminate many foods that are usually high on peoples' favorite foods lists, such as ice cream and meat. Although grains, fruits, and vegetables are nutrient-dense foods, eating them repeatedly and without fat can cause "diet boredom."

Dietary Supplements for Weight Loss

Many overweight and obese people are attracted to dietary supplements for weight loss because they believe promoters' claims that their products are "magic bullets" for shedding unwanted weight quickly and effortlessly.[69] Although several different types of weight-loss supplements are available, these products generally have not been scientifically tested in humans for safety and effectiveness.

In 2004, FDA banned the sale of most dietary supplements that contained the natural stimulant ephedra (*eh-feh'-dra*) or ephedra-related compounds, after the agency received reports of serious side effects and even deaths resulting from use of these products. The death in 2003 of Steve Bechler, Baltimore Orioles baseball player, was linked to ephedra (Fig. 10.22). Table 10.8 presents science-based findings about some popular weight-loss supplements, including their potential usefulness and safety concerns. At this point, medical experts do not recommend any dietary supplement for weight loss.[69]

Analyzing Advertising Hype for Weight-Loss Supplements

Maybe you have heard or read remarkable claims for weight-loss products such as "Lose weight while you sleep," "Lose 30 pounds in just 30 days," and "Eat anything you want and still lose weight." In general, advertising claims that a product promises quick and easy weight loss are too good to be true. According to an investigation conducted by the Federal Trade Commission (FTC) in 2001, 55% of the 300 advertisements for weight-loss products included false or misleading claims.[70]

The FTC study identified several features, including typical claims, for popular weight-loss products and services. The agency's report also provided reasons why you should be skeptical of such features when they are used in magazine ads, in television infomercials, or on Internet websites. According to the FTC, you should be wary of claims that the product or service:

- *Causes rapid and extreme weight loss*. Ads commonly use outrageous claims such as "Lose up to 18 pounds in one week!" to attract consumers. The use of the modifier "up to" means that the person using the product could lose considerably less than 18 pounds a week.

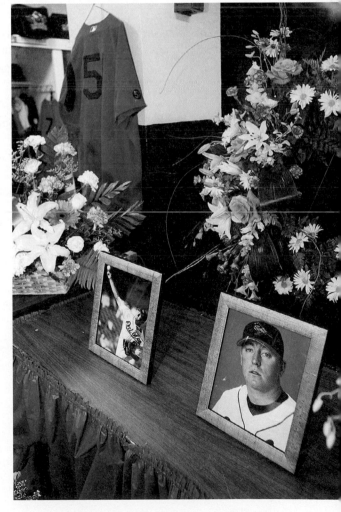

Figure 10.22 Toxic herbal supplement. In 2003, Baltimore Orioles pitcher Steve Bechler's death was linked to ephedra. Bechler had taken a large dose of an ephedra-containing supplement a few hours before he died.

TABLE 10.8 *Summary of Selected Weight-Loss Supplements*

Supplement	Usefulness	Side Effects/Safety Concerns (Usual Doses)
Beta-hydroxy-betamethylbutyrate	May decrease adipose tissue and increase lean body mass, but more research is needed	None reported
Chinese diet pills, Chaso Diet Capsules, Chaso Genpi	Not determined	Linked to illness and deaths in Japan May contain the active drug fenfluramine
Chitosan	Doubtful	May cause gastrointestinal discomfort including nausea, constipation, and intestinal gas
Chromium picolinate	May enhance weight loss to a small extent	None reported, but may damage DNA
*Green Tea or Extracts**	May enhance weight loss to a small extent	Concentrated extracts linked to severe liver damage
Ephedrine (ma huang, ephedra, ephedra sinica, sida cordifolia, pinellia, and ephedrine with caffeine)	Ephedrine-containing products promote short-term weight loss but also increase risk of serious side effects. Ephedra-containing dietary supplements are banned in the United States.	May cause rapid heart rate, elevated blood pressure, dizziness, sweating, headache, and sleep disturbances Linked to heart attacks, strokes, and deaths
*GHB (gamma hydroxybutyrate, liquid ecstasy, GBL)***	GHB is illegal in the United States, except for FDA-approved studies.	May cause nausea, vomiting, delusions, seizures, breathing difficulties, and coma Linked to more than 45 deaths in the United States
Garcinia cambogia (hydroxycitric acid, HCA)	Conflicting results, but overall evidence does not suggest usefulness	May cause headache and gastrointestinal discomfort
Glucomannan	May be effective, but more research is needed	None reported
Guar gum	Not effective	May cause diarrhea and intestinal gas
Hoodia	Not effective	Vomiting, increased blood pressure and heart rate, signs of liver damage
Human Chorionic Gonadotropin (hCG)	Not effective	Unknown
Pyruvate	Not effective	None reported
Spirulina (blue-green algae)	Not effective	Unknown

Sources: Pittler MH, Ernst E: Dietary supplements for body-weight reduction: A systematic review. *American Journal of Clinical Nutrition* 79:529, 2004.

Saper RB and others: Common dietary supplements for weight loss. *American Family Physician* 70:1731, 2004.

*Hursel R and others: The effects of green tea on weight loss and weight management: a meta-analysis. *International Journal of Obesity* advance online publication, 14 July 2009; doi:10.1038/ijo.2009.135; Sarma DN and others: Safety of green tea extracts: a systematic review by the US Pharmacopeia. *Drug Safety* 31(6): 469, 2008.

**Nordenberg T: The death of the party: All the rave, GHB's hazards go unheeded. *FDA Consumer* 34:14, 2000.

- *Requires no need to change dietary patterns or physical activity.* Principles of energy balance do not support claims such as "Lose weight without dieting or strenuous exercise" and "Eat as much as you want—the more you eat, the more you'll lose." Regular exercise and moderate energy intake are necessary for weight loss and long-term maintenance.
- *Results in permanent weight loss.* Claims such as "Discover the secret to permanent weight loss" and "Lose weight and keep it off" often appear in ads. These claims target consumers who have lost weight but gained it back and are wary of weight-loss products. Long-term weight loss is difficult to achieve without calorie reduction and regular exercise, and claims that permanent weight loss can result simply from using a product are questionable.[70]

- *Is scientifically proven or doctor endorsed.* Some ads claim their product or service has been "clinically tested," "scientifically proven," or "physician recommended." Scientific testing of the product or service supposedly occurred at "respected" or "leading" medical centers or universities. However, most ads do not provide information about testing sites or journals where the results were published. Such information is critical for assessing the reliability of claims. Endorsements by "doctors" or medical professionals can be misleading. A doctor could be someone with a bogus doctorate degree (Ph.D.) or a Ph.D. in a nonscientific field. Moreover, consumers need to be aware that the "professionals" pictured or featured in the ads may be models or fictional characters.
- *Includes a money-back guarantee.* Consumers should recognize that a product does not necessarily work just because it is guaranteed. The FTC frequently sues companies that fail to return money to dissatisfied consumers as their ads guaranteed.
- *Is safe or natural.* Ads may include safety-related claims, such as "proven 100% safe" or "safe, immediate weight loss." Additionally, the term "natural" often accompanies safety claims, implying that "natural" weight-loss products are safer than prescribed weight-loss treatments. Despite such assurances, weight-loss supplement manufacturers usually have little scientific evidence to support safety claims, particularly concerning long-term use of their products. Furthermore, "natural" does not indicate safety. Mushrooms are natural, but many species of the fungi are highly toxic and even deadly.
- *Is supported by satisfied customers.* Ads for weight-loss products or services typically feature testimonials from satisfied users. The assumption is that if the product worked for the person providing the testimonial, it should work for anyone. According to the FTC, testimonials generally provide little reliable information about what consumers can expect from using the product.
- *Displays before-and-after photos.* Many ads use photos of "satisfied" customers to support claims that their weight-loss products are effective. In the typical "before" photo, the subject has poor posture, no smile, unkempt hair, and unfashionable, unflattering clothing. In the "after" photo, the person stands with his or her shoulders held back and abdomen tucked in. Additionally, the subject is usually smiling and appears more attractive than in the "before" photo. If you read carefully, you may find disclaimers in small print, such as "results not typical," at the bottom of the "after" photo.

The FTC presents an ad for a mythical product called "FatFoe" at its interactive website (http://wemarket4u.net/fatfoe/). The ad includes typical features of weight-loss product advertising, such as a physician's endorsement and guarantee.

Concept **Checkpoint**

40. What is a "fad" diet? List at least four typical features of fad diets.
41. Why do fad diets and dietary supplements promoted for weight loss appeal to overfat people?
42. Identify at least four popular weight-loss supplements and indicate whether each supplement is safe and effective.
43. Discuss at least three features or claims that are commonly used in ads for weight-loss products or services.

underweight describes person with a BMI of less than 18.5

10.9 Gaining Weight

In 2003–2006, 2.6% of Americans who were 20 to 39 years of age were underweight.[71] An **underweight** individual has a BMI that is less than 18.5. Factors that contribute to underweight include genetics, lifestyle practices, chronic diseases, and psychological disturbances.

It is often difficult to pinpoint a cause of underweight; multiple factors contribute to having a lower-than-average body weight. Individuals who inherit higher resting metabolic rates, tall body frames, or both may find it difficult to gain weight. Excessive physical activity can result in low body weight. Compared to sedentary adults, the bodies of rapidly growing, physically active children and adolescents have higher energy needs. If these children do not consume enough energy, they can lose weight. Chronic diseases such as cancer, tuberculosis, AIDS, and *inflammatory bowel disease* often result in severe weight loss that is difficult to treat. Some people who suffer from depression fail to eat enough food to support their energy needs, and they lose weight as a result.

If a person's BMI was within the healthy range before excessive weight loss occurred, an evaluation by a physician may be necessary to determine the cause or causes of the loss, especially when the underweight person has not tried to shed pounds. A thorough medical examination can rule out possible reasons for unintentional weight loss, such as hormonal imbalances, depression, cancer, and infectious or digestive tract diseases.

Many underweight individuals want to gain weight, especially muscle mass. For an underweight person, gaining weight can be just as challenging as losing weight is for an overfat person. To gain weight, underweight adults can gradually increase their consumption of calorie-dense foods, especially those high in healthy fats. Fatty fish, such as salmon; olives; avocados; seeds; low-fat cheeses; nuts and nut butters; bananas; and granola made with dried fruit, seeds, and nuts are high-calorie nutritious food choices with low saturated-fat content. Additionally, underweight people can replace beverages such as soft drinks with more nutritious calorie sources, such as 100% fruit juices, smoothies, and milk shakes made with peanut butter and fat-reduced ice cream. Encouraging a regular meal and snack schedule also aids in weight gain and maintenance.

Sometimes people who are underweight are too busy to eat, and as a result, their caloric intakes are too low to support weight gain. If physical activity habits contribute to their inability to increase their weight, underweight people can find ways to be less active. If their weight remains low, underweight persons can add muscle mass through a *resistance-training* (weight-lifting) program, but they must increase their calorie intake to support the additional exercise. Otherwise, gaining muscle tissue is not likely to occur.

In many instances, healthy underweight people may have to accept their body builds. Furthermore, they can realize the health benefits of being lean and the sheer enjoyment of being able to eat a variety of foods without gaining weight. For the typical slim person, the passage of time is usually all that is necessary for weight gain to occur, as the aging process is often accompanied with increasing body fat.

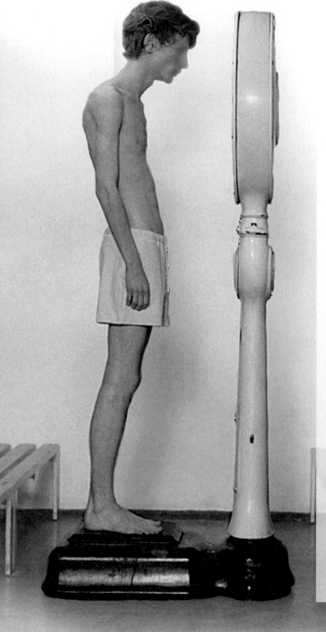

Many underweight individuals are interested in gaining weight, especially muscle mass.

Concept **Checkpoint**

44. List at least three health conditions that are often associated with underweight.
45. Discuss at least three measures an underweight person can take to gain lean mass safely.

Chapter 10 Highlight

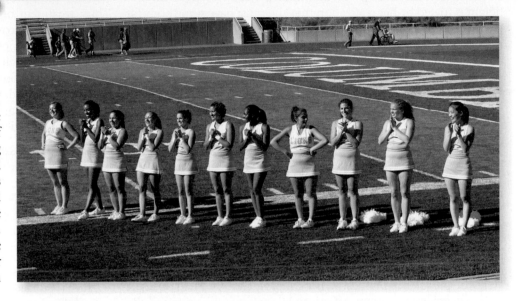

EATING DISORDERS: OVER THE DEEP EDGE

By the time she was a junior in high school, Emily Manoff was on top of her world. She had been freshman class president, captain of the cheerleading squad, and a homecoming "maid." Although she was academically and socially successful, Emily sensed that her peers were jealous of her. Also, she was concerned about her weight—130 pounds. At 5'2", she had a BMI (23.8) within the healthy range. Nevertheless, Emily began an effort to lose some weight after she overheard a teacher commenting that her cheerleading uniform was too tight.

At first, Emily's food choices were healthy, but soon she began skipping breakfast. Eventually, she stopped eating every other day, and when she did eat, she ate mostly fruit, vegetables, and some bagels with cream cheese. She avoided milk but drank lots of diet soft drinks. Occasionally, she would *binge eat*, that is, lose control over her restrictive eating practices. During such food binges, Emily consumed large amounts of fat-free ice cream and sugar-coated cereal. However, she did not practice *purging*, self-induced vomiting and other techniques intended to prevent macronutrients from being absorbed by the digestive tract.

While limiting her food intake, Emily increased her calorie output. She burned calories during intense cheerleading workouts that lasted 90 minutes every day after school. Following the exhausting workouts, she would run around the school's track, thinking to herself, "I may pass out any second"—yet she continued to run.

As Emily lost weight, people began to take notice of her appearance and she received compliments. According to Emily, "The positive attention fueled continued dieting . . . it [dieting] took me over." Although she was hungry all the time, she suppressed the urge to eat. When her weight loss became excessive, her parents were very concerned about her health. Although Emily agreed to see therapists to obtain counseling, at that point, she was not ready to be helped.

After graduating from high school, Emily moved to Florida, a considerable distance from her family, so she could be a singer in a band. A few months after making the move, she woke up in the middle of the night. Her heart was racing, and she thought she was having a heart attack. She called her mother and cried, "I can't live like this anymore." Fearing her daughter was going to die, Emily's mother flew to Florida and brought her home. At this point, Emily weighed about 90 pounds. She finally realized she wanted to live, and to live, she had to eat.

When Emily returned home, she threw out the bathroom scale. She promised herself not to skip meals, and she limited her exercise regimen to an hour a day. Within a few months, her weight climbed to 120 pounds. Although she felt her body was getting

(continued)

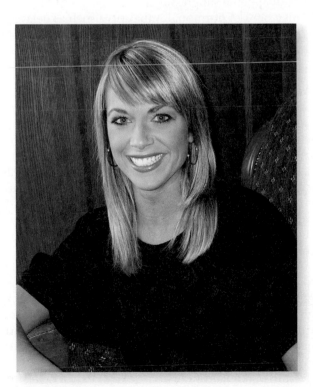

| Emily Manoff

back to normal, she decided to obtain counseling to help deal with the emotional and physical changes she was experiencing.

Today, Emily is healthy, employed as a nanny for three children, married, and attending college part time. Emily loves being around children. Her motivation to maintain a healthy weight for her height is fueled by her realization that she must have some body fat to become pregnant someday. Her advice: "The decisions you're making now affect you forever. Take care of your body; nurture it, and remember—not everyone is meant to be a supermodel!"

Emily suffered from *anorexia nervosa*, a serious eating disorder that is more common among young women than among young men. Fortunately, she was able to recover completely from this disorder. Many people who suffer from anorexia nervosa do not regain healthy body weights; some even die as a result of starvation.

What is an eating disorder? How can you distinguish quirky eating behaviors from harmful eating disorders? What are the typical signs of eating disorders? How are eating disorders treated? By reading this "Highlight," you will find the answers to these questions.

Disordered Eating or Eating Disorder?

With the prevalence of obesity rising rapidly in the United States, it is not surprising that many American adolescents and young adults are concerned about their body shape and weight. Furthermore, the media constantly bombards us with images of the "ideal" body. Television shows and movies often portray thin women or muscular men as happy and successful. Excessive concern about body size and social pressure to avoid weight gain can lead to *disordered eating*, chaotic and abnormal food-related practices such as skipping meals, limiting food choices, following fad diets, and bingeing on food. Disordered eating behaviors are temporary and often occur when a person is under a lot of stress or wants to lose weight to improve his or her appearance. When a person adopts disordered eating behaviors as a lifestyle, the practices can become harmful and difficult-to-treat *eating disorders*.

Eating disorders are psychological disturbances that lead to certain physiological changes and serious health complications. According to the American Psychiatric Association, females are more likely to develop eating disorders than males.[72] In most cases, eating disorders develop during adolescence or early adulthood, but these conditions may begin at any age. A person who has an eating disorder typically experiences problems adjusting to the demands of work and school as well as those involving relationships.

The causes of eating disorders are unknown, but genetic, social, and psychological factors contribute to their development. Risk factors for eating disorders include being a female, having low self-esteem, experiencing sexual abuse as a child, being teased

eating disorders psychological disturbances that lead to certain physiological changes and serious health complications

anorexia nervosa (AN) severe psychological disturbance characterized by self-imposed starvation

about weight, dieting repeatedly to lose weight, having a perfectionist personality, and being in a dysfunctional family.[72] Mood and anxiety disorders as well as substance abuse often accompany these conditions, but it is not clear whether eating disorders cause psychological problems or are the result of mental disturbances. Thus, treatment of eating disorders is complex, involving more than just dietary counseling.

If you or someone you know has an eating disorder, it is important to seek help for the condition as early as possible—before the behavior becomes highly ingrained or the affected person's life is at risk. In academic environments, professional help is commonly available at student health centers and student guidance/counseling facilities on college campuses.

Anorexia Nervosa Anorexia nervosa (AN) is a severe psychological disturbance characterized by self-imposed starvation that results in malnutrition and low body weight. In developed countries, AN affects about 1 in 200 women.[73] An estimated 0.3% to 3.7% of American females suffer from anorexia nervosa.[72] Although males also develop AN, females comprise most cases. People suffering from AN

- Maintain BMIs of 17.5 or less.
- Have distorted body images. Patients deny they are too thin and they are overly concerned about becoming fat.
- Are obsessed with losing weight.
- Avoid "fattening foods."
- Engage in one or more of the following practices:
  - self-induced vomiting
  - abuse of laxatives or diuretics
  - excessive exercise regimens
  - use of appetite suppressants
- Display signs of hormonal imbalances such as delayed puberty, loss of menstrual periods in females, and loss of sexual interest and functioning in males.
- Are depressed and anxious.[74]

Young women suffering from AN have lower-than-normal estrogen levels that not only result in failure to menstruate but can also accelerate bone loss and cause premature osteoporosis. Other physical signs of the condition include severe constipation; widespread delicate, dense, white hairs on the skin (*lanugo hair*); and shrunken breasts and buttocks. People with AN often wear layers of clothing to keep warm, because they lack adequate subcutaneous fat and they want to hide their extremely thin appearances.

Effective treatment for AN usually involves a team of health professionals, including registered dietitians, physicians, nurses, and mental health counselors, who are specially trained to treat the condition. Dietitians work with patients to restore healthy weight and promote healthy attitudes toward food and gaining weight. Additionally, dietitians are sources of accurate food and nutrition information for patients with AN and other eating disorders. A key goal of treatment is for patients to achieve and maintain healthy BMIs.

People suffering from AN have a high risk of dying from starvation, electrolyte imbalances, or suicide.[75] Five percent of people with AN eventually die as a result of the disorder.[75] Although nearly 50% of patients fully recover from AN, the illness becomes chronic in about 20% of cases. AN patients who binge eat and then follow up binges with *purging* activities, such as self-induced vomiting or laxative abuse, are more likely to have poor long-term outcomes.[76] On the other hand, patients who do not binge eat or purge and have good relationships with their parents are more likely to recover.

Bulimia Nervosa   An estimated 1.0 to 4.2% of the U.S. population has **bulimia nervosa,** a condition characterized by cyclic episodes of overeating (bingeing) and calorie-restrictive dieting.[72] As in cases of anorexia nervosa, females are more likely to have bulimia nervosa than males. People with "bulimia" often consume cakes, cookies, ice cream, and other high-fat high-carbohydrate foods during binges. After a binge, the person attempts to *purge* the calories consumed during binges by vomiting and abusing laxatives, diuretics, or enemas. Another way a bulimic person attempts to avoid gaining weight after a binge is by exercising excessively.

People with bulimia frequently induce vomiting by thrusting fingers deep into their mouths and, as a result, scrape their knuckles. Thus, characteristic signs of bulimia nervosa are bite marks and scars on the knuckles. Dentists often identify people who practice bulimia because the acid in vomit erodes the enamel on the surfaces of teeth, especially the backs of teeth.

The practice of inducing vomiting leads to many of the health problems associated with bulimia nervosa. Repeated vomiting can cause

- Blood chemistry abnormalities; blood potassium can drop dramatically, altering heartbeat and increasing risk of sudden death.
- Swelling of the salivary glands in the mouth as a result of infection or irritation.
- Tears and bleeding of the esophagus.

Unlike people who have anorexia nervosa, people with bulimia are often difficult to identify by their appearances, because they tend to have BMIs in the normal or overweight range. Furthermore, they usually hide their binge-purge behaviors from others. Many people with the condition lie about their food-related behaviors to family and friends, and they resort to shoplifting groceries because they cannot afford to buy such large amounts of food. Persons with bulimia nervosa often have low self-esteem, and they feel guilty and depressed after a binge. The compelling need to binge and purge eventually becomes a preoccupation for people with bulimia, and as a result, they become less involved in social activities and more isolated. Some people show behavioral characteristics of both anorexia nervosa and bulimia nervosa, because the illnesses can overlap. About half of the women diagnosed as having anorexia nervosa eventually develop signs of bulimia.

Effective treatment for bulimia nervosa, as for anorexia nervosa, requires a team of medical professionals who have experience treating eating disorders. A key goal of treatment is having patients with bulimia develop a plan to eat normally.[77] Dietitians can help people with the disorder by providing reliable

bulimia nervosa eating disorder characterized by cyclic episodes of bingeing and calorie-restrictive dieting

nutrition information and suggestions for developing healthy eating patterns. For example, patients may be encouraged to keep a food diary to monitor their food intake and help identify situations that trigger binge episodes. Psychotherapy can also help patients learn to change unhealthy beliefs about themselves, accept themselves, and use alternative methods—other than bingeing—to cope with stressful situations. Additionally, patients may need to take certain prescribed medications, particularly antidepressants. Up to 60% of people with bulimia nervosa improve with treatment.[74]

Other Eating Disorders   Some people have eating disorders that are not classified as anorexia nervosa or bulimia nervosa. The prevalence of *night eating syndrome* (*NES*) and *binge-eating disorder* (*BED*) is difficult to estimate, but these conditions may be as common as anorexia nervosa and bulimia nervosa.[77] People with NES and BED experience episodic food binges that are not followed by purging. A person with NES consumes more than 50% of his or her daily calorie intake during the evening or overnight.[77] The condition is also characterized by sleep disturbances, including waking up during the night to binge eat. Obesity is often associated with NES as well as BED.

For people with BED and NES, stressful events and feelings of loneliness, anxiety, depression, anger, isolation, and frustration can trigger a food binge. During binges, a person with BED typically isolates him- or herself and consumes large quantities of calorie-dense foods, such as ice cream, cookies, sweets, and potato chips. While bingeing, the person may feel better, but after the episode of overeating, this individual usually feels depressed, ashamed, guilty, and disgusted with him- or herself.

People who experienced sexual and physical abuse as children are at risk of BED.[78] The condition may develop in people who never learned to express and deal appropriately with their negative

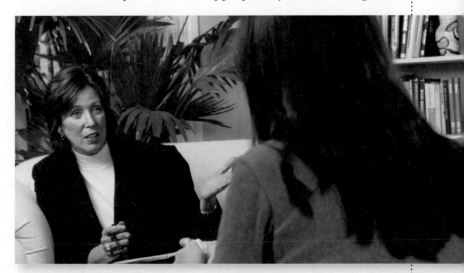

Psychotherapy can help patients with eating disorders learn to change unhealthy beliefs about themselves.

feelings. Treatment for BED usually includes individual and group therapy. A major goal of treatment is to reduce the patient's frequency of binges. In therapy, the BED patient learns how to eat in response to hunger rather than emotional needs or external factors, such as the presence of food. Some experts feel that learning to eat all foods—but in moderation—is an effective behavioral goal for binge eaters. This practice may prevent people with BED from feeling deprived and frustrated. Antidepressants may also be helpful, because such medications can improve the patient's negative moods that often trigger food binges.

Female Athlete Triad An estimated 62% of female athletes and 33% of male athletes have eating disorders.[79] Females participating in appearance-based competitive sports that require low body mass, such as gymnastics, swimming, and distance running, are at risk

of developing the **female athlete triad.** This condition is characterized by low energy intakes, abnormal menstrual cycles, and bone mineral irregularities.[79] Severe food restriction and chronic emotional stress can result in lower blood estrogen levels that, in turn, can cause the absence of menstrual cycles. Furthermore, estrogen is needed to maintain bone mineral mass. Thus, young women with low estrogen levels have bones that are less dense and weaker than normal. As a result, these women have an increased risk of bone fractures such as "stress" fractures.

Patients with symptoms of the female athlete triad should seek treatment from a multidisciplinary team of health professionals. The goal of treatment is improving the nutritional state of the patient to reverse the signs and symptoms of her disordered eating practices. However, highly competitive athletes may not be willing to accept necessary treatment plans. Until she recovers, the female athlete may need to decrease the time she spends in training or the intensity of her workouts by 10 percent.[80]

> **female athlete triad** condition characterized by low energy intakes, abnormal menstrual cycles, and bone mineral irregularities

CHAPTER REFERENCES

See Appendix I.

SUMMARY

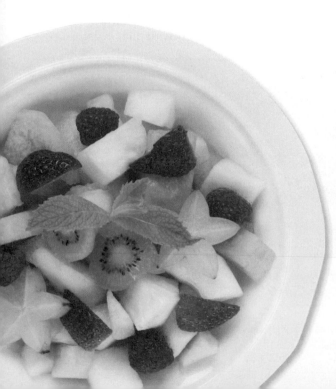

The prevalence of overweight and obesity has reached epidemic proportions in the United States and throughout the world. Over two-thirds of American adults were either overweight or obese in 2007 to 2008; about one-third of the adults were obese. The prevalence of obese American infants, children, and adolescents has risen sharply over the past 25 years.

The body is composed of two major compartments: total body fat and fat-free mass. Overfat people have excessive adipose tissue. Percentage of body fat is associated with risks of obesity-related diseases. According to certain standards, a man is overweight when his body is 22 to 25% fat; a woman is overweight when her body is 32 to 37% fat. A man is obese when fat comprises 26% or more of his body; a woman is obese when fat makes up 38% or more of her body.

In addition to percentage of body fat, medical experts use BMI to determine whether one's weight is healthy. BMIs of 18.5 to 24.9 are healthy; BMIs of 25.0 to 29.9 are in the overweight range. Persons with BMIs of 30.0 or more are obese.

Biological fuels are foods and beverages that contain macronutrients and the nonnutrient alcohol. Under normal conditions, human cells metabolize primarily glucose and fatty acids, but small amounts of amino acids are also used for energy. Cells release the energy stored in biological fuels by breaking bonds within the molecules. Cells obtain only about 40% of the energy that was in macronutrients by forming ATP. Cells release the remaining energy as heat.

Basal or resting metabolism, physical activity, TEF, and NEAT account for total energy use by the body. Metabolism accounts for the largest share of an average person's daily energy needs. Various factors including thyroid hormone, body composition, gender, and age influence the metabolic rate. Physical activity is energy use by skeletal muscle movement. TEF is the increase in energy needs that occurs during digestion, absorption, and processing of nutrients in food. NEAT is energy use for involuntary skeletal muscle activities, such as shivering.

Energy balance is a state in which a person's calorie intake from food and beverages equals his or her calorie output for metabolism, physical activity, TEF, and NEAT. Negative energy balance occurs when calorie output is greater than calorie intake, resulting in weight loss. Positive energy balance occurs when calorie intake is greater than calorie output, resulting in weight gain.

People with BMIs greater than 25 have increased risks of CVD, hypertension, type 2 diabetes, and certain cancers. Compared to people with healthy BMIs, obese people are more likely to die prematurely from all causes. Body fat distribution is associated with obesity-related diseases. Excessive central-body fat (apple shape) is associated with increased risks of CVD, type 2 diabetes, and hypertension. Waist circumferences that exceed 40 inches (men) or 35 inches (women) are linked to obesity-related diseases.

There is no simple cause for obesity. From a physiological standpoint, eating behavior is complex and largely involves interactions among the nervous, endocrine, and digestive systems, as well as fat tissue. Dietary and inherited factors also influence body weight. Additionally, overfat people may have inherited genes for "thrifty metabolisms." According to the set-point theory, the body's fat content is genetically predetermined. The set point may protect the body from losing weight and explain why weight loss is so difficult to achieve and maintain.

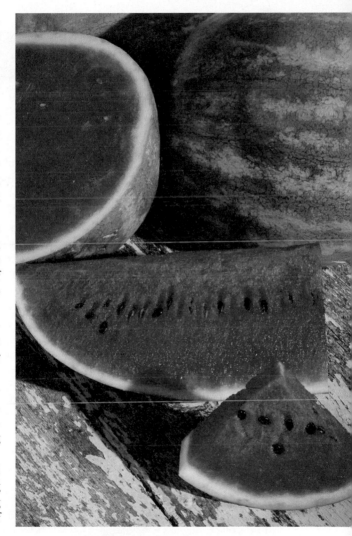

Environmental factors, such as food advertising, can have a powerful influence on food choices and appetite. The increased consumption of oversized portions of restaurant foods may be partly responsible for the obesity epidemic. The environment also influences people's patterns of physical activity. According to experts with the American College of Sports Medicine and the American Heart Association, healthy adults under 65 years of age should perform 30 minutes of moderate-intensity physical activity five days of the week.

A reliable weight-loss plan is safe and effective, and the plan should meet the dieter's nutritional, psychological, and social needs. Successful weight loss and long-term weight maintenance involve four key elements: motivation, caloric reduction, regular physical activity, and behavior modification.

A pound of adipose tissue supplies about 3500 kcal. If energy output exceeds calorie intake by about 500 kcal per day, a person can expect to lose a pound of fat per week. The healthiest way to lower total calorie intake is to reduce consumption of added sugars, fats, and alcohol. A dieter's goal should be reducing total calorie intake while obtaining all essential nutrients.

Members of the National Weight Control Registry have lost weight and maintained their lower weights by eating a low-calorie, low-fat, high-carbohydrate diet; maintaining the same diet regimen every day; eating regular meals, including breakfast; weighing themselves frequently; exercising at least 60 minutes daily; and eating a limited variety of nutritious foods.

At present, the FDA has approved three medications for weight loss. Orlistat can improve weight loss to a small degree, when it is combined with a plan that includes calorie restriction and regular exercise. Bariatric surgeries reduce the stomach volume of people with extreme obesity.

People can lose weight while following fad diets, but they usually regain much of the weight that was lost when they resume their prior eating and other lifestyle habits. Achieving a healthy body weight and maintaining that weight requires making lifestyle changes that a person adopts for the rest of his or her life. No dietary supplement is recommended for weight loss.

Underweight can be caused by various factors, such as genetics, excessive physical activity, and certain diseases. To gain weight, an underweight person generally needs to increase portion sizes, eat more calorie-dense foods, and reduce physical activity, if excessive.

Disordered eating, involving temporary chaotic and abnormal food-related practices, often occurs when a person is under a lot of stress or wants to lose weight. When a person adopts disordered eating behaviors as a lifestyle, the practices can become harmful and difficult-to-treat eating disorders. Eating disorders are psychological disturbances that lead to behavioral changes and serious health complications. Anorexia nervosa, bulimia nervosa, or "eating disorders not otherwise specified," such as binge-eating disorder, are major types of eating disorders. The causes of eating disorders are unknown, but genetic, social, and psychological factors contribute to their development. Risk factors include being a female, having low self-esteem, experiencing sexual abuse as a child, being teased about weight, dieting repeatedly to lose weight, having a perfectionist personality, and being in a dysfunctional family. Treatment of eating disorders is complex, involving more than just dietary counseling. It is important to seek help for the condition as early as possible—before the behavior becomes highly ingrained or the affected person's life is at risk.

Recipe for Healthy Living

Did You Make That Dip?!

When it's time to entertain your friends, you can make a fiesta dip that will disappear quickly and provide plenty of compliments too. Fresh cilantro and dried cumin give recipes a distinctive "Mexican" flavor. Bean dip recipes often include canned refried beans and cheeses that are high in fat. This lower-fat version uses canned red beans and reduced-fat cheese. You can save time by using canned fat-free "refried" beans (yes, there is such a product). You can also substitute commercially prepared salsa for the home-made version, but you may find that making salsa with fresh ingredients is worth the extra effort. If you like a hotter salsa, use jalapeño peppers instead of mild green chili peppers. When preparing hot peppers, be careful to avoid touching your eyes or the inside of your nose until after you have thoroughly washed your hands with soap and water. The peppers contain *capsaicin*, the highly irritating chemical used in pepper spray that causes intense burning when in contact with mucous membranes.

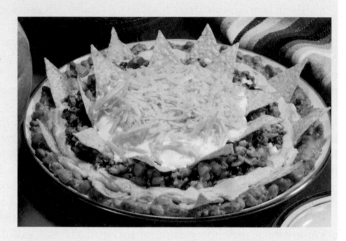

This recipe makes approximately eight ¼-cup servings. Each serving (without tortilla) supplies approximately 122 kcal, 7 g protein, 4.8 g fat, 19.0 mg vitamin C, 65 mcg folate, 400 mg potassium, 285 mg sodium, 1.4 mg iron, and 4.0 g fiber.

SALSA LAYER INGREDIENTS:

1 large, fresh ripe tomato
¼ medium onion, finely chopped
1 clove garlic, finely minced
1 4-oz can of mild green chilies (peeled and diced)
3 Tbsp chopped fresh cilantro leaves

GUACAMOLE LAYER INGREDIENTS:

1 ripe, black-
  skinned avocado
  (slightly soft)
juice of ½ lime
⅛ tsp dried cumin
  (a spice)
⅛ tsp ground
  black pepper

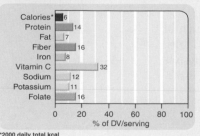

Fat 42%
Protein 23%
Carbohydrate 35%

	% of DV/serving
Calories*	6
Protein	14
Fat	7
Fiber	16
Iron	8
Vitamin C	32
Sodium	12
Potassium	11
Folate	16

*2000 daily total kcal

OTHER LAYERS:

1 14-oz to
  16-oz can
  red beans
1 cup shredded
  fat-reduced cheddar cheese
⅓ cup fat-free plain yogurt (optional)

PREPARATION STEPS:

1. Cover an 8" dinner plate with a sheet of heavy-duty aluminum foil.

2. Wash cilantro in cool water and shake off excess water. Wash tomato, avocado, and lime in cool water. Set cilantro and fruits aside on paper towels.

3. Use a sharp knife to *mince* (finely chop) onion, garlic, and cilantro on a cutting board. Place in small bowl.

4. Add chilies to the onion, garlic, and cilantro mixture. Stir gently until well mixed.

5. *Dice* (cut into small pieces) tomato and add to minced ingredients. You've made *salsa*.

6. To make guacamole, remove skin and seed from avocado. In a small bowl, dice avocado into small pieces and sprinkle with lime juice. Mash avocado and lime mixture. Add cumin and black pepper to avocado mixture, stir, and set aside.

7. Drain juice from beans and rinse them with cool water. Mash beans with the back of a large spoon; bean mixture will be lumpy.

8. Spread mashed beans evenly on the plate, leaving about ¾" from the edge of the plate free of beans.

9. Cover beans with individual layers of salsa and guacamole, and top with shredded cheese. If desired, place yogurt in the center as a low-fat substitute for sour cream and top with the cheese.

10. Loosely cover layered dip with clear plastic wrap and refrigerate.

11. To serve, spoon dip on pieces of soft tortillas.

Personal *Dietary* Analysis

1. Consider your eating behaviors.

a. Explain how your emotional state influences your eating behaviors. For example, do you eat certain foods when you feel happy, "stressed out," or depressed? Which foods do you eat under these circumstances? Describe a situation in which you ate in response to an emotional state instead of being hungry.

b. Discuss the influence that food advertising has on your eating practices.

c. Besides emotional state and food advertising, what other factors influence your eating habits?

2. Estimate your energy requirement by using one of the following formulas; choose the appropriate formula for your gender group.

Men 19 Years and Older:

Estimated Energy Requirement (EER) = 662 − (9.53 × AGE) + PA × (15.91 × WT + 539.6 × HT)

Women 19 Years and Older:

Estimated Energy Requirement (EER) = 354 − (6.91 × AGE) + PA × (9.36 × WT + 726 × HT)

The variables in the formulas are as follows:

AGE = age in years

PA = physical activity estimate (see Table 10.3)

WT = weight in kg (lb ÷ 2.2)

HT = height in meters (inches ÷ 39.4)

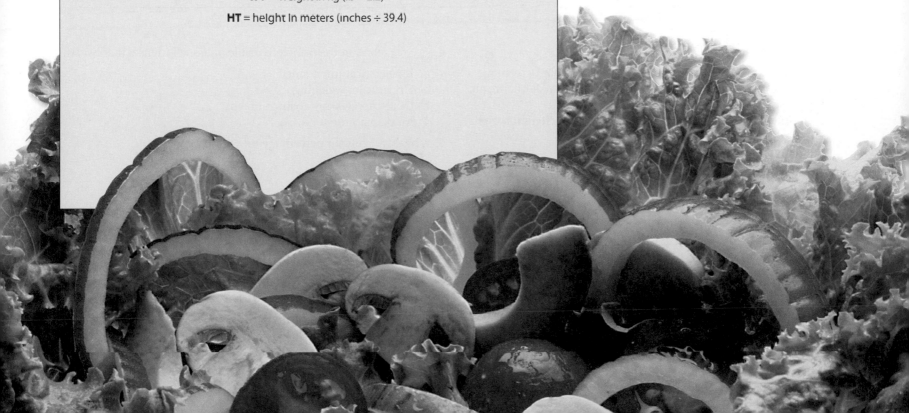

CRITICAL THINKING

1. Kim and Kevin weigh the same and have similar swimming skills. While in a swimming pool, Kim floats easily when she extends her arms and legs in the water. When Kevin extends his arms and legs and tries to float in the pool, he sinks. Why is Kim able to float more easily than Kevin?

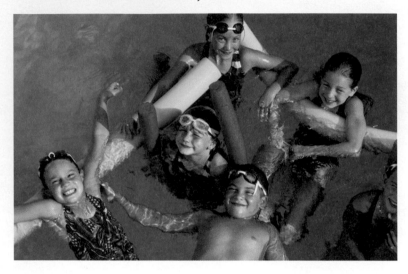

2. Why does your body "warm up" when you exercise?

3. An advertisement for a weight-loss supplement claims that the mixture of herbs in the product increases the metabolic rate by 150%. Explain why you would or would not recommend this product to someone who wants to lose weight.

4. Explain why it is usually difficult to pinpoint a *cause* of obesity.

5. Why are most people who lose weight unable to maintain the lower body weight over time?

6. If your BMI is within the overweight or obese range, discuss your reasons for being interested or not interested in losing weight. If you want to lose weight, what lifestyle changes will you make?

7. If your BMI is within the underweight range, discuss your reasons for being interested or not interested in gaining weight. If you want to gain weight, what lifestyle changes will you make?

8. If your BMI is in the healthy range, discuss steps you can take to maintain a healthy body weight as you grow older.

PRACTICE TEST

Select the best answer.

1. Body mass index (BMI) is
   a. a standard used to calculate a person's body fat percentage.
   b. based on a relationship between weight and risk of chronic disease.
   c. gradually being replaced by more reliable height/weight tables.
   d. None of the above is correct.

2. _____ cells are specialized to store fat.
   a. Carcinoma
   b. Megaloblastic
   c. Neural
   d. Adipose

3. _____ fat deposits are under the abdominal muscles.
   a. Subcutaneous
   b. Visceral
   c. Cellulite
   d. Bulimic

4. _____ relies on the principle that lean tissue is denser than water.
   a. Bioelectrical impedance
   b. Underwater weighing
   c. Dual-energy X-ray absorptiometry
   d. Air displacement

5. A healthy body fat percentage for women is
   a. 3–10%.
   b. 23–31%.
   c. 32–37%.
   d. 40–50%.

6. For the typical active person, basal metabolism accounts for _____ of the body's total energy use.
   a. 10–20%
   b. 21–49%
   c. 60–75%
   d. over 75%

7. Basal metabolism includes energy needs for

   a. breathing and circulating blood.
   b. performing physical activity.
   c. digesting food.
   d. absorbing nutrients.

8. Which of the following statements is true?

   a. Women generally have higher metabolic rates than men.
   b. Thyroid hormone levels influence BMR.
   c. A person who has more muscle mass will have a lower BMR than someone with less muscle tissue.
   d. When a person has a fever, his or her BMR drops below normal.

9. Negative energy balance occurs when

   a. the body needs more calories than the diet supplies.
   b. fat storage in the body increases.
   c. energy intake is higher than energy output.
   d. the thermic effect of food equals NEAT.

10. _____ is a hormone that reduces hunger and inhibits fat storage in the body.

   a. Coumadin
   b. Leptin
   c. Ghrelin
   d. Dexadrin

11. Members of the National Weight Control Registry tend to

   a. skip breakfast regularly.
   b. follow low-carbohydrate/high-protein diets.
   c. exercise 2 to 3 times per week.
   d. eat meals regularly, including breakfast.

12. Joseph's BMI is 23. When he is under a lot of stress, he eats a large amount of empty-calorie foods. Soon after eating these foods, he goes to a bathroom and makes himself vomit. Based on this information, Joseph probably has

   a. diarexia psychosis.
   b. anorexia nervosa.
   c. cystic fibrosis.
   d. bulimia nervosa.

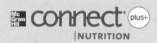

Additional resources related to the features of this book are available on ConnectPlus® Nutrition. Ask your instructor how to get access.

Answers to Chapter 10 Quiz *Yourself*

1. You can determine whether you have an unhealthy amount of body fat simply by measuring your waistline. **True.** (p. 367)

2. The best way to lose weight and keep it off is to follow a low-carbohydrate, high-fat diet, such as the Atkins diet. **False.** (p. 387)

3. As people age, their muscle cells turn into fat cells. **False.** (p. 360)

4. When a person consumes more carbohydrates than needed, the excess is converted to fat and stored in fat cells. **True.** (p. 364)

5. Cellulite is a unique type of fat that can be eliminated by taking certain dietary supplements. **False.** (p. 354)

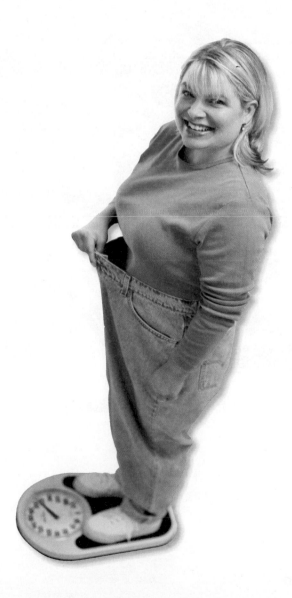

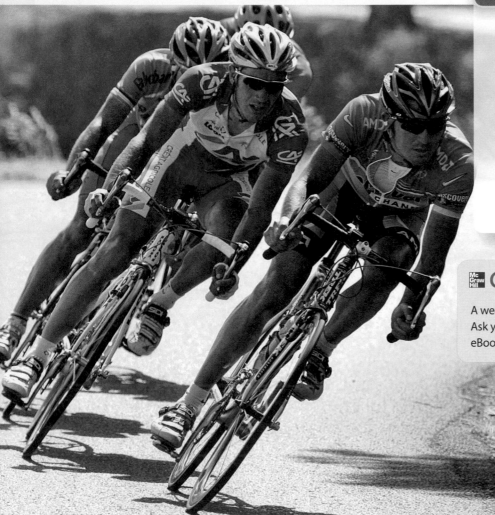

CHAPTER **11**

Nutrition for Physically Active Lifestyles

Chapter Learning Outcomes

After reading Chapter 11, you should be able to

1. List five health benefits of a physically active lifestyle.

2. Differentiate between anaerobic and aerobic use of energy, and identify advantages and disadvantages of each.

3. Plan nutritionally adequate, high-carbohydrate menus.

4. Estimate an athlete's energy and protein needs.

5. List at least five ergogenic aids that athletes often use, and describe their effects on health and physical performance.

6. Design a personal fitness regimen that suits your interests and lifestyle.

connect plus+ | **NUTRITION**   **www.mcgrawhillconnect.com**

A wealth of proven resources are available on ConnectPlus® Nutrition! Ask your instructor about ConnectPlus, which includes an interactive eBook, an adaptive learning program and much, much more!

BICYCLING FOR WEEKS through quaint villages and over steep mountains in France; swimming for miles in the chilly English Channel while being buffeted by waves; lifting metal disks that weigh more than the weight lifter—the extent to which some people push their bodies is truly amazing. Superior athletes seem to thrive on performing grueling physical feats that require extraordinary stamina, strength, and energy. Millions of Americans admire competitive athletes for their physical accomplishments and enjoy watching them perform. Many Americans, however, lead *sedentary* lives; that is, their daily activities do not require much muscular exertion. In 2009, about 50% of adults in the United States did not obtain recommended amounts of moderate or vigorous physical activity.[1] Even when Americans have the time, many chose not to be physically active (Fig.11.1). In 2008, approximately 25% of adults reported that they had not participated in leisure-time physical activity during the past month.[2]

The human body is designed for **physical activity,** movement that results from skeletal muscle contraction. Most of the physical activities you perform each day are *unstructured*, for example, shopping for groceries or doing household tasks. **Exercise** refers to physical activities that are usually planned and structured for a particular purpose, such as having fun or increasing muscle mass. Both forms of physical activity can benefit your health.

Physical fitness is the ability to perform moderate- to vigorous-intensity activities without becoming excessively fatigued. A *physically fit* person has the strength, endurance, flexibility, and balance to meet the physical demands of daily living, exercise, and sports. Proper nutrition is essential for optimal physical fitness and sports performance.

Regardless of whether you aspire to be a world-class athlete or simply want to be healthier, regular exercise should be a part of your daily routine. Physically inactive people do not have to perform high-intensity structured workouts daily to improve their health. According to recommendations of the

(continued)

Quiz *Yourself*

What is ATP? How much protein is needed for optimal muscular development? Are there any dietary supplements that can improve muscle strength and endurance safely? To test your nutrition and fitness knowledge, take the following quiz. The answers are on page 431.

1. People who exercise regularly can reduce their risk of type 2 diabetes. _____ T _____ F

2. Sports drinks are not useful for fluid replacement. _____ T _____ F

3. Protein is the body's preferred fuel for muscular activity. _____ T _____ F

4. Heatstroke is a serious illness that requires immediate professional medical treatment. _____ T _____ F

5. While at rest, skeletal muscles metabolize more glucose than fat for energy. _____ T _____ F

physical activity movement resulting from contraction of skeletal muscles

exercise physical activities that are usually planned and structured for a purpose

physical fitness ability to perform moderate- to vigorous-intensity activities without becoming excessively fatigued

Figure 11.1 Leisure-time physical activity. Many people choose to be sedentary when they have time to be physically active.

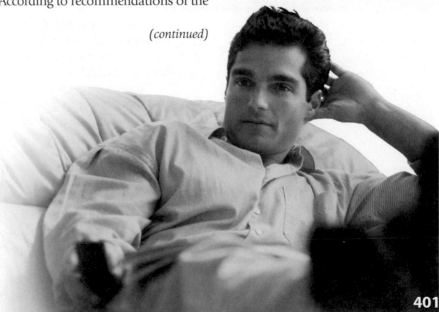

American College of Sports Medicine and the American Heart Association, healthy adults under 65 years of age should perform:

- moderate-intensity physical activity for 30 minutes daily, 5 days a week,

or

- vigorous-intensity physical activity 20 minutes a day, 3 days a week,

and

- eight to 10 strengthening exercises (eight to 12 repetitions of each exercise) twice a week.[3]

By reading Chapter 11, you will learn about the benefits of a physically active lifestyle, different cellular energy systems, and dietary practices that are appropriate for athletes and other physically active people. Chapter 11 also provides practical tips for planning an exercise routine that you can follow for a lifetime.

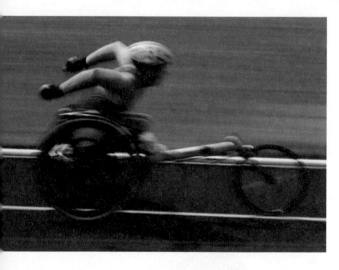

11.1 Benefits of Regular Exercise

Millions of Americans suffer from chronic illnesses that can be prevented or improved by exercising more often. People who exercise regularly can help reduce their risks of serious chronic conditions, including cardiovascular disease, type 2 diabetes, hypertension, obesity, osteoporosis, and certain cancers.[4] Maintaining a physically active lifestyle is one of the most important steps that people can take to improve their health. In 2008, the U.S. Department of Health and Human Services issued the *2008 Physical Activity Guidelines for Americans* (http://www.health.gov/paguidelines/). These guidelines provide evidence-based physical activity recommendations to help Americans reduce the risk of chronic diseases that contribute to millions of premature deaths each year.[5]

Determining the Intensity of Physical Activity

As Figure 11.2 illustrates, you can gain physical as well as psychological benefits by performing moderate-intensity physical activity regularly. Furthermore, you may achieve even greater health benefits by increasing the duration, frequency, and intensity (physical effort) of your exercise routine.

Intensity refers to the level of exertion used to perform an activity. Duration and type of physical activity, as well as body weight, influence the intensity of skeletal muscle movement. Thus, activities such as walking and bicycling can be classified as either moderate- or vigorous-intensity physical activity, depending on the rate at which the activities are performed as well as the weight of the person performing them. See http://www.cdc.gov/physicalactivity/everyone/measuring/index.html for examples of physical activities that are generally classified as moderate or vigorous intensity.

There are a few ways to determine the intensity of exercise. One way is to judge your level of exertion based on physical signs, such as breathing rate and sweat production. While exercising at the moderate-intensity level, you should be aware of your muscular effort, but you should also be able to chat with an exercise partner comfortably.

A popular method of estimating the intensity of exercise is to use a percentage of your *age-related maximum heart rate*. To calculate your age-related maximum heart rate, subtract your age from 220, the age-related maximum heart rate. (Some experts suggest using a slightly lower age-related maximum heart rate for women.) Your **target heart rate zone** is the range of heart rate that reflects the intensity of your exertion during physical activity. For moderate-intensity physical activity, your target heart rate zone should be

target heart rate zone heart rate range that reflects intensity of physical exertion

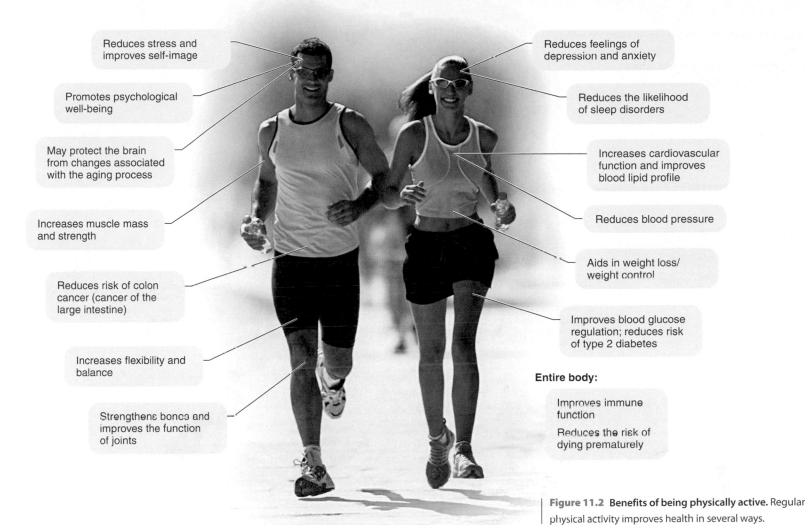

Reduces stress and improves self-image

Promotes psychological well-being

May protect the brain from changes associated with the aging process

Increases muscle mass and strength

Reduces risk of colon cancer (cancer of the large intestine)

Increases flexibility and balance

Strengthens bones and improves the function of joints

Reduces feelings of depression and anxiety

Reduces the likelihood of sleep disorders

Increases cardiovascular function and improves blood lipid profile

Reduces blood pressure

Aids in weight loss/ weight control

Improves blood glucose regulation; reduces risk of type 2 diabetes

Entire body:

Improves immune function

Reduces the risk of dying prematurely

Figure 11.2 Benefits of being physically active. Regular physical activity improves health in several ways.

50 to 70% of your age-related maximum heart rate.[6] To determine your moderate-intensity "zone," take your age-related maximum heart rate and multiply this figure by 0.50 and 0.70. For example, the age-related maximum heart rate of a 20-year-old person is 200 beats per minute (220 minus 20). Multiply 200 beats per minute (bpm) by 0.50 to calculate the 50% value and multiply 200 bpm by 0.70 to obtain the 70% level. This person's target heart rate zone for moderate-intensity activities is 100 to 140 bpm.

Moderate-intensity physical activities expend 3.5 to 7.0 kcal/min.[7] To "burn" (*oxidize* or *metabolize*) more energy and give your heart a more vigorous workout, you can engage in physical activities that expend more than 7 kcal/min. Such physical activities usually require considerable muscular effort and result in significant increases in breathing rate and perspiration. Examples of vigorous physical activities include jogging, running, aerobic dancing, swimming laps, and bicycling uphill.

To exercise vigorously, your target heart rate should be 70 to 85% of your age-related maximum heart rate.[6] To calculate this range, follow the same formula that you used to determine the range for moderate-intensity activity, except that you need to change "0.50 and 0.70" to "0.70 and 0.85." A 20-year-old person, for example, would have an estimated maximum age-related heart rate of 200 bpm, and the 70 to 85% levels would range from 140 to 170 bpm. If you have any serious health problems, ask your physician to help you determine your target zone.

You can measure your heart rate (pulse) easily, by finding the *radial artery* in your wrist. Locate the radial artery by gently placing your index and middle fingers on the underside of your wrist by the thumb, as shown in Figure 11.3. Count your pulse for 10 seconds, and then multiply that number by 6 to determine your heart rate for 1 minute. Your heart rate begins to decline as soon as you stop exercising, so you need to practice taking your pulse while still working out.

Figure 11.3 Finding the radial artery. To locate the radial artery, gently place your index and middle fingers on the underside of your wrist, by the thumb, as shown.

Figure 11.4 Physical activity pyramid. Educators with the Department of Kinesiology and Health at Georgia State University developed this pyramid to help people add more physical activity into their daily routines.

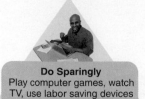

Do Sparingly
Play computer games, watch TV, use labor saving devices like escalators

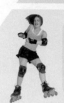

**Recreational Activities
(2-3 days/week)**
Golf, bowling, baseball, soccer, hiking, in-line skating, dancing, canoeing, yoga, martial arts

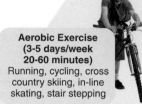 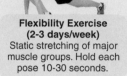 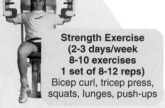

**Aerobic Exercise
(3-5 days/week
20-60 minutes)**
Running, cycling, cross country skiing, in-line skating, stair stepping

**Flexibility Exercise
(2-3 days/week)**
Static stretching of major muscle groups. Hold each pose 10-30 seconds.

**Strength Exercise
(2-3 days/week
8-10 exercises
1 set of 8-12 reps)**
Bicep curl, tricep press, squats, lunges, push-ups

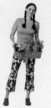 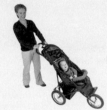

**Physical Activity
(Most days of the week
Accumulate 30+ minutes)**
Take the stairs, garden, wash and wax your car, rake leaves, mow the lawn, walk to do your errands, walk the dog, clean your house, play with your kids

aerobic exercise physical activities that involve sustained, rhythmic contractions of large muscle groups

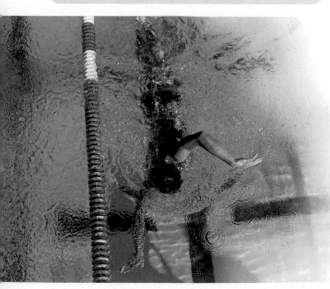

Aerobic exercise involves sustained, rhythmic contractions of large muscle groups in the legs and arms.

Physical Activity Pyramid

Educators with the Department of Kinesiology and Health at Georgia State University developed a physical activity pyramid to help people add more physical activity into their daily routines (Fig. 11.4). This pyramid presents various activities that need to be performed regularly and provides practical suggestions for increasing the intensity of various routine activities. For example, you will exert more physical effort and expend more energy if you use stairs instead of elevators or "jog" instead of "walk" the dog.

Low-intensity, unstructured physical activities that involve usual daily living activities, such as routine household chores, form the foundation of the physical activity pyramid. The next level of the activity pyramid recommends adding *aerobic* exercise to foundation activities at least three times a week. **Aerobic exercise** involves sustained, rhythmic contractions of large muscle groups in the legs and arms. Such activities raise your heart rate, giving your heart a more effective workout. Running, jogging, rapid walking, and swimming are aerobic activities. Additionally, the second level of the pyramid recommends performing resistance and stretching exercises at least two times a week to increase muscle mass, strength, and flexibility. Resistance exercises, such as weight lifting, can also increase bone mass. The third level of the pyramid encourages regularly performing recreational activities that are physical, such as yoga and dancing. The top of the pyramid depicts activities that expend little energy, such as watching television or using a personal computer. The pyramid recommends spending little time being sedentary. The Chapter 11 "Highlight" provides information concerning how to design a more formal physical fitness plan.

Concept **Checkpoint**

1. What is the difference between physical activity and exercise?
2. Define physical fitness.
3. List at least five health benefits of performing moderate-intensity exercise regularly.
4. To obtain some health benefits, what is the minimum amount of time an adult should spend engaging in exercise each day?
5. What are at least two benefits of performing resistance exercise regularly?
6. Calculate the target heart rate range for a 24-year-old person performing moderate-intensity physical activity.

 ## 11.2 Energy for Muscular Work

To move, muscles must contract, and to contract, muscles must have a source of energy. Under normal conditions, most cells, including muscle cells, metabolize a mixture of biological fuels, especially glucose and fatty acids. Muscle cells also metabolize a small amount of amino acids from proteins to obtain energy.[8]

Energy Metabolism

Cells obtain energy by means of a complex series of chemical reactions that progressively break down (*catabolize*) macronutrients and alcohol to release the energy that is stored within them. Cells lose much of this energy as heat, but they capture some of the energy in *high-energy compounds* such as **adenosine triphosphate (ATP)**. ATP forms when an *inorganic phosphate* group (P_i) bonds with **adenosine diphosphate (ADP)** and traps energy in the process (Fig. 11.5). Note in Figure 11.5 that ADP has two inorganic phosphate groups and ATP has three inorganic phosphate groups.

Glucose is the most useful biological fuel, because the simple sugar can be catabolized when free oxygen (O_2) is unavailable (**anaerobic**) or available (**aerobic**). Catabolic processes involve *oxidation*, the removal of electrons from compounds to create new compounds. During **glycolysis** (*glyco* = carbohydrate [particularly sugar]; *lysis* = breakdown), the first stage of glucose oxidation, glucose is degraded to form

> **adenosine triphosphate (ATP)** high-energy compound, major direct energy source for cells
>
> **adenosine diphosphate (ADP)** high-energy compound, by-product of ATP use
>
> **anaerobic** conditions that lack free oxygen
>
> **aerobic** conditions that require free oxygen
>
> **glycolysis** first stage of glucose oxidation

Figure 11.5 ATP. Cells capture and store energy by forming ATP from ADP and inorganic phosphate (P_i).

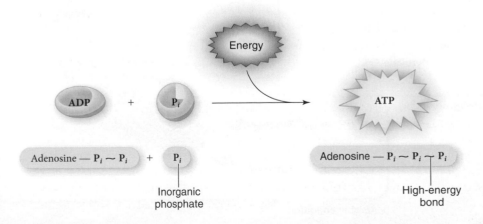

pyruvate compound that results from anaerobic breakdown of glucose

mitochondria organelles that generate energy from macronutrients

pyruvate under anaerobic conditions (Fig. 11.6a). Glycolysis produces a small amount of ATP.

If oxygen is available, pyruvate undergoes further oxidation in a stepwise series of chemical pathways called *aerobic respiration*. Pyruvate moves from the fluid within cells (cytoplasm) into **mitochondria** (Fig. 11.6b). Mitochondria are often referred to as "powerhouses," because much of the energy stored in glucose or other biological fuels is released within these organelles. In mitochondria, pyruvate undergoes complete degradation, and as a result, cells generate more ATP than during glycolysis. Furthermore, carbon dioxide (CO_2) and ATP are produced. Oxygen is a key player in this phase of the process, because the element bonds to hydrogen atoms that were released from pyruvate, forming water (H_2O) (see Fig. 11.6b). When cells completely oxidize glucose to release energy, the end products are simply CO_2 and H_2O. Most of the CO_2 is exhaled, and the H_2O produced metabolically can help maintain proper body water volume. Besides glucose, triglycerides (fat), amino acids, and alcohol are also sources of ATP. Figure 11.7 summarizes the pathways that dietary protein, carbohydrate, and fat follow during energy metabolism. For more detailed illustrations of the metabolic pathways that biological fuels undergo, see Appendix D.

How Do Cells Use ATP?

ATP is the primary source of direct energy for all cells. ATP is often referred to as "energy currency," because it functions like money. Just as you save money until it is needed to make a purchase, your cells save energy in ATP until it is needed to power cellular work.

When a cell needs some energy to drive a chemical reaction, it uses an enzyme to break the bond between the last two phosphate groups of ATP (Fig. 11.8). This process releases energy (*ATP-energy*) and reforms ADP and P_i. Thus, cells can recycle their supplies of ADP and P_i. Cells do not store much ATP, so they must constantly replace their supply of the high-energy compound by recycling ADP and P_i.

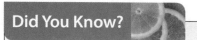

Did You Know?

Human cells can convert certain amino acids into glucose, but the cells are unable to make glucose from fatty acids.

Figure 11.6 Obtaining energy. (*a*) During glycolysis, the first stage of glucose oxidation, cells degrade glucose into pyruvate under anaerobic conditions. (*b*) If oxygen is available, pyruvate moves from the cytoplasm into mitochondria. Pyruvate undergoes further degradation in mitochondria, forming CO_2, H_2O, and ATP, at certain points.

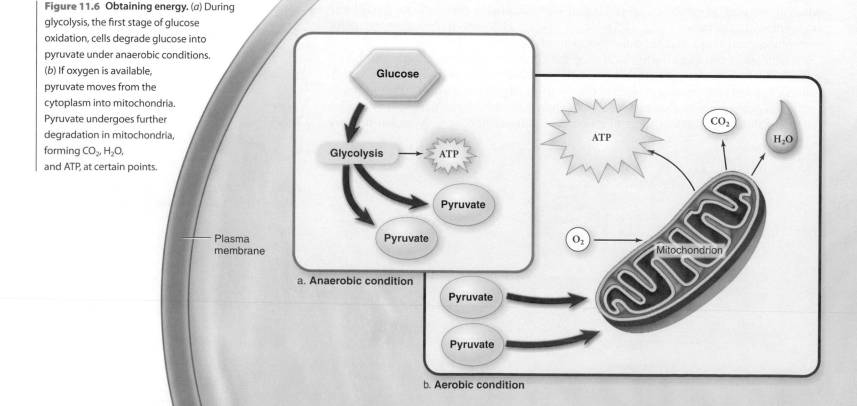

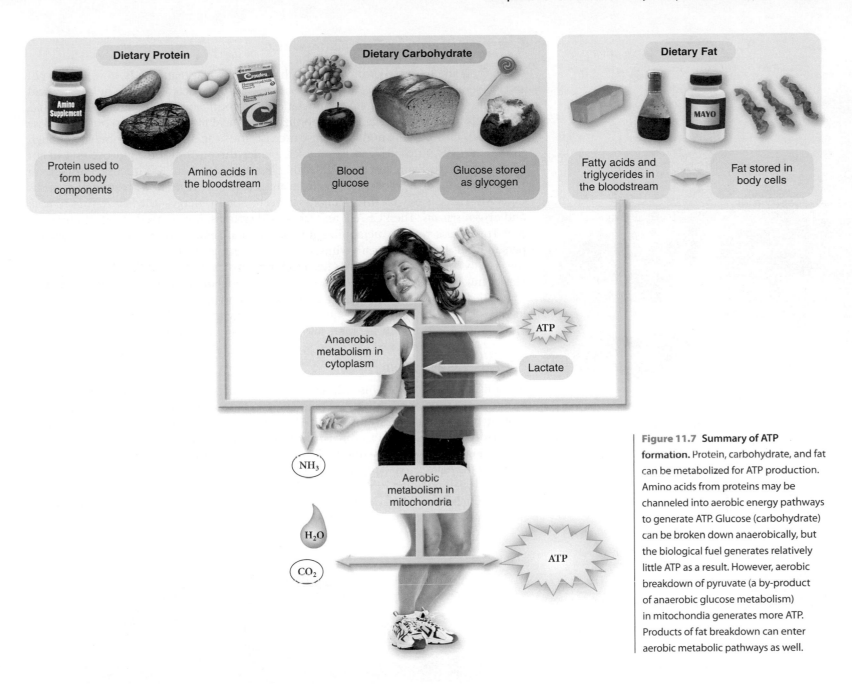

Figure 11.7 Summary of ATP formation. Protein, carbohydrate, and fat can be metabolized for ATP production. Amino acids from proteins may be channeled into aerobic energy pathways to generate ATP. Glucose (carbohydrate) can be broken down anaerobically, but the biological fuel generates relatively little ATP as a result. However, aerobic breakdown of pyruvate (a by-product of anaerobic glucose metabolism) in mitochondia generates more ATP. Products of fat breakdown can enter aerobic metabolic pathways as well.

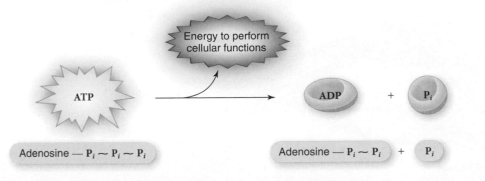

Figure 11.8 Energy from ATP. When a cell needs energy to drive a chemical reaction, it uses an enzyme to break the bond between the last two phosphate groups of ATP, releasing energy and reforming ADP and P_i.

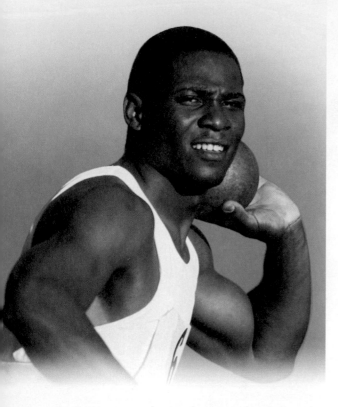

During a brief bout of intense anaerobic exercise, glucose is a major source of energy for working muscles.

Energy Systems for Exercising Muscles

Gram for gram, fat supplies more energy than carbohydrate. Fatty acids, however, are not a very useful fuel for intense, brief exercise, such as a 100-meter sprint. Why? A fatty acid molecule has fewer oxygen atoms in relation to carbon atoms than a glucose molecule. Thus, cells need more oxygen to metabolize a fatty acid molecule than to burn a glucose molecule. During a brief bout of intense exercise, the heart and lungs do not have enough time to deliver much oxygen to muscles. Under these conditions, glucose is a major source of energy. For physical activities that last longer and are less intense, muscles can use more fat for energy, because the lungs are able to supply them with enough oxygen.

Muscle cells rely on three major systems to obtain energy—the *PCr-ATP, lactic acid,* and *oxygen systems.* The PCr-ATP and lactic acid systems do not need oxygen to produce ATP. Thus, these systems metabolize glucose under anaerobic conditions, such as when a person holds his or her breath while sprinting or lifting a heavy load. As the duration of the activity increases, muscle cells need to form considerably more ATP. To meet this demand, muscle cells depend heavily on the oxygen system to metabolize glucose and fat.

The three energy-releasing systems do not function independently of each other during intense physical exertion; each contributes ATP-energy to power intense muscular activity.[9] The following sections provide more information about these major energy systems.

PCr-ATP Energy System

A resting muscle cell contains only a small amount of ATP that can be used immediately. Muscle cells have another type of high-energy compound—**phosphocreatine (PCr)**—that enables the cells to produce more ATP quickly under anaerobic conditions. To make the ATP, cells break down PCr into *creatine* and P_i, releasing energy to form ATP from ADP and P_i (Fig. 11.9a). Cells do not use PCr directly to power their activities; the compound provides the energy to resupply ATP.

By breaking down PCr to form ATP, muscle cells can obtain enough energy to function during intense events lasting only a few seconds.[10] However, the PCr-ATP system can be activated instantly, replenishing ATP fast enough to meet the energy demands of the

Figure 11.9 PCr. Muscle cells break down PCr into creatine and inorganic phosphate, releasing energy to form ATP from ADP and P_i (*a*). When the intense activity stops and there is no need to maintain high levels of ATP, an inorganic phosphate group bonds with creatine to recycle PCr (*b*).

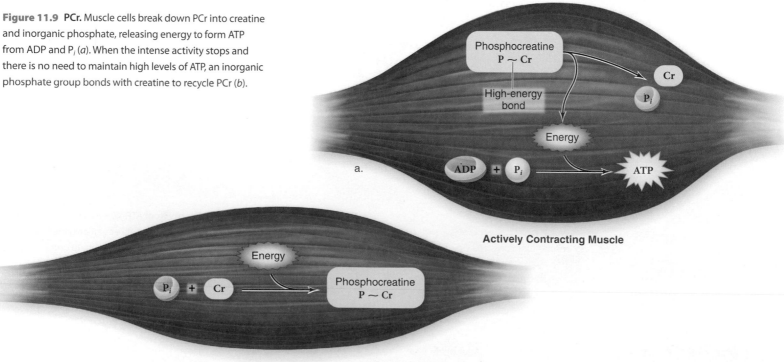

swiftest and most powerful muscle movements, such as jumping, lifting, throwing, and sprinting. When the intense activity stops and there is no need to maintain high levels of ATP, an inorganic phosphate group bonds with creatine to recycle PCr (see Fig. 11.9b). Muscle cells, however, do not make or store much PCr.

Lactic Acid Energy System

When physical activity lasts longer than a few seconds, the PCr-ATP energy system cannot keep up with the demand for energy, and muscle cells must metabolize glucose to generate more ATP. The immediate source of glucose for working muscles is glycogen that is stored in muscles. The liver also helps supply glucose for muscles by degrading glycogen and releasing glucose molecules into the bloodstream.

In anaerobic conditions, muscle cells metabolize glucose to pyruvate and then convert pyruvate to **lactic acid** (Fig. 11.10.1). The degradation of glucose to lactic acid produces a small amount of ATP—only enough to sustain maximum physical exertion for 30 to 40 seconds.[11] Lactic acid accumulates in muscles and converts to a related substance, *lactate*. Although certain muscle cells can use lactate as a fuel, some of the compound enters the bloodstream (Fig. 11.10.2). The liver removes lactate from blood and can convert the compound into glucose (Fig. 11.10.3). The liver may then release the glucose into the bloodstream to help meet muscles' demand for fuel or use the simple sugar to make glycogen (Fig. 11.10.4).

phosphocreatine (PCr) high-energy compound used to reform ATP under anaerobic conditions

lactic acid compound formed from pyruvate during anaerobic metabolism

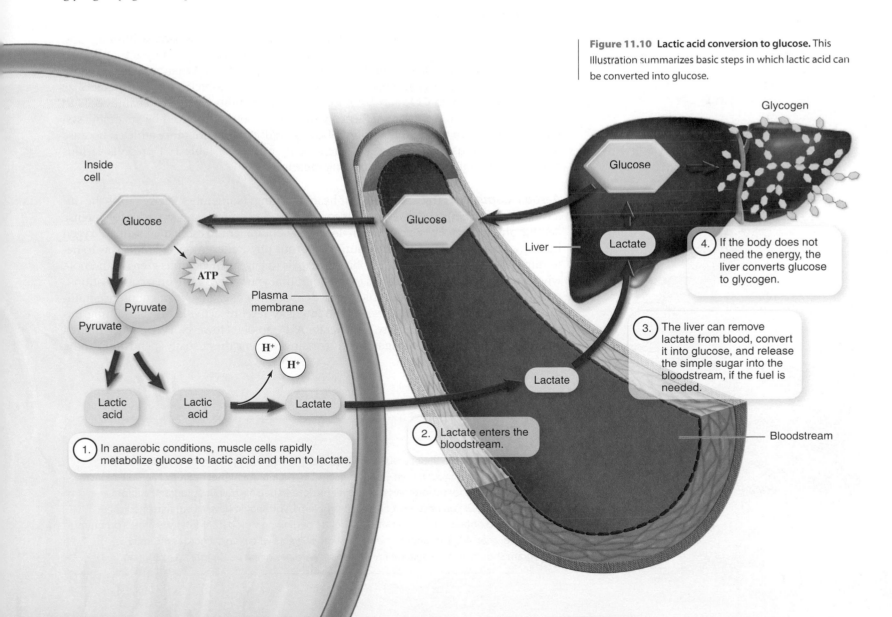

Figure 11.10 Lactic acid conversion to glucose. This illustration summarizes basic steps in which lactic acid can be converted into glucose.

Even well-trained athletes experience muscle fatigue as the time they spend performing intense muscular exertion increases. This marathon runner collapsed as she crossed the finish line of the 28th Annual U.S. Marine Corps Marathon. *Photo: LCPL Richard A. Burkdall, USMC.*

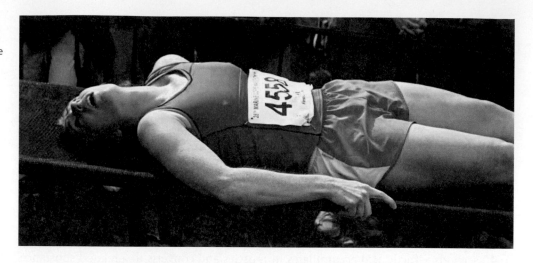

Hydrogen ions (H⁺) form as a result of the conversion of lactic acid to lactate. The accumulation of H⁺ in muscle tissue contributes to muscle acidity, a condition that can lead to muscle fatigue and declining physical performance.

Oxygen Energy System

You would not be able to enjoy activities such as walking at a fast pace, swimming laps, playing a game of soccer or basketball, or other continuous types of physical activity, if your muscles depended only on the anaerobic energy systems. When muscle cells have plenty of oxygen, such as during low- to moderate-intensity exercise, they can metabolize glucose completely to CO_2 and H_2O. In fact, the availability of oxygen enables cells to produce about 18 times more ATP-energy than the amount produced by anaerobic systems. The ability to obtain this amount of energy is useful for endurance athletes, because it allows their muscle cells to contract repeatedly for hours. Table 11.1 presents various energy sources for resting and contracting muscles.

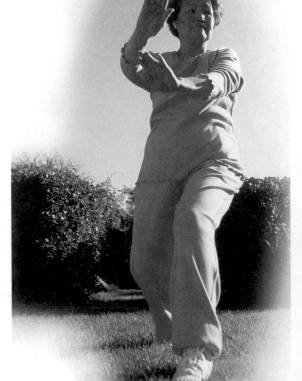

Aerobic Capacity   The ability of your heart and lungs (sometimes referred to as the *cardiorespiratory system*) to deliver oxygen to muscles determines your capacity for intense aerobic physical activity. Scientists can use special equipment to estimate maximal oxygen intake (*aerobic capacity* or *VO₂max*) during vigorous physical exertion. A simple way to determine if you are nearing your aerobic capacity is to engage in vigorous exercise and note when your breathing rate increases to the point that you cannot carry on a conversation.

You can increase your aerobic exercise capacity by engaging in an endurance training program that gradually increases the intensity level of activities. Such training improves your muscle cells' ability to generate ATP rapidly. However, even highly trained athletes experience muscle fatigue after increasing the time they usually spend performing intense muscular exertion.

Did You Know?

As people grow older, their aerobic capacities decline with each passing decade. By being physically active, however, even elderly persons can maintain a higher degree of aerobic capacity than their sedentary counterparts. It is never too late to begin a training program to improve physical fitness. If you have existing health problems, you should have a complete medical checkup and obtain your physician's "OK" before beginning a moderate-intensity fitness program. Men older than 40 years and women older than 50 years who plan a vigorous-intensity program should also consult their physician for help designing a safe, effective program.

TABLE 11.1 *Energy Sources for Muscles**

Source/System	When in Use	Examples of Activities
ATP	At all times	All types
Phosphocreatine (PCr)	All exercise initially; short bursts of exercise thereafter	Shot put, high jump, bench press
Carbohydrate		
Anaerobic	High-intensity exercise, especially lasting 30 seconds to 2 minutes	200-yard sprint
Aerobic	Exercise lasting 2 minutes to 3 hours or more; the higher the intensity of exercise, the greater the use	Basketball, swimming, jogging
Fat	At rest	Sitting
	Exercise lasting more than a few minutes; low- to moderate-intensity physical activities	30-minute brisk walk
Protein	Low amounts during all exercise, slightly more during endurance exercise, especially when carbohydrate fuel is lacking	Long-distance running

* Note that at any given time, more than one energy system is operating. Adapted from: Wardlaw GM, Smith AM: *Contemporary Nutrition*. 7th ed. New York: McGraw-Hill, 2009.

Fat or Carbohydrate for Fueling Exercise?

The intensity of a physical activity largely influences the relative amounts of fatty acids and glucose that muscles metabolize for energy. Glucose supplies only about 40% of the energy needed to sustain a person who is resting or engaged in very light to light activities, such as watching TV, typing, and walking. Fat is the primary fuel muscles use while resting or engaged in low- to moderate-intensity physical activities.[12] During high-intensity exercise, the rate of fat oxidation decreases while that of glucose oxidation increases. The chart in Figure 11.11 illustrates rough estimates of carbohydrate and fat metabolism during six forms of exercise.

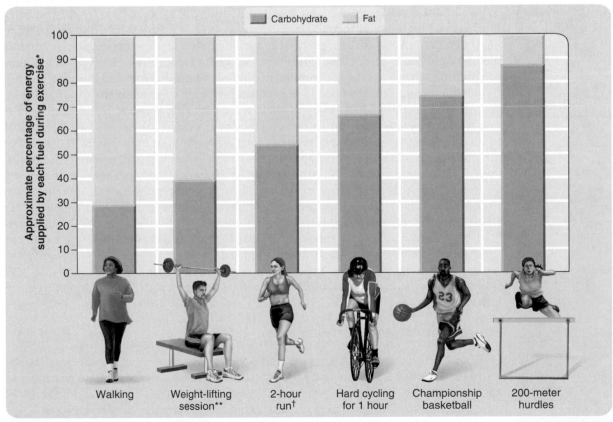

Figure 11.11 Rough estimates of energy use during exercise. The intensity of an exercise largely influences the relative amounts of macronutrients that muscles metabolize for energy.

*Protein supplies a minor percentage of energy.
**Fat use generally is higher because much of the time spent weight lifting is for rest periods.
†The values shown are for a runner consuming carbohydrate during the run; more fat and less carbohydrate would be used if carbohydrates were not consumed.

An individual's level of training influences the ratio of glucose to fatty acids that his or her muscles use during exercise. Trained endurance athletes tend to oxidize more fat when exercising at the same intensity than untrained persons.[13] As a result, muscle cells of trained athletes "spare" glycogen; that is, they conserve their supply of glucose. By sparing their glycogen supplies, athletes can enhance their capacity to exercise longer.

Concept **Checkpoint**

7. How is glycogen used during exercise?
8. How is ATP formed? How do cells use ATP?
9. Explain how each energy system supplies ATP for muscles. Which energy systems operate under anaerobic conditions?
10. How can you improve your aerobic capacity?
11. When is fat a major source of energy for muscles?

genetic endowment inherited physical characteristics that can affect physical performance

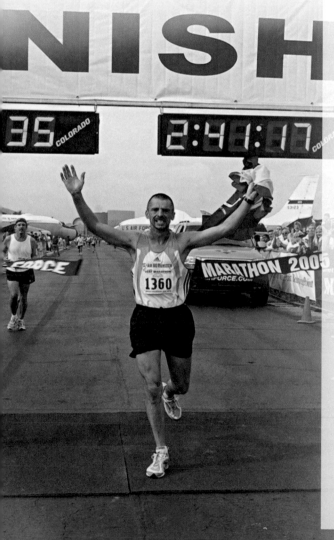

Optimizing an athlete's diet may provide a competitive advantage.

11.3 General Dietary Advice for Athletes

Athletes often manipulate their diets to lose or gain weight, increase their muscular strength, and prevent or delay fatigue during exercise. Although an athlete's diet plays a major role in determining if he or she finishes first or last in a competitive event, *genetic endowment* and *physical training* are the most crucial factors that influence athletic performance.[10] **Genetic endowment** refers to inherited physical characteristics that can affect an athlete's physical performance, such as body size, shape, and composition. Regardless of how well an athlete eats, if this person lacks the physical traits that are necessary for success in his or her chosen sport, the athlete will find it difficult to compete effectively. Athletes must also be highly motivated to compete and engage in a well-designed intensive training program to maximize their physical capabilities. Nevertheless, optimizing an athlete's diet may provide a competitive advantage, especially for sporting events in which hundredths of a second can mean the difference between finishing first and finishing second.

Athletes and coaches often believe misinformation concerning the value of dietary supplements, certain foods, and fad diets for optimizing physical health and performance. Such beliefs can lead to diet-related practices that are useless and a waste of money. In some cases, however, these practices are harmful or even deadly.

Sports nutrition focuses on applying nutrition principles and research findings to improving athletic performance. This section of Chapter 11 provides specific dietary recommendations that are appropriate for athletes and other physically active people. If you would like additional information on sports nutrition, contact a registered dietitian. Other reliable sources of sports nutrition include websites of the American College of Sports Medicine (www.acsm.org), Centers for Disease Control and Prevention (http://www.cdc.gov/physicalactivity/index.html), and the journal *The Physician and Sportsmedicine* (www.physsportsmed.com). If you are interested in studying sports nutrition, check with your academic advisor to determine whether your college or university offers sports nutrition courses.

Energy for Athletic Performance

Compared to nonathletes, athletes generally need more energy to support their physically active lifestyles. Athletes who do not consume enough food energy can lose muscle mass and bone density, experience fatigue and menstrual problems (females), and be at risk of injury.[14] Thus, low energy intakes can hinder an athlete's chances of performing well.

Male athletes who train or compete aerobically for more than 90 minutes daily need at least 50 kcal/kg/day; their female counterparts need 45 to 50 kcal/kg/day.[15] Thus, athletes may require 3000 kcal/day or more to support their energy needs and maintain their weight. Table 11.2 presents three sample daily menus that are nutritionally adequate;

TABLE 11.2 *Sample Daily 3000, 4000, and 5000 kcal Menus*

3000 kcal 65% carbohydrate 21% fat 17% protein	4000 kcal 66% carbohydrate 23% fat 14% protein	5000 kcal 66% carbohydrate 22% fat 15% protein
Breakfast	**Breakfast**	**Breakfast**
Fat-free milk, 1 cup	Fat-free milk, 1 cup	Fat-free milk, 1 cup
Cheerios, 2 cups	Cheerios, 2 cups	Cheerios, 2 cups
Bagel, 1	Bran muffins, 2	Bran muffins, 2
Cherry preserves, 1 tsp	Orange, 1	Orange, 1
Oat bran muffin, 1		
Low-fat cream cheese, 1 Tbsp		
Snack	**Snack**	**Snack**
Oatmeal-raisin cookies, 2	Chopped dates, ¾ cup	Low-fat plain yogurt, 1 cup
		Chopped dates, 1 cup
Lunch	**Lunch**	**Lunch**
Chicken breast, skinless roasted, 2 oz	Macaroni and cheese, 2½ cups	Chicken enchilada, 1
Whole-wheat bread, 2 slices	Romaine lettuce, 1 cup	Romaine lettuce, 1 cup
Provolone cheese, 1 oz	Garbanzo beans, 1 cup	Garbanzo beans, 1 cup
Mayonnaise, 1 tsp	Grated carrots, ½ cup	Shredded carrots, ¾ cup
Raisins, ⅓ cup	French dressing, 2 Tbsp	Chopped celery, ½ cup
Cranberry juice, 1½ cups	Apple juice, 1 cup	Seasoned croutons, 1 oz
Low-fat vanilla yogurt, 1 cup		French dressing, 2 Tbsp
		Whole-wheat bread, 2 slices
		Soft margarine, 1 Tbsp
Snack	**Snack**	**Snack**
Banana, 1	Whole-wheat bread, 2 slices	Banana, 1
Oatmeal-raisin cookie, 1	Margarine, 1 tsp	Bagel, 1
	Grape jelly, 2 Tbsp	Cream cheese, 1 Tbsp
Dinner	**Dinner**	**Dinner**
Lean broiled beef, sirloin, 3 oz	Skinless, roasted turkey breast, 2 oz	Lean broiled beef, sirloin, 5 oz
Romaine lettuce, 1 cup	Mashed potatoes, 2 cups	Mashed potatoes, 2 cups
Garbanzo beans, 1 cup	Peas and onions, 1 cup	Soft margarine, 2 tsp
Italian dressing, 2 Tbsp	Soft margarine, 2 tsp	Spinach egg noodles, 1½ cups cooked
Spinach egg noodles, 1½ cups cooked	Mango, 1	Grated parmesan cheese, 2 Tbsp
Soft margarine, 1 tsp	Fat-free milk, 1 cup	Green beans, 1 cup
Green beans, 1 cup		Oatmeal-raisin cookies, 3
Fat-free milk, ½ cup		
	Snack	**Snack**
	Pasta, 1 cup cooked	Air-popped popcorn, 2 cups
	Parmesan cheese, 2 Tbsp	Raisins, ⅓ cup
	Cranberry juice, 1 cup	Cranberry juice, 2 cups

Adapted from: Wardlaw GM, Hampl JS: *Perspectives in nutrition*. New York: McGraw-Hill, 2007.

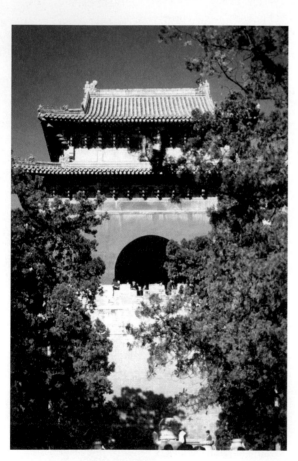

| Ming Tombs at Beijing Pavilions.

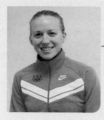

REAL *People*
REAL *Stories*

Sarah Haskins

Sarah Haskins' love of sports and athletic competition began when she learned to swim and compete in swim meets as a 5-year-old. By the time she was 9, she was competing in local swim meets and winning them. Swimming was not the only sport in which Sarah excelled. During her junior year in high school, she finished first in her state as a cross-country runner. Sarah's success as an athlete enabled her to earn an athletic scholarship to the University of Tulsa, where she majored in elementary education.

In 2000, Sarah watched televised events of the Summer Olympics and became intrigued with the women's triathlon—a grueling combination of continuous sports activity that is comprised of swimming almost a mile (1.5 km), bicycling 24.8 miles (40 km), and running 6.2 miles (10 km). Sarah was so interested in the sport, she became determined to become an Olympic athlete. Over the next few years, she trained for the triathlon and competed in women's triathlon events held in the United States and other countries. By 2004, she was one of the top 125 female triathlon athletes in the world and one of only three women accepted by the U.S. Olympic Training Center in Colorado to prepare for the 2008 Summer Olympic Games in Beijing, China. During the Summer Olympics, Sarah finished in 11th place among the 45 women who completed the triathlon event.

Before competing in Beijing, Sarah and the other U.S. Olympic athletes generally ate foods that had been pre-prepared in the United States and then shipped to China. In Beijing, an American chef finished preparing the foods, and the items were served to the athletes in a special cafeteria. The registered dietitian who planned diets for U.S. Olympic athletes while they trained in Colorado was also in China for the Olympics. Two days before members of the U.S. women's triathlon team were to compete, the dietitian used a microwave oven in a hotel room to heat pre-prepared meals for the athletes. According to Sarah, the food was "good, but not gourmet. At least we weren't going to get sick eating something unfamiliar. When you go into major competition, you want 'normalcy' as much as possible." Elite competitive athletes such as Sarah need to consume nutritious diets that supply enough energy to sustain their extensive workout regimes. Sarah is 5' 7" and weighs 130 pounds. To maintain her weight and meet her energy needs during heavy training periods, she consumes at least 3500 kilocalories daily. Sarah's typical high-intensity training diet includes baked chicken, yogurt, peanut butter, oatmeal, salads, and fresh fruit. Even when she is not training intensively, her diet is well-balanced and supplies enough energy for her to maintain a healthy weight.

Sarah loves teaching children and talking to them about the importance of being physically active and setting meaningful goals in life. She tells her young audiences, "If you set a goal, with hard work that goal can be achieved. If you fall short of your goal, it's important not to get discouraged and give up. Just reevaluate your goal and change it, if necessary. The 'journey' is what's important, not necessarily the end results. While making the journey, you grow, learn, and become a stronger person!"

supply approximately 3000, 4000, and 5000 kcal/day; and provide ample amounts of carbohydrate. The Chapter 11 "Real People, Real Stories" feature is about Sarah Haskins, an elite Olympic athlete who must maintain a relatively high calorie intake because she trains throughout the year.

How can athletes tell if they are consuming enough energy? One way is to have them keep accurate food records and use the information to estimate their daily calorie intakes. Athletes can also monitor their body weights and have their skinfold thicknesses measured regularly. If their weights were within the healthy BMI range before training and they start to lose weight during training, the individuals should consume more food until they regain their pretraining weights. Consuming an additional 500 to 700 kcal/day, especially by eating calorie- and nutrient-dense foods such as nuts and dried fruit, is a healthy way for anyone to boost his or her calorie intake. Athletes who gain too much body fat can increase their energy output by spending more time in training. Overfat athletes can also reduce their food intake by about 200 to 500 kcal/day until they are in the healthy body mass index (BMI) range. In general, a good way to reduce energy intake is to limit portions of fatty foods. Chapter 3 provides general information to help you plan nutritious menus.

For most physically active people, fat should supply 20 to 35% of energy, which is within the range recommended for the general population.[16] Trained endurance athletes may adapt to long-term, very-high-fat diets (65% or more of total energy) without harming their performance.[17] Nevertheless, the bulk of scientific evidence does not support the use of high-fat diets for athletes.[14] Furthermore, very-low-fat diets (< 20% of total energy from fat) are not beneficial for athletic performance.[14]

Focusing on Carbohydrate Intake

Recommended diets for athletes should supply adequate amounts of energy from carbohydrates. To maintain adequate muscle glycogen, athletes should consume 6 to 10 grams of carbohydrate per kilogram of body weight daily.[14] Glycogen depletion is a major cause of fatigue during endurance exercise. By consuming several servings of grains, starchy vegetables, and fruits daily, an athlete can obtain enough carbohydrate to maintain adequate liver and muscle glycogen stores.

To calculate your recommended range of carbohydrate intake, multiply your weight in kilograms by 6 and then by 10. For example, a 145-pound (66 kg) female athlete should consume between 396 and 660 g of carbohydrate each day. If she requires 3000 kcal/day to maintain her weight and physical activity level and she consumes 60% of her energy from carbohydrates, she will obtain about 450 g of carbohydrate, which is within the recommended range.

It is important to keep in mind that there is no "one size fits all" diet plan that specifies amounts of carbohydrate-rich foods for pre-event, event, or post-event meals and snacks. Diets for athletes should be individualized and based on factors such as the athlete's sex, body size and weight, sport and training level, and exposure to environmental conditions, as well as personal experiences and food preferences. Furthermore, athletes should test any dietary strategies during practices or trials—several days or weeks before a competitive event.

Pre-Event Meals and Snacks

About 3 to 4 hours before competing, athletes should consider eating a meal that supplies 200 to 300 g of carbohydrate, because such meals can

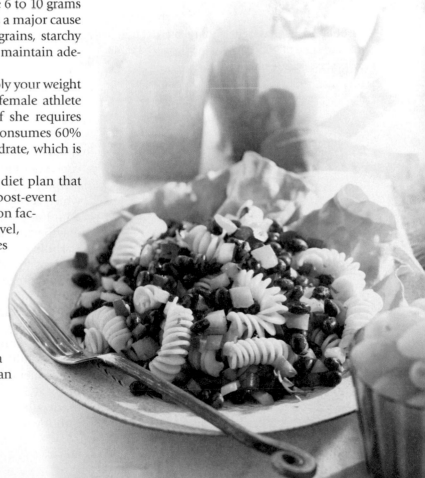

TABLE 11.3 *High-Carbohydrate, Low-Fat Pre-Event Meals*

Meal A	Meal B	Meal C
Instant oatmeal, cinnamon-flavored, 2 packets Fat-free milk, 8 oz	Pasta salad, 1½ cups* French bread, 4 ounces Soft margarine, 1 Tbsp	Cornflakes, ready-to-eat cereal, 1½ cup Fat-free milk, 8 oz Banana, medium
Canned peaches, light syrup, sliced, 1 cup	Apple juice, 8 oz	Orange juice, 8 oz
Orange juice, 8 oz Raisin bread, toasted 2 slices Soft margarine Jelly, 2 Tbsp	Frozen yogurt, 1 cup	English muffin, toasted Soft margarine, 1 Tbsp Jelly, 2 Tbsp Nutty energy bar*

* See Chapter 11 "Recipes for Healthy Living."

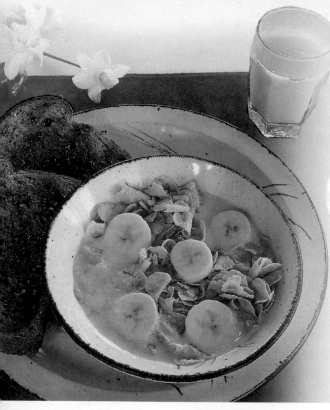

About 3 to 4 hours before performing vigorous exercise, athletes can eat a low-fat meal that supplies 200 to 300 g of carbohydrate.

carbohydrate (glycogen) loading practice of manipulating physical activity and dietary patterns to increase muscle glycogen stores

improve performance.[14] Table 11.3 provides some menu ideas for high-carbohydrate, low-fat pre-event meals that supply approximately 200 g of carbohydrate. Eating fatty foods such as sausage, bacon, sauces, and gravies is not recommended because they take longer to empty from the stomach than low-fat foods.[10] Although some nutritionists advise athletes to exclude high-fiber foods from pre-event meals, there is a lack of scientific evidence to support this recommendation. Nevertheless, athletes can have different responses to eating high-fiber diets prior to events; individuals who react negatively may find it necessary to avoid eating high-fiber foods until after competing.

High-carbohydrate, low-fat food choices for pre-event meals or snacks include cereal with fat-free milk, bagels, dried fruit, pretzels and a sports drink, cooked oatmeal with fruit, pasta, baked potato topped with yogurt, and toasted bread with jelly. Table 11.4 presents commonly eaten foods that are high in carbohydrate and relatively low in fat. Food eaten about an hour before competing should be blended or liquid to promote rapid stomach emptying. Examples of such foods are low-fat smoothies or liquid meal-replacement formulas, such as "instant breakfast" products.

The longer the period before the start of an event, the larger the meal can be, because there will be more time for the stomach to empty and some digestion to occur prior to the activity. Many athletes, however, are anxious before competing and may experience nausea and vomiting if they eat at this time. Other athletes feel comfortable consuming a high-carbohydrate, low-fat meal or snack prior to an event.

What Is Carbohydrate (Glycogen) Loading? A healthy person stores about 6 g of glycogen per kilogram of body weight. Therefore, an individual who weighs 165 pounds (75 kg) stores about 450 g of glycogen. This amount of glycogen supplies 1800 kcal, which is enough energy to enable the person to bicycle at 13 mph for about 4 hours and 15 minutes. Endurance athletes who have more muscle glycogen at the start of an event may be able to exercise longer than those who do not have as much muscle glycogen. **Carbohydrate** or **glycogen loading** involves manipulating dietary and physical activity patterns a few days before an event to increase muscle glycogen stores well above the normal range. The practice helps delay fatigue in athletes participating in events lasting more than 90 minutes.[18]

According to one type of carbohydrate loading technique that lasts for 7 days before an event, an athlete trains intensely during the first day to deplete his or her muscle glycogen stores. Over the next 3 days, the person gradually reduces the duration of his or her daily aerobic workouts (tapering), and during this period, the athlete eats a mixed diet that contains moderate amounts of carbohydrate (about 300 g/day). During the next 3 days, the athlete can exercise lightly or rest. The athlete also switches from a moderate-carbohydrate to a high-carbohydrate diet—one that supplies 400 to 700 g of carbohydrate/day.

TABLE 11.4 *Energy and Macronutrient Contents of Selected Foods*

Food and Amount	kcal	Carbohydrate (g)	Protein (g)	Fat (g)
Macaroni, plain, cooked, 1 cup	221	43.20	8.12	1.30
Spaghetti, cooked, 1 cup	220	42.83	8.12	1.30
Rice, instant, white, cooked, 1 cup	194	41.16	4.60	0.58
Egg noodles, cooked, 1 cup	221	40.26	7.26	3.31
Baked potato, ½ large	139	31.62	3.74	0.19
Corn, canned, drained, 1 cup	133	30.49	4.30	1.64
Bagel, ½, 4″ diam.	144	28.04	5.51	0.84
Grapes, 1 cup	104	27.33	1.09	0.24
Banana, 1 med. (approx. 7″ long)	105	26.95	1.29	0.39
Baked beans, ½ cup	119	26.85	6.03	0.47
Crackers, 6 rectangular saltines	154	25.53	3.32	4.09
Orange juice, unsweetened, 1 cup	110	25.05	1.99	0.69
Cornflakes, 1 cup	101	24.28	1.88	0.03
Pretzels, 1 oz	108	22.61	2.93	0.75
Cooked oatmeal, plain, 1 cup	129	22.44	5.43	2.13
Apple, 1 med. (approx. 3″ diam.)	72	19.06	0.36	0.23
Yogurt, low-fat, plain, 1 cup	154	17.25	12.86	3.80
English muffin, ½	67	13.11	2.53	0.51
Bread, white, 1 slice	66	12.65	2.19	0.82
Fat-free milk, 1 cup	83	12.15	8.26	0.20
Tortilla, corn, ready-to-cook, 6″ diam. (1)	58	12.12	1.48	0.65
Soy milk, 1 cup	127	12.08	10.98	4.70

Source: USDA: *USDA national nutrient database for standard reference, release 19.* 2006. www.nal.usda.gov/fnic/foodcomp/search/

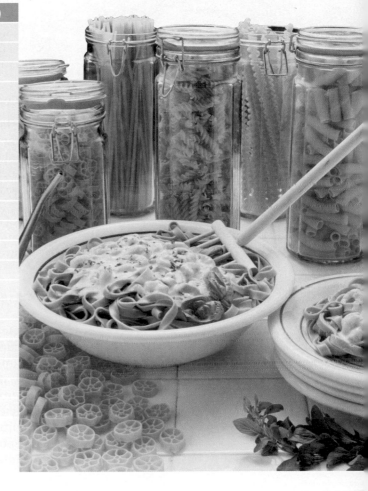

About 3 g of water are incorporated into muscle tissue along with each gram of glycogen. Thus, carbohydrate loading adds water to muscles. Although this fluid aids in maintaining proper hydration status, some individuals experience muscle stiffness and unwanted weight gain as a result of carbohydrate loading. Athletes who would like to determine whether a carbohydrate-loading regimen helps their performance should try the regimen during training to experience its effects. Rather than promote carbohydrate loading, many nutrition and human performance experts simply recommend that athletes routinely follow a high-carbohydrate diet and consume certain forms of carbohydrate during prolonged exercise.

Consuming Carbohydrate During Events

When athletes exercise vigorously for longer than 60 minutes, their glycogen supplies become depleted. At this point, athletes report they have "hit the wall"; that is, they feel unable to maintain a competitive pace. While performing prolonged physical activity, athletes can delay reaching "the wall" by consuming 30 to 60 g of carbohydrate per hour of activity.[14]

Sports drinks are a convenient way to obtain a source of glucose during lengthy and vigorous physical activities. Commercially available sports drinks are usually sweetened with nutritive sweeteners such as sucrose, glucose, fructose, or maltodextrin. Such beverages typically provide 15 to 27 g of carbohydrate per 12-ounce serving. Foods or

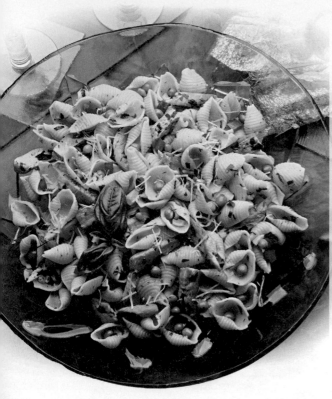

During a post-event meal, starchy foods, such as pasta, can be served to boost an athlete's carbohydrate consumption.

drinks that are concentrated sources of fructose are not recommended, because large amounts of this particular simple sugar may cause gastrointestinal upset. In addition to supplying carbohydrate, sports drinks contain water and electrolytes, such as sodium, that can benefit athletes during prolonged physical effort. Sports gels are also good sources of simple carbohydrate, but they generally supply very little fluid. Therefore, it is important for athletes who consume these products to drink enough water to maintain proper hydration during endurance events.

Consuming Carbohydrates During Exercise Recovery

After completing exhaustive physical activity, trained athletes can replenish nearly all of their glycogen stores within a few days, provided they rest and eat a high-carbohydrate diet. During a post-event meal, starchy foods such as whole-grain bread, mashed potatoes, rice, and pasta can be served to boost athletes' carbohydrate consumption. A pasta recipe is included in the Chapter 11 "Recipes for Healthy Living."

Athletes who train intensely each day need to consume 8 to 10 g of carbohydrate/kg of body weight to replenish their muscle glycogen stores.[10] To restore their supply of muscle glycogen quickly after an event, athletes can consume sports drinks, candy, sugar-sweetened soft drinks, and fruit or fruit juices.

What About Protein?

One of the most controversial topics in nutrition is the amount of protein needed to support athletic performance. Many athletes are convinced that consuming ample amounts of protein from animal foods and taking protein or amino acid supplements is necessary to improve their physical performance and body build. The adult RDA for protein is 0.8 g/kg of body weight.[16] A review of the nutritional practices of elite athletes indicated that individuals training for aerobic sports consumed 1.1 to 3.0 g of protein/kg of body weight per day (g/kg/day), whereas those training for anaerobic sports, such as weight lifting, consumed 1.1 to 3.2 g/kg/day.[15] Are such high-protein intakes recommended or even necessary?

Under normal conditions, carbohydrate and fat are the primary fuels for cellular activity, and protein provides no more than 15% of the body's energy needs. Thus, protein is not a major biological fuel. During prolonged physical activity, muscles lose some protein because they metabolize certain amino acids for energy.[19] To spare protein so the nutrient can be used for muscle tissue growth and repair instead of for energy, it is very important for physically active people to consume adequate amounts of carbohydrate and fat.

After strenuous exercise, muscle cells repair damaged muscle tissue by using available amino acids to synthesize new proteins. Thus, having adequate amounts of amino acids in muscle tissue promotes positive nitrogen balance after exercise.[20, 21] After engaging in intense physical activity, athletes may be able to enhance protein synthesis in their muscles by eating protein-rich foods.[19, 22, 23] Compared to nonathletes, however, the typical athlete consumes more food to meet his or her increased energy needs and, as a result, obtains plenty of dietary protein.[23] Therefore, healthy active Americans who eat varied diets that supply adequate energy do not need to take protein or amino acid supplements.[24] If people consume excess protein from foods or supplements and they do not need the energy, the amino acids in these proteins will not be used for building or repairing muscles. Instead, the body converts the extra amino acids into fat for storage in adipose tissue.

Protein: Recommendations for Athletes

Despite conventional wisdom that athletes have higher protein requirements than nonathletes, there are no specific protein RDAs for endurance or resistance athletes. A recent report published by the Institute of Medicine states that "no additional dietary protein is suggested for healthy adults who undertake resistance or endurance exercise."[16] Nevertheless, the RDA for protein may not apply to athletes involved in training or competition. According to joint recommendations issued by the Academy of Nutrition and Dietetics, Dietitians of Canada, and the American College of Sports Medicine, endurance and resistance athletes should consume 1.2 to 1.4 g of protein/kg of body weight/day and 1.2 to 1.7 g of protein/kg of body weight/day, respectively.[14] Although these amounts of protein are considerably higher than the RDAs for nonathletes, they do not appear to be harmful for *healthy* physically active people.

Raising the Bar?

"Lasting energy," "fast fuel," "optimal energy"—such claims are used to promote so-called "energy" bars, gels, and drinks. Energy or sports bars are essentially cookies made from soy and milk proteins that are fortified with vitamins, minerals, and fiber. Sugary syrups hold these ingredients together. *High-protein* energy bars may appeal to athletes who think proteins are a source of energy and enhance muscular development. However, proteins are not a major biological fuel, and they are not "quick energy" sources, because the liver must process amino acids before they can be used for energy. Moreover, eating more protein than the body needs does not build muscle tissue. People need to follow a resistance training program to enlarge their skeletal muscles safely.

Granola bars, fruit-filled cookies, and fresh or dried fruits are less expensive and more natural sources of energy and nutrients than energy or sports bars. You can make your own "energy" bars by following the recipe in the Chapter 11 "Recipes for Healthy Living." If you prefer to eat commercial energy bars, check the products' Nutrition Facts panels to determine amounts of carbohydrates and other nutrients that are in a serving. By eating several energy bars daily, you may ingest high amounts of iron, vitamin A, and other micronutrients. Therefore, consider energy bars as occasional snacks and not as meal replacements. Table 11.5 presents approximate energy and macronutrient contents per 100 g of various popular energy bars and gels.

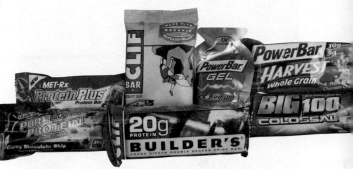

High-protein energy bars may appeal to athletes who think proteins are a source of energy and enhance muscular development.

> **caffeine** naturally occurring stimulant drug

TABLE 11.5 *Popular Energy Bars and Gels: Energy and Macronutrient Contents/100 g*

Product	Energy kcal/100 g	Carbohydrates g/100 g	Protein g/100 g	Fat g/100 g
PowerBar Performance (cookies & cream)	370	66.2	12.3	4.6
PowerBar ProteinPlus (cookies & cream)	385	48.7	29.5	7.7
PowerBar PowerGel (vanilla)	268	65.9	0	0
Luna Bar (peanut butter cookies)	375	47.9	28.8	12.5
Clif Bar (chocolate chip)	368	66.2	28.8	7.4
Clif Shot (vanilla gel)	312	78.1	0	0
Balance Bar (chocolate)	400	44.0	28.0	12.0
Balance CarbWell (chocolate peanut butter)	400	44.0	28.0	16.0

Sources: Clif Bar & Company, www.clifbar.com/; Luna Bar, www.lunabar.com/index_main.cfm; Balance Bar Food Company, www.balance.com/; Power Bar, www.powerbar.com/

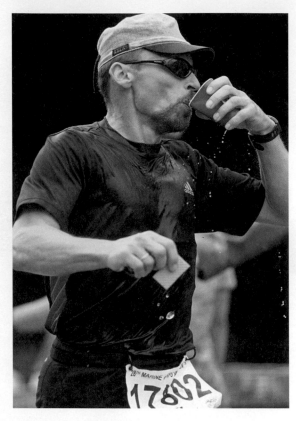

To reduce the risk of heat illnesses, athletes and other physically active people should replace fluid losses that occur during prolonged exertion.

TABLE 11.6 *Heat-Related Illnesses: Signs and Symptoms*

Heat cramps
• Painful muscle spasms

Heat exhaustion
• Muscle ("heat") cramps
• Low-grade fever
• Heavy sweating
• Weakness
• Light-headedness or dizziness
• Lack of interest in doing things
• Headache
• Nausea

Heatstroke
• Severe weakness
• High fever (over 104°F)
• Lack of sweating
• Rapid, shallow breathing
• Irritability and confusion
• Coma

Energy drinks usually contain sugars and a lot of **caffeine,** a stimulant drug that is naturally in coffee and tea. When consumed in moderate amounts, caffeine can increase alertness and decrease fatigue.[25] Some energy drinks also contain the amino acid *taurine* and herbal substances such as ginseng. Although the body uses taurine, the compound is not required by humans. Ginseng may enhance the stimulating effects of caffeine.[26] The "Ergogenic Aids" section of Chapter 11 provides more information about caffeine, ginseng, and some other substances that are promoted for enhancing physical performance.

Focusing on Fluids

The Adequate Intake (AI) for total water intake is approximately 11 cups (2.7 L) and 15.5 cups (3.7 L) for young women and men, respectively. Athletes generally require more water than nonathletes to keep their bodies cool during muscular activity. Many factors, however, influence a person's hydration status. Among athletes in particular, differences in sports, fitness levels, and environmental conditions affect fluid needs. For example, sweating can cause runners to lose 3 to 8 cups (750 to 2000 ml) of water per hour.[27] Even a small degree of dehydration can lead to declines in an athlete's endurance, strength, and overall performance. Moreover, body temperature rises when dehydration occurs, increasing the risk of heat-related illness.

Heat-Related Illness

As the environmental temperature and humidity increase, the evaporation of sweat from skin slows, and the body has difficulty cooling itself by perspiring. Ineffective sweating contributes to fatigue, makes the heart work harder, and raises the risk of *heat-related illness*. Table 11.6 presents three major types of heat-related illness and their common signs and symptoms.

Many athletes are familiar with **heat cramps.** These painful muscle *spasms* (involuntary contractions) can affect any muscle, but they usually occur in the back, abdominal, or calf muscles. The cause of heat cramps is unclear, but the spasms may partially result from the loss of electrolytes in sweat.[10] Treatment of heat cramps includes resting, drinking juice or a sports drink, and gently stretching and massaging the affected muscles.[28]

Heat exhaustion can occur after heavy exercise in warm conditions, especially when fluid and salt intakes have been inadequate. A person suffering from heat exhaustion experiences heat cramps, sweats excessively, and has a body temperature of around 102°F.[29] Other signs of the illness include cool, moist, gray-colored skin and rapid, weak pulse. To treat heat exhaustion, move the victim to a cool or shady place and have the person lie on his or her back with legs slightly elevated. Furthermore, cool the person by fanning, spraying with cool water, or giving a cool sponge bath. It is also very important to have the victim drink cool water or a sports drink. People with heat exhaustion should be monitored closely, because the condition can rapidly develop into *heatstroke*.

Heatstroke is the most dangerous form of heat-related illness. Signs of heatstroke include elevated body temperature (often more than 104°F); lack of sweating; rapid, shallow breathing; irritable and confused behavior; and loss of consciousness (coma).[30] Heatstroke is a medical emergency that needs to be treated by trained medical staff. If you suspect that a person has heatstroke, summon emergency medical assistance immediately (dial 911) and move the victim to a cool environment. While waiting for professional medical care to arrive, you can give the patient cool water to drink (if he or she is conscious) and spray the person with cool water.

Replenishing Fluids

To reduce the risk of heat illnesses, athletes and other physically active people should avoid exercising under extremely hot, humid conditions and should replace fluid losses that occur during prolonged exertion. According to recommendations recently established by the International Marathon Medical Directors Association (IMMDA), thirst protects athletes from consuming too little or too much fluid.[31] Experts with this organization no longer recommend drinking fluids even if you are not thirsty, because this practice can lead to water intoxication (*hyponatremia*). However, athletes should avoid losing more than 2% of their body weight during exercise.[27]

To estimate the amount of fluids needed to replace water loss during exercise (*rehydration*), athletes can weigh themselves prior to exercising and then calculate 2% of their body weight (0.02 × weight). After working out, athletes should weigh themselves again. If the difference between preexercise and postexercise body weights is more than 2%, fluid replacement is necessary during such activities. For example, if you weigh 150 pounds, 2% of that weight is 3 pounds (0.02 × 150). Therefore, you should drink enough watery fluids to avoid losing 3 or more pounds when you train or compete. In general, you can replace each pound that you lose during exercise by drinking 1½ pints (3 cups) of water.[10] For example, if your usual weight is 150 pounds and you weigh 149 pounds immediately after exercising, you have lost 1 pound of body water during the activity. The next time you exercise under similar conditions, you can consume 3 cups of water during the activity to maintain your body's water balance. Why do you need to drink 50% more fluids than you have lost in sweat? After exercise, rehydration may stimulate the kidneys to produce more urine than normal; thus, you need to drink the extra watery fluids to achieve proper hydration. As noted in Chapter 9, alcoholic beverages have a diuretic effect on the body and are not recommended for rehydration.

Do I Need a Sports Drink?

Sports drinks provide some nutritional benefits beyond those of plain water. These beverages usually contain simple carbohydrates, a source of energy that can enhance performance during endurance activities. Recommended products contain about 21 g of carbohydrate per 12-ounce serving, or about 6% carbohydrate by weight. Drinks with sugar contents above 10%, such as soft drinks or fruit juices, are not recommended because they may cause intestinal discomfort. Sodium and other electrolytes in sports beverages help maintain blood volume, enhance the absorption of water and carbohydrate from the intestinal tract, and stimulate thirst.

Should you drink water or a sports drink during competition? According to the Association of International Marathons and Road Races (IMMDA), sports drinks are necessary when workouts or events last longer than 30 minutes.[31] Although electrolytes are lost in sweat, the quantities lost in shorter periods can be easily replaced by consuming foods and beverages, such as water or fruit juice, after the event.

It is possible to drink too much water and develop water intoxication (see Chapter 9). Endurance athletes, especially poorly trained individuals, may compete at relatively low exercise intensities for prolonged periods. Under these conditions, the athletes do not sweat as much; therefore, they do not need to replace as much water as better-trained athletes who exercise at higher intensities. Regardless of training level, athletes who drink too much water can dilute the level of sodium in their blood and develop serious and even deadly side effects. Although sports

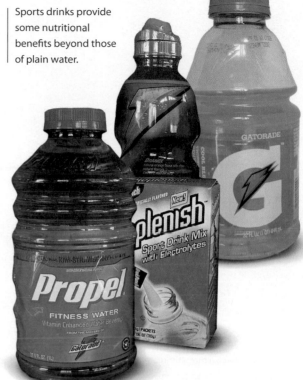

Sports drinks provide some nutritional benefits beyond those of plain water.

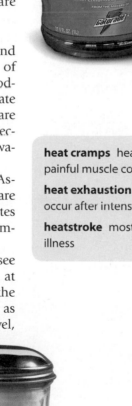

heat cramps heat-related illness characterized by painful muscle contractions

heat exhaustion heat-related illness that can occur after intense exercise

heatstroke most dangerous form of heat-related illness

Food & Nutrition *tip*

Compared to commercially available sports drinks, dilute fruit juices with added sugar and salt are less expensive sources of water, sodium, and simple sugars. You can prepare your own "sports" drink by adding ¼ cup of orange juice, ¼ cup of sugar, and ⅛ tsp of table salt to 30 oz of water or club soda. Pour the beverage into a quart pitcher, cover, and refrigerate until needed.

drinks generally contain sodium, these beverages are mostly water; therefore, consuming excessive amounts of sports drinks can contribute to fluid overload. To avoid water intoxication, athletes should drink water according to their thirst. If an athlete gains weight while exercising, he or she may be retaining too much fluid.

Antioxidant Vitamins

During aerobic physical activities, skeletal muscles use more oxygen and generate more free radicals than resting muscle tissue.[32] Exercise can produce a temporary imbalance between free radical generation and the ability of antioxidants to counteract them. Scientific evidence suggests that such *oxidative stress* may contribute to muscle fatigue and damage. Nevertheless, results of studies that examined whether antioxidant vitamin supplements enhanced athletic performance generally concluded that performance was not improved, unless there was a preexisting deficiency of those particular vitamins.

Findings of some scientific studies indicate that free radicals generated during intense exercise may stimulate the body's natural antioxidant defense system. Thus, the oxidative stress produced during exercise might have benefits, and blocking this process by taking antioxidant vitamin supplements may not be desirable.[32, 33]

Currently, antioxidant vitamin supplements are not recommended for athletes.[32] Athletes should be cautious about taking such supplements based on anecdotes or advertising claims, because there is not enough scientific evidence concerning the long-term effects of using these products. Rather than experiment on themselves with antioxidant supplements, athletes should follow diets that contain foods naturally rich in antioxidants, such as fruits, vegetables, whole-grain breads and cereals, and vegetable oils.

Iron

The body needs iron to produce red blood cells, transport oxygen, and obtain energy. Thus, iron deficiency can negatively affect athletic performance. Young female athletes are likely to develop iron deficiency because of their menstrual blood losses—bleeding is a cause of iron deficiency. Athletes who follow low-calorie or vegetarian (especially vegan) diets are also at risk of iron deficiency, because their food choices may be low in iron. Additionally, distance runners may develop low iron status, because intense prolonged workouts can lead to gastrointestinal bleeding.

In the early phase of their training, endurance athletes often develop *sports anemia*, a temporary condition that results from an increase in the liquid portion of blood (*plasma*), rather than iron deficiency.[10] The effects of sports anemia on physical performance are unknown. Nevertheless, it can be difficult to differentiate between sports anemia and true iron deficiency anemia. It is a good idea for athletes, especially females, to have their iron status checked at the beginning of a training season and at least once during midseason. If an athlete is iron deficient, a physician needs to determine the cause and prescribe treatment.

Calcium

Athletes, especially those who are total vegetarians or restrict their consumption of dairy products to lose weight, can have marginal or low calcium intakes. This practice may result in weak bones that fracture easily, as well as in osteoporosis later in life. Additionally, female athletes who have irregular or no menstrual cycles may be deficient in the hormone estrogen. Although weight-bearing exercise, such as jogging, improves bone density, estrogen is also necessary for maintaining healthy bones. Female athletes who develop menstrual cycle abnormalities should consult a physician to determine the cause. Decreasing the amount of training or gaining weight may restore a regular menstrual pattern. For information about the *female athlete triad*, see the Chapter 10 "Highlight"; Chapter 9 provides information about osteoporosis.

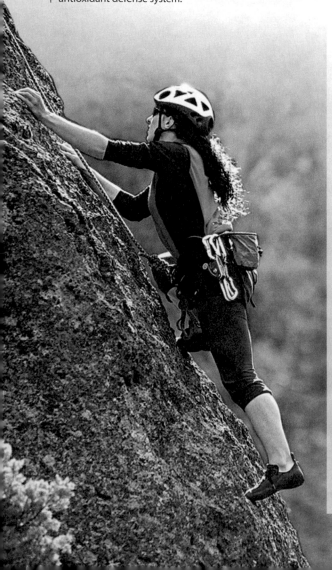

Intense exercise may stimulate the body's natural antioxidant defense system.

Concept **Checkpoint**

12. What are some practical ways to assess whether an athlete's energy intake is adequate?
13. Why should athletes be concerned about their carbohydrate intakes before, during, and after prolonged intense physical activity?
14. Identify at least five high-carbohydrate/low-fat foods.
15. Explain why athletes do not need to take protein or amino acid supplements.
16. Why should athletes be concerned about their bodies' fluid status?
17. What are major signs and symptoms of heat cramps, heat exhaustion, and heatstroke?
18. When is consuming a sports drink a better choice than plain water for rehydration?
19. Explain why you would or would not recommend that an athlete take antioxidant supplements.
20. Explain why iron deficiency can impair an athlete's physical performance.
21. For young female athletes, what is the significance of having irregular or no menstrual cycles for bone health?

 # 11.4 Ergogenic Aids: Separating Fact from Fiction

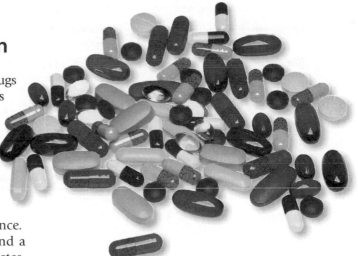

Athletes often use **ergogenic aids**—foods, devices, dietary supplements, and even drugs ("doping")—to improve their physical performance. Bee pollen, dried adrenal glands from cattle, seaweed, freeze-dried liver flakes, and ginseng are among the dietary supplements that athletes consume as they hope to gain the competitive edge over their rivals. However, no reliable scientific evidence supports the effectiveness of most dietary supplements purported to have ergogenic effects. Nevertheless, many athletes firmly believe in the value of the performance-enhancing aids that they use. In many instances, the perceived benefits are more likely to result from the placebo effect than from actual physiological changes (see Chapter 2).

A few dietary substances and practices can enhance physical performance. These ergogenic aids include sufficient water and electrolytes, carbohydrates, and a balanced and varied diet consistent with MyPlate recommendations. For athletes, meeting carbohydrate and fluid needs—along with overall nutrient needs—is the most important ergogenic aid.

Athletes should be skeptical of claims made for any substance until its ergogenic effects and long-term safety have been determined by researchers who are not associated with the supplement industry. Rather than searching for a "magic bullet" to enhance their performance, athletes should concentrate their efforts on improving their dietary habits, training routines, and sports techniques. Nutrient supplements should be used for specific dietary deficiencies, such as preventing iron deficiency or boosting calcium intakes.

Table 11.7 summarizes science-based findings regarding caffeine, carnitine, creatine, and some other dietary supplements and ergogenic aids that are popular among athletes. It is important to note that certain dietary supplements are known to be unsafe, and the use of others is restricted or banned by major athletic organizations. For example, in 2004 the U.S. Food and Drug Administration (FDA) banned the use of ephedrine-containing supplements. Ephedrine (ephedra, ma huang) increases central nervous system activity, but the drug can cause serious, even deadly side effects. The following section discusses the ergogenic properties of caffeine.

ergogenic aids foods, devices, dietary supplements, or drugs used to improve physical performance

TABLE 11.7 *Evaluation of Some Popular Ergogenic Supplements/Aids*

Substance	Claim	Current Science-Based Findings Concerning Claims	Side Effects
Caffeine	Enhances fat metabolism Increases alertness	Consuming 3 to 9 mg of caffeine/kg of body weight about 1 hour before events may benefit certain athletes	High doses can cause nervousness, shakiness, and sleep disturbances. Intakes of more than 600 mg (6 to 8 cups of coffee) can produce levels of caffeine in urine that are banned by the National Collegiate Athletic Association (NCAA).
Creatine	Enhances muscular endurance and strength Increases lean muscle mass	May enhance performance of sprinters and weight lifters	High doses may cause kidney damage, especially in persons with kidney disease.
Sodium bicarbonate (baking soda)	Reduces lactic acid accumulation	May enhance performance	May cause nausea and vomiting
Beta-hydroxy-beta-methylbutyrate (HMB)	Decreases protein metabolism, increasing muscle mass	May increase muscle mass, but evidence is weak	None reported, but results of long-term use are unknown
Branched chain amino acids	Provide energy for muscles	May enhance muscle recovery after intense physical activity	None reported
Glucosamine	Aids in repairing damaged joints	Mixed results, but generally no beneficial results	None reported
Chromium	Increases lean mass	No benefit	Toxic level: intakes above 400 mcg daily
Coenzyme Q_{10}	Enhances cardiac function, delays fatigue	No benefit	Long-term safety is unknown.
Bee pollen	Shortens muscle recovery time Increases muscular strength and endurance	No benefit	May cause allergic reactions in sensitive persons
Ginseng	Combats fatigue and improves stamina	May have mild stimulant effects	Results of most clinical studies (200 to 1600 mg/day) indicate that ginseng does not improve physical performance, but more research is needed.
Anabolic steroids	Increase muscle mass and strength	Increase protein synthesis In the United States, legal use requires physician's prescription.	Side effects include: bloody liver cysts; increased risk of cardiovascular disease, hypertension, and reproductive problems; mood swings and aggressive behavior ("roid rage"); sleep disturbances. Banned by many sports organizations
Gamma hydroxybutyric acid (GHB)	Increases muscle mass by acting like an anabolic steroid	Illegal—FDA has not approved GHB for production or sale in the United States.	Vomiting, dizziness, shakiness, and seizures May cause death
Human growth hormone	Increases muscle mass and fat metabolism	Most studies indicate no benefit.	May increase height as well as size of the heart and other internal organs Very dangerous, can be deadly International Olympic Committee bans the use of growth hormone.
DHEA and androstenedione ("andro")	Increases the body's steroid production	No benefit	May be dangerous Banned by International Olympic Committee In 2004, the FDA warned companies to stop manufacturing products that contain "andro."

Sources: Byrd-Bredbenner and others: *Perspectives in nutrition*. New York: McGraw-Hill, 2009; Ahrendt DM: Ergogenic aids: Counseling the athlete. *American Family Physician* 63:913, 2001; Kiwdwe D, Pantuso T: Panax ginseng. *American Family Physician* 68:1539, 2003; Hsu C-C and others: American ginseng supplementation attenuates creatine kinase level induced by submaximal exercise in human beings. *World Journal of Gastroenterology* 11:5327, 2005; Liang MT and others: Panax notoginseng supplementation enhances physical performance during endurance exercise. *Journal of Strength and Conditioning Research* 19:108, 2005; U.S. Department of Health and Human Services: *HS launches crackdown on products containing andro.* 2004. www.fda.gov/bbs/topics/news/2004/hhs_031104.html

Caffeine

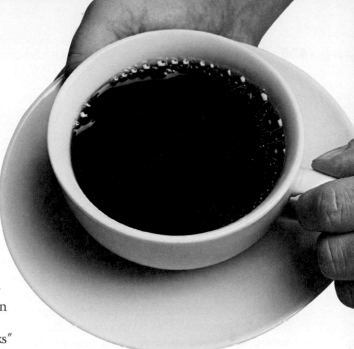

Worldwide, caffeine is the most widely used ergogenic aid. Caffeine raises the level of fatty acids in blood, and as a result, exercising muscles can use more fat for energy. Caffeine also enhances the ability of skeletal and heart muscles to contract and increases mental alertness. Although consuming even small amounts of caffeine may help endurance athletes, the National Collegiate Athletic Association (NCAA) limits the amount of caffeine that athletes can have in their bodies during competition. Athletes who have more than 15 micrograms of caffeine per milliliter (mcg/ml) of their urine can be banned.[34] Nevertheless, the World Anti-Doping Agency (WADA) does not prohibit the use of caffeine.[35]

People who are not regular caffeine consumers may experience shakiness, rapid heart rate, sleep disturbances, diarrhea, and frequent urination after ingesting relatively high amounts of the stimulant drug. Caffeine is addictive; discontinuing its use results in *withdrawal*, temporary unpleasant side effects, especially headache.

It is important to understand that the quick "energy" boost provided by "energy drinks" is a result of caffeine or other stimulants contained in the products.[36] Nevertheless, energy drinks also provide calories if they are sweetened with added sugars. Table 11.8 compares the caffeine and calorie contents of popular beverages, including an energy drink ("Red Bull"). Note that an 8.5-ounce serving of brewed coffee supplies more caffeine but fewer kilocalories than the same amount of the energy drink. However, amounts of caffeine in brewed coffee can vary widely, depending on preparation methods. "Stay awake" pills and chewing gums are concentrated sources of caffeine that can be purchased without a prescription.

Caffeine raises the level of fatty acids in blood, and as a result, exercising muscles can use more fat for energy.

Concept **Checkpoint**

22. Why do many athletes use ergogenic aids?

23. Identify three ergogenic aids that have been banned by at least one athletic association.

24. Identify at least three foods or beverages that are rich sources of caffeine.

25. Discuss the ergogenic effects that caffeine can have on the body.

TABLE 11.8 *Caffeine Content of Selected Beverages*

Beverage and Amount	kcal	Caffeine (mg)
Coffee, Starbucks Coffee Grande, 16 oz*	5	330
Coffee, brewed from grounds, unsweetened, 8 oz	2	95
Red Bull, 8.3-oz can	115	76
Coffee, instant plain, prepared, 8 oz	5	62
Cola with caffeine, 12-oz can	136–151	29–99
Mountain Dew, 12-oz can**	170	54
Tea, brewed, unsweetened, 8 oz	2	47
Tea, ready-to-drink, 12-oz can	89	11
Chocolate drink, 8 oz	120	2

*Starbucks beverages: Nutrition information. www.starbucks.com/retail/nutrition_beverages.asp, Accessed: August 31, 2009.
**Brands: http://pepsiproductfacts.com, Accessed August 31, 2009.
Source: USDA: USDA national nutrient database for standard reference, release 21. 2008. www.nal.usda.gov/fnic/foodcomp/search/

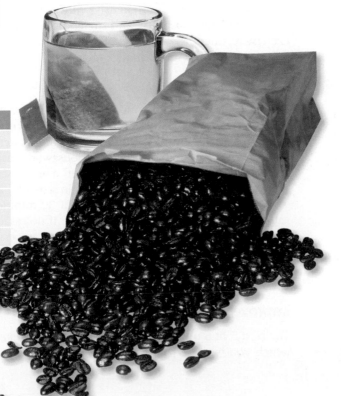

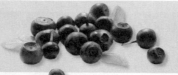

Chapter 11 Highlight

DEVELOPING A PERSONAL PHYSICAL FITNESS PLAN

According to guidelines established by the American College of Sports Medicine and the American Heart Association, healthy adults under 65 years of age should perform moderate-intensity aerobic activity for 30 minutes daily, 5 days a week.[3] Adults who would like to do more physically intense workouts can perform vigorous activities 20 minutes a day, 3 days a week. In addition to the aerobic activities, adults should perform strength-training exercises twice each week.

Most healthy people can gradually increase their level of physical activity. Sedentary men who are 40 years of age or older, physically inactive women who are 50 years of age or older, and people who have existing health problems may want to discuss their fitness goals with their physicians before beginning a fitness program. Health problems that require a preliminary medical evaluation are obesity, cardiovascular disease (or family history of CVD), hypertension, type 2 diabetes (or family history), shortness of breath after mild exertion, and arthritis. Additionally, pregnant women should check with their physicians before starting an exercise regimen.

When developing your personal physical fitness plan, first consider your fitness goals. For example, if you want to lose weight, how much do you want to lose and how many weeks will it take to lose that amount? Do you want to focus more on strengthening your muscles or on improving your aerobic capacity? Then determine when you can work out and whether you'll need to join a fitness facility such as a gym or purchase special equipment, such as hand-held weights. For a comprehensive fitness program, make sure to include aerobic, resistance, and stretching activities in your weekly exercise regimen. The following fitness plan has three stages: initial, improvement, and maintenance phases.

Initiation

The first 3 to 6 weeks of your new exercise program is the *initiation* stage. Start by incorporating short periods of physical activity into your daily routine. For example, you can walk more often, take the stairs instead of the elevator, and do more housework, gardening, or other activities that cause you to "huff and puff" a bit. Furthermore, you can strive to reduce the time that you spend in sedentary activities.

The goal is to accumulate a total of 30 minutes of moderate-intensity types of activity 5 days a week. If necessary, the time that you spend engaging in the activity each day can occur in three short intervals lasting at least 10 minutes. If you do not have 30 minutes to spend on exercising, try increasing the intensity of the activities during shorter bouts of exercise to obtain some health benefits.

Improvement and Maintenance

The next 5 or 6 months of the program is the *improvement* stage, in which you increase the intensity and duration of exercises. When

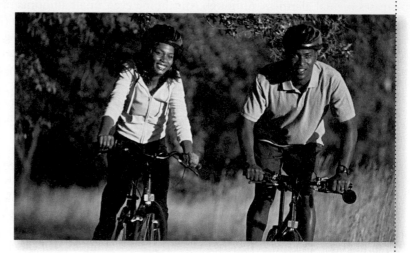

you begin the improvement phase, exercise at an intensity that is near the lower end of your target heart rate zone. As you progress and become more physically fit, you can increase the intensity by exercising at a higher heart rate.

By the end of the improvement stage, you may notice that you have reached your goals, and you do not seem to be making further gains in your fitness. This plateau marks the beginning of your *maintenance* stage. At this point, you can evaluate your personal fitness plan, and if you would like to make new goals, this is the time to develop them. If you are satisfied with your fitness level, continue with your present program. Discontinuing exercise gradually results in *detraining*, declining physical fitness.

Components of a Workout Regimen

Ideally, you should establish a regular time for exercising that fits into your daily routine. To be effective, your aerobic workout program needs to include the following components:

1. **Warm-up** Warming up muscles can increase your joints' range of motion (flexibility) and may decrease your risk of injury. Stretching for 5 to 10 minutes is a good way to warm up. Start with smaller muscle groups such as the arms and progressively work toward stretching larger muscle groups in the legs and abdomen. Hold your position in the stretch for 15 seconds and do not bounce. If stretching causes pain, stop immediately. "No pain, no gain" is not true—pain is an indication of injury. Another way to warm up is to perform 5 to 10 minutes of the anticipated activity but at a low intensity. For example, if you walk for fitness, warm up by walking at a slower pace.
2. **Aerobic workout** To obtain substantial health benefits, you should engage in some form of aerobic activity regularly. A comprehensive aerobic workout emphasizes the *type, duration, frequency, intensity,* and *progression* of exercise.
   - **Type:** The kinds of exercise you choose should increase your heart and breathing rates and involve rhythmic

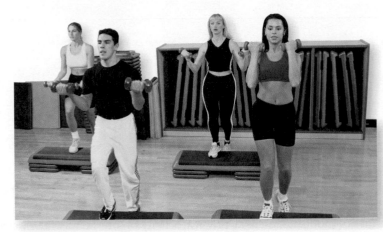

To obtain substantial health benefits, people should engage in some form of aerobic activity regularly.

movements of large muscle groups in the legs. Examples include brisk walking, running, swimming, and cycling. If you swim, add some *weight-bearing activities*, such as walking, to your fitness plan. Weight-bearing exercises place stress on your bones, increasing their strength.

- **Duration:** Duration is the amount of time spent in an exercise session. A session should generally last at least 20 to 30 minutes, depending on intensity, not including time spent warming up and cooling down. Ideally, the exercise session should be continuous (without stopping), but multiple 10-minute bouts of moderate to intense activity with rest periods in between are also acceptable.
- **Frequency:** The frequency of exercise describes the number of times that the activity is performed, generally on a weekly basis. To derive significant health benefits, the frequency of aerobic exercise should be at least five times per week. By exercising daily, you can enjoy even greater benefits.
- **Intensity:** Health benefits can occur when you achieve at least a moderate level of intensity during exercise.
- **Progression:** Progression, the final component of a comprehensive fitness plan, refers to the gradual increase in the frequency, intensity, and duration of exercise that occurs over a period.

3. **Cool-down** To cool down, you can repeat the same stretches you performed during warming up. Stretch for 5 to 10 minutes. Cooling down may prevent injury and reduce muscle soreness.

What About Strength (Resistance) Training?

Strength training, such as weight lifting, is an important part of a comprehensive physical fitness plan. Strength training should be done at least 2 days per week. To start, warm up by stretching for 5 to 10 minutes. Then perform a group of 8 to 10 exercises that strengthen major muscle groups of the upper body and lower body. Cool down for 5 to 10 minutes at the end of each session.

Fitness centers have machines that provide resistance for various muscle groups. For resistance training outside of gymnasiums or fitness clubs, you can purchase simple elastic exercise cords designed to increase muscular strength (Fig. 11.12). For increasing upper arm

strength, a set of inexpensive handheld weights can be kept in a convenient location for performing resistance exercise regularly, such as near the TV. The weights should allow you to perform at least one set of 8 to 15 repetitions. When you can do more than 15 repetitions with relative ease, consider increasing the weight slightly.

Mixing It Up

To make your exercise routine more enjoyable, include several types of physical activity in your weekly regimen. For example, jogging one day might be followed by swimming the next day. Adding variety to a program not only keeps you from becoming bored with your workouts but also strengthens different muscle groups in your body and reduces your risk of injury. Additionally, invite a friend or relative to be your exercise partner. Having an exercise partner may provide additional motivation and encouragement to exercise regularly.

Some overfat people do not experience significant weight loss while following an exercise regimen. However, they still benefit from regular physical activity. Initially, exercise programs for obese people should emphasize non-weight-bearing activities, such as swimming, water aerobics, and bicycling. As obese people lose weight and become more fit, they can add weight-bearing activities to their plans.

Whatever physical activities you choose to include in your fitness program, they should be enjoyable and easy to incorporate into your routine. You can apply the dietary principles of variety, balance, and moderation to your exercise routine:

- **Variety:** Perform several different activities to exercise different muscle groups.
- **Balance:** For overall fitness, balance your exercise regimen by including activities that build cardiovascular endurance, muscular strength, and flexibility.
- **Moderation:** Focus on exercising to keep fit without overdoing it and injuring yourself. You do not need to work out vigorously every day to become healthier.

To learn more about the health benefits of physical fitness, determine your level of fitness, or develop a personal fitness program, access the following websites:

www.shapeup.org
www.fitness.gov
www.presidentschallenge.org

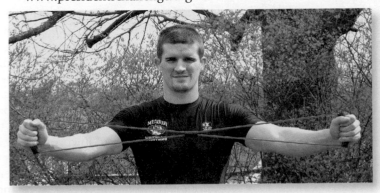

Figure 11.12 Increasing muscle strength. This individual is using a simple rubber exercise cord to increase muscular strength.

CHAPTER REFERENCES

See Appendix 1.

SUMMARY

Many Americans lead sedentary lives. People can manage their weight more effectively and reduce their risk of developing the major causes of death and disability by engaging in at least 30 minutes of moderate-intensity physical activity on most days of the week. Furthermore, most people can achieve even greater health benefits by increasing the duration, frequency, and intensity of their physical activities.

Regular physical activity reduces the risk of dying prematurely and developing heart disease, diabetes, and high blood pressure. Additionally, regular exercise builds and maintains healthy bones, muscles, and joints; helps reduce blood pressure in people who have high blood pressure; reduces the risk of developing certain cancers; aids weight-control efforts; helps older adults become stronger and reduces their risk of falls; reduces risk of sleep disorders, depression, and anxiety; and promotes psychological well-being. Millions of Americans suffer from chronic illnesses that can be prevented or improved by exercising more often.

ATP is the major form of energy used by cells. Phosphocreatine (PCr) can rapidly reform ATP from its breakdown product ADP, but PCr supplies are limited. To generate ATP, muscle cells can metabolize carbohydrate, fat, and protein. In muscle cells, glucose molecules are broken down through a series of steps to yield lactic acid (in anaerobic conditions) or CO_2 plus H_2O (in aerobic conditions).

The proportions of macronutrients used for energy largely depend on the intensity of the physical activity. Fat is a key aerobic fuel for muscle cells, especially at low-intensity exercise. At rest and during light activity, muscles burn primarily fat for energy needs. In comparison, little protein generally is used to fuel muscles. During brief bouts of intense physical effort, the cardiorespiratory system is unable to deliver adequate oxygen to muscles. Under such anaerobic conditions, muscle cells metabolize glucose rather than fat for energy, but their ability to sustain the release of energy for intense activity is limited. Muscle cells can obtain far more energy when in aerobic conditions.

Sports nutrition focuses on applying nutrition principles and research findings to improving athletic performance. Athletes often manipulate their diets to enhance their body contours, increase their muscular strength, and prevent or delay fatigue during exercise. Although diet is important, genetic endowment and physical training are the most crucial factors that influence athletic performance.

A high-carbohydrate diet can be beneficial for athletes, and carbohydrate-rich foods should form the foundation of pre-event meals. Many athletes consume more protein than they require. Despite marketing claims, protein supplements are unnecessary. By eating their usual food choices, most athletes can meet their protein needs.

Physically active people need to be concerned about their fluid intakes. Fluid replacement should be based on thirst and loss of body weight while exercising. Consuming a source of electrolytes, such as a sports drink, can be helpful, especially when the duration of intense exercise exceeds 30 minutes. It is important to avoid overconsumption of water because of the risk of water intoxication.

Athletes often ingest certain substances, including herbal products, because they believe these substances have ergogenic effects. Scientific evidence, however, does not suggest that most of these substances are effective. Furthermore, long-term safety of many ergogenic aids has not been determined, and use of some substances is restricted or banned by various athletic organizations.

According to guidelines established by the American College of Sports Medicine and the American Heart Association, healthy adults under 65 years of age should perform

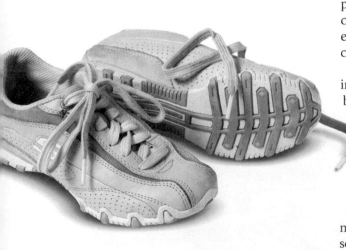

moderate-intensity aerobic activity for 30 minutes daily, 5 days a week. Adults who would like to do more physically intense workouts can perform vigorous activities 20 minutes a day, 3 days a week. In addition to aerobic activities, adults should perform strength training exercises twice weekly. The three components of an aerobic workout are warming up, performing the moderate or vigorous intensity activity, and cooling down.

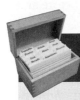

Recipes for Healthy Living

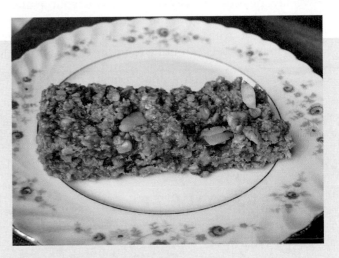

Nutty Energy Bars

You can use the following recipe to make your own "energy bars." This recipe makes eight 4" × 2" bars. Each bar supplies approximately 253 kcal, 8 g protein, 13 g fat, 26 g carbohydrate, 3 g fiber, and 4.9 mg iron.

INGREDIENTS:

Oil cooking spray
1 egg, large
1½ cups instant oats, dry
¼ cup almonds, slivered
¼ cup enriched wheat flour
½ cup smooth peanut butter
1 Tbsp vegetable oil
½ cup honey
½ tsp ground cinnamon
1 tsp vanilla

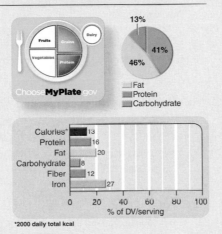

	% of DV/serving
Calories*	13
Protein	16
Fat	20
Carbohydrate	8
Fiber	12
Iron	27

*2000 daily total kcal

Fat 13%
Protein 41%
Carbohydrate 46%

PREPARATION STEPS:

1. Preheat oven to 350°.

2. Spray "nonstick" oil on the inside bottom and sides of an 8" × 8" pan.

3. Crack open the egg, drop the egg's contents into a medium-size bowl, and discard the shell. Using a fork, beat the egg until its yolk is completely mixed with the egg white.

4. Add remaining ingredients to the egg and stir until well blended. Mixture will be thick, like cookie dough.

5. Using a large spoon, press dough into the bottom of the pan, covering the inside of the pan evenly.

6. Bake for 12 to 14 minutes.

7. Cool completely before cutting into eight 2" × 4" bars.

Spiral Pasta Salad

Athletes often rely on pasta dishes to help maintain or replenish their glycogen supplies. There are many different forms of pasta, including shells, tubes, and twisted pieces called "rotini." This quick and easy pasta salad recipe uses rotini mixed with fresh green pepper, tomato, onion, and garlic. The recipe makes two 1-cup servings. Each serving supplies approximately 270 kcal, 46 g carbohydrate, 8 g protein, 2.5 g fiber, 6 g fat, 2 mg iron, 135 mg potassium, and 140 mcg folate.

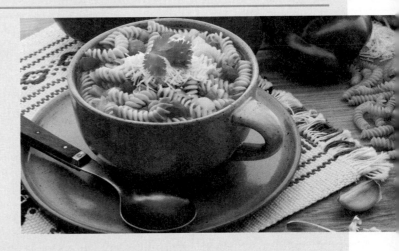

INGREDIENTS:

4 oz rotini pasta (1⅓ cups uncooked)
1 small garlic clove, minced
1 Tbsp finely chopped onion
⅓ cup chopped green pepper
⅓ cup chopped tomato
2 Tbsp lite mayonnaise-type salad dressing
pinch of black pepper
Parmesan cheese, grated, 1 Tbsp (optional)

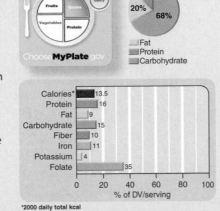

Fat 12%
Protein 20%
Carbohydrate 68%

	% of DV/serving
Calories*	13.5
Protein	16
Fat	9
Carbohydrate	15
Fiber	10
Iron	11
Potassium	4
Folate	35

*2000 daily total kcal

PREPARATION STEPS:

1. Prepare rotini according to package directions but do not add salt to boiling water.

2. Drain cooked rotini.

3. Gently mix rotini with other ingredients. Top with grated cheese, if desired. Serve hot or cold.

CRITICAL THINKING

1. Using the recommendations of the National College of Sports Medicine and the American Heart Association, analyze your weekly physical activity habits. Does your participation in various physical activities meet the minimum recommendations? If not, which physical activities are you willing to include in your weekly routine to improve your fitness level?

2. Calculate your target heart rate zone for moderate-intensity as well as vigorous-intensity activities.

3. Why do human cells rely far more on glucose and fat for energy than on protein?

4. Your neighbor is planning to run in a marathon. What advice would you give him or her concerning fluid intake before and during the event?

5. One of your friends is a competitive athlete. She tells you that she ordered a mixture of amino acids from a manufacturer's website. According to testimonials posted at the site, the dietary supplement improves athletic performance. What would you tell her about the general effectiveness of such products?

PRACTICE TEST

Select the best answer.

1. Miranda is physically fit. She has
   a. an increased risk of osteoporosis.
   b. the strength, endurance, and flexibility to meet the demands of daily living.
   c. a greater need for vitamins and minerals than other women.
   d. None of the above is correct.

2. During glycolysis, the body
   a. converts two fatty acid molecules into one glucose molecule.
   b. synthesizes one amino acid molecule from one carbon dioxide molecule and two oxygen molecules.
   c. breaks down one glucose molecule to form two pyruvate molecules.
   d. metabolizes fatty acids into carbon monoxide and peroxide.

3. A _____ physical activity generally requires a high degree of exertion.
   a. vigorous
   b. basic
   c. moderate
   d. precise

4. Aerobic activities
   a. enable muscles to use less oxygen than normal.
   b. do not require voluntary muscular contractions.
   c. force muscle cells to use more vitamins and minerals for energy.
   d. involve sustained, rhythmic contractions of certain large skeletal muscles.

5. Which of the following statements is true?
   a. Resistance exercises do not help build bone mass.
   b. Sedentary activities do not require much energy to perform.
   c. Anaerobic energy systems need large quantities of oxygen to produce ATP.
   d. All of the above are correct.

6. Amy is studying quietly. Under these conditions, her muscles are using primarily _____ for energy.
   a. fat
   b. glucose
   c. amino acids
   d. ketone bodies

7. Carbohydrate loading
   a. provides a competitive edge for award-winning sprinters, bodybuilders, and weight lifters.
   b. involves manipulating dietary patterns and physical activities prior to an endurance event.
   c. often results in short-term weight loss and positive energy balance.
   d. is generally recommended for long-term weight control for athletes.

8. Which of the following foods is high carbohydrate and low fat?
   a. dried fruit
   b. pretzels
   c. toast spread with strawberry jam
   d. All of the above are correct.

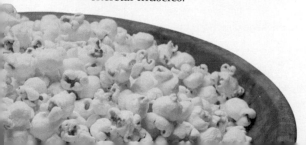

9. Caffeine
   a. is the most widely used ergogenic aid in the world.
   b. reduces the level of fatty acids in blood.
   c. is nonaddictive.
   d. decreases mental alertness.

10. Drinking at least 6 liters of water daily
    a. is recommended by the National Academy of Sciences.
    b. is necessary for healthy persons even if they are not thirsty.
    c. can result in water intoxication.
    d. improves athletic performance.

11. Which of the following beverages contains caffeine?
    a. Red Bull
    b. tea
    c. chocolate milk
    d. All of the above are correct.

12. Under aerobic conditions, cells break down glucose to form
    a. carbon dioxide and water.
    b. acetyl Co-A and sorbitol.
    c. beta-carotene and glutamine.
    d. phosphocreatine and ADP.

13. Human cells release most of the energy stored in carbohydrates, fats, and amino acids as
    a. electricity.
    b. phosphocreatine.
    c. ATP.
    d. heat.

14. To obtain energy under aerobic conditions, cells need
    a. ribose.
    b. oxygen.
    c. methionine.
    d. alanine.

15. _____ is an immediate and direct source of energy for cells.
    a. LDP
    b. Glycogen
    c. ATP
    d. Phospholipid

16. Which of the following activities is not a usual component of an aerobic workout?
    a. lifting weights
    b. cooling down
    c. moderate-intensity activity
    d. warming up

Answers to Chapter 11 Quiz *Yourself*

1. People who exercise regularly can reduce their risk of type 2 diabetes. **True.** (p. 402)

2. Sports drinks are not useful for fluid replacement. **False.** (p. 421)

3. Protein is the body's preferred fuel for muscular activity. **False.** (p. 418)

4. Heatstroke is a serious illness that requires immediate professional medical treatment. **True.** (p. 420)

5. While at rest, skeletal muscles metabolize more glucose than fat for energy. **False.** (p. 411)

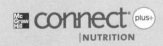

Additional resources related to the features of this book are available on ConnectPlus® Nutrition. Ask your instructor how to get access.

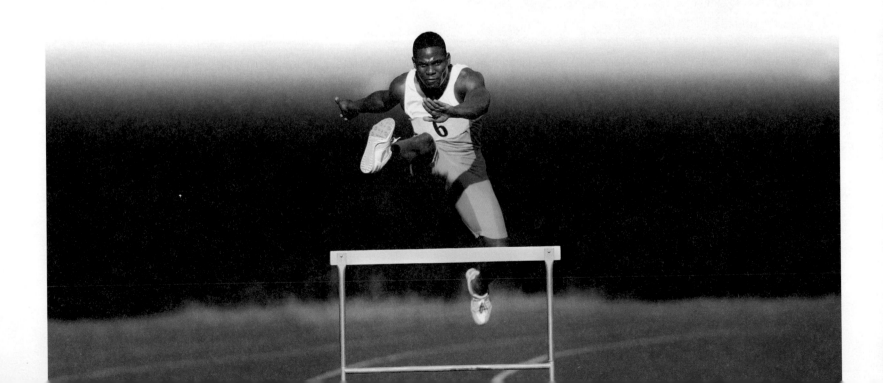

Food Safety Concerns

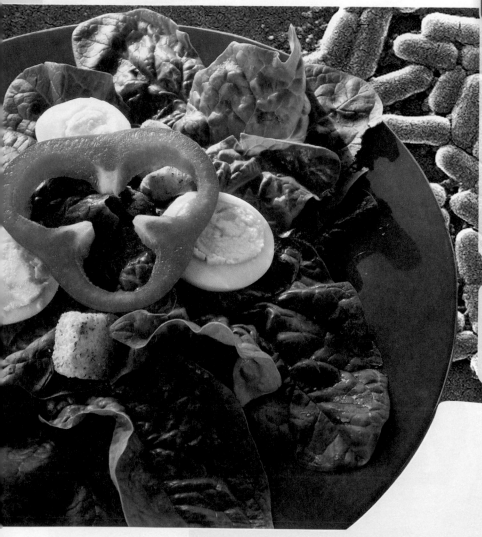

Chapter Learning Outcomes

After reading Chapter 12, you should be able to

1. List some common types and sources of microbes that can cause food-borne illness.
2. Identify the government's role in protecting the food supply.
3. Describe procedures that can reduce the risk of food-borne illness.
4. Identify various food preservation methods.
5. List at least three functions of food additives.
6. Identify sources of contaminants in food.
7. Discuss the pros and cons of pesticide use.

McGraw Hill **connect** plus+ | NUTRITION **www.mcgrawhillconnect.com**

A wealth of proven resources are available on ConnectPlus® Nutrition! Ask your instructor about ConnectPlus, which includes an interactive eBook, an adaptive learning program and much, much more!

A FEW DAYS before Labor Day in 2006, graduate student Jill Kohl bought a package of raw baby spinach and used about half of the bag to prepare a large spinach salad. About 3 or 4 days after eating the salad, she developed a fever, body aches, severe intestinal cramps, and bloody diarrhea. After being taken to a hospital emergency room, Jill was admitted and hospitalized for two and a half weeks. The seriously ill young woman spent much of that time in the intensive care unit. At one point, her kidneys stopped functioning properly and her physicians feared she would die. Jill survived the terrible ordeal and today feels "back to normal." By the end of 2006, 205 confirmed cases of the illness, including three deaths, had occurred in the United States.

After conducting their detective work, public health investigators determined that Jill and the other victims had something in common—they had eaten raw baby spinach processed and packed at a company in San Juan Bautista, California. The culprit lurking in the spinach was a type of bacteria called *E. coli* O157:H7. **Bacteria** are simple, single-cell microorganisms. Some bacteria, such as *E. coli* O157:H7, cause infectious diseases in humans. Experts with the U.S. Food and Drug Administration and Centers for Disease Control and Prevention identified cattle or wild pig manure as possible sources of the bacteria that tainted the baby spinach leaves. The manure might have been in water used to irrigate the spinach fields or spread on the spinach fields. Public health experts, however, were unable to determine the origin of the bacterial contamination.[1]

Since 2006, more widespread serious outbreaks of **food-borne illnesses** have occurred in the United States. In the spring of 2008, more than 1400 people were sickened after eating raw tomatoes and raw jalapeño and serrano peppers imported from Mexico.[2] Later that year and into early 2009, over 700 Americans became ill and 9 people may have died after eating products made with peanut butter.[3] Investigators determined that the peanut butter had been produced by a single facility in Georgia. The discovery of the source of the infection resulted in one of the largest nationwide food recalls in United States history—over 2000 different products that contained the peanut butter were removed from store shelves, and consumers were warned to discard the items if they had them in their homes. Strains of *Salmonella*, a type of bacteria, were responsible for both of these nationwide illness outbreaks.

Infections spread through the ingestion of food or beverages are common, debilitating, and sometimes life-threatening diseases for millions of people around the world. Each year,

(continued)

Quiz *Yourself*

Which foods are most likely to be responsible for food-borne illness? How can you reduce the risk of contracting one of these illnesses? Which government agencies monitor the safety of the U.S. food supply? After reading Chapter 12, you will learn answers to these questions. Test your knowledge of food safety by taking the following quiz. The answers are found on page 465.

1. Aflatoxins are the most common sources of food-borne illness in the United States. _____ T _____ F

2. In the United States, foods such as ready-to-eat cereals, commercially canned vegetables, and orange juice are common sources of food-borne illness. _____ T _____ F

3. Certain fungi, such as button mushrooms, are safe to eat. _____ T _____ F

4. The Environmental Protection Agency (EPA) regulates the proper use of pesticides in the United States. _____ T _____ F

5. The best way to tell if a food is safe to eat is to smell it. _____ T _____ F

bacteria simple single-celled microorganisms

food-borne illness infection caused by microscopic disease-causing agents in food

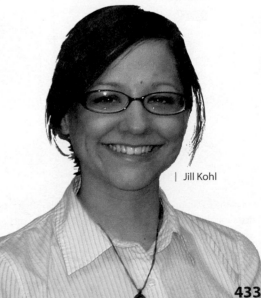
Jill Kohl

an estimated 76 million Americans become sick from various food-borne illnesses.[4] Of those persons who contract such ailments, 325,000 require hospitalization and over 5000 die. There are more than 250 food-borne illnesses; preventing these diseases is a major U.S. public health objective.

Food-borne as well as water-borne illnesses can occur when microscopic agents (*microbes*) or their toxic by-products enter food or water and they are consumed. In the United States, water-borne disease-causing microbes are not major health threats. Therefore, Chapter 12 focuses primarily on food-borne illness, including common sources of these infections in the United States. Additionally, Chapter 12 presents safe food handling practices and examines the safety of our food supply.

12.1 Protecting Our Food

The United States has one of the safest food supplies in the world, primarily the result of a team effort conducted by cooperating federal, state, and local agencies that regulate and monitor the production and distribution of food. The Food and Drug Administration (FDA) of the U.S. Department of Health and Human Services and the U.S. Department of Agriculture (USDA) are the key federal agencies that protect consumers by regulating the country's food industry. Other team members include the Environmental Protection Agency (EPA), the Centers for Disease Control and Prevention (CDC), the Federal Trade Commission (FTC), and state and local governments.

To help protect our food supply, the FDA performs many important tasks, such as regulating nearly all domestic and imported food sold in interstate commerce and enforcing federal food safety laws. Additionally, the FDA establishes standards for safe food manufacturing practices, such as Hazard Analysis and Critical Control Point (HACCP) programs. HACCP is a science-based, systematic approach to preventing food-borne illness by predicting which hazards are most likely to occur in a food production facility. When a hazard is identified, food manufacturers can then take appropriate measures to prevent the illness. If necessary, FDA officials can take certain enforcement actions, such as requesting that a food manufacturer recall an unsafe item, so that it is removed from store shelves. Another important function of the FDA is educating the general public about safe food handling practices.

Although the FDA oversees the safety of most foods, the USDA's Food Safety and Inspection Service (FSIS) enforces food safety laws for domestic and imported meat and poultry products. FSIS staff inspect beef, poultry, and other food animals for diseases before and after slaughter, and the agency also ensures that meat and poultry processing plants meet federal standards. Additionally, FSIS staff collect and analyze food samples to check for the presence of microbial and other unwanted and potentially harmful material in foods. If a food hazard is identified, FSIS officials can ask meat and poultry processors to recall their unsafe products. Additionally, food safety experts with FSIS conduct programs and publish a magazine (*be FoodSafe*) to educate people about proper food handling practices. For more information, visit the FSIS website at www.fsis.usda.gov/.

The EPA oversees the quality of our drinking water. EPA staff establish safe drinking water standards and assist state officials in their efforts to monitor water quality. Furthermore, EPA staff regulate toxic substances and wastes to prevent their entry into foods and the environment.

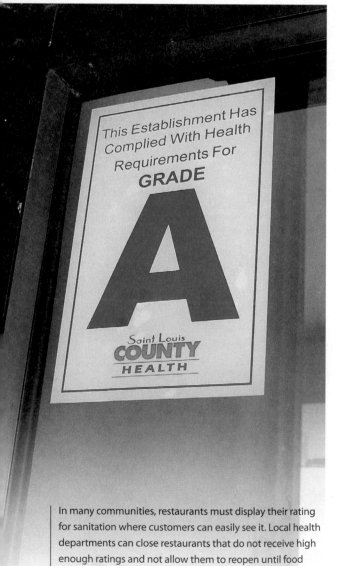

In many communities, restaurants must display their rating for sanitation where customers can easily see it. Local health departments can close restaurants that do not receive high enough ratings and not allow them to reopen until food safety hazards have been corrected.

State and local officials work with the FDA and other federal agency staff to implement national food safety standards for foods produced and sold within their state's borders. Local health departments, for example, are responsible for inspecting restaurants, grocery stores, dairy farms, and local food processing companies. In many communities, restaurants are required to post their sanitation rating where customers can easily see it. Local health departments can close restaurants that do not receive high enough ratings and prevent them from reopening until food safety hazards have been corrected.

After you obtain foods and bring them into your home, it becomes your responsibility to reduce the risk of food-borne illness by handling the items properly. However, if you suspect that something you consumed made you or a family member very sick, you should contact your physician for treatment. The physician may decide to report the case of food-borne illness to local public health officials, so they can investigate and determine the source of your infection.

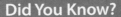

Did You Know?

You cannot always rely on your senses to judge the wholesomeness of a food. A food can taste, smell, and appear safe to eat, but it may contain pathogens and/or their toxic by-products.

Concept **Checkpoint**

1. Discuss the roles of the FDA, FSIS, and EPA in protecting the U.S. food supply.
2. How do local health departments protect consumers from food-borne illness?

 ## 12.2 Microbes in Food

For thousands of years, people have used certain microbes to produce a variety of foods, including hard cheeses, raised breads, pickled foods, and alcoholic beverages. When microorganisms metabolize nutrients in food, they often secrete substances that alter the color, texture, taste, and other characteristics of the food in beneficial and desirable ways. Other kinds of microbes grow and multiply in food, but their metabolic by-products spoil the food, making it unfit for human consumption. Disease-causing microbes are referred to as **pathogens**. When pathogens are in food, they can make the item unsafe to eat.

A **contaminated food** (or beverage) is no longer wholesome—pure or safe for human consumption. Contamination generally occurs when something that may or may not be harmful enters food or beverages unintentionally. Such contaminants include pathogens, insect parts, residues of compounds used to kill insects that destroy food crops, and metal fragments from food processing equipment. The following section discusses how pathogens can contaminate our food.

pathogens disease-causing microbes

contaminated food item that is impure or unsafe for human consumption

food intoxication illness that results when poisons produced by certain microbes contaminate food and irritate the intestinal tract

Pathogens

Many kinds of food-borne pathogens infect the digestive tract, inflaming the tissues and causing an "upset stomach" within a few hours after being ingested. A few types of food-borne pathogens multiply in the human intestinal tract, enter the bloodstream, and cause general illness when they invade other tissues. Other pathogens do not sicken humans directly, but these microbes contaminate food and secrete poisons (toxins). When the contaminated food is eaten, the toxins irritate the intestinal tract and cause a type of food-borne illness called **food intoxication** (or food poisoning).

The microbes that cause food-borne illness can live practically anywhere—in air, water, soil, and sewage, and on various surfaces. Our skin, nasal passages, and large intestines have vast colonies of various kinds of microbes, some of which can be

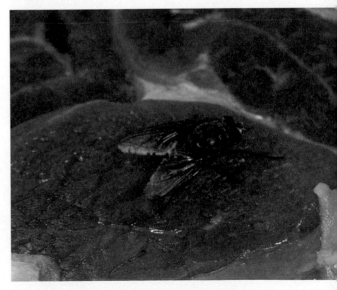

To reduce your risk of food-borne illness, keep flies, cockroaches, and other vermin away from your food.

cross-contamination unintentional transfer of pathogenic microbes from one food to another

pasteurization process that kills the pathogens in foods and beverages as well as many microbes responsible for spoilage

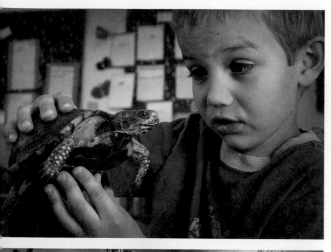

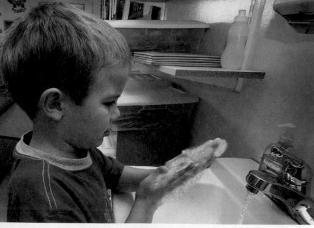

People who touch turtles or other potential *Salmonella* carriers should wash their hands thoroughly after handling the animals.

pathogenic. Animals, including cats, dogs, reptiles, cattle, and poultry, can also harbor harmful microbes on and in their bodies, especially in their intestinal tracts. Because pathogens are found throughout your environment, there are numerous ways that the microbes can contaminate your food. To reduce your risk of food-borne illness, you need to be aware of how pathogens can enter foods. The "Preventing Food-Borne Illness" section of this chapter discusses specific steps you can take to reduce the chances of contracting or spreading food-borne illness.

Common Routes for Transmitting Pathogens

One common route for transmitting harmful microbes involves *vermin*, animals that often live around sewage or garbage, such as flies, cockroaches, mice, and rats. When vermin land on or crawl across filth, they pick up pathogens on their feet. When the vermin come in contact with food, they can transfer the pathogens to humans. To reduce your risk of food-borne illness, keep flies, cockroaches, and other vermin away from your food.

Poor personal hygiene practices frequently transfer microbes to food. People can contaminate their hands with pathogens when they come in contact with feces, such as while using the toilet or changing a baby's soiled diaper. Furthermore, animals harbor pathogens in their feces as well as on their skin and fur. If children prepare or eat foods after stroking animals at petting zoos or playing with pets, they can transmit these microbes to themselves or others. Thus, it is important for people to wash their hands before preparing or eating foods. Children (and many adults) often need to be reminded to wash their hands.

Improper food handling frequently results in food-borne illness. A common practice is failing to wash cutting boards and food preparation utensils after they come in contact with raw meat or poultry. The contaminated boards and utensils are then used to prepare other foods. As a result of this practice, **cross-contamination** is likely to occur, because the pathogens in one food are transferred to another food, contaminating it. If that food is eaten raw, such as carrots in a salad, it carries a high risk of food-borne illness. Failing to cook foods properly can also increase the likelihood of food-borne illness. **Pasteurization** is a special heating process used by many commercial food producers to kill pathogens. In the United States, for example, most juices and milk have been pasteurized before they are marketed. The "Food Preservation" section of Chapter 12 discusses other ways of preserving foods.

High-Risk Foods

Not all foods are likely to harbor pathogens. To survive and multiply, most microbes need warmth, moisture, and a source of nutrients, and some also require oxygen. In general, high-risk foods are warm, moist, and protein-rich, and they have a neutral or slightly acidic pH. Many of the foods we eat every day, such as meats, eggs, milk, and products made from milk, fit this description. Table 12.1 presents some high-risk foods and the primary food-borne pathogens they may contain.

Concept **Checkpoint**

3. Discuss at least three ways pathogens can contaminate human foods.
4. With regard to food preparation, what is cross-contamination?
5. What is pasteurization?
6. Discuss conditions that favor the survival and multiplication of food-borne pathogens.
7. Identify at least four foods that are high risk for supporting pathogens.

TABLE 12.1   *Summary of Some High-Risk Foods and Their Primary Pathogens*

Raw or Undercooked Animal Food	Typical Menu Item	Common Pathogens
Beef	Rare hamburger	*Salmonella* species
	Steak tartare	*E. coli* O157:H7
	Carpaccio	
Pork	Sausage	*Trichinella*
	Pork roast	
Poultry	Chicken, turkey, duck	*Salmonella* species
		Campylobacter jejuni
Eggs	Quiche, hollandaise sauce, eggs Benedict, homemade mayonnaise, meringue pies, mousse, tiramisu, chicken croquettes, rice balls, stuffing, French toast, crab cakes, eggnog, Caesar salad, homemade ice creams and frozen custards	*Salmonella enteritidis*
Raw fish/finfish	Sushi; lightly cooked fish; raw-marinated, cold-smoked fish; cerviche, tuna carpaccio	*Anisakis* *Vibrio parahaemolyticus*
Shellfish	Oysters	*Vibrio vulnificus* and other
	Clams	*Vibrio* species
		Hepatitis A
		Norovirus
Milk and milk products	Raw or unpasteurized milk, some soft cheeses such as Camembert and Brie	*Listeria monocytogenes* *Salmonella* species *Campylobacter jejuni,* *E. coli* O157:H7

Source: FDA: *Annex 3–Hazard Analysis for Managing Food Safety: A Manual for the Voluntary Use of HACCP Principles for Operators of Food Service and Retail Establishments,* Updated 2009. http://www.fda.gov/Food/FoodSafety/RetailFoodProtection/ManagingFoodSafetyHACCPPrinciples/Operators/ucm078069.htm

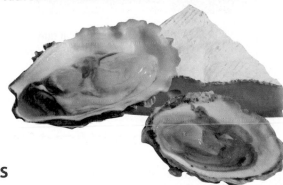

12.3 Food-Borne Illness

Signs and symptoms of food-borne (and water-borne) illnesses generally involve the digestive tract and include nausea, vomiting, diarrhea, and intestinal cramps. However, most pathogens have an *incubation period*, a length of time in which they grow and multiply in food or the digestive tract before they can cause illness. Thus, if you develop signs and symptoms of a food-borne illness, you might have difficulty identifying the source of the infection or intoxication. Was the vomiting and diarrhea that you experienced at 3 A.M. the result of eating soft-cooked eggs for breakfast 18 hours earlier or the sliced deli chicken you ate for lunch 2 days ago?

Various factors influence whether an individual becomes ill after consuming a food or beverage that has been contaminated with a pathogen or toxin. The number of pathogenic microbes in a food or the amount of toxin it contains can contribute to the risk and severity of a food-borne illness. Furthermore, individuals vary in their vulnerability to many food-borne pathogens. In general, high-risk groups are pregnant women, very young children, the elderly, and persons who suffer from serious chronic illnesses or weakened immune systems.

In most cases, otherwise healthy individuals who suffer from common types of food-borne illness recover completely and without professional medical care within a few days. However, vomiting, diarrhea, and other signs of illness can be so severe, the patient requires hospitalization. You should consult a physician when an intestinal disorder is accompanied by one or more of the following signs: fever (oral temperature above 101.5°F), bloody bowel movements, prolonged vomiting that reduces fluid intake, diarrhea that lasts more than 3 days, or dehydration.[5]

Many people mistakenly report that they have the "stomach *flu*," when they actually are suffering from a food- or water-borne illness. "Flu," or *influenza*, is an infectious disease caused by specific viruses that invade the respiratory tract. Influenza is characterized by coughing, fever, weakness, and body aches. On the other hand, food-borne illness primarily affects the digestive system and not the respiratory system. Intestinal cramps, diarrhea, and vomiting are *not* typical signs and symptoms of influenza, and coughing is not a usual sign of a food-borne illness. Thus, it is inaccurate to call a bout of diarrhea and intestinal cramps the "stomach flu."

Did You Know?

Honey, even commercially processed brands of the sweetener, should not be fed to infants because it may contain *Clostridium botulinum* spores. The spores can grow in an infant's intestinal tract, produce toxin, and cause botulism (see Chapter 5). Older children and adults can consume honey safely, because their immune systems prevent the spores from growing.

Concept **Checkpoint**

8. Identify at least three typical signs and symptoms of food-borne illness.
9. When should a person suffering from a food-borne illness seek professional medical help?
10. Discuss the differences between a food-borne illness and "the flu."

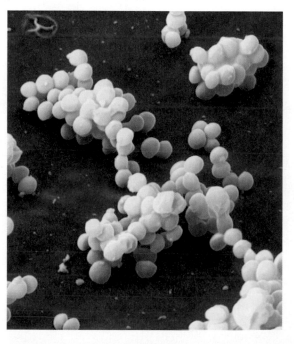

Improperly cooked or handled meat, poultry, eggs, and foods made with eggs are common sources of *Staphylococcus aureus*. The bacteria produce a toxin that results in food-borne illness.

12.4 Common Food-Borne Pathogens

The major kinds of pathogens are bacteria, viruses, protozoans, and fungi. In the United States, *bacteria* and *viruses* are responsible for most cases of food-borne illness. The following sections take a closer look at some of the major pathogens that can cause food-borne illness.

Bacteria

Bacteria are single-cell microorganisms that do not have the complex array of organelles that plant and animal cells contain. Some bacteria can live without oxygen, such as in canned or vacuum-packed foods. Other types of bacteria transform into inactive resistant forms called *spores* when living conditions are less than ideal. If the environment becomes more hospitable, the spores revert to the active bacterial state.

Many kinds of bacteria are pathogens that cause food-borne illness, including forms of *Campylobacter, Clostridium, Escherichia, Listeria, Salmonella* and *Staphylococcus* (*kam'-pih-low-bak'-ter, klo-strid'-e-um, esh'-ear-i'-ke-ah, lis-te'-re-ah, sal'-mo-nell-ah, staff'-il-lo-cawk'-kiss*). Some types of pathogenic bacteria do not cause infections when they are consumed in food, but these microbes produce toxins that cause food intoxication. Table 12.2 summarizes some general information about common bacterial sources of food-borne illness in the United States.

TABLE 12.2 *Common Sources of Food-Borne Illness: Bacteria*

Bacterium	High-Risk Foods	Approx. Time of Onset	Typical Signs and Symptoms
Bacillus cereus (toxin)	Meat, poultry, and starchy foods (rice, potatoes, puddings, some soups)	6–15 hours	Abdominal cramps, watery diarrhea, nausea
Campylobacter jejuni	Raw, undercooked poultry; raw milk; contaminated water	2–5 days	Diarrhea (often bloody), abdominal cramping, vomiting, fever
Clostridium botulinum (toxin)	Vacuum-packed foods, improperly canned foods, garlic-in-oil mixtures Honey may contain spores.	18–36 hours	Vomiting, diarrhea, blurry or double vision, difficulty swallowing, muscular weakness Can be fatal
Clostridium perfringens (toxin)	Cooked meat, poultry, casseroles, gravies	8–22 hours	Watery diarrhea, severe abdominal cramps
Escherichia coli O157:H7 (toxin)	Raw ground beef, raw seed sprouts, raw leafy greens, fresh fruit, raw milk, unpasteurized juices, foods contaminated with feces	2 hours to 6 days	Intestinal cramps, diarrhea, bloody diarrhea, kidney failure Can be fatal
Listeria monocytogenes	Raw meat and poultry, raw milk, fresh soft cheese made from raw milk, liver paté, smoked seafood, deli meats and salads, hot dogs, produce	Unknown but probably more than 12 hours for GI tract signs and symptoms; probably a few days to 3 weeks for invasive disease	Fever, muscular aches, vomiting, diarrhea In pregnant women, the infection can lead to stillbirth (birth of a dead fetus) or premature birth.
Salmonella species	Raw or undercooked meat, poultry, seafood, and eggs; raw seed sprouts; raw vegetables, unpasteurized juice	6 hours–2 days	Nausea, vomiting, fever, chills, headache, abdominal cramps, diarrhea Infection can be fatal in infants, the elderly, and people suffering from chronic illness.
Shigella species	Raw vegetables, herbs, and other foods that were contaminated as a result of poor food handling practices	12–50 hours	Abdominal cramps, fever, diarrhea that may contain blood and mucus
Staphylococcus aureus (toxin)	Meats, poultry, and eggs; foods made with eggs, such as potato, egg, macaroni, and egg salads; certain homemade ice creams, custards, and cream-filled pastries Cooked foods are often contaminated as a result of improper food handling practices.	1–6 hours	Diarrhea, nausea, vomiting, abdominal cramps, weakness
Vibrio vulnificus	Raw oysters, clams, crabs and other raw or undercooked seafood	16 hours	Vomiting, diarrhea, abdominal cramps
Yersinia enterocolitica	Raw vegetables, undercooked pork, contaminated water, unpasteurized milk	1–2 days	Diarrhea, fever, vomiting, abdominal pain

Sources: Nester EW and others: *Microbiology: a human perspective*. 6th ed. New York: McGraw-Hill, 2009.

U.S. Food and Drug Administration: *Bad Bug Book: Introduction:*

Foodborne Pathogenic Microorganisms and Natural Toxins Handbook, updated June 2009. http://www.fda.gov/Food/FoodSafety/FoodborneIllness/FoodborneIllnessFoodbornePathogensNaturalToxins/BadBugBook/default.htm. Accessed: August 1, 2011.

TABLE 12.3 *Common Sources of Food-Borne Illness: Viruses*

Virus	High-Risk Foods	Approx. Time of Onset	Typical Signs and Symptoms
Norovirus	Food or water that has been contaminated with infected feces, enabling the virus to be spread person-to-person	1–2 days	Vomiting; watery, nonbloody diarrhea; abdominal cramps; nausea; low-grade fever (occasionally)
Rotavirus	Food or water that has been contaminated with infected feces Most children have been infected by 5 years of age.	2 days	Fever, abdominal pain, vomiting, watery diarrhea Worldwide, thousands of children die each year as a result of rotavirus infection.
Hepatitis A (HAV)	Food or water that has been contaminated with HAV from feces	2 to 6 weeks	Fever, loss of appetite, nausea, vomiting, diarrhea, muscle aches, general weakness May have signs of liver inflammation, such as jaundice (indicated by yellow discoloration of skin and whites of eyes), liver enlargement, and dark-colored urine Most people recover after a few weeks, but in rare cases, the illness is deadly.

Sources: Centers for Disease Control and Prevention: *Norovirus technical fact sheet*. Last reviewed May 2011. http://www.cdc.gov/ncidod/dvrd/revb/gastro/norovirus-factsheet.htm. Accessed: August 1, 2011. Centers for Disease Control and Prevention: *Rotavirus*. Updated April 2011. http://www.cdc.gov/rotavirus/clinical.html. Accessed: August 1, 2011. Centers for Disease Control and Prevention: *Hepatitis A information for health professionals*. Page updated June 2009. http://www.cdc.gov/hepatitis/HAV/HAVfaq.htm#. Accessed: August 1, 2011.

Viruses

Viruses are another common source of food-borne infection (Table 12.3). A **virus** is simply a piece of genetic material coated with protein (Fig. 12.1). Viruses must invade a living cell to produce more viruses. Unlike certain bacteria, viruses do not secrete toxins, and therefore, they do not cause food intoxication. Contaminated food or water, however, can transmit viruses to humans and cause food infection.

Vaccines that protect against hepatitis A and rotaviral infections are available. A vaccine to prevent norovirus infections is in development.

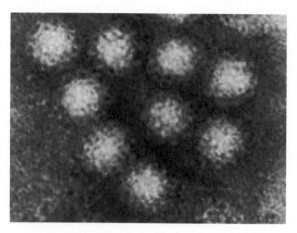

Figure 12.1 *Norovirus.* A virus, such as this *Norovirus*, is simply a piece of genetic material coated with protein.

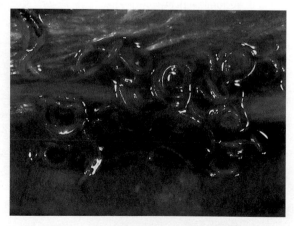

Figure 12.2 *Anisakis. Anisakis* is a type of worm that can be transferred to humans who eat raw or undercooked fish or squid.

Parasites

A **parasite** is an organism that lives in or on another living thing, often deriving nourishment from its host. Some parasites, such as *Giardia* (*jee-ar'-de-ah*) and *Cryptosporidium* (*krip'-toe-spo-rid'-ee-um*), are **protozoans** (*pro-toe-zoe'-ans*), single-celled microorganisms that have a more complex cell structure than bacteria. Protozoans are often responsible for causing traveler's diarrhea; the Chapter 12 "Highlight" discusses this condition.

In addition to protozoans, food-borne parasites include types of worms such as *Trichinella* (*trick'-ah-nell'-ah*) and *Anisakis* (*ah'-ni-sa'-kis*) (Fig. 12.2). Table 12.4 provides information about parasites that can cause food-borne infections. Most Americans who become infected with parasites that are common in the United States recover when they receive proper treatment. Nevertheless, some infected persons suffer long-term health problems and even die as a result of the illnesses.

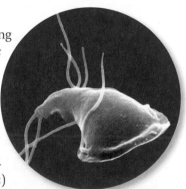

Giardia is a parasitic protozoan, a single-celled microorganism that has a more complex cell structure than bacteria.

Fungi

Fungi such as molds, yeast, and mushrooms are simple life forms that live on dead or decaying organic matter. Certain fungi, such as button mushrooms and the mold in blue cheese, are beneficial and edible. Other fungi are responsible for spoiling foods, such as bread molds, or causing respiratory problems or allergic reactions in sensitive people.[6] A serious concern is the toxicity of several varieties of wild mushrooms. Cases of severe

TABLE 12.4 *Common Sources of Food-Borne Illness: Parasites*

Parasite	High-Risk Foods	Approx. Time of Onset	Typical Signs and Symptoms
Cryptosporidium	Foods prepared with contaminated water or by people whose hands were contaminated with infected feces	2–10 days	Profuse, watery diarrhea; abdominal pain; fever; nausea; vomiting; weight loss
Giardia	Consumption of contaminated water, including water from lakes, streams, swimming pools High-risk groups include travelers to certain countries, hikers, and people who swim in or camp by lakes and streams.	1–2 weeks	Diarrhea, abdominal pain, loss of appetite
Toxoplasma	Raw or partially cooked infected meat, especially pork, lamb, or deer meat Accidentally ingesting infected cat feces	Difficult to determine because of uncertain timing of exposure	Fever, headache, muscle aches, rash Pregnant women should avoid contact with cat feces, because the parasite can infect their unborn offspring, causing eye or brain damage.
Trichinella	Raw or undercooked infected meat, especially pork, bear, seal, and walrus meat	1–2 days	Initially: nausea, vomiting, diarrhea, fatigue, fever, abdominal discomfort Later: headaches, chills, cough, eye swelling, muscle and joint pain In severe cases, death can occur.
Anisakis	Raw or undercooked infected seafood	1 hour to 2 weeks	Tickling sensation in throat during or after eating raw/undercooked fish or squid; vomiting or coughing up the worm may prevent infection. In severe cases, severe abdominal pain that may be mistaken for appendicitis.

Sources: FDA: *Bad bug book: Foodborne pathogenic microorganisms and natural toxins handbook.* Updated July 2009. http://www.fda.gov/Food/FoodSafety/FoodborneIllness/FoodborneIllnessFoodborne-PathogensNaturalToxins/BadBugBook/ucm070753.htm; CDC: *Cryptosporidiosis: disease.* Updated March 2011. http://www.cdc.gov/parasites/crypto/; CDC: *Parasites- giardia.* Updated March 2011. http://www.cdc.gov/parasites/giardia/index.html ; Nester EW and others: *Microbiology: A Human Perspective,* 6th ed. New York: McGraw-Hill, 2009; CDC: Parasites-*Trichinellosis (also known as trichinosis).* Updated 2010. http://www.cdc.gov/parasites/trichinellosis/index.html ; CDC: *Anisakiasis.* Modified 2010. http://www.cdc.gov/parasites/anisakiasis/index.html. Accessed: August 1, 2011.

illness and death have been reported as a result of people picking and eating toxic wild mushrooms after mistaking them for edible varieties (Fig. 12.3). Nevertheless, fungi are not a major source of food-borne illness in the United States.

Certain molds produce *aflatoxins,* substances that can cause severe illness, particularly liver damage, and even death when consumed. Tree nuts, peanuts, and corn that are stored under warm, humid conditions can become sources of aflatoxins. In some regions of the world, especially Africa and Southeast Asia, people often eat foods that are contaminated with aflatoxin-producing molds. Rates of liver cancer are high in these places. Thus, medical researchers think there is an association between exposure to aflatoxins and development of liver cancer. No outbreaks of food-borne intoxication caused by aflatoxins have been reported among the U.S. population.[7]

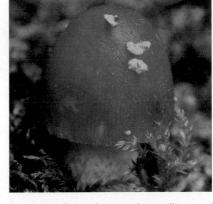

Figure 12.3 Deadly mushrooms. Severe illness and even death can occur if people pick and eat toxic mushrooms, such as this *Amanita* mushroom.

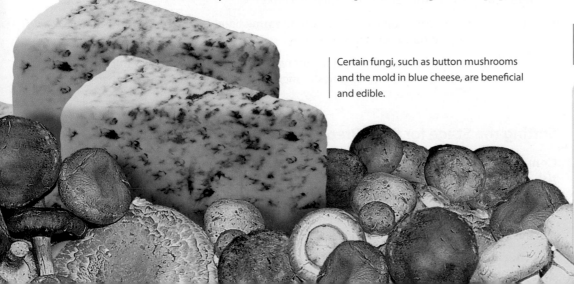

Certain fungi, such as button mushrooms and the mold in blue cheese, are beneficial and edible.

virus microbe consisting of a piece of genetic material coated with protein

parasite organism that lives in or on another organism, often deriving nourishment from its host

protozoans single-celled microorganisms that have complex cell structures

fungi simple organisms that live on dead or decaying organic matter

Concept **Checkpoint**

11. Identify at least three bacterial sources of food-borne illness in the United States.
12. Identify three viruses that are sources of food-borne illness in the United States.
13. Identify three parasites that can cause food- or water-borne illness in the United States.
14. What are aflatoxins?

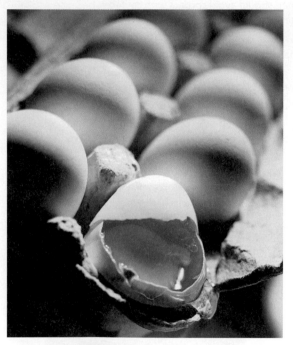

Before purchasing eggs, open the carton and check the eggs. Do not buy cartons that have any cracked eggs.

 # 12.5 Preventing Food-Borne Illness

In many instances, you cannot control the safety of foods that are prepared in restaurants or other places outside your home. However, you can greatly reduce your risk of food-borne illness by following some important rules, most of which require changing risky food selection, preparation, and storage practices.

Purchasing Food

To reduce your risk of food-borne illness:

- When shopping in a supermarket, select frozen foods and highly perishable foods, such as meat, poultry, or fish, last.

- Check "best by" dates on packaged perishable foods. Choose meats and other animal products with the latest dates.

- Do not buy food in damaged containers; for example, avoid containers that leak, bulge, or are severely dented, or jars that are cracked or have loose or bulging lids.

- Open egg cartons and examine eggs; do not buy cartons that have cracked eggs.

- Purchase only pasteurized milk, cheese, and fruit and vegetable juices (check the label).

- Purchase only the amount of produce needed for a week's menus. The longer you keep fresh fruits and vegetables, the more likely they are to spoil.

- Pack meat, fish, and poultry in separate plastic bags, so their drippings do not contaminate each other and your other groceries.

- After shopping for food, take groceries home immediately. Refrigerate or freeze meat, fish, egg, and dairy products promptly.

- Store whole eggs in their cartons, even if your refrigerator has a place for storing eggs. Egg cartons are designed to keep eggs fresh longer than a refrigerator's egg compartment.

Setting the Stage for Food Preparation

Contaminated hands and food preparation surfaces spread pathogens. To reduce the risk of food-borne illness:

- Wash hands thoroughly with very warm, soapy water for at least 20 seconds before and after touching food. If clean water for handwashing is not available, use sanitizing hand wipes.

- Use a fresh paper towel or clean hand towel to dry hands. Reserve dish towels for drying pots, pans, and cooking utensils that are not washed and dried in a dishwasher.

- Before preparing food, clean food preparation surfaces, including kitchen counters, cutting boards, dishes, knives, and other food preparation equipment with hot, soapy water. You can kill most pathogens when you clean and *sanitize* food preparation surfaces with a solution made by adding a tablespoon of bleach to 1 gallon of water. However, avoid getting the bleach solution on colored fabrics or surfaces that can be damaged by bleach (granite, for example).

- The FDA recommends cutting boards with unmarred surfaces made of easy-to-clean, nonporous materials, such as plastic, marble, or glass. If you prefer to use wooden cutting boards, make sure they are made of a nonabsorbent hardwood, such as oak or maple, and have no obvious seams or cracks.

- Replace cutting boards when they become streaked with cuts, because these grooves can be difficult to clean thoroughly and may harbor bacteria.

- If possible, have a cutting board reserved for meats, fish, and poultry; have another cutting board for fruits and vegetables; and have a third board for breads. Clean all cutting boards in the dishwasher or with hot, soapy water. You can also sanitize cutting boards with a dilute bleach solution.

- Sanitize food preparation surfaces and equipment that have come in contact with raw meat, fish, poultry, and eggs as soon as possible to destroy pathogens that may be present. In addition, sanitize kitchen sponges and wash kitchen towels frequently.

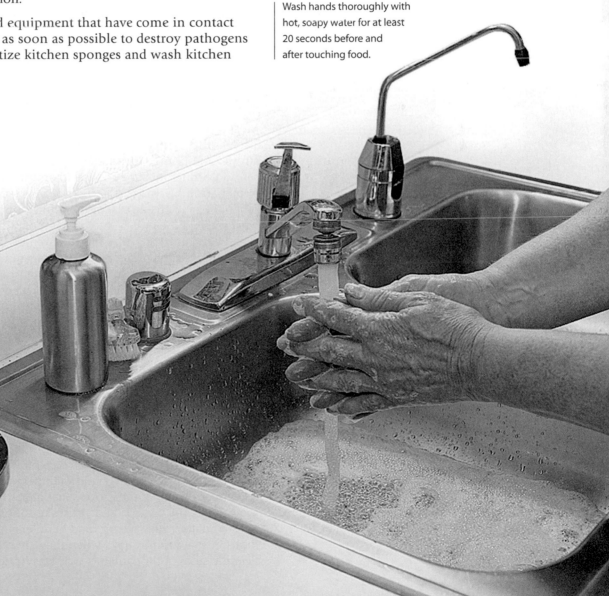

Wash hands thoroughly with hot, soapy water for at least 20 seconds before and after touching food.

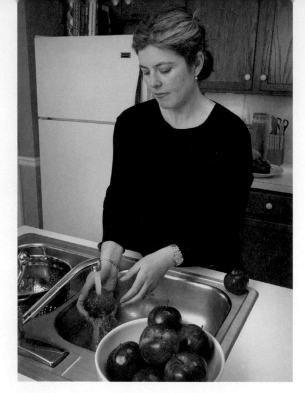

Wash produce in water before eating or preparing it.

Preparing Food

To reduce your risk of food-borne illness:

- Do not use foods from containers that leak, bulge, or are severely dented or from jars that are cracked or have loose or bulging lids.

- Do not use foods from containers that have damaged safety seals, because the food they contain may have been contaminated.

- Do not taste or use food that spurts liquid or has a bad odor when the can is opened.

- Read product labels to determine whether foods need to be refrigerated after their packages are opened.

- Before preparing fresh produce, carefully wash the foods under running water to remove dirt and bacteria clinging to the surface. Bacteria can be sticky, so scrub the peel with a vegetable brush if it is to be eaten. Even if you plan to remove the skin or peel, wash the produce before you cut it.

- Avoid eating moldy foods. Mold does not grow well on low-moisture foods. Thus, small amounts of mold on hard cheeses and on firm fruits and vegetables can be removed by cutting away the mold along with at least 1 inch of food that surrounds the moldy area.[6]

- **When in doubt, throw the food out.**

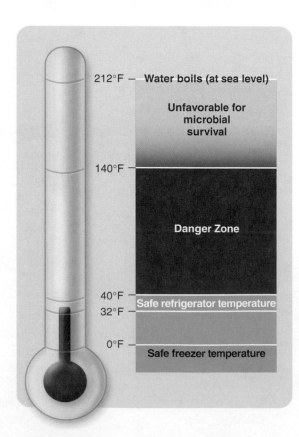

Figure 12.4 Temperature guide for food safety. Most pathogenic microbes grow well when the temperature of risky food is between 40°F and 140°F—the "danger zone."

Maintaining the Proper Temperature of Foods

Most microbes grow well when the temperature of a high-risk food is between 40°F and 140°F—the "danger zone" (Fig. 12.4).[8] Cooking foods to the proper temperature destroys food-borne viruses and bacteria, such as *Norovirus* and *E. coli* O157:H7. To be safe, a product must be cooked to an internal temperature that is high enough to destroy harmful pathogens and certain bacterial toxins. Using a meat thermometer is a reliable way to ensure that meat, poultry, thick pieces of fish, and egg-containing dishes have reached the proper internal temperature without overcooking. When you remove veal, beef, lamb, or pork from the oven or grill, allow it to "rest" for 3 minutes before carving. While the meat "rests," its temperature remains constant or rises slightly, which helps kill microorganisms. Table 12.5 indicates recommended minimum internal temperatures for cooking these foods.

Meat thermometers must be used properly. In general, the thermometer should be placed in the thickest part of the muscle tissue, away from bone, fat, or gristle (Fig. 12.5). If the thermometer is inserted incorrectly or placed in the wrong area, the reading may not accurately reflect the internal temperature of the product.

Microwave cooking can result in uneven heating that does not destroy microbes in the cool spots. While cooking a food in a microwave oven, keep the dish covered, and stop the oven occasionally to stir the food. Stirring the food reduces uneven heating. Cook the food until it reaches 165°F. Microwave cooking is not recommended for stuffed foods, because during cooking, the temperature of the stuffing may not be high enough to kill pathogens.[9]

Chilling food slows the growth of microbes in the items, but some bacteria can grow even at proper refrigeration temperatures. Freezing does not kill bacteria or inactive viruses in food; the process just halts the microbes' ability to multiply. As frozen food thaws, the bacteria and viruses resume their activities and can cause illness.

A major challenge for food handlers involves keeping large amounts of high-risk foods at safe temperatures when they are served from a single container. Food that is near the sides of the container may stay hotter or colder than food that is near or in the

TABLE 12.5 *USDA Recommended Safe Minimum Internal Temperatures*

Food	Safe Minimum Internal Temperature (°F)
Beef steaks and roasts	145
Fish	145
Pork	145
Ground beef, pork, lamb, and veal	160
Egg dishes	160
Poultry products	165

Source: U.S. Department of Agriculture, Safe minimum cooking temperature. http://www.foodsafety.gov/keep/charts/mintemp.html

Figure 12.5 Meat thermometer. Using a meat (food) thermometer is a reliable way to ensure that the cooked item has reached the proper internal temperature.

center of the container. As shown in Figure 12.6, chilled foods should be kept covered and served from a shallow container filled with ice. Hot foods should be kept covered and be served from shallow, heated pans. The best simple advice to follow: "Keep hot foods hot and cold foods cold."

To reduce your risk of food-borne illness:

• Always thaw high-risk foods in the refrigerator, under cold running water, or in a microwave oven.

• Cook foods immediately after thawing. Do not refreeze.

• Marinate food in the refrigerator, and if marinating meat, fish, or poultry, discard the marinade.

• Do not remove cold foods from the refrigerator or hot foods from the stove until it is time to serve them.

Did You Know?

Have you heard about the "5-second rule"? Supposedly, food that drops on the floor will not pick up microbes if it is picked up within 5 seconds. A study determined that this is a food-related myth. As soon as food touches a contaminated surface such as a floor, microbes adhere to it.[10]

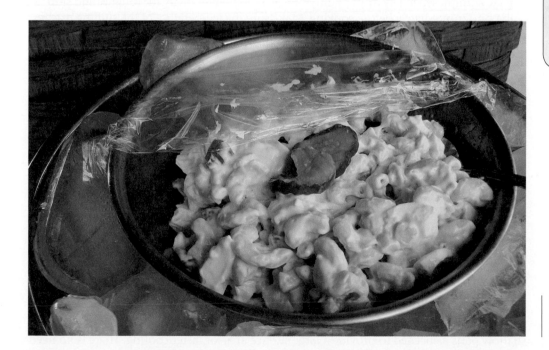

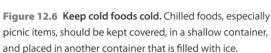

Figure 12.6 Keep cold foods cold. Chilled foods, especially picnic items, should be kept covered, in a shallow container, and placed in another container that is filled with ice.

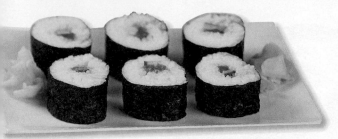

Eating raw fish, such as some forms of sushi, can be safe for most healthy people if the fish is very fresh before being commercially frozen and then thawed.

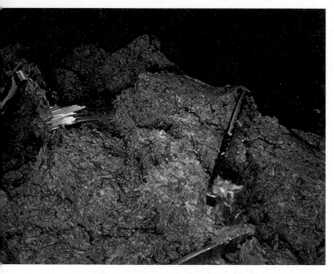

Prior to being ground up, the surface of a chunk of meat, fish, or poultry may contain relatively harmless concentrations of pathogens. The grinding process mixes the pathogens throughout the meat.

Raw Fish

Eating raw fish, such as sushi, can be safe for most healthy people if the fish is very fresh before being commercially frozen and then thawed. While frozen, the fish must maintain an internal temperature of 10°F for 7 days. The freezing step is important because very cold temperatures can kill parasites that are often in fish tissues. If you choose to eat uncooked fish, purchase it from reputable establishments that have high standards for quality and sanitation. Nevertheless, it is prudent to not eat any raw animal products, including fish.

Ground Meats, Poultry, and Fish

Ground meats, poultry, and fish are highly perishable and must be thoroughly cooked to avoid being a source of food-borne illness. The interior portion of an intact piece of raw animal flesh is free of bacteria, because the tissues are not exposed to air. However, ground meats, fish, and poultry products are often contaminated with microbes. Prior to being ground up, the surface of a chunk of meat, fish, or poultry may contain relatively harmless concentrations of pathogens. The grinding process, however, mixes the pathogens throughout the meat. At the same time, grinding the meat greatly increases its surface area, exposing more of the protein-rich tissues to microbes in air. Furthermore, the meat grinder can be a source of pathogens and spread them to the food product, especially if the machine was not properly cleaned after its last use. The particles of food that remained in the grinder can provide food for pathogenic microorganisms. Therefore, surfaces that touch ground meats should be cleaned carefully.

To reduce your risk of food-borne illness:

- Cook beef, poultry, pork, thick pieces of fish, and egg-containing dishes thoroughly, using a meat thermometer to check for doneness.

- Cook eggs until the yolk and white have solidified and no "runniness" remains.

- Heat alfalfa and other types of sprouts until they are steaming, because fresh sprouts may be contaminated with pathogenic bacteria.

- Remember that properly cooked seafood should not be shiny but be firm and flake easily when touched with a fork.

- Bake stuffing separately from poultry or wash the poultry cavity thoroughly and stuff the bird immediately before cooking. Make sure the temperature of the stuffing reaches 165°F. After cooking, transfer the stuffing to a clean bowl for serving or storage.

- Serve meat, poultry, and fish on a clean plate. Never use the same plate that held the raw product. For example, when grilling hamburgers, do not put cooked items on the plate that was used to carry the raw meat to the grill.

- Give picnic foods special attention, because outdoor temperatures may favor rapid bacterial growth. Keep cold salads and desserts on ice. Meats should be cooked completely at a picnic site. Do not partially cook foods in advance and plan to finish cooking them at the picnic.

Storing and Reheating Food

After food is cooked, careless food handling continues to set the stage for the growth of pathogens. Food-borne pathogens thrive at "room temperature," temperatures that are between 60°F and 110°F. A common practice is to let hot or cold foods remain on the table at room temperature for a few hours. Although you may not feel like clearing the table after eating, it is a good idea to cover leftovers and refrigerate or freeze them as soon as you have finished eating, or within 2 hours. If environmental temperatures are above 90°F, refrigerate the leftovers within 1 hour.[11] Do this by separating the food into as many shallow pans as needed to provide a large surface area for faster cooling. There is no need to let hot foods cool before chilling or freezing them.

To reduce your risk of food-borne illness, follow these food storage tips:

- Check your refrigerator's temperature regularly to make sure it stays below 41°F. Keep the refrigerator as cold as possible without freezing milk and lettuce.

- Cook ground meats and poultry soon after purchasing. If this is not possible, freeze the ground items.

- Note that raw fish, shellfish, and poultry are highly perishable. It is best to cook these foods or freeze them the day they are purchased.

- Use refrigerated ground meat and patties within 1 to 2 days, and use frozen meat and patties within 3 to 4 months after purchasing them. Table 12.6 presents recommended time limits for refrigeration and freezer storage of foods. Foods that are stored in the freezer for longer than recommended periods often develop unappealing flavors. Note that ground meats are more perishable than intact cuts of meat.

- Use refrigerated leftovers within 4 days. "Recipe for Healthy Living" at the end of Chapter 12 features a chilled chicken salad recipe that uses leftover chicken.

- Reheat leftovers to 165°F; reheat gravy to a rolling boil to kill pathogenic bacteria that may be present.

TABLE 12.6 *Cold Storage Time Limits for Perishable Foods*

Product	Storage Period in Refrigerator (40°F)	Storage Period in Freezer (0°F)
Fresh meat		
Ground meat	1–2 days	3–4 months
Steaks and roasts	3–5 days	6–12 months
Fresh pork		
Chops	3–5 days	4–6 months
Ground	1–2 days	3–4 months
Roasts	3–5 days	4–6 months
Cured meats		
Luncheon meat (deli sliced or open package)	3–5 days	1–2 months
Unopened package	2 weeks	1-2 months
Sausage	1–2 days	1–2 months
Gravy	1–2 days	2–3 months
Fresh fish		
Lean (such as cod, flounder, haddock)	1–2 days	Up to 6 months
Fatty (such as perch, salmon)	1–2 days	2–3 months
Fresh chicken or turkey (whole)	1–2 days	12 months
Parts	1–2 days	9 months
Giblets	1–2 days	3–4 months
Dairy products		
Cheese (swiss, brick, processed cheese)	3–4 weeks	(Not recommended)
Milk	5 days	1 month
Ice cream, ice milk	—	2–4 months
Eggs		
Fresh, in shell	3 weeks	—
Hard-cooked	1 week	—

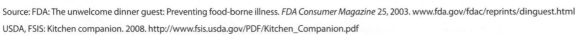

Source: FDA: The unwelcome dinner guest: Preventing food-borne illness. *FDA Consumer Magazine* 25, 2003. www.fda.gov/fdac/reprints/dinguest.html

USDA, FSIS: Kitchen companion. 2008. http://www.fsis.usda.gov/PDF/Kitchen_Companion.pdf

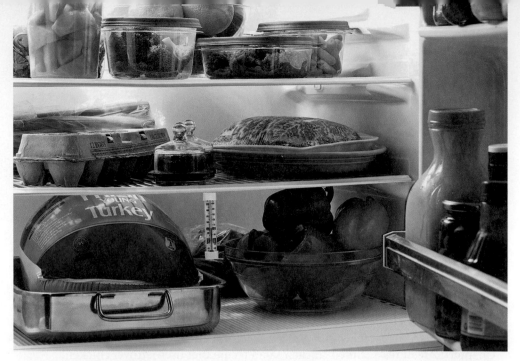

Figure 12.7 Storing risky foods in the refrigerator. In this photograph, can you identify two risky foods that are improperly stored? What can be done to store the foods safely?

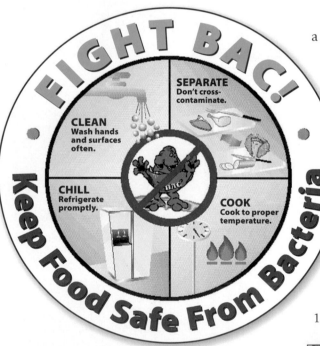

Food safety educators at the USDA condensed food safety rules into four simple actions as a part of their Fight BAC! program.

Cross-contamination is a threat not only during food preparation; it can also become a problem during food storage. Therefore, keep all foods, including leftovers, covered while they are in the refrigerator. This practice can prevent drippings from foods that are often contaminated, such as raw chicken, from tainting other foods. Furthermore, store raw meats, fish, poultry, and shellfish on lower shelves of the refrigerator, so they are separated from foods that are to be eaten raw. Examine Figure 12.7. Can you find two examples of improperly stored refrigerated foods?

Food safety educators at the USDA condensed these rules into four simple actions as a part of their Fight BAC! program (see www.fightbac.org):

1. **CLEAN.** Wash hands and surfaces often.
2. **SEPARATE.** Do not cross-contaminate.
3. **COOK.** Cook to proper temperatures.
4. **CHILL.** Refrigerate promptly.

In addition to the "Fight BAC!" website, you can find reliable information about food-borne illness at www.foodsafety.gov and www.homefoodsafety.org/index.jsp. For general food safety questions, you can call FDA's food safety hotline at 1-888-723-3366.

Concept **Checkpoint**

15. List at least four rules for reducing the risk of food-borne illness when you purchase foods and beverages.
16. List at least five rules for reducing the risk of food-borne illness when you prepare and cook foods.
17. List at least three rules for reducing the risk of food-borne illness when you store cooked foods.
18. Explain why ground meat and poultry often are sources of food-borne illness.
19. What preparation step can be taken to make fish safer to eat raw?
20. What temperature range encourages rapid multiplication of pathogens?
21. What are the USDA's four simplified actions for reducing the risk of food-borne illness?

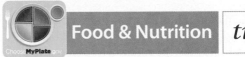

Food & Nutrition *tips*

- Be alert for signs of unsafe food handling practices when you eat out.

- Make sure tabletops, dishes, and eating utensils are clean.

- Make sure servers who handle food directly are wearing gloves.

- Check custard, pudding, pies, and salad bar foods to make sure they are chilled and kept on ice.

- Make sure hot foods are served hot or served from a heated food bar.

- If your serving of meat, poultry, or fish does not appear to be thoroughly cooked, ask the waiter to return the item to the kitchen to be heated again.

- Be wary of perishable foods in vending machines, especially those selling sandwiches. These tips also apply to foods prepared for dormitory residents.

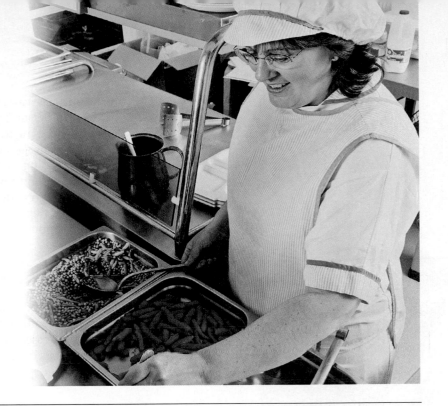

 ## 12.6 Food Preservation

If nothing is done to preserve a fresh food, the item soon undergoes various chemical changes that eventually result in spoilage. Preserving food extends its shelf life. **Shelf life** refers to the period of time that a food can be stored before it spoils. Heating is one of the oldest ways to preserve foods. Heat can kill or deactivate pathogens, and the process also destroys naturally occurring enzymes in foods that can contribute to food spoilage.

Fermentation is an ancient method of food preservation that is still used to produce a variety of foods, including yogurt, wine, pickles, and sauerkraut. The fermentation process involves adding certain bacteria or yeast to food. These microbes use sugars in the food to make acids and alcohol, chemicals that hinder the growth of other types of bacteria and yeast that can spoil food.

For centuries, people preserved meats, fruits, and other foods that had high water contents by adding salt or sugar to them. To grow, bacteria need plenty of water; yeasts and molds can grow when less water is available. Adding sugar or salt to foods draws water out of cells, including bacteria, fungi, protozoans, and worms. As a result, these pathogens are less likely to survive in sugary or salty foods. Drying reduces a food's water content. Dried fruits such as raisins, for example, have a longer shelf life than grapes, their natural counterparts.

> **shelf life** period of time that a food can be stored before it spoils
>
> **fermentation** process used to preserve or produce a variety of foods, including pickles and wine

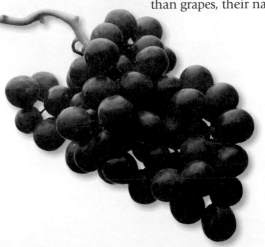

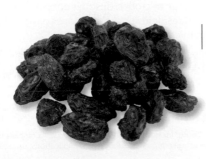

Can you explain why dried fruits such as raisins have a longer shelf life than grapes, their natural counterparts?

sterilization process that kills or destroys all microorganisms and viruses

Today, we can add pasteurization, refrigeration, freezing, canning, irradiation, additives, and *aseptic* processing to the list of food preservation techniques (Table 12.7). Aseptic processing involves sterilizing a food and its package separately, before the food enters the package. The **sterilization** process destroys all microorganisms and viruses. After undergoing aseptic packaging, boxes of sterile foods and beverages, such as milk or juices, can remain free of microbial growth for several years while sitting on supermarket or pantry shelves. However, once the containers of these products are opened, the foods or beverages have the same shelf life as their counterparts that have not undergone aseptic processing.

Home-Canned Foods

When food is canned, commercial food production methods require heating the food to certain temperatures for specified times. Thus, unless the can or jar has been damaged, properly processed canned foods should be free of pathogens. Certain home-canned foods, however, may contain the microorganism *Clostridium botulinum (C. botulinum)* that causes

TABLE 12.7 *Summary of Food Preservation Methods*

Method	Means of Effectiveness	Examples of Foods
Heating (cooking, pasteurization, aseptic processing)	Kills or deactivates spoilage and pathogenic microbes, destroys enzymes that result in food spoilage	Most foods
Adding salt/sugar	Binds water, decreasing the amount available for microbes	Ham, bacon, fish, pickled foods
Smoking	Kills spoilage microbes, destroys enzymes that result in food spoilage	Meats, fish
	Smoking is a method of heating. The process involves salting food before smoking and refrigerating or freezing the food after smoking.	
Curing	Retards the growth of *C. botulinum* and stabilizes the flavor of the food	Luncheon meats, smoked fish
	Additives such as sodium nitrate and nitrite are used to cure meat, fish, or poultry.	
Chilling/freezing	Slows molecular movement, retarding microbial and enzymatic activity	Most foods
Drying (dehydration)	Removes much of the moisture in food that microbes need to survive	Fruit, herbs, meat jerkies, seeds
Fermenting	Produces acids and alcohol that interfere with the survival of unwanted microbes	Alcoholic beverages, yogurt, cheeses, soy sauce
Canning	Kills spoilage microbes, destroys enzymes in food that result in spoilage, removes oxygen that certain microbes need to survive	Meat, fish, poultry, fruits, vegetables, milk
Irradiating	Destroys most pathogens, delays sprouting (potatoes)	Spices, raw meat and poultry, fresh fruits and vegetables

Sources: Hilderbrand KS: *Smoking fish at home—safely.* PNW 238, 2003. extension.oregonstate.edu/catalog/pdf/pnw/pnw238.pdf

National Center for Home Food Preservation: *USDA Complete Guide to Home Canning, 2009 revision.* http://www.uga.edu/nchfp/publications/publications_usda.html

botulism or its toxin. The home-canning process may kill *C. botulinum* bacteria in the food, but their spores or toxin may remain. That is why home-canned, *low-acid* foods such as beans and corn should be boiled for 10 minutes before eating. Foods made with vinegar, tomatoes, or citrus juices are usually high-acid foods, and as a result, such items are not likely to be sources of *C. botulinum*. The botulinum toxin is highly poisonous; never taste a home-canned low-acid food before boiling it. For more information about proper home canning of foods, obtain a copy of the U.S. Department of Agriculture's *Complete Guide to Home Canning* (http://www.uga.edu/nchfp/publications/publications_usda.html) or contact a food and nutrition specialist at your community's university extension office.

Irradiation

The process of food irradiation preserves food by using a high amount of energy to kill pathogens such as *Salmonella* and *E. coli* O157:H7 (Fig. 12.8). The processes used to irradiate foods do not make the items radioactive. The energy passes through the food, as in microwave cooking, and no radioactive material is left behind. The energy is strong enough to destroy the genetic material as well as cell membranes or cell walls of insects and microbes. As a result, irradiation is a highly effective way of killing insects and microorganisms that may be in foods. However, irradiation is not always an effective way to destroy viruses.[13] It is important to recognize that even when foods, especially meats, have been irradiated, once their packaging has been opened, the foods can still become contaminated.

Irradiation extends the shelf life of spices, dry vegetable seasonings, meats, seeds, shell eggs, and fresh fruits and vegetables. Except for dried seasonings, packages that contain irradiated foods must be labeled with the international food irradiation symbol, the Radura, and include a statement indicating the product has been treated by irradiation (Fig. 12.9).

Irradiation of food is not a new technology; in 1963, U.S. food manufacturers were given approval to irradiate wheat flour. Today, France, Israel, Russia, and China are among the countries that use irradiation to preserve various foods. Nevertheless, some consumer groups claim that irradiation diminishes the nutritional value of food and leads to the formation of harmful compounds, such as **carcinogens,** cancer-causing substances. According to medical experts with the World Health Organization (WHO), FDA, and CDC, irradiated foods are safe to eat.[13] Furthermore, irradiation causes few or no nutritive losses. Despite such assurances, many Americans are skeptical about the safety of irradiated foods, and they avoid purchasing such products.

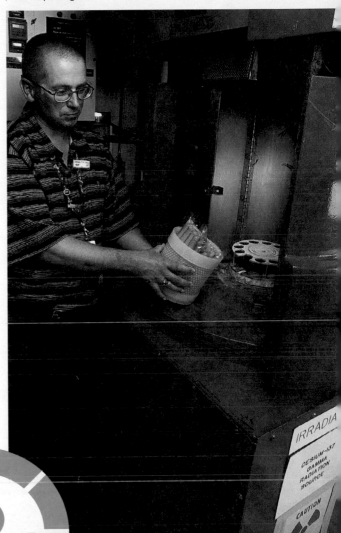

Figure 12.8 **Irradiating food.** U.S. Department of Agriculture microbiologist Glenn Boyd places a batch of hot dogs into the gamma radiation source to rid them of food-borne pathogens.

Figure 12.9 **Radura symbol.** The Radura symbol indicates the food in this package has been irradiated.

carcinogens cancer-causing substances

Concept **Checkpoint**

22. Define *shelf life*.
23. Identify four methods of food preservation and explain how each method extends the shelf life of foods.
24. What preparation step can be taken to make home-canned, low-acid foods safe to eat?
25. What is a carcinogen?

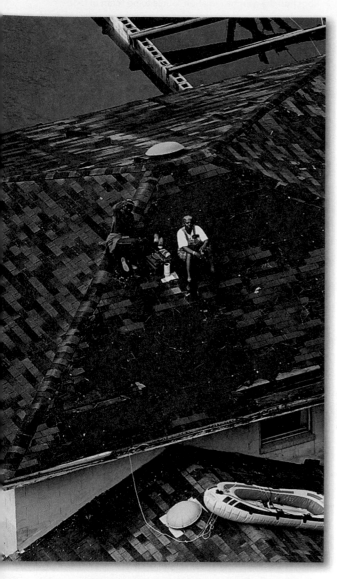

This aerial photo shows people waiting to be rescued from the roof of a house that was surrounded by floodwater in New Orleans, Louisiana, on August 30, 2005. After Hurricane Katrina struck New Orleans, thousands of people were saved after they moved to their roofs or attics.

 ## 12.7 Preparing for Disasters

In late August 2005, Hurricane Katrina devastated the central Gulf Coast region of the United States. At least 1800 individuals lost their lives and more than 250,000 people were displaced from their homes as a result of the hurricane. Media coverage of the storm's aftermath showed desperate conditions as people lived in their attics or on their roofs, waiting to be rescued. What steps can you take to have enough water and food available to survive hurricanes, earthquakes, or other serious emergency situations?

A supply of clean water and wholesome food is necessary for surviving disasters such as hurricanes and earthquakes. The Chapter 12 "Highlight" provides instructions for sanitizing water. The following recommendations may help sustain you and your loved ones for several days:

- Store at least 1 gallon of water per person per day. Ideally, you should have at least a 3- to 5-day supply of drinking water, or at least 5 gallons of water for each person in a household. Children and breastfeeding women may need more than 1 gallon of water per day. Also, more water may be necessary for people living in warm climates. Furthermore, store extra water for food preparation, personal hygiene, dishwashing, and pets.

- Water should be maintained in a cool place and in sturdy plastic bottles with tight-fitting lids.

- Avoid storing water in areas where toxic substances, such as gasoline and pesticides, are stored. Over time, toxic vapors from these products may penetrate the plastic and contaminate the water.

- Change stored water every 6 months.

- Drink only bottled, boiled, or treated water until you are certain the public water supply is safe.

- If you have time to prepare, fill a bathtub with water to use if it becomes necessary. The water, however, will need to be sanitized before being consumed.

- If you drink bottled water, make sure the seal has not been broken.

If your emergency water supply is inadequate, you can consume melted ice cubes from the freezer, canned fruit juices, and water drained from an undamaged water heater. Water stored in the tank of the toilet (not the bowl) is also fit to drink. Pets can drink toilet bowl water that has not been treated with a toilet bowl sanitizer. Water in swimming pools and spas can be used for personal hygiene needs but not for drinking. Never drink water from car radiators, home heating systems, or water beds. Alcoholic beverages contribute to dehydration and therefore should be avoided.

Emergency Food Supply

A disaster can easily disrupt your access to safe food; therefore, you should store at least a 3-day supply of food for emergency use. Choose foods that have a long storage life, require no refrigeration, and can be eaten without cooking, such as canned meats, fruits, and vegetables. If you have pets, you should also keep a supply of pet foods. Table 12.8 lists foods that can be included in your emergency food supply. Also store a manual can opener, paper plates, and eating utensils.

If stored under proper conditions, unopened canned or boxed foods will remain fresh for about 2 years. Before storing food, use a permanent marking pen to write the date on the package. You should use and replace foods before they lose their freshness or reach their expiration dates. An ideal food storage location is a cool, dry, dark place. Do not store foods near gasoline, oil, paints, or petroleum-based solvents, because some food products absorb their odors. You can protect foods from rodents and insects by storing them in airtight containers or plastic storage bins.

If you have no electricity, consume perishable food in your refrigerator or freezer before using your emergency food supply. However, discard cooked foods after they have been at room temperature for 2 hours. Do not eat food that appears or smells spoiled or is from cans that are leaking or bulging.

To prepare meals safely after a disaster, you will need to store

- A camp stove or charcoal grill.

- Fuel for cooking, such as charcoal. **Never** cook food on a camp stove or charcoal grill indoors. The fumes contain *carbon monoxide*, an odorless deadly gas.

- Matches.

- Cooking and eating utensils.

- Paper plates, cups, and towels.

- Heavy-duty aluminum foil.

For more information about emergency preparedness, visit the Centers for Disease Control and Prevention's website: www.bt.cdc.gov/disasters/.

TABLE 12.8 *Foods to Store for Emergency Situations*

- Canned meats, fish, fruits, and vegetables
- Canned fruit juices
- Unopened boxes of cereal, low-salt crackers, and trail mix
- Prewrapped fruit-filled granola bars
- Peanut or other nut butters
- Raisins and other dried fruit
- Dry milk powder
- Baby foods

Concept **Checkpoint**

26. Develop an emergency food and water supply plan for your home. Identify at least five foods that are appropriate for an emergency food supply.

27. In case public water supplies are disrupted, identify at least three sources of drinking water in homes that are safe for humans. Identify at least two sources of water that are unsafe to drink.

food additive any substance that becomes incorporated into food during production, packaging, transport, or storage

color additives dyes, pigments, or other substances that provide color to food

12.8 Food Additives

A **food additive** is any substance that becomes incorporated into food during production, packaging, transport, or storage. Food manufacturers incorporate *direct* or *intentional additives* into their products for various reasons. Such additives may make food easier to process, more nutritious, able to stay fresh longer, or better tasting. Most additives are added to influence a food's sensory characteristics, including taste or color.

Many direct food additives help maintain the safety of foods by limiting the growth of bacteria that cause food-borne illness. Other additives protect against the action of enzymes that can lead to undesirable changes in the food's color and taste. Such unwanted chemical changes occur when enzymes that are naturally in certain foods are exposed to the oxygen in air. *Antioxidant additives*, including vitamins E and C and a variety of *sulfites*, can prevent oxygen from reacting with these enzymes. **Color additives** are dyes, pigments, or other substances that provide color to foods, drugs, or cosmetics, such as beta-carotene in margarine and FD&C (Food, Drug, & Cosmetic) Red No. 40 in cherry-flavored cough

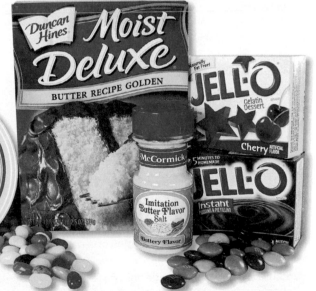

Color additives are dyes, pigments, or other substances that provide color to foods, drugs, or cosmetics.

Did You Know?

Sulfites are sulfur-containing food additives that limit the growth of food spoilage microbes and prevent enzymatic browning of certain foods, such as pieces of fruit and vegetables. Some people, however, are sensitive or allergic to sulfites, and they can have severe reactions when they ingest the compounds. The FDA requires manufacturers who add sulfites to foods and beverages to indicate on their products' package labels that these chemicals are among the ingredients.

Food Additives Amendment U.S. legislation that requires evidence that a new food additive is safe before it can be marketed for use

Generally Recognized as Safe (GRAS) ingredients thought to be safe

Delaney Clause component of the 1958 Food Additives Amendment that prevents manufacturers from adding carcinogenic compounds to food

syrup. Table 12.9 lists common types of direct food additives (including color additives), their uses, examples of products that contain the additives, and names of specific additives.

Indirect additives, such as compounds from a food's wrapper or container, can enter food as it is packaged, transported, or stored. Indirect additives, however, have no purpose. The FDA and certain international organizations regulate *all* food additives to ensure that processed foods and their packaging are safe.[14]

Food Safety Legislation: Food Additives

By the 1950s, hundreds of ingredients were being added to foods during processing. Many of these substances had long histories of being safe; others were deemed safe after undergoing scientific testing. In 1958, the U.S. Congress enacted the **Food Additives Amendment.** According to this amendment, an ingredient that had been in use prior to 1958 was **Generally Recognized as Safe (GRAS)** when qualified experts generally agreed that the substance was safe for its intended use. The Food Additives Amendment excluded GRAS substances from being defined as food additives.[15] Thus, modern food manufacturers can include substances on the GRAS list as ingredients without testing them for safety or getting prior approval from the FDA.

As a result of the 1958 Food Additives Amendment, the manufacturer of a *new* food additive (one developed after 1958) must provide evidence of the substance's safety to the FDA before the additive can be used.[16] When evaluating the safety of a newly developed food additive, FDA experts consider the chemical composition and characteristics of the substance, the amount of the substance that Americans would typically ingest, and the additive's effects on the body. If the additive is safe in amounts that people are likely to consume, FDA experts establish a level of the substance that can be added to foods.

According to the **Delaney Clause** of the Food Additives Amendment, food manufacturers cannot add a new compound that causes cancer at *any* level of intake. Thus, if an

TABLE 12.9 *Common Types of Direct Food Additives*

Type of Additive	Functions	Typical Products	Examples of Specific Ingredients
Preservatives	Prevent food spoilage	Jellies, beverages, baked goods, cured meats, cereals, snack foods	Ascorbic acid, citric acid, sodium benzoate, calcium propionate, sodium erythorbate, BHA, BHT, EDTA, sulfites
Sweeteners	Add sweetness	Processed foods, beverages, baked goods, sugar substitutes	Sucrose, glucose, mannitol, corn syrup, aspartame, sucralose
Flavors and spices	Add specific flavors	Puddings, pie fillings, gelatins, cake mixes, candies, soft drinks	Natural flavorings, artificial flavorings, spices
Flavor enhancers	Enhance flavors already present	Snack foods	Monosodium glutamate (MSG), hydrolyzed soy protein
Nutrients	Replace nutrients lost during processing, boost levels of nutrients naturally in food	Flour, grains, cereals, margarine, juice, energy bars	Thiamin hydrochloride, riboflavin, niacin, niacinamide, folic acid, beta-carotene, ascorbic acid
Emulsifiers	Keep oily and watery ingredients from separating	Salad dressings, peanut butter, chocolate, frozen desserts	Soy lecithin, mono- and diglycerides, polysorbates
Leavening agents	Promote rising of certain baked goods	Baked goods	Baking soda, monocalcium phosphate, calcium carbonate
Stabilizers, thickeners, binders	Provide uniform texture and improve "mouth feel"	Frozen desserts, puddings, sauces	Gelatin, pectin, guar gum, carregeenan
Color additives	Enhance natural colors, provide color to colorless and "fun" foods as well as medications and cosmetics	Processed foods, including candies, snack foods, margarine, cheese, soft drinks, gelatin, drug capsules, cough syrup, lipstick	FD&C Blue No. 1, FD&C Red No. 40, beta-carotene, caramel color

Modified from: International Food Information Council and U.S. Food and Drug Administration: *Food ingredients and colors.* 2004. www.cfsan.fda.gov/~dms/foodic.html

additive causes cancer, even though very high doses may be necessary to cause the disease, no amount of the additive is considered to be safe, and none is allowed in food. Evidence for cancer risk could come from either laboratory animal or human studies. The FDA allows very few exceptions to this clause.

The FDA cannot ban **unintentional food additives**—various industrial chemicals, pesticide residues, and mold toxins—from foods, even though some of these contaminants may be carcinogenic. The Food Quality Protection Act of 1996 established the safety standard of "a reasonable certainty of no harm" for pesticide residues in foods. As a result of this act, the "no risk" provision of the Delaney Clause does not apply to pesticide residues. However, the Delaney Clause remains in effect for food additives.[17] The following section discusses chemical contaminants and other unintentional food additives.

Did You Know?

According to the results of numerous scientific studies, food additives do not cause hyperactivity or learning disabilities in children. However, a small percentage of preschool children may be allergic to FD&C Yellow No. 5, so this color additive must be listed on the package label if it is used as an ingredient.[14]

Other Substances in Foods

Various substances can accidentally enter food during processing. Although such contaminants can blend into a food, they are not food additives. Common biological and physical food contaminants are insect parts, rodent feces or urine, dust and dirt, and bits of metal or glass from machinery used to process food. Although some of these substances may not be harmful to health, most people find it unappealing to have filth and other unintentional ingredients in their foods.

According to the Federal Food, Drug, and Cosmetic Act, adulterated food contains objectionable and unsanitary material, and it cannot be distributed. However, the FDA permits very small amounts of unavoidable, naturally occurring substances such as dirt and insect parts in foods, because they are not harmful when consumed in minute amounts. The FDA established guidelines concerning amounts (*action levels*) of certain materials that are permitted in specific foods, such as mold and rodent hairs in paprika or insect eggs in canned orange juice. According to the FDA, "…it is economically impractical to grow, harvest, or process raw products that are totally free of non-hazardous, naturally occurring, unavoidable defects. Products harmful to consumers are subject to regulatory action whether or not they exceed the action levels."[18]

Chemical contaminants also enter foods unintentionally. Toxic metals, such as lead, cadmium, and mercury, are naturally in our environment, and these elements may also be in our food. Poisonous human-made compounds such as *benzene* and *polychlorinated biphenols (PCBs)* are in the environment as well. Toxic metals or poisonous compounds resulting from human manufacturing practices can pollute sources of water used by consumers (well water, for example). Americans who drink water from municipal supplies can be assured that the water is analyzed regularly to determine its concentrations of toxic substances. However, people who rely on privately owned wells should have the water tested routinely.

Common biological and physical food contaminants include rodent feces or urine.

unintentional food additives substances that are accidentally in foods

What Is Benzene?

Late in 2005, the FDA received reports that low levels of benzene had been detected in some soft drinks that contained ascorbic acid (vitamin C) and a group of food additives called benzoate (*ben'-zo-ate*) salts. Benzene is a cancer-causing agent present in the environment from natural and manufactured sources. After receiving the reports, the FDA's Center for Food Safety and Applied Nutrition (CFSAN) surveyed benzene levels in soft drinks. The survey's findings indicated that the vast majority of beverages sampled, including those containing both benzoate salts and ascorbic acid, contained either no detectable amounts of benzene or amounts that were very low and within the

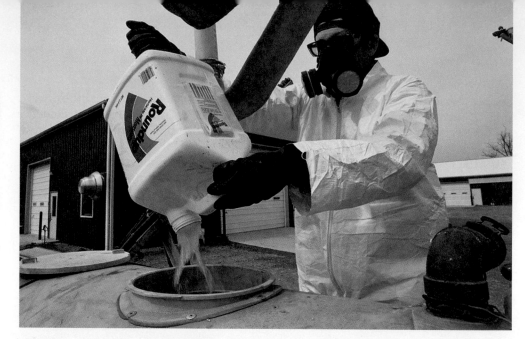

Herbicides are the most widely used type of pesticide in agriculture. Note the protective gear worn by this farmworker as he handles an herbicide.

pesticide substance that people use to kill or control unwanted insects, weeds, or other organisms

insecticides substances used to control or kill insects

rodenticides substances used to kill mice and rats

herbicides substances used to destroy weeds

fungicides substances used to limit the spread of fungi

tolerances maximum amounts of pesticide residues that can be in or on each treated food crop

range allowed by the U.S. water standard.[19] Thus, FDA scientists concluded that the levels of benzene in soft drinks did not pose a safety concern. Nevertheless, agency officials determined it was necessary to contact beverage manufacturers to ensure that processing conditions avoid or minimize benzene formation.

What Are Pesticides?

A **pesticide** is any substance that people use to control or kill unwanted insects, weeds, rodents, fungi, or other organisms. There are several different kinds of pesticides. **Insecticides** control or kill insects; **rodenticides** kill mice and rats; **herbicides** destroy weeds; and **fungicides** limit the spread of fungi, such as mold and mildew. Over 1 *billion* tons of pesticides are used in the United States annually.[20] Herbicides are the most widely used type of pesticide in agriculture.[20]

Pesticide Residue Tolerances The use of pesticides in modern farming practices has helped increase crop yields, reduce food costs, and protect the quality of many agricultural products. However, many pesticides leave small amounts (*pesticide residues*) in or on treated crops, including fruits, vegetables, and grains, even when they are applied correctly. Concentrations of pesticide residues often decrease as food crops are washed, stored, processed, and prepared. Nevertheless, some of these substances may remain in fresh produce, such as apples or peaches, as well as in processed foods, such as canned applesauce or peaches.

The EPA regulates the proper use of pesticides. The agency can limit the amount of a pesticide that is applied on crops, restrict the frequency or location of the pesticide's application, or require the substance be used only by specially trained, certified persons. The EPA also sets pesticide **tolerances,** maximum amounts of pesticide residues that can be in or on each treated food crop. A pesticide tolerance includes a margin of safety, so the maximum pesticide residue that is allowed to be in or on a food is much lower than amounts that can cause negative health effects.[20]

Nonchemical Methods of Pest Management Although the EPA focuses on chemical methods of managing pests, the agency also promotes nonchemical pest management techniques that may be safer for humans and the environment. Integrated Pest Management (IPM) involves using a variety of methods for controlling pests while limiting damage to the environment. IPM methods include growing pest-resistant crops, using predatory wasps to control crop-destroying insects, and trapping adult insect pests before they can reproduce. Biologically based pesticides, such as sex hormones (*pheromones*) that attract pesky insects to predators or traps and viruses that infect insects and weeds, are

Did You Know?

Lead is a highly toxic mineral that may be in candies imported from Mexico and traditional ethnic folk remedies, especially *greta*, *azarcon*, *ghasard*, and *ba-baw-san*. Therefore, it is prudent to avoid ingesting these candies or folk remedies.

becoming increasingly popular among farmers (Figure 12.10). Such methods are often safer for humans than traditional chemical pesticides.

It is important to note that IPM permits the use of chemical pesticides but only as needed to enhance the effects of nonchemical methods. Studies suggest that IPM techniques generally increase crop yields and economic profits, while reducing the use of chemical pesticides.[20] As IPM programs become more widely adopted, conventional farmers will depend less on the use of chemical pesticides.

Fruits and vegetables grown without use of pesticides are available and may bear an "organic" label (see Chapter 3 for information about organic foods). These products generally are more expensive than those grown using pesticides, and they are not necessarily safer or more nutritious than conventionally produced foods.

How Safe Are Pesticides? Pesticides used in agriculture have both beneficial and unwanted effects. Pesticides help protect the food supply and make food crops available at reasonable cost. Nevertheless, pesticides have the potential to harm humans, animals, or the environment because they are designed to kill or otherwise negatively affect organisms. If a pesticide is applied improperly to cropland, it may remain in the soil, be taken up by plant roots, decompose to other compounds, or enter groundwater and waterways. Winds may carry pesticides in air and dust to distant locations. Each path can be a route to the human food chain (Fig. 12.11).

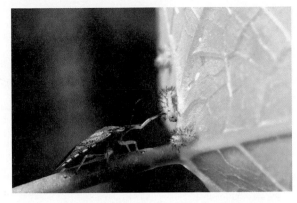

Figure 12.10 Helpful insect. The spined soldier bug (left) makes a meal of a Mexican bean beetle larva. Bean beetle larvae are devastating pests of snap beans and soybeans. The spined soldier bug's pheromone may help farmers control many insects that eat crops.

Figure 12.11 Pesticide pathways. If a pesticide is applied improperly to cropland, it may remain in the soil, be taken up by plant roots, decompose to other compounds, or enter groundwater and waterways. Winds may carry pesticides in air and dust to distant locations. Each path can be a route to the human food chain.

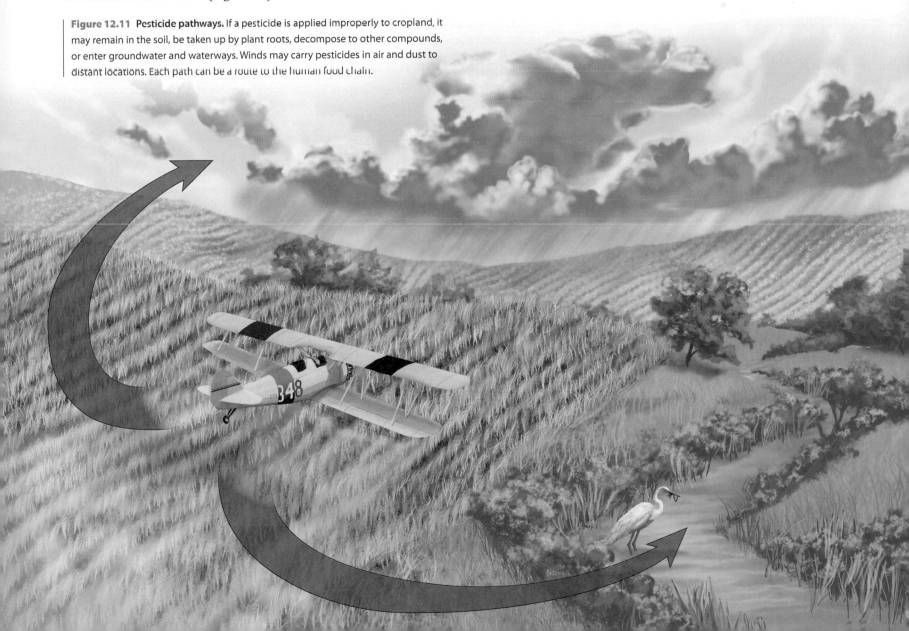

The potential harmful effects of a pesticide in food depend on the particular chemical and how effectively the body can eliminate it, its concentration in the food, how much and how often it is eaten, and the consumer's vulnerability to the substance. Tolerable amounts of pesticide residues on or in foods are extremely small. However, it is possible that regular exposure to small amounts of these chemicals may enable the substances to accumulate in the body and produce toxicity or initiate cancer.[21] Health experts have studied rates of cancers among people who have close contact with pesticides, such as farmers and pesticide applicators. Among the people who applied pesticides, the likelihood of developing lip cancer was elevated. The risk of prostate cancer was also elevated but primarily among applicators with a family history of this type of cancer.[22] Environmental health experts will continue to monitor the effects of pesticides on humans.

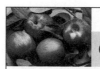

Concept **Checkpoint**

28. What is a food additive? What is the difference between direct and indirect food additives?
29. What is a color additive?
30. What is the GRAS list?
31. Explain the role of the Delaney Clause in protecting the U.S. food supply.
32. What is an unintentional food additive? Provide at least three examples of such additives.
33. What is a pesticide? Provide at least three examples of types of pesticides.
34. Define *integrated pest management* and provide an example of this method.
35. Which U.S. agency regulates the use of pesticides?
36. What is a pesticide tolerance?
37. Explain how pesticides can enter the human food chain.

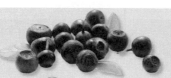

Chapter 12 Highlight

AVOIDING "THE REVENGE"

If you like traveling to foreign countries and enjoy sampling exotic cuisines in these places, one thing you do not need to encounter is *travelers' diarrhea (TD)*. Also referred to as "Montezuma's Revenge" and "Tut's Tummy," TD can ruin your vacation. By taking some precautions, however, your digestive system can stay healthy while you travel abroad.

TD results from consuming food or water contaminated with pathogens. The illness is characterized by the abrupt onset of abdominal cramps and loose or watery bowel movements. Additional symptoms may include nausea, vomiting, intestinal bloating, and fever. TD generally lasts 3 to 5 days without treatment, but signs and symptoms may persist in a small percentage of infected travelers.

Unless precautions are taken, TD is likely to occur during or shortly after traveling in regions where sanitary water supplies are

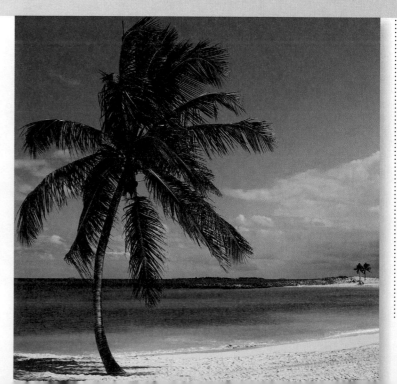

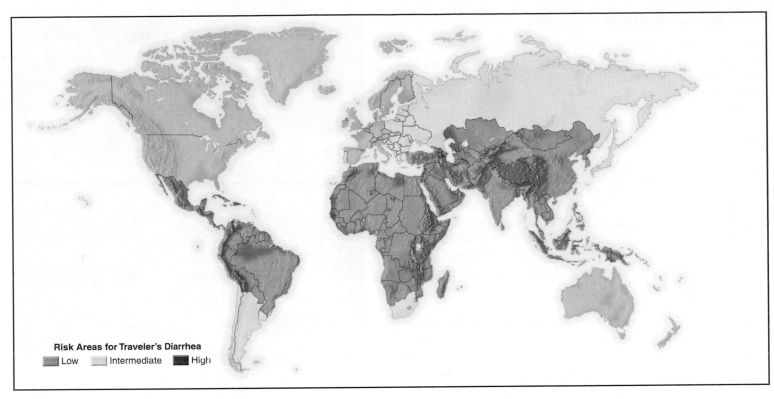

| **Figure 12.12 Areas of risk for travelers' diarrhea.** This map presents regions of the world where the risks are low, intermediate, and high.

not always available, people who prepare food have less than ideal personal hygiene practices, and untreated human feces are used for fertilizer. Health experts estimate that bacterial pathogens are responsible for 80% to 90% of cases of TD.[23] Parasitic protozoans such as *Giardia* and *Cryptosporidium* ("Crypto") account for about 10% of TD cases. When travelers suffer from persistent symptoms, the illness is likely to be the result of a parasitic rather than a bacterial infection.

Thirty to seventy percent of travelers will develop TD, depending on their destinations.[23] However, it is important to note that a trip to every foreign destination is likely to include the risk of TD. Figure 12.12 presents regions of the world where the risks are low, intermediate, and high. Low-risk countries include the United States, Canada, Australia, New Zealand, Japan, and countries in Northern and Western Europe. Intermediate-risk countries include those in Eastern Europe, South Africa, and some of the Caribbean islands. High-risk areas generally have high-density populations, widespread pollution, and inadequate water treatment systems.[24] These regions include Mexico and other Central American countries, and most of Asia, the Middle East, Africa, and South America.

Reducing Your Risk of TD

Experts at the CDC recommend several approaches for reducing your risk of TD. These include following instructions regarding food and beverage selection, avoiding contact with contam-

inated waterways, sanitizing drinking water, and using medications that may prevent TD.

Carry a small container of an alcohol-based (at least 60% alcohol) hand cleaner with you. Before you eat, wash your hands with the hand cleaner. When you visit places where risk of contracting TD is moderate to high, avoid consuming food or beverages purchased from street vendors. Before you eat meat or other high-risk foods, make sure they are fully cooked and served hot. Avoid raw foods that have been washed in water, such as fresh fruits, raw vegetables, and salads. Do not eat fresh fruit without peeling it first. Avoid water, ice, and beverages diluted with water or ice, such as reconstituted fruit juices and iced drinks. Do not drink fresh fluid milk or milk products that have not been pasteurized. Safe beverages include those that are bottled and sealed; bottled beer and wine may also be safe to drink. If boiled water is used to make tea and coffee, these beverages may be safe to consume. Use bottled water to wash hands, brush teeth, and take medication.

TD can be spread when pathogens from human or animal feces are in sources of water, including swimming pools, lakes, rivers, and other bodies of water. Accidentally swallowing even small amounts of contaminated water can cause illness. Swimming pools that contain chlorinated water may be safe places to swim, if the disinfectant and pH levels are properly maintained. However, some pathogens are resistant to levels of chlorine commonly used to disinfect swimming pools. Thus, you should also avoid swallowing chlorinated swimming pool water.

How Can I Sanitize Drinking Water?

Boiling is the most reliable method to make impure water safe to drink.[24] Water should be boiled for 1 minute, covered, and allowed to cool to room temperature without adding ice. To inactivate microbes at altitudes greater than 6562 feet, water should be boiled for 3 minutes.

Chemical Disinfection Disinfection methods kill large numbers of microorganisms, reducing the likelihood of infection. Chemical disinfection with chlorine (in household bleach) or iodine is an alternative method of sanitizing water when boiling water is not practical. Iodine and chlorine are available in tablets and drops, but iodine is not recommended for long-term use.[24] To reduce the risk of TD, follow the manufacturer's instructions for sanitizing water with these chemicals. Keep in mind, however, that chemical disinfection is not a reliable method of killing Crypto.

Filtering Water Microstrainer filters can remove bacteria and protozoans from drinking water, but they may not remove viruses (Fig. 12.13). To destroy viruses, you should disinfect the water with iodine or chlorine after using microstrainer filters. Filters collect organisms from water, so wash your hands with sanitized water after handling used filters. A travelers' guide to buying water filters can be found at the following government website: http://www.cdc.gov/parasites/crypto/gen_info/filters .html.

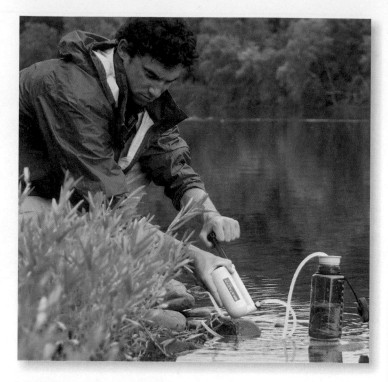

Figure 12.13 Microstrainer filters. Microstrainer filters can remove bacteria and protozoans from drinking water, and some types of these devices can remove certain viruses.

Preventive Medications

Before you leave the United States to enter a high-risk region, see your physician for his or her recommendations for preventing TD. You can also take medications that contain bismuth subsalicylate (BSS), the active ingredient in Pepto-Bismol, to reduce the risk of TD. Side effects of BSS commonly include nausea, constipation, and blackening of the tongue and bowel movements. BSS is not recommended for children under 3 years of age, and the medication should be avoided by people who are allergic to aspirin or have certain chronic conditions. Therefore, check with your physician before taking BBS along when you travel to other countries.

Treating TD

Because pathogenic bacteria are often the cause of TD, antibiotics are the primary method of treating the condition. In the United States, physicians often prescribe antibiotics for their patients to bring with them when they travel out of the country. When used in combination with antibiotics, *antimotility* agents can be helpful. These medications, such as loperamide, the active ingredient in Imodium, slow the muscular activity of the digestive tract and can provide relief from the diarrhea associated with TD.

Dehydration can be a serious complication of TD. To prevent dehydration, it is important for people suffering from TD to replace fluids and electrolytes lost by vomiting and diarrhea. However, travelers should remember to use only beverages that are in sealed containers, including carbonated soft drinks. If fluid loss is severe, it is best to obtain professional medical treatment.

CHAPTER REFERENCES

See Appendix I.

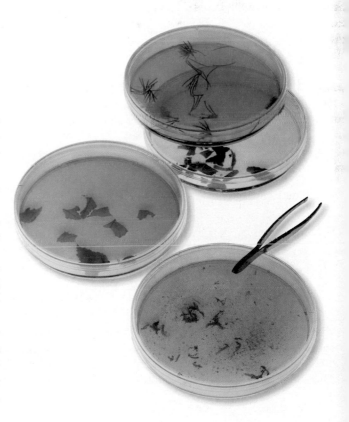

SUMMARY

In the United States, an estimated 76 million people become ill from various food-borne illnesses each year. Food-borne illness occurs when microscopic pathogens or their toxic by-products enter food (or beverages) and are consumed. Many kinds of pathogens infect the digestive tract; other types of food-borne pathogens do not sicken humans directly, but these microbes secrete toxins into food. When the food is eaten, the toxins irritate the intestinal tract and cause food intoxication.

The United States has one of the safest food supplies in the world, primarily the result of a team effort conducted by cooperating federal, state, and local agencies that regulate and monitor the production and distribution of food. The FDA and the USDA are the key federal agencies that protect consumers by regulating the country's food industry. Other team members include the EPA, the CDC, the FTC, and state and local governments.

People use certain microbes to produce a variety of foods, including hard cheeses, raised breads, pickled foods, and alcoholic beverages. When microorganisms metabolize nutrients in food, they often secrete substances that alter the color, texture, taste, and other characteristics of the food in beneficial and desirable ways. Other kinds of microbes grow and multiply in food, but their metabolic by-products spoil the food, making it unfit for human consumption. When pathogens are in food, they can make the item unsafe to eat. Food contaminants include pathogens, insect parts, residues of compounds used to kill insects that destroy food crops, and metal fragments from food processing equipment.

The microbes that cause food-borne illness can live practically anywhere. Common routes for transmitting harmful microbes to food involve vermin, poor personal hygiene practices, and improper food preparation and storage practices.

To grow, most microbes need warmth, moisture, and a source of nutrients, and some microorganisms also need oxygen. In general, high-risk foods are warm, moist, and protein-rich, and they have a neutral or slightly acidic pH. Such foods include meat, poultry, milk and milk products, and eggs.

Many factors influence whether an individual becomes ill after eating food or drinking a beverage that has been contaminated with a pathogen. The number of pathogens in a food or the amount of toxin it contains can contribute to the risk and severity of a food-borne illness. Furthermore, people vary in their vulnerability to many food-borne pathogens. In general, high-risk groups are pregnant women, very young children, the elderly, and persons who suffer from serious chronic illnesses or weakened immune systems.

Signs and symptoms of food- or water-borne illnesses primarily involve the digestive tract and include nausea, vomiting, diarrhea, and intestinal cramps. In most cases, otherwise healthy persons who suffer from common types of food-borne illness recover completely within a few days. Medical treatment should be obtained when an intestinal disorder is accompanied by fever, bloody bowel movements, prolonged vomiting and diarrhea, and/or dehydration.

The major kinds of pathogens are bacteria, viruses, protozoans, and fungi. In the United States, bacteria and viruses are responsible for most cases of food-borne illness. Bacteria are single-cell microorganisms. Some bacteria can live without oxygen; other types of bacteria transform into spores when living conditions are less than ideal. A virus is simply a piece of genetic material coated with protein. Viruses must invade a living cell to produce more viruses. A parasite is an organism that lives in or on another organism, often deriving nourishment from its host. Fungi such as molds, yeast, and mushrooms are simple life forms that live on dead or decaying organic matter.

People can reduce their risk of food-borne illness by following some important rules, most of which require changing risky food selection, preparation, and storage practices. Cooking foods is an effective way to destroy pathogens. After food is cooked, however, careless food handling sets the stage for the growth of pathogens. A simple rule to follow is this: "Keep hot foods hot and cold foods cold." Other simple rules include these: wash hands and surfaces often, do not cross-contaminate, heat foods to proper temperatures, and chill foods promptly.

For centuries, people preserved foods by heating, adding salt or sugar, fermenting, and drying. More modern methods of food preservation include pasteurization, refrigeration, freezing, canning, aseptic processing, using preservative additives, and irradiation. According to medical experts, irradiated foods are safe to eat, but many Americans avoid purchasing such products.

Direct food additives can make food easier to process, more nutritious, able to stay fresh longer, better tasting, or more attractive in appearance. An indirect food additive is a substance that becomes incorporated into food during production, packaging, transport, or storage. The 1958 Food Additives Amendment established the GRAS list and requires the manufacturer of a new food additive to provide evidence of the substance's safety to the FDA before the additive can be marketed for use. According to the Delaney Clause of the Food Additives Amendment, food manufacturers cannot add a new compound that causes cancer at *any* level of exposure.

Unintentional food additives are substances that accidentally are in foods, such as dirt, rodent hairs, pesticide residues, and metals that enter the food and water from the environment. A pesticide is any substance that people use to kill or control unwanted insects, weeds, rodents, or other organisms. The use of pesticides in modern agricultural practices has helped increase crop yields, reduce food costs, and protect the quality of many agricultural products. The EPA regulates the proper use of pesticides and sets pesticide tolerances. IPM methods control agricultural pests while limiting damage to the environment.

Agricultural pesticides have both beneficial and unwanted effects. Pesticides help protect the food supply and make food crops available at reasonable cost. Nevertheless, these substances may harm humans, animals, or the environment. The potentially harmful effects of pesticide residues in food depend on the particular chemical, its concentration in the food, how much and often it is eaten, and the consumer's vulnerability to the substance. Environmental health experts continually monitor the effects of pesticides on humans.

Traveler's diarrhea (TD) results from consuming food or water contaminated with pathogens. TD is likely to occur during or shortly after travel in regions where sanitary water supplies are lacking, people who prepare food have less than ideal personal hygiene practices, and untreated human feces are used for fertilizer. To reduce the risk of TD, follow instructions regarding safe food and beverage selection, avoid contact with contaminated waterways, sanitize drinking water, and use medications that may prevent the condition.

Recipe for Healthy Living

Very Easy Chicken Salad

Chicken that is properly prepared, cooked, and stored is a safe, nutritious, economical food. A good way to use up day-old cooked chicken is to make chicken salad. This recipe is unusual, because it includes seedless grapes and sunflower seeds. (You can substitute day-old cooked turkey for the chicken and chopped apple or dried apricots for the grapes.)

The chicken salad recipe makes approximately three 1-cup servings. A serving of this salad supplies approximately 320 kcal, 23 g protein, 19 g fat, 3.3 g fiber, and 190 mg sodium.

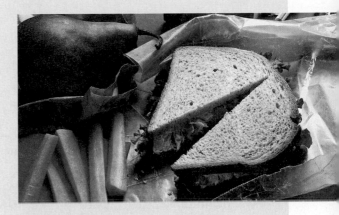

INGREDIENTS:

1¼ cups cooked and chilled, skinless, boneless chicken meat (approximately 1 whole chicken breast)

1 medium stalk celery, washed and chopped

½ cup raw onion, skinned and finely chopped

½ cup washed seedless red or green grapes, halved

½ cup unsalted roasted sunflower seeds

⅛ tsp curry powder

⅛ tsp ground black pepper

¼ cup low-fat mayonnaise-type salad dressing

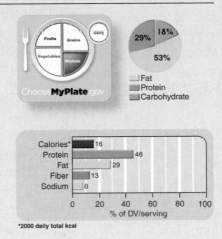

Fat
Protein
Carbohydrate

Calories*	16
Protein	46
Fat	29
Fiber	13
Sodium	0

% of DV/serving

*2000 daily total kcal

PREPARATION STEPS:

1. Cut chicken into small pieces and place in a large bowl.

2. Add the rest of the ingredients to the chicken and gently mix until well blended.

3. Serve on a bed of washed romaine lettuce leaves or as a sandwich filling.

CRITICAL THINKING

1. Prepare a food safety checklist that can be used in your household.

2. Consider your usual food preparation practices. After having read Chapter 12, list any food preparation practices you have that are unsafe.

3. Consider your usual food storage practices. After having read Chapter 12, list any of your food storage practices that are unsafe.

4. For lunch on Monday, you visited a restaurant and ordered a hamburger, French fries, baked beans, and a container of orange juice. Two days later, you developed nausea, vomiting, fever, chills, headache, abdominal cramps, and diarrhea. You suspect Monday's lunch made you sick. Considering the foods that you ate for lunch on Monday, which one was the most likely source of your infection? Why? Which food-borne pathogen was the most likely suspect for causing the intestinal disorder? In the future, what steps can you take to reduce the likelihood that the food will make you sick again?

5. Develop a pamphlet to educate consumers about food-borne illness.

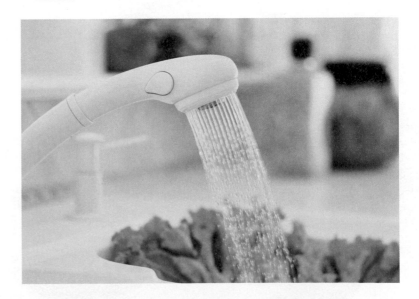

PRACTICE TEST

Select the best answer.

1. _____ are disease-causing microbes.

   a. Pathogens
   b. Toxins
   c. Teratogens
   d. Oxidants

2. The _____ is the primary government agency that oversees the safety of most foods in the United States.

   a. Food and Drug Administration (FDA)
   b. Agricultural Research Service (ARS)
   c. Centers for Disease Control and Prevention (CDC)
   d. Environmental Protection Agency (EPA)

3. Which of the following foods is most likely to support the growth of pathogens?

   a. overripe bananas
   b. pasteurized milk
   c. raw ground meat
   d. commercially canned tomato soup

4. Food-borne illnesses are usually characterized by

   a. flulike signs and symptoms.
   b. coughing, sneezing, and respiratory inflammation.
   c. megaloblastic anemia and nervous system defects.
   d. abdominal cramps, diarrhea, and vomiting.

5. In the United States, common sources of food-borne illness include all of the following, except

   a. *Norovirus.*
   b. *Staphylococcus aureus.*
   c. fungi.
   d. *Salmonella.*

6. Aflatoxins are

   a. responsible for 30% of food-borne illnesses in the United States.
   b. harmful compounds produced by certain molds.
   c. a type of parasitic worm.
   d. medications that are effective against viral toxins.

7. Which of the following practices can help reduce the growth of food-borne pathogens?

   a. washing hands before preparing food
   b. keeping cold foods cold and hot foods hot
   c. cooking foods to proper internal temperatures
   d. All of the above are correct.

8. Which of the following substances are not direct food additives?

   a. sulfites
   b. enrichment nutrients
   c. pesticide residues
   d. All of the above are correct.

9. Irradiation of food is

   a. an untested technology.
   b. not recommended, because the process increases nutrient losses.
   c. widely used in France, Russia, and China.
   d. a common method of food preservation in the United States.

10. Which of the following food preservation processes effectively destroys microbes?

    a. freezing
    b. sterilization
    c. smoking
    d. All of the above are correct.

11. _____ is the commercial heating process that destroys harmful bacteria in milk and fruit juices.

    a. Sporulation
    b. Sedimentation
    c. Detoxification
    d. Pasteurization

12. When you travel to countries outside the United States, you can reduce your risk of "travelers' diarrhea" by

    a. eating whole fresh fruits and vegetables.
    b. avoiding water that has not been bottled and sealed.
    c. purchasing foods from street vendors.
    d. consuming ice with beverages.

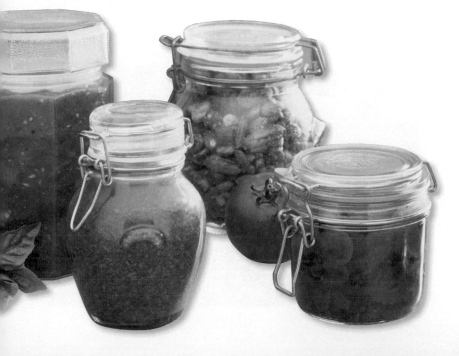

13. A _____ is a substance that kills weeds.

    a. rodenticide
    b. herbicide
    c. fungicide
    d. paracide

14. Which of the following temperatures is recommended for storing chilled foods in a refrigerator?

    a. 40°F
    b. 50°F
    c. 60°F
    d. 70°F

15. To reduce the risk of food-borne illness, raw poultry should be cooked to an internal temperature of at least

    a. 125°F
    b. 145°F
    c. 165°F
    d. 185°F

16. _____ is the most reliable method of making water that contains pathogens safe to drink.

    a. Detoxification
    b. Straining
    c. Boiling
    d. Carbonation

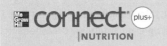

Additional resources related to the features of this book are available on ConnectPlus® Nutrition. Ask your instructor how to get access.

Answers to Chapter 12 Quiz Yourself

1. Aflatoxins are the most common sources of food-borne illness in the United States. **False.** (p. 441)

2. In the United States, foods such as ready-to-eat cereals, commercially canned vegetables, and orange juice are common sources of food-borne illness. **False.** (p. 436)

3. Certain fungi, such as button mushrooms, are safe to eat. **True.** (p. 440)

4. The Environmental Protection Agency (EPA) regulates the proper use of pesticides in the United States. **True.** (p. 456)

5. The best way to tell if a food is safe to eat is to smell it. **False.** (p. 435)

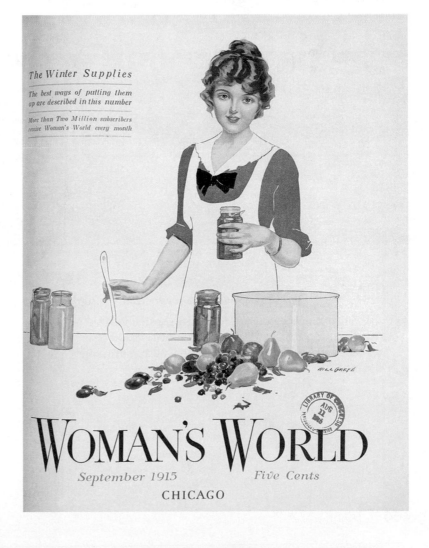

Nutrition for a Lifetime

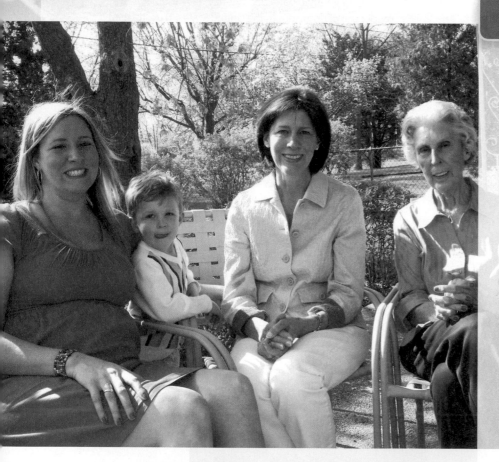

Chapter Learning Outcomes

After reading Chapter 13, you should be able to

1. List major physiological changes that occur during pregnancy and identify typical nutrition-related discomforts of pregnancy.

2. Identify the range of weight that healthy adult women should gain during pregnancy.

3. Discuss the effects that pregnancy-induced hypertension and gestational diabetes can have on pregnancy.

4. Identify nutrients that may need to be supplemented during pregnancy.

5. Describe the physiological processes involved in lactation and breastfeeding.

6. Compare the nutritional composition of infant formula with breast milk, and identify at least three advantages of breastfeeding.

7. Explain the rationale for delaying the introduction of solid foods to infants until they are 4 to 6 months of age.

8. Summarize practical suggestions for encouraging healthy eating habits among children.

9. Identify some major nutrition-related health concerns facing American children and teenagers.

10. Identify at least three physiological changes that occur during the normal aging process.

11. Discuss how the aging process can affect an individual's nutrient needs.

THIS PORTRAIT FEATURES four generations of an American family. Three-year-old Dylan stands next to his young mother, who is pregnant with his "little" brother, Jackson. The preschooler's grandmother is in the center of the picture. Dylan's great-grandmother is sitting next to his grandmother, on the right side of the photo. Thanks to technological and medical advances that occurred during the twentieth century, Dylan and Jackson have an excellent chance of enjoying healthy, long lives.

If you are a woman, are you pregnant? Do you already have children? If you have children, were they breastfed or formula fed? Do you live with and help care for an elderly parent or grandparent? These may seem to be personal questions, but many undergraduate college students do not fit the stereotype of being 18 to 22 years of age, having no children, and residing away from home.

Most of the nutrition recommendations presented in this textbook apply to people who are "adults"—loosely defined as the period when a person is 19 to 70 years of age.[1] Chapter 13 focuses on the differing nutrition needs and health concerns of people who are in specific *life stages*. These particular life stages are the **prenatal period** or pregnancy, the time between conception and birth; **lactation** (milk production for breastfeeding); infancy; childhood; adolescence; and the older adult period that generally spans from 70 years of age until death.

Why is it necessary to learn some basic information about nutrition-related concerns during various life stages? If you do not have children, you may become a parent in the future. If your parents and grandparents are relatively young and vigorous now, you can expect them to experience declining physical functioning as they grow older. Finally, you need to recognize that most of these changes are normal and will affect you as well.

Today in the United States, many of the leading causes of death are chronic diseases, such as heart disease and cancer. Long-term health-related practices, including dietary and physical activity habits, often contribute to the development of these diseases. Whether you enjoy overall good health or suffer from one or more disabling physical ailments as you grow older depends not only on your lifestyle choices but also on several other factors, including your heredity, relationships, environment, income, education level, and access to health care.

Quiz *Yourself*

What steps can young women take to prepare for pregnancy? Compared to breast milk, do infant formulas provide the same health benefits for infants? When is the best time to begin feeding solid foods to infants? Which nutrients are most likely to be deficient in diets of older adults? While reading Chapter 13, you will learn answers to these questions. Test your knowledge of nutrition during various life stages by taking the following quiz. The answers are found on page 509.

1. During pregnancy, a mother-to-be should double her food intake because she's "eating for two." _____ T _____ F

2. The natural size of a woman's breasts is not a factor in determining her ability to breastfeed her baby. _____ T _____ F

3. Experts with the American Academy of Pediatrics recommend parents should add solid foods to the infant's diet within the first month after a baby is born. _____ T _____ F

4. Over the past 35 years, the prevalence of obesity has increased among American school-age children. _____ T _____ F

5. Compared to younger persons, older adults have lower risks of nutritional deficiencies. _____ T _____ F

prenatal period time between conception and birth; pregnancy

lactation milk production

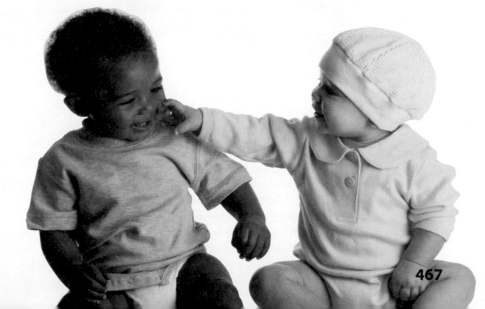

467

conception moment when a sperm enters an egg (fertilization)

uterus female reproductive organ that protects the developing organism during pregnancy

embryo human organism from 14 days to 8 weeks after conception

fetus human organism from 8 weeks after conception until birth

13.1 From Fertilized Egg to Newborn

"It's positive!" Each day, the results of pregnancy testing are a source of excitement, relief, or concern for thousands of women. An estimated 50% of pregnancies are unplanned in the United States.[2] Therefore, all sexually active women of childbearing age should be aware of their likelihood of becoming pregnant. Regardless of whether a pregnancy is planned or not, dietary practices before and during pregnancy play a major role in the course of the pregnancy and the primary outcome—a healthy infant.

The prenatal period (*gestation*) encompasses the time from **conception**, the moment a male sperm cell enters a female egg cell, until the birth of a *full-term* infant, about 38 to 42 weeks later. During the first 2 weeks after conception, the fertilized egg (*ovum*) divides repeatedly, forming a mass of cells that enters the woman's **uterus**, the female reproductive organ that protects the developing organism. The mass of cells buries itself into the nutrient-rich lining of the uterus and continues to develop. For the next 6 weeks, the rapidly dividing mass of cells, called an **embryo**, increases in size and forms organs. Eight weeks after conception, the developing human being is referred to as a **fetus** (Fig. 13.1).

The prenatal period is often divided into three stages or *trimesters*. During the first trimester, the embryo/fetus develops most of its organs, and by the end of this period, the fetus can move. The first trimester is a critical stage in human development because nutrient deficiencies or excesses and exposure to toxic compounds, such as alcohol, are most likely to have devastating effects on the embryo/fetus. However, many women who are in their first trimester do not realize they are pregnant.

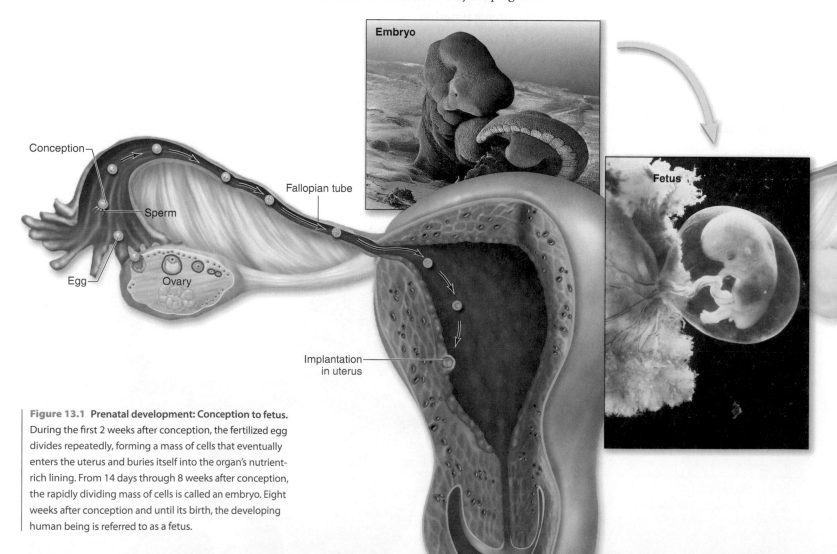

Figure 13.1 Prenatal development: Conception to fetus. During the first 2 weeks after conception, the fertilized egg divides repeatedly, forming a mass of cells that eventually enters the uterus and buries itself into the organ's nutrient-rich lining. From 14 days through 8 weeks after conception, the rapidly dividing mass of cells is called an embryo. Eight weeks after conception and until its birth, the developing human being is referred to as a fetus.

As the second trimester begins, the fetus is still very tiny, about 2½ to 3 inches in length, and weighs only about an ounce. However, the fetus is beginning to look more like a human infant—it has fully formed arms, hands, fingers, legs, feet, and toes. The fetus's organs continue to grow and mature in their ability to function. As the fetus moves around, its mother becomes increasingly aware of its presence within her body.

By the beginning of the third trimester, the fetus is approximately 12 inches long and weighs about 1½ to 2 pounds. During this trimester, the fetus will nearly double in length and multiply its weight by three to four times. Thus, the fetus usually weighs about 6 to 8 pounds and is 19 to 21 inches long by the time it is full-term and ready to be born.

Throughout the prenatal period, the embryo/fetus depends entirely on its mother for survival. During most of the pregnancy, the expectant mother nourishes her embryo/fetus through the **placenta,** the organ of pregnancy that connects the uterus to the embryo/fetus via the *umbilical cord* (see Fig. 13.1). The role of the placenta is to transfer nutrients and oxygen from the mother's bloodstream to the embryo/fetus. Additionally, the placenta transfers wastes from the embryo/fetus to the mother's bloodstream, so her body can eliminate them. Unfortunately, the placenta does not filter many microbes and toxic substances, such as alcohol and nicotine, from the mother's blood. Thus, agents of infection and harmful chemicals can pass through the placenta, enter the embryo/fetus, and cause disease, birth defects, or embryonic/fetal death.

A fetus generally needs to spend at least 37 weeks developing within the uterus to be physiologically mature enough to survive after birth without the need for special care. A fetus's weight depends on the supply of nutrients that it receives through the placenta.[3] If the placenta fails to grow properly, the developing fetus is likely to be born too soon and be lighter than average at birth.

Low-Birth-Weight and Preterm Newborns

Birth weight is a major factor that determines whether a baby is healthy and survives his or her first year of life. **Low-birth-weight (LBW) infants** generally weigh less than 5½ pounds at birth. In 2009, about 8.2% of infants born in the United States were low birth weight.[4] Pregnant females who are 45 to 54 years of age or under 15 years of age are more likely to give birth to low-birth-weight infants than women in other age groups.[5] Additionally, women who smoke during pregnancy are at risk to have LBW babies.[6]

Low birth weight is often associated with *premature* or *preterm births*. In 2009, approximately 12.2% of births in the United States were **preterm;** that is, they occurred before the 37th week of pregnancy.[4] Preterm birth and LBW are one of the leading causes of death among American infants who are less than 28 days of age.[7] In 2009, about 2% of births were *very preterm*, that is, the infants were born before 32 weeks of gestation. Very preterm infants are more likely to have serious health problems or die soon after birth than babies delivered after 32 weeks of pregnancy.[8]

A very preterm infant who is born after about 26 weeks of pregnancy may survive if cared for in a hospital nursery for high-risk newborns (Fig. 13.2). However, the tiny infant's body will not have stores of fat and certain minerals that normally accumulate during the last month of pregnancy. Additionally, very preterm babies are likely to have conditions that complicate their medical care and food intake, such as breathing difficulties and weak sucking and swallowing abilities.

Concept **Checkpoint**

1. When is an embryo referred to as a fetus?
2. What is the role of the placenta?
3. What is a major factor that determines whether a newborn baby is healthy and survives its first year of life?
4. What is a preterm birth?

> **placenta** organ of pregnancy that connects the uterus to the embryo/fetus via the umbilical cord
>
> **low-birth-weight (LBW) infant** infant generally weighing less than 5½ pounds at birth
>
> **preterm** describes infant born before 37 weeks of pregnancy

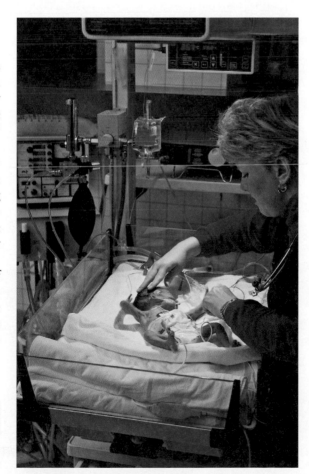

Figure 13.2 Very preterm infant. A very preterm infant may survive if cared for in a hospital nursery for such high-risk newborns.

13.2 Pregnancy

During pregnancy, a woman's body undergoes major physiological changes, such as increased blood volume, breast size, and levels of several hormones. These adaptations enable her body to nourish and maintain the developing embryo/fetus, as well as produce milk for her infant after its birth. However, some of the physical changes cause discomfort for the pregnant woman.

Common Nutrition-Related Signs of Pregnancy

In the first trimester, most women experience physical signs that they are pregnant, such as enlarged breasts and "morning sickness." Other common nutrition-related signs as well as complaints of pregnancy include extreme tiredness, swollen feet, constipation, and heartburn. In most cases, such discomforts do not create serious complications and they resolve within a few months.

Breast Changes

During pregnancy, hormones signal the breasts to increase in size in preparation for lactation. The mother's pituitary gland in the brain produces **prolactin,** a hormone that stimulates the development of milk-producing tissue in the breasts. However, a pregnant woman's breasts do not form milk, because high levels of progesterone, a hormone that helps maintain pregnancy, inhibit milk production.[9] After birth, the level of progesterone drops rapidly, essentially removing the "brakes" from the breasts' ability to produce milk.

Morning Sickness

A common sign of pregnancy is **morning sickness,** nausea that is sometimes accompanied by vomiting. The name "morning sickness" is misleading because the queasy feeling can occur at any time of the day. The cause of this unpleasant condition is unclear, but it may be the result of the pregnant woman's body adapting to higher levels of female hormones. Additionally, emotional stress and certain foods can contribute to nausea. The condition generally begins early in the first trimester, and most women are no longer affected by the sixteenth week of pregnancy.[10] However, some women experience nausea and vomiting occasionally throughout their pregnancies.

To help control mild morning sickness, pregnant women can avoid odors and foods, such as fried or greasy foods, that trigger nausea. Some women find that eating crackers and drinking some water helps reduce the likelihood of feeling nauseated, especially before they get out of bed in the morning. Furthermore, eating smaller but more frequent meals and nutritious snacks can be helpful.

If the nausea and vomiting contribute to weight loss of more than 2 pounds, the pregnant woman should contact her physician for treatment. Morning sickness that persists beyond the fourth month of pregnancy should also be brought to the attention of a physician. During pregnancy, excessive vomiting is harmful because it can lead to dehydration and nutritional deficiencies.

Fatigue in Pregnancy

Early in pregnancy, the mother's blood volume expands to approximately 150% of normal. The number of red blood cells, however, increases by only 20 to 30%, and this change occurs more gradually. As a result, the pregnant woman develops *physiological*

prolactin hormone that stimulates milk production after delivery

morning sickness nausea and vomiting associated with pregnancy

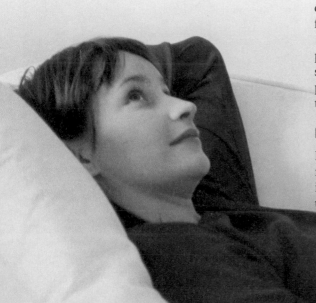

anemia, a condition characterized by a lower concentration of red blood cells in the bloodstream. This form of anemia is a normal response to pregnancy, rather than the result of inadequate nutrient intake. Nevertheless, physiological anemia may be responsible for the extreme tiredness experienced by pregnant women during their first trimester. As their red blood cell numbers increase, expectant mothers report having more energy, especially during the second trimester. By the third trimester, however, most pregnant women are easily fatigued again, possibly because carrying a rapidly growing fetus is physically demanding.

What Is Edema?

High levels of certain hormones can cause various tissues to retain fluid during pregnancy. Although the extra fluid causes some minor swelling (edema), especially in the hands and feet, the condition is normal. In most cases, mild edema does not require treatment such as restricting salt intake or taking diuretics. Edema, however, can be a sign of trouble if hypertension and the appearance of extra protein in the urine accompany the swelling. The "Pregnancy-Induced Hypertension (PIH)" section of Chapter 13 discusses hypertension during pregnancy.

Digestive Tract Discomforts

During pregnancy, certain hormones produced by the placenta relax muscles of the digestive tract. As a result, intestinal movements slow down and digested material takes longer to pass through the tract, increasing the likelihood of constipation (see the "Fiber and the Digestive Tract" section of Chapter 5). To help prevent constipation, pregnant women should consume adequate amounts of fiber and fluids. During pregnancy, the Adequate Intake (AI) for fiber is 28 g/day, and the AI for total water is 3 L/day.[1] If constipation still persists after making these dietary changes, the pregnant woman should discuss this concern with her physician.

Heartburn is another common complaint of pregnant women. As the fetus grows, the uterus pushes upward in the mother's abdominal cavity and applies pressure on her stomach (Fig. 13.3). When this occurs, stomach acid can enter the esophagus, causing

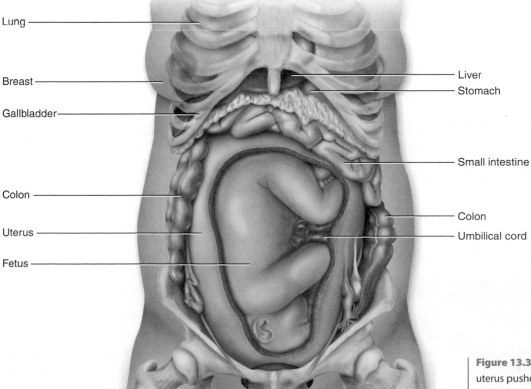

Lung
Breast
Gallbladder
Colon
Uterus
Fetus

Liver
Stomach
Small intestine
Colon
Umbilical cord

Figure 13.3 Heartburn during pregnancy. As the fetus grows, the uterus pushes upward and applies pressure to the pregnant woman's stomach, contributing to heartburn.

TABLE 13.1 *Comparing Selected DRIs: 25-Year-Old Nonpregnant and Pregnant Women*

Energy/ Nutrient	Nonpregnant	Pregnant
Kilocalories	Estimated Energy Requirement (EER)	First trimester = EER + 0
		Second trimester = EER + 340
		Third trimester = EER + 452
Protein*	46 g/day	71 g/day
Vitamin C*	75 mg/day	85 mg/day
Thiamin*	1.1 mg/day	1.4 mg/day
Niacin*	14 mg/day	18 mg/day
Folate*	400 mcg/day	600 mcg/day
Vitamin D*	15 mcg/day	15 mcg/day
Calcium*	1000 mg/day	1000 mg/day
Iron*	18 mg/day	27 mg/day
Iodine*	150 mcg/day	220 mcg/day

* RDA

Source of data: Institute of Medicine: *Dietary Reference Intakes.* Available from Nutrient recommendations: Dietary Reference Intakes (DRIs). http://ods.od.nih.gov/Health_Information/Dietary_Reference_Intakes.aspx

heartburn (see the Chapter 4 "Highlight"). To help avoid heartburn, the pregnant woman can consume smaller meals, avoid lying down after eating, eat less fatty foods, and learn to identify and avoid foods that seem to contribute to heartburn. If heartburn continues to be bothersome, the woman should consult her physician and discuss other ways to treat the condition.

Pregnancy: General Dietary Recommendations

Ideally, women of childbearing age should take steps to ensure good health before becoming pregnant. For example, women can analyze the nutritional adequacy of their diets and choose to eat foods that correct any marginal or deficient intakes. Prior to pregnancy, sedentary women can begin an exercise regimen; overweight or obese women can lose some excess weight; and women who smoke can join smoking cessation programs. The time to remedy faulty lifestyle practices and increase chances of having a healthy pregnancy and baby is long before pregnancy occurs.

During pregnancy, the mother-to-be should follow a diet that meets her own nutritional needs as well as those of her developing offspring. Depending on the trimester, an expectant woman's requirements for energy (calories), protein, and many other nutrients are greater than her needs prior to pregnancy. Nevertheless, a pregnant woman does not need to double her usual food intake just because she is "eating for two." Table 13.1 compares Recommended Dietary Allowances (RDA) for energy and selected nutrients that apply to healthy 25-year-old nonpregnant and pregnant women.

Energy Needs

In the first trimester, a pregnant woman's daily energy requirement (*Estimated Energy Requirement* or *EER*) is essentially the same as a nonpregnant woman's, because the embryo/fetus is quite small (see Table 13.1). However, the fetus grows rapidly during the second and third trimesters, and the pregnant woman requires more energy and nutrients to support its growth as well as her own body's needs. During the second trimester, the expectant mother should consume approximately 340 more kilocalories per day than her prepregnancy EER. Throughout the third trimester, she should add about 450 kcal per day to her prepregnancy EER (see Table 13.1). If a woman is physically active during her pregnancy, she may need to increase her kilocalorie intake by even more than these levels. Why? As the pregnant woman gains weight, her muscles require more energy to move her body. The average expectant mother, however, reduces her physical activity level during the third trimester, conserving energy.

Folate and Iron Needs

A pregnant woman's requirements for folate and iron are 50% higher than those of a nonpregnant woman. It is important for women to enter pregnancy with adequate folate status, because embryos need the vitamin to support rapid cell division. As discussed in Chapter 8, pregnant women who are folate deficient have high risk of giving birth to infants with neural tube defects, such as spina bifida (see Fig. 8.26). To obtain adequate folate, women of childbearing age as well as pregnant women should include rich food sources of folate in their diets, such as green leafy vegetables, and take a vitamin/mineral supplement that supplies at least 400 mcg of *folic acid*, a form of folate.

As the pregnant woman's blood volume expands, her need for iron increases because her body must make more hemoglobin for the extra red blood cells. Additionally, the woman's body transfers iron to the fetus to build its stores of the mineral. If women fail to meet their iron needs during pregnancy, their iron stores can be severely depleted, and they can develop iron deficiency anemia. Pregnant women who are iron deficient have high risk of giving birth prematurely and having low-birth-weight infants.[11]

Even when their diets include good sources of iron such as red meats and enriched cereals, pregnant women often need a supplemental source of iron. Thus, most physicians recommend special prenatal multiple vitamin/mineral supplements that contain iron for their pregnant patients.

Menu Planning for Pregnant Women

Rather than view pregnancy as a time to splurge by eating energy-dense empty-calorie foods, the mother-to-be should obtain the extra calories from nutrient-dense foods. For example, drinking an additional cup of fat-free milk, eating a bowl of an enriched whole-grain cereal, and taking a prenatal supplement each day can supply extra kilocalories as well as protein, fiber, and micronutrients. Table 13.2 presents a day's meals and snacks for a sedentary 25-year-old woman who is in her second trimester of pregnancy. Her prepregnancy EER was 2000 kcal, so her sample menu is based on MyPlate recommendations for 2400 kcal, enough to cover her increased EER during this trimester.

Is Fish Safe to Eat During Pregnancy?

Fish and shellfish (e.g., clams, shrimp, and crabs) are excellent sources of many minerals, omega-3 fatty acids, and high-quality protein. However, most fish and shellfish contain very small amounts of methylmercury, a compound that contains the toxic mineral mercury.[12] For most healthy adults, ingesting amounts of methylmercury that are generally in fish and shellfish is not thought to be harmful. Certain kinds of fish and shellfish, however, contain higher levels of methylmercury than others. When a pregnant woman eats these foods, the methylmercury in them can eventually reach the developing fetus and damage its nervous system. According to recommendations issued by the U.S. Food and Drug Administration (FDA) and the Environmental Protection Agency (EPA), women who may become pregnant, are pregnant, or are breastfeeding their babies should

- Eat up to 12 ounces of various fish and shellfish per week that generally contain small amounts of mercury, such as shrimp, canned light tuna, salmon, pollock, and catfish. (Albacore tuna contains more methylmercury than canned light tuna, but eating up to 6 ounces of albacore tuna per week is allowed.)

- Avoid eating types of fish that often contain high amounts of methylmercury, particularly shark, swordfish, king mackerel, and tilefish.

The FDA and the EPA also recommend that caregivers should not feed fish that contain high amounts of methylmercury to young children because their nervous systems are still developing.

What About Cravings?

The stereotype of a pregnant woman who craves pickles and ice cream is not simply a myth. Cravings are common during this stage of life. However, ask pregnant women to identify the foods they crave, and you are likely to get a variety of responses. The causes of cravings are unknown, but they may be responses to the hormonal changes associated with pregnancy or to the emotional state of the mother-to-be. In other instances, specific food cravings may simply reflect the pregnant woman's family traditions. Unless food cravings contribute to excess weight gain, they are generally harmless.

Some women develop **pica**, the craving of nonfood items such as laundry starch, chalk, cigarette ashes, and soil. Some studies have linked pica with iron and zinc deficiency, but it is not clear if pica is the result or the cause of such deficiencies. Pregnant

TABLE 13.2 *Sample Menu for a 25-Year-Old Pregnant Woman (Second Trimester)*

Breakfast

¾ cup cooked oatmeal, made with ½ cup fat-free milk and sprinkled with ¼ cup raisins

½ cup calcium-fortified orange juice

Mid-morning snack

½ cup calcium-fortified orange juice

1 rectangular graham cracker

2 Tbsp peanut butter

Lunch

Cheese sandwich

    2 slices whole-grain bread

    1 slice American cheese

    2 slices tomato

    ¼ cup leaf lettuce

    2 tsp mayonnaise-type low-calorie salad dressing

1 cup apple slices

1 cup fat-free milk

½ cup orange sherbet

Mid-afternoon snack

    1 whole-grain English muffin, toasted

    1 Tbsp soft margarine

    2 tsp jelly

    ½ cup fat-free milk

Dinner

    Broiled salmon filet, 5 oz

    1¼ cups mixed salad greens

    1 Tbsp low-calorie Italian dressing

    ½ cup enriched white rice

    1 cup steamed broccoli

    2 small dinner rolls

    1 Tbsp soft margarine

Evening snack

    1 cup frozen yogurt

pica craving nonfood items

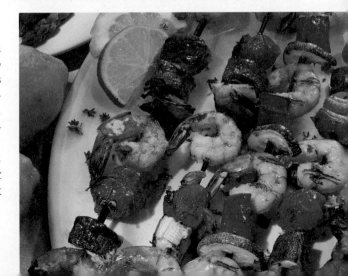

TABLE 13.3 *Distribution of Weight Gain During Pregnancy*

Tissue	Approximate Pounds
Maternal	
Blood	3
Breasts	2
Uterus	2
Fat, protein, and retained fluid	11
Fetus	7.5
Placenta	1.5
Amniotic fluid*	2.0

* Protective fluid that surrounds fetus.

Source: March of Dimes, www.marchofdimes.com/pnhec/159_153.asp

women should refrain from practicing pica, especially eating clay or soil. Soil may contain substances that interfere with the absorption of minerals in the intestinal tract. Furthermore, eating soil can be harmful because the dirt may be contaminated with toxic substances, such as lead and pesticides, and pathogenic microbes.

Weight Gain During Pregnancy

Nearly all pregnant women experience weight gain. In fact, gaining an appropriate amount of weight is crucial during pregnancy. How much weight a woman should gain depends on her prepregnancy weight. According to experts with the American College of Obstetricians and Gynecologists (ACOG), women who were underweight prior to pregnancy should gain 28 to 40 pounds; women whose prepregnancy weights were within the healthy range can expect to gain 25 to 35 pounds.[13] Women who were overweight before they became pregnant should gain 15 to 25 pounds, and obese women should gain at least 15 pounds during pregnancy. The recommendations are higher for women who are pregnant with more than one fetus. For example, a healthy woman who is carrying twins may gain as much as 45 pounds during pregnancy.[14] In 2009, experts with the Institute of Medicine (IOM) issued new weight gain guidelines for obese pregnant women. According to the experts, the obese women should limit their weight gain to 11 to 20 pounds.

In 2006, 21% of women in the United States gained more than 40 pounds during pregnancy.[4] Women who gain excess weight during pregnancy are likely to retain the extra pounds long after their babies are born.[15] Furthermore, expectant mothers who gain excessive amounts of weight are more likely to give birth to *high-birth-weight* (*HBW*) *babies*.[15] HBW newborns generally weigh more than 8.8 pounds. When compared to newborns with healthy weights, HBW infants have higher risk of being injured during the birth process and of having birth defects. Furthermore, HBW infants are more likely to develop obesity, diabetes, and hypertension at some point in their lives.[16] In 2006, about 8% of babies born in the United States were HBW.[4]

Underweight women who do not gain enough weight during pregnancy are at risk of having preterm or low-birth-weight (LBW) infants. Underweight pregnant women should try to reach healthy weights by the end of the first trimester and then meet the recommended weight-gain goals. Obese women have a greater risk of developing hypertension as well as type 2 diabetes during pregnancy. Obese pregnant women are also at risk of giving birth to HBW babies.[15] However, women should not try to lose weight while they are pregnant because calorie restriction may harm the fetus.

Accounting for the Weight Gain

It is important to understand that much of the weight a woman gains during a healthy pregnancy is not body fat. By the end of a full-term pregnancy, the average fetus weighs about 7½ pounds, and the placenta and amniotic fluid that surrounds the fetus account for about 3½ pounds. The remaining weight is comprised of tissues and fluids the mother's body gains during pregnancy (*maternal weight* gain). Table 13.3 indicates the typical distribution of weight that is gained during this life stage.

Rate of Weight Gain

For an expectant mother, the rate of the weight gain is important, as well as the amount of weight gained. Most pregnant women add up to 4 pounds of weight during the first trimester. Throughout the rest of their pregnancies, women typically gain at a faster rate, 3 to 4 pounds *each* month. Figure 13.4 charts the course of weight gain in a healthy pregnancy. Note how the rate reaches a steady pace of about 1 pound/week during the second and third trimesters.

Figure 13.4 Rate of weight gain: Healthy pregnancy. This chart illustrates the rate of maternal weight gain that typically occurs during a healthy pregnancy.

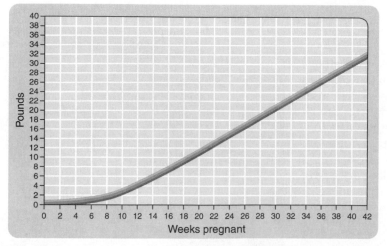

The Importance of Prenatal Care

Ideally, women of childbearing age should plan for pregnancy and receive dietary advice before becoming pregnant. If this is not possible, *prenatal care* should begin early in pregnancy, because many medical problems that may occur during this life stage can be diagnosed and treated before the health of the mother or her fetus are threatened. **Prenatal care** is specialized to meet the health care needs of pregnant women. Routine prenatal health care includes measuring and monitoring the pregnant woman's weight, blood pressure, blood glucose level, and uterine growth. The prenatal health care provider may also discuss various concerns with the expectant mother, such as morning sickness, safe types of physical activity, what to expect during the birth process, and basic infant care skills. Additionally, the health care provider can advise the pregnant woman to make appropriate lifestyle choices, such as avoiding the use of tobacco, alcohol, and illegal substances. Women who receive adequate prenatal care are more likely to have good pregnancy outcomes, including babies who have healthy birth weights, than women who do not receive such care.[17]

During pregnancy, it is important for a woman to decide whether she will breastfeed her baby. Pregnant women who decide to breastfeed their babies should inform their physicians and learn as much as they can about breastfeeding early in their pregnancy.

Gestational Diabetes

According to estimates, 3 to 8% of pregnant women in the United States develop type 2 diabetes during pregnancy (*gestational diabetes*). When a woman has gestational diabetes, her fetus receives too much glucose and converts the excess into fat. Thus, women with this form of diabetes often give birth to high-birth-weight babies. After birth, these infants often have difficulty controlling their own blood glucose levels and are at risk of becoming overweight as children.

Gestational diabetes can be detected during routine prenatal care. Diet and exercise are usually necessary to treat the condition, but in some cases, insulin injections are required. After giving birth, the women who developed diabetes during pregnancy generally experience a decline in their blood glucose levels to normal values. However, women who have experienced gestational diabetes have higher risk of developing type 2 diabetes later in life. For more information about diabetes, see Chapter 5.

Pregnancy-Induced Hypertension (PIH)

Rapid weight gain, especially after the fifth month of pregnancy, could be a sign of a serious type of hypertension called **pregnancy-induced hypertension (PIH)**. PIH is commonly referred to as preeclampsia (*pre-e-klamp'-see-a*). Preeclampsia is characterized by sudden, dramatic increase in weight that is due to edema, particularly of the hands, calves, and face; hypertension; and protein in urine.[18] If a woman suffering from preeclampsia develops convulsions, her condition is called eclampsia (*e-klamp'-see-a*). In the United States, eclampsia is the second leading cause of death among pregnant women.[19]

Hypertension is a common complication of pregnancy. In the United States, 6 to 8% of pregnant women develop high blood pressure.[19] Pregnant women who have high risk of PIH are those who are under 20 or over 40 years of age, are overweight or obese, have a history of diabetes or hypertension, and are carrying more than one fetus.

Most American women have normal pregnancies and deliver healthy infants, but some women experience serious health problems such as PIH. At present, the only effective treatment for PIH is delivering the fetus, but infants born before the 24th week of pregnancy are unlikely to survive. If the fetus is older than 24 weeks, its mother may

Major signs of preeclampsia include sudden weight gain, elevated blood pressure, edema, and protein in urine.

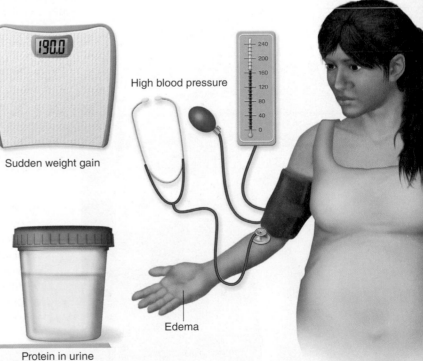

Sudden weight gain

High blood pressure

Edema

Protein in urine

be hospitalized for treatment. This practice helps physicians monitor the mother's condition and enables the fetus to mature until it has a better chance of surviving after a premature birth.

Drug Use

Exposure to alcohol and tobacco is harmful to the embryo/fetus. Women who drink alcohol during pregnancy are at risk of having a child with a fetal alcohol spectrum disorder such as FAS (see Fig. 6.30). Scientists do not know if there is a "safe" amount of alcohol that pregnant women can consume; therefore, women of childbearing age who are sexually active or pregnant should avoid alcoholic beverages. The Chapter 6 "Highlight" provides more information about fetal alcohol spectrum disorder.

Compared to pregnant women who do not smoke cigarettes, expectant mothers who smoke have higher risk of giving birth too early and having LBW babies. Furthermore, expectant mothers who smoke cigarettes may increase the risk of having babies with birth defects or that die of *sudden infant death syndrome (SIDS)*. SIDS is the sudden, unexplained death of an infant younger than 1 year of age and the leading cause of death for babies between 1 month and 1 year of age.[20]

The use of illegal drugs, herbal supplements, and medications during pregnancy can also harm the embryo/fetus. Ideally, the time to quit abusing illegal drugs is before pregnancy. Pregnant women should consult their physicians before using herbal supplements or taking any drugs, even over-the-counter medications.

What About Physical Activity?

Women can derive many benefits from being physically active during pregnancy, including enhanced muscle tone and strength, reduced edema, and improved mood and sleep. Most pregnant women can continue their prepregnancy exercise regimens, especially those that included low- or moderate-intensity activities. However, the exercise routine should not result in weight loss. Recommended activities generally include walking, cycling, swimming, or light aerobics. Pregnancy is not the time to begin an intense fitness regimen or perform high-risk physical activities. Activities that are risky and should be avoided include downhill skiing; contact sports such as judo, soccer, and basketball; and scuba diving.[21] Pregnant women should discuss their physical activity practices and needs with their physicians. Some expectant women, such as those experiencing PIH or premature labor contractions, may need to restrict their physical activity.

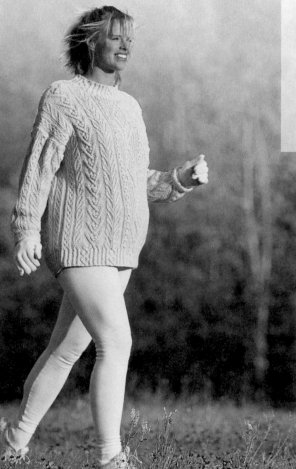

Most pregnant women can continue their prepregnancy exercise regimens, especially those that included low- or moderate-intensity activities.

Concept **Checkpoint**

5. Identify at least three different nutrition-related signs of pregnancy.

6. According to recommendations of the American College of Obstetricians and Gynecologists, how much weight should a woman at a healthy weight gain during pregnancy; how much weight should she gain if she was underweight before becoming pregnant? How much weight should she gain if she was overweight or obese before pregnancy?

7. Why is having adequate folate and iron status important for pregnant women?

8. Discuss the harmful effects that a pregnant woman's alcohol consumption and cigarette smoking can have on her embryo/fetus.

13.3 Infant Nutrition

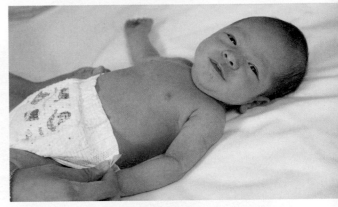

Rapid physical growth characterizes infancy, the life stage that extends from birth to about 2 years of age. During the first 4 to 6 months of life, a healthy baby doubles its birth weight, and by 1 year of age, an infant's birth weight has tripled. Additionally, an infant's length increases by 50% during its first year of life. Thus, if a baby girl weighs 7 pounds and is 20 inches long at birth, you would expect her to weigh 21 pounds and be 30 inches long by her first birthday (Fig. 13.5).

Compared to older children, an infant needs more energy and nutrients per pound of body weight to support its rapid growth.[1] If an infant's diet lacks adequate energy and nutrients, the baby's growth may slow or even stop. The following sections take a closer look at infant nutrition, including breastfeeding and other infant feeding practices.

Breast Milk Is Best Milk

Two hundred years ago, if a new mother was unable to breastfeed her baby, the child faced certain death—unless a woman who was producing breast milk could be located to suckle (*nurse*) the infant. Today, a new mother can choose to nurse her baby or feed the child an **infant formula,** a synthetic food that simulates human milk. Although both foods provide adequate nutrition for young babies, breastfeeding provides benefits beyond nutrition for the new mother as well as her infant.

Human milk is uniquely formulated to meet the nutrient needs of a newborn baby. During the first couple of days after giving birth, the new mother's breasts produce **colostrum** (*co-loss'-trum*), a yellowish fluid that does not look like milk. (Some women report that colostrum leaked from their breasts late in the pregnancy.)[22] By the end of the first week of lactation, colostrum has undergone a transition to *mature milk*. If you compare the appearance of mature human milk to cow's milk, you will notice that breast milk is more watery than cow's milk and may have a slightly bluish color.

If they are unaware that colostrum is secreted by breasts soon after birth, women may think something is wrong with their ability to produce milk. However, colostrum is a very important first food for babies, because the fluid contains antibodies and immune system cells that can be absorbed by the infant's immature digestive tract. Colostrum also contains a substance that encourages the growth of a type of bacteria, *Lactobacillus bifidus* (*L. bifidus*), in the infant's GI tract. Such biologically active substances help an infant's body fight infections and hasten the maturation of the baby's immune system. Thus, breastfed infants, especially those who are exclusively breastfed, have lower risks of allergies and gastrointestinal, respiratory, and ear infections than formula-fed infants.[23] Furthermore, breastfed babies are less likely to develop childhood asthma, leukemia, obesity, sudden infant death syndrome (SIDS), and type 1 diabetes than infants who are not breastfed.

Human milk is a rich source of lipids, including cholesterol, and fatty acids such as linoleic acid, *arachidonic acid (AA)*, and *docosahexaenoic acid (DHA)*. An infant's nervous system, especially the brain and eyes, depends on AA and DHA for proper development. Furthermore, the fat in breast milk helps supply the energy needed to maintain the infant's overall growth.

The practice of breastfeeding also provides some important advantages for parents, particularly the new mother. Breastfeeding is more convenient and economical than using infant formula. Human milk is readily available; there is no need to purchase cans of infant formula and have them on hand. As milk leaves the breast, it is always fresh, free of bacteria, and ready-to-feed without mixing, bottling, or warming. Because human milk production requires a considerable amount of energy, lactating women can lose the extra body fat gained during pregnancy faster than mothers who use infant formula. Additionally, women who breastfeed their babies

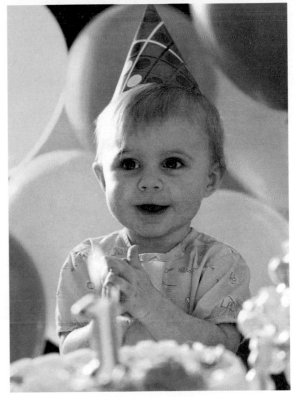

Figure 13.5 Growth rates during infancy. A healthy newborn baby (*a*) grows rapidly during its first year. During the first 4 to 6 months of life, a baby doubles its birth weight, and by 1 year of age, an infant's birth weight has tripled (*b*). Additionally, an infant's length increases by 50% during its first year of life.

infant formula synthetic food that simulates human milk

colostrum initial form of breast milk that contains anti-infective properties

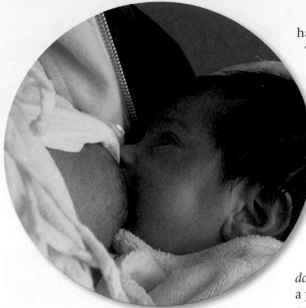

American infants who are breastfed have a lower infant mortality rate than American babies who are not.

oxytocin hormone that elicits the "let-down" response and causes the uterus to contract

have lower risks of breast cancer (before menopause) and ovarian cancer than women who do not breastfeed. Some of these benefits depend on whether a woman breastfeeds exclusively, that is, provides no other foods, and the number of months the mother nurses her infant. Table 13.4 lists these and several other advantages of breastfeeding.

The Milk Production Process—Lactation

When an infant suckles, nerves in the mother's nipple signal her brain to release prolactin and **oxytocin** (*ox-e-tose'-in*) into her bloodstream. Prolactin stimulates specialized cells in breasts to form milk. These cells carry out the lactation process by synthesizing some nutrients and removing others from the mother's bloodstream and adding them to her milk. Oxytocin plays a different role in establishing successful lactation. This hormone signals breast tissue to "let down" milk. The *let-down reflex* enables milk to travel in several tubes (ducts) to the nipple area. A reflex is a physical response that is automatic and not under conscious control. When let-down occurs, the infant removes the milk by continued sucking (Fig. 13.6). Shortly before the flow of milk begins, the lactating woman often feels a tingling sensation in her nipples, a signal that let-down is occurring.

Embarrassment, emotional stress and tension, pain, and fatigue can easily block the let-down reflex. For example, if a lactating mother is tense or upset, let-down does not occur, and her infant will not be able to obtain milk when it suckles. When this happens, the hungry infant becomes frustrated and angry, and the mother may respond by becoming even more tense and upset, setting up a vicious cycle. At this point, new mothers often give up breastfeeding, reporting that they tried to suckle their babies but were unable to "produce" milk.

Lactating women need to be aware of the connection between their emotional state and failure to let down. To smooth the path to successful lactation, it helps if new mothers are in a comfortable, relaxed environment when they breastfeed their babies.

Did You Know?

When a new mother breastfeeds her newborn immediately after delivery, oxytocin signals her uterus to contract, reducing the risk of excessive uterine bleeding.

TABLE 13.4   *Advantages of Breastfeeding*

Advantages for Infants

Human milk

- Is free of bacteria as it leaves the breast.
- Supplies antibodies and immune cells.
- Is easily digested.
- Reduces risk of food allergies, especially to proteins in infant formulas and cow's milk.
- Changes in composition over time to meet the changing needs of a growing infant.
- Contains zinc, iron, and other minerals in highly absorbable forms.
- Decreases risks of ear, intestinal, and respiratory infections.
- May reduce the risk of asthma, obesity, and type 1 diabetes in childhood.

Advantages for New Mothers

Breastfeeding

- Reduces uterine bleeding after delivery.
- Promotes shrinkage of the uterus to its prepregnancy size.
- Decreases the risk of breast cancer (before menopause) and ovarian cancer.
- May promote maternal weight loss.
- May enhance bonding with the infant.
- Is less expensive and more convenient than feeding infant formula.

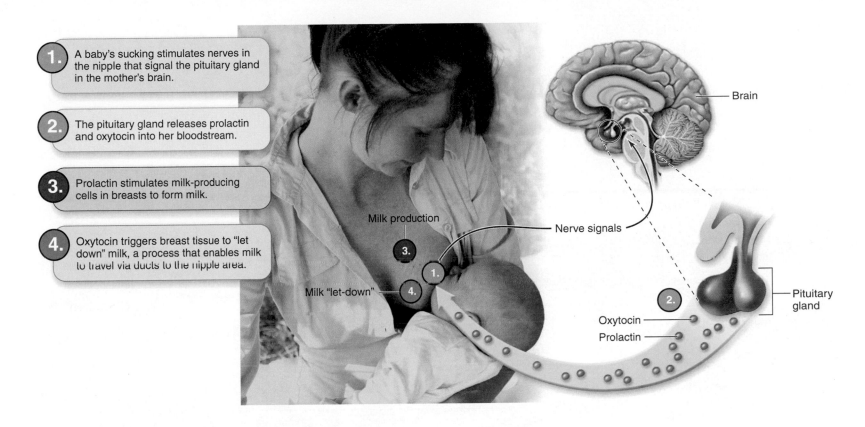

1. A baby's sucking stimulates nerves in the nipple that signal the pituitary gland in the mother's brain.

2. The pituitary gland releases prolactin and oxytocin into her bloodstream.

3. Prolactin stimulates milk-producing cells in breasts to form milk.

4. Oxytocin triggers breast tissue to "let down" milk, a process that enables milk to travel via ducts to the nipple area.

Milk production

Milk "let-down"

Brain

Nerve signals

Pituitary gland

Oxytocin

Prolactin

Figure 13.6 Breastfeeding. Milk formation and release ("let down") rely on sensations of an infant sucking on the mother's nipple, as well as signals from her nerves and hormones.

When lactation and breastfeeding are well established, the let-down response often occurs without the need for suckling. For example, the mother's let-down reflex may be triggered just by thinking about nursing her infant or hearing it cry.

Breastfeeding is a skill, and like other skills, it takes some practice to fully master. Thus, it may take a few weeks for the new mother to feel comfortable with the process. By persevering, she and her baby are likely to become a successful breastfeeding team.

Typically, a lactating woman produces over 3 cups of milk per day.[9] It is important to recognize that milk production relies on "supply and demand." The more the infant suckles (demand), the more milk its mother's breasts produce (supply). However, if milk is not fully removed from the breasts, milk production soon ceases. This is likely to occur when infants are not hungry because they have been given baby food and formula to supplement breast milk feedings.

Dietary Planning for Lactating Women

Milk production requires approximately 800 kcal every day. However, the lactating woman's daily energy needs can be met by adding only about 300 to 400 kcal to her prepregnancy EER. The difference between the energy needed for milk production and the recommended energy intake can enable the new mother to lose the extra body fat she accumulated during pregnancy. This loss is more likely to occur if she continues breastfeeding her baby for 6 months or more and increases her physical activity level. A woman, for example, who needed 2000 kcal before becoming pregnant would require about

Did You Know?

The size of a woman's breasts does not influence her ability to breastfeed her infant. However, certain surgical procedures used to enlarge or decrease breast size can disrupt the nerves and milk-producing tissue in the breasts. Women who had surgery to alter their breasts may be able to produce milk after giving birth, but their infants' growth rates should be monitored to make sure the babies are obtaining enough milk.[24]

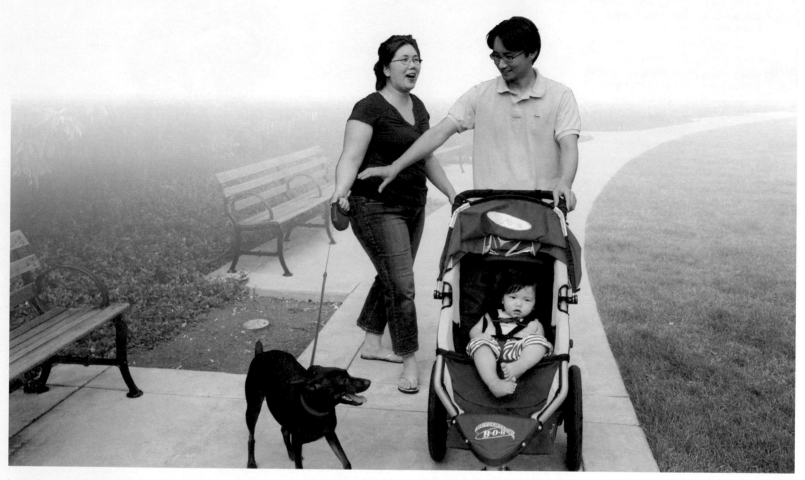

Figure 13.7 Vitamin D and infants. Exposing an infant's skin to some direct sunlight enables the baby's body to form vitamin D.

2400 to 2600 kcal daily during lactation. To help plan meals and snacks that are nutritionally adequate, she can follow recommendations at www.choosemyplate.gov.

No special foods are necessary to sustain milk production. However, a lactating woman should drink fluids every time her infant suckles to help her maintain adequate milk volume and keep her body properly hydrated. For as long as she breastfeeds her baby, the lactating mother should limit her intake of alcohol- and caffeine-containing beverages because her body secretes these drugs into her milk. A woman who breastfeeds her baby should also check with her physician before using any medications, even over-the-counter and herbal products, because such substances may also end up in her breast milk.

Is Breast Milk a Complete Food?

Dietitians and pediatricians generally recommend that new mothers breastfeed their infants exclusively during their babies' first 6 months of life.[23, 25] It is not necessary to supplement young infants' diets with other fluids, such as water, infant formula, and juices, or with solid foods, such as baby food.[25] After an infant reaches 6 months of age, breastfeeding should continue, but the infant can also be offered some appropriate solid foods. Breastfeeding may be combined with infant foods until the child's first birthday. However, there is no reason why children cannot be breastfed for longer periods. Throughout the world, many mothers continue to nurse their babies well past the babies' first birthdays, but in the United States, this practice is uncommon.

Although breast milk is highly nutritious, it is not a complete food for all infants. Human milk may contain inadequate amounts of vitamins D and B-12, and the minerals iron and fluoride. The American Academy of Pediatrics (AAP) recommends all breastfed infants be given a supplement that supplies 400 IU of vitamin D per day until they are consuming that amount of the vitamin from food or infant formula. Exposing the infant to some sun can also help meet part of the child's vitamin D needs (Fig. 13.7). If a lactating woman is a total vegetarian and she does not consume a source of vitamin B-12, she should consult her physician concerning the need for vitamin B-12 supplementation. When breastfed infants are about 6 months old, they should also be consuming some iron-containing solid foods, because the amount of iron in their mother's milk may no longer meet their needs. Furthermore, a fluoride supplement may be necessary for breast-fed babies. Before giving any dietary supplements to their baby, parents or caregivers should discuss their infant's nutritional needs with the child's physician.

A question commonly asked is whether the breastfed infant needs additional water, especially in hot weather. Human milk provides adequate water intake for *healthy* infants who are exclusively breastfed.[25] However, it is important to obtain prompt professional medical care to prevent a baby from becoming dehydrated, particularly if the infant is suffering from diarrhea, vomiting, or fever.

Quitting Too Soon

Nearly all healthy women are physically capable of breastfeeding their infants. In 2008, about 75% of American women started breastfeeding their babies soon after birth.[26] Within 2 days of birth, almost 25% of the breastfed babies were also consuming formula. By the time the infants were 6 months old, 43% continued to be breastfed. By their first birthday, only about 24% of the babies were still being nourished with their mother's milk.

Women who breastfeed their newborns often stop the practice within 6 months. There are many reasons why women discontinue nursing their infants too soon. New mothers often quit because they lack information about and support for breastfeeding their babies. Some women discontinue breastfeeding because of uncertainty over how much milk their babies are consuming. Baby bottles are marked to indicate ounces, so a mother who bottle-feeds her infant can easily measure the amount of formula consumed. A lactating mother, however, has to observe her baby for cues indicating the child is full. When a breastfeeding baby is no longer interested in nursing and stops, its mother has to assume the infant is satisfied with the feeding. A well-nourished breastfed infant will gain weight normally and generally have six or more wet diapers as well as one or two soft bowel movements per day. Parents or caregivers who are concerned about their infants' food intake or nutritional status should consult their physician immediately.

Many new mothers discontinue breastfeeding before their babies are 6 months old because they need to return to work and have caregivers feed their babies. Although lactating women can learn to express milk from their breasts and preserve it for later feedings, many workplaces do not have comfortable, private facilities for women to express milk and then store it safely.

To enhance the likelihood that a nursing mother continues to breastfeed, it is helpful to enlist the support of a female relative or friend who has successfully breastfed her children. Furthermore, the woman's partner needs to understand and appreciate the function of the human breast as a source of nearly perfect nourishment for infants. New mothers are unlikely to begin and continue nursing their babies without their partners' support. La Leche League is an international organization dedicated to providing education and support for breastfeeding women (1-877-4-LALECHE or www.llli.org). Also, hospitals may employ lactation consultants or specialists. Lactation consultants are often nurses who are trained to provide information and advice about breastfeeding. For more information about breastfeeding, visit http://www.cdc.gov/breastfeeding/.

Did You Know?

In the United States, newborns are given an injection of vitamin K to protect them against excessive bleeding.

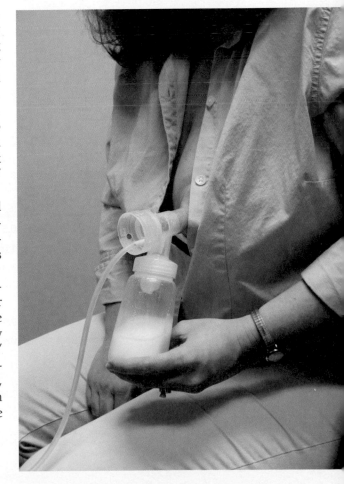

This mother is using an electric device to express milk in a private room at her workplace. She will chill the milk and give it to her baby's caregiver for bottle-feeding.

Infant Formula Feeding

Not every woman wants or is able to breastfeed her baby. Infant formulas are a safe and nutritionally adequate source of nutrients for babies who are not breastfed (Fig. 13.8). To produce artificial milk for babies, infant formula manufacturers alter cow's milk to improve its digestibility and nutrient content. Infant formulas generally contain heat-treated proteins from cow's milk, lactose and/or sucrose, and vegetable oil. Infant formulas generally lack cholesterol, but some of these products have the fatty acids DHA and AA added to them. Vitamins and minerals are added to the product, and in some instances, infant formula contains higher levels of micronutrients than human milk. Although infant formulas mimic the water, macronutrient, and micronutrient content of human milk, their compositions are not identical to human milk (Table 13.5). Formula manufacturers have been unable to duplicate human antibodies and other unique immune system factors that are in breast milk.

An interesting feature of human milk is that its fat content changes during each feeding, which usually lasts about 20 minutes. In the beginning of the session, the mother's milk is low in fat, but as her infant continues to suckle, the fat content of her milk gradually increases.[27] The higher fat content of the "hind milk" may make the baby feel satisfied and, as a result, discontinue feeding. Infant formulas, however, have uniform composition; that is, they do not change their fat content during a feeding session. Thus, the mother or infant caregiver is more likely to control the amount of formula the baby consumes, possibly leading to overfeeding. Nevertheless, the overall energy content of human milk is about the same as that of infant formulas (about 20 kcal per ounce).

Experts with the AAP recommend that caregivers provide an iron-fortified infant formula for babies who are not breastfed. Not all infant formulas contain iron, so it is important to read the product's label before purchasing it. Formula-fed babies may also need a source of fluoride, but caregivers should check with their infants' physicians before providing a supplement containing the mineral. For babies who are allergic to infant formulas made from cow's milk proteins, similar products made with soy or other proteins are available.

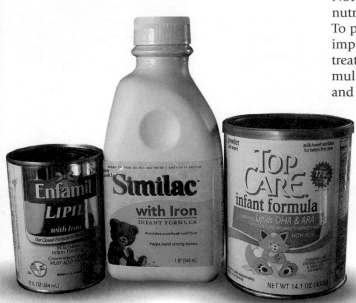

Figure 13.8 Infant formulas. Infant formulas provide a safe and nutritionally adequate source of nutrients for babies who are not breastfed.

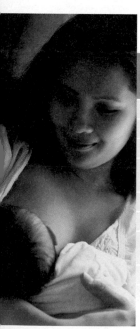

TABLE 13.5 *Comparing Approximate Compositions of Human Milk, Cow's Milk, and Iron-Fortified Infant Formulas (per Ounce)*

Milk or Iron-Fortified Formula	Energy (kcal/oz)	Protein (g/oz)	Carbo-hydrate (g/oz)	Fat (g/oz)	Choles-terol (mg/oz)	Iron (mg/oz)	Calcium (mg/oz)
Human milk	22.5	0.32	2.12	1.35	4.00	0.01	10.0
Cow's milk, whole	20.1	1.08	1.60	1.08	3.00	0.01	34.0
Cow's milk, fat-free	10.8	1.08	1.56	0.03	1.00	0.01	38.0
Cow's milk protein-based formulas							
Similac	20.0	0.41	2.10	1.08	1.00	0.36	16.0
Enfamil	20.0	0.42	2.19	1.07	0.00	0.36	16.0
Soy protein-based formulas							
ProSobee	20	0.50	2.13	1.07	0.00	0.36	21.0
Isomil	20	0.49	2.04	1.09	0.00	0.36	21.0

Source of data: U.S. Department of Agriculture, Agricultural Research Service. *What's in the foods you eat search tool, 2.0.* www.ars.usda.gov/Services/docs.htm?docid=7783

What About Cow's Milk?

Why not feed fresh fluid cow's milk to an infant? Cow's milk is too high in minerals and protein and does not contain enough carbohydrate to meet an infant's nutrient needs (see Table 13.5). In addition, infants have more difficulty digesting **casein** (*kay'-seen*), the major protein in cow's milk, than the major proteins in human milk. Cow's milk can also contribute to intestinal bleeding and iron deficiency.[28] Thus, whole cow's milk should not be fed to infants until they are 1 year of age.[25] Furthermore, fat-reduced and fat-free cow's milk are too low in energy to be given to most children until they are 2 years of age.

Allergies   Allergies are immune system responses to the presence of foreign proteins in the body. Allergies to proteins in foods, especially cow's milk proteins, often begin in infancy and may persist through childhood. Signs and symptoms of food allergies typically include the following:

- Vomiting, diarrhea, intestinal gas and pain, bloating, or constipation
- Itchy, swollen, or reddened skin
- Runny nose and breathing difficulties, such as asthma

Compared to breastfed infants, formula-fed babies have a greater risk of food allergies. When a woman has a personal or family history of food allergies, she may be able to prevent her children from developing such allergies if she breastfeeds her babies exclusively for 6 months. Infants rarely develop allergic reactions to food proteins that enter breast milk from the mother's bloodstream.

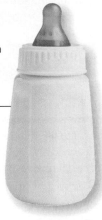

Food & Nutrition *tip*

Do not heat infant formula or human milk in a microwave oven. The heat can destroy immune factors in human milk and create hot spots that can scald an infant's tongue.

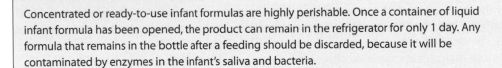

Did You Know?

Concentrated or ready-to-use infant formulas are highly perishable. Once a container of liquid infant formula has been opened, the product can remain in the refrigerator for only 1 day. Any formula that remains in the bottle after a feeding should be discarded, because it will be contaminated by enzymes in the infant's saliva and bacteria.

Introducing Solid Foods

Before 6 months of age, babies' nutritional needs can generally be met with human milk and/or infant formula. According to AAP experts, solid foods should not be introduced to infants until they are about 6 months of age. At this age, many infants need the additional calories supplied by solid foods. Breastfed babies may also need a dietary source of iron, because their stores of the mineral are usually exhausted about 6 months after birth. Nevertheless, caregivers should continue to provide human milk or iron-fortified infant formula as the foundation of the baby's diet for the first year.

Many new parents are anxious to start feeding their young infants solid food. However, babies are not physically mature enough to consume solids before they are 4 to 6 months of age. For example, a baby's kidney functions are quite limited until the child is about 4 to 6 weeks of age. Additionally, an infant's digestive tract cannot readily digest starch before the child is about 3 months old.

Infants are born with the **extrusion reflex,** an involuntary response that occurs when a solid or semisolid object is placed in an infant's mouth. As a result of this reflex, a young baby thrusts its tongue forward, pushing the object out of its mouth. Thus, trying to feed the infant solid foods is a messy, frustrating process, as the child automatically pushes the food out of its mouth. Liquid foods, such as breast milk or infant formula, do not elicit the extrusion reflex, so the baby swallows fluids.

As the infant reaches 4 to 6 months of age, the extrusion reflex disappears, and the child has developed the physiological abilities to digest, metabolize, and excrete a wider range of foods. Moreover, a 6-month-old infant can usually sit up with back support and coordinate muscular control over his or her mouth and neck movements. These signs

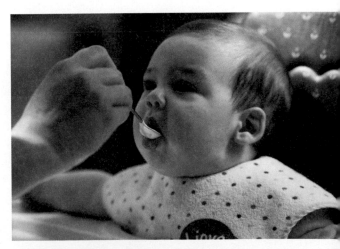

casein major protein in cow's milk

extrusion reflex involuntary response in which a young infant thrusts its tongue forward when a solid or semisolid object is placed in its mouth

weaning gradual process of shifting from breastfeeding or bottle-feeding to drinking from a cup and eating solid foods

Did You Know?

Many parents think adding solid foods to infants' diets helps babies sleep through the night. Actually, this developmental milestone generally occurs around 3 to 4 months of age, regardless of what infants are eating.

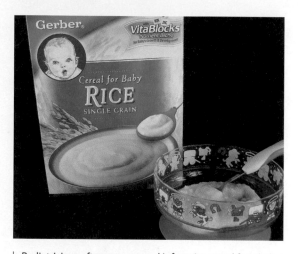

Pediatricians often recommend infant rice cereal for a baby's first solid food because it is fortified with iron and may not cause allergies.

Single-food items, such as carrots or peas, are more nutrient-dense choices for feeding infants than mixed dinners and desserts.

indicate the baby is ready physically to eat solid foods, is less likely to choke on such foods, and can turn his or her head away from food when full.

Weaning is the gradual process of shifting an infant from breastfeeding or bottle-feeding to drinking from a cup and eating solid foods. Pediatricians often recommend introducing an iron-fortified infant cereal made from rice as the first solid food. After feeding the infant cereal for the first time, caregivers should offer the food to the baby for at least 4 days and observe the infant for signs and symptoms of food allergy. If the infant appears to tolerate rice cereal, caregivers can add a new food to the baby's diet, such as another type of baby cereal or a cooked, strained vegetable. As each new food is introduced, caregivers should wait 2 to 4 days before adding a different food to the child's diet.[29] If the infant develops diarrhea, vomiting, or a rash during this period, he or she may be allergic to the new food.

Is is a good idea to avoid giving mixed foods such as casseroles or commercially prepared baby food "dinners" to infants. If the baby has an allergic response after eating a food mixture, it will be difficult to determine which ingredient was responsible. Serving mixed foods is acceptable when the child has eaten each ingredient individually without having an allergic response.

Infants who have a high risk of food allergy have a parent or sibling who has a history of allergies, including food allergy. Foods that are associated with allergic responses in infants include egg whites, chocolate, nuts, and cow's milk. Therefore, caregivers should not offer these foods to high-risk babies under 6 months of age. Many babies outgrow food allergies during childhood, but some children remain allergic to the foods through adulthood.

Many varieties of strained baby food are available at the supermarket. Single-food items, such as carrots or peas, are more nutrient-dense choices for feeding infants than mixed dinners and desserts. Most brands have no added salt, but some fruit desserts contain a lot of added sugar. As an alternative, caregivers can prepare their own baby food by taking plain, unseasoned cooked foods and pureeing them in a blender. If a large amount of the item is blended, the pureed food can be poured into an ice cube tray, covered with a plastic bag, and frozen. When it is feeding time, an ice cube portion of the baby food can be popped out of the tray and warmed. The Chapter 13 "Recipes for Healthy Living" feature includes an applesauce recipe that both children and adults will enjoy.

At about 6 to 8 months of age, the baby's first set of teeth, the "primary teeth," begin to appear. These teeth are important for proper nutrition because they help the

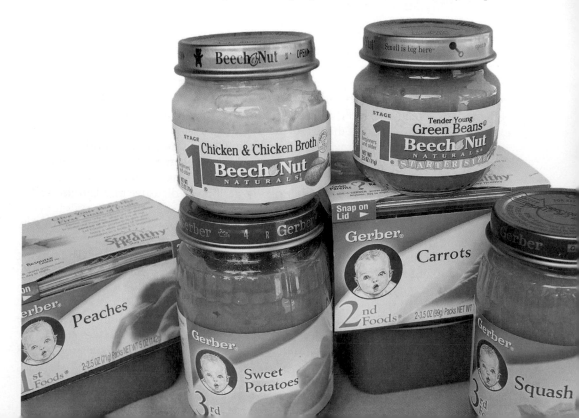

child bite and chew food. By 8 to 12 months of age, most infants can use their fingers to pick up and chew "finger foods" such as crackers, toast, and cooked string beans. Babies can also hold a bottle and practice drinking from a special cup ("sippy cup") that has a lid with a spout (Fig. 13.9). Babies need to practice self-feeding skills, even if it means playing with food and creating messes. By about 10 months of age, many infants are mastering self-feeding and making the transition from baby foods to menu items the rest of the family enjoys.

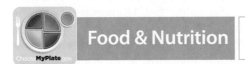

Food & Nutrition *tips*

When feeding solid foods to an infant:

- Use a baby-sized spoon—a small spoon with a broad handle.

- Hold the infant comfortably on your lap, as for breastfeeding or bottle-feeding, but in a more upright position to ease swallowing.

- Add some breast milk or infant formula to the cereal, and place a small dab of the semisolid food on the spoon's tip. Gently place the spoon on the infant's tongue and tilt it so the food slides onto the tongue. If the infant spits it out, do not continue with the feeding.

- Expect the infant to take only two or three bites during these early feeding sessions.

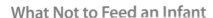

What Not to Feed an Infant

By the end of the first year, an infant should be consuming many different foods—grain products, meats, fruits, and vegetables—along with breast milk or infant formula. Introducing a baby to various foods helps the child learn about different tastes, odors, and textures. However, certain foods and beverages are not appropriate for infants. Avoid feeding an infant these things:

- **Honey.** This product may contain spores of *Clostridium botulinum* that can produce a potentially fatal toxin in children who are under 1 year old (see Chapter 12).
- **Excessive infant formula or human milk.** Depending on their age, most infants need less than 30 ounces of human milk or infant formula daily. A child who drinks too much milk may not eat enough solid foods that contain nutrients lacking in milk.
- **Semisolid baby cereal in a baby bottle that has the nipple opening enlarged.** This practice contributes to overfeeding and does not help the child learn self-feeding skills.
- **Candy, flavored gelatin water, or soft drinks.** These items provide few micronutrients.
- **Small pieces of hard or coarse foods.** Foods such as hot dogs (unless finely cut into sticks, not coin shapes), whole nuts, grapes, chunks of cooked meat, raw carrots, popcorn, and peanut butter can cause choking. Caregivers should supervise meals to keep young children from stuffing too much food in their mouths.
- **Excessive amounts of apple or pear juice.** The fructose and *sorbitol*, a sugar alcohol, contained in these juices can lead to diarrhea. Also, if the infant drinks fruit juice or fruit drinks rather than breast milk or infant formula, the child may not be receiving adequate amounts of calcium and other essential minerals.
- **Unpasteurized (raw) milk.** Raw milk may be contaminated with bacteria or viruses.
- **Goat's milk.** Goat's milk is low in iron, folate, and vitamins C and D.

Baby Bottle Caries

At bedtime, many caregivers place infants in their cribs with a baby bottle containing formula, juice, or a sugar-sweetened drink. This practice is not recommended, because the sleepy infant sucks slowly, allowing the carbohydrate-containing fluid to bathe the child's

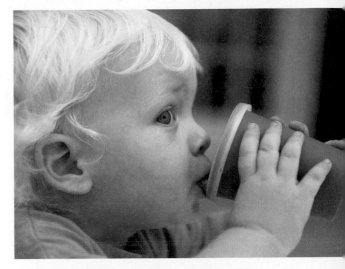

Figure 13.9 Learning to drink from a cup. After a baby learns to hold a bottle, the child can practice holding a "sippy cup" and learn how to drink from it.

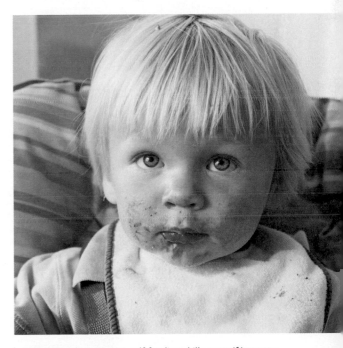

Babies need to practice self-feeding skills, even if it means playing with food and creating messes.

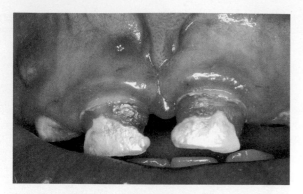

Figure 13.10 Baby bottle caries. This infant has baby bottle caries. To reduce the risk of baby bottle caries, infants should be given only water in a baby bottle at bedtime.

teeth and provide a source of nutrients for bacteria that stick to teeth. These bacteria produce acids that dissolve tooth enamel, causing cavities to form in the teeth (*dental caries*). Dentists often refer to this condition as "baby bottle caries" (Fig. 13.10). To reduce the risk of baby bottle caries, infants should be given only water in their bedtime bottles.

Monitoring an Infant's Growth

During routine "well baby" checkups, a health professional usually measures the infant's length, weight, and *head circumference* (Fig. 13.11). Head circumference measurements assess brain growth, which occurs at a rapid rate during the first 18 months of life. The three values are then compared to those indicating typical growth patterns displayed on growth charts available at the Centers for Disease Control and Prevention website (www.cdc.gov/growthcharts/). The charts display percentile divisions; a percentile ranks the child's size among other children who are the same age and gender. If an infant boy's length, for example, is at the 90th percentile according to the length-for-age chart, he is the same length as or taller than 90% of the other boys his age. Furthermore, this child is the same length as or shorter than 10% of boys his age. If the infant's rate of growth slows down too much or is higher than normal, the child's physician should investigate whether a medical or nutritional problem is responsible for the unusual measurements.

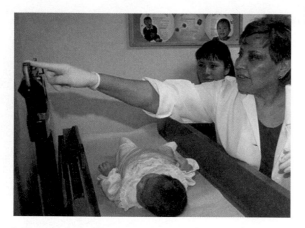

Figure 13.11 Measuring growth rates during infancy. During routine "well baby" checkups, a health professional usually measures the infant's length, weight, and head circumference.

Concept **Checkpoint**

9. What is the "let-down reflex"?
10. How does lactation affect a new mother's energy needs?
11. What is colostrum, and why is it a valuable first food for breastfed babies?
12. Dietitians and other health experts recommend that infants be breastfed exclusively during their first ____ months of life.
13. List at least five benefits that infants derive from breastfeeding.
14. Identify at least three benefits that women derive from breastfeeding their babies.
15. Compare the energy, macronutrient, and calcium contents of an ounce of human milk with those of an ounce of cow's milk.
16. Identify at least three physiological indications that an infant is ready to eat solid foods.
17. Describe three ways that a qualified health care practitioner can monitor an infant's growth.

13.4 Childhood

Childhood can be divided into the preschool period (2 to 5 years of age) and the school-age period (6 to 11 years of age). The rapid growth rate that characterizes the first 12 months of life tapers off quickly during the preschool years and proceeds at a slow but steady rate until the end of childhood. If an average infant's growth rate did not slow down, he or she might weigh about 190 pounds and be about 5'7" tall by 3 years of age! However, the average 3-year-old weighs about 32 pounds and is about 3 feet in height.

The preferred growth standard for children who are 2 to 20 years of age is the *body mass index (BMI)-for-age*. The BMI-for-age is a number calculated from the child's height and weight. BMI charts for children are both sex- and age-specific (see Appendix G). An *overweight* child has a BMI-for-age that is at or above the 85th percentile and lower than

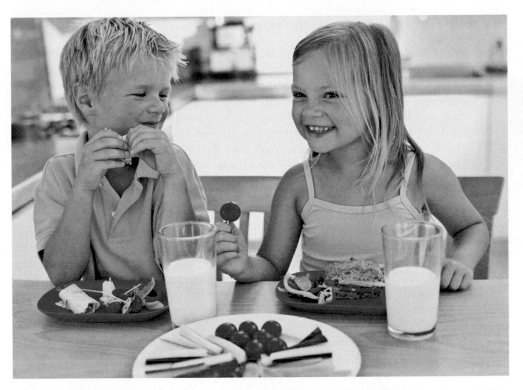

Figure 13.12 Age-appropriate portion sizes. Healthy young children should not be expected to eat adult-size portions of food. Each of these children is eating half a sandwich, a reasonable amount for their age.

TABLE 13.6 *Preschool Children: Daily Food Plan Based on MyPlate Recommendations*

Energy/Food Group	2 Years	3 to 5 Years
Kilocalories*	1000	1400
Grains	3 oz	5 oz
Vegetables	1 cup	1½ cups
Fruits	1 cup	1½ cups
Dairy	2 cups	2½ cups
Protein foods	2 oz	4 oz

* Kilocalorie estimates are based on age and 30 to 60 minutes of physical activity.

Source: U.S. Department of Agriculture: *MyPlate*. www.choosemyplate .gov/myplate/index.aspx. Accessed: August 5, 2011.

the 95th percentile for children of the same age and sex.[30] An *obese* child has a BMI-for-age that is at or above the 95th percentile for children of the same age and sex.

As the growth rate slows after infancy, preschoolers' appetites decrease because they do not need as much food. Parents and other caregivers must recognize that a 3-year-old child should not be expected to eat as eagerly as he or she did as an infant. Furthermore, children do not have the stomach capacity to eat adult-size portions of foods (Fig. 13.12). When planning meals and snacks for children who eat relatively little food, caregivers should emphasize nutrient-dense foods, such as lean meats, low-fat dairy products, whole-grain cereals, fruits, nuts, and vegetables. Although many ready-to-eat cereals are sweetened with sugar, it is not necessary to eliminate such foods. Caregivers, however, should read product labels and choose varieties with less added sugar. Additionally, it is important to monitor children's intake of sweets, because sugary items can crowd out more nutritious foods from their diets.

Table 13.6 presents a day's food group selections, based on MyPlate recommendations, that are appropriate for children who are 2 to 5 years of age. Recall that fish and seafood are in the protein foods group. Caregivers should include fish in children's meals regularly, especially fish that are rich sources of omega-3 fatty acids, such as salmon.

Snacks

Snacking is not necessarily a bad habit, especially if snacks are nutrient dense and fit into the child's overall diet. Preschool children have relatively small stomachs, so nutritious snacks can be offered at midmorning or midafternoon, when the child is likely to become hungry between meals. A 4- or 5-year-old child can safely eat raw vegetables without fear of choking. Thus, a platter of raw or lightly cooked carrots; broccoli flowerets; slices of green, yellow, and red peppers; and mushrooms served as a snack may be accepted. Nutritious dips, such as the yogurt dip in the Chapter 13 "Recipes for Healthy Living," may make raw vegetables more appealing to children. Table 13.7 lists some nutritious snacks that children tend to like.

TABLE 13.7 *Nutritious Snacks*

- Peanut butter spread on graham crackers
- Fruit smoothies (see Chapter 9 "Recipes for Healthy Living")
- Fruit salad (or cut-up fruit)
- Mini-pizzas (half an English muffin, topped with tomato sauce and Mozzarella cheese, and heated in toaster oven or microwave oven)
- Plain, low-fat yogurt topped with granola or fresh fruit
- Pasta salad
- Peanuts, cashews, or sunflower seeds
- Fruitpops
- Leftovers (pizzas, macaroni and cheese, lasagna)
- Quick breads, such as banana bread
- Cheese melted on whole-wheat crackers
- Dried fruit
- Trail mix
- Ready-to-eat cereal
- Vegetable sticks dipped in hummus

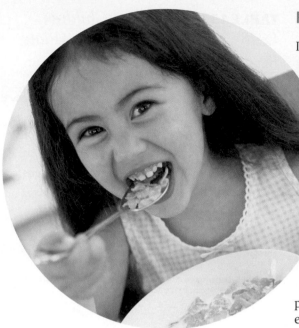

It is not unusual for children to have "food jags," periods in which they insist on eating a particular food, such as cereal and milk.

Fostering Positive Eating Behaviors

Parents often refer to their preschool children as "picky eaters" because the youngsters do not eat everything offered to them. Furthermore, it is not unusual for children to have "food jags," periods in which they refuse to eat a food that they liked in the past, or want to eat only a particular food, such as peanut butter and jelly sandwiches or cereal and milk. Picky eating and food jags may be expressions of a child's growing need for independence. Caregivers should avoid nagging, forcing, and bribing children to eat. Instead, caregivers can offer the children a variety of healthy foods each day and allow the youngsters to choose which items and how much to eat.

Many children, especially preschool children, resist eating new foods. The temperature, appearance, texture, and taste of a food influence whether children will sample it. For example, young children often reject lumpy or hot-temperature foods. Sometimes children object to having foods mixed together such as in stews and casseroles, even though they like the ingredients when served separately. It is not unusual for young children to dislike vegetables that have strong flavors or odors, such as broccoli, onions, and asparagus. The idea of eating vegetables may become more appealing when children help grow, select, or prepare fresh produce. Nevertheless, it is important to recognize that everyone, including a child, is entitled to dislike certain foods.

The social atmosphere can make mealtimes enjoyable or unbearable, which in turn influences a child's desire to eat. Mealtimes should be happy, social occasions to enjoy healthful foods with parents or other caregivers. The kitchen table should not become a battleground in which adults use threats or bribes to force children to eat unfamiliar foods. For example, avoid telling a child, "You'll just sit there until you clean your plate" or "You can have a cupcake if you eat your peas." When a child refuses to eat, have the youngster remain at the table for a while. If the child continues to be disinterested in eating, remove the food and wait until the next scheduled meal or snack.

Healthy children are not in danger of starving if they skip a meal. A child who is not hungry at mealtimes may have eaten a snack before the meal at a friend's home. If a child's lack of appetite persists, caretakers should consult the child's physician to rule out illness.

Eating vegetables may become more appealing when children help grow, select, or prepare fresh produce.

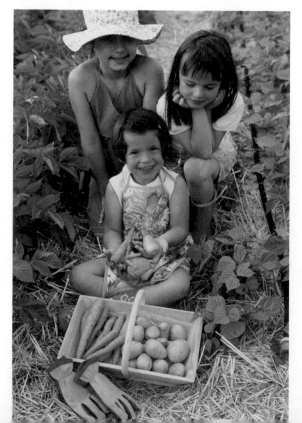

Common Food-Related Concerns

Nutrition-related problems that often affect preschool children are iron deficiency, dental caries, food allergies, and obesity. Additionally, vegetarian diets can also pose problems if they are not planned to meet children's nutrient needs.

Iron Deficiency

Iron deficiency can lead to decreased physical stamina and learning ability, and resistance to infection. The best way to prevent iron deficiency in children is to provide foods that are good sources of iron, such as lean meat and enriched breads and cereals. Milk and other dairy products are poor sources of iron, so caregivers may need to limit daily servings of foods from this food group. Preschool children should consume 2 cups/day of fat-free or low-fat milk or equivalent dairy products.[31] Chapter 9 provides more information about iron deficiency.

Dental Caries

Many preschool children have had one or more dental caries by the time they enter school. If dental caries are not treated, jaw pain, gum infection, and tooth loss can occur. The following tips can help reduce the risk of dental caries in children:

- Brush teeth with a pea-sized amount of fluoride-containing toothpaste twice daily.
- Provide routine pediatric dental care.

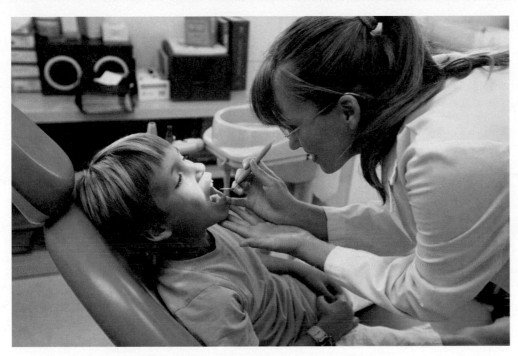

| To reduce the risk of dental caries, children should receive regular dental checkups.

- Provide fluoridated drinking water.
- Avoid eating sticky, sugary snacks, especially between meals.
- If preschoolers want to chew gum, have them chew sugarless gum to reduce the risk of dental caries.[32]

Allergies

Although any food can trigger allergic reactions among preschool children, the most common food *allergens* are peanuts, tree nuts (e.g., walnuts and pecans), fish, shellfish, milk, eggs, soybeans, and wheat. A child who is extremely allergic to a food may have an adverse reaction just by being in the room where that food is being cooked or eaten. For a small number of children, avoiding foods that produce allergic responses is a matter of life and death.

The best treatment for a food allergy is avoiding exposure to the problem food. Parents and other caregivers must learn to read the lists of ingredients on labels to determine whether products contain foods an allergic child should avoid. Furthermore, caregivers should inform adults who have contact with the child about the youngster's need to avoid the offending food. A registered dietitian can assist caregivers in planning menus that meet the allergic child's nutrient needs.

Obesity

The prevalence of obesity among American preschool children increased from 13.1% in 2000 to 14.4% in 2010.[33] Obesity among preschoolers is a major public health concern. Childhood obesity is an early risk factor for type 2 diabetes, hypertension, and obesity later in life. Obese children are more likely to mature into obese adults than children who have healthy body weights.[34]

There is no single cause of excess body fat in children, but researchers have identified factors that are associated with the development of the condition. These factors include having a family history of excess body fat, high birth weight, and obese family members. Furthermore, youngsters who spend a lot of time at sedentary activities and

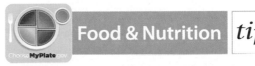

Food & Nutrition *tips*

- Foods with bright colors, crisp textures, and sweet or mild flavors usually appeal to children. When planning meals, consider including foods with these attractive characteristics.

- As a parent, you may want to consider having the "one bite policy." According to this policy, your child should try at least one bite of each new food provided at mealtimes. If you do not like a particular food that is offered, you should follow the "one-bite policy" as well. Taste the item—you may discover that you like it.

- To stimulate your child's appetite, try serving food on a small colorful plate that is designed to appeal to young children.

- Keep in mind that you are your children's role model for food choices and physical activity habits. If you eat a variety of nutrient-dense foods and are physically active, your children are likely to eat such foods and be active as well.

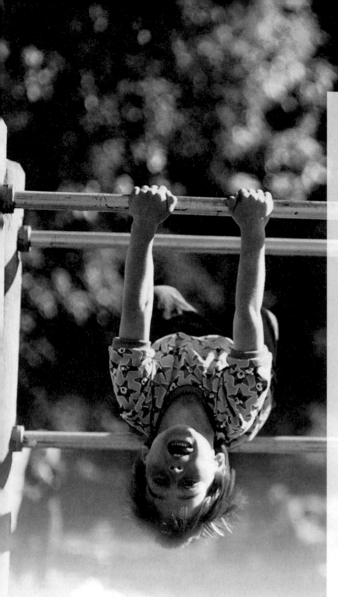

To help reduce the likelihood that young children become obese, caregivers need to provide opportunities for youngsters to be physically active.

consuming too many energy-dense empty-calorie foods and beverages are also at risk of gaining excess fat in childhood.[35]

Medical experts have not determined the best long-term treatment program for obese children.[36] A major challenge is *preventing* the condition in childhood without negatively affecting normal growth and development. To help reduce the likelihood that young children become too fat, caregivers need to promote healthy eating practices for all family members and provide opportunities for youngsters to be physically active.

Concept **Checkpoint**

18. What is a "food jag"?
19. Discuss effects that iron deficiency can have on children.
20. List at least three steps caregivers can take to reduce the risk of dental caries in children.
21. List at least four foods that commonly trigger allergic responses in children.
22. Identify at least four factors that contribute to obesity among preschool children.

13.5 School-Age Children

By the time children are 6 years of age, many have adopted diets that are not nutritionally adequate.[37] Compared to preschoolers, older children often skip breakfast, and they typically consume more foods away from home, larger portions of food, and more fried foods and sweetened beverages. School-age children also tend to reduce their intakes of dairy products as well as fruits and vegetables, except fried potatoes. As a result, diets of many school-age children provide too much sodium while supplying inadequate amounts of other minerals, particularly calcium and potassium.[37] Table 13.8 presents a day's food recommendations for healthy school-age children, based on MyPlate. The www .choosemyplate.gov website has a special series of web pages for children who are 6 to

TABLE 13.8 *Six- to 11-Year-Old Children: Daily Food Plan Based on MyPlate Recommendations*

Energy/ Food Group	Age/Sex 6 Years		Age 7–8 Years	Age/Sex 9 Years		Age 10–11 Years
	Girls	Boys	Both	Girls	Boys	Both
Kilocalories*	1400	1600	1600	1600	1800	1800
Grains	4 oz	5 oz	5 oz	5 oz	6 oz	6 oz
Vegetables	1.5 cups	2 cups	2 cups	2 cups	2.5 cups	2.5 cups
Fruits	1.5 cups	1.5 cups	1.5 cups	1.5 cups	1.5 cups	1.5 cups
Dairy	2 cups	3 cups	3 cups	3 cups	3 cups	3 cups
Protein foods	4 oz	5 oz	5 oz	5 oz	5 oz	5 oz

* Kilocalorie estimates are based on age, sex, and 30 to 60 minutes of physical activity. Source: U.S. Department of Agriculture: *MyPlate.* www.choosemyplate.gov/myplate/index.aspx. Accessed: August 5, 2011.

11 years of age. Children can visit the website and play the interactive "Blast Off Game." To test the game, visit http://www.choosemyplate.gov/kids/kids_game.html.

Caregivers can help improve children's diets by encouraging youngsters to eat breakfast regularly. Children who routinely eat breakfast are more likely to have better diets and healthier body weights than children who skip this meal.[38] Breakfast menus do not need to feature traditional fare such as bacon, eggs, waffles, or pancakes. For example, leftovers from the previous night's dinner can be eaten for breakfast. Convenient "fast breakfasts" that school-age children can prepare quickly include ready-to-eat cereal with milk and fruit, cottage cheese and fruit, a peanut butter and jelly sandwich, or yogurt topped with trail mix or pieces of fresh fruit.

Parents and other caregivers need to be concerned about foods that are available at school and obtain answers to the following questions. What kinds of foods are offered for school breakfasts and lunches? Does the school have vending machines accessible to youngsters? If so, what kinds of foods and beverages are sold from these machines? Do

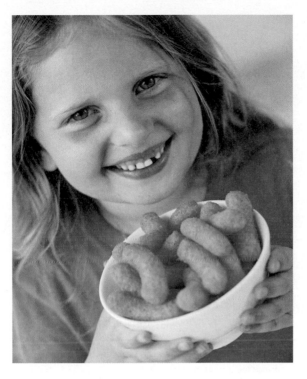

Parents and other caregivers need to be concerned about their children's food choices.

Children need at least 60 minutes of moderate-intensity physical activity, ideally every day.

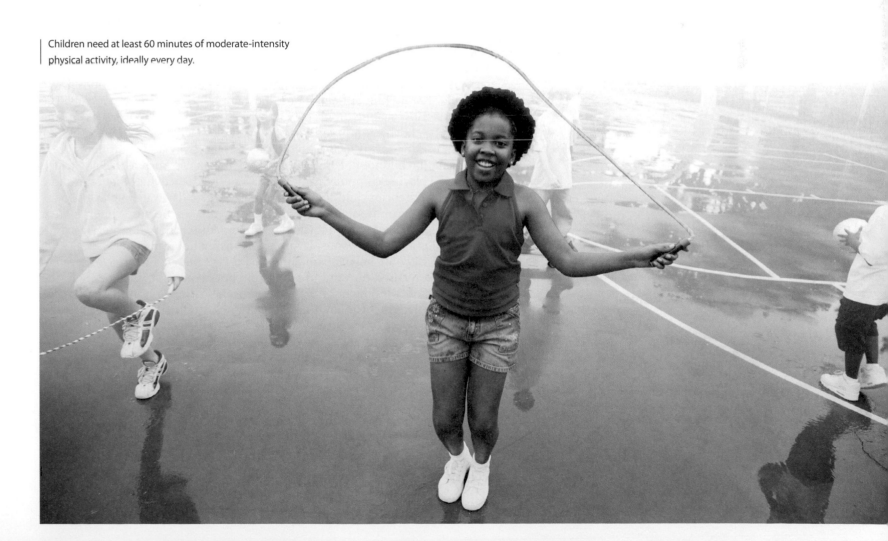

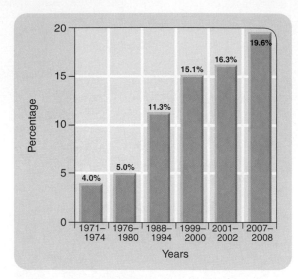

Figure 13.13 **Prevalence of obesity among American children aged 6 to 11 years, 1971–1974 through 2007–2008.** In 2007–2008, the percentage of obesity among American children 6 to 11 years of age was much higher than the percentage obtained in similar national surveys conducted about 35 years earlier.

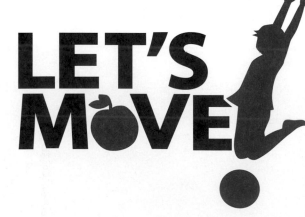

vending machines offer competitively priced nutrient-dense foods? What can be done to ensure that the machines and the school's cafeteria provide nutritious foods that children will eat? Furthermore, what efforts are being made to teach children about proper nutrition while they are in school?

Common Nutrition-Related Concerns

Public health experts are alarmed about the increasing prevalence of obesity among school-age children in the United States. The following sections take a closer look at the problems associated with excess body fat during childhood and at other nutrition-related concerns, such as multiple vitamin/mineral supplements and vegetarianism.

Obesity

In the United States, the prevalence of obesity among school-age children has risen dramatically since the early 1970s. Almost 20% of 6- to 11-year-old children were obese in 2007–2008.[39] This percentage is much higher than those obtained in similar national surveys conducted about 35 years earlier (Fig. 13.13).

Obese children often have higher than normal blood pressure, cholesterol, and glucose levels.[34] Obese youngsters are also more likely to have low self-esteem, sleep apnea, heartburn, and musculoskeletal problems. Such children are at risk to develop hypertension, heart disease, and type 2 diabetes later in life. Furthermore, obese children are likely to be obese as adults.

In most cases, no single factor is responsible for causing obesity in childhood. Obesity tends to "run in families," but genetics does not account for all individual differences in body weight. Environmental factors—such as frequent consumption of fast foods, easy access to energy-dense foods, and lack of safe areas for playing outdoors—also contribute to excess body fat in childhood.

Caregivers may need to limit the obese child's intakes of empty-calorie foods. These items often replace more nutrient-dense or lower-calorie foods in children's diets. The "Food & Nutrition Tips" feature on page 493 provides some suggestions for improving children's food-related behaviors, regardless of their body weights.

Aside from making poor dietary choices, physical inactivity also contributes to excessive weight gain in childhood. For many children, media use, such as viewing television programs and playing computer games, replaces physical activities that burn more energy. The average American child spends about 4.5 hours a day watching television.[40] Television viewing also contributes to increased energy intakes, because children often snack and eat meals while watching TV. Child health experts recommend caregivers limit children's TV viewing and video game playing to less than 2 hours per day.[41]

In 2010, First Lady Michelle Obama introduced *Let's Move!*, a comprehensive national program that focused on ways to reduce the prevalence of child obesity in the United States. A major component of the program is increasing opportunities for children to be physically active.[42] Children need at least 60 minutes of moderate-intensity physical activity most days of the week—ideally, every day.[43] Table 13.9 presents common physical activities that children usually enjoy. It is important to assess an overfat youngster's daily physical activity level and encourage the child to be more physically active. Caregivers can ask their children's teachers about opportunities for youngsters to be physically active while they are in school. For example, how often do children participate in the school's physical education classes? Are boys and girls active during recess? If children are not obtaining enough physical activity during the day, their caregivers can enroll them in after-school sports or community-based exercise programs. Being physically active will help children not only to attain healthy body weights but also to *maintain* healthy body weights later in life.

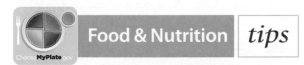

Food & Nutrition *tips*

The following tips can help you improve your child's diet:

- Guide your family's food choices instead of dictating what they eat.

- Eat meals together as a family as often as possible.

- If necessary, reduce the amount of fat, especially saturated and trans fat, in your family's diet.

- Do not place your child on a restrictive diet, unless the diet is recommended by the child's physician.

- Avoid using food as a reward or punishment.

- Encourage the child to drink water instead of sugar-sweetened beverages.

- Keep healthy snacks (such as fat-free or low-fat milk, fresh fruit, and vegetables) on hand.

- Serve at least 5 servings of fruits and vegetables each day.

- Discourage eating meals or snacks while watching TV.

- Encourage the child to eat a nutrient-dense breakfast daily.

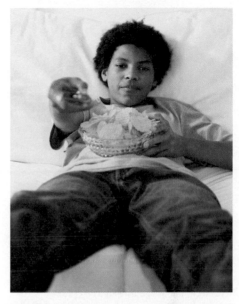

Caregivers should discourage children from eating while watching TV.

Parents and other caregivers are primary role models for children. Before trying to alter their children's weight, caregivers should evaluate their own weights, as well as eating and physical activity practices. Often, everyone in a family reaps healthful benefits from eating more meals prepared and eaten at home and becoming more physically active.

When helping a child lose weight, caregivers should avoid scolding or nagging the youngster because doing so can make the child rebel against adults, feel unloved and depressed, and dislike his or her body shape. As a result of harboring such negative feelings, an obese child may become vulnerable to developing disordered eating practices or eating disorders.

Vegetarianism

Vegetarian diets can be nutritionally adequate for children, but careful planning is necessary to make sure youngsters obtain enough energy, high-quality protein, vitamin B-12, iron, calcium, and zinc. Nuts, seeds, ready-to-eat cereals, and fortified soy milk can supply some of the nutrients that tend to be low in vegan diets. Additionally, vegan children will need a source of vitamin D, such as regular sun exposure. For more information about vegetarianism, see Chapter 7.

Do Children Need Multiple Vitamin/Mineral Supplements?

In general, multiple vitamin/mineral supplements are not necessary for healthy children who eat a variety of foods from all food groups, including ready-to-eat cereals that are fortified with micronutrients. However, children's diets may supply inadequate amounts of vitamin D, iron, and zinc, especially if youngsters eat few or no rich food sources of these nutrients. Children who refuse to eat meat or who follow vegan diets may benefit from taking a children's multiple vitamin/mineral supplement. Regardless of one's age, taking nutrient supplements is no substitute for eating a varied and nutritious diet.

TABLE 13.9 *Popular Physical Activities for Children*

- Dancing
- Playing tag
- Jumping rope
- Biking
- Shooting hoops with a basketball
- Swimming
- Rollerblading
- Playing soccer or "kickball"
- Skateboarding

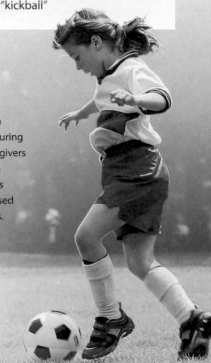

If children are not obtaining enough physical activity during the day, their caregivers can enroll them in after-school sports or community-based exercise programs.

Concept **Checkpoint**

23. Discuss how young children's eating patterns often change when they enter school.
24. Identify at least three health consequences of obesity during childhood.
25. How much physical activity is recommended for school-age children?
26. List at least three tips for improving diets of school-age children.

adolescence life stage in which a child matures physically into an adult

 # 13.6 Adolescence

Adolescence is the life stage in which a child matures physically into an adult. During adolescence, the reproductive organs increase in size and begin functioning properly. Furthermore, individuals attain their full height by the end of adolescence.[44] During this life stage, youth also develop emotionally, intellectually, and socially as they prepare for their adult roles.

Healthy adolescents learn to function independently of their adult caregivers. Thus, youths face a variety of lifestyle choices, including decisions regarding eating and physical activity habits. Such decisions often set the stage for the quality of their health in adulthood. For many teens, however, pressure to conform to fads and be influenced by other adolescents ("peer pressure") negatively affects their diets and overall health.

Puberty signals the end of childhood. Most boys begin puberty when they are between 10 and 12 years of age; most girls begin puberty between 8 and 10 years of age.[44] Puberty is a period characterized by dramatic physical changes, including increases in height and weight, known as the adolescent "growth spurt."

Most girls begin their growth spurt between 10 and 13 years of age. Boys begin their growth spurt later than girls—generally when they are between 12 and 15 years of age. Girls usually begin menstruating during their growth spurt. A girl's skeletal growth is almost complete about 2 years after her first menstrual period, whereas boys typically continue to gain stature until they are in their early twenties. The timing of puberty and growth spurts can vary widely, primarily due to genetic, environmental, and nutritional factors. Figure 13.14 shows a group of adolescents who are about the same age but are at different stages of physical maturity.

When their growth spurts begin, adolescents eat more to support their higher energy needs. If maturing boys and girls choose to eat nutritious foods and maintain a high level of physical activity, they can take advantage of their increased hunger and gain lean body mass without gaining excess body fat. The MyPlate food guide can provide the basis for healthy adolescents to plan nutritionally adequate meals and snacks (Table 13.10).

Figure 13.14 Different rates of physical maturity. Although these adolescents are about the same age, they are in different stages of physical maturity.

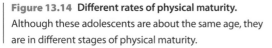

TABLE 13.10 *Adolescents: Daily Food Plan Based on MyPlate Recommendations*

Energy/ Food Group	Age/Sex 12–18 Years Girls	Age/Sex 12–13 Years Boys	Age/Sex 14 Years Boys	Age/Sex 15 Years Boys	Age/Sex 16–18 Years Boys
Kilocalories*	2000	2200	2400	2600	2800
Grains	6 oz	7 oz	8 oz	9 oz	10 oz
Vegetables	2.5 cups	3 cups	3 cups	3.5 cups	3.5 cups
Fruits	2 cups	2 cups	2 cups	2 cups	2.5 cups
Dairy	3 cups	3 cups	3 cups	3 cups	3 cups
Protein foods	5.5 oz	6 oz	6.5 oz	6.5 oz	7 oz

* Kilocalorie estimates are based on age, sex, and 30 to 60 minutes of physical activity. Source: U.S. Department of Agriculture: *MyPlate.* www.choosemyplate.gov/myplate/index.aspx. Accessed: August 5, 2011.

Did You Know?

Many teenagers are plagued by *acne*—pimples, blackheads, and reddening of the skin—that often occurs on the face, upper back, and chest. Many people think acne is caused by eating certain foods, especially greasy foods and chocolate. However, no scientific evidence links specific foods with acne. According to physicians who treat skin disorders (*dermatologists*), hormonal changes normally associated with puberty cause acne.[45]

Nutrition-Related Concerns of Adolescents

Many people establish their future eating habits and physical activity practices when they are teenagers. According to results of nationwide surveys, the majority of youth are not following recommendations of the Dietary Guidelines. In 2009, about 80% of high school students had not eaten fruits and vegetables five or more times/day and only about 14% of the students had consumed at least three glasses of milk/day during the 7 days preceding the survey.[46]

Adolescents whose diets rely heavily on energy-dense foods purchased at fast-food restaurants or vending machines may be setting the stage for the development of obesity, type 2 diabetes, heart disease, and other serious chronic diseases. Obesity, eating disorders, and low iron and calcium intakes are major nutrition-related concerns of adolescents. Youth, especially teenage girls, are at risk of developing disordered eating practices and eating disorders. You can learn more about eating disorders by reading the Chapter 10 "Highlight."

Obesity

In the United States, the prevalence of obesity is rising rapidly among adolescents. In 2007–2008, 18.1% of 12- to 19-year-old American youth were obese.[39] This figure is much higher than those obtained in similar surveys conducted between 1971–1974 and 1980 (Fig. 13.15). Compared to adolescents whose BMIs are in the healthy range, obese youth are more likely to mature into obese adults.

Although the prevalence of obesity has increased for all American children over the past few decades, rates vary among youngsters of different ethnic/racial groups. In 2007–2008, 14.5% of non-Hispanic white girls between 12 and 19 years of age were obese.[39] However, 17.4% of the Mexican-American girls and 29.2% of the black girls in this age group were obese. Mexican-American boys are more likely to obese than non-Hispanic white or black, non-Hispanic boys. Reasons for these disparities are unclear.

Physical inactivity contributes to overweight and obesity among adolescents. Teenagers need to perform at least 60 minutes of moderate-intensity physical activity at least 5 days/week.[43] According to results of the 2009 National Youth Risk Behavior Survey, 63% of the participants in the survey did not obtain recommended amounts of physical activity during 5 or more days of the week that preceded the survey.[46]

Many American teens spend much of their leisure time using a computer, playing video games, or watching television. In 2009, almost 25% of high school students

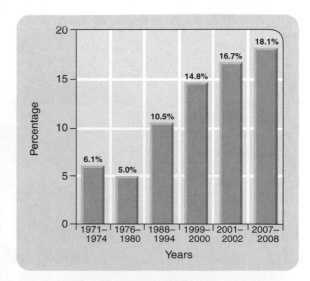

Figure 13.15 **Prevalence of obesity among American adolescents aged 12 to 19 years, for selected years 1971–1974 through 2007–2008.** In 2007–2008, the percentage of obesity among American children 12 to 19 years of age was much higher than the percentage obtained in similar national surveys conducted about 35 years earlier.

reported using a computer for purposes other than schoolwork, or playing video or computer games, for 3 or more hours/day during the week before the survey.[46] Furthermore, about 33% of the students watched television for 3 or more hours/day. Experts with the American Academy of Pediatrics recommend that teenagers limit their television and video use to no more than 2 hours daily.[41]

Excess Body Fat and Atherosclerosis   Although it is unusual for young adults to have heart attacks or strokes, the process of atherosclerosis begins in childhood and continues during adolescence.[47] High blood glucose, cholesterol, and blood pressure levels are major risk factors for atherosclerosis. The prevalence of type 2 diabetes and hypertension is increasing among obese American adolescents.[36, 48] Thus, medical experts are concerned that many overfat teenagers with type 2 diabetes, elevated blood cholesterol, or hypertension will develop atherosclerosis prematurely.

Weight Loss for Adolescents   In many cases, overweight teenagers who are experiencing their growth spurt do not need to lose weight because their lengthening skeletons eventually add inches to their height. However, these youth may need to slow their rate of weight gain, so they are less likely to be overfat when their skeletal growth stops. Before embarking on a weight-loss program, overfat teens should be evaluated by a physician to determine how much weight they should lose. After the assessment, the physician can refer the overweight or obese adolescent to a registered dietitian for specific help in planning a calorie-reduced diet.

Appropriate weight-loss diets for overfat teenagers should provide adequate amounts of essential nutrients while providing just enough energy to support normal growth. Caregivers and health professionals should encourage heavy teenagers to achieve gradual weight loss without relying on fad diets, disordered eating behaviors, or diet pills. To avoid regaining lost weight, formerly overfat teens must be motivated to continue practicing healthy eating habits and maintaining a high degree of physical activity for the rest of their lives.

Iron and Calcium Intakes

Adolescent boys may become iron deficient during their growth spurt because their iron intakes do not keep up with their bodies' needs for the mineral. Adolescent girls are also at risk of iron deficiency, especially if their diets lack iron-rich foods and they have heavy menstrual blood losses. Iron deficiency leads to increased fatigue and decreased ability to concentrate and learn. Teenagers need to understand why iron is important for good health and incorporate reliable food sources of the mineral in their diets (see Chapter 9). Over the last 20 years, many adolescents have switched from drinking milk to drinking soft drinks. Dietitians and other nutrition experts are concerned that many adolescents have inadequate calcium intakes because of this practice. Inadequate calcium intake during adolescence is associated with decreased bone mass and increased likelihood of bone fractures later in life. To encourage youth to consume adequate amounts of calcium, parents or other caregivers should explain the importance of the mineral to bone health and provide calcium-rich foods and beverages during meals and snacks. Adolescents should consume 3 cups/day of fat-free or low-fat milk or equivalent dairy products daily. Furthermore, teenagers need to be aware that physical activity can strengthen bones, whereas smoking cigarettes is a risk factor for *osteoporosis*, a condition characterized by loss of bone density. To learn more about this condition, see the "What Is Osteoporosis?" section of Chapter 9.

Vegetarianism

Some teenagers adopt vegetarian diets as a way of defining their identity and asserting independence from their caregivers. Although vegetarian diets can be healthy alternatives to the

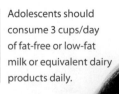

Adolescents should consume 3 cups/day of fat-free or low-fat milk or equivalent dairy products daily.

typical American diet, some youth use vegetarianism to mask disordered eating behaviors (see the Chapter 10 "Highlight").[49] When planning their diets, teenage vegans need to include foods that supply adequate amounts of calcium, iron, and zinc, and vitamins D and B-12. For information to help plan well-balanced, nutritionally adequate diets, teens can use the recommendations of the MyPlate food guide that are appropriate for their age, sex, and physical activity level. Chapter 7 discusses vegetarianism in more detail.

Concept **Checkpoint**

27. At what age does the adolescent growth spurt usually occur in boys? At what age does the growth spurt generally occur in girls?
28. Identify at least three health consequences that obese adolescents are likely to experience.
29. Why are intakes of iron and calcium important during adolescence?

 ## 13.7 Nutrition for Older Adults

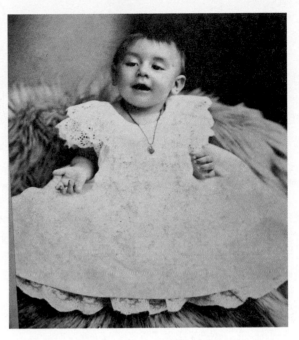

George John Blum of St. Louis, Missouri, circa 1900. In 1900, the life expectancy of a baby born in the United States was only 47 years.

In 1900, the life expectancy of a baby born in the United States was only 47 years. **Life expectancy** is the length of time a person born in a specific year, such as 1900, can expect to live. One hundred years ago, the top three leading causes of death for Americans were pneumonia, influenza, and other infectious diseases. By 2009, life expectancy in the United States rose to almost 80 years.[50] Major factors that contributed to increased life expectancy during the past century include improved diets, housing conditions, and public sanitation, as well as advances in medicine.

life expectancy length of time an average person born in a specific year can expect to live

According to the 2010 U.S. census, 13% of the U.S. population were 65 years of age or older when the census was conducted.[51] By 2050, government experts estimate that about 21% of Americans will be in this age group. Americans who are the "oldest old"—85 years of age or older—comprise one of the fastest-growing segments of the U.S. population. In 2000, 1.5% of Americans were in that age group. By 2010, 1.8% of the population were 85 years of age or older. By 2050, about 5% of Americans will be 85 years of age or older.

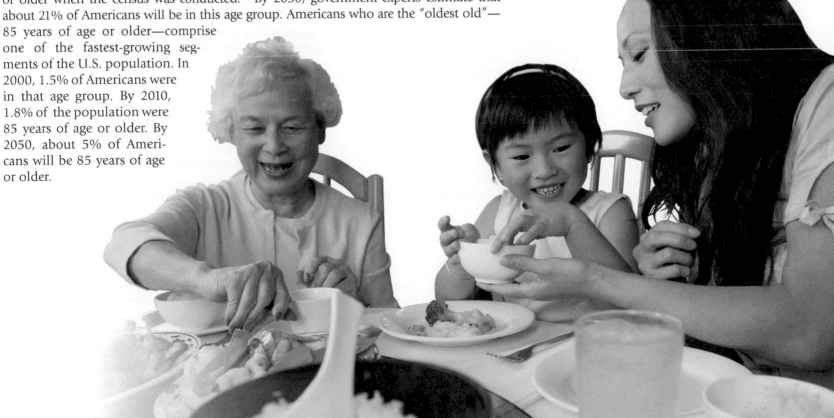

Although more Americans are living longer than their ancestors, they are not necessarily living well. Chronic diseases are among the leading causes of death in the United States (see Figure 1.3). These diseases are associated with lifestyles that include smoking, eating a poor diet, and being physically inactive.[52]

The Aging Process

The aging process begins at conception and is characterized by numerous predictable physical changes. By the time you are 65 years of age, you will have reached the final life stage, *older adulthood*. What causes people to age is unclear. Scientists who study the aging process have learned that cell structure and function inevitably decline with time, leading to many of the physiological changes shown in Table 13.11. Eventually, most cells lose the ability to regenerate their internal parts, and they die. As more and more cells in an organ die, the organ loses its functional capacity, and as a result, other organs fail and body systems are adversely affected. When this happens, the person soon dies. **Senescence** (*se-ness'-enz*) refers to declining organ functioning and increased vulnerability to disease that occurs after a person reaches physical maturity.

Extending the Human Life Span

Life span refers to the maximum number of years an organism such as a human can live. To date, the longest documented human life span is 122 years (Fig. 13.16). Some scientists think the human life span can be lengthened considerably just by making certain dietary changes. The Chapter 13 "Highlight" takes a closer look at the role of diet and longevity.

Growing old is a normal and natural process. Your body ages, regardless of dietary and other health-related practices you follow. Nevertheless, scientists have found a

senescence declining organ functioning and increased vulnerability

life span maximum number of years an organism can live

TABLE 13.11 *Aging: Normal Physiological Changes*

Body System	Changes
Digestive	Reduced saliva, gastric acid, and intrinsic factor secretion; increased heartburn and constipation
Skin, hair, and nails (integument)	Graying hair; drier skin and hair; skin loses elasticity and forms wrinkles; skin bruises easily
Musculoskeletal	Bone-forming cells become less active, resulting in bone loss that can lead to tooth loss and bones that fracture easily; fractures heal more slowly; joints become stiff and painful; muscle mass declines, resulting in loss of strength and stamina
Nervous	Decreased brain weight, reduced production of neurotransmitters, delayed transmission of nervous impulses, loss of short-term memory, and reduced sensory abilities (e.g., vision, hearing, smell, and taste)
Lymphatic (immune)	Reduced functioning resulting in increased vulnerability to cancer and infections
Circulatory	Hardening of the arteries, reduced cardiac output, increased risk of blood clots
Endocrine	Decreased production of reproductive, growth, and thyroid hormones
Respiratory	Reduced lung capacity, increased vulnerability to respiratory infections
Urinary	Increased loss of functional kidney cells, resulting in decreased blood filtration rate; loss of bladder control
Reproductive	Men: Decreased male hormone production and sperm count Women: Declining female hormone production, cessation of menstrual cycles, and loss of fertility

strong genetic component to human longevity. If you have ancestors who are very old or lived to be 90 years of age or more, you may have inherited "longevity genes." If your ancestors were not so fortunate, to some extent, you can control the rate at which you age. How? By making responsible healthy lifestyle decisions while you are still young, such as selecting a nutritious diet, exercising regularly, and avoiding tobacco. Your focus should not be simply on living longer but on living longer *and* healthier.

Older Adults: Common Nutrition-Related Concerns

Compared to younger persons, older adults have greater risk of nutritional deficiencies because of physiological changes associated with the normal aging process. Other factors that can influence an older person's nutritional status include illnesses, medications, low income, and lack of social support. Diets of older adults, particularly older women, often provide inadequate amounts of vitamins D, A, C, and B-12 and minerals such as calcium, iron, and zinc.[53] Results of a survey of over 1700 older adults indicated that subjects often failed to consume recommended amounts of grain and dairy products, vegetables, and fruits.[54] Furthermore, most subjects were overfat, with BMIs equal to or greater than 25. The following sections discuss some of the major health concerns that often affect the nutritional status of older adults. Some of these conditions have been discussed in previous chapters.

Changes in Body Weight

As the human body ages, its need for energy decreases.[1] In senescence, muscle mass declines as some muscle cells shrink or die. The loss of muscle mass leads to a decrease in muscular strength and basal metabolism. The aging body typically loses lean tissue and gains fat tissue. Increased body fat results from overeating and lack of physical activity, but even athletic men and lean women usually gain some central body fat after they are 50 years of age. Being overfat may increase the bone density of older adults and result in stronger bones,[55] but having too much body fat increases the risk of type 2 diabetes, hypertension, cardiovascular disease, and osteoarthritis. For more information about overweight and obesity, see Chapter 10.

People who are over 70 years of age are at risk of nutrient deficiencies, because their food intake tends to decrease as their metabolic rates and physical activity levels decline. Despite having lower energy needs, however, older adults need the same or even higher amounts of vitamins and minerals. Meeting micronutrient needs while eating less food can be difficult for older persons to accomplish.

After reaching 70 years of age, it is not unusual for people to lose some weight. Several factors can contribute to weight loss among older adults (Table 13.12). Elderly persons may eat less because they have lost the ability to taste and smell food. Loss of teeth and difficulty swallowing can also result in decreased food consumption. Declines in normal *cognitive* functioning (thought processes) resulting from conditions such as Alzheimer's disease or reduced blood flow to the brain can contribute to poor nutritional status. People who lack normal cognitive functioning may be unable to make decisions

TABLE 13.12 *Reduced Food Intake Among Older Adults: Contributing Factors*

- Reduced ability to taste and smell food
- Difficulty swallowing
- Loss of teeth
- Loss of normal cognitive function
- Lack of income
- Depression
- Reduced mobility and flexibility

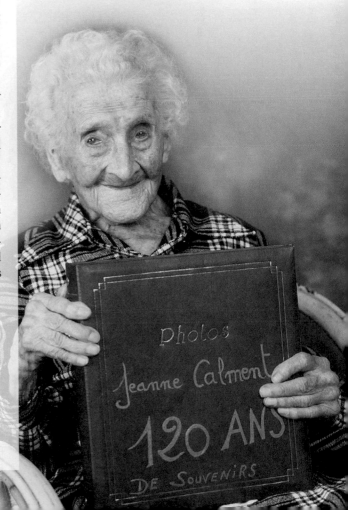

Figure 13.16 Oldest human being. When the French woman Jeanne Calment died in 1997 at 122 years of age, she was documented as the world's longest-living human being.

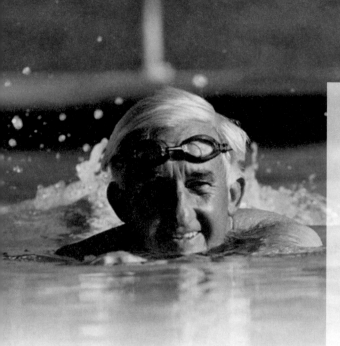

regarding planning nutritious meals, as well as to shop for and prepare food. Conditions that interfere with mobility and flexibility, such as arthritis and osteoporosis, can also interfere with food shopping and preparation activities. Social and economic factors often play a role in reduced food intake. Many older people live alone and on fixed incomes, circumstances that are associated with depression and inability to afford adequate amounts of nutritious food. In many instances, very old people refuse to eat and, as a result, lose considerable amounts of weight, a situation that hastens their death.

For older adults who find that food no longer tastes "good," adding more spices may improve the taste of food and, as a result, stimulate weak appetites. Efforts to make mealtimes social events, such as inviting friends to share potluck meals together, can enhance older adults' mental outlooks and spark their interest in eating. Older adults can increase or maintain their weight by consuming energy-dense snacks between meals, such as cheese, milkshakes, nuts, or oatmeal cookies. If weight loss becomes significant, a physician should be consulted to determine the cause.

Figure 13.17 **It's never too late.** Most older adults can benefit from performing aerobic and strength-training activities regularly.

Physical Inactivity

Many of the undesirable physical changes we associate with growing old are the result of a lifetime of physical inactivity. Regardless of a person's age, a physically active lifestyle increases muscle strength and mobility, improves balance, slows bone loss, and boosts emotional well-being. Most older adults can benefit from performing aerobic and strength-training activities regularly (Fig. 13.17). Before embarking on a program to increase physical fitness, however, sedentary older adults should consult their physicians concerning appropriate activities.

Did You Know?

You are never too old to gain some benefits from aerobic and strength-training exercise. Any form of physical activity, even performing household chores, can help extend an older person's longevity.[56]

Tooth Loss

In the 1950s, surveys of Americans indicated that the majority of older adults had lost all their natural teeth. Since then, the percentage of older adults who retain all or most of their teeth has increased in the United States. Adults should have 28 natural teeth. In 2007–2009, about 8% of Americans who were 18 years of age or older had lost all of their teeth.[57] Moreover, approximately 25% of Americans who were 65 years or older had lost all their natural teeth. Tooth loss is related to long-term poor dental hygiene, cigarette smoking, and poor dietary practices. By following recommended dental hygiene practices, obtaining regular dental care, and avoiding tobacco use, you can greatly increase your chances of keeping most of your teeth as you age.

Excessive tooth loss can lead to faulty eating habits. People who lack teeth often avoid crisp or chewy foods, such as fresh fruits, vegetables, whole-grain cereals, and meat. According to results of an 8-year study involving nearly 32,000 men, subjects who had lost all or several teeth consumed less dietary fiber, vitamin E, and polyunsaturated fat than those who had maintained most of their teeth.[58] Although dentures that replace natural teeth can enable some people to chew normally, many older adults do not like to wear them because they can be uncomfortable. When a person has difficulty chewing food, serving soft foods such as ground meats, cooked vegetables, pureed fruits, and puddings can stimulate the individual's appetite.

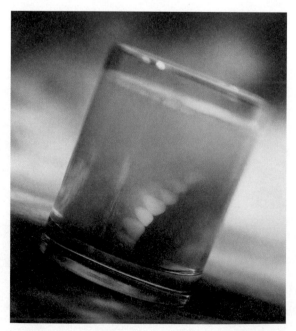

Although dentures that replace natural teeth can enable some people to chew normally, many older adults do not like to wear them because they can be uncomfortable.

Intestinal Tract Problems

Constipation is a major complaint of older adults. By increasing their intakes of fiber-rich foods, such as whole-grain products and vegetables, older adults may be able to have more regular bowel movements (see the "Fiber" section of Chapter 5). Dehydration contributes to constipation, so older persons should make sure their fluid intake is adequate.

As a person ages, his or her stomach secretes less hydrochloric acid (HCl) and intrinsic factor. These changes can contribute to poor absorption of vitamin B-12 and the development of vitamin B-12 deficiency and pernicious anemia. Older adults may be able to meet their vitamin B-12 needs by eating foods fortified with the micronutrient or taking vitamin B-12 supplements. Some older adults, however, must take injections of the B vitamin to prevent pernicious anemia (see Chapter 8). Older persons are also at risk of iron deficiency because reduced stomach acid production may hinder iron absorption. Furthermore, many older adults take aspirin regularly, and this practice can cause intestinal bleeding that can lead to iron deficiency anemia. Intestinal ulcers and cancer can also cause blood loss from the digestive tract. The discovery of blood in bowel movements needs to be reported to a physician—regardless of one's age.

Many older adults take one or more prescription drugs daily. Although such medications can improve health and quality of life of elderly persons, some drugs interfere with the body's absorption and/or use of certain nutrients. Additionally, older adults often take one or more dietary supplements regularly. According to results of a national survey conducted in 2005–2006, about 55% of women and 43% of men aged 57 through 87 years reported that they currently used at least one dietary supplement regularly.[59] Nutrient supplements, such as multivitamin/multimineral supplements, were the most widely used type of dietary supplement. Certain dietary supplements, including herbal products, can reduce or amplify the effects of prescribed medications. Therefore, older adults should notify their physicians about their use of all dietary supplements. A few foods also interfere with prescribed drugs. Grapefruit juice, for example, can alter the potency of certain medications that are used to lower blood pressure or cholesterol.

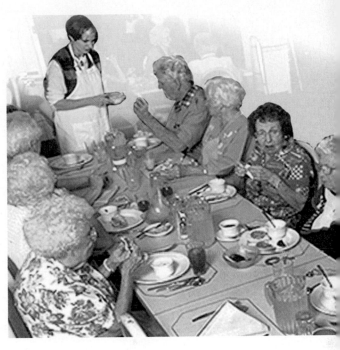

Older adults dining together at senior apartments in Nevada City, California.

Depression in Older Adults

In 2006, 18% of women and 10% of men age 65 and over reported having symptoms of depression.[60] Situations that contribute to depression among the elderly population include coping with chronic illness or loss of mobility, and isolation and loneliness as family members and friends die or move away. If the depressed person loses interest in cooking and eating, weight loss and nutrient deficiencies are likely to occur. In many instances,

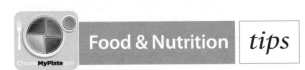

Food & Nutrition *tips*

The following suggestions can help caregivers improve nutrient intakes of elderly persons:

- Emphasize nutrient-dense foods when planning daily menus.
- Try new foods, seasonings, and ways of preparing foods.
- Have easy-to-prepare nutrient-dense foods on hand for times when the older person is too tired to cook large meals.
- Serve meals in well-lit or sunny areas, and plan appealing meals by using foods with different flavors, colors, shapes, textures, and smells.
- Plan occasions for the older adult to share cooking responsibilities and eat meals with friends or relatives.
- Encourage the older person to eat at a senior center whenever possible. Investigate community resources for helping the older adult obtain groceries, cook, or manage other daily care needs.
- Encourage the older adult to be physically active.
- If biting and chewing are difficult for an elderly person, chop, grind, or blend tough or crisp foods.
- Prepare extra amounts of soup, stew, or casserole, so leftovers can be frozen for future meals.

TABLE 13.13 *Daily Food Plan Based on MyPlate Recommendations for Healthy Persons Aged 70 Years*

Energy/Food Group	Females (5' 5", 130 lb)	Males (5' 7", 150 lb)
Kilocalories*	1800	2200
Grains	6 oz	7 oz
Vegetables	2.5 cups	3 cups
Fruits	1.5 cups	2 cups
Dairy	3 cups	3 cups
Protein foods	5 oz	6 oz

* Based on 30 to 60 minutes of physical activity.

depression can be managed with medication, but social support and psychological counseling may be necessary as well. Without proper treatment, depressed persons are at risk of alcoholism and suicide. In fact, you may be surprised to learn that suicide rates of American men 75 years of age and older are higher than rates for men of other age groups.[61]

Dietary Planning in Older Adulthood

MyPlate can provide the basis for planning nutritionally adequate meals and snacks for healthy older adults (Table 13.13). However, amounts of foods recommended in these diet plans may not provide enough vitamin D and vitamin B-12 for elderly persons. By regularly consuming fortified and/or enriched foods, older adults can increase their intakes of these micronutrients. In many instances, older adults can also benefit from taking a daily multiple vitamin/mineral supplement.

Friends, relatives, and health care personnel should be alert for indications of poor nutrient intakes among older people, especially those who are at risk and live in nursing homes or other long-term care facilities. For example, family members can make sure the older adult's nutrient needs are met by visiting the person's residence during mealtimes, observing the foods that are offered, and, if necessary, helping the older adult eat. Additionally, monitoring the elderly individual's weight can indicate whether long-term food intake has been adequate. Older adults who live at home may need help planning nutritionally adequate diets. In these instances, registered dietitians can be consulted to provide personalized dietary advice.

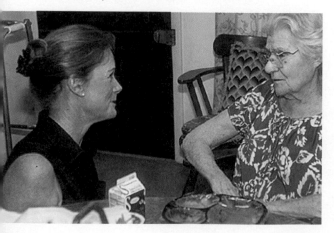

Figure 13.18 Meals on Wheels. Many communities in the United States offer the Meals on Wheels program in which volunteers deliver nutritious meals prepared at a senior center to qualified, homebound older adults.

Community Nutrition Services for Older Adults

In the United States, most large communities offer special nutrition programs for independent-living older adults, such as congregate meals and home-delivered meals. The home-delivered meal program may be called Meals on Wheels if it is sponsored by the local private or public agencies (Fig. 13.18). The Chapter 1 "Highlight" provides more information about these popular community-based nutrition services for older adults.

You can obtain information regarding locally available nutrition services for older people from medical clinics, private practitioners, hospitals, and health maintenance organizations in your area. To learn more about nutrition-related programs for older adults, visit the following websites: National Institute on Aging, www.nia.nih.gov/; American Geriatrics Society, www.americangeriatrics.org/; and Administration on Aging, www. aoa.gov/.

Concept **Checkpoint**

30. What is the difference between life expectancy and life span?

31. Identify at least five physiological changes that are associated with the normal aging process.

32. Explain why nutrient needs for older adults are often higher than those for younger persons.

33. List at least four nutrients that are often lacking in diets of older adults.

34. Suggest at least three ways caregivers can improve nutrient intakes of older persons.

35. What is Meals on Wheels?

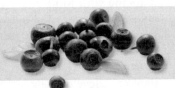

Chapter 13 Highlight

IN SEARCH OF THE FOUNTAIN

In 1513, Spanish explorer Juan Ponce de León (Fig. 13.19) sailed to the southeastern coastal region of North America and discovered an area he named "Land of Flowers" (Florida). Ponce de León was on a mission to find gold, but he was also eager to locate a natural spring that supposedly had magical powers. According to Native-Americans in the area, elderly people who drank the spring's water regained their youthful looks and vigor. Unfortunately, Ponce de León never found gold or the mythical "fountain of youth" in Florida. Nevertheless, many older adults still seek ways to combat aging, especially by taking certain hormones and dietary supplements promoted for their age-defying properties. Older Americans spend considerable amounts of money on such products, some of which may be harmful in the long run.[62] Promoters of antiaging formulas or therapies claim their treatments can stop, and even reverse, the process of aging. Is there any reliable scientific evidence to support claims that you can take something to stay young longer?

Claims that a nutritional fountain of youth exists are simply not true. Currently, scientific evidence does not support the use of antiaging therapies that include taking megadoses of vitamins or dietary supplements that contain *DHEA* (*dehydroepiandrosterone*). In the United States, DHEA is classified as a dietary supplement, but the substance is produced by the body and has hormonal activity. Levels of DHEA decline steadily through adulthood, and some of the changes associated with the aging process, such as weight gain, dry skin, reduced muscle mass, and decreased bone density, are thought to be associated with reductions of the hormone in the body. However, more long-term research is needed to

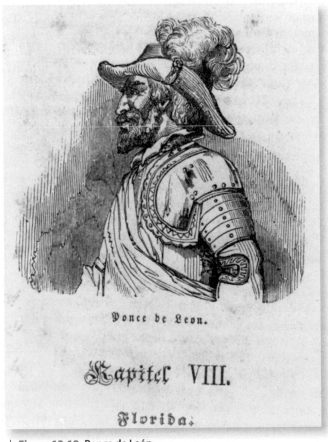

| **Figure 13.19** Ponce de León.

determine whether the DHEA hormone replacement can provide some health benefits to aging persons.[63] At this point, there is no way to prevent aging from following its natural course in humans.[64] Nevertheless, researchers are conducting experiments to better understand the process of aging and the keys to longevity.

According to *biogerontologists,* scientists who study the biology of aging, longevity results from the body's ability to maintain and repair the damage done by a lifetime of exposure to the environment and the effects of everyday "wear and tear."[65] Some multicellular organisms are able to live longer when they can improve their abilities to repair damage to their DNA, reduce the toxicity of free radicals, and replace nonfunctioning cells. Antioxidants reduce the toxic effects of free radicals (see Chapter 8), and organisms produce a variety of antioxidants to control free radical production. In scientific laboratories, a species of tiny flies commonly called "fruit flies" had their genes for antioxidant synthesis modified by genetic engineering. As a result, these fruit flies lived longer than nongenetically modified fruit flies.[66] Although the genetically engineered flies provide intriguing evidence that it is possible to extend the normal life expectancy of an organism by modifying its DNA, the production of a genetically engineered human being raises numerous ethical concerns.

One area of biogerontological research that shows some promise is the use of *calorie restriction (CR)* to extend longevity. Since the 1930s, scientists have studied the effects of CR on the health and life spans of various species of multicellular organisms. According to the research findings, CR can increase life spans of various organisms, including rodents, fish, flies, and worms.[67] Despite the growing body of scientific evidence, researchers do not fully understand how CR enhances longevity. Moreover, there are no long-term studies that examine the effects of consuming a high-quality but calorie-restricted diet in humans.

In a 6-month study involving 48 healthy men, subjects who followed a nutritious but very low-calorie diet (about 900 kcal/day) experienced reductions in body temperature, fasting insulin levels, and signs of reduced DNA damage.[68] These physiological adaptations to such calorie-restricted diets may be biological indicators of a lengthening human life span, but at present, no one is certain of their significance.

Some scientists hypothesize that prolonged CR is not necessary for achieving life-extending benefits. In a small study of 16 nonobese adults, participants fasted every other day for 3 weeks.[69] Results of this study indicated that the subjects lost weight and total body fat, but they did not develop most of the physiological changes associated with lengthening the life span. Furthermore, the subjects reported being hungry on fasting days, indicating people may be unlikely to follow the diet for the long run. Even if scientists provide evidence that any form of CR adds some years to the human life span, would you be interested in reducing your food intake to such a drastic extent? How enjoyable would your life be if you ate only 900 kcal daily? What is important to you—how long you can live, or how *well* you live?

The science of biogerontology is still in its beginning stages; researchers have much to learn about the aging process before they can develop safe ways to enhance longevity. We already know that you can reduce your risk of dying prematurely from chronic diseases such as heart disease, hypertension, type 2 diabetes, and many forms of cancer by adopting healthy lifestyles. Rather than wait until the fountain of youth becomes a reality, you can take charge of your health now by consuming a nutritionally adequate diet, obtaining regular moderate- to vigorous-intensity physical activity, maintaining a healthy weight, avoiding tobacco products, limiting your alcohol consumption, and having regular physical checkups.

CHAPTER REFERENCES

See Appendix I.

SUMMARY

The leading causes of death for Americans are chronic diseases—heart disease, cancer, and stroke. Lifestyles, especially dietary practices and physical activity patterns, contribute to the development of these chronic conditions. Other factors that influence a person's overall health include heredity, relationships, environment, income, education level, and access to health care.

Embryonic/fetal life is characterized by rapid rates of cell division, resulting in a dramatic increase in cell numbers. The first trimester of pregnancy is a critical stage in human development because inadequate or excessive nutrient intakes as well as exposure to toxic compounds can have devastating effects on the embryo/fetus during this period. The placenta is the organ of pregnancy that transfers nutrients and oxygen from the mother's bloodstream to her embryo/fetus. The placenta also transfers wastes from the embryo/fetus to the mother's bloodstream so her body can eliminate them. Infectious agents and harmful chemicals can pass through the placenta, enter the embryo/fetus, and cause disease, birth defects, or embryonic/fetal death.

Women of childbearing age should take steps to ensure they are in good health prior to becoming pregnant. During pregnancy, the woman's body undergoes various physiological changes. These changes enable her body to nourish and maintain the developing fetus, as well as to produce milk for her infant after its birth. A pregnant woman should follow a diet that meets her own nutritional needs as well as those of her developing offspring. During the second and third trimester, the pregnant woman's energy needs increase beyond her prepregnancy energy requirement. Additionally, needs for certain vitamins and minerals increase during pregnancy. The mother-to-be can use MyPlate to develop nutritionally adequate daily menus, but she may also need to take a prenatal vitamin/mineral supplement.

Women whose prepregnancy weights were within the healthy range can expect to gain 25 to 35 pounds during pregnancy. Women who gain excess weight during pregnancy may retain the extra weight long after delivery. Most women gain up to 4 pounds during the first trimester; they gain 3 to 4 pounds each month during the second and third trimesters.

Monitoring weight gain is an important aspect of prenatal care. Rapid weight gain, especially after the fifth month of pregnancy, could be a sign of pregnancy-induced hypertension (PIH). Underweight women who do not gain enough weight during pregnancy are at risk of having preterm or low-birth-weight infants. Obese women have greater risk of developing hypertension and type 2 diabetes during pregnancy. However, women should not try to lose weight while they are pregnant.

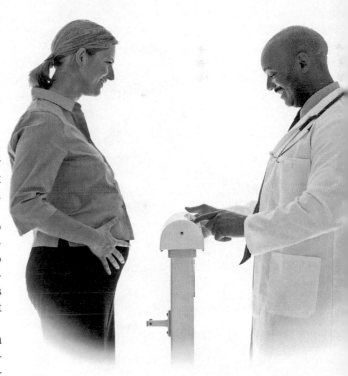

Breast milk is the best first food for infants because it is uniquely formulated to meet the nutrient needs of a newborn human being. Furthermore, human milk contains biologically active substances that help an infant's immune system. Compared to babies who are not breastfed, breastfed infants have lower risks of allergies and of gastrointestinal, respiratory tract, and ear infections. Women who breastfeed their babies can also derive some important benefits from the practice, such as losing extra fat gained during pregnancy.

Prolactin stimulates the development of milk-producing tissue in the breasts of a pregnant woman. After delivery, this hormone stimulates milk production. When an infant suckles, nerves in the nipple signal the mother's brain to release prolactin and oxytocin into her bloodstream. Oxytocin is necessary for the let-down reflex and causes the uterus to contract. Milk production relies on "supply and demand." If the breasts are not emptied fully, milk production soon ceases. To support milk production, the lactating mother needs about 400 to 500 extra kilocalories daily.

Growth is very rapid during infancy; birth weight doubles in 4 to 6 months, and length increases by 50% in the first year. Health care practitioners can assess growth in infants and children by measuring body weight, height (or length), and head circumference over time. For the first 6 months, the infant's nutrient needs can be met by human milk or iron-fortified infant formula. Breastfed babies need vitamin D and possibly iron and fluoride supplements.

Most infants do not need solid foods before 6 months of age. At this age, the child's GI tract can digest complex foods, the baby can sit up with support, he or she no longer has the extrusion reflex, and the risk of developing food allergies has decreased. The first solid food offered to babies should be an iron-fortified infant cereal. Other foods should be added one at a time, and the child should be observed for allergy signs and symptoms. Whole cow's milk should not be fed to babies until they are 1 year of age.

It is normal for a preschooler's appetite to decline as the child's growth rate tapers off. Additionally, it is not unusual for preschool children to be "picky eaters" or embark

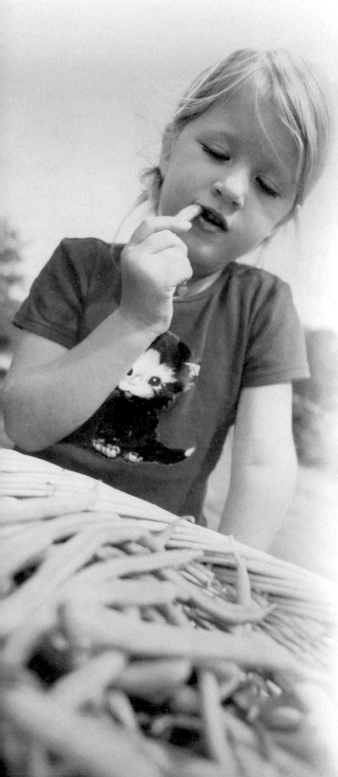

on "food jags." Caregivers should avoid nagging, forcing, and bribing children to eat but instead offer a variety of healthy food choices and allow the child to choose what and how much to eat. Nutrition-related problems that often affect preschool children are iron deficiency, dental caries, obesity, and food allergies.

School-age children often skip breakfast, and they tend to consume more foods away from home, larger portions of food, and more fried foods and sweetened beverages. Children who eat breakfast are more likely to have better diets and healthier body weights than children who skip this meal. Diets of many school-age children fail to supply recommended amounts of calcium and potassium while providing too much sodium.

Public health experts are very concerned about the increasing prevalence of obesity among children in the United States. Overfat children have higher risks of elevated blood pressure, cholesterol, and glucose levels than children whose weights are within the healthy range. Overfat children may also have higher risk of hypertension, heart disease, and type 2 diabetes later in life. Such children are also more likely to have low self-esteem and become obese as adults.

A young child matures physically into an adult during adolescence. Adolescents face a variety of lifestyle choices, including decisions regarding eating and physical activity habits. For many teens, pressure to conform to fads and be influenced by other adolescents negatively affects their diets and overall health. Obesity, eating disorders, and low iron and calcium intakes are major nutrition-related concerns of adolescents.

The aging process is characterized by numerous predictable physical changes. Senescence refers to declining organ functioning and increased vulnerability to disease that occurs after a person reaches physical maturity. Aging is not a disease, and diseases that often accompany old age are not an inevitable aspect of aging. Many of the chronic ailments that are associated with senescence can be managed, delayed, and even prevented. Although genetics play a role in determining longevity, lifestyle practices and environmental conditions influence a person's rate of aging. People may be able to live longer and healthier by making responsible healthy lifestyle decisions while they are still young.

Compared to younger persons, older adults have greater risk of nutritional deficiencies because of physiological changes associated with the normal aging process. Other factors that can influence an older person's nutritional status include illnesses, tooth loss, medications, low income, depression, and lack of social support. Diets of older adults, particularly older women, often provide inadequate amounts of vitamins D, A, C, and B-12 and minerals such as calcium, iron, and zinc. Friends, relatives, and health care personnel should be alert for indications of poor nutrient intakes among older people, especially those who live in nursing homes or other long-term care facilities.

According to biogerontologists, longevity results from the body's ability to maintain and repair the damage done by a lifetime of exposure to the environment and the effects of everyday "wear and tear." Little credible scientific evidence exists to support the use of antiaging therapies that include taking hormones or megadoses of vitamins and antioxidants. At this point, there is no way to prevent aging from following its natural course in humans. Nevertheless, researchers are conducting experiments to better understand the process of aging and the keys to longevity.

Recipes for Healthy Living

Homemade Applesauce

It takes a little bit of work, but once you've eaten homemade applesauce, you're unlikely to eat commercially prepared applesauce again. This version has no added sugar, salt, or spices and is suitable for infants to eat. If you're not making the sauce for a baby, you may want to add a dash of cinnamon to it. You'll need a 2-quart saucepan with a lid and a strainer.

To make applesauce for a baby, cook the apples and strain the sauce. Spoon it into a clean ice cube tray, tightly cover the tray with a freezer plastic bag, and place in freezer. Whenever you want to feed your baby some applesauce, just pop one of the cubes out of the tray and heat it gently in a small saucepan. Apricots, pears, and peaches can be substituted for apples. This recipe makes approximately eight ice cube-sized servings. Each serving supplies approximately 36 kcal, 3.2 mg vitamin C, 74 mg potassium, and 1.6 g fiber.

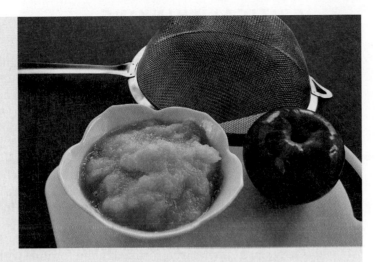

INGREDIENTS:

4 medium apples
(2¾" diam.), preferably
Jonathan apples
2 Tbsp water

PREPARATION STEPS:

1. Wash apples in warm water.

2. Peel skin from apples.

3. Cut small pieces of apple away from the core, avoiding any seeds, and place the fruit in a saucepan.

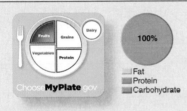

4. Add water to saucepan. Cover the saucepan with its lid and cook on high heat for about 2 minutes.

5. Reduce heat to simmer, and cook fruit for about 10 minutes. Stir occasionally with a large spoon, mashing the fruit.

6. Place strainer over a small bowl. Spoon cooked fruit into the strainer and mash it through the strainer. If sauce is lumpy, return it to the strainer and repeat the straining process.

7. Serve the applesauce while warm, or cover and refrigerate it. You can also freeze the sauce in an ice cube tray as described previously.

Vegetable Dip

You can make low-fat versions of fruit or vegetable dips by replacing sour cream or mayonnaise in recipes with plain, low-fat yogurt. This vegetable dip recipe makes approximately five ¼-cup servings of dip. Each serving provides approximately 46 kcal, 3 g protein, 2 g fat, 90 mg calcium, 160 mg sodium, and 120 mg potassium

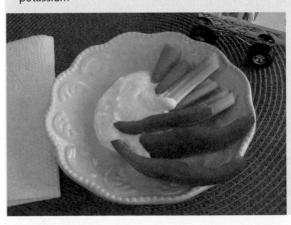

INGREDIENTS:

1 cup plain, low-fat yogurt
3 Tbsp calorie-reduced ranch dressing
¼ tsp curry powder (optional)

PREPARATION STEPS:

1. In a small bowl, combine yogurt with the dressing and stir until well blended.

2. Refrigerate until ready to serve.

3. Serve chilled in a bowl that is surrounded with fresh pieces of raw vegetables.

4. Discard any remaining dip.

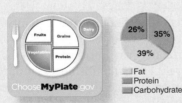

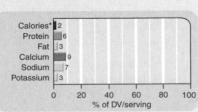

CRITICAL THINKING

1. One of your friends just found out that she is pregnant. Although her BMI is within the healthy range, she is concerned about gaining too much weight during pregnancy. What advice would you provide concerning the need to gain some weight during this life stage? If your friend's prepregnancy weight was 125 pounds, how much weight would be appropriate for her to gain during pregnancy?

2. Your pregnant friend wants your advice concerning whether she should breastfeed or formula-feed her baby. After reading Chapter 13, what information would you provide to help your friend decide to breastfeed?

3. Olivia is a healthy 2-month-old baby. Olivia's mother, Kara, wants to replace Olivia's iron-fortified infant formula with the same fresh fluid 2% milk that she drinks. What advice would you give to Kara concerning the appropriateness of making such a decision?

4. Marcus is 3 years old and his BMI is in the overweight range. His caregivers are also overweight, but they seem to be concerned about Marcus's excess body weight. What advice would you provide his caregivers to help Marcus achieve a healthy BMI?

5. Are your parents, grandparents, and great-grandparents still alive? If any of your ancestors died before they were 60 years of age, can you identify their causes of death and factors that contributed to their deaths? What lifestyle changes can you make now that can help you achieve a longer, healthier lifetime?

6. Use MyPlate to design a day's menu for a 70-year-old woman who obtains 30 to 60 minutes of physical activity daily.

PRACTICE TEST

Select the best answer.

1. The embryo/fetus develops most of its organs during the
   a. preconception period.
   b. first trimester.
   c. second trimester.
   d. third trimester.

2. The placenta cannot
   a. transfer nutrients from the mother's bloodstream to the embryo/fetus.
   b. eliminate waste products from the embryo/fetus.
   c. prevent all toxic substances from reaching the embryo/fetus.
   d. transfer oxygen from the mother's bloodstream to the embryo/fetus.

3. During the first trimester, a pregnant woman's daily energy requirement is _____ her daily energy needs before she became pregnant.
   a. 300 kcal lower than
   b. about the same as
   c. 300 kcal higher than
   d. 500 kcal higher than

4. Women with prepregnancy weights within the healthy range should gain _____ during pregnancy.
   a. 10–20 pounds
   b. 20–25 pounds
   c. 25–35 pounds
   d. 35–50 pounds

5. Preeclampsia is a form of _____ that can develop during pregnancy.
   a. hypertension
   b. diabetes
   c. hypertriglyceridemia
   d. anemia

6. Which of the following statements is true?
   a. A woman's energy needs are higher during the first trimester than at any other time in pregnancy.
   b. Using infant formula to bottle-feed a baby is more convenient and less expensive than breastfeeding a baby.
   c. Oxytocin is necessary for the "let-down" reflex to occur.
   d. The American Pediatric Association recommends feeding fresh whole milk to infants when they are 6 months of age.

7. A healthy infant who weighs 6.5 pounds at birth can be expected to weigh _____ pounds by her first birthday.
   a. 13.0
   b. 16.5
   c. 19.5
   d. 23.5

8. Breastfed infants are _____ than babies who are fed infant formula.
   a. more likely to have diarrhea
   b. less likely to have cystic fibrosis
   c. more likely to have respiratory infections
   d. less likely to have ear infections

9. Infants are physically ready to start eating solid foods when they are _____ of age.
    a. 4 to 6 weeks
    b. 4 to 6 months
    c. 6 to 12 months
    d. 12 to 14 months

10. Pediatricians often recommend ____ as the first solid food offered to an infant.
    a. iron-fortified infant rice cereal
    b. mixed baby food dinners
    c. French fries
    d. cooked egg whites

11. Which of the following foods is not a common source of food allergens?
    a. peanuts
    b. eggs
    c. milk
    d. applesauce

12. Which of the following factors is associated with increased risk of obesity during childhood?
    a. having a family history of obesity
    b. eating 3 to 5 servings of fresh fruit daily
    c. being a low-birth-weight infant
    d. All of the above are correct.

13. Which of the following factors can influence an older person's nutritional status?
    a. illnesses
    b. medications
    c. income level
    d. All of the above are correct.

Answers to Chapter 13 Quiz *Yourself*

1. During pregnancy, a mother-to-be should double her food intake because she's "eating for two." **False.** (p. 472)

2. The natural size of a woman's breasts is not a factor in determining her ability to breastfeed her baby. **True.** (p. 479)

3. Experts with the American Academy of Pediatrics recommend adding solid foods to the infant's diet within the first month after a baby is born. **False.** (p. 483)

4. Over the past 35 years, the prevalence of obesity has increased among American school-age children. **True.** (p. 492)

5. Compared to younger persons, older adults have lower risks of nutritional deficiencies. **False.** (p. 499)

14. Which of the following practices has been scientifically shown to extend the human life span?
    a. taking antioxidant supplements
    b. eating a high-protein diet
    c. performing vigorous physical exercise
    d. None of the above is correct.

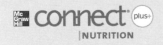

Additional resources related to the features of this book are available on ConnectPlus® Nutrition. Ask your instructor how to get access.

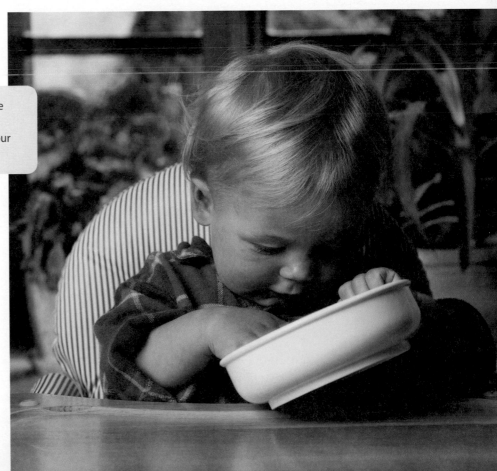

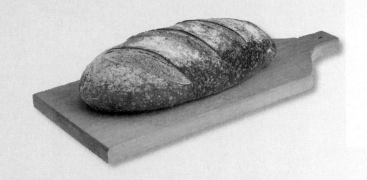

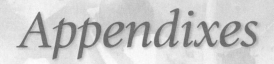

Appendixes

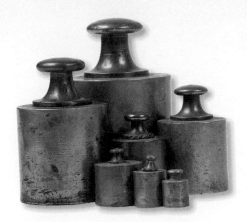

English-Metric Conversions and Metric-to-Household Units

English-Metric Conversions

Length

English (USA)	Metric
inch (in)	= 2.54 cm, 25.4 mm
foot (ft)	= 0.30 m, 30.48 cm
yard (yd)	= 0.91 m, 91.4 cm
mile (statute) (5280 ft)	= 1.61 km, 1609 m
mile (nautical) (6077 ft, 1.15 statute mi)	= 1.85 km, 1850 m

Metric	English (USA)
millimeter (mm)	= 0.039 in (thickness of a dime)
centimeter (cm)	= 0.39 in
meter (m)	= 3.28 ft, 39.4 in
kilometer (km)	= 0.62 mi, 1091 yd, 3273 ft

Weight

English (USA)	Metric
grain	= 64.80 mg
ounce (oz)	= 28.35 g
pound (lb)	= 453.60 g, 0.45 kg
ton (short—2000 lb)	= 0.91 metric ton (907 kg)

Metric	English (USA)
milligram (mg)	= 0.002 grain (0.000035 oz)
gram (g)	= 0.04 oz ($^1/_{28}$ of an oz)
kilogram (kg)	= 35.27 oz, 2.20 lb
metric ton (1000 kg)	= 1.10 tons

Volume

English (USA)	Metric
cubic inch	= 16.39 cc
cubic foot	= 0.03 m^3
cubic yard	= 0.765 m^3
teaspoon (tsp)	= 5 ml
tablespoon (tbsp)	= 15 ml
fluid ounce	= 0.03 liter (30 ml)*
cup (c)	= 237 ml
pint (pt)	= 0.47 liter
quart (qt)	= 0.95 liter
gallon (gal)	= 3.79 liters

Metric	English (USA)
milliliter (ml)	= 0.03 oz
liter (L)	= 2.12 pt
liter	= 1.06 qt
liter	= 0.27 gal

1 liter ÷ 1000 = 1 milliliter or 1 cubic centimeter (10^{-3} liter)*
1 liter ÷ 1,000,000 = 1 microliter (10^{-6} liter)

*1 ml = 1 cc

Metric and Other Common Units

Unit/Abbreviation	Other Equivalent Measure
milligram/mg	$^1/_{1000}$ of a gram
microgram/µg	$^1/_{1,000,000}$ of a gram
deciliter/dl	$^1/_{10}$ of a liter (about ½ cup)
milliliter/ml	$^1/_{1000}$ of a liter (5 ml is about 1 tsp)
International Unit/IU	Crude measure of vitamin activity generally based on growth rate seen in animals

Fahrenheit-Celsius Conversion Scale

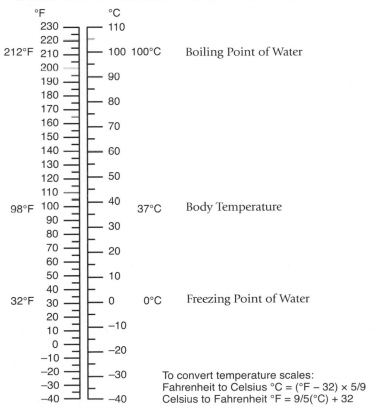

212°F — 100 100°C — Boiling Point of Water
98°F — 37°C — Body Temperature
32°F — 0°C — Freezing Point of Water

To convert temperature scales:
Fahrenheit to Celsius °C = (°F − 32) × 5/9
Celsius to Fahrenheit °F = 9/5(°C) + 32

Household Units

3 teaspoons	= 1 tablespoon
4 tablespoons	= ¼ cup
5⅓ tablespoons	= ⅓ cup
8 tablespoons	= ½ cup
10⅔ tablespoons	= ⅔ cup
16 tablespoons	= 1 cup
1 tablespoon	= ½ fluid ounce

1 cup	= 8 fluid ounces
1 cup	= ½ pint
2 cups	= 1 pint
4 cups	= 1 quart
2 pints	= 1 quart
4 quarts	= 1 gallon

Appendix B
Canada's Food Guide

The information in this appendix includes advice on dietary patterns, as well as regulations that apply to food labeling. Previous *Recommended Nutrient Intakes* (*RNIs*) for nutrients have been replaced by the Dietary Reference Intakes (DRIs) that apply to Canadian and U.S. citizens. These are listed on the inside back cover. Both Canadian and American scientists worked on the various DRI committees, coming up with a set of harmonized Dietary Reference Intakes for both countries.

Summary of the Nutrition Recommendations for Canadians

The Canadian federal department responsible for helping Canadians maintain and improve their health is Health Canada. The Office of Nutrition Policy and Promotion is within the Health Products and Food Branch of Health Canada and focuses on nutrition. Health Canada's National Dietary Guidance programs have been in existence since the 1930s and have always relied on scientific and other related evidence. Since 1977, a pattern of eating that meets nutrient needs and reduces the risk of chronic diseases has been promoted. In the 1990s, dietary guidance included *Canada's Guidelines for Healthy Eating* and *Food Guide to Healthy Eating* as well as *Nutrition for a Healthy Pregnancy* and *Nutrition for Healthy Term Infants*. The *Recommended Nutrient Intakes* (*RNI*), a Canadian version of the RDA, was published in 1990.

In 1995, the U.S. Institutes of Medicine (IOM) brought together Canadian and American scientists to work on various committees that came up with a set of harmonized Dietary Reference Intakes for both countries. The DRIs replaced the previous RNIs, and a new set of recommendations (EAR, AI, RDA, UL) similar to those in the United States were adopted in Canada. Adoption of the DRIs in Canada led to a review and subsequent revision of *Canada's Food Guide to Healthy Eating* and *Guidelines for Healthy Eating*.

The revised *Canada's Food Guide* (Fig. B.1) was released in early 2007. The basic message to Canadians is to "Eat Well" with *Canada's Food Guide*. Learning more about *Canada's Food Guide* will help Canadians know how much food they need, what types of foods are better for them, and the importance of physical activity in their day.

In addition, if Canadians have the amount and type of food recommended and follow the tips included in *Canada's Food Guide*, this will help them:

- Meet their needs for vitamins, minerals, and other nutrients.

- Reduce their risk of obesity, type 2 diabetes, heart disease, certain types of cancer, and osteoporosis.

- Contribute to their overall health and vitality.

Canada's Food Guide (Fig. B.1) places foods into four groups: vegetables and fruits; grain products; milk and alternatives; and meat and alternatives. *Canada's Food Guide* also includes information on the recommended number of Food Guide Servings per day, examples of what one Food Guide Serving consists of, and how to make each Food Guide Serving count within each food group (Fig. B.2). Recommendations are also included about the types and amounts of

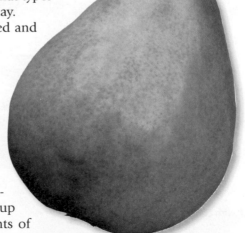

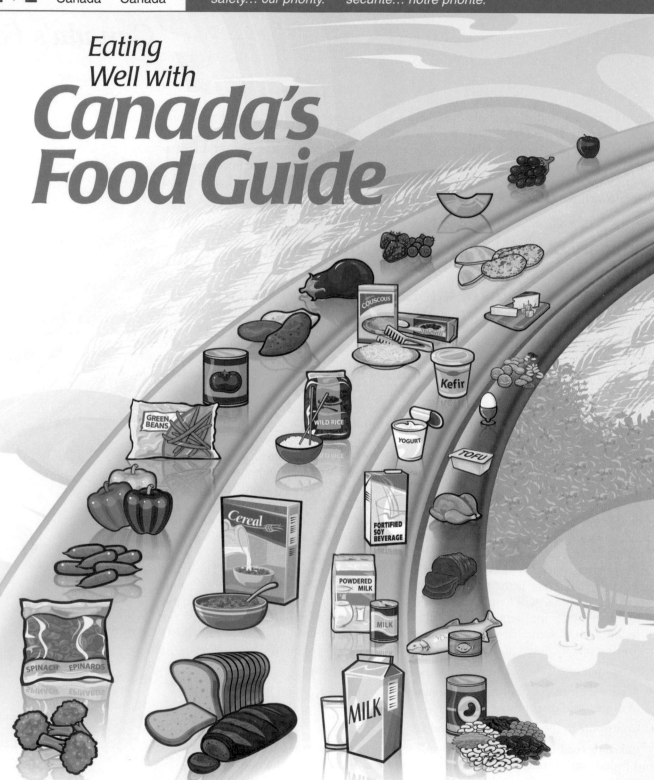

| **Figure B.1** Eating Well with *Canada's Food Guide*.

Figure B.2 Information about Food Guide Servings from *Canada's Food Guide*.

Recommended Number of *Food Guide Servings* per Day

	Children			Teens		Adults			
Age in Years	**2-3**	**4-8**	**9-13**	**14-18**		**19-50**		**51+**	
Sex	Girls and Boys			**Females**	**Males**	**Females**	**Males**	**Females**	**Males**
Vegetables and Fruit	4	5	6	7	8	7-8	8-10	7	7
Grain Products	3	4	6	6	7	6-7	8	6	7
Milk and Alternatives	2	2	3-4	3-4	3-4	2	2	3	3
Meat and Alternatives	1	1	1-2	2	3	2	3	2	3

The chart above shows how many Food Guide Servings you need from each of the four food groups every day.

Having the amount and type of food recommended and following the tips in *Canada's Food Guide* will help:

• Meet your needs for vitamins, minerals and other nutrients.

• Reduce your risk of obesity, type 2 diabetes, heart disease, certain types of cancer and osteoporosis.

• Contribute to your overall health and vitality.

What is One Food Guide Serving?
Look at the examples below.

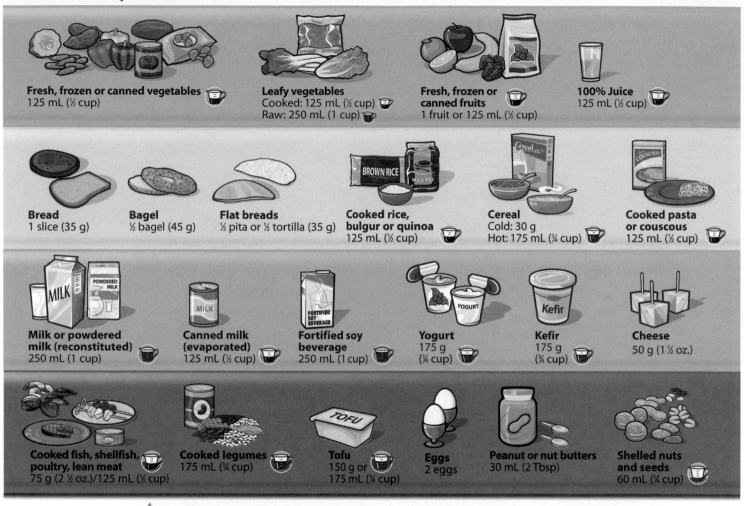

Fresh, frozen or canned vegetables
125 mL (½ cup)

Leafy vegetables
Cooked: 125 mL (½ cup)
Raw: 250 mL (1 cup)

Fresh, frozen or canned fruits
1 fruit or 125 mL (½ cup)

100% Juice
125 mL (½ cup)

Bread
1 slice (35 g)

Bagel
½ bagel (45 g)

Flat breads
½ pita or ½ tortilla (35 g)

Cooked rice, bulgur or quinoa
125 mL (½ cup)

Cereal
Cold: 30 g
Hot: 175 mL (¾ cup)

Cooked pasta or couscous
125 mL (½ cup)

Milk or powdered milk (reconstituted)
250 mL (1 cup)

Canned milk (evaporated)
125 mL (½ cup)

Fortified soy beverage
250 mL (1 cup)

Yogurt
175 g
(¾ cup)

Kefir
175 g
(¾ cup)

Cheese
50 g (1 ½ oz.)

Cooked fish, shellfish, poultry, lean meat
75 g (2 ½ oz.)/125 mL (½ cup)

Cooked legumes
175 mL (¾ cup)

Tofu
150 g or
175 mL (¾ cup)

Eggs
2 eggs

Peanut or nut butters
30 mL (2 Tbsp)

Shelled nuts and seeds
60 mL (¼ cup)

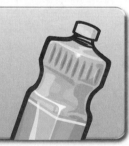

Oils and Fats

- Include a small amount – 30 to 45 mL (2 to 3 Tbsp) – of unsaturated fat each day. This includes oil used for cooking, salad dressings, margarine and mayonnaise.
- Use vegetable oils such as canola, olive and soybean.
- Choose soft margarines that are low in saturated and trans fats.
- Limit butter, hard margarine, lard and shortening.

| **Figure B.2**   *(continued)*

oils and fats to consume, along with guidance to enjoy a variety of foods and to satisfy your thirst with water. *Canada's Food Guide* uses a sample meal to explain how to use the guide (Fig. B.3) and emphasizes the importance of being physically active every day (Fig. B.4). A Canadian Nutrition Facts label is highlighted with the message to "Read the label" (see Fig. B.4). This food guide also includes specific nutrition advice for different ages and stages (Fig. B.5). "My Food Guide" is a Web-based interactive tool that will help you personalize the information found in *Canada's Food Guide*. Check out "My Food Guide" at http://www.hc-sc.gc.ca/fn-an/food-guide-aliment/myguide-monguide/index-eng.php.

Make each Food Guide Serving count...
wherever you are – at home, at school, at work or when eating out!

▶ **Eat at least one dark green and one orange vegetable each day.**
- Go for dark green vegetables such as broccoli, romaine lettuce and spinach.
- Go for orange vegetables such as carrots, sweet potatoes and winter squash.

▶ **Choose vegetables and fruit prepared with little or no added fat, sugar or salt.**
- Enjoy vegetables steamed, baked or stir-fried instead of deep-fried.

▶ **Have vegetables and fruit more often than juice.**

▶ **Make at least half of your grain products whole grain each day.**
- Eat a variety of whole grains such as barley, brown rice, oats, quinoa and wild rice.
- Enjoy whole grain breads, oatmeal or whole wheat pasta.

▶ **Choose grain products that are lower in fat, sugar or salt.**
- Compare the Nutrition Facts table on labels to make wise choices.
- Enjoy the true taste of grain products. When adding sauces or spreads, use small amounts.

▶ **Drink skim, 1%, or 2% milk each day.**
- Have 500 mL (2 cups) of milk every day for adequate vitamin D.
- Drink fortified soy beverages if you do not drink milk.

▶ **Select lower fat milk alternatives.**
- Compare the Nutrition Facts table on yogurts or cheeses to make wise choices.

▶ **Have meat alternatives such as beans, lentils and tofu often.**

▶ **Eat at least two Food Guide Servings of fish each week.***
- Choose fish such as char, herring, mackerel, salmon, sardines and trout.

▶ **Select lean meat and alternatives prepared with little or no added fat or salt.**
- Trim the visible fat from meats. Remove the skin on poultry.
- Use cooking methods such as roasting, baking or poaching that require little or no added fat.
- If you eat luncheon meats, sausages or prepackaged meats, choose those lower in salt (sodium) and fat.

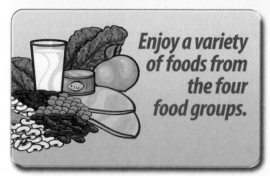

Enjoy a variety of foods from the four food groups.

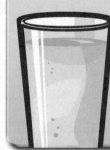

Satisfy your thirst with water!

Drink water regularly. It's a calorie-free way to quench your thirst. Drink more water in hot weather or when you are very active.

* Health Canada provides advice for limiting exposure to mercury from certain types of fish. Refer to www.healthcanada.gc.ca for the latest information.

| **Figure B.2**   *(continued)*

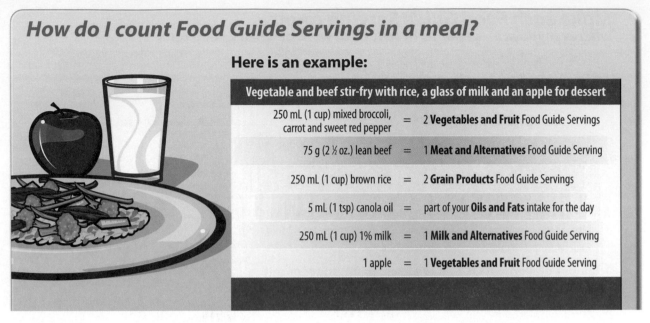

How do I count Food Guide Servings in a meal?

Here is an example:

Vegetable and beef stir-fry with rice, a glass of milk and an apple for dessert		
250 mL (1 cup) mixed broccoli, carrot and sweet red pepper	=	2 **Vegetables and Fruit** Food Guide Servings
75 g (2 ½ oz.) lean beef	=	1 **Meat and Alternatives** Food Guide Serving
250 mL (1 cup) brown rice	=	2 **Grain Products** Food Guide Servings
5 mL (1 tsp) canola oil	=	part of your **Oils and Fats** intake for the day
250 mL (1 cup) 1% milk	=	1 **Milk and Alternatives** Food Guide Serving
1 apple	=	1 **Vegetables and Fruit** Food Guide Serving

| **Figure B.3** How to count Food Guide Servings in a meal.

How to Read the Canadian Nutrition Label

The Regulations provide for the optional declaration of the number of Calories both from fat and from saturates plus *trans*. Recommendations on the % of Calories from fat apply to the total diet rather than to an individual food. Therefore, inclusion of the % of Calories from fat in the Nutrition Facts table may be confusing and is not permitted.

The Nutrition Facts table provides information on saturated and *trans* fatty acids, shown to raise serum cholesterol levels. The declaration of the other groups of fatty acids, monounsaturates, omega-3, and omega-6 polyunsaturates, is optional unless claims are made, in which case all three must be declared.

Potassium is not included as a mandatory nutrient of the Nutrition Facts table because it is not considered to be a nutrient of general public health importance. The declaration of potassium, however, is mandatory when a claim is made for the sodium or salt content of a food that contains an added potassium salt.

Daily Value is a comparison standard comprised of
(*a*) vitamin or mineral amounts referred to in the definition of a recommended daily intake for that vitamin or mineral
(*b*) nutrient amounts referred to in the definition of reference standard for that nutrient

Nutrition Facts
Per 1 cup (264g)

Amount	% Daily Value
Calories 260	
Fat 13g	**20%**
Saturated Fat 3g + *Trans* Fat 2g	**25%**
Cholesterol 30mg	
Sodium 660mg	**28%**
Carbohydrate 31g	**10%**
Fibre 0g	**0%**
Sugars 5g	
Protein 5g	

Vitamin A 4%	Vitamin C 2%
Calcium 15%	Iron 4%

g = gram
mg = milligram

Serving size is stipulated for various foods.

The amount of vitamins and minerals is expressed as a percentage of the Daily Value per serving of stated size.

Eat well and be active today and every day!

The benefits of eating well and being active include:

- Better overall health.
- Lower risk of disease.
- A healthy body weight.
- Feeling and looking better.
- More energy.
- Stronger muscles and bones.

Be active

To be active every day is a step towards better health and a healthy body weight.

Canada's Physical Activity Guide recommends building 30 to 60 minutes of moderate physical activity into daily life for adults and at least 90 minutes a day for children and youth. You don't have to do it all at once. Add it up in periods of at least 10 minutes at a time for adults and five minutes at a time for children and youth.

Start slowly and build up.

Eat well

Another important step towards better health and a healthy body weight is to follow *Canada's Food Guide* by:

- Eating the recommended amount and type of food each day.
- Limiting foods and beverages high in calories, fat, sugar or salt (sodium) such as cakes and pastries, chocolate and candies, cookies and granola bars, doughnuts and muffins, ice cream and frozen desserts, french fries, potato chips, nachos and other salty snacks, alcohol, fruit flavoured drinks, soft drinks, sports and energy drinks, and sweetened hot or cold drinks.

Read the label

- Compare the Nutrition Facts table on food labels to choose products that contain less fat, saturated fat, trans fat, sugar and sodium.
- Keep in mind that the calories and nutrients listed are for the amount of food found at the top of the Nutrition Facts table.

Nutrition Facts
Per 0 mL (0 g)

Amount	% Daily Value
Calories 0	
Fat 0 g	0 %
Saturates 0 g	0 %
+ Trans 0 g	
Cholesterol 0 mg	
Sodium 0 mg	0 %
Carbohydrate 0 g	0 %
Fibre 0 g	0 %
Sugars 0 g	
Protein 0 g	

Vitamin A	0 %	Vitamin C	0 %
Calcium	0 %	Iron	0 %

Limit trans fat

When a Nutrition Facts table is not available, ask for nutrition information to choose foods lower in trans and saturated fats.

Take a step today...

✓ Have breakfast every day. It may help control your hunger later in the day.

✓ Walk wherever you can – get off the bus early, use the stairs.

✓ Benefit from eating vegetables and fruit at all meals and as snacks.

✓ Spend less time being inactive such as watching TV or playing computer games.

✓ Request nutrition information about menu items when eating out to help you make healthier choices.

✓ Enjoy eating with family and friends!

✓ Take time to eat and savour every bite!

For more information, interactive tools, or additional copies visit Canada's Food Guide on-line at:
www.healthcanada.gc.ca/foodguide

or contact:
Publications
Health Canada
Ottawa, Ontario K1A 0K9
E-Mail: publications@hc-sc.gc.ca
Tel.: 1-866-225-0709
Fax: (613) 941-5366
TTY: 1-800-267-1245

Également disponible en français sous le titre :
Bien manger avec le Guide alimentaire canadien

This publication can be made available on request on diskette, large print, audio-cassette and braille.

| **Figure B.4** Recommendations to eat well and be active from *Canada's Food Guide*.

Advice for different ages and stages...

Children

Following *Canada's Food Guide* helps children grow and thrive.

Young children have small appetites and need calories for growth and development.

- Serve small nutritious meals and snacks each day.

- Do not restrict nutritious foods because of their fat content. Offer a variety of foods from the four food groups.

- Most of all... be a good role model.

Women of childbearing age

All women who could become pregnant and those who are pregnant or breastfeeding need a multivitamin containing **folic acid** every day. Pregnant women need to ensure that their multivitamin also contains **iron**. A health care professional can help you find the multivitamin that's right for you.

Pregnant and breastfeeding women need more calories. Include an extra 2 to 3 Food Guide Servings each day.

Here are two examples:

- Have fruit and yogurt for a snack, or

- Have an extra slice of toast at breakfast and an extra glass of milk at supper.

Men and women over 50

The need for **vitamin D** increases after the age of 50.

In addition to following *Canada's Food Guide*, everyone over the age of 50 should take a daily vitamin D supplement of 10 µg (400 IU).

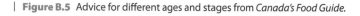

| **Figure B.5** Advice for different ages and stages from *Canada's Food Guide*.

Templates for Canadian "Nutrition Facts" Tables

Bilingual Label

Nutrition Facts
Valeur nutritive
Per 125 mL (87 g) / 0par 125 mL (87 g)

Amount Teneur	% Daily Value % valeur quotidienne
Calories / Calories 80	
Fat / Lipids 0.5 g	1 %
Saturated / saturés 0 g + *Trans* / trans 0 g	0 %
Cholesterol / Cholestérol 0 mg	
Sodium / Sodium 0 mg	0 %
Carbohydrate / Glucides 18 g	6 %
Fibre / Fibres 2 g	8 %
Sugars / Sucres 2 g	
Protein / Protéines 3 g	
Vitamin A / Vitamine A	2 %
Vitamin C / Vitamine C	10 %
Calcium / Calcium	0 %
Iron / Fer	2 %

English Label

Nutrition Facts
Per 125 mL (87 g)

Amount	% Daily Value
Calories 80	
Fat 0.5 g	1 %
Saturated 0 g + *Trans* 0 g	0 %
Cholesterol 0 mg	
Sodium 0 mg	0 %
Carbohydrate 18 g	6 %
Fibre 2 g	8 %
Sugars 2 g	
Protein 3 g	
Vitamin A 2 %	Vitamin C 10 %
Calcium 0 %	Iron 2 %

French Label

Valeur nutritive
par 125 mL (87 g)

Teneur	% valeur quotidienne
Calories 80	
Lipids 0,5 g	1 %
saturés 0 g + trans 0 g	0 %
Cholestérol 0 mg	
Sodium 0 mg	0 %
Glucides 18 g	6 %
Fibres 2 g	8 %
Sucres 2 g	
Protéines 3 g	
Vitamine A 2 %	Vitamine C 10 %
Calcium 0 %	Fer 2 %

g = gram
mg = milligram

New Canadian Nutrition Facts Label for Children Under Two Years of Age

Nutrition Facts
Per 1 jar (126 mL)

	Amount
Calories	110
Fat	0g
Sodium	10 mg
Carbohydrate	27g
Fibre	4g
Sugars	18g
Protein	0g
% Daily Value	
Vitamin A 6%	Vitamin C 45%
Calcium 2%	Iron 2%

g = gram
mg = milligram

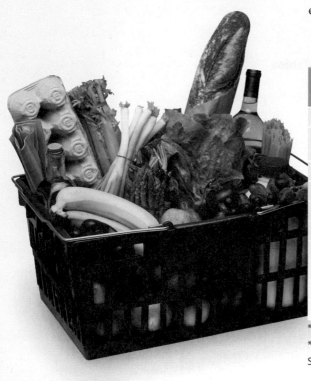

Daily Values

The daily values for vitamins and minerals are based on the 1983 Recommended Nutrient Intakes for Canadians.

Dietary Constituent	Daily Values*
Fat	**65 g**
The sum of saturated fatty acids and trans fatty acids	**20 g**
Cholesterol	**300 mg**
Carbohydrate	**300 g**
Fibre	**25 g**
Sodium	**2400 mg**
Calcium	**1100 mg**
Iron	**14 mg**
Vitamin A	**1000 RE****
Vitamin C	**60 mg**

* For persons 2 years of age and older.

**RE = retinol equivalents

Source: Health Canada. The % Daily Value. http://www.hc-sc.gc.ca/fn-an/label-etiquet/nutrition/cons/dv-vq/info-eng.php#

Approved Nutrient Content Claims for Canada

The following is a sample of approved nutrient content claims for food labels.

Energy

- *Free of energy:* The food provides less than 5 Calories or 21 kilojoules per reference amount and serving of stated size.
- *Low in energy:* The food provides 40 Calories or 167 kilojoules or less per reference amount and serving of stated size.
- *Reduced in energy:* The food is processed, formulated, reformulated, or otherwise modified so that it provides at least 25% less energy per reference amount of a similar food.
- *Lower in energy:* The food provides at least 25% less energy per reference amount of a similar food.
- *Source of energy:* The food provides at least 100 Calories or 420 kilojoules per reference amount and serving of stated size.
- *More energy:* The food provides at least 25% more energy, totalling at least 100 more Calories or 420 more kilojoules per reference amount of a similar food.

Protein

- *Low in protein:* The food contains no more than 1 gram of protein per 100 grams of the food.
- *Source of protein:* The food has a protein rating of 20 or more, as determined by official method FO-1, *Determination of Protein Rating,* October 15, 1981, (*a*) per reasonable daily intake; or (*b*) per 30 grams combined with 125 milliliters of milk, if the food is a breakfast cereal.

- *Excellent source of protein:* The food has a protein rating of 40 or more, as determined by official method FO-1, *Determination of Protein Rating,* October 15, 1981, (*a*) per reasonable daily intake; or (*b*) per 30 grams combined with 125 milliliters of milk, if the food is a breakfast cereal.

- *More protein:* The food (*a*) has a protein rating of 20 or more, as determined by official method FO-1, *Determination of Protein Rating,* October 15, 1981, (i) per reasonable daily intake, or (ii) per 30 grams combined with 125 milliliters of milk, if the food is a breakfast cereal; and (*b*) contains at least 25% more protein, totalling at least 7 grams more, per reasonable daily intake compared to the reference food of the same food group or the similar reference food.

Fat

- *Free of fat:* The food contains less than 0.5 grams of fat per reference amount and serving of stated size.

- *Low in fat:* The food contains 3 grams or less of fat per reference amount and serving of stated size and, if the reference amount is 30 grams or 30 milliliters or less, per 50 grams.

- *Reduced in fat:* The food is processed, formulated, reformulated, or otherwise modified so that it contains at least 25% less fat than the reference amount of a similar food.

- *Lower in fat:* The food contains at least 25% less fat per reference amount of the food, than the reference amount of the reference food of the same food group.

- *100% fat-free:* The food (*a*) contains less than 0.5 grams of fat per 100 grams; (*b*) contains no added fat.

- *No added fat:* The food contains no added fats or oils set out in Division 9, or added butter or ghee, or ingredients that contain added fats or oils, or butter or ghee.

- *Free of saturated fatty acids:* The food contains less than 0.2 grams saturated fatty acids and less than 0.2 grams *trans* fatty acids per reference amount and serving of stated size.

- *Low in saturated fatty acids:* (1) The food contains 2 grams or less of saturated

fatty acids and *trans* fatty acids combined per reference amount and serving of stated size. (2) The food provides 15% or less energy from the sum of saturated fatty acids and *trans* fatty acids.

- *Reduced in saturated fatty acids:* The food is processed, formulated, reformulated, or otherwise modified without increasing the content of *trans* fatty acids, so that it contains at least 25% less saturated fatty acids per reference amount of the food than the reference amount of the similar reference food.

- *Lower in saturated fatty acids:* The food contains at least 25% less saturated fatty acids and the content of *trans* fatty acids is not higher per reference amount of the food, than the reference amount of the reference food of the same food group.

- *Free of* trans *fatty acids:* The food contains less than 0.2 grams of *trans* fatty acids per reference amount and serving of stated size.

- *Reduced in* trans *fatty acids:* The food is processed, formulated, reformulated, or otherwise modified without increasing the content of saturated fatty acids, so that it contains at least 25% less *trans* fatty acids per reference amount of the food than the reference amount of the similar reference food.

- *Lower in* trans *fatty acids:* The food contains at least 25% less *trans* fatty acids and the content of saturated fatty acids is not higher per reference amount of the food compared to the reference amount of a similar food.

- *Source of omega-3 polyunsaturated fatty acids:* The food contains 0.3 grams or more of omega-3 polyunsaturated fatty acids per reference amount and serving of stated size.

- *Source of omega-6 polyunsaturated fatty acids:* The food contains 2 grams or more of omega-6 polyunsaturated fatty acids per reference amount and serving of stated size.

Cholesterol

- *Free of cholesterol:* The food contains less than 2 milligrams of cholesterol per reference amount and serving of stated size.

- *Low in cholesterol:* The food contains 20 milligrams or less of cholesterol per reference amount and serving of stated size (if the reference amount is 30 grams or 30 milliliters or less, per 50 grams).

- *Reduced in cholesterol:* The food is processed, formulated, reformulated, or otherwise modified so that it contains at least 25% less cholesterol per reference amount of a similar food.

- *Lower in cholesterol:* The food contains at least 25% less cholesterol per reference amount of a similar food.

Sodium or Salt

- *Free of sodium or salt:* The food contains less than 5 milligrams of sodium per reference amount and serving of stated size.

- *Low in sodium or salt:* The food contains 140 milligrams or less of sodium per reference amount and serving of stated size.

- *Reduced in sodium or salt:* The food is processed, formulated, reformulated, or otherwise modified so that it contains at least 25% less sodium per reference amount of a similar food.

- *Lower in sodium or salt:* The food contains at least 25% less sodium per reference amount of the food.

- *No added sodium or salt:* The food contains no added salt, other sodium salts, or ingredients that contain sodium that functionally substitute for added salt.

- *Lightly salted:* The food contains at least 50% less added sodium than the sodium added to a similar reference food.

Sugars

- *Free of sugars:* The food contains less than 0.5 milligrams of sugars per reference amount and serving of stated size.

- *Reduced in sugars:* The food is processed, formulated, reformulated, or otherwise modified so that it contains at least 25% less sugars, totalling at least 5 grams less, per reference amount of the food.

- *Lower in sugars:* The food contains at least 25% less sugars, totalling at least 5 grams less, per reference amount of the food.

- *No added sugars:* The food contains no added sugars, no ingredients containing added sugars, or ingredients that contain sugars that functionally substitute for added sugars.

Fibre

- *Source of fibre:* The food contains 2 grams or more (*a*) of fibre per reference amount and serving of stated size, if no fibre or fibre source is identified in the statement or claim; or (*b*) of each identified fibre or fibre from an identified fibre source per reference amount and serving of stated size, if a fibre or fibre source is identified in the statement or claim.

- *High source of fibre:* The food contains 4 grams or more (*a*) of fibre per reference amount and serving of stated size, if no fibre or fibre source is identified in the statement or claim; or (*b*) of each identified fibre or fibre from an identified fibre source per reference amount and serving of stated size, if a fibre or fibre source is identified in the statement or claim.

- *Very high source of fibre:* The food contains 6 grams or more (*a*) of fibre per reference amount and serving of stated size, if no fibre or fibre source is identi-

fied in the statement or claim; or (*b*) of each identified fibre or fibre from an identified fibre source per reference amount and serving of stated size, if a fibre or fibre source is identified in the statement or claim.

- *More fibre:* The food contains at least 25% more fibre, totalling at least 1 gram more, if no fibre or fibre source is identified in the statement or claim, or at least 25% more of an identified fibre or fibre from an identified fibre source, totalling at least 1 gram more, if a fibre or fibre source is identified in the statement or claim compared to reference amount of a similar food.

Light and Lean

- *Light in energy or fat:* The food meets the conditions set out for the subject "reduced in energy" or "reduced in fat."

- *Lean:* The food (*a*) is meat or poultry that has not been ground, a marine or fresh water animal or a product of any of these; and (*b*) contains 10% or less fat.

- *Extra lean:* The food (*a*) is meat or poultry that has not been ground, a marine or fresh water animal or a product of any of these; and (*b*) contains 7.5% or less fat.

Approved Health Claims for Nutrition Labels

If a manufacturer follows specific guidelines addressing both the nutrients noted in the claim and guidelines pertaining to other nutrients in a food, the following health claims can be made:

- A healthy diet containing foods high in potassium and low in sodium may reduce the risk of high blood pressure, a risk factor for stroke and heart disease.

- A healthy diet, adequate calcium and vitamin D intake, and regular physical activity help to achieve strong bones and may reduce the risk of osteoporosis.

- A healthy diet low in saturated and *trans* fats may reduce the risk of heart disease.

- A healthy diet rich in a variety of vegetables and fruit may help reduce the risk of some types of cancer.

- Foods very low in starch and fermentable sugars can make the following health claims:
  - Won't cause cavities;
  - Does not promote tooth decay;
  - Does not promote dental caries; or is
- Non-cariogenic.

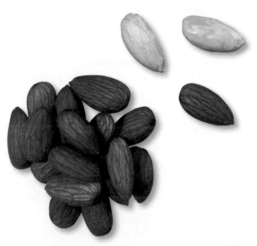

Appendix C
Daily Values Table

Nutrition Facts

Serving Size 1 cup (38 g)
Servings Per Container 18

Amount Per Serving

Calories 100
Calories from Fat 20

	% Daily Value*
Total Fat 2g	**3**%
Saturated Fat 0g	0%

The Daily Values used on food labels in the United States, with a comparison to the latest RDAs and other nutrient standards*

Dietary Constituent	Unit of Measure	Current Daily Values for People Over 4 Years of Age	RDA or Other Current Daily Dietary Standard Males 19 Years Old	Females 19 Years Old
Total fat**	g	65	—	—
Saturated fatty acids**	"	20	—	—
Protein**	"	50	56	46
Cholesterol‡	mg	300	—	—
Total carbohydrate**	g	300	130	130
Fiber	"	25	38	25
Vitamin A†	µg (RAEs)	1500	900	700
Vitamin D†	µg	10	15	15
Vitamin E†	mg	14 20	15	15
Vitamin K	µg	80	120	90
Vitamin C	mg	60	90	75
Folate	µg	400	400	400
Thiamin	mg	1.5	1.2	1.1
Riboflavin	"	1.7	1.3	1.1
Niacin	"	20	16	14
Vitamin B-6	"	2	1.3	1.3
Vitamin B-12	µg	6	2.4	2.4
Biotin	mg	0.3	0.03	0.03
Pantothenic acid	"	10	5	5
Calcium	"	1000	1000	1000
Phosphorus	"	1000	700	700
Iodine	µg	150	150	150
Iron	mg	18	8	18
Magnesium	"	400	400	310
Copper	"	2	0.9	0.9
Zinc	"	15	11	8
Sodium	"	2400	1500	1500
Potassium	"	3500	4700	4700
Chloride	"	3400	2300	2300
Manganese	"	2	2.3	1.8
Selenium	µg	70	55	55
Chromium	"	120	35	25
Molybdenum	"	75	45	45

Abbreviations: g = gram, mg = milligram, µg = microgram, RAEs = retinol activity equivalents, ATE = alpha tocopherol equivalent

*Daily Values are generally set at the highest nutrient recommendation in a specific age and gender category. Many Daily Values exceed current nutrient standards. This is in part because aspects of the Daily Values were originally developed using estimates of nutrient needs published in 1968. The Daily Values have yet to be updated to reflect the current state of knowledge.
**These Daily Values are based on a 2000 kcal diet.
† Converted from IUs.
‡ Based on recommendation of U.S. Dietary Guidelines

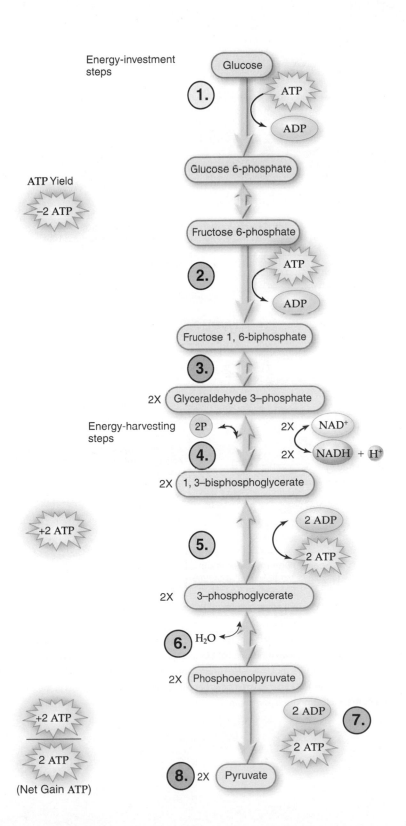

Figure D.1 Glycolysis, step by step. This metabolic pathway begins with glucose and ends with pyruvate. Net gain of two ATP molecules can be calculated by subtracting those used during the energy-investment steps from those produced during the energy-harvesting steps. Text in boxes explains the reactions.

1. Adding phosphate to glucose using ATP produces an activated molecule.

2. Rearrangement, followed by a second addition of phosphate using ATP, produces fructose 1, 6-biphosphate.

3. The 6-carbon molecule is split into two 3-carbon-phosphate molecules.

4. Oxidation, followed by the addition of phosphate produces 2 NADH + 2H$^+$ molecules and two 3-carbon-phosphate-phosphate molecules.

5. Removal of 2 phosphate groups by 2 ADP molecules produces 2 ATP molecules and two 3-carbon-phosphate molecules.

6. Removal of water produces two 3-carbon-phosphate molecules.

7. Removal of 2 phosphate groups by 2 ADP molecules produces 2 ATP molecules.

8. Pyruvate is the end product of the glycolysis pathway. Generally pyruvate enters mitochondria for further breakdown.

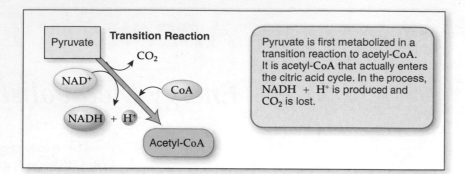

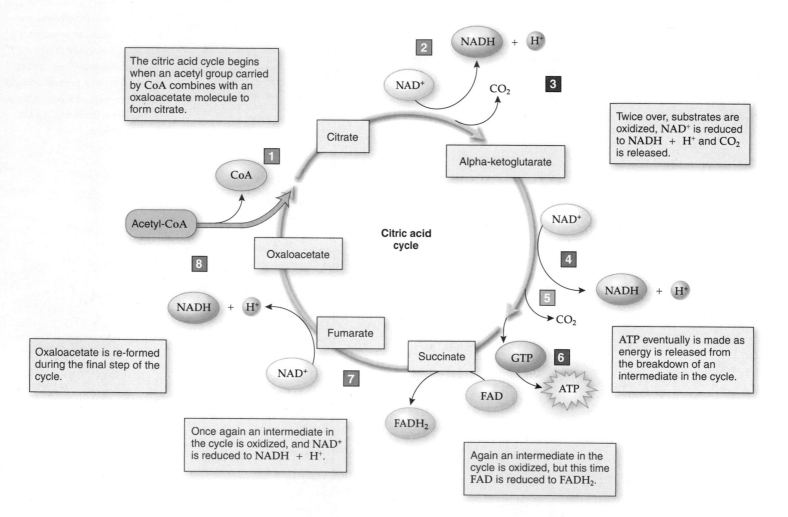

Intermediates of the citric acid cycle, such as oxaloacetate, can leave the cycle and go on to form other compounds, such as glucose.

Figure D.2 The transition reaction and the citric acid cycle. The net result of one turn of this cycle of reactions (steps 1–8) is the oxidation of an acetyl group to two molecules of CO_2 and the formation of three molecules of $NADH + H^+$ and one molecule of $FADH_2$. One GTP molecule also results, which eventually forms ATP. The citric acid cycle turns twice per glucose molecule. Note that oxygen does not participate in any of the steps in the citric acid cycle. It instead participates in the electron transport chain.

Figure D.3   Simplified depiction of electron transfer in energy metabolism. High-energy compounds, such as glucose, give up electrons and hydrogen ions to NAD^+ and FAD. The $NADH + H^+$ and $FADH_2$ that are formed transfer these electrons and hydrogen ions, using specialized electron carriers, to oxygen to form water (H_2O). The energy yielded by the entire process is used to generate ATP from ADP and P_i.

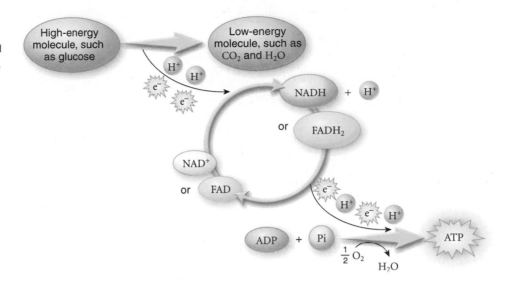

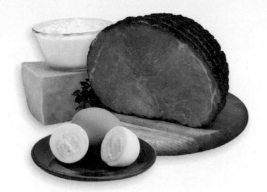

Histidine (His)
(essential)

Tryptophan (Trp)
(essential)

Glycine (Gly)

Methionine (Met)
(essential)

Leucine (Leu)
(essential)

Alanine (Ala)

Arginine (Arg)
(essential in infancy)

Lysine (Lys)
(essential)

Proline (Pro)

Glutamic Acid (Glu)

Aspartic Acid (Asp)

Serine (Ser)

Phenylalanine (Phe)
(essential)

Isoleucine (Ile)
(essential)

Tyrosine (Tyr)

Glutamine (Gln)

Asparagine (Asn)

Threonine (Thr)
(essential)

Valine (Val)
(essential)

Cysteine (Cys)

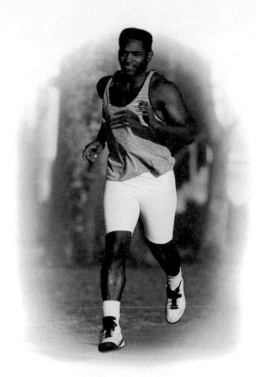

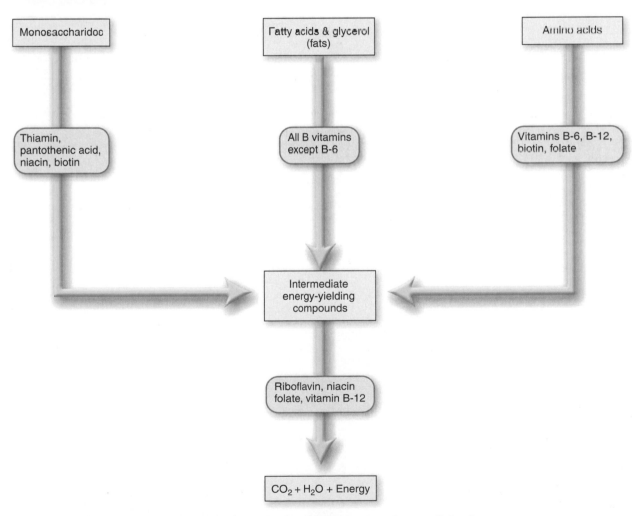

| Figure F.1 The metabolism of monosaccharides, fats, and amino acids for energy requires several vitamins.

Appendix G

Body Mass Index-for-Age Percentiles

2 to 20 years: Boys
Body mass index-for-age percentiles

NAME _____

RECORD # _____

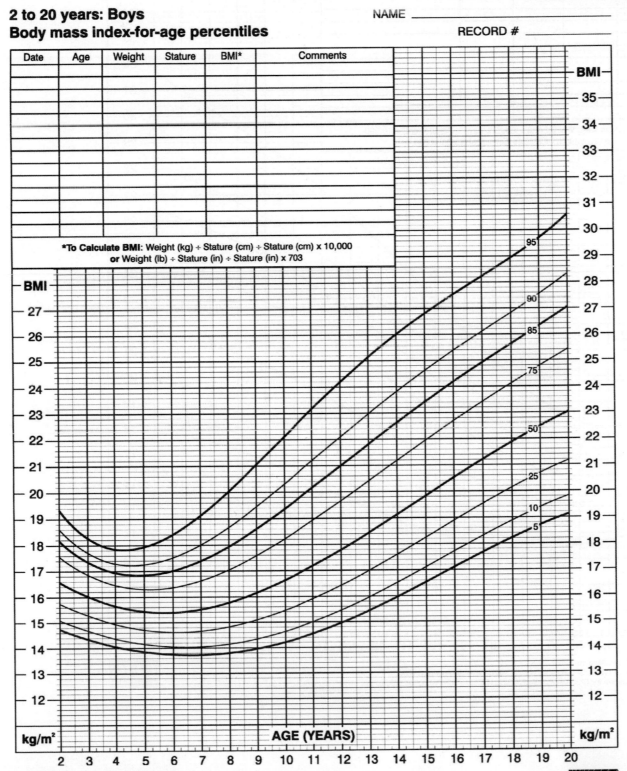

*To Calculate BMI: Weight (kg) ÷ Stature (cm) ÷ Stature (cm) x 10,000
or Weight (lb) ÷ Stature (in) ÷ Stature (in) x 703

Published May 30, 2000 (modified 10/16/00).
SOURCE: Developed by the National Center for Health Statistics in collaboration with
the National Center for Chronic Disease Prevention and Health Promotion (2000).

2 to 20 years: Girls
Body mass index-for-age percentiles

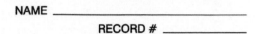

NAME _____

RECORD # _____

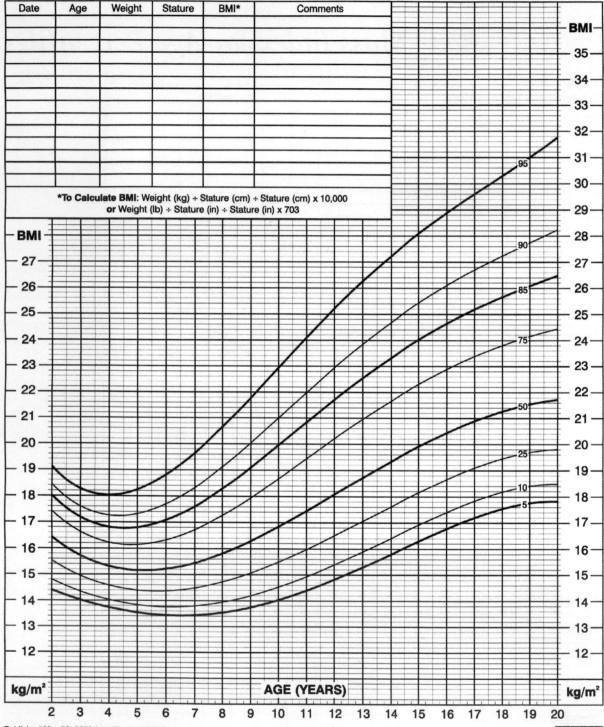

*To Calculate BMI: Weight (kg) ÷ Stature (cm) ÷ Stature (cm) x 10,000
or Weight (lb) ÷ Stature (in) ÷ Stature (in) x 703

AGE (YEARS)

Published May 30, 2000 (modified 10/16/00).
SOURCE: Developed by the National Center for Health Statistics in collaboration with
the National Center for Chronic Disease Prevention and Health Promotion (2000).

Appendix H

Answers to Concept Checkpoint Questions and Practice Test Questions

Concept Checkpoint Answers

Chapter 1

1. Heart disease, some types of cancer, stroke, and type 2 diabetes are among the 10 leading causes of death that are diet related.

2. Answers will vary but should include factors shown in Figure 1.1.

3. The six major classes of nutrients are carbohydrates, fats and other lipids, proteins, vitamins, minerals, and water.

4. The smallest functional living unit in the body is the cell.

5. The key features that indicate a substance is an essential nutrient include the following: a deficiency disease results when the substance is missing from the diet; the deficiency disease is corrected when the missing substance is added to the diet; and scientists can identify the nutrient's specific roles in the body and explain why abnormalities occurred when the substance was missing from the diet.

6. A phytochemical is a substance made by plants.

7. According to the DSHEA, a dietary supplement is a product (excluding tobacco) that contains a vitamin, a mineral, an herb or other plant product, an amino acid, or a dietary substance that supplements the diet by increasing total intake.

8. A risk factor is a personal characteristic that increases chances of developing a chronic disease.

9. Answers will vary but should include lifestyle factors such as diet; alcohol, tobacco, and other drug use; and physical activity patterns.

10. Americans eat less red meat and eggs, and more fish and poultry, than in 1970. The diet supplies more grain and cereal products, but refined grain foods make up the majority of these products. Americans are eating additional servings of fruit, but not enough to meet recommended amounts. Today, Americans eat higher amounts of vegetables than in the past, but choices tend to lack variety. Over the past 60 years, milk consumption declined and carbonated soft drink intake increased dramatically.

11. The main objectives of *Healthy People 2020* encourage ways for Americans to attain higher quality, longer lives that are free of preventable disease, disability, injury, and premature death; achieve health equity by eliminating disparities to improve the health of all groups; create social and physical environments that promote good health for all; and promote quality of life, healthy development, and healthy behaviors across all life stages.

12. Scientists generally use liters, grams, and meters to report volume, weight, and length.

13. A 154-pound person weighs 70 kg. To obtain the answer, divide 154 by 2.2 (70 kg).

14. To estimate the number of kilocalories in the slice of bread, add the number of kilocalories contributed by carbohydrate (13 g × 4 kcal = 52 kcal), fat (1 g × 9 kcal = 9 kcal), and protein (3 g × 4 kcal – 12 kcal). The answer is 73 kcal/slice.

15. Carbohydrates, fats, and proteins are macronutrients; vitamins and minerals are micronutrients.

16. Answers will vary but should be taken from the key nutrition-related concepts listed in Table 1.7.

17. An empty-calorie food contributes a large portion of its energy from solid fat, added sugar, and/or alcohol in relation to its supply of micronutrients. A nutrient-dense food contains more vitamins and minerals in relation to its fat, sugar, and/or alcohol contents.

18. The physiological dose of a nutrient is the amount that is within the range of safe intake and enables the body to function optimally. A megadose is generally defined as an amount of a vitamin or mineral that is at least 10 times the recommended amount of the nutrient. Megadose amounts of certain nutrients can be toxic.

Chapter 2

1. Epidemiology is the study of the occurrence, distribution, and causes of health problems in a population.

2. A control group is used to compare results of having a treatment against those of not having a treatment.

3. A prospective study follows a large group of healthy people over time to determine whether those with a certain characteristic develop a disease and those without that characteristic remain disease free. A retrospective study follows a group of people who already suffer from a disease and compares them to a group of people with similar characteristics who do not have the disease.

4. A placebo is a fake treatment, such as a sham pill, injection, or medical procedure. Providing placebos to members of the control group enables scientists to compare the extent of the treatment's response with that of the placebo.

5. In a double-blind study, both the investigators and the subjects are not aware of the subjects' assignments in treatment or control groups.

6. A peer-reviewed article is one that has been critically analyzed by a group of "peers." If peers agree that a study was well conducted, its results are fairly represented, and the research is of interest

to the journal's readers, these scientists are likely to recommend that the journal's editors publish the article.

7. Conflicting research findings often result from differences in the ways various studies are designed and results analyzed. For example, the numbers, ages, and physical conditions of subjects; the type and length of the study; the amount of the treatment provided; and the statistical tests used to analyze results typically vary among studies. Other factors, such as genetic and lifestyle differences among human subjects, can influence the results of nutrition research.

8. A testimonial is a personal endorsement of a product. Anecdotes are reports or personal experiences.

9. Answers will vary but should be clues that indicate a source of nutrition information is unreliable.

10. Answers will vary but should include points presented in Table 2.1.

11. Although some states regulate and license people who call them-selves nutritionists, consumers cannot always rely on someone who refers to him- or herself as a "nutritionist" because there are no standard legal definitions for this descriptor. Registered dietitians are college-trained professionals who have extensive knowledge of foods, nutrition, and dietetics, the application of nutrition and food information to treat many health-related con-ditions. The title "registered dietitian" is legally protected.

12. Consumers may find reliable nutrition experts, including reg-istered dietitians, among faculty members in universities or colleges. Registered dietitians may also be listed in telephone directories. Other ways to find registered dietitians include con-tacting the local dietetic association, calling the dietary depart-ment of a local hospital, or visiting the Academy of Nutrition and Dietetics' website (www.eatright.org) or the Dietitians of Canada's website (www.dietitians.ca).

Chapter 3

1. RDAs are standards for recommending daily intakes of several nutrients. RDAs meet the nutrient needs of nearly all healthy individuals (about 98%) in a particular life stage/gender group. In some instances, scientists set AIs for certain nutrients because they do not have enough information to establish RDAs for them. An AI represents a group's average daily intake that appears to be adequate for health.

2. To establish an RDA for a nutrient, nutrition scientists first determine its estimated average requirement. Then scientists add a "margin of safety" amount to the EAR that allows for individual variations in nutrient needs and helps maintain tissue stores.

3. The EER is more specific than RDAs or AIs because it takes into account the person's physical activity level, height, and weight, as well as sex and life stage. Furthermore, the EER does not include an additional number of kilocalories to serve as a margin of safety.

4. Dietitians refer to DRIs as standards for planning nutritious diets for groups of people and evaluating the nutritional adequacy of a population's diet. Pharmaceutical companies refer to DRIs when developing formulas that replace breast milk or regular foods.

For nutrition labeling purposes, the FDA uses RDAs to develop Daily Values (DVs).

5. Answers will vary but should include grains, such as products made from wheat, rice, and oats. Pasta, noodles, and flour torti-llas are grains because wheat flour is their main ingredient. Corn is a type of grain; therefore, cornmeal and popcorn are usually grouped with grains.

6. Enrichment is the addition of iron and certain B vitamins to cereal grain products such as flour and rice. Fortification is the addition of nutrients to food.

7. Foods generally classified as dairy include forms of fluid milk, yogurt, hard cheese, cottage cheese, ice cream, pudding, frozen yogurt, and ice milk.

8. Dry beans are protein-rich foods that can substitute for meats.

9. One-half cup of dried fruit is nutritionally equivalent to 1 cup of fresh fruit. Therefore, 1 cup of dried apricots is nutritionally equivalent to 2 cups of fresh apricots.

10. Eggs and nuts are protein-rich foods that can substitute for meats.

11. Solid fats are hard at room temperature, such as beef fat, butter, lard, and shortening.

12. Maintain caloric balance over time to achieve and sustain a healthy weight and focus on consuming nutrient-dense foods and beverages.

13. A healthy Asian American should reduce his or her sodium intake to less than 2300 mg/day.

14. Women of childbearing age should be concerned about their in-take of iron and folic acid.

15. Replace solid fats with oils.

16. Your diet should have less than 10% of total calories from satu-rated fat.

17. Limit cholesterol intake to less than 300 mg/day.

18. At least one-half of your grains should be whole grains.

19. An African American should limit his or her sodium intake to 1500 mg/day.

20. According to information in the Highlight of Chapter 6, moder-ate alcohol consumption is one standard drink/day for women and no more than two standard drinks/day for men.

21. Calcium, vitamin D, potassium, and dietary fiber are nutrients that Americans tend to consume in limited amounts.

22. Answers will vary but should include five of the following tips: make at least half of your grains foods whole grains; vary veg-etable choices; make half of your plate fruits and vegetables; fo-cus on fruit; consume sources of calcium; choose lean protein sources; find your balance between food and physical activity; and keep food safe to eat.

23. Answers may vary but should include comparing dietary intakes against recommended amounts of foods and beverages within one's diet pattern. Furthermore, a response can involve using the interactive tracking features at the www.choosemyplate.gov web-site to monitor food and nutrient intakes.

24. An empty calorie food is high in added solid fat, added sugar, or alcohol.

25. The Exchange System focuses on the energy, protein, carbohydrate, and fat content of foods. Unlike the MyPlate food groupings, classification of foods into exchange lists is based on energy and macronutrient contribution.

26. Answers may vary but should discuss how %DVs can be confusing, because a goal is to obtain at least 100% of the DVs for fiber, vitamins, and minerals each day. On the other hand, a goal should be to consume less than 100% of the DV for total fat, cholesterol, and sodium each day. Many fresh or raw foods do not have labels indicating %DVs. Therefore, people may underestimate their intakes of nutrients if they rely on nutrition labels for the information.

27. Information provided on food labels and dietary supplements can be used to compare ingredients as well as energy and nutrient contributions of similar products.

28. A health claim describes the relationship between a food, food ingredient, or dietary supplement and the reduced risk of a nutrition-related condition. Examples of health claims can vary but students can use the ones listed in Table 3.7. A structure/function claim describes the role a nutrient or dietary supplement plays in maintaining a structure, such as "calcium strengthens bone," or in promoting a normal function, such as "fiber aids bowel regularity." Examples of nutrient claims can vary but students can use the ones listed in Table 3.8.

29. The FDA is responsible for taking action against any unsafe dietary supplement after it reaches the market. The agency receives, monitors, and evaluates reports from consumers and their health care providers concerning unwanted side effects that may have resulted from taking dietary supplements. If the evidence indicates that a dietary supplement is harmful, the FDA may issue a consumer alert. If necessary, the FDA can take legal action against companies that do not comply with the agency's orders or regulations.

30. Organic foods are those produced without the use of antibiotics, hormones, synthetic fertilizers and pesticides, genetic improvements, or ionizing radiation. According to the USDA, organic food is produced by farmers who emphasize the use of renewable resources and the conservation of soil and water to enhance the quality of the environment.

31. The Nutrition Facts panels on food labels, nutrient analysis software programs, and government websites can be reliable sources of information about the energy and nutrient contents of foods and beverages.

Chapter 4

1. Electrons are negatively charged particles that surround the nucleus; protons are positively charged particles in the nucleus of an atom. An element is a substance that cannot be broken down into distinctive components under usual conditions. A chemical bond is an attraction that forms when atoms interact. A molecule results from the formation of chemical bonds. A compound is a molecule that contains two or more different elements. A solution is an evenly distributed mixture of two compounds. The solvent is the primary compound of a solution, and the solute is the substance dissolved in the solvent.

2. An ion is an atom or group of atoms that has an electrical charge because it has gained or lost one or more electrons.

3. Acids are substances that lose H^+ when dissolved in water; bases are substances that remove and accept H^+ when dissolved in water.

4. The pH of a watery solution refers to its hydrogen ion concentration.

5. A chemical reaction is a process that changes the arrangement of atoms in molecules.

6. Enzymes are proteins that initiate or facilitate (catalyze) chemical reactions.

7. Enzymes are sensitive to environmental conditions, including pH, temperature, and the presence of certain vitamins and minerals.

8. A cell is the smallest living functional unit in an organism. An organelle is a structure within the cell that has specific functions. DNA is a molecule that provides coded instructions for synthesizing proteins. A tissue is comprised of cells usually joined together that have similar characteristics and functions.

9. Homeostasis is an internal chemical and physical environment that supports life and good health.

10. Answers will vary but should include information from Table 4.2.

11. Answers will vary but should relate to Figure 4.21 and begin with the mouth and end with the anus.

12. Examples of mechanical digestion include the biting and grinding actions of teeth and the muscular contractions of the GI tract. Chemical digestion includes actions of enzymes and HCl.

13. Answers may vary but should include four of the following known tastes for humans: sweet, salty, bitter, sour, and umami.

14. Choking can occur while eating if the epiglottis does not function properly and food enters the windpipe (trachea).

15. Mucus protects the stomach lining from being damaged by acid, so Sara is at risk of developing stomach ulcers.

16. Peristalsis and segmentation, normal muscular movements of the digestive tract, keep food and chyme from becoming stuck in the tract.

17. The gastroesophageal sphincter keeps stomach contents from backing up into the esophagus.

18. The three sections of the small intestine are the duodenum, jejunum, and ileum. Most nutrient digestion and absorption takes place in the upper portion of the small intestine, primarily in the jejunum.

19. Removal of the pancreas would reduce nutrient digestion because the pancreas produces digestive enzymes.

20. Answers will vary but should include transport proteins or pumping mechanisms within the absorptive cell's plasma membrane, diffusion, or plasma membrane "swallowing" large substances.

Chapter 5

1. The major function of carbohydrate in the body is to provide a source of energy.

2. The three most important dietary monosaccharides are glucose, fructose, and galactose.

3. Glucose is blood sugar; sucrose is table sugar; lactose is milk sugar; and maltose is malt sugar. Maltose is comprised of two glucose molecules; glucose and galactose comprise lactose; and glucose and fructose comprise sucrose.

4. A nutritive sweetener provides energy, whereas a nonnutritive sweetener does not provide energy in the amounts typically used to sweeten foods.

5. The parents should give their child the beverage sweetened with sucralose because the sweetener does not provide phenylalanine.

6. Starch and glycogen are both storage forms of polysaccharides, but starch is in plant foods and glycogen is primarily in liver and muscle tissue.

7. Most forms of dietary fiber are indigestible carbohydrates. Oat bran and oatmeal, beans, apples, carrots, oranges and other citrus fruits, and psyllium seeds are rich sources of soluble fiber; whole-grain products, including brown rice, contain high amounts of insoluble fiber.

8. A minor amount of starch is digested in the mouth by the action of salivary amylase. Starch digestion stops soon after the food enters the acid environment of the stomach. In the small intestine, pancreatic amylase breaks down remaining starch molecules into maltose molecules. The enzyme maltase splits each maltose molecule into two glucose molecules. The glucose molecules are absorbed by small intestinal cells; they enter the bloodstream and travel to the liver via the portal vein. In the small intestine, sucrase splits the sucrose molecules in the grape jelly into glucose and fructose molecules. These monosaccharides are absorbed by small intestinal cells and eventually enter the hepatic portal vein and travel to the liver. The fiber in the crackers was not digested. The fiber moves through her intestinal tract and may be fermented by bacteria in her large intestine or contribute to her feces.

9. Soluble fiber is viscous fiber, because it usually forms a semisolid mass in the intestinal tract that is rapidly fermented by bacterial action. Insoluble or fermentation-resistant fiber does not break down completely, and as a result, contributes to softer and easier-to-eliminate bowel movements.

10. A ketone body is a chemical that results from the incomplete breakdown of fat. Cells form ketone bodies when they must use greater-than-normal amounts of fat for energy. Under these conditions, there is not enough glucose available for cells to metabolize the fat efficiently, and excessive ketone bodies form as a result.

11. Insulin helps regulate blood glucose levels because the hormone enables glucose to enter most cells. The hormone enhances energy storage by promoting fat, glycogen, and protein production. Glucagon opposes insulin's effects by promoting the breakdown of glycogen. This process releases glucose into the bloodstream and, as a result, boosts the blood glucose level back to normal. Glucagon also stimulates liver and kidney cells to produce glucose from certain amino acids, the basic molecules that make up proteins. Furthermore, glucagon stimulates the breakdown of triglyceride into glycerol and fatty acids. As a result, glycerol and fatty acids rapidly enter into the bloodstream.

12. Regular soft drinks are the primary source of added sugars in the typical American's diet.

13. Fruit juice is a better choice because juice is a natural product that contains nutrients and phytochemicals in fruit. "Orange-Ade" is not a nutritionally equivalent substitute for orange juice, because it may contain only 10% fruit juice.

14. To estimate the grams of starch in the serving of the cereal, subtract the amount of starch and sugars in a serving (15 grams) from the amount of total carbohydrates (44 grams), and the remainder is the amount of starch (29 grams).

15. Answers will vary but should be the signs and symptoms listed in Table 5.9.

16. To reduce her risk of developing type 2 diabetes, Erika should avoid overweight, be physically active, and eat a "prudent" diet.

17. Answers may vary but should include signs presented in Table 5.10.

18. Lactose intolerance is a condition characterized by the inability to digest lactose completely.

19. Answers will vary but should include increasing one's intake of plant foods, especially whole-grain breads and cereals.

20. Eating soluble fiber can reduce the risk of cardiovascular disease by reducing blood cholesterol levels. The liver recycles the cholesterol from bile that is absorbed by the intestinal tract to make new bile. Soluble fiber interferes with the absorption of bile salts in the intestinal tract. As a result, the liver must use other sources of cholesterol, such as blood cholesterol, to produce bile. The insoluble fiber in food attracts water and swells in the digestive tract, forming a large soft mass that applies pressure to the inner muscular walls of the large intestine, stimulating the muscles to push the residue quickly through the tract. As a result, people are less likely to strain while having bowel movements than people whose diets lack fiber.

21. A person can read the Nutrition Facts panel to determine the carbohydrate and fiber content in a serving of food.

Chapter 6

1. Major lipids include fatty acids, triglycerides, phospholipids, and cholesterol.

2. A saturated fatty acid has each carbon within the fatty acid chain completely filled with hydrogen atoms. An unsaturated fatty acid has two neighboring carbons within the chain that are missing two hydrogen atoms. Monounsaturated fatty acids have one double bond within the carbon chain; polyunsaturated fatty acids have two or more double bonds within the carbon chain.

3. Answers will vary but will relate to Figure 6.5.

4. Alpha-linolenic acid and linoleic acid are essential fatty acids.

5. Trans fats are unsaturated fatty acids that have at least one trans double bond. The trans shape enables the hydrocarbon chain to be relatively straight. Foods that are rich sources of trans fat contain partially hydrogenated fat, such as shortening and stick margarine.

6. An omega-3 fatty acid has the first double bond in the polyunsaturated fatty acid's carbon chain appearing at the third carbon, when you start counting carbons at the omega end of the molecule. Alpha-linolenic acid, eicosapentaenoic acid (EPA), and docosahexaenoic acid (DHA) are omega-3 fatty acids.

7. Egg yolk or whole egg would keep the oil and milk emulsified.

8. Cholesterol is found only in animal foods. Egg yolk, liver, meat, poultry, whole milk, cheese, and ice cream are rich sources of cholesterol. Cholesterol is a component of every cell membrane; cells use cholesterol to synthesize vitamin D, bile, and steroid hormones.

9. Answers will vary but should follow the steps outlined in Figure 6.11 and the summary of lipid digestion and absorption presented in Figure 6.13.

10. Fat contributes 34% of the typical American's total energy intake.

11. The AMDR for fat is 20 to 35% of total calories.

12. According to *Dietary Guidelines for Americans 2010*, adults should consume less than 10% of their total calories from saturated fatty acids, limit their cholesterol intake to 300 mg/day, and keep trans fats as low as possible.

13. Fat contributes about 66% of the energy in the chips (100 kcal ÷ 150 kcal).

14. Atherosclerosis is a long-term disease process in which plaques build up inside arterial walls. Arteriosclerosis is a condition that results from atherosclerosis and is characterized by loss of arterial flexibility. A thrombus is a fixed bunch of clots that remains in place. An embolus is a thrombus or part of a plaque that breaks free and travels through the bloodstream. Atherosclerosis can occur when something in the bloodstream irritates the lining of an artery. The body's immune system responds by producing inflammation within the artery. Inflammation can stimulate healing, but the process can also trigger certain cells within the arterial wall to deposit cholesterol and other substances under the artery's lining. As a result, arterial plaque forms. Plaque interferes with or blocks circulation in the affected area. Plaque also roughens the normally smooth surface that lines the artery. The rough lining slows blood flow in the area and makes clots more likely to form. If a plaque ruptures, repairing the damage also involves clot formation, and such blood clots can be life threatening.

15. American Heart Association guidelines recommend limiting total fat intake to 25 to 35% of total calories and reducing trans fat intake to less than 1% of total energy.

16. Answers will vary but should relate to information about risk factors presented in Table 6.3.

17. According to this information, Bernard has a low risk of CVD because his HDL cholesterol level is high.

18. The liver releases high-sensitivity C-reactive protein in response to infection and inflammation. Elevated CRP may be a marker for atherosclerosis, which means it may be an early warning sign for the condition. A lipoprotein profile can provide information about blood levels of HDL, LDL, and triglycerides.

19. Answers will vary but should include reducing intakes of meats; foods made from whole milk; and crackers, cakes, cookies, pies, and other high-fat processed foods. Increasing intakes of most nuts, fatty fish, and sources of polyunsaturated oils can increase intakes of unsaturated fats.

20. Answers will vary but should include sources of omega-3 fatty acids (in Table 6.5), and vegetable oils and whole grains as major sources of omega-6 fatty acids.

21. Elevated blood levels of homocysteine levels may injure arterial walls and contribute to atherosclerosis. However, more research is needed to clarify the role of this compound and the development of atherosclerosis.

22. A statin is a prescription drug that reduces elevated blood lipid levels. Statins interfere with the liver's metabolism of cholesterol, effectively reducing LDL cholesterol and/or triglyceride levels as a result.

Chapter 7

1. The amino acid is the chemical unit that makes up a protein.

2. Answers may vary but may include cell development and maintenance, and the production of enzymes, antibodies, certain hormones, structural and contractile components, and blood-clotting factors. Additionally, proteins transport nutrients and oxygen in the bloodstream, help maintain acid-base and fluid balance, and can be used for energy.

3. The three groups that make up an amino acid are the amino or nitrogen-containing group, R group, and acid group.

4. A carbon skeleton is the part of an amino acid that remains after the amino group is removed.

5. Twenty amino acids are needed to make human proteins. Nine of these amino acids are essential.

6. A high-quality or complete protein contains all essential amino acids in amounts that will support protein deposition in muscles and other tissues or support a young child's growth. A low-quality protein lacks one or more essential amino acids.

7. Most animal proteins are sources of high-quality proteins. Quinoa and processed soy proteins are also good sources of high-quality protein. Other plant foods, particularly fruits, vegetables, and grains, are sources of low-quality proteins.

8. Tryptophan, threonine, lysine, methionine, and cysteine are often the limiting amino acids in foods.

9. Answers will vary but should include key steps noted in Figure 7.6.

10. A protein undergoes denaturation when it is exposed to various conditions that alter the macronutrient's natural folded and coiled shape. Deamination is the removal of the nitrogen-containing group from an amino acid. Transamination is the transfer of an amino group from an amino acid to a receiving compound such as a carbon skeleton.

11. Negative balance occurs during starvation, serious illnesses, and severe injuries. Positive balance occurs during periods of rapid growth such as pregnancy, infancy, and puberty, and when people are recovering from illness or injury. Performing weight-training activities also leads to nitrogen retention.

12. To calculate the answer, convert the woman's weight to kilograms by dividing 143 pounds by 2.2 (65 kg). Multiply her weight in kilograms (65) by 0.8 grams of protein/kg to calculate her RDA for protein (52 g).

13. Answers will vary but should follow the path illustrated in Figure 7.10.

14. Common signs and symptoms of food allergy are hives, swollen or itchy lips, skin flushing, eczema, difficulty swallowing, wheezing and difficulty breathing, and abdominal pain, vomiting, and diarrhea. Common signs and symptoms of celiac disease are abdominal bloating, chronic diarrhea, weight loss, and poor growth in children.

15. They must provide their children with a special diet that is very low in phenylalanine.

16. The AMDR for adult protein intake is 10 to 35% of energy from protein.

17. Americans generally eat about the same amount of protein that they did in the early 1900s. Americans, however, now consume more protein from meat, fish, and poultry than from plant foods.

18. Answers will vary based on individual food intakes but should include tips for reducing saturated fat intakes.

19. Answers will vary but should include reading the ingredient list to determine animal or soy sources of protein in the product.

20. Substituting high-quality proteins refers to replacing meat, fish, or poultry with eggs, soy products, or protein-rich dairy products such as cheese and yogurt. Extending high-quality protein refers to preparing dishes that incorporate small amounts of animal proteins with much larger amounts of plant proteins. Spaghetti with meat sauce is an example of a dish that extends high-quality protein in meat with more low-quality proteins in pasta.

21. The recipe does not provide a complementary mixture of proteins because fruit is not a good source of plant proteins to combine with peanuts.

22. Answers will vary but should include nuts, dry beans, quinoa, or seeds to complement the cereal protein.

23. Semivegetarians consume small amounts of meat, fish, or poultry, whereas other vegetarians do not eat animal flesh.

24. Plant-based diets may not contain enough energy, high-quality protein, omega-3 fatty acids, vitamins B-12 and D, and minerals zinc, iron, and calcium to meet a person's nutritional needs.

25. Children have higher protein and energy needs per pound of body weight than adults do. Since plant foods add bulk to the diet, vegan children are more likely to eat far less food than adult vegans because they become full sooner during meals. Thus, very young vegans may be unable to eat enough plant foods to meet their protein and energy needs.

26. People suffering from alcoholism, anorexia nervosa, or certain intestinal tract disorders are at risk of protein undernutrition. People with low incomes, especially elderly persons, are also at risk of protein deficiency.

27. Protein-energy malnutrition results when diets lack sufficient protein as well as energy.

28. According to this information, the child probably suffers from protein-energy malnutrition because of the parental neglect and presence of muscular wasting and abdominal edema.

29. Consuming supplements that contain large amounts of specific amino acids may upset intestinal cells' ability to absorb other amino acids. Little is known about the long-term safety of using protein and amino acid supplements. Excessive amounts of methionine and tyrosine can be toxic.

Chapter 8

1. Vitamins are complex organic compounds that regulate metabolic reactions. The body cannot synthesize most vitamins; vitamins naturally occur in commonly eaten foods; signs and symptoms of deficiency disease eventually occur when a vitamin is missing from the diet; if the deficiency disorder is treated early, good health is restored by supplying the missing vitamin.

2. Foods generally contain much smaller amounts of vitamins than of macronutrients; the body requires vitamins in much smaller amounts than macronutrients; and the body does not use vitamins directly for energy.

3. A provitamin is a vitamin precursor—a substance that does not function as a vitamin until the body converts it into an active form. An antioxidant is a substance that protects other compounds from oxidizing agents. A radical is a substance with an unpaired electron; radicals are highly reactive.

4. The federally regulated enrichment program specifies amounts of thiamin, riboflavin, niacin, folic acid, and iron that manufacturers must add to their refined flour and other milled grain products. Fortification involves the addition of one or more vitamins (and/or other nutrients) to a wide array of commonly eaten foods during manufacturing. The vitamins that are added may or may not be in the food naturally.

5. Answers will vary but should relate to information concerning food preparation, such as cooking methods and food storage practices.

6. Answers will vary, but the table should include vitamins A, D, E, and K and conform to information provided in Table 8.2.

7. Answers will vary, but the table should include all B vitamins, vitamin C, and choline, and should conform to information provided in Table 8.7.

8. Taking megadoses of vitamins can produce drug-like effects in the body, including unpleasant and even dangerous side effects.

9. Answers will vary, but should include three of the following: flushing of the skin, itchy skin, GI tract upsets, and liver damage.

10. High doses of vitamin B-6 have been associated with sensory nerve damage. The damage is reversible—after affected people stop taking excessive amounts of the vitamin.

11. Routine vitamin C supplementation does not protect against infection by common cold viruses, but the practice may shorten the duration of cold symptoms.

12. There is no clear scientific evidence that taking antioxidants, such as vitamins C and E, prevents healthy people from developing macular degeneration.

Chapter 9

1. Water is a major solvent, and the nutrient often participates directly in chemical reactions. Water's other physiological roles include transporting substances, removing waste products, lubricating tissues, and regulating body temperature and acid-base balance. Additionally, water is a major component of blood, saliva, sweat, tears, mucus, and the fluid in joints.

2. Osmosis is the diffusion of water through a selectively permeable membrane.

3. Extracellular water contains higher concentrations of sodium and chloride ions than intracellular water. Intracellular water contains higher concentrations of potassium and phosphate ions than extracellular water.

4. The body obtains water by consuming various foods and liquids, such as fruit juice, milk, soup, coffee, tea, soft drinks, tap water, and plain or flavored bottled water. Cells also form some water as a metabolic by-product of metabolism. The body loses water in urine, perspiration, exhaled air, feces, vomit, and insensible perspiration.

5. If the body cannot regulate its water balance, cells can shrink, swell, and even die.

6. In response to dehydration, the posterior pituitary gland releases antidiuretic hormone that stimulates kidneys to conserve water. Additionally, the adrenal glands secrete aldosterone, a hormone that signals kidneys to reduce the elimination of sodium in urine. As a result, the kidneys return the mineral to the general circulation. Because water follows sodium, it is conserved as well.

7. The AI for total water intake is approximately 11 cups (2.7 L) for young women and approximately 15.5 cups (3.7 L) for young men.

8. A diuretic is a substance that increases urine production. Alcohol and caffeine have diuretic effects on the body.

9. Signs and symptoms of dehydration include weight loss, fatigue, thirst, loss of muscular strength and endurance, severe weakness, and coma.

10. Signs and symptoms of water intoxication may include dizziness, headache, confusion, inability to coordinate muscular movements, bizarre behavior, seizures, and coma.

11. Answers may vary, but may include inorganic structural components of tissues, such as calcium and phosphorus in bones and teeth. Minerals may also function as inorganic ions, such as calcium ions (Ca^{++}) that participate in blood clotting and sodium ions (Na^+) that help maintain fluid balance. Some ions, such as magnesium (Mg^{++}) and copper (Cu^{++}), are cofactors for chemical reactions. Many minerals are components of various enzymes, hormones, or other organic molecules, such as cobalt in vitamin B-12, iron in hemoglobin, and sulfur in the amino acids methionine and cysteine.

12. A mineral nutrient is classified as a major mineral if humans require 100 mg or more per day, or a trace mineral if humans require less than 100 mg/day. Table 9.3 lists major and trace minerals.

13. Refining foods can result in mineral losses. Minerals are water soluble and can be lost by leaching into watery cooking fluids.

14. The bioavailability of minerals depends largely on the body's need for the micronutrient. Additionally, minerals from animal foods are often better absorbed than minerals in plant foods.

15. The enrichment program requires the addition of iron to grain products.

16. Osteoporosis is a chronic disease characterized by low bone mass and reduced bone structure. People with osteoporosis have weak bones that are susceptible to fractures that can be costly to treat and result in disability and death, particularly among elderly persons.

17. Answers may vary, but should relate to risk factors listed in Table 9.6.

18. Prehypertension is a condition characterized by persistent systolic blood pressure readings of 120 to 139 mm Hg and diastolic readings of 80 to 89 mm Hg. Hypertension is characterized by persistent systolic values ≥140 mm Hg and diastolic values ≥90 mm Hg. Risk factors for hypertension include advanced age, African-American ancestry, obesity, physical inactivity, smoking cigarettes, and excess alcohol and sodium intakes. Table 9.10 presents major risk factors for hypertension.

19. The Dietary Approaches to Stop Hypertension (DASH) diet is low in sodium, total fat, saturated fat, and cholesterol; and high in fruits, vegetables, and low-fat dairy products. Other lifestyle changes that can reduce blood pressure include losing excess body fat and increasing physical activity.

20. Answers should conform to information in Table 9.4.

21. Iron deficiency is a condition characterized by low blood iron levels that are not low enough to result in severe health problems. Iron deficiency anemia occurs when oxygen transport in blood is impaired, generally because there are not enough red blood cells to carry the oxygen or because red blood cells do not contain enough hemoglobin. Signs and symptoms of

iron deficiency anemia include conditions listed in Table 9.16. People who are likely to develop iron deficiency include those who have lost substantial amounts of blood and young women who exclude meat and enriched bread and cereal products from their diets. Additionally, others at risk of iron deficiency are women of childbearing age (who generally lose some iron during menstruation), pregnant women, and infants born to women who are iron deficient.

22. Hemochromatosis is an inherited disorder in which the body absorbs too much iron. Signs and symptoms include joint pain, fatigue, lack of energy, abdominal pain, loss of sex drive, abnormal bronze skin color, and heart problems. The condition is treated by avoiding iron supplements and periodically having blood removed.

23. In humans, zinc deficiency results in dwarfism, mental retardation, iron deficiency anemia, underdeveloped sexual organs, and delays in sexual maturation.

24. Goiter is an enlarged thyroid gland. Cretinism occurs in infants born to women who were iodine deficient during pregnancy. The condition is characterized by permanent brain damage, reduced intellectual functioning, and growth retardation. Cretinism can be prevented by including a source of iodine in diets of pregnant women.

25. Rich food sources of selenium include Brazil nuts, fish, whole-grain products, and meats (see Table 9.19).

26. Chromium may enhance insulin's action on cell membranes and facilitate the entry of glucose into cells.

27. Answers will vary but should conform to information presented in Table 9.14.

28. Answers will vary but should include arsenic, boron, lithium, nickel, silicon, or vanadium.

29. Answers will vary but should conform to information provided in Table 9.20.

Chapter 10

1. Total body fat includes adipose cells and fat in cell membranes, nervous tissue, and certain bones. Fat-free mass is comprised of body water; mineral-rich tissues such as bones and teeth; and protein-rich tissues, including muscles and organs.

2. When food is plentiful, adipose cells remove excess fat from the bloodstream for storage. As the amount of fat stored in adipose cells increases, the size of each cell expands, and the body gains weight. The body can produce more fat cells during periods of rapid growth and in response to overeating.

3. Body fat stores energy. Additionally, fat cells secrete numerous proteins, some of which have roles in regulating food intake, glucose metabolism, and immune responses.

4. Subcutaneous fat helps insulate the body against cold temperatures and protects muscles and bones from bumps and bruises. Subcutaneous fat also provides body contours.

5. Visceral fat is an adipose tissue deposit that lies under abdominal muscles and forms a protective "apron" for abdominal organs.

6. Cellulite is lumpy-appearing skin, but it is not a unique type of fat. Scientists have no clear understanding of why cellulite occurs, but it may simply be subcutaneous fat held in place by irregular bands of connective tissue.

7. Adult adipose tissue has a yellowish or creamy white appearance and may be referred to as "white fat." Brown fat is richly supplied with blood and contains more mitochondria, the energy-generating organelles, than white fat tissue. Brown fat cells use fat for generating heat, whereas white fat cells store fat.

8. Answers will vary but may include "underwater weighing" and measuring dual-energy x-ray absorptiometry, air displacement, bioelectrical impedance, and skinfold thicknesses. For many of the techniques, drawbacks include cost and size of equipment needed to measure body fat.

9. The average healthy young woman has more body fat than the average healthy young man because she needs the extra fat for hormonal and reproductive purposes.

10. He has a healthy percentage of body fat.

11. To estimate daily basal metabolic needs of a 185-pound woman, first convert the woman's weight to kilograms by dividing 185 pounds by 2.2 (approximately 84 kg). Then multiply 84 kg by 0.9 kcal to determine the amount of energy expended for metabolism in an hour (approximately 76 kcal/hr). Multiply 76 kcal/hour by 24 hours to obtain the amount of energy expended for basal metabolic needs in a day (1824 kcal).

12. The four major ways the body uses energy are basal metabolism, physical activity, TEF, and NEAT.

13. For most people, metabolism uses the most energy each day.

14. Answers will vary but may include body composition, gender, body surface area, age, calorie intake, fever, stimulants, pregnancy, milk production after childbirth, and recovery after exercise.

15. Physical activity level can be easily altered.

16. TEF refers to the relatively small amount of energy needed to digest foods and beverages as well as to absorb and further process the macronutrients. TEF increases after meals. Energy needs for physical activity are related to skeletal muscle movements.

17. NEAT is nonexercise activity thermogenesis. NEAT refers to involuntary skeletal muscle activity and includes shivering, fidgeting, maintaining muscle tone, and maintaining body posture when not lying down.

18. A person gains weight when in positive energy balance.

19. Positive energy balance is desirable for pregnant women and during periods of growth, such as during fetal development, infancy, childhood, and adolescence.

20. Weight loss is characterized by negative energy balance.

21. This woman is likely to be overweight.

22. Answers will vary but should include conditions listed in Table 10.5.

23. The stigma of obesity is the negative attitude that many people have toward obese persons, such as characterizing overfat people as lazy, stupid, and sloppy.

24. Central-body obesity ("apple shape") is more likely to pose serious health risks than having excess fat below the waist, or a pear-shaped fat distribution. Central-body fat distribution is associated with increased risks of type 2 diabetes and CVD.

25. Measuring a person's waist circumference is a quick and easy way to determine whether body fat distribution is likely to result in serious chronic health problems.

26. Hunger is an uncomfortable feeling that drives a person to consume food. Satiety is the sense that enough food or beverages have been consumed to satisfy hunger.

27. Adipose cells secrete leptin, a hormone that reduces hunger and inhibits fat storage in the body. The stomach secretes ghrelin that stimulates eating behavior.

28. Thrifty genes could benefit people during periods of food deprivation, such as famine.

29. According to the set-point theory, the body's fat content (and, therefore, body weight) is genetically predetermined. The set point acts like a home thermostat, except that it regulates body weight instead of temperature.

30. Hunger is a drive to eat food, whereas appetite is a desire to eat appealing food.

31. Answers will vary but should include food marketing and sensory appeal, such as appearance, taste, and odor. Our work and home environments influence whether we are sedentary or physically active by providing opportunities to be active.

32. Answers will vary but should include socioeconomic factors, such as low income and education levels; psychological factors, such as mood and self-esteem; and societal factors, such as factors that influence young American women to idealize underweight.

33. The four key elements necessary for weight loss and maintenance are motivation, calorie reduction, regular physical activity, and behavior modification.

34. Answers will vary but should include points listed in Table 10.6.

35. Before joining a weight-loss group or plan, consumers should find out how much the program costs and how often they will need to pay for the program. Consumers should ask whether they need to sign a contract and the length of the contract. Do special foods or supplements need to be purchased? If nutrition counseling is provided, what are the credentials of the persons providing nutrition counseling and information? Furthermore, does the plan emphasize the importance of making lifestyle changes? Does the program's advertising include questionable weight-loss claims and deceptive testimonials?

36. Answers will vary but should include these: eat a low-calorie, low-fat, high-carbohydrate diet; maintain the same diet regimen every day of the week; eat regular meals, including breakfast almost every day; weigh themselves at least once a week; exercise for at least 60 minutes daily; and eat a limited variety of nutritious foods.

37. When orlistat is taken along with a meal, the medication reduces fat digestion by about 30%.

38. Roux-en-Y and gastric banding procedures are the two most common forms of bariatric surgery performed in the United States. Bariatric surgeries are effective because they reduce the size of the stomach. As a result, patients can consume only small portions of food at a time. Gastric banding is easier to perform, safer than other types of bariatric surgery, and relatively easy to reverse.

39. Liposuction is a surgical method of reducing the size of local fat deposits by suctioning excess fat out of the body. Risks of liposuction are infection, permanent dimpling of the skin at the suctioning site, and the production of tiny clumps of fat or blood clots that can be deadly, if they enter the bloodstream.

40. A fad diet is a trendy dietary practice that has widespread appeal among a population; after a period, people lose interest in the practice and it becomes no longer fashionable. Fad diets typically promote rapid weight loss without calorie restriction and increased physical activity; limit food selections to be from only a few food groups and dictate specific diet rituals; require buying a book or various gimmicks; use outlandish and unscientific claims to support their usefulness, rely on testimonials from famous people; connect the diet to trendy places; and do not emphasize the need to change eating habits and physical activity patterns.

41. Many overweight and obese people are attracted to fad diets and dietary supplements for weight loss because they believe promoters' claims that the diets or products are "magic bullets" for shedding unwanted weight quickly and effortlessly.

42. Answers will vary but should include supplements presented in Table 10.8.

43. Answers will vary but should include features or claims that the product or service causes rapid and extreme weight loss; requires no need to change dietary patterns or physical activity; results in permanent weight loss; is scientifically proven or doctor endorsed; includes a money-back guarantee; is safe; is supported by satisfied customers; displays before-and-after photos; and provides disclaimers in small print, such as "Results not typical" at the bottom of the ad or with an "after" photo.

44. Chronic diseases such as cancer, tuberculosis, AIDS, inflammatory bowel disease, depression, and hormonal imbalances can result in severe weight loss that is difficult to treat.

45. To gain weight, underweight adults can gradually increase their consumption of calorie-dense foods, especially those high in healthy fats. Eating regular meals and snacks also aids in weight gain and maintenance. If excess physical activity habits contribute to the inability to gain weight, underweight people can find ways to be less active. Furthermore, underweight individuals can add muscle mass by following resistance-training programs regularly, but their calorie intake must support extra energy demands of those programs.

Chapter 11

1. Physical activity is any movement that results from skeletal muscle contraction. Exercise refers to physical activities that are usually planned and structured for a particular purpose.

2. Physical fitness is the ability to perform moderate- to vigorous-intensity activities without becoming excessively fatigued.

3. Answers will vary but should include benefits indicated in Figure 11.2.

4. According to the American College of Sports Medicine and the American Heart Association, healthy adults under 65 years of age should engage in at least 30 minutes of moderate-intensity physical activity five days a week or 20 minutes of vigorous-intensity physical activity 3 days a week. Additionally, adults should include eight to 10 strengthening exercises twice a week.

5. Performing resistance exercises regularly can increase muscle mass, strength, and flexibility. Resistance exercises can also increase bone mass.

6. To calculate the target heart rate range of a 24-year-old person performing moderate-intensity activity, subtract the person's age (24) from 220 to obtain 196, the age-related maximum heart rate. Moderate-intensity activity raises the heart rate to 50 to 70% of the age; therefore, multiply 196 × .50 to obtain the lower limit of the range (98 bpm), and 196 × .70 to obtain the upper limit of the range (approximately 137 bpm). Thus, the heart rate range for this individual is 98 to 137 bpm.

7. Muscle cells break down glycogen to provide a source of glucose during exercise.

8. ATP is formed as a result of glycolysis and aerobic respiration. Some ATP is also formed by the breakdown of triglycerides, amino acids, and alcohol. Muscle cells also use phosphocreatine to produce ATP quickly under anaerobic conditions.

9. Muscle cells rely on the PCr-ATP, lactic acid, and oxygen systems to obtain energy. The PCr-ATP system forms ATP by breaking down PCr into creatine and P_i. The energy that is released helps synthesize ATP from ADP and P_i. In anaerobic conditions, muscle cells metabolize glucose to pyruvate and then convert pyruvate to lactic acid. The degradation of glucose to lactic acid produces a small amount of ATP. Lactic acid accumulates in muscles and converts to a related substance, lactate. Although certain muscle cells can use lactate as a fuel, some of the compound enters the bloodstream. The liver removes lactate from blood and can convert the compound into glucose. The oxygen system metabolizes glucose completely to CO_2 and H_2O, resulting in the production of far more ATP-energy than the amount produced by anaerobic systems. The PCr-ATP and lactic acid systems do not need oxygen to produce ATP.

10. Individuals can increase their aerobic exercise capacity by engaging in endurance-training programs that gradually increase the intensity level of activities. Such training improves muscle cells' ability to generate ATP rapidly.

11. Fat is a major energy source for muscles while one is resting or engaged in low- to moderate-intensity physical activities.

12. Practical ways to assess whether an athlete's energy intake is adequate include having the athlete keep accurate food records and use the information to estimate his or her daily calorie intakes. An athlete can also monitor his or her body weight and have skinfold thicknesses measured regularly.

13. Carbohydrate intake contributes to glycogen stores; glycogen depletion is a major cause of fatigue during endurance exercise. To maintain adequate muscle glycogen, athletes should consume 6 to 10 g of carbohydrate per kilogram of body weight daily. By consuming several servings of grains, starchy vegetables, and fruits daily, an athlete can obtain enough carbohydrate to maintain adequate liver and muscle glycogen stores.

14. Answers will vary but should include grains, starchy vegetables, and fruits. Also, see Table 11.4 for high-carbohydrate, low-fat foods.

15. Compared to nonathletes, the typical athlete consumes more food to meet his or her increased energy needs, and, as a result, obtains plenty of dietary protein. Therefore, healthy active Americans who eat varied diets that supply adequate energy do not need to take protein or amino acid supplements. If people consume excess protein from foods or supplements and they do not need the energy, the amino acids in these proteins will not be used for building or repairing muscles. Instead, the body converts the extra amino acids into fat for storage in adipose tissue.

16. Dehydration and overhydration detract from optimal physical performance and can cause serious health problems.

17. Answers will vary but should include signs and symptoms listed in Table 11.6.

18. According to the IMMDA, sports drinks are necessary when workouts or events last longer than 30 minutes. Although electrolytes are lost in sweat, the quantities lost in shorter periods can be easily replaced by consuming foods and beverages, such as water or fruit juice, after the event.

19. The practice of taking antioxidant supplements may not be helpful and could be harmful. Results of studies that examined whether antioxidant vitamin supplements enhanced athletic performance generally concluded that performance was not improved, unless there was a preexisting deficiency of those particular vitamins. Free radicals generated during intense exercise may stimulate the body's natural antioxidant defense system. Thus, the oxidative stress produced during exercise might have benefits, and blocking this process by taking antioxidant vitamin supplements may not be desirable.

20. Iron deficiency can negatively affect athletic performance because the body needs iron to produce red blood cells, transport oxygen, and obtain energy.

21. Female athletes who have irregular or no menstrual cycles may lack adequate amounts of the hormone estrogen. Although

weight-bearing exercise, such as jogging, improves bone density, estrogen is necessary for maintaining healthy bones. Female athletes who develop menstrual cycle abnormalities should consult a physician to determine the cause.

22. Athletes often use ergogenic aids to improve their physical performance, because they hope to gain the competitive edge over their sports rivals.

23. Answers will vary but should include ephedra-containing supplements, caffeine (high intakes), anabolic steroids, human growth hormone, and DHEA.

24. Coffee, energy drinks, caffeinated soft drinks, chocolate, and tea (see Table 11.8).

25. Caffeine raises the level of fatty acids in blood, and as a result, exercising muscles can use more fat for energy. Caffeine also enhances the ability of skeletal and heart muscles to contract and increases mental alertness.

Chapter 12

1. The FDA regulates nearly all domestic and imported food sold in interstate commerce and enforces federal food safety laws. Additionally, the FDA establishes standards for safe food manufacturing practices, such as Hazard Analysis and Critical Control Point (HACCP) programs. FDA officials can take certain enforcement actions, such as requesting that a food manufacturer recall an unsafe item, so that it is removed from store shelves. The FDA also educates the general public about safe food handling practices. The Food Safety and Inspection Service (FSIS) enforces food safety laws for domestic and imported meat and poultry products. Additionally, FSIS staff collect and analyze food samples to check for the presence of microbial and other unwanted and potentially harmful material in foods. FSIS officials can ask meat and poultry processors to recall unsafe products. FSIS also conducts programs and publishes a magazine to educate people about proper food handling practices. The EPA oversees drinking water quality and assists state officials in their efforts to monitor water quality. Furthermore, EPA staff regulate toxic substances and wastes to prevent their entry into foods and the environment.

2. Local health departments are responsible for inspecting restaurants, grocery stores, dairy farms, and local food processing companies.

3. Three common ways harmful microbes are transmitted to food are by vermin, poor personal hygiene practices, and improper food handling.

4. Cross-contamination occurs when pathogens in one food are transferred to another food, contaminating it.

5. Pasteurization is a special heating process used by many commercial food producers to kill pathogens.

6. To survive and multiply, most microbes need warmth, moisture, and a source of nutrients, and some also require oxygen.

7. In general, high-risk foods are warm, moist, and protein rich, and they have a neutral or slightly acidic pH (see Table 12.1).

8. Signs and symptoms of food-borne illnesses generally involve the digestive tract and include nausea, vomiting, diarrhea, and intestinal cramps.

9. People who suffer from a food-borne illness should consult a physician when an intestinal disorder is accompanied by one or more of the following signs: fever (oral temperature above 101.5°F), bloody bowel movements, prolonged vomiting that reduces fluid intake, diarrhea that lasts more than 3 days, or dehydration.

10. Food-borne illness generally causes gastrointestinal tract symptoms, whereas influenza is primarily a respiratory tract infection.

11. Answers will vary but should include bacteria listed in Table 12.2.

12. Answers will vary but should include viruses listed in Table 12.3.

13. Answers will vary but should include parasites listed in Table 12.4.

14. Aflatoxins are poisonous substances produced by certain molds.

15. Answers will vary but should include points under the "Purchasing Food" section of Chapter 12.

16. Answers will vary but should include points under the "Setting the Stage for Food Preparation" and "Preparing Food" sections of Chapter 12.

17. Answers will vary but should include points under the "Storing and Reheating Food" section of Chapter 12.

18. Ground meats and poultry are often sources of food-borne illness because grinding increases the surface area of the protein-rich food, exposing it to contaminants.

19. Raw fish should be frozen for recommended amounts of time before being eaten.

20. The "danger zone" for rapid pathogen multiplication is between 40°F and 140°F.

21. The USDA's Fight BAC! program recommends four simplified actions: clean, separate, cook, and chill.

22. Shelf life is the period of time that a food can be stored before it spoils.

23. Answers will vary but should include methods highlighted in Table 12.7.

24. Boiling home-canned, low-acid foods for 10 minutes can make them safe to eat.

25. A carcinogen is a cancer-causing substance.

26. Answers will vary but should include points made under the "Preparing for Disasters" section of Chapter 12. Table 12.8 lists foods that can be stored safely for emergency situations.

27. Safe sources of drinking water include bottled water, an undamaged water heater, toilet tanks (not bowls), melted water from ice cubes, and fruit juices. Water from pools, spas, radiators, heating systems, and water beds is unsafe to drink.

28. A food additive is a substance added to food that influences the product's characteristics. Direct food additives may maintain the safety of foods, prevent undesirable changes, or improve taste or color of foods. Indirect additives, such as compounds from

a food's wrapper or container, can enter food as it is packaged, transported, or stored. Indirect additives have no purpose.

29. Color additives are dyes, pigments, or other substances that provide color to foods, drugs, or cosmetics.

30. Food ingredients that had been in use prior to 1958 were listed as Generally Recognized as Safe (GRAS), when qualified experts generally agreed that the substance was safe for its intended use. Food manufacturers can include substances on the GRAS list as ingredients without testing them for safety or getting prior approval from the FDA.

31. According to the Delaney Clause, food manufacturers cannot add a new compound that causes cancer at any level of intake. Thus, if an additive causes cancer, even though very high doses may be necessary to cause the disease, no amount of the additive is considered to be safe, and none is allowed in food. Evidence for cancer risk could come from either laboratory animal or human studies. The FDA allows very few exceptions to this clause.

32. An unintentional food additive is a substance that accidentally enters food during processing. Common biological and physical food contaminants are insect parts, rodent feces or urine, dust and dirt, and bits of metal or glass from machinery used to process food.

33. A pesticide is any substance that people use to control or kill unwanted insects, weeds, rodents, fungi, or other organisms. Types of pesticides include insecticides, rodenticides, herbicides, and fungicides.

34. Integrated Pest Management involves using a variety of methods for controlling pests while limiting damage to the environment. IPM methods include growing pest-resistant crops, using predatory wasps to control crop-destroying insects, trapping adult insect pests before they can reproduce, and using biologically based pesticides.

35. The EPA regulates the use of pesticides.

36. A pesticide tolerance is the maximum amount of pesticide residue that can be in or on each treated food crop. A pesticide tolerance includes a margin of safety, so the maximum pesticide residue that is allowed to be in or on a food is much lower than amounts that can cause negative health effects.

37. Once a pesticide is applied to cropland, it may remain in the soil, be taken up by plant roots, decompose to other compounds, or enter groundwater and waterways. Winds may carry pesticides in air and dust to distant locations, where the toxic material can land on food crops.

Chapter 13

1. Eight weeks after conception, the developing human being is referred to as a fetus.

2. The role of the placenta is to transfer nutrients and oxygen from the mother's bloodstream to the embryo/fetus. Additionally, the placenta transfers wastes from the embryo/fetus to the mother's bloodstream, so her body can eliminate them.

3. Birth weight is a major factor that determines whether a baby is healthy and survives his or her first year of life.

4. A preterm birth is defined as one that occurs before 37 weeks of pregnancy.

5. Answers will vary but should include enlarged breasts, "morning sickness," tiredness, swollen feet, constipation, and heartburn.

6. Women whose prepregnancy weights were within the healthy range can expect to gain 25 to 35 pounds. Underweight women should gain 28 to 40 pounds; overweight women should gain 15 to 25 pounds during pregnancy. Obese women should gain at least 15 pounds during pregnancy. The recommendations are higher for women who are pregnant with more than one fetus.

7. Pregnant women who are folate deficient have a high risk of giving birth to infants with neural tube defects, such as spina bifida. Pregnant women who are iron deficient can develop iron deficiency anemia, a condition that increases the risk of giving birth prematurely and having low-birth-weight (LBW) infants.

8. Women who drink alcohol during pregnancy are at risk of having a child with a fetal alcohol spectrum disorder. Compared to pregnant women who do not smoke cigarettes, expectant mothers who smoke have higher risk of giving birth too early and having LBW babies. Furthermore, expectant mothers who smoke cigarettes may increase the risk of having babies with birth defects or that die of sudden infant death syndrome.

9. In response to an infant sucking on its mother's nipple, the brain releases oxytocin, a hormone that signals breast tissue to "let down" milk. The let-down reflex enables milk to travel in several tubes to the nipple area. When let-down occurs, the infant removes the milk by continued sucking.

10. Lactation increases a new mother's energy needs by about 300 to 400 kcal more than her prepregnancy energy needs.

11. Colostrum is the first secretion of the breasts that occurs after delivery. Colostrum is a very important first food for babies, because the fluid contains antibodies and immune system cells that can be absorbed by the infant's immature digestive tract. Colostrum also contains a substance that encourages the growth of a type of bacteria in the baby's intestinal tract that reduces the risk of infection.

12. New mothers should exclusively breastfeed their babies for the first 6 months of life.

13. Answers will vary but should include points in Table 13.4.

14. Answers will vary but should include points in Table 13.4.

15. Compared to whole cow's milk, human milk provides about the same amount of energy, less protein and calcium, and more carbohydrate and fat.

16. Signs indicating a baby is ready physically to eat solid foods include these: loss of the extrusion reflex; physiological maturity to digest, metabolize, and excrete a wider range of foods; ability to sit up with back support and coordinate muscular control over mouth and neck movements.

17. A qualified health care practitioner can monitor an infant's growth by monitoring weight, length, and head circumference measurements.

18. A food jag is a period in which the child refuses to eat a food that was liked in the past or in which the child wants to eat only a particular food.

19. In children, iron deficiency can lead to decreased physical stamina, learning ability, and resistance to infection.

20. Answers will vary but should include brushing teeth with a pea-sized amount of fluoride-containing toothpaste twice daily; providing routine pediatric dental care; offering fluoridated drinking water; not eating sticky, sugary snacks, especially between meals; and offering sugarless chewing gum.

21. Foods that commonly trigger allergic responses in children are peanuts, tree nuts, fish, shellfish, milk, eggs, soybeans, and wheat.

22. Factors that contribute to obesity among children include spending too much time on sedentary activities; consuming too many energy-dense empty-calorie foods and beverages; and having a family history of obesity, high birth weight, and obese family members.

23. Compared to preschoolers, older children often skip breakfast, and they typically consume more foods away from home, larger portions of food, and more fried foods and sweetened beverages. School-age children also tend to consume less milk and fewer fruits and vegetables, except fried potatoes.

24. Answers will vary but should include having higher-than-normal blood pressure, cholesterol, and glucose levels. Obese children are also more likely to have low self esteem, sleep apnea, musculoskeltal problems, and heartburn than children who have healthy body weights. Obese children are at risk of hypertension, heart disease, obesity, and type 2 diabetes later in life.

25. Children need at least 60 minutes of moderate-intensity physical activity, most days of the week.

26. Answers will vary but should include encouraging children to eat breakfast and other tips from the "Food & Nutrition Tips" feature in the "School-Age Children" section of Chapter 13.

27. Boys usually begin their growth spurt when they are between 12 and 15 years of age. Most girls begin their growth spurt between 10 and 13 years of age.

28. Obese teenagers are at risk of developing type 2 diabetes, elevated blood cholesterol, and hypertension.

29. Iron deficiency leads to increased fatigue and decreased ability to concentrate and learn. Inadequate calcium intake during adolescence is associated with decreased bone mass and increased likelihood of bone fractures later in life.

30. Life expectancy is the length of time a person born in a specific year, such as 1900, can expect to live. Life span refers to the maximum number of years a human can live.

31. Answers will vary but should include points listed in Table 13.11.

32. Compared to younger persons, older adults have greater risk of nutritional deficiencies because of physiological changes associated with the normal aging process. Other factors that can influence an older person's nutritional status include illnesses, medications, low income, and lack of social support.

33. Diets of older adults, particularly older women, often provide inadequate amounts of vitamins D, A, C, and B-12 and minerals such as calcium, iron, and zinc.

34. Caregivers can improve nutrient intakes of older persons by adding more spices to foods, making mealtimes social events, and serving energy-dense snacks between meals, such as cheese, milkshakes, nuts, or oatmeal cookies. If the elderly person has difficulty chewing, serving soft items such as ground meats, cooked vegetables, pureed fruits, and puddings can increase food intake. The "Food & Nutrition Tips" feature in the "Nutrition for Older Adults" section of Chapter 13 presents more suggestions for improving nutrient intakes of elderly persons.

35. Meals on Wheels is a program that offers home-delivered meals for older adults who are homebound.

Answers to Practice Test Questions

Chapter 1

1. b	2. a	3. d	4. d	5. b
6. a	7. c	8. d	9. b	10. c
11. a	12. c	13. a	14. b	15. c
16. b				

Chapter 2

1. d	2. b	3. a	4. d	5. c
6. d	7. a	8. c	9. b	10. d
11. c	12. a			

Chapter 3

1. a	2. d	3. c	4. a	5. d
6. a	7. d	8. d	9. b	10. a
11. c	12. b	13. a	14. c	15. b
16. a				

Chapter 4

1. a	2. d	3. b	4. c	5. d
6. a	7. b	8. b	9. d	10. b
11. a	12. d	13. b	14. d	15. c
16. b				

Chapter 5

1. b	2. c	3. a	4. d	5. b
6. c	7. b	8. b	9. c	10. b
11. a	12. c	13. b	14. b	

Chapter 6

1. a	2. b	3. c	4. a	5. b
6. d	7. b	8. c	9. b	10. c
11. c	12. b	13. d		

Chapter 7

1. b	2. c	3. a	4. a	5. b
6. d	7. c	8. a	9. d	10. c
11. d	12. c	13. a		

Chapter 8

1. d	2. c	3. a	4. d	5. d
6. a	7. b	8. a	9. b	10. c
11. c	12. a	13. b	14. c	15. d
16. a				

Chapter 9

1. c	2. b	3. d	4. d	5. a
6. c	7. d	8. a	9. b	10. c
11. b	12. a			

Chapter 10

1. b	2. d	3. b	4. b	5. b
6. c	7. a	8. b	9. a	10. b
11. d	12. d			

Chapter 11

1. b	2. c	3. a	4. d	5. b
6. a	7. b	8. d	9. a	10. c
11. d	12. a	13. d	14. b	15. c
16. a				

Chapter 12

1. a	2. a	3. c	4. d	5. c
6. b	7. d	8. c	9. c	10. b
11. d	12. b	13. b	14. a	15. c
16. c				

Chapter 13

1. b	2. c	3. b	4. c	5. a
6. c	7. c	8. d	9. b	10. a
11. d	12. a	13. d	14. d	

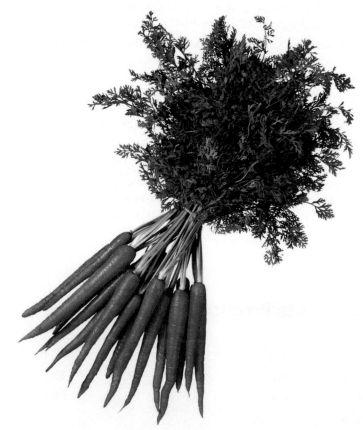

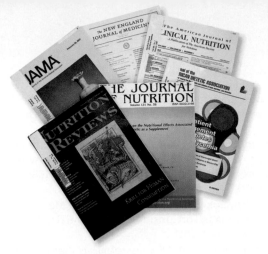

Chapter 1

1. Putnam J and others: U.S. per capita food supply trends: More calories, refined carbohydrates, and fats. *FoodReview* 25(2):2, 2002.

2. Kant AK and others: Dietary patterns predict mortality in a national cohort: The National Health Interview Surveys, 1987 and 1992. *Journal of Nutrition* 134(7):1793, 2004.

3. U.S. Department of Health and Human Services, U.S. Department of Agriculture. (Released January 31, 2011) *Dietary Guidelines for Americans, 2010* http://www.cnpp.usda.gov/DGAs2010-PolicyDocument .htm Accessed: July 1, 2011

4. Dietary Supplement Health and Education Act of 1994. Public Law 103–417, 103rd Congress. http://ods.od.nih.gov/About/DSHEA_ Wording.aspx Accessed: July 2, 2011

5. Kochanek KD and others: Deaths: Preliminary data for 2009. *National Vital Statistics Reports* 59, 2011 http://www.cdc.gov/nchs/data/nvsr/ nvsr59/nvsr59_04.pdf Accessed: July 2, 2011

6. Beliveau R, Gingras D: Role of nutrition in preventing cancer. *Canadian Family Physician* 53, 2007.

7. American Cancer Society: *Diet and physical activity: What's the cancer connection?* American Cancer Society, (Last revised October 2010). http://www.cancer.org/Cancer/CancerCauses/DietandPhysicalActivity/ diet-and-physical-activity Accessed: July 2, 2011

8. Allshouse J: In the long run. *Amber Waves*, p. 49. Economic Research Service, U.S. Department of Agriculture, 2004.

9. O'Leary N: Soft drink consumption continues to decline. *AdWeek* March 30, 2010. http://www.adweek.com/news/advertising-branding/ soft-drink-consumption-continues-decline-107218 Accessed: July 2, 2011

10. Schulze MB and others: Sugar-sweetened beverages, weight gain, and incidence of type 2 diabetes in young and middle-aged women. *Journal of the American Medical Association* 292(8):927, 2004.

11. Farah H, Buzby J: U.S. food consumption up 16 percent since 1970. *Amber Waves*. U.S. Department of Agriculture, Economic Research Service, November 2005.

12. Food and Drug Administration and National Institutes of Health. *Healthy People 2020*. http://www.healthypeople.gov/2020/about/new2020.aspx Accessed: July 2, 2011

13. Duffey KJ, Popkin BM: Energy density, portion size, and eating occasions: Contributions to increased energy intake in the United States, 1977–2006. *PLoS Medicine* 8(6):e1001050. doi:10.1371/journal .pmed.1001050

14. What is a megadose and why do you recommend against taking megadoses of vitamins? *Johns Hopkins Medical Letter Health After 50* 13(6):8, 2001.

15. Fletcher RH, Fairfield KM: Vitamins for chronic disease prevention in adults. *Journal of the American Medical Association* 287(23):3127, 2002.

16. Huang H-Y and others: The efficacy and safety of multivitamin and mineral supplement use to prevent cancer and chronic disease in adults: A systematic review for a National Institutes of Health State-of-the-Science Conference. *Annals of Internal Medicine* 145(5):372, 2006.

17. American Dietetic Association: Position of the American Dietetic Association: Functional foods. *Journal of the American Dietetic Association* 109(4):735, 2009.

18. United Nations (UN), UN News Service: *World population to reach 9.1 billion in 2050, UN projects.* 2005. http://www.un.org/apps/news/storyAr .asp?NewsID=13451&Cr=population&Cr1= Accessed: July 2, 2011

19. United Nations, UN News Service: *Number of world's hungry to top 1 billion this year—UN food agency.* June 19, 2009. http://www.un.org/apps/news/ story.asp?NewsID=31197&Cr=hunger&Cr1=# Accessed: July 2, 2011

20. Black RE and others: Maternal and child undernutrition: Global and regional exposures and health consequences. *The Lancet* 371(9608): 243–60, 2008.

21. Knoll Rajaratnam J and others: Neonatal, postneonatal, childhood and under-5 mortality for 187 countries, 1970–2010: A systematic analysis of progress towards Millennium Development Goal 4. *The Lancet* May 24, 2010 DOI:10.1016/S0140-6736(10)60703-9

22. World Health Organization: WHO, nutrition experts take action on malnutrition. March 16, 2011. http://www.who.int/nutrition/pressnote_ action_on_malnutrition/en/ Accessed: July 3, 2011

23. U.S. Census Bureau: *Income, Poverty and Health Insurance Coverage in the United States: 2009.* (2010) http://www.census.gov/newsroom/releases/ archives/income_wealth/cb10-144.html Accessed: July 3, 2011

24. U.S. Department of Health and Human Services: *The 2011 HHS Poverty Guidelines.* http://aspe.hhs.gov/poverty/11poverty.shtml Accessed: July 3, 2011

25. U.S. Department of Agriculture: *Food insecurity in the United States.* http://www.ers.usda.gov/Briefing/FoodSecurity/ Accessed: July 3, 2011

26. U.S. Department of Agriculture, Food and Nutrition Service: *WIC The Special Supplemental Nutrition Program for Women, Infants, and Children. Nutrition Program Facts.* Updated 2009. http://www.fns.usda.gov/wic/ WIC-Fact-Sheet.pdf Accessed: July 3, 2011

27. United Nations Children's Fund: *Nutrition and micronutrients.* ND. http:// www.unicef.org/supply/index_39993.html Accessed: July 3, 2011

28. United Nations Children's Fund: *Supply annual report 2010,* 2011 http:// www.unicef.org/supply/index_report.html Accessed: July 3, 2011

29. Committee on Identifying and Assessing Unintended Effects of Genetically Engineered Foods on Human Health. *Safety of genetically engineered foods: Approaches to assessing unintended health effects,* National Research Council, 2004.

30. Thomson JA: Genetically modified crops—paying a positive role in sustainable development in Africa. *South African Medical Journal* 96(6):509, 2006.

Chapter 2

1. Kraut A: *Dr. Joseph Goldberger & the war on pellagra*. Office of NIH History. http://history.nih.gov/exhibits/Goldberger/index.html Accessed: July 4, 2011

2. Simoni RD and others: Copper as an essential nutrient and nicotinic acid as the anti-black tongue (pellagra) factor: The work of Conrad Arnold Elvehjem. *Journal of Biological Chemistry* 277(34):e22, 2002.

3. Marshall BJ and others: Pyloric Campylobacter infection and gastroduodenal disease. *Medical Journal of Australia* 142(8):439, 1985.

4. Centers for Disease Control and Prevention: *National Diabetes Fact Sheet, 2011*. 2011. http://www.cdc.gov/diabetes/pubs/pdf/ndfs_2011.pdf Accessed: July 4, 2011

5. Centers for Disease Control and Prevention: *Breast cancer rates by race and ethnicity*. http://www.cdc.gov/cancer/breast/statistics/race.htm Accessed: July 4, 2011

6. Rossignol A: *Principles and Practice of Epidemiology*. Boston: McGraw-Hill, 2007.

7. Benedetti F and others: How placebos change the patient's brain. *Neuropsychopharmacology* 36(1):339–354, 2011.

8. Nagata C: Factors to consider in the association between isoflavone intake and breast cancer risk. *Journal of Epidemiology* 20(2):83, 2010.

9. McCracken M and others: Cancer incidence, mortality, and associated risk factors among Asian Americans of Chinese, Filipino, Vietnamese, Korean, and Japanese ethnicities. *CA: A Cancer Journal for Clinicians* 57:190, 2007.

10. American Cancer Society: *What are the risk factors for breast cancer?* http://www.cancer.org/Cancer/BreastCancer/DetailedGuide/breast-cancer-risk-factors Accessed: July 4, 2011

11. U.S. Federal Trade Commission: Marketers of unproven weight-loss products ordered to pay nearly $2 million. 2010. http://www.ftc.gov/opa/2010/01/diet.shtm Accessed: July 11, 2011

12. Kennedy J: Herb and supplement use in the US adult population. *Clinical Therapeutics* 27, 2005.

13. Bardia A and others: Use of herbs among adults based on evidence-based indications: Findings from the National Health Interview Survey. *Mayo Clinic Proceedings* 82:561, 2007.

14. Rock CL: Multivitamin-mineral supplements: Who uses them? *American Journal of Clinical Nutrition* 85:277S, 2007.

15. Food and Drug Administration: *Overview of dietary supplements*. Updated October, 2009. http://www.fda.gov/Food/DietarySupplements/ConsumerInformation/ucm110417.htm Accessed: July 4, 2011

16. National Center for Complementary and Alternative Medicine: *Using dietary supplements wisely*. Updated March 2010. http://nccam.nih.gov/health/supplements/wiseuse.htm Accessed: July 4, 2011

17. National Center for Complementary and Alternative Medicine: *The use of complementary and alternative medicine in the United States*. http://nccam.nih.gov/news/camstats/2007/camsurvey_fs1.htm Accessed: July 4, 2011

18. Kelly JP and others: Recent trends in use of herbal and other products. *Archives of Internal Medicine* 165:281, 2005.

19. Goldin BR, Gorach SL: Clinical indications for probiotics: An overview. *Clinical Infectious Diseases* 46:S96, 2008.

20. National Institutes of Health, Office of Dietary Supplements: *Dietary supplements: Background information*. Reviewed June 2011. http://ods.od.nih.gov/factsheets/DietarySupplements.asp Accessed: July 4, 2011

21. Food and Drug Administration: *Dietary supplements*. Last updated July 3, 2011. http://www.fda.gov/Food/DietarySupplements/default.htm Accessed: July 4, 2011

22. Food and Drug Administration: *FDA News Release: FDA issues dietary supplements final rule*. Updated May 2009. http://www.fda.gov/NewsEvents/Newsroom/PressAnnouncements/2007/ucm108938.htm Accessed: July 4, 2011

23. Food and Drug Administration: *FDA 101: Product recalls*. May 2010. http://www.fda.gov/downloads/ForConsumers/ConsumerUpdates/UCM143332.pdf Accessed: July 4, 2011

24. Food and Drug Adminstration: *FDA 101: Dietary supplements*. Posted 2008. http://www.fda.gov/ForConsumers/ConsumerUpdates/ucm050803.htm Accessed: July 4, 2011

25. American Academy of Allergy Asthma & Immunology: *Allergy & Asthma Advocate*, Summer 2006. http://www.aaaai.org/patients/advocate/2006/summer/herbal.asp Accessed: July 4, 2011

26. Mast C: Supplement sales continue strong growth trajectory in 2010. *Nutrition Business Journal*, January 2011. http://newhope360.com/print/supplements/supplement-sales-continue-strong-growth-trajectory-2010 Accessed: July 4, 2011

27. Liu RH: Potential synergy of phytochemicals in cancer prevention: Mechanism of action. *Journal of Nutrition* 134:3479S, 2004.

Chapter 3

1. Food Marketing Institute: *Supermarket facts: Industry overview 2010*. http://www.fmi.org/facts_figs/?fuseaction=superfact Accessed: July 6, 2011

2. Martinez S: Food product introductions buck long-term trend. *Amber Waves* 8 (2):44. USDA Agricultural Research Service, 2010. http://www.ers.usda.gov/AmberWaves/June10/Indicators/InTheLongRun.htm Accessed: July 6, 2011

3. Institute of Medicine: *Dietary Reference Intakes for vitamin C, vitamin E, selenium, and carotenoids*. Washington, DC: National Academies Press, 2000.

4. Otten JJ and others (eds): *Dietary Reference Intakes: The essential guide to nutrient requirements*. Institute of Medicine of the National Academies. Washington, DC: National Academies Press, 2006.

5. Barr SI and others: Interpreting and using the Dietary Reference Intakes in dietary assessment of individuals and groups. *Journal of the American Dietetic Association* 102(6):780, 2002.

6. FDA provides guidance on "whole grain" for manufacturers. *FDA News*, P06–23 (updated 2009). http://www.fda.gov/NewsEvents/Newsroom/PressAnnouncements/2006/ucm108598.htm Accessed: July 6, 2011

7. U.S. Department of Agriculture: Choose MyPlate: *What counts as a cup of fruit?* (Last modified June 2011). http://www.choosemyplate.gov/foodgroups/fruits_counts.html# Accessed: July 6, 2011

8. Centers for Disease Control and Prevention: *Eat a variety of fruits & vegetables every day*. http://www.fruitsandveggiesmatter.gov/qa/index.html#14 Accessed: July 6, 2011

9. U.S. Department of Agriculture: Choose MyPlate: *What are oils?* (Last modified June 2011). http://www.choosemyplate.gov/foodgroups/oils.html Accessed: July 6, 2011

10. U.S. Departments of Health and Human Services and Agriculture: *Dietary Guidelines for Americans 2010*. 2011. http://health.gov/dietaryguidelines/2010.asp Accessed: July 6, 2011

11. U.S. Department of Agriculture. Science and Education Administration: *Food*. Home and Garden Bulletin No. 228. Washington, DC: GPO, 1979.

12. U.S. Department of Agriculture: *Choose MyPlate.gov* 2011. http://www.choosemyplate.gov/ Accessed: July 6, 2011

13. U.S. Department of Agriculture: *Physical activity.* http://www.choosemyplate.gov/foodgroups/physicalactivity.html Accessed: July 10, 2011

14. Guenther PM and others: Diet quality of low-income and higher-income Americans in 2003–04 as measured by the Healthy Eating Index–2005. U.S. Department of Agriculture, *Nutrition Insight 42, 2008.* http://www.cnpp.usda.gov/Publications/NutritionInsights/Insight42.pdf Accessed: July 6, 2011

15. Neithercott T: Understanding exchanges. *Diabetes Forecast*, August 2009. http://forecast.diabetes.org/magazine/features/understanding-exchanges Accessed: July 6, 2011

16. U.S. Food and Drug Administration, Center for Food Safety and Applied Nutrition: *How to understand and use the Nutrition Facts label.* Updated March 2011. http://www.fda.gov/Food/LabelingNutrition/ConsumerInformation/ucm078889.htm#see6 Accessed: July 6, 2011

17. U.S. Food and Drug Administration: *New menu and vending machine labeling requirements.* Updated June, 2011. http://www.fda.gov/Food/LabelingNutrition/ucm217762.htm Accessed: July 10, 2011

18. Urban LE and others: The accuracy of stated energy contents of reduced-energy, commercially prepared foods. *Journal of the American Dietetic Association* 110(1):116, 2010.

19. Earles K: *Sustainable agriculture: An introduction.* National Sustainable Agricultural Service, 2005. https://attra.ncat.org/attra-pub/PDF/sustagintro.pdf Accessed: July 6, 2011

20. U.S. Department of Agriculture, National Organic Program: *Background information.* Updated 2008. http://www.ams.usda.gov/AMSv1.0/getfile?dDocName=STELDEV3004443&acct=nopgeninfo Accessed: July 6, 2011

21. Comis D: No shortcuts in checking soil health. *Agricultural Research* 55(6):4, 2007. Accessed: July 6, 2011

22. Environmental Protection Agency: *Pesticides and Food: Healthy, Sensible Food Practices.* Updated February 2011. http://www.epa.gov/pesticides/food/tips.htm Accessed: July 6, 2011

23. U.S. Department of Agriculture, Economic Research Service: *Organic agriculture: Organic market overview.* Updated 2009. http://www.ers.usda.gov/briefing/organic/demand.htm Accessed: July 6, 2011

24. Organic Trade Association: *U.S. Organic Product Sales Reach $26.6 Billion in 2009.* 2010. http://www.organicnewsroom.com/2010/04/us_organic_product_sales_reach_1.html Accessed: July 6, 2011

25. U.S. Food and Drug Administration, Animal & Veterinary: *Animal cloning.* Updated 2010. http://www.fda.gov/AnimalVeterinary/SafetyHealth/AnimalCloning/default.htm Accessed: July 6, 2011

26. Dangour AD and others: Nutritional quality of organic foods: A systematic review. *American Journal of Clinical Nutrition* July 29, 2009 DOI: 10.3945/ajcn.2009.28041

27. U.S. Department of Agriculture, Alternative Farming Systems Information Center: *Should I purchase organic foods?* Last modified 2010. http://www.nal.usda.gov/afsic/pubs/faq/BuyOrganicFoodsIntro.shtml Accessed: July 6, 2011

Chapter 4

1. Saladin KS: *Anatomy & physiology.* 6th ed. Boston: McGraw-Hill Publishing Company, 2012.

2. Widmaier E and others: *Vander's human physiology.* 12th ed. Boston: McGraw-Hill Publishing Company, 2010.

3. Seeley RR and others: *Essentials of anatomy & physiology.* 9th ed. Boston: McGraw-Hill Publishing Company, 2011.

4. Prescott LM and others: *Microbiology.* 8th ed. Boston: McGraw-Hill Publishing Company, 2011.

5. Goldin BR, Gorbach SL: Clinical indications for probiotics: An overview. *Clinical Infectious Diseases* 46:S96-100, 2008.

6. American Gastroenterological Association: *Understanding constipation.* 2008. http://www.gastro.org/patient-center/digestive-conditions/constipation Accessed: July 10, 2011

7. The Cleveland Clinic Information Center: *Nausea and vomiting.* 2009. http://my.clevelandclinic.org/symptoms/nausea/hic_nausea_and_vomiting.aspx Accessed: July 10, 2011

8. American Gastroenterological Association: *Understanding heartburn and reflux disease.* 2008. http://www.gastro.org/patient-center/digestive-conditions/heartburn-gerd Accessed: July 10, 2011

9. American Society for Gastrointestinal Endoscopy: *Understanding upper endoscopy.* ND. www.asge.org/PatientInfoIndex.aspx?id=378 Accessed: July 10, 2011

10. National Digestive Diseases Information Clearinghouse: *Irritable bowel syndrome.* 2007. http://www.digestive.niddk.nih.gov/ddiseases/pubs/ibs/index.aspx Accessed: July 10, 2011

11. Mayo Clinic.com: *Irritable bowel syndrome.* 2009. www.mayoclinic.com/invoke.cfm?id=DS00106& Accessed: July 11, 2011

Chapter 5

1. Economic Research Service, U.S. Department of Agriculture: U.S. per capita loss-adjusted food availability: Sweeteners by individual caloric sweetener 2010. http://www.ers.usda.gov/Data/FoodConsumption/app/loss_adjusted.aspx Accessed: July 5, 2011

2. Tanzi MG, Gabay MP: Association between honey consumption and infant botulism. *Pharmacotherapy* 22(11):1479, 2002.

3. Centers for Disease Control and Prevention, National Center for Zoonotic, Vector-Borne, and Enteric Diseases. *Botulism.* 2010. http://www.cdc.gov/nczved/dfbmd/disease_listing/botulism_gi.html#8 Accessed: July 5, 2011

4. American Dietetic Association: Position of the American Dietetic Association: Use of nutritive and nonnutritive sweeteners. *Journal of the American Dietetic Association* 104(2):255, 2004.

5. Swithers SE and others: High-intensity sweeteners and energy balance. *Physiology & Behavior* 100(1):55, 2010.

6. Soffritti M and others: First experimental demonstration of the multipotential carcinogenic effects of aspartame administered in the feed to Sprague-Dawley rats. *Environmental Health Perspectives* 114(3):379, 2006.

7. U.S. Food and Drug Administration: *FDA Statement on European Aspartame Study.* Updated 2010. http://www.fda.gov/Food/FoodIngredientsPackaging/FoodAdditives/ucm208580.htm Accessed: July 12, 2011

8. FDA provides guidance on "whole grain" for manufacturers. *FDA News*, P06–23. Updated 2009. http://www.fda.gov/NewsEvents/Newsroom/PressAnnouncements/2006/ucm108598.htm Accessed: July 11, 2011

9. Otten JJ and others, eds.: *Dietary Reference Intakes: The essential guide to nutrient requirements.* Washington, DC: National Academies Press, 2006.

10. U.S. Department of Agriculture, Agricultural Research Service: *Nutrient intakes from food: Mean amounts consumed per individual, by gender and age, in the United States, 2007–2008.* http://www.ars.usda.gov/SP2UserFiles/Place/12355000/pdf/0708/Table_1_NIN_GEN_07.pdf Accessed: July 10, 2011

11. U.S. Department of Agriculture: *Choose MyPlate.gov* 2011. http://www.choosemyplate.gov/ Accessed: July 6, 2011

12. U.S. Department of Agriculture, Agricultural Research Service, Nutrient Data Laboratory: *USDA database for the added sugars content of selected foods, release 1.* 2006. http://www.ars.usda.gov/SP2UserFiles/Place/12354500/Data/Add_Sug/addsug01.pdf Accessed: July 11, 2011

13. Welsh JA and others: Consumption of added sugars is decreasing in the United States. *American Journal of Clinical Nutrition* ajcn.018366; First published online July 13, 2011.

14. O'Leary N: Soft drink consumption continues to decline. *AdWeek* March 30, 2010. http://www.adweek.com/news/advertising-branding/soft-drink-consumption-continues-decline-107218 Accessed: July 2, 2011

15. Gaesser GA: Carbohydrate quantity and quality in relation to body mass index. *Journal of the American Dietetic Association* 107(10):1768, 2007.

16. Rosen LA and others: Effects of cereals on postprandial glucose, appetite regulation and voluntary energy intake at subsequent lunch; focusing on rye products. *Nutrition Journal* 10:7, 2011.

17. Saris WH: Sugars, energy metabolism, and body weight control. *American Journal of Clinical Nutrition 78(Suppl):* 850S–857S, 2003.

18. Rolls BJ: Plenary lecture 1 dietary strategies for the prevention and treatment of obesity. *Proceedings of the Nutrition Society* 69(1): 70, 2010.

19. Wolff E, Dansinger M: Soft drinks and weight gain: How strong is the link? *Medscape Journal of Medicine* 10(8):189, 2008.

20. Jennings A and others: Diet quality is independently associated with weight status in children aged 9-10 years. *Journal of Nutrition* 141(3): 453, 2011.

21. Centers for Disease Control and Prevention: Beverage consumption among high school students—United States, 2010. *Morbidity Mortality Weekly Report* 60(23):778, 2011.

22. Yanovski S: Sugar and fat: Cravings and aversions. *Journal of Nutrition,* 133 (3):835S, 2003.

23. Benton D: The plausibility of sugar addition and its role in obesity and eating disorders. *Clinical Nutrition* 29(3):288, 2010.

24. Dennis EA and others: Beverage consumption and adult weight management: A review. *Eating Behaviors* 10(4):237, 2009.

25. Hu FB, Malik VS: Sugar-sweetened beverages and risk of obesity and type 2 diabetes: Epidemiologic evidence. *Physiology and Behavior* 100(1):47, 2010.

26. U.S. Department of Agriculture, Economic Research Service: *U.S. per capita loss-adjusted food availability: Total calories.* http://www.ers.usda.gov/data/foodconsumption/app/reports/displayCommodities.aspx?reportName=Total%20Calories&id=36#startForm Accessed: July 18, 2011

27. Report of the expert committee on the diagnosis and classification of diabetes mellitus. *Diabetes Care* 26(Suppl 1):S5, 2003.

28. Centers for Disease Control and Prevention: *National diabetes fact sheet, 2011.* 2011. http://www.cdc.gov/diabetes/pubs/pdf/ndfs_2011.pdf Accessed: July 11, 2011

29. National Institutes of Health, National Diabetes Information Clearinghouse: *What diabetes is.* 2008. http://www.diabetes.niddk.nih.gov/dm/pubs/type1and2/what.aspx Accessed: July 18, 2011

30. Yeung WG and others: Enterovirus infection and type 1 diabetes mellitus: Systematic review and meta-analysis of observational molecular studies. *British Medical Journal* 2011:342:d35 doi:10.1136/bmj.d35

31. Luopajärvi K and others: Enhanced levels of cow's milk antibodies in infancy in children who develop type 1 diabetes later in childhood. *Pediatric Diabetes* 9(5):434, 2008.

32. Poston L and others: Obesity in pregnancy: Implications for the mother and lifelong health of the child. A consensus statement. *Pediatric Research* 69(2):175, 2011.

33. Mayo Clinic: *A1C test.* http://www.mayoclinic.com/health/a1c-test/MY00142 Accessed: July 16, 2011

34. American Diabetes Association: *Weight loss.* http://www.diabetes.org/food-and-fitness/fitness/weight-loss/?utm_source=WWW&utm_medium=DropDownFF&utm_content=WeightLoss&utm_campaign=CON Accessed: July 18, 2011

35. National Institutes of Health, National Diabetes Information Clearinghouse: Diabetes prevention program. http://diabetes.niddk.nih.gov/dm/pubs/preventionprogram/ Accessed: July 19, 2011

36. Esposito K and others: Prevention of type 2 diabetes by dietary patterns: A systematic review of prospective studies and meta-analysis. *Metabolic Syndrome and Related Disorders* 8(6):471, 2010.

37. Song Y and others: A prospective study of red meat consumption and type 2 diabetes in middle-aged and elderly women: The women's health study. *Diabetes Care* 27(9):2108, 2004.

38. de Munter JSL and others: Whole grain, bran, and germ intake and risk of type 2 diabetes: A prospective cohort study and systematic review. *PLOS Medicine* 4(8):135, 2007.

39. Johnson RJ and others: Potential role of sugar (fructose) in the epidemic of hypertension, obesity and the metabolic syndrome, diabetes, kidney disease, and cardiovascular disease. *American Journal of Clinical Nutrition* 86:899, 2007.

40. National Institute of Diabetes and Digestive and Kidney Diseases: *Hypoglycemia.* Publication No. 09–3926, 2008. http://diabetes.niddk.nih.gov/dm/pubs/hypoglycemia/ Accessed: July 16, 2011

41. Bakris GL: Current perspectives on hypertension and metabolic syndrome. *Journal of Managed Care Pharmacy* 13(5):S3, 2007.

42. Grundy SM and others: Diagnosis and management of the metabolic syndrome: An American Heart Association/National Heart, Lung, and Blood Institute scientific statement: Executive summary. *Circulation* 112:e285, 2005.

43. National Center for Biotechnology Information: Metabolic syndrome. *PubMed Health.* 2010. http://www.ncbi.nlm.nih.gov/pubmedhealth/PMH0004546/ Accessed: July 19, 2011

44. National Institutes of Health, National Heart Lung and Blood Institute: *Metabolic syndrome: What is metabolic syndrome?* Revised April 2011. http://www.nhlbi.nih.gov/health/dci/Diseases/ms/ms_whatis.html

45. National Institute of Diabetes and Digestive and Kidney Diseases: *Lactose intolerance.* NIH Publication No. 06–2751, 2009. http://digestive.niddk.nih.gov/ddiseases/pubs/lactoseintolerance/index.htm Accessed: July 16, 2011

46. Montalto M and others: Management and treatment of lactose malabsorption. *World Journal of Gastroenterology* 12(2):187, 2006.

47. National Institute of Mental Health: *Attention deficit hyperactivity disorder.* Last revised July 5, 2011. http://www.nimh.nih.gov/health/publications/attention-deficit-hyperactivity-disorder/complete-index.shtml Accessed: July 16, 2011

48. Centers for Disease Control and Prevention: *Attention-Deficit/Hyperactivity Disorder (ADHD), Data & statistics.* Updated 2010. http://www.cdc.gov/ncbddd/adhd/data.html Accessed: July 16, 2011

49. World Health Organization: *Cancer: World cancer day 2011.* http://www.who.int/cancer/en/index.html Accessed: July 16, 2011

50. Centers for Disease Control and Prevention: *Facts about colorectal cancer.* Last updated January 2011. http://www.cdc.gov/cancer/colorectal/basic_info/facts.htm Accessed: July 16, 2011

51. Park Y and others: Dietary fiber intake and risk of colorectal cancer: A pooled analysis of prospective cohort studies. *Journal of the American Medical Association* 294(22):2849, 2005.

52. Egeberg R and others: Intake of whole grain products and risk of colorectal cancers in the Diet, Cancer, and Health cohort study. *British Journal of Cancer* 103(5):730, 2010.

53. Centers for Disease Control and Prevention: *Colorectal (colon) cancer: Colorectal cancer prevention.* Updated July 14, 2011. http://www.cdc.gov/cancer/colorectal/basic_info/prevention.htm Accessed: July 19, 2011

54. American Dietetic Association: Position of the American Dietetic Association: Health implications of dietary fiber. *Journal of the American Dietetic Association* 108(10):1716, 2008.

55. Webb D: Glycemic index: Gateway to good health or grand waste of time? *Environmental Nutrition* 25(1): 1, 6, 2002.

56. Barclay AW and others: Glycemic index, glycemic load, and chronic disease risk—a meta-analysis of observational studies. *American Journal of Clinical Nutrition* 87(3):627, 2008.

57. Foster-Powell K and others: International table of glycemic index and glycemic load values. *American Journal of Clinical Nutrition* 76(1):5, 2002.

58. Denova-Gutierrez E and others: Dietary glycemic index, dietary glycemic load, blood lipids, and coronary heart disease. *Journal of Nutrition and Metabolism* Published online 2010 February 28. doi: 10.1155/2010/170680

59. Jenkins DJ and others: Effect of low-glycemic index or a high-cereal fiber diet on type 2 diabetes: A randomized trial. *Journal of the American Medical Association* 300(23):2742, 2008.

60. Saul N and Maryniuk MD: Using the glycemic index in diabetes management. *American Journal of Nursing* 110(7):68, 2010.

Chapter 6

1. Shikany JM and others: Is dietary fat "fattening"? A comprehensive research synthesis. *Critical Reviews in Food Science and Nutrition* 50(8):699, 2010.

2. McTiernan A and others: Weight, physical activity, diet, and prognosis in breast and gynecological cancers. *Journal of Clinical Oncology* 28(26):4074, 2010.

3. Siri-Tarino and others: Saturated fatty acids and risk of coronary heart disease: Modulation by replacement nutrients. *Current Atherosclerosis Reports* 12(6):384, 2010.

4. Hunter JE and others: Cardiovascular disease risk of dietary stearic acid compared with trans, other saturated, and unsaturated fatty acids: A systemic review. *American Journal of Clinical Nutrition* 91(1):46, 2010.

5. Otten JJ and others (eds.): *Dietary Reference Intakes: The essential guide to nutrient requirements.* Washington, DC: National Academies Press, 2006.

6. Remig V and others: Trans fat in America: A review of their use, consumption, health implications, and regulation. *Journal of the American Dietetic Association* 110(4):585, 2010.

7. Brouwer IA and others: Effect of animal and industrial trans fatty acids on HDL and LDL cholesterol levels in humans—a quantitative review. *PLoS One* 5(3):e9434, 2010.

8. American Heart Association: *Knowing your fats.* Updated 2010. http://www.heart.org/HEARTORG/GettingHealthy/NutritionCenter/Knowing-Your-Fats_UCM_305976_Article.jsp Accessed: July 20, 2011

9. Sundram K and others: Stearic-acid rich interesterified fat and trans fat raise the LDL/HDL ratio and plasma glucose relative to palm olein in humans. *Nutrition & Metabolism* 4:3, 2007.

10. Astrup A and others: The role of reducing intakes of saturated fat in the prevention of cardiovascular disease: Where does the evidence stand in 2010? *American Journal of Clinical Nutrition* 93(4): 684, 2011.

11. Zeisel SH: Nutritional genomics: Defining the dietary requirement and effects of choline. *Journal of Nutrition* 141(3):531, 2011.

12. Penry JT and Manore MM: Choline: An important micronutrient for maximal endurance-exercise performance? *International Journal of Sports Nutrition, Exercise, and Metabolism* 18(2):191, 2008.

13. Rodriguez NR and others: Position of the American Dietetic Association, Dietitians of Canada, and the American College of Sports Medicine: Nutrition and athletic performance. *Journal of the American Dietetic Association* 109(3):509, 2009.

14. Oregon State University, Linus Pauling Institute: *Choline.* Updated 2009. http://lpi.oregonstate.edu/infocenter/othernuts/choline// Accessed: July 20, 2011

15. Plat J, Mensink RP: Plant stanol and sterol esters in the control of blood cholesterol levels: Mechanism and safety aspects. *American Journal of Cardiology* 96(1A):15D, 2005.

16. U.S. Department of Agriculture: *Nationwide food consumption survey, Food and nutrient intakes by individuals in the United States, 1 day, 1987–88.* http://www.ars.usda.gov/SP2UserFiles/Place/12355000/pdf/8788/nfcs8788_rep_87-i-1.pdf Accessed: July 20, 2011

17. U.S. Department of Agriculture, Agricultural Research Service: *Nutrient intakes from food: Mean amounts consumed per individual, by gender and age, in the United States, 2007–2008.* http://www.ars.usda.gov/SP2UserFiles/Place/12355000/pdf/0708/Table_1_NIN_GEN_07.pdf Accessed: July 20, 2011

18. U.S. Departments of Health and Human Services and Agriculture: *Dietary Guidelines for Americans 2010.* 2011. http://www.health.gov/dietaryguidelines/dga2010/DietaryGuidelines2010.pdf Accessed: July 21, 2011

19. American Heart Association: AHA statistics update: Heart disease and stroke statistics—2010 update. 2009. http://circ.ahajournals.org/content/early/2009/12/17/CIRCULATIONAHA.109.192667 Accessed: July 20, 2011

20. Kochanek KD and others: Deaths: Preliminary data for 2009. *National Vital Statistics Reports* 59, 2011 http://www.cdc.gov/nchs/data/nvsr/nvsr59/nvsr59_04.pdf Accessed: July 2, 2011

21. National Heart Lung and Blood Institute: *Atherosclerosis: Who is at risk for atherosclerosis?* ND. http://www.nhlbi.nih.gov/health/dci/Diseases/Atherosclerosis/atherosclerosis_risk.html Accessed: July 21, 2011

22. Abraham JM, Cho L: The homocysteine hypothesis: Still relevant to the prevention and treatment of cardiovascular disease? *Cleveland Clinic Journal of Medicine,* 77(12):911, 2010.

23. Centers for Disease Control and Prevention: *National diabetes fact sheet, 2011.* http://www.cdc.gov/diabetes/pubs/pdf/ndfs_2011.pdf Accessed: July 16, 2011

24. Centers for Disease Control and Prevention: *Smoking & tobacco use.* Updated March 2011. http://www.cdc.gov/tobacco/data_statistics/fact_sheets/health_effects/effects_cig_smoking/index.htm Accessed: July 21, 2011

25. Centers for Disease Control and Prevention: *Smoking & tobacco use: Health effects of secondhand smoke.* March 2011. http://www.cdc.gov/tobacco/data_statistics/fact_sheets/secondhand_smoke/health_effects/index.htm Accessed: July 21, 2011

26. Shoji T and others: Small dense low-density lipoprotein cholesterol concentration and carotid atherosclerosis. *Atherosclerosis* 202(2):582, 2009.

27. Thanassoulis G and others: Associations of long-term and early adult atherosclerosis risk factors with aortic and mitral valve calcium. *Journal of the American College of Cardiology* 55(22):2491, 2010.

28. Centers for Disease Control and Prevention, National Center for Health Statistics: *FastStats: Cholesterol.* Updated February 2011. http://www.cdc.gov/nchs/fastats/cholest.htm Accessed: July 22, 2011

29. Mayo Clinic: *How important is the cholesterol ratio?* 2010. http://www.mayoclinic.com/health/cholesterol-ratio/AN01761 Accessed: July 20, 2011

30. Fernandez ML, Webb D: The LDL to HDL cholesterol ratio as a valuable tool to evaluate coronary heart disease risk. *Journal of the American College of Nutrition* 27(1):1, 2008.

31. National Institutes of Health: C-reactive protein. *MedLinePlus.* Last updated June 2011. http://www.nlm.nih.gov/medlineplus/ency/article/003356.htm Accessed: July 20, 2011

32. Fernandez ML, West KL: Mechanisms by which dietary fatty acids modulate plasma lipids. *Journal of Nutrition* 135(9):2075, 2005.

33. Eckel RH and others: Understanding the complexity of trans fatty acid reduction in the American diet. *Circulation* 115(16):2231, 2007.

34. De Caterina R: n-3 Fatty acids in cardiovascular disease. *New England Journal of Medicine* 364:2439, 2011.

35. Harris WS and others: Omega-6 fatty acids and risk for cardiovascular disease: A science advisory from the American Heart Association Nutrition Subcommittee of the Council on Nutrition, Physical Activity, and Metabolism; Council on Cardiovascular Nursing; and Council on Epidemiology and Prevention. *Circulation* 119(6):902, 2009.

36. Djoussé L, Gaziano JM: Egg consumption and risk of heart failure in the Physician's Health Study. *Circulation* 117(4):512, 2008.

37. Mayo Clinic: *Butter vs. margarine: Which is better for my heart?* 2010. http://www.mayoclinic.com/print/butter-vs-margarine/AN00835/METHOD=print Accessed: July 22, 2011

38. National Institutes of Health, National Center for Alternative and Complementary Medicine: *Garlic.* 2010. http://nccam.nih.gov/health/garlic/ataglance.htm Accessed: July 22, 2011.

39. American Dietetic Association: Position of the American Dietetic Association: Fat replacers. *Journal of the American Dietetic Association* 105(2):266, 2005.

40. Nestel PJ and others: Management of dyslipidaemia: Evidence and practical recommendations. *Australian Family Physician* 37(7):521, 2008.

41. National Institutes of Health, National Institute on Alcohol Abuse and Alcoholism. *Alcohol: A women's health issue.* Rev. 2008. http://pubs.niaaa.nih.gov/publications/brochurewomen/women.htm Accessed: July 22, 2011

42. Substance Abuse and Mental Health Services Administration: *Results from the 2009 National Survey on Drug Use and Health: Volume I: Summary of National Findings.* 2010. http://oas.samhsa.gov/NSDUH/2k9NSDUH/2k9Results.htm#3.1 Accessed: July 22, 2011

43. Centers for Disease Control and Prevention: *Alcohol & Public Health.* Last update June 17, 2011. http://www.cdc.gov/alcohol/index.htm Accessed: July 22, 2011

44. Centers for Disease Control and Prevention: *Vital signs: Binge drinking by age, US, 2009.* 2010. http://www.cdc.gov/vitalsigns/BingeDrinking/Risk-large.html#age Accessed: July 22, 2011

45. Hasin DS and others: Prevalence, correlates, disability, and comorbidity of DSM-IV alcohol abuse and dependence in the United States. *Archives of General Psychiatry* 64(7):830, 2007.

46. American Cancer Society: *Alcohol use and cancer.* 2010. http://www.cancer.org/Cancer/CancerCauses/DietandPhysicalActivity/alcohol-use-and-cancer Accessed: July 22, 2011

47. King DE and others: Adopting moderate alcohol consumption in middle-age: Subsequent cardiovascular events. *American Journal of Medicine* 121(3):201, 2008.

48. Leifert WR and Abeywardena MY: Cardioprotective actions of grape polyphenols. *Nutrition Research* 28(11):729, 2008.

Chapter 7

1. Shier D and others: *Hole's human anatomy & physiology.* 12th ed. Boston: McGraw-Hill Publishing Company, 2010.

2. Reeds PJ: Dispensable and indispensable amino acids for humans. *Journal of Nutrition* 130:1835S, 2000.

3. Food and Nutrition Board: *Dietary Reference Intakes for energy, carbohydrate, fiber, fat, fatty acids, cholesterol, protein, and amino acids (macronutrients).* Institute of Medicine of the National Academies, Washington, DC: National Academies Press, 2005.

4. Oelke EA and others: Quinoa. *Alternative Field Crops Manual.* University of Wisconsin-Extension, University of Minnesota: Center for Alternative Plant & Animal Productions, and the Minnesota Extension Service. ND. http://www.hort.purdue.edu/newcrop/afcm/quinoa.html. Accessed: July 22, 2011

5. Young VR: Soy protein in relation to human protein and amino acids nutrition. *Journal of the American Dietetic Association* 91(7):828, 1991.

6. Messina MJ: Legumes and soybeans: Overview of their nutritional profiles and health effects. *American Journal of Clinical Nutrition* 70(Suppl):439S, 1999.

7. Tomé D, Bos C: Dietary protein and nitrogen utilization. *Journal of Nutrition* 130(7):1868S, 2000.

8. Layman DK: Dietary Guidelines should reflect new understandings about adult protein needs. *Nutrition & Metabolism* 2009, 6:12 doi:10.1186/1743-7075-6-12

9. Cleveland Clinic: *Sulfite sensitivity.* 2010. http://my.clevelandclinic.org/disorders/sulfite_sensitivity/hic_Sulfite_Sensitivity.aspx Accessed: July 22, 2011

10. American Academy of Allergy, Asthma, and Immunology (AAAAI): *Allergy statistics.* ND. http://www.aaaai.org/media/statistics/allergy-statistics.asp#foodallergy Accessed: July 22, 2011

11. Niggemann B, Gruber C: Unproven diagnostic procedures in IgE-mediated allergic diseases. *Allergy* 59(8):806, 2004.

12. Center for Food Safety and Applied Nutrition: *Food Allergen Labeling and Consumer Protection Act of 2004.* (Title II of Public Law 108–282). 2004. http://www.fda.gov/Food/LabelingNutrition/FoodAllergensLabeling/GuidanceComplianceRegulatoryInformation/ucm106187.htm Accessed: July 22, 2011

13. National Institutes of Health, National Digestive Diseases Information Clearinghouse: *Celiac disease.* September 2008. http://digestive.niddk.nih.gov/ddiseases/pubs/celiac/celiac.pdf Accessed: July 22, 2011

14. National Institutes of Health, U.S. Department of Health and Human Services, National Human Genome Research Institute: *Learning about phenylketonuria (PKU).* Last reviewed 2010. http://www.genome.gov/pfv.cfm?pageID=25020037 Accessed: July 22, 2011

15. Centers for Disease Control and Prevention: *After the baby arrives: Health: Newborn screening.* Last updated 2010. http://www.cdc.gov/ncbddd/pregnancy_gateway/after.html Accessed: July 22, 2011

16. U.S. Department of Agriculture, Agricultural Research Service: *Nutrient intakes from food: Mean amounts consumed per individual, by gender and age, in the United States, 2007–2008.* http://www.ars.usda.gov/SP2UserFiles/Place/12355000/pdf/0708/Table_1_NIN_GEN_07.pdf Accessed: July 23, 2011

17. Hiza HAB and others: *Nutrient content of the U.S. food supply, 2005.* U.S. Department of Agriculture, Center for Nutrition Policy and Promotion. Home Economics Research Report Number 58. March 2008. http://www.cnpp.usda.gov/Publications/FoodSupply/FoodSupply2005Report.pdf Accessed: July 24, 2011

18. U.S. Department of Agriculture: *Food groups: Protein foods.* Last modified June 2011. http://www.choosemyplate.gov/foodgroups/proteinfoods.html Accessed: July 23, 2011

19. American Dietetic Association: Position of the American Dietetic Association: Vegetarian diets. *Journal of the American Dietetic Association* 109(7):1266, 2009.

20. Robinson-O'Brien R and others: Adolescent and young adult vegetarianism: Better dietary intake and weight outcomes but increased risk of disordered eating behaviors. *Journal of the American Dietetic Association* 109(4):648, 2009.

21. Craig WJ: Health effects of vegan diets. *American Journal of Clinical Nutrition* 89(5):1627S, 2009.

22. American Dietetic Association: Position of the American Dietetic Association, Dietitians of Canada, and the American College of Sports Medicine: Nutrition and Athletic Performance. *Journal of the American Dietetic Association* 109:509, 2009.

23. Watanabe F: Vitamin B-12 sources and bioavailability. *Experimental Biology & Medicine* 232:1266, 2007.

24. Anon: Neurologic impairment in children associated with maternal dietary deficiency of cobalamin—Georgia, 2001. *Morbidity and Mortality Weekly Report* 52(4):61, 2003.

25. American Cancer Society: *What are the risk factors for colorectal cancer?* Last revised March 2011. http://www.cancer.org/Cancer/ColonandRectumCancer/DetailedGuide/colorectal-cancer-risk-factors Accessed: July 24, 2011

26. American Cancer Society: *What are the risk factors for prostate cancer?* Last revised June 2011. http://www.cancer.org/Cancer/ProstateCancer/DetailedGuide/prostate-cancer-risk-factors Accessed: July 24, 2011

27. American Cancer Society: *What are the risk factors for pancreatic cancer?* Last revised June 2011. http://www.cancer.org/Cancer/PancreaticCancer/DetailedGuide/pancreatic-cancer-risk-factors Accessed: July 24, 2011

28. American Cancer Society: *What are the risk factors for stomach cancer?* Last revised June 2011. http://www.cancer.org/Cancer/StomachCancer/DetailedGuide/stomach-cancer-risk-factors Accessed: July 24, 2011

29. Weikert C and others: The relation between dietary protein, calcium and bone health in women: Results from the EPIC-Potsdam Cohort. *Annals of Nutrition & Metabolism* 49:312, 2005.

30. Weigle DS and others: A high-protein diet induces sustained reductions in appetite, ad libitum caloric intake, and body weight despite compensatory changes in diurnal plasma leptin and ghrelin concentrations. *American Journal of Clinical Nutrition* 82(1):41, 2005.

31. World Health Organization: *Global health observatory: Underweight in children.* ND. http://www.who.int/gho/mdg/poverty_hunger/underweight/en/index.html Accessed: July 24, 2011

32. Lemon PW and others: Protein requirements and muscle mass/strength changes during intensive training in novice bodybuilders. *Journal of Applied Physiology* 73(2):767, 1992.

33. Williams MH: *Nutrition for health, fitness, & sport.* 8th ed. New York: McGraw-Hill, 2007.

34. U.S. Department of Agriculture, Food Safety and Inspection Service. *Fact sheets: Food labeling: Food product dating.* Last modified April 2011. www.fsis.usda.gov/Fact_Sheets/Food_Product_Dating/index.asp Accessed: July 23, 2011

Chapter 8

1. Bartholomew, M: James Lind's *Treatise of the Scurvy* (1753). *Postgraduate Medicine* 78:695, 2002.

2. Zeisel SH: Importance of methyl donors during reproduction. *American Journal of Clinical Nutrition* 89(20):673S, 2009.

3. What is a megadose and why do you recommend against taking megadoses of vitamins? *Johns Hopkins Medical Letter Health After 50*, p. 8, August 2001.

4. Food and Nutrition Board: *Dietary Reference Intakes for vitamin C, vitamin E, selenium, and carotenoids.* Washington, DC: National Academy Press, 2000.

5. Vandamme EJ: Production of vitamins, coenzymes and related biochemicals by biotechnological processes. *Journal of Chemical Technology & Biotechnology* 53(4):313, 1992.

6. Murphy SP and others: Multivitamin-multimineral supplements' effect on total nutrition intake. *American Journal of Clinical Nutrition* 85(suppl):280S, 2007.

7. Rock CL: Multivitamin-multimineral supplements: Who uses them? *American Journal of Clinical Nutrition* 85(suppl):277S, 2007.

8. Hernandez A: Personal communication. Kelloggs' Consumer Affairs Department, 2007.

9. U.S. Department of Agriculture, Agricultural Research Service: *Nutrient intakes from food: Mean amounts consumed per individual, by gender and age, in the United States, 2007–2008.* http://www.ars.usda.gov/SP2UserFiles/Place/12355000/pdf/0708/Table_1_NIN_GEN_07.pdf Accessed: July 25, 2011

10. Office of Dietary Supplements: *Dietary supplement fact sheet: Vitamin C.* Last reviewed June 2011. http://ods.od.nih.gov/factsheets/VitaminC-HealthProfessional/ Accessed: July 27, 2011

11. Food and Drug Administration, Center for Devices and Radiological Health, CDRH Consumer Information: *Microwave oven radiation.* Updated June 2011. http://www.fda.gov/Radiation-EmittingProducts/ResourcesforYouRadiationEmittingProducts/ucm252762.htm Accessed: July 25, 2011

12. Office of Dietary Supplements: *Dietary supplement fact sheet: Vitamin A and carotenoids.* 2006. http://ods.od.nih.gov/factsheets/VitaminA-HealthProfessional/ Accessed: July 25, 2011

13. World Health Organization: *Micronutrient deficiencies: Vitamin A deficiency.* ND. http://www.who.int/nutrition/topics/vad/en/index.html Accessed: July 25, 2011

14. Zile MH: Function of vitamin A in vertebrate embryonic development. *Journal of Nutrition* 131:705, 2001.

15. Sale TA, Stratman E: Carotenemia associated with green bean ingestion. *Pediatric Dermatology* 21(6):657, 2004.

16. Holick MF: Vitamin D deficiency. *New England Journal of Medicine* 357:266, 2007.

17. National Institutes of Health, Office of Dietary Supplements: *Dietary Supplement Fact Sheet: Vitamin D.* Last reviewed June 2011. http://ods.od.nih.gov/factsheets/VitaminD-HealthProfessional/ Accessed: July 25, 2011

18. Hanley DA, Davison KS: Vitamin D insufficiency in North America. *Journal of Nutrition* 135:332, 2005.

19. Cardinal RN and Gregory CA: Osteomalacia and vitamin D deficiency in a psychiatric rehabilitation unit: Case report and survey. *BMC Research Notes* 2: 82, 2009.

20. National Institutes of Health, Office of Dietary Supplements: *Dietary Supplement Fact Sheet: Vitamin E.* Updated June 2011. http://ods.od.nih.gov/factsheets/VitaminE-HealthProfessional/ Accessed: July 25, 2011

21. Linus Pauling Institute, Oregon State University, Micronutrient Information Center: *Vitamin K.* Updated May 2008. http://lpi.oregonstate.edu/infocenter/vitamins/vitaminK/ Accessed: July 26, 2011

22. Food and Nutrition Board: *Dietary Reference Intakes for thiamin, riboflavin, niacin, vitamin B-6, folate, vitamin B-12, pantothenic acid, biotin, and choline.* Washington, DC: National Academy Press, 1998.

23. National Institutes of Health, Office of Dietary Supplements: *Dietary Supplement Fact Sheet: Vitamin B6.* Updated 2007. http://ods.od.nih.gov/factsheets/VitaminB6-HealthProfessional/ Accessed: July 26, 2011

24. McDowell MA and others: Blood folate levels: The latest NHANES results. *NCHS Data Brief No. 6*, May 2008.

25. Office of Dietary Supplements: *Dietary supplement fact sheet: Folate.* Updated April 2009. http://ods.od.nih.gov/factsheets/Folate-HealthProfessional/ Accessed: July 26, 2011

26. Mason JB: Folate, cancer risk, and the Greek god, Proteus: A tale of two chameleons. *Nutrition Reviews* 67(4):206, 2009.

27. Centers for Disease Control and Prevention: Spina bifida homepage: Facts. Last updated March 2011. http://www.cdc.gov/ncbddd/spinabifida/facts.html Accessed: July 26, 2011

28. Centers for Disease Control and Prevention: *Anencephaly.* Last reviewed February 2011. http://www.cdc.gov/ncbddd/birthdefects/Anencephaly.html Accessed: July 26, 2011

29. Centers for Disease Control and Prevention: Spina bifida: Data and statistics. Updated March 2011. http://www.cdc.gov/ncbddd/spinabifida/data.html Accessed: July 26, 2011

30. Petrini JR and others: Use of supplements containing folic acid among women of childbearing age—United States, 2007. *Morbidity and Mortality Weekly Report* 57(01): 5, 2008.

31. Dali-Youcef N, Andrès R: An update on cobalamin deficiency in adults. *Quarterly Journal of Medicine* 102(1):17, 2008.

32. Allen LH: How common is vitamin B-12 deficiency? *American Journal of Clinical Nutrition* 89(Suppl):693S, 2009.

33. National Institutes of Health, Office of Dietary Supplements: *Dietary Supplement Fact Sheet: Vitamin B 12.* Last reviewed June 2011. http://ods.od.nih.gov/factsheets/VitaminB12-HealthProfessional/ Accessed: July 27, 2011

34. Codazzi D and others: Coma and respiratory failure in a child with severe vitamin B(12) deficiency. *Pediatric Critical Care Medicine* 6:483, 2005.

35. Taylor EN and others: Dietary factors and the risk of incident kidney stones in men: New insights after 14 years of follow-up. *Journal of the American Society of Nephrology* 15:3225, 2004.

36. Quadri P and others: Homocysteine, folate, and vitamin B-12 in mild cognitive impairment, Alzheimer disease, and vascular dementia. *American Journal of Clinical Nutrition* 80:114, 2004.

37. Tucker KL and others: High homocysteine and low B vitamins predict cognitive decline in aging men: The Veterans Affairs Normative Aging Study. *American Journal of Clinical Nutrition* 82:627, 2005.

38. Hemilä H and others: Vitamin C for preventing and treating the common cold. *Cochrane Database of Systematic Reviews* 3:CD000980, 2007.

39. Riccioni G and others: Antioxidant vitamin supplementation in cardiovascular diseases. *Annals of Clinical and Laboratory Science* 37(1):89, 2007.

40. Engelhart MJ and others: Dietary intake of antioxidants and risk of Alzheimer disease. *Journal of the American Medical Association* 287:3223, 2002.

41. Chandrashekhar CD and others: Antioxidants in central nervous system diseases: Preclinical promise and translational challenges. *Journal of Alzheimers Disease* 15(3):473, 2008.

42. Lee KW and others: Vitamin C and cancer chemoprevention: Reappraisal. *American Journal of Clinical Nutrition* 78:1074, 2003.

43. Golde DW: Vitamin C in cancer. *Integrative Cancer Therapies* 2:158, 2003.

44. Heaney ML and others: Vitamin C antagonizes the cytotoxic effects of antineoplastic drugs. *Cancer Research* 68(19):8031, 2008.

45. Ford ES and others: Brief communication: The prevalence of high intakes of vitamin E and the use of supplements among U.S. adults. *Annals of Internal Medicine* 143:116, 2005.

46. Coleman HR and others: Age-related macular degeneration. *Lancet* 372(9652):1835, 2008.

47. Wong IYH and others: Prevention of age-related macular degeneration. *International Ophthalmology* 31(10):73, 2011.

48. U.S. Preventive Services Task Force: *Routine vitamin supplementation to prevent cancer and cardiovascular disease: Recommendations and rationale.* Agency for Healthcare Research and Quality, Rockville, MD, June 2003. http://www.uspreventiveservicestaskforce.org/3rduspstf/vitamins/vitaminsrr.htm#discussion Accessed: July 27, 2011

49. Liu RH: Health benefits of fruit and vegetables are from additive and synergistic combinations of phytochemicals. *American Journal of Clinical Nutrition* 78:517S, 2003.

50. American Cancer Society: *Cancer Facts & Figures 2011.* www.cancer.org Accessed: July 27, 2011

51. U.S. Department of Health and Human Services, National Institutes of Health, National Cancer Institute. *What You Need to Know About Cancer^TM: Risk factors.* http://www.cancer.gov/cancertopics/wyntk/cancer/page3 Accessed: July 27, 2011

52. Béliveau R and Gingras D: Role of nutrition in preventing cancer. *Canadian Family Physician* 53:1905, 2007.

53. American Cancer Society: *ACS guidelines on nutrition and physical activity for cancer prevention.* Last reviewed June 2011. http://www.cancer.org/Healthy/EatHealthyGetActive/ACSGuidelinesonNutritionPhysicalActivityforCancerPrevention/acs-guidelines-on-nutrition-and-physical-activity-for-cancer-prevention-diet-activity-cancer-risk Accessed: July 27, 2011

54. American Cancer Society: *ACS guidelines on nutrition and physical activity for cancer prevention: Common questions about diet and cancer.* Last revised May 2011. http://www.cancer.org/Healthy/EatHealthyGetActive/ACSGuidelinesonNutritionPhysicalActivityforCancerPrevention/acs-guidelines-on-nutrition-and-physical-activity-for-cancer-prevention-diet-cancer-questions Accessed: July 27, 2011

55. American Cancer Society: *Body weight and cancer risk*. 2010. http://www.cancer.org/Cancer/CancerCauses/DietandPhysicalActivity/BodyWeightandCancerRisk/body-weight-and-cancer-risk-effects Accessed: July 27, 2011

56. NIH State-of-the Science Panel: National Institutes of Health State-of-the-Science Conference Statement: Multivitamin/mineral supplements and chronic disease prevention. *American Journal of Clinical Nutrition* 85(Suppl):257S, 2007.

57. Lin J and others: Vitamins C and E and beta carotene supplementation and cancer risk: A randomized controlled trial. *Journal of the National Cancer Institute* 101(1):14, 2009.

Chapter 9

1. Centers for Disease Control and Prevention: Hyperthermia and dehydration-related deaths associated with intentional rapid weight loss in three collegiate wrestlers—North Carolina, Wisconsin, and Michigan, November–December 1997. *Morbidity and Mortality Weekly Report* 47:105, 1998. http://www.cdc.gov/mmwr/preview/mmwrhtml/00051388.htm

2. Saladin KS: *Anatomy & physiology*. 6th ed. Boston: McGraw-Hill Publishing Company, 2012.

3. Negoianu D and Goldfarb S: Just add water. *Journal of the American Society of Nephrology* 19(6):1041, 2008.

4. Food and Nutrition Board, Institute of Medicine: *Dietary Reference Intakes for water, potassium, sodium, chloride, and sulfate*. Washington, DC: National Academy Press, 2004.

5. Valtrin H: "Drink at least eight glasses of water a day." Really? Is there evidence for "8×8"? *American Journal of Physiological Regulation and Integrative Comparative Physiology* 283:R993, 2002.

6. Verster JC: The alcohol hangover—A puzzling phenomenon. *Alcohol & Alcoholism* 43(2):124, 2008.

7. Casa DJ and others: American College of Sports Medicine roundtable on hydration and physical activity: Consensus statements. *Current Sports Medicine Reports* 4:115, 2005.

8. Yeates KE and others: Salt and water: A simple approach to hyponatremia. *Canadian Medical Association Journal* 170:365, 2004.

9. Centers for Disease Control and Prevention: *2008 statistics for water fluoridation status*. Last modified August 2010. http://www.cdc.gov/fluoridation/statistics.htm Accessed: July 27, 2011

10. U.S. Department of Health and Human Services: *Bone health and osteoporosis: A report of the Surgeon General*. Rockville, MD: U.S. Department of Health and Human Services, Office of the Surgeon General, 2004. http://www.surgeongeneral.gov/library/bonehealth/content.html

11. Montgomery H and others: Finding whole grains and calcium rich food sources on supermarket shelves. *Forum for Family and Consumer Issues* 9: SSN 1540 5273, 2004. http://www.ncsu.edu/ffci/publications/2004/v9-n2-2004-october/ar-2-finding.php Accessed: July 28, 2011

12. Guéguen L, Pointillart A: The bioavailability of dietary calcium. *Journal of the American College of Nutrition* 19:119S, 2000.

13. National Institute of Arthritis and Musculoskeletal and Skin Diseases: *Calcium supplements: What to look for*. Reviewed January 2011. http://www.niams.nih.gov/Health_Info/Bone/Bone_Health/Nutrition/calcium_supp.asp Accessed: July 28, 2011

14. U.S. Department of Agriculture, Agricultural Research Service: *Nutrient intakes from food: Mean amounts consumed per individual, by gender and age, in the United States, 2007–2008*. http://www.ars.usda.gov/SP2UserFiles/Place/12355000/pdf/0708/Table_1_NIN_GEN_07.pdf Accessed: July 27, 2011

15. Office of Dietary Supplements, National Institutes of Health: *Calcium*. Reviewed June 2011. http://ods.od.nih.gov/factsheets/Calcium-HealthProfessional/ Accessed: July 27, 2011

16. National Osteoporosis Foundation: *Fast facts*. ND. http://www.nof.org/node/40 Accessed: July 27, 2011

17. National Institutes of Health, National Institute of Arthritis and Musculoskeletal and Skin Diseases: *Osteoporosis: Warning signs and diagnosis*. Last reviewed January 2011. http://nihseniorhealth.gov/osteoporosis/warningsignsanddiagnosis/02.html Accessed July 27, 2011

18. Jackson RD and others: Calcium plus vitamin D supplementation and the risk of fractures. *New England Journal of Medicine* 354:669, 2006.

19. Warburton DER and others: Health benefits of physical activity: The evidence. *Canadian Medical Journal* 174:801, 2006.

20. American Medical Association: *Putting away the salt shaker*. 2006. http://www.ama-assn.org/amednews/2006/08/28/edsa0828.htm Accessed: July 27, 2011

21. Appel LJ and others: Dietary approaches to prevent and treat hypertension: A scientific statement from the American Heart Association. *Hypertension* 47:296, 2006.

22. Keenan NL, Rosendorf KA: Prevalence of hypertension and controlled hypertension—United States, 2005–2008. *Morbidity and Mortality Weekly Report* 60(1):94, 2011.

23. Jago R and others: Prevalence of abnormal lipid and blood pressure values among an ethnically diverse population of eighth-grade adolescents and screening implications. *Pediatrics* 117:2065, 2006.

24. National Heart, Lung, and Blood Institute, National Institutes of Health: *Your guide to lowering high blood pressure: Categories for blood pressure levels in adults*. ND. http://www.nhlbi.nih.gov/hbp/detect/categ.htm Accessed: July 28, 2011

25. Khaw K-T and others: Blood pressure and urinary sodium in men and women: The Norfolk Cohort of the European Prospective Investigation into Cancer (EPIC-Norfolk). *American Journal of Clinical Nutrition* 80:1397, 2004.

26. U.S. Departments of Health and Human Services and Agriculture: *Dietary Guidelines for Americans 2010*. 2011. http://www.health.gov/dietaryguidelines/dga2010/DietaryGuidelines2010.pdf Accessed: July 21, 2011

27. Doorenbos CJ, Vermeij CG: Danger of salt substitutes that contain potassium in patients with renal failure. *British Medical Journal* 325:35, 2003.

28. National Heart, Lung, and Blood Institute, National Institutes of Health: *Your guide to lowering high blood pressure: Do vitamin mineral supplements such as potassium, calcium or magnesium help lower blood pressure?* ND. http://www.nhlbi.nih.gov/hbp/prevent/factors/supls.htm Accesssed: July 28, 2011

29. Office of Dietary Supplements, National Institutes of Health: *Magnesium*. 2009. http://ods.od.nih.gov/factsheets/Magnesium-HealthProfessional/ Accessed: July 28, 2011

30. Food and Nutrition Board: *Dietary Reference Intakes for vitamin A, vitamin K, arsenic, boron, chromium, copper, iodine, iron, manganese, molybdenum, nickel, silicon, vanadium, and zinc*. Washington, DC: National Academy Press, 2000.

31. Ghosh K: Non-haematological effects of iron deficiency—A perspective. *Indian Journal of Medical Sciences* 60:30, 2006.

32. World Health Organization: *Miconutrient deficiencies: Iron deficiency anemia*. ND. http://www.who.int/nutrition/topics/ida/en/ Accessed: July 28, 2011

33. Centers for Disease Control and Prevention: *Iron deficiency*. Last updated February 2011. http://www.cdc.gov/nccdphp/dnpa/nutrition/nutrition_for_everyone/iron_deficiency/index.htm Accessed: July 28, 2011

34. Kazal LA: Prevention of iron deficiency in infants and toddlers. *American Family Physician* 66:1217, 2002.

35. Tenebein M: Unit-dose packaging of iron supplements and reduction of iron poisoning in young children. *Archives of Pediatric and Adolescent Medicine* 159: 557, 2005.

36. Office of Dietary Supplements, National Institutes of Health: *Dietary supplement fact sheet: Iron*. Reviewed August 2007. http://ods.od.nih.gov/factsheets/Iron-HealthProfessional/ Accessed: July 28, 2011

37. National Institute of Diabetes and Digestive and Kidney Diseases: *Hemochromatosis*. NIH Publication No. 07–4621, National Digestive Diseases Information Clearinghouse, 2007. http://digestive.niddk.nih.gov/ddiseases/pubs/hemochromatosis/ Accessed: July 28, 2011

38. Prasad A: Zinc deficiency. *British Medical Journal* 326:409, 2003.

39. Prasad AS and others: Zinc deficiency in sickle cell disease. *Clinical Chemistry* 21:582, 1975.

40. Office of Dietary Supplements, National Institutes of Health: *Dietary supplement fact sheet: Zinc*. Reviewed June 2011. http://ods.od.nih.gov/factsheets/Zinc-HealthProfessional/ Accessed: July 28, 2011

41. Carpenter KJ: David Marine and the problem of goiter. *Journal of Nutrition* 135:675, 2005.

42. Office of Dietary Supplements, National Institutes of Health: *Dietary supplement fact sheet: Iodine*. Updated June 2011. http://ods.od.nih.gov/factsheets/Iodine-HealthProfessional/

43. Office of Dietary Supplements, National Institutes of Health: *Selenium*. Updated November, 2009. http://ods.od.nih.gov/factsheets/Selenium-HealthProfessional/ Accessed: July 28, 2011

44. Office of Dietary Supplements, National Institutes of Health: *Chromium*. 2005. http://ods.od.nih.gov/factsheets/Chromium-HealthProfessional/ Accessed: July 28, 2011

45. Whittaker P and others: Mutagenicity of chromium picolinate and its components in *Salmonella typhimurium* and L5178Y mouse lymphoma cells. *Food and Chemical Toxicology* 43:1619, 2005.

46. International Bottled Water Association: *Bottled water 2009*. 2010. http://www.bottledwater.org/files/2009BWstats.pdf Accessed: July 28, 2011

47. Environmental Protection Agency: *Water health series: Bottled water basics*. 2005. http://water.epa.gov/aboutow/ogwdw/upload/2005_09_14_faq_fs_healthseries_bottledwater.pdf Accessed: July 28, 2011

48. U.S. Food and Drug Administration: Food facts from the U.S. Food and Drug Administration. Last updated May 2011. http://www.fda.gov/Food/ResourcesForYou/Consumers/ucm046894.htm Accessed: July 28, 2011

49. U.S. Department of Health and Human Services: *Bisphenol A (BPA) information for parents*. ND. http://www.hhs.gov/safety/bpa Accessed: July 28, 2011

Chapter 10

1. National Institutes of Health, National Heart Lung and Blood Institute: *Aim for a healthy weight: What is overweight and obesity?* ND. http://www.nhlbi.nih.gov/health/public/heart/obesity/lose_wt/index.htm Accessed: July 29, 2011

2. National Institutes of Health, National Heart Lung and Blood Institute: *Classification of overweight and obesity by BMI, waist circumference, and associated disease risks*. ND. http://www.nhlbi.nih.gov/health/public/heart/obesity/lose_wt/bmi_dis.htm Accessed: July 29, 2011

3. Yanovski JA: Rapid weight gain during infancy as a predictor of adult obesity. *American Journal of Clinical Nutrition* 77:1350, 2003.

4. Ogden CL, Carroll MD: National Center for Health Statistics: *Prevalence of overweight, obesity, and extreme obesity among adults: United States, trends 1960–62 through 2007–2008*. Updated June 2011. http://www.cdc.gov/nchs/data/hestat/obesity_adult_07_08/obesity_adult_07_08.htm Accessed: July 29, 2011

5. Ogden C, Carroll M: National Center for Health Statistics: *Prevalence of obesity among children and adolescents: United States, trends 1963–1965 through 2007–2008*. 2010. http://www.cdc.gov/nchs/data/hestat/obesity_child_07_08/obesity_child_07_08.htm Accessed: July 29, 2011

6. National Center for Health Statistics: *Prevalence of overweight, infants and children less than 2 years of age: United States, 2003–2004*. Last updated April 2010. http://www.cdc.gov/nchs/data/hestat/overweight/overweight_child_under02.htm Accessed: July 29, 2011

7. U.S. Department of Health and Human Services: *Healthy People 2020: Nutrition and weight status*. http://healthypeople.gov/2020/topicsobjectives2020/ objectiveslist.aspx?topicId=29 Accessed: July 29, 2011

8. Centers for Disease Control and Prevention: *Overweight and obesity: Economic consequences: National estimated cost of obesity*. Updated March 2011. http://www.cdc.gov/obesity/causes/economics.html Accessed: July 29, 2011

9. World Health Organization: *Obesity and overweight*. Updated March 2011. http://www.who.int/mediacentre/factsheets/fs311/en/index.html Accessed: July 29, 2011

10. Weiss EC and others: Weight-control practices among U.S. adults, 2001–2002. *American Journal of Preventive Medicine* 31:18, 2006.

11. Wing RR, Phelan S: Long-term weight loss maintenance. *American Journal of Clinical Nutrition* 82:222S, 2005.

12. Williams MH: *Nutrition for health, fitness, and sport*. 9th ed. New York: McGraw-Hill, 2010.

13. Naaz A and others: Loss of cyclin-dependent kinase inhibitors produces adipocyte hyperplasia and obesity. *The FASEB Journal* 18:1925, 2004.

14. Trayhurn P: Adipose tissue in obesity—An inflammatory issue. *Endocrinology* 146:1003, 2005.

15. Avram MM: Cellulite: A review of its physiology and treatment. *Journal of Cosmetic and Laser Therapy* 6:181, 2004.

16. Saladin KS: *Anatomy & Physiology*. 6th ed. Boston: McGraw-Hill Publishing Company, 2012.

17. Bray GA, Champagne CM: Dietary patterns may modify central adiposity. *Journal of the American Dietetic Association* 109:1354, 2009.

18. Tiraby C and others: Acquirement of brown fat cell features by human white adipocytes. *Journal of Biological Chemistry* 278:33370, 2003.

19. Garcia AL and others: Improved prediction of body fat by measuring skinfold thickness, circumferences, and bone breadths. *Obesity Research* 13:626, 2005.

20. Food and Nutrition Board, National Institute of Health: *Dietary Reference Intakes for energy, carbohydrate, fiber, fat, fatty acids, cholesterol, protein, and amino acids (macronutrients)*. Washington, DC: National Academies Press, 2005.

21. Hyperthyroidism. *Medline Plus, Medical Encyclopedia.* Updated 2010. http://www.nlm.nih.gov/medlineplus/ency/article/000356.htm Accessed: July 30, 2011

22. Knudsen N and others: Small differences in thyroid function may be important for body mass index and the occurrence of obesity in the population. *Journal of Clinical Endocrinology & Metabolism* 90:4019, 2006.

23. Roberts SB, Dallal GE: Energy requirements and aging. *Public Health Nutrition* 8:1028, 2005.

24. Weinsier RL and others: Do adaptive changes in metabolic rate favor weight regain in weight-reduced individuals? An examination of the set-point theory. *American Journal of Clinical Nutrition* 72:1088, 2000.

25. Haugen HA and others: Variability of measured resting metabolic rate. *American Journal of Clinical Nutrition* 78:1141, 2005.

26. Hajhosseini L and others: Changes in body weight, body composition and resting metabolic rate (RMR) in first-year university freshmen students. *Journal of the American College of Nutrition* 25:123, 2006.

27. Racette SB and others: Weight changes, exercise, and dietary patterns during freshmen and sophomore years of college. *Journal of American College Health* 53:245, 2005.

28. National Institutes of Health, National Heart Lung and Blood Institute: *Assessing your weight and health risk.* ND. http://www.nhlbi.nih.gov/health/public/heart/obesity/lose_wt/risk.htm Accessed: July 29, 2011

29. Flegal K and others: Excess deaths associated with underweight, overweight, and obesity. *Journal of the American Medical Association* 293:1861, 2005.

30. Jackson Y and others: Summary of the 2000 Surgeon General's Listening Session: Toward a national action plan on overweight and obesity. *Obesity Research* 10:1299, 2002.

31. Virji A, Murr MM: Caring for patients after bariatric surgery. *American Family Physician* 73:1403, 2006.

32. Cedergren MI: Maternal morbid obesity and the risk of adverse pregnancy outcome. *Obstetrics & Gynecology* 103:219, 2004.

33. Friedman KE and others: Weight stigmatization and ideological beliefs: Relation to psychological functioning in obese adults. *Obesity Research* 13.907, 2005.

34. Hamdy O and others: Metabolic obesity: The paradox between visceral and subcutaneous fat. *Current Diabetes Review* 2(4):367, 2006.

35. Barnett AH: The importance of treating cardiometabolic risk factors in patients with type 2 diabetes. *Diabetes & Vascular Disease Research* 5(1):9, 2008.

36. Klein S: The case of visceral fat: Argument for the defense. *Journal of Clinical Investigation* 113:1530, 2004.

37. National Heart, Lung, and Blood Institute: *The practical guide: Identification, evaluation, and treatment of overweight and obesity in adults.* HIH Publication 00–4084, 2000. http://www.nhlbi.nih.gov/guidelines/obesity/prctgd_b.pdf

38. Klein S and others: Waist circumference and cardiometabolic risk. *Diabetes Care* 30(6):1647, 2007.

39. Wasan KM, Looije NA: Emerging pharmacological approaches to the treatment of obesity. *Journal of Pharmacy and Pharmaceutical Sciences* 8:259, 2005.

40. Jequier E: Leptin signaling, adiposity, and energy balance. *Annals of the New York Academy of Sciences* 967:379, 2002.

41. Ello-Martin JA and others: The influence of food portion size and energy density on energy intake: Implications for weight management. *American Journal of Clinical Nutrition* 82:236S, 2005.

42. Jequier E: Pathways to obesity. *International Journal of Obesity and Related Metabolic Disorders* 26:S12, 2002.

43. Wylie-Rosett J and others: Carbohydrates and increases in obesity: Does the type of carbohydrate make a difference? *Obesity Research* 12:124S, 2004.

44. Ledikwe JH and others: Portion sizes and the obesity epidemic. *Journal of Nutrition* 135:905, 2005.

45. U.S. Department of Agriculture, Agricultural Research Service: *Nutrient intakes from food: Mean amounts consumed per individual, by gender and age, in the United States, 2007–2008.* http://www.ars.usda.gov/SP2UserFiles/Place/12355000/pdf/0708/Table_1_NIN_GEN_07.pdf Accessed: July 27, 2011

46. Centers for Disease Control and Prevention, National Center for Chronic Disease Prevention and Health Promotion: *U.S. physical activity statistics.* 2010. http://apps.nccd.cdc.gov/PASurveillance/StateSumResultV.asp Accessed: July 30, 2011

47. American College of Sports Medicine and the American Heart Association: *Guidelines for healthy adults under age 65.* 2007. http://www.acsm.org/AM/Template.cfm?Section=Home_Page&TEMPLATE=/CM/HTMLDisplay.cfm&CONTENTID=7764 Accessed: July 30, 2011

48. Jakicic JM, Otto AD: Physical activity considerations for the treatment and prevention of obesity. *American Journal of Clinical Nutrition* 82:226, 2005.

49. Whitaker RC: Predicting preschooler obesity at birth: The role of maternal obesity in early pregnancy. *Pediatrics* 114:e29, 2004.

50. Esposito L and others: Developmental perspectives on nutrition and obesity from gestation to adolescence. *Preventing Chronic Disease* 6(3), 2009. http://www.cdc.gov/pcd/issues/2009/jul/09_0014.htm Accessed: August 18, 2009

51. Healton CG and others: Smoking, obesity, and their co-occurrence in the United States: Cross sectional analysis. *British Medical Journal* 333:25, 2006.

52. Zhang Q, Wang Y: Trends in the association between obesity and socioeconomic status in U.S. adults: 1971–2000. *Obesity Research* 12.1622, 2004.

53. Atlantis E, Baker M: Obesity effects on depression: A systematic review of epidemiological studies. *International Journal of Obesity* 32(6):881, 2008.

54. Bish CL and others: Diet and physical activity behaviors among Americans trying to lose weight: 2000 Behavioral Risk Factor Surveillance System. *Obesity Research* 13:596, 2005.

55. Klein S and others: Weight management through lifestyle modification for the prevention and management of type 2 diabetes: Rationale and strategies. A statement of the American Diabetes Association, the North American Association for the Study of Obesity, and the American Society for Clinical Nutrition. *American Journal of Clinical Nutrition* 80:257, 2004.

56. Kruger J and others: Attempting to lose weight: Specific practices among U.S. adults. *American Journal of Preventive Medicine* 269:402, 2004.

57. U.S. Departments of Health and Human Services (USDHHS) and Agriculture (USDA): *Dietary Guidelines for Americans 2010.* 2011. http://www.health.gov/dietaryguidelines/dga2010/DietaryGuidelines2010.pdf Accessed: July 21, 2011

58. Rolls BJ and others: What can intervention studies tell us about the relationship between fruit and vegetable consumption and weight management? *Nutrition Reviews* 62:1, 2004.

59. Hu FB and others: Television watching and other sedentary behaviors in relation to risk of obesity and type 2 diabetes mellitus in women. *Journal of the American Medical Association* 289:1785, 2003.

60. Irwin ML and others: Estimation of energy expenditure from physical activity measures: Determinants of accuracy. *Obesity Research* 9:517, 2001.

61. Raynor HA and others: Amount of food group variety consumed in the diet and long-term weight loss maintenance. *Obesity Research* 13:883, 2005.

62. Phelan S and others: Are the eating and exercise habits of successful weight losers changing? *Obesity* 14:710, 2006.

63. Hollywood A, Ogden J: Taking orlistat: Predicting weight loss over 6 months. *Journal of Obesity*, 2011: doi:10.1155/2011/806896.

64. O'Brien PE and others: Obesity, weight loss, and bariatric surgery. *Medical Journal of Australia* 183:310, 2005.

65. National Institutes of Health: *Medical encyclopedia: Gastric bypass surgery.* Updated February 12, 2009. http://www.nlm.nih.gov/medlineplus/ency/article/007199.htm Accessed: August 23, 2009

66. Guller U and others: Safety and effectiveness of bariatric surgery: Roux-en-Y gastric bypass is superior to gastric banding in the management of morbidly obese patients. *Patient Safety in Surgery* 3(10), doi:10.1186/1754-9493-3-10, 2009.

67. Personal communication: Professor Dee Anna Glaser, M.D., Director of Cosmetic & Laser Surgery, Department of Dermatology, Saint Louis University, St. Louis Missouri, July 11, 2006.

68. Hession M and others: Systematic review of randomized controlled trials of low-carbohydrate vs. low-fat/low-calorie diets in the management of obesity and its comorbidities. *Obesity Reviews* 10:36, 2009.

69. Saper RB and others: Common dietary supplements for weight loss. *American Family Physician* 70:1731, 2004

70. Federal Trade Commission, Bureau of Consumer Protection: *Weight loss advertising: An analysis of current trends.* 2002. http://www.ftc.gov/bcp/reports/weightloss.pdf Accessed: July 31, 2011

71. Fryar CD, Ogden CL: *Prevalence of underweight among adults: United States, 2003–2006.* 2009. http://www.cdc.gov/nchs/data/hestat/underweight/underweight_adults.htm Accessed: July 31, 2011

72. American Psychiatric Association: Treatment of patients with eating disorders, 3rd. ed. 2006. http://www.psychiatryonline.com/pracGuide/pracGuideChapToc_12.aspx Accessed: July 31, 2011

73. Torpy JM and others: Anorexia nervosa. *Journal of the American Medical Association* 295:2684, 2006.

74. Nicholls D, Viner R: Eating disorders and weight problems. *British Medical Journal* 330:950, 2005.

75. Gucciardi E and others: Eating disorders. *BMC Women's Health* 4:S21 2004.

76. Steinhausen H-C: The outcome of anorexia nervosa in the 20th century. *American Journal of Psychiatry* 159:1284, 2002.

77. Henry BW, Ozier AD: Position of the American Dietetic Association: Nutrition intervention in the treatment of anorexia nervosa, bulimia nervosa, and other eating disorders. *Journal of the American Dietetic Association* 106:2073, 2006.

78. Striegel-Moore RH and others: Abuse, bullying, and discrimination as risk factors for binge eating disorder. *American Journal of Psychiatry* 159:1902, 2002.

79. Bonci CM and others: National Athletic Trainers' Association position statement: Preventing, detecting, and managing disordered eating in athletes. *Journal of Athletic Training* 43(1):80, 2008.

80. Birch K: Female athlete triad. *British Medical Journal* 330:244, 2006.

Chapter 11

1. Centers for Disease Control and Prevention: *Prevalence and trends data-physical activity 2009.* http://apps.nccd.cdc.gov/brfss/list.asp?cat=PA&yr=2009&qkey=4418&state=All Accessed: July 31, 2011

2. Centers for Disease Control and Prevention: *1988–2008 no leisure-time physical activity trend chart.* 2010 http://www.cdc.gov/nccdphp/dnpa/physical/stats/leisure_time.htm Accessed: July 31, 2011

3. American College of Sports Medicine and the American Heart Association: *Guidelines for healthy adults under age 65.* http://www.acsm.org/AM/Template.cfm?Section=Home_Page&TEMPLATE=/CM/HTMLDisplay.cfm&CONTENTID=7764 Accessed: August 1, 2011

4. Centers for Disease Control and Prevention: *Physical activity and health: The benefits of physical activity.* Last updated February 2011. http://www.cdc.gov/physicalactivity/everyone/health/index.html Accessed: August 1, 2011

5. U.S. Department of Health and Human Services: *2008 Physical activity guidelines for Americans summary.* 2008. http://www.health.gov/paguidelines/guidelines/summary.aspx Accessed: August 1, 2011

6. Centers for Disease Control and Prevention: *Target heart rate and estimated maximum heart rate.* http://www.cdc.gov/physicalactivity/everyone/measuring/heartrate.html Accessed: August 1, 2011

7. U.S. Department of Labor: *OSHA technical manual.* ND. http://www.osha.gov/dts/osta/otm/otm_iii/otm_iii_4.html Accessed: August 1, 2011

8. Sherman WM: Metabolism of sugars and physical performance. *American Journal of Clinical Nutrition* 62:228S, 1995.

9. Gastin PB: Energy system interaction and relative contribution during maximal exercise. *Sports Medicine* 31:725, 2001.

10. Williams MH: *Nutrition for health, fitness, and sport.* 9th ed. New York: McGraw-Hill, 2010.

11. Saladin KS: *Anatomy and physiology.* 6th ed. New York: McGraw-Hill, 2012.

12. Van Loon LJC and others: The effects of increasing exercise intensity on muscle fuel utilization in humans. *Journal of Physiology* 536:295, 2001.

13. Holloszy JO and others: The regulation of carbohydrate and fat metabolism during and after exercise. *Frontiers Bioscience* 3:D1011, 1998.

14. American Dietetic Association: Position of the American Dietetic Association, Dietitians of Canada, and the American College of Sports Medicine—Nutrition and athletic performance. *Journal of the American Dietetic Association* 109:509, 2009.

15. Economos CD and others: Nutritional practices of elite athletes: Practical recommendations. *Sports Medicine* 16:381, 1993.

16. Otten JJ and others (eds.): Institute of Medicine of the National Academies: *Dietary Reference Intakes: The essential guide to nutrient requirements.* National Academies Press: Washington, DC, 2006.

17. Lambert EV and others: High-fat diet versus habitual diet prior to carbohydrate loading: Effects of exercise metabolism and cycling performance. *International Journal of Sports Nutrition and Exercise Metabolism* 11:209, 2001.

18. Wismann J, Willoughby D: Gender differences in carbohydrate metabolism and carbohydrate loading. *Journal of the International Society of Sports Nutrition* 3(1):28, 2006.

19. Rennie MJ, Tipton KD: Protein and amino acid metabolism during and after exercise and the effects of nutrition. *Annual Review of Nutrition* 20:457, 2000.

20. Tipton KD, Wolfe RR: Protein and amino acids for athletes. *Journal of Sports Science* 22:65, 2004.

21. Gibala MJ: Nutritional supplementation and resistance exercise: What is the evidence for enhanced skeletal muscle hypertrophy? *Canadian Journal of Applied Physiology* 25:524, 2000.

22. Maughan R: The athlete's diet: Nutritional goals and dietary strategies. *Proceedings of the Nutrition Society* 61:87, 2002.

23. Fielding RA, Parkington J: What are the dietary protein requirements of physically active individuals? New evidence on the effects of protein utilization during post-exercise recovery. *Nutrition in Clinical Care* 5:191, 2002.

24. Lemon PW: Beyond the zone; protein needs of active individuals. *Journal of the American College of Nutrition* 19:513S, 2000.

25. Burke LM: Caffeine and sports performance. *Applied Physiology, Nutrition, and Metabolism* 33:1319, 2008.

26. A guide to the best and worst drinks. *Consumer Reports on Health*, p. 8, July 2006.

27. Coyle EF: Fluid and fuel intake during exercise. *Journal of Sports Science* 22:39, 2004.

28. MayoClinic.com: *Heat cramps: First aid.* 2010. http://www.mayoclinic.com/health/first-aid-heat-cramps/FA00021 Accessed: August 1, 2011

29. MayoClinic.com: *Heat exhaustion: First aid.* 2010. http://www.mayoclinic.com/health/first-aid-heat-exhaustion/FA00020 Accessed: August 1, 2011

30. MayoClinic.com: *Heat stroke: First aid.* 2010. http://www.mayoclinic.com/health/first-aid-heatstroke/FA00019 Accessed: August 1, 2011

31. Association of International Marathons and Road Races: *IMMDA's revised fluid recommendations for runners & walkers.* 2006. http://www.aims-association.org/guidelines_fluid_replacement.htm Accessed: August 1, 2011

32. Powers SK and others: Dietary antioxidants and exercise. *Journal of Sports Sciences* 22:81, 2004.

33. Nieman DC and others: Vitamin E and immunity after the Kona Triathlon World Championship. *Medicine and Science in Sports and Exercise* 36:1328, 2004.

34. National Collegiate Athletic Association: *NCAA banned drug list.* http://www.ncaa.org/wps/wcm/connect/public/NCAA/Student-Athlete+Experience/NCAA+banned+drugs+list Accessed: August 1, 2011

35. World Anti-Doping Agency: *The World Anti-Doping Code. The 2009 prohibited list, international standard.* Last updated May 2011. http://www.wada-ama.org/World-Anti-Doping-Program/Sports-and-Anti-Doping-Organizations/The-Code/ Accessed: August 1, 2011

36. University Extension, Iowa State University: *To your health.* 2007. http://www.extension.iastate.edu/NR/rdonlyres/7E800DD4-0456-42BE-9E45-33C07335DE6D/52821/ToYourHealthApril07.pdf Accessed: August 1, 2011

37. U.S. Department of Health and Human Services: *Healthy People 2020: Physical activity.* http://healthypeople.gov/2020/topicsobjectives2020/objectiveslist.aspx?topicId=33 Accessed: July 31, 2011

Chapter 12

1. U.S. Food and Drug Administration: FDA finalizes report on 2006 spinach outbreak. *FDA News Release*, March 23, 2007. Last updated May 2009. http://www.fda.gov/NewsEvents/Newsroom/PressAnnouncements/2007/ucm108873.htm Accessed: July 13, 2011

2. Centers for Disease Control and Prevention: Outbreak of *Salmonella* serotype Saintpaul infections associated with multiple raw produce items—United States, 2008. *Mortality and Morbidity Weekly Report* 57(34):929, 2008.

3. Centers for Disease Control and Prevention: Multistate outbreak of *Salmonella* infections associated with peanut butter and peanut butter-containing products—United States, 2008–2009. *Mortality and Morbidity Weekly Report* 58(04):85, 2009.

4. National Institute of Allergy and Infectious Diseases: *Foodborne diseases.* Updated 2010. http://www.niaid.nih.gov/topics/foodborne/pages/default.aspx Accessed: July 13, 2011

5. Centers for Disease Control and Prevention: *Foodborne illness: Frequently asked questions.* 2005. http://www.cdc.gov/ncidod/dbmd/diseaseinfo/files/foodborne_illness_FAQ.pdf Accessed: July 13, 2011

6. USDA Food Safety and Inspection Service: Safe food handling: *Molds on food: Are they dangerous?* Modified 2010. http://www.fsis.usda.gov/Fact_Sheets/Molds_On_Food/index.asp Accessed: July 13, 2011

7. Food and Drug Administration: *Bad bug book: Foodborne pathogenic microorganisms and natural toxins handbook.* Updated 2009. http://www.fda.gov/Food/FoodSafety/FoodborneIllness/FoodborneIllnessFoodbornePathogensNaturalToxins/BadBugBook/ucm071020.htm Accessed: July 13, 2011

8. U.S. Department of Health and Human Services: *Keep foods safe: Cook.* ND. http://www.foodsafety.gov/keep/basics/cook/index.html Accessed: August 1, 2011

9. U.S. Department of Agriculture, Food Safety and Inspection Service: Appliances and thermometers: *Microwave ovens and food safety.* Last modified May 2011. http://www.fsis.usda.gov/Fact_Sheets/Microwave_Ovens_and_Food_Safety/index.asp Accessed July 13, 2011

10. Picklesimer P: Scientists weigh in on the 5-second rule. *ACES News.* University of Illinois at Champaign–Urbana, College of Agricultural, Consumer and Environmental Sciences, 2003. http://www.aces.uiuc.edu/news/stories/news2467.html Accessed: July 13, 2011

11. U.S. Department of Agriculture, Food Safety and Inspection Service: *Food safety information: Basics for handling food safely.* Revised June 2011. http://www.fsis.usda.gov/PDF/Basics_for_Safe_Food_Handling.pdf Accessed: July 13, 2011

12. U.S. Department of Agriculture, Food Safety and Inspection Service: Keeping food safe during an emergency. *Fact sheets: Emergency preparedness.* 2006. http://www.fsis.usda.gov/Fact_Sheets/Keeping_Food_Safe_During_an_Emergency/index.asp Accessed: July 13, 2011

13. Centers for Disease Control and Prevention, Division of Bacterial and Mycotic Diseases: *Food irradiation.* 2005. http://www.cdc.gov/ncidod/dbmd/diseaseinfo/foodirradiation.htm Accessed: July 13, 2011

14. International Food Information Council and U.S. Food and Drug Administration: *Food ingredients and colors.* Last updated May 2011. http://www.fda.gov/Food/FoodIngredientsPackaging/ucm094211.htm Accessed: July 13, 2011

15. Center for Food Safety and Applied Nutrition, U.S. Food and Drug Administration: *Frequently asked questions about GRAS.* 2004. Update May 2011. http://www.fda.gov/Food/GuidanceComplianceRegulatoryInformation/GuidanceDocuments/FoodIngredientsandPackaging/ucm061846.htm Accessed: July 13, 2011

16. Meadows M: A century of ensuring safe foods and cosmetics. *FDA Consumer Magazine* 40:6, 2006.

17. Congressional Research Service Report for Congress, Pesticide Legislation: *Food Quality Protection Act of 1996 (P.L. 104–170) II 96–759 ENR.* http://www.ncseonline.org/nle/crsreports/pesticides/pest-8a.cfm#The%20Delaney%20Clause Accessed: July 13, 2011

18. Center for Food Safety and Applied Nutrition, U.S. Food and Drug Administration: *The food defect action levels: Levels of natural or unavoidable defects in foods that present no health hazards for humans.* Updated 2005. http://www.fda.gov/Food/GuidanceComplianceRegulatoryInformation/GuidanceDocuments/Sanitation/ucm056174.htm Accessed: July 13, 2011

19. Food and Drug Administration: *FDA statement: Benzene in soft drinks.* 2006. Updated June 2009. http://www.fda.gov/NewsEvents/Newsroom/PressAnnouncements/2006/ucm108636.htm Accessed: July 13, 2011

20. Environmental Protection Agency: *Pesticides: Topical & chemical fact sheets.* The EPA and food security. Last updated February 2011. http://www.epa.gov/pesticides/factsheets/securty.htm Accessed: July 13, 2011

21. Centers for Disease Control and Prevention: *Fourth national report on human exposure to environmental chemicals.* Updated June 2011. http://www.cdc.gov/exposurereport/pdf/FourthReport.pdf Accessed: July 13, 2011

22. Blair A and others: Disease and injury among participants in the Agricultural Health Study. *Journal of Agricultural Safety and Health* 11:141, 2005.

23. Centers for Disease Control and Prevention: *Traveler's Health Yellow Book: Traveler's diarrhea.* Last reviewed July 1, 2011. http://wwwnc.cdc.gov/travel/yellowbook/2012/chapter-2-the-pre-travel-consultation/travelers-diarrhea.htm Accessed: July 13, 2011

24. Centers for Disease Control and Prevention: *Traveler's Health Yellow Book: Water disinfection for travelers.* Last reviewed July 1, 2011. http://wwwnc.cdc.gov/travel/yellowbook/2012/chapter-2-the-pre-travel-consultation/water-disinfection-for-travelers.htm Accessed: July 13, 2011

Chapter 13

1. Otten JJ and others (eds.): Institute of Medicine: *Dietary Reference Intakes: The essential guide to nutrient requirements.* Washington, DC: National Academies Press, 2006.

2. Centers for Disease Control and Prevention: *Unintended pregnancy prevention.* 2010. http://www.cdc.gov/reproductivehealth/UnintendedPregnancy/index.htm Accessed: August 3, 2011

3. Thame M and others: Fetal growth is directly related to maternal anthropometry and placental volume. *European Journal of Clinical Nutrition* 58:894, 2004.

4. Hamilton BE and others: Births: Preliminary data for 2009. *National Vital Statistics Reports* 59(3):1, 2010.

5. Hamilton BE and others: Births: Preliminary data for 2007. *National Vital Statistics Reports* 57(12):1, 2009.

6. Centers for Disease Control and Prevention: *2004 Surgeon General's Report: The health consequences of smoking.* 2004. http://www.cdc.gov/tobacco/data_statistics/sgr/2004/index.htm Accessed: August 3, 2011

7. MacDornan MF, Mathews TJ: Recent trends in infant mortality in the United States. *NCSH Data Brief No. 9.* 2008. http://www.cdc.gov/nchs/data/databriefs/db09.pdf Accessed: August 3, 2011

8. Tucker J, McGuire W: Epidemiology of preterm birth. *British Medical Journal* 329:675, 2004.

9. Neville MC, McManaman JL: Milk secretion and composition. In *Neonatal nutrition and metabolism.* 2nd ed. Thureen P, Hay W (eds.) Cambridge University Press, 2006.

10. U.S. National Library of Medicine and National Institutes of Health: Morning sickness. *MedLine Plus.* Updated 2009. http://www.nlm.nih.gov/medlineplus/ency/article/003119.htm Accessed: August 3, 2011

11. Scholl TO: Iron status during pregnancy: Setting the stage for mother and infant. *American Journal of Clinical Nutrition* 81:1218S, 2005.

12. U.S. Environmental Protection Agency and Food and Drug Administration: *What you need to know about mercury in fish and shellfish.* 2009. http://www.fda.gov/Food/FoodSafety/Product-SpecificInformation/Seafood/FoodbornePathogensContaminants/Methylmercury/ucm115662.htm Accessed: August 3, 2011

13. American College of Obstetricians and Gynecologists: *Nutrition during pregnancy.* 2010. http://www.acog.org/publications/patient_education/bp001.cfm Accessed: August 3, 2011

14. American College of Obstetricians and Gynecologists: *Having twins.* 2004. http://www.acog.org/publications/patient_education/bp092.cfm

15. American Dietetic Association: Position of the American Dietetic Association and American Society for Nutrition: Obesity, reproduction, and pregnancy outcomes. *Journal of the American Dietetic Association* 109:918, 2009.

16. Jannson N and others: Maternal hormones linking maternal body mass index and dietary intake to birth weight. *American Journal of Clinical Nutrition* 87:1743, 2008.

17. Centers for Disease Control and Prevention: Recommendations to improve preconception health and health care—United States: A report of the CDC/ATSDR Preconception Care Work Group and the Select Panel on Preconception Care. *Morbidity and Mortality Weekly Report* 55(No. RR-6):1, 2006.

18. Seely EW, Maxwell C: Chronic hypertension in pregnancy. *Circulation* 115:e188, 2007.

19. National Heart Lung and Blood Institute: *High blood pressure in pregnancy.* ND. http://www.nhlbi.nih.gov/health/public/heart/hbp/hbp_preg.htm Accessed: August 3, 2011

20. National Institutes of Health, National Institute of Child Health & Human Development: *Safe Sleep for Your Baby: Reduce the Risk of Sudden Infant Death Syndrome (SIDS).* Updated 2009. http://www.nichd.nih.gov/publications/pubs/safe_sleep_gen.cfm Accessed: August 3, 2011

21. American College of Obstetricians and Gynecologists: *Exercise during pregnancy.* 2003. http://www.acog.org/publications/patient_education/bp119.cfm Accessed: August 3, 2011

22. Neville MC: Personal communication. November 2006

23. American Dietetic Association: *Position paper: Promoting and supporting breastfeeding.* 2009. *Journal of the American Dietetic Association* 109:1926, 2009.

24. Hurst N: Breastfeeding after breast augmentation. *Journal of Human Lactation* 19:70, 2003.

25. American Academy of Pediatrics, Policy Statement: Breastfeeding and the use of human milk. *Pediatrics* 115:496, 2005.

26. Centers for Disease Control and Prevention: *Breastfeeding Among U.S. Children Born 2000–2008, CDC National Immunization Survey.* Last updated August 1, 2011. http://www.cdc.gov/breastfeeding/data/NIS_data/index.htm Accessed: August 3, 2011

27. Saarela T and others: Macronutrient and energy contents of human milk fractions during the first six months of lactation. *Acta Paediatricia* 94(9):1176, 2005.

28. Fomon SJ: Infant feeding in the 20th century: Formula and beikost. *Journal of Nutrition* 131:409S, 2001.

29. American Dietetic Association: *Introducing solid foods.* ND. http://www.eatright.org/Public/content.aspx?id=8049 Accessed: August 3, 2011

30. Centers for Disease Control and Prevention: *Basics about childhood obesity.* Last updated April 2011. http://www.cdc.gov/obesity/childhood/basics.html Accessed: August 4, 2011

31. U.S. Department of Agriculture: *How much food from the dairy group is needed daily?* http://www.choosemyplate.gov/foodgroups/dairy_amount.aspx Accessed: July 13, 2011

32. Touger-Decker R, van Loveren C: Sugars and dental caries. *American Journal of Clinical Nutrition* 78:881S, 2003.

33. Centers for Disease Control and Prevention: *Table 20D, 2010 Pediatric nutrition surveillance; national summary of growth indicators by age: Children aged less than 5 years.* 2010. http://www.cdc.gov/pednss/pednss_tables/html/pednss_national_table20.htm Accessed: August 4, 2011

34. Centers for Disease Control and Prevention: *Overweight and obesity: Basics about childhood obesity.* Last updated April 2011. http://www.cdc.gov/obesity/childhood/basics.html Accessed: August 4, 2011

35. Centers for Disease Control and Prevention: *Overweight and obesity: A growing problem.* Last updated April 2011. http://www.cdc.gov/obesity/childhood/problem.html Accessed: August 4, 2011

36. Goran MI and others: Obesity and risk of type 2 diabetes and cardiovascular disease in children and adolescents. *Journal of Clinical Endocrinology & Metabolism* 88:1417, 2003.

37. American Academy of Pediatrics, Committee on Nutrition: Prevention of pediatric overweight and obesity. *Pediatrics* 112:424, 2003.

38. Rampersaud GC and others: Breakfast habits, nutritional status, body weight, and academic performance in children and adolescents. *Journal of the American Dietetic Association* 105:743, 2005.

39. Ogden C, Carroll M: National Center for Health Statistics: *Prevalence of obesity among children and adolescents: United States, trends 1963–1965 through 2007–2008.* 2010. http://www.cdc.gov/nchs/data/hestat/obesity_child_07_08/obesity_child_07_08.htm Accessed: July 29, 2011

40. Centers for Disease Control and Prevention: *Overweight and obesity: A growing problem—what causes childhood obesity?* Updated April 2011. http://www.cdc.gov/obesity/childhood/causes.html Accessed: August 4, 2011

41. Centers for Disease Control and Prevention: *Overweight and obesity: Strategies and solutions. Updated April 2011.* http://www.cdc.gov/obesity/childhood/solutions.html Accessed: August 4, 2011

42. Let's Move! ND. http://www.letsmove.gov/learn-facts/epidemic-childhood-obesity Accessed: August 4, 2011

43. Centers for Disease Control and Prevention: *Physical activity for everyone.* Updated March 2011. http://www.cdc.gov/physicalactivity/everyone/guidelines/children.html Accessed: August 4, 2011.

44. Saladin KS: *Anatomy & Physiology.* 6th ed. Boston: McGraw-Hill Publishing Company, 2012.

45. American Academy of Dermatologists: *Frequently asked questions about acne.* ND. http://www.skincarephysicians.com/acnenet/FAQ.html#1 Accessed: August 4, 2011

46. Centers for Disease Control and Prevention: *Adolescent and school health: Youth Risk Behavior Surveillance System (YRBSS).* Updated June 2011. http://www.cdc.gov/healthyyouth/yrbs/index.htm Accessed: August 4, 2011

47. McMahan CA and others: Pathobiological determinants of atherosclerosis in youth risk scores are associated with early and advanced atherosclerosis. *Pediatrics* 118:1447, 2006.

48. Sorof JM and others: Overweight, ethnicity, and the prevalence of hypertension in school-aged children. *Pediatrics* 113:475, 2004.

49. Position of the American Dietetic Association and Dietitians of Canada: Vegetarian diets. *Journal of the American Dietetic Association* 103:748, 2003.

50. Kochanek KD and others: Deaths: Preliminary data for 2009. *National Vital Statistics Reports* 59(4):1, 2011.

51. U.S. Census Bureau: *Facts for features: Older Americans month: May 2011.* Released March 2011. http://www.census.gov/newsroom/releases/archives/facts_for_features_special_editions/cb11-ff08.html Accessed: August 4, 2011

52. Mokdad AH and others: Actual causes of death in the United States, 2000. *Journal of the American Medical Association* 291:1238, 2004.

53. Chernoff R: Micronutrient requirements in older women. *American Journal of Clinical Nutrition* 81:1240S, 2005.

54. Foote JA and others: Older adults need guidance to meet nutritional recommendations. *Journal of the American College of Nutrition* 19:628, 2000.

55. Pesonen J and others: High bone mineral density among perimenopausal women. *Osteoporosis International* 16:1899, 2005.

56. Manini TM and others: Daily activity energy expenditure and mortality among older adults. *Journal of the American Medical Association* 296(2):171, 2006.

57. Centers for Disease Control and Prevention: *Edentulism. Health Data Interactive* http://205.207.175.93/HDI/TableViewer/tableView.aspx?ReportId=110 Accessed: August 4, 2011

58. Hung H-C and others: Tooth loss and dietary intake. *Journal of the American Dental Association* 134:1185, 2003.

59. Qato DM and others: Use of prescription and over-the-counter medications and dietary supplements among older adults in the United States. *Journal of the American Medical Association* 300(24):2867, 2008.

60. Federal Interagency Forum on Aging Related Statistics: *Older Americans 2010: Key indicators of well being.* 2010. http://www.agingstats.gov/agingstatsdotnet/Main_Site/Data/2010_Documents/Docs/OA_2010.pdf Accessed: August 4, 2011

61. Centers for Disease Control and Prevention: *Suicide: Facts at a glance.* 2010. http://www.cdc.gov/ViolencePrevention/pdf/Suicide_DataSheet-a.pdf

62. U.S. General Accounting Office: Antiaging products pose potential for physical and economic harm. Special Committee on Aging, GAO-01-1129, 2001.

63. Genazzani AD and others: Might DHEA be considered a beneficial replacement therapy in the elderly? [Current Opinion]. *Drugs & Aging,* 24(3):173, 2007.

64. Olshansky SJ and others: Position statement on human aging. *Journals of Gerontology, Series A, Biological Sciences and Medical Sciences* 57:B292, 2002.

65. Rattan SIS: Anti-ageing strategies: Prevention or therapy? *EMBO Reports* 6:S25, 2005.

66. Johnson FB and others: Molecular biology of aging. *Cell* 96:291, 1999.

67. Heilbronn LK, Ravussin E: Calorie restriction and aging: A review of the literature and implications for studies in humans. *American Journal of Clinical Nutrition* 78:361, 2003.

68. Heilbronn LK and others: Effect of 6-month calorie restriction on biomarkers of longevity, metabolic adaptation, and oxidative stress in overweight individuals: A randomized controlled trial. *Journal of the American Medical Association* 295:1539, 2006.

69. Heilbronn LK and others: Alternate-day fasting in nonobese subjects: Effects on body weight, body composition, and energy metabolism. *American Journal of Clinical Nutrition* 81:69, 2005.

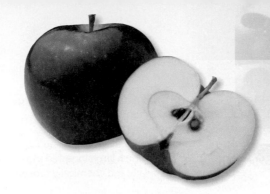

Glossary

A

absorption   process by which substances are taken up from the GI tract and enter the bloodstream or the lymph

Acceptable Macronutrient Distribution Ranges (AMDRs)   macronutrient intake ranges that are nutritionally adequate and may reduce the risk of diet-related chronic diseases

acids   substances that donate hydrogen ions

acid-base balance   maintaining the proper pH of body fluids

acid group   acid portion of a compound

added sugars   sugars added to foods during processing or preparation

adenosine diphosphate (ADP)   high-energy compound, by-product of ATP use

adenosine triphosphate (ATP)   high-energy compound that stores energy, major direct energy source for cells

Adequate Intakes (AIs)   dietary recommendations that assume a population's average daily nutrient intakes are adequate because no deficiency diseases are present

adipose cells   fat cells; specialized cells that store fat

adolescence   life stage in which a child matures physically into an adult

aerobic   conditions that require free oxygen

aerobic exercise   physical activities that involve sustained, rhythmic contractions of large muscle groups

air displacement   method of estimating body composition by determining body volume

aldosterone   hormone that participates in sodium and water conservation

alpha-linolenic acid   an essential fatty acid

alpha-tocopherol   vitamin E

alternative sweeteners   substances that sweeten foods while providing few or no kilocalories

amino acids   nitrogen-containing chemical units that comprise proteins

amino or nitrogen containing group   portion of an amino acid that contains nitrogen

anaerobic   conditions that lack free oxygen

anatomy   scientific study of cells and other body structures

anecdotes   reports of personal experiences

anemia   disorder characterized by too few red blood cells and poor oxygen transport in blood

anencephaly   type of neural tube defect in which the brain does not form properly or is missing

anorexia nervosa (AN)   severe psychological disturbance characterized by self-imposed starvation

antibodies   infection-fighting proteins

antidiuretic hormone (ADH)   hormone that participates in water conservation

antioxidant   substance that protects other compounds from being damaged or destroyed by certain factors

appetite   desire to eat appealing food

arteries   vessels that carry blood away from the heart

arteriosclerosis   condition that results from atherosclerosis and is characterized by loss of arterial flexibility

ascorbic acid   vitamin C

atherosclerosis   long-term disease process in which plaques build up inside arterial walls

B

bacteria   simple single-celled microorganisms

bariatric medicine   medical specialty that focuses on the treatment of obesity

basal metabolism   minimal number of calories the body uses to support vital activities after fasting and resting for 12 hours

bases   substances that accept hydrogen ions

beriberi   thiamin deficiency disease

beta-carotene   carotenoid that the body can convert to vitamin A

bile   emulsifier that aids lipid digestion

bioavailability   extent to which the digestive tract absorbs a nutrient and how well the body uses it

bioelectrical impedance   technique of estimating body composition in which a device measures the conduction of a weak electrical current through the body

biological activity   describes vitamin's degree of potency or effects in the body

body mass index (BMI)   numerical value of relationship between body weight and risk of certain chronic health problems associated with excess body fat

buffer   substance that can protect the pH of a solution

bulimia nervosa   eating disorder characterized by cyclic episodes of bingeing and calorie-restrictive dieting

C

caffeine   naturally occurring stimulant drug

calcitonin   hormone secreted by the thyroid gland when blood calcium levels are too high

Calorie   *See* kilocalorie

capillaries   smallest blood vessels

carbohydrate (glycogen) loading   practice of manipulating physical activity and dietary patterns to increase muscle glycogen stores

carbohydrates   class of nutrients that is a major source of energy for the body

carcinogens   cancer-causing substances

cardiovascular disease (CVD)   group of diseases that affect the heart and blood vessels

carotenemia   yellowing of the skin that results from excess beta-carotene in the body

carotenoids   yellow-orange pigments in fruits and vegetables

case-control study   study in which individuals who have a health condition are compared with individuals with similar characteristics who do not have the condition

casein   major protein in cow's milk

cell   smallest living functional unit in an organism

central-body obesity   condition characterized by excessive abdominal fat

chemical bond   attraction that holds atoms together

chemical reactions   processes that change the atomic arrangements of molecules

chemistry   study of the composition and characteristics of matter and changes that can occur to it

cholecystokinin (CCK)   hormone that stimulates the gallbladder to release bile and pancreas to secrete digestive enzymes

cholesterol   lipid found in animal foods and precursor for steroid hormones, bile, and vitamin D

choline   water-soluble compound in lecithin

chylomicron   lipoprotein formed by small intestinal cells that transports lipids in the bloodstream

chyme   mixture of gastric juice and partially digested food

coenzyme   small molecule that interacts with enzymes, enabling the enzymes to function

cofactor   ion or molecule that catalyzes chemical reactions

cohort study   study that measures variables of a group of people over time

collagen   fibrous protein that gives strength to connective tissues

color additives   dyes, pigments, or other substances that provide color to food

colostrum   initial form of breast milk that contains anti-infective properties

complementary combinations   mixing certain plant foods to provide all essential amino acids without adding animal protein

complex carbohydrates (polysaccharides)   compounds comprised of 10 or more monosaccharides bonded together

compounds   molecules that contain two or more different elements in specific proportions

conception   moment when a sperm enters an egg (fertilization)

connective tissue   type of cells that hold together, protect, and support organs

contaminated food   item that is impure or unsafe for human consumption

control group   group being studied that does not receive treatment

coronary artery disease (CAD)   a major form of CVD

correlation   relationship between two variables

cretinism   condition affecting infants of women who were iodine deficient during pregnancy

cross-contamination   unintentional transfer of pathogenic microbes from one food to another

cytochromes   group of proteins involved in the release of energy from macronutrients

D

Daily Values (DVs)   set of nutrient intake standards developed for labeling purposes

deamination   removal of the nitrogen-containing group from an amino acid

deficiency disease   state of health that occurs when a nutrient is missing from the diet

dehydration   body water depletion

Delaney Clause   component of the 1958 Food Additives Amendment that prevents manufacturers from adding carcinogenic compounds to food

denaturation   altering a protein's natural shape and function by exposing it to conditions such as heat, acids, and physical agitation

diabetes mellitus (diabetes)   group of serious chronic diseases characterized by abnormal glucose, fat, and protein metabolism

diastolic pressure   pressure in an artery that occurs when the ventricles relax between contractions

diet   usual pattern of food choices

dietary fiber (fiber)   indigestible plant material; most types are polysaccharides

Dietary Reference Intakes (DRIs)   various energy and nutrient intake standards for Americans

dietary supplements   nutrient preparations, certain hormones, and herbal products

digestion   process by which large ingested molecules are mechanically and chemically broken down

disaccharide   simple sugar comprised of two monosaccharides

diuretic   substance that increases urine production

diverticula   abnormal, tiny sacs that form in wall of colon

DNA   molecule that contains coded instructions for synthesizing proteins

double-blind study   experimental design in which neither the participants nor the researchers are aware of each participant's group assignment

dual-energy X-ray absorptiometry (DXA)   technique of estimating body composition that involves scanning the body with multiple low-energy X-rays

duodenum   first segment of the small intestine

E

eating disorders   psychological disturbances that lead to certain physiological changes and serious health complications

edema   accumulation of fluid in tissues

electrolytes   ions that conduct electricity when they are dissolved in water

electrons   small, negatively charged particles that surround the nucleus of an atom

element   each type of atom; substance that cannot be separated into simpler substances by ordinary chemical or physical means

embolus   thrombus or part of a plaque that breaks free and travels through the bloodstream

embryo   human organism from 14 days to 8 weeks after conception

empty-calorie   describes food or beverage that is a poor source of micronutrients in relation to its energy value

empty-calorie allowance   daily amount of energy remaining after a person consumes recommended amounts of foods from the major food groups

emulsifier   substance that helps water-soluble and water-insoluble compounds mix with each other

energy   capacity to perform work

energy density   energy value of a food in relation to the food's weight

energy equilibrium   calorie intake equals calorie output

energy intake   calories from foods and beverages that contain macronutrients and alcohol

energy output   calories cells use to carry out their activities

enrichment   addition of iron and certain vitamins to cereal grain products

enterohepatic circulation   process that recycles cholesterol (bile salts) in the body

enzymes   compounds that speed up chemical reactions

epidemiology   study of the occurrence, distribution, and causes of health problems in populations

epiglottis   flap of tissue that folds down over the windpipe to keep food from entering the respiratory system during swallowing

epinephrine   hormone produced by adrenal glands; also called adrenalin

epithelial cells   cells that form protective tissues that line the body

epithelial tissue   cells that line every body surface

ergogenic aids   foods, devices, dietary supplements, or drugs used to improve physical performance

esophagus   tubular structure of the GI tract that connects the pharynx with the stomach

essential amino acids   amino acids the body cannot make or make enough of to meet its needs

essential fatty acids   lipids that must be supplied by the diet

essential nutrient   nutrient that must be supplied by food

Estimated Average Requirement (EAR)   amount of a nutrient that meets the needs of 50% of healthy people in a life stage/gender group

Estimated Energy Requirement (EER)   average daily energy intake that meets the needs of a healthy person maintaining his or her weight

estrogen   hormone needed for normal bone development and maintenance

Exchange System   method of classifying foods into numerous lists based on macronutrient composition

exercise   physical activities that are usually planned and structured for a purpose

extracellular water   water that surrounds cells or is in blood

extrusion reflex   involuntary response in which a young infant thrusts its tongue forward when a solid or semisolid object is placed in its mouth

F

fad   trendy practice that has widespread appeal for a period, then becomes no longer fashionable

fat-free mass   lean tissues

fat-soluble vitamins   vitamins A, D, E, and K

female athlete triad   condition characterized by low energy intakes, abnormal menstrual cycles, and bone mineral irregularities

fermentation   process used to preserve or produce a variety of foods, including pickles and wine

fetus   human organism from 8 weeks after conception until birth

folic acid and **folacin** forms of folate

food additive any substance that becomes incorporated into food during production, packaging, transport, or storage

Food Additives Amendment U.S. legislation that requires evidence that a new food additive is safe before it can be marketed for use

Food and Nutrition Board (FNB) group of nutrition scientists who develop DRIs

food-borne illness infection caused by microscopic disease-causing agents in food

food insecurity situation in which individuals or families are concerned about running out of food or not having enough money to buy more food

food intoxication illness that results when poisons produced by certain microbes contaminate food and irritate the intestinal tract

fortification addition of one or more nutrients to foods during their manufacturing process

fructose monosaccharide in fruits, honey, and certain vegetables; "levulose" or "fruit sugar"

fungi simple organisms that live on dead or decaying organic matter

fungicides substances used to limit the spread of fungi

G

galactose monosaccharide that is a component of lactose

gastroesophageal sphincter section of esophagus next to the stomach that controls the opening to the stomach

gastrointestinal (GI) tract muscular tube that extends from the mouth to the anus

gene portion of DNA

Generally Recognized As Safe (GRAS) ingredients thought to be safe

genetic endowment inherited physical characteristics that can affect physical performance

genetic modification techniques that alter an organism's DNA

ghrelin hormone that stimulates eating behavior

glucagon hormone that helps regulate blood glucose levels

glucose monosaccharide that is a primary fuel for muscles and other cells; "dextrose" or "blood sugar"

glycemic index (GI); glycemic load (GL) standards that indicate the body's insulin response to a carbohydrate-containing food

glycogen storage polysaccharide in animals

glycogenolysis glycogen breakdown

glycolysis first stage of glucose oxidation

goitrogens compounds that inhibit iodide metabolism by the thyroid gland

H

H⁺ hydrogen ion chemical formula

heartburn backflow of irritating stomach contents into the esophagus

heat cramps heat-related illness characterized by painful muscle contractions

heat exhaustion heat-related illness that can occur after intense exercise

heatstroke most dangerous form of heat-related illness

heme iron form of iron in hemoglobin and myoglobin

hemoglobin iron-containing protein in red blood cells that transports oxygen

hemolysis disintegration of red blood cells

hepatic portal vein vein that collects nutrients from the intestinal tract and delivers them to the liver

herbicides substances used to destroy weeds

hereditary hemochromatosis common inherited disorder characterized by excess iron absorption

high-density lipoprotein (HDL) lipoprotein that transports cholesterol away from tissues and to the liver, where it can be eliminated

high-quality (complete) protein protein that contains all essential amino acids in amounts that support the deposition of protein in tissues and the growth of a young person

high-sensitivity C-reactive protein (hs-CRP) protein produced primarily by the liver in response to inflammation; a marker for CVD

homeostasis maintenance of an internal chemical and physical environment that is critical for good health and survival

homocysteine amino acid that may play a role in the development of atherosclerosis

hormones chemical messengers that convey information to target cells and regulate body processes and responses

hunger uncomfortable feeling that drives a person to consume food

hydration water status

hydrocarbon chain chain of carbon atoms bonded to each other and to hydrogen atoms

hydrogenation food manufacturing process that adds hydrogen atoms to liquid vegetable oil, forming trans fats

hydrophilic part of molecule that attracts water

hydrophobic part of molecule that avoids water and attracts lipids

hypercalcemia condition characterized by higher-than-normal concentration of calcium in blood

hyperglycemia abnormally high blood glucose level

hypoglycemia condition that occurs when the blood glucose level is abnormally low

hypertension abnormally high blood pressure levels that persist

hyperthermia very high body temperature

hypothesis possible explanation about an observation that guides scientific research

I

ileum last segment of the small intestine

infant formula synthetic food that simulates human milk

insecticides substances used to control or kill insects

insoluble fiber forms of dietary fiber that generally do not dissolve in water

insulin hormone that helps regulate blood glucose levels

intracellular water water that is inside cells

intrinsic factor substance produced in the stomach that facilitates intestinal absorption of vitamin B-12

ion atom or group of atoms that has a positive or negative charge

iron deficiency condition characterized by low body stores of iron

J

jejunum middle segment of the small intestine

K

keratin tough protein found in hair, nails, and the outermost layers of skin

ketone bodies chemicals that result from incomplete fat breakdown

kilocalorie or **Calorie** heat energy needed to raise the temperature of 1 liter of water 1° centigrade; measure of food energy

kwashiorkor form of undernutrition that results from consuming adequate energy and insufficient high-quality protein

L

lactase enzyme that splits lactose molecule

lactation milk production

lacteal lymph vessel in villus that absorbs most lipids

lactic acid compound formed from pyruvate during anaerobic metabolism

lactoovovegetarian vegetarian who consumes milk products and eggs for animal protein

lactose disaccharide comprised of a glucose and a galactose molecule; "milk sugar"

lactose intolerance inability to digest lactose properly

lactovegetarian vegetarian who consumes milk and milk products for animal protein

legumes plants that produce pods with a single row of seeds

leptin hormone that reduces hunger and inhibits fat storage in the body

life expectancy length of time an average person born in a specific year can expect to live

life span maximum number of years an organism can live

lifestyle way of living

linoleic acid an essential fatty acid

lipases enzymes that break down lipids

lipids class of nutrients that do not dissolve in water

lipolysis fat breakdown

lipoprotein water-soluble structure that transports lipids through the bloodstream

lipoprotein lipase enzyme in capillary walls that breaks down triglycerides

liposuction surgical method of reducing the size of local fat deposits

low-birth weight (LBW) infant describes infant generally weighing less than 5½ pounds at birth

low-density lipoprotein (LDL) lipoprotein that carries cholesterol into tissues, including arterial plaques

low-quality (incomplete) protein protein that lacks or has inadequate amounts of one or more of the essential amino acids

lumen open space within a structure such as the small intestine

lymph fluid in the lymphatic system

M

macronutrients nutrients needed in gram amounts daily and that provide energy; carbohydrates, proteins, and fats

major minerals essential mineral elements required in amounts of 100 mg or more per day

malnutrition state of health that occurs when the body is improperly nourished

maltose disaccharide comprised of two glucose molecules; "malt sugar"

marasmus starvation

megadose generally defined as 10 times the recommended amount of a vitamin or mineral

metabolic syndrome condition that increases risk of type 2 diabetes and CVD

metabolic water water formed by cells as a metabolic by-product

metabolism the sum of all chemical reactions occurring in living cells

micronutrients vitamins and minerals

minerals elements that are found in the earth's crust

mitochondria organelles that generate energy from macronutrients

moderation obtaining adequate amounts of nutrients while balancing calorie intake with calorie expenditure

molecule matter that forms when two or more atoms interact and are held together by a chemical bond

monoglyceride single fatty acid attached to a glycerol backbone

monosaccharide simple sugar that is the basic molecule of carbohydrates

monounsaturated fatty acid fatty acid that has one double bond within the carbon chain

morning sickness nausea and vomiting associated with pregnancy

mucus fluid that lubricates and protects certain cells

myocardial infarction heart attack

myoglobin iron-containing protein in muscle cells that controls oxygen uptake from red blood cells

MyPlate USDA's interactive Internet dietary and menu planning guide

N

negative energy balance calorie intake is less than calorie output

negative nitrogen balance state in which the body loses more nitrogen than it retains

neural tube embryonic structure that eventually develops into the brain and spinal cord

nitrogen balance (equilibrium) balancing nitrogen intake with nitrogen losses

nonessential amino acids group of amino acids that the body can make

nonexercise activity thermogenesis (NEAT) involuntary skeletal muscular activities such as fidgeting

nonheme iron form of iron in vegetables, grains, meats, and supplements

nonnutritive sweeteners group of synthetic compounds that are intensely sweet tasting compared to sugar

nutrient-dense describes food or beverage that has more vitamins and minerals in relation to its energy value

nutrients chemicals necessary for proper body functioning

nutrition scientific study of nutrients and how the body uses these substances

nutritive sweeteners substances that sweeten and contribute energy to foods

O

obesity condition characterized by excess body fat

omega-3 fatty acid type of polyunsaturated fatty acid

omnivore organism that can digest and absorb nutrients from plants, animals, fungi, and bacteria

organ collection of tissues that function in a related fashion

organ system collection of organs that work together to perform a major function

organelles structures in cells that perform specialized functions

organic foods foods produced without the use of antibiotics, hormones, synthetic fertilizers and pesticides, genetic improvements, or spoilage-killing radiation

osmosis movement of water through a selectively permeable membrane

osteoblasts bone cells that add bone to where the tissue is needed

osteoclasts bone cells that tear down bone tissue

osteomalacia adult rickets; condition characterized by poorly mineralized (soft) bones

osteoporosis chronic disease characterized by bones with low mass and reduced structure

overweight having extra weight from bone, muscle, body fat, and/or body water

ovovegetarian vegetarian who eats eggs for animal protein

oxidizing agent or **oxidant** substance that removes electrons from atoms or molecules

oxytocin hormone that elicits the "let-down" response and causes the uterus to contract

P

pancreatic amylase enzyme secreted by pancreas that breaks down starch into maltose molecules

pancreatic lipase digestive enzyme that removes two fatty acids from each triglyceride molecule

parasite organism that lives in or on another organism, often deriving nourishment from its host

parathyroid hormone (PTH) hormone secreted by parathyroid glands when blood calcium levels are too low

pasteurization process that kills the pathogens in foods and beverages as well as many microbes responsible for spoilage

pathogens disease-causing microbes

peer review expert critical analysis of a research article before it is published

pellagra niacin deficiency disease

pepsin gastric enzyme that breaks down proteins into polypeptides

peptide bond chemical attraction that connects two amino acids together

peptides small chains of amino acids

peristalsis type of muscular contraction of the gastrointestinal tract

pernicious anemia condition caused by the lack of intrinsic factor and characterized by vitamin B-12 deficiency, nerve damage, and megaloblastic RBCs

pesticide substance that people use to kill or control unwanted insects, weeds, or other organisms

pH measure of the acidity or alkalinity of a solution

phosphocreatine (PCr) high-energy compound used to reform ATP under anaerobic conditions

phospholipid type of lipid needed to make cell membranes and for proper functioning of nerve cells

physical activity   movement resulting from contraction of skeletal muscles

physical fitness   ability to perform moderate- to vigorous-intensity activities without becoming excessively fatigued

physiological dose   amount of a nutrient that is within the range of safe intake and enables the body to function optimally

physiology   scientific study of the functioning of cells and other body structures

phytochemicals   compounds made by plants that are not nutrients

pica   practice of eating nonfood items

placebo   fake treatment, such as a sham pill, injection, or medical procedure

placebo effect   response to a placebo

placenta   organ of pregnancy that connects the uterus to the embryo/fetus via the umbilical cord

polypeptides   proteins comprised of 50 or more amino acids

polyunsaturated fatty acid   fatty acid that has two or more double bonds within the carbon chain

positive energy balance   calorie intake is greater than calorie output

positive nitrogen balance   state in which the body retains more nitrogen than it loses

pregnancy-induced hypertension (PIH)   type of hypertension that can develop during pregnancy

prehypertension   persistent systolic blood pressure readings of 120 mm Hg to 139 mm Hg and diastolic readings of 80 mm Hg to 89 mm Hg

prenatal care   specialized health care for pregnant women

prenatal period   time between conception and birth; pregnancy

preterm   describes infant born before the 37th week of pregnancy

prolactin   hormone that stimulates milk production after delivery

prooxidant   substance that promotes free radical production

protein turnover   cellular process of breaking down proteins and recycling their amino acids

proteins   large, complex organic molecules made up of amino acids

protons   positively charged particles in the nucleus of an atom

protozoans   single-celled microorganisms that have complex cell structures

pseudoscience   presentation of information masquerading as factual and obtained by scientific methods

pyruvate   compound that results from anaerobic breakdown of glucose

Q

quackery   promotion of useless medical treatments

R

R group (side chain)   part of amino acid that determines the molecule's physical and chemical properties

radical   substance with an unpaired electron

Recommended Dietary Allowances (RDAs)   standards for recommending daily intakes of several nutrients

requirement   smallest amount of a nutrient that maintains a defined level of health

resting metabolic rate (RMR)   body's rate of energy use a few hours after resting and eating

retinol (preformed vitamin A)   most active form of vitamin A in the body

rhodopsin   vitamin A–containing protein that is needed for vision in dim light

rickets   vitamin D deficiency disorder in children

risk factor   personal characteristic that increases a person's chances of developing a disease

rodenticides   substances used to kill mice and rats

S

salivary amylase   enzyme secreted by salivary glands that begins starch digestion

salt   substance that forms when an acid combines with a base

satiety   feeling that enough food has been eaten to delay the next eating episode and/or reduce subsequent food intake

saturated fatty acid   fatty acid that has each carbon atom within the chain filled with hydrogen atoms

scurvy   vitamin C deficiency disease

selectively permeable membrane   barrier that allows the passage of certain substances and prevents the movement of other substances

senescence   declining organ functioning and increased vulnerability

set-point theory   scientific notion that body fat content is genetically predetermined

shelf life   period of time that a food can be stored before it spoils

simple diffusion   molecular movement from a region of higher to lower concentration

skinfold thickness measurements   technique of estimating body composition in which calipers are used to measure the width of skinfolds at multiple body sites

solubility   describes how easily a substance dissolves in a liquid solvent

soluble fiber   forms of dietary fiber that dissolve or swell in water

solute   lesser component of a solution that dissolves in solvent

solution   evenly distributed mixture of two or more compounds

solvent   primary component of a solution

spina bifida   type of neural tube defect in which the spine does not form properly before birth, and it fails to enclose the spinal cord

starch   storage polysaccharide in plants

sterilization   process that kills or destroys all microorganisms and viruses

sterols/stanols   types of lipids made by plants

sucrase   enzyme that splits sucrose molecule

sucrose   disaccharide comprised of a glucose and a fructose molecule; "table sugar"

sugars   group of simple carbohydrates

syndrome   group of signs and symptoms that occur together and indicate a specific health problem

systolic pressure   maximum blood pressure within an artery that occurs when the ventricles contract

T

target heart rate zone   heart rate range that reflects intensity of physical exertion

teratogen   an agent that causes birth defects

testimonial   personal endorsement of a product

tetrahydrofolic acid (THFA)   folate coenzyme

thermic effect of food (TEF)   energy used to digest foods and beverages as well as absorb and further process the macronutrients

thrombus   fixed bunch of clots that remains in place

thyroid hormone   hormone that regulates the body's metabolic rate

tissues   masses of cells that have similar characteristics and functions

Tolerable Upper Intake Level (Upper Level or UL)   standard representing the highest average amount of a nutrient that is unlikely to be harmful when consumed daily

tolerances   maximum amounts of pesticide residues that can be in or on each treated food crop

total body fat   essential fat and adipose tissue

total water intake   water in beverages and foods

trace minerals   essential mineral elements required in amounts that are less than 100 mg per day

trans fats   unsaturated fatty acids that have a *trans* double bond

transamination   transfer of the nitrogen-containing group from an unneeded amino acid to a carbon skeleton to form an amino acid

treatment group   group being studied that receives a treatment

triglyceride   lipid that has three fatty acids attached to a three-carbon compound called glycerol

U

underwater weighing technique of estimating body composition that involves comparing weight on land to weight when completely submerged in a tank of water

underweight describes person with a BMI of less than 18.5

unintentional food additives substances that are accidentally in foods

unsaturated fatty acid fatty acid that is missing hydrogen atoms and has one or more double bonds within the carbon chain

urea waste product of amino acid metabolism

uterus female reproductive organ that protects the developing organism during pregnancy

V

variable personal characteristic or other factor that changes and can influence an outcome

vegan vegetarian who eats only plant foods

vegetarians people who eat plant-based diets

veins vessels that return blood to the heart

very-low density lipoprotein (VLDL) lipoprotein that carries much of the triglycerides in the bloodstream

villi (singular, villus) tiny, fingerlike projections of the small intestinal lining that participate in digesting and absorbing food

virus microbe consisting of a piece of genetic material coated with protein

vitamin complex organic molecule that regulates certain metabolic processes

W

water intoxication condition that occurs when too much water is consumed in a short time period or the kidneys have difficulty filtering water from blood

water-soluble vitamins thiamin, riboflavin, niacin, vitamin B-6, pantothenic acid, folate, biotin, vitamin B-12, and vitamin C

weaning gradual process of shifting from breastfeeding or bottle feeding to drinking from a cup and eating solid foods

Wernicke-Korsakoff syndrome degenerative brain disorder resulting from thiamin deficiency that occurs primarily among alcoholics

X

xerophthalmia condition affecting the eyes that results from vitamin A deficiency

Photo Credits

Chapter 1

Opener: © Blend Images/Getty Images RF; Figure **1.1:** © Getty Images RF; **1.2 both:** © RubberBall Productions RF; **Page 5:** © Greg Kuchik/Getty Images RF; **Page 6 (Red Onion):** © C Squared Studios/Getty Images RF; **Page 6 (Garlic):** © Stockdisc/PunchStock RF; **Page 6 (Carrots):** © Photodisc/Getty Images RF; **Page 7 (Apple):** © Burke/Triolo Productions/Getty Images RF; **Page 7 (Black Grapes):** © PhotoAlto/PunchStock RF; **Page 7 (Red Grapes):** © Jules Frazier/Getty Images RF; **Page 7 (Strawberry):** © Burke/Triolo Productions/Getty Images RF; **Page 7 (Chile Pepper):** © Royalty Free/Corbis RF; **Page 7 (Peppers & Broccoli):** © Photodisc/Getty Images RF; **Page 7 (Coffee Beans):** © Photodisc/PunchStock RF; **Page 7 (Lemon):** © Photodisc/Getty Images RF; **Page 7 (Oranges and Juice):** © Royalty Free/Corbis RF; **Page 8:** © Nancy R. Cohen/Getty Images RF; **Page 9 (Milk):** © The McGraw-Hill Companies, Inc./Christopher Kerrigan, photographer; **Page 9 (Soda):** © Pixtal/SuperStock RF; **Page 9:** U.S. Dept. of Health and Human Services; **Page 10:** © Royalty Free/Corbis RF; **Page 11 (Ruler):** © Amos Morgan/Getty Images RF; **Page 11 (Scales):** © Burke/Triolo/Brand X Pictures/JupiterImages RF; **Page 12:** © Wendy Schiff; **1.5a:** © Ed Carey/Cole Group/Getty Images RF; **1.5b-d:** © The McGraw-Hill Companies, Inc./Christopher Kerrigan, photographer; **Page 13 (Pumpkin Pie):** © Royalty Free/Corbis RF; **1.6 left:** © The McGraw-Hill Companies, Inc./Christopher Kerrigan, photographer; **1.6 right:** © Pixtal/SuperStock RF; **Page 14 (Lettuce):** © Royalty Free/Corbis RF; **Page 15 (Strawberries):** © Burke/Triolo Productions/Getty Images RF; **Page 15 (Brownies):** © Michael Lamotte/Cole Group/Getty Images RF; **1.9 left:** © PhotoDisc/PunchStock RF; **1.9 right:** © The McGraw-Hill Companies, Inc./Michael Scott, photographer; **Page 17 (Supplements):** © Nancy R. Cohen/Getty Images RF; **Page 17 (Spread):** © Wendy Schiff; **1.10:** © The McGraw-Hill Companies, Inc./Lars A. Niki, photographer; **Page 18 (Locusts):** © IT Stock/Alamy RF; **1.12:** © Digitial Vision/PunchStock RF; **1.13:** Courtesy of the Centers for Disease Control/Dr. Lyle Conrad RF; **1.14:** © Getty Images RF; **1.15:** USDA Photo by Ken Hammond; **1.16:** © Comstock/Alamy RF; **Page 23 (Kernels):** © Don Farrall/Getty Images RF; **Page 23-24 (Strawberries):** © Burke/Triolo Productions/Getty Images RF; **Page 25 (Muffin), Page 26 (Cookies):** © Wendy Schiff; **Page 27:** © Photodisc/

Getty Images RF; **Page 29 (Raspberries):** © PhotoAlto/PunchStock RF; **Page 29 (Kale):** © Stockdisc/PunchStock RF; **Page 29 (Eggs):** © Image Source/PunchStock RF; **Page 29 (Peas):** © Burke/Triolo Productions/Getty Images RF; **Page 29 (Coke):** © Royalty Free/Corbis RF

Chapter 2

Opener: Courtesy of the Waring Historical Library, MUSC, Charleston, S.C.; **Page 31 (Cabbage):** © Burke Triolo Productions/Getty Images RF; **Page 31 (Potatoes):** © Ingram Publishing/Alamy RF; **Page 32:** Centers for Disease Control; **2.1:** © NIBSC/Photo Researchers, Inc.; **2.3:** Russ Hanson/ARS/USDA; **2.5:** Stephen Ausmus/ARS/USDA; **Page 38:** © Siede Preis/Getty Images RF; **Page 39:** © Getty Images RF; **Page 40:** © Wendy Schiff; **2.8:** © The McGraw-Hill Companies, Inc./Andrew Resek, photographer; **Page 43 (Labels):** © Wendy Schiff; **2.9 both:** WHO; **Page 44:** © Stockdisc/PunchStock RF; **2.10:** © Wendy Schiff; **Page 47:** © Photodisc/PunchStock RF; **Page 48 top, Page 49 (Label):** © Wendy Schiff; **Page 49 (Pills):** © The McGraw-Hill Companies, Inc./Jill Braaten, photographer; **Page 50 (Pills):** © C Squared Studios/Getty Images RF; **Page 50 (Plant):** © Brand X Pictures/PunchStock RF; **Page 50 (Ginger):** © Stockbyte/Getty Images RF; **Page 51 (Tea):** © Mitch Hrdlicka/Getty Images RF; **Page 51 (Plant):** Jennifer Anderson/USDA-NRCS Plants Database; **Page 53:** © Photodisc/Getty Images RF; **Page 55 (Soup), Page 55 (Tea):** © Wendy Schiff; **Page 56:** © Photodisc/Getty Images RF; **Page 57:** © Wendy Schiff

Chapter 3

Opener: © Ryan McVay/Getty Images RF; **Page 59:** © Digitial Vision/PunchStock RF; **Page 62:** © Wendy Schiff; **Page 63 top:** © D. Hurst/Alamy RF; **Page 63 bottom:** © Wendy Schiff; **Page 64 left:** © Digital Vision/Getty Images RF; **Page 64 right:** © PhotoDisc/Getty Images RF; **Page 64 (bottom):** © Cordelia Molloy/Photo Researchers, Inc.; **3.4:** © The McGraw-Hill Companies, Inc./Christopher Kerrigan, photographer; **Page 65 (bottom):** U.S. Dept. of Agriculture; **Page 66 (Salt):** © C Squared Studios/Getty Images RF; **Page 66 (Wine), Page 66 (Bread):** © Jules Frazier/Getty Images RF; **Page 66 (Cheese):** © PhotoDisc/Getty Images RF; **3.5, 3.6, 3.7:** U.S. Dept. of Agriculture; **Page 70 (Dice):**

© The McGraw-Hill Companies, Inc./Christopher Kerrigan, photographer; **Page 70 (Mouse):** © Royalty Free/Corbis RF; **Page 70 (Ball):** © Radlung & Associates/Getty Images RF; **Page 71 (Baseball):** © Ryan McVay/Getty Images RF; **Page 71 (Yo yo):** © PhotoDisc/Getty Images RF; **Page 71 (Soap):** © The McGraw-Hill Companies, Inc./Christopher Kerrigan, photographer; **Page 71 top:** © Wendy Schiff; **Page 72 top:** © C Squared Studios/Getty Images RF; **Page 72 bottom:** © Photodisc/Getty Images RF; **Page 73, 3.10, 3.11, Page 78, 3.13, 3.14:** © Wendy Schiff; **Page 81:** © Royalty Free/Corbis RF; **Page 82 bottom:** © Keith Ovregaard/Cole Group/Getty Images RF; **3.15, 3.16:** © 2009 Oldways Preservation & Exchange Trust, http://oldwayspt.org; **Page 84 bottom:** © Burke/Triolo Productions/Getty Images RF; **Page 85 (Noodles):** © Wendy Schiff; **Page 85 (Bagel):** © Photodisc/PunchStock RF; **Page 87 (Fruit Salad), Page 87 (Lassi):** © Wendy Schiff; **Page 89:** © Royalty Free/Corbis RF; **Page 90:** © D. Hurst/Alamy RF; **Page 91 (Ham):** © Royalty Free/Corbis RF; **Page 91 (Egg):** © The McGraw-Hill Companies, Inc./Ken Karp, photographer; **Page 91 (USDA):** U.S. Dept. of Agriculture

Chapter 4

Opener: © The McGraw-Hill Companies, Inc./Joanne Brummett, artwork ; **4.3a,b:** © Wendy Schiff; **4.5 (Lemon and Wine):** © Burke/Triolo Productions/Getty Images RF; **4.5 (Cola):** © Royalty Free/Corbis RF; **4.5 (Tomato and Banana):** © Stockdisc/PunchStock RF; **4.5 (Coffee):** © Royalty Free/Corbis RF; **4.5 (Milk):** © The McGraw-Hill Companies, Inc./Bob Coyle, photographer; **4.5 (Egg):** © Siede Preis/Getty Images RF; **4.5 (Baking Soda):** © The McGraw-Hill Companies, Inc./Stephen Frisch, photographer; **4.5 (Ammonia):** © The McGraw-Hill Companies, Inc./Jacques Cornell, photographer; **4.5 (Oven cleaner):** © The McGraw-Hill Companies, Inc./Ken Karp, photographer; **Page 96 bottom left:** © The McGraw-Hill Companies, Inc./Stephen Frisch, photographer; **4.6a,b, 4.8:** © Wendy Schiff; **Page 106 left:** © Royalty Free/Corbis RF; **Page 106 right:** © Brand X Pictures/PunchStock RF; **4.28:** © Gladden Willis, M.D./Visuals Unlimited; **Page 112 top:** © Lee W. Wilcox; **Page 112 bottom, Page 113 left:** © Wendy Schiff; **Page 113 right:** © Jim Arbogast/Getty Images/RF **Page 114:** © The McGraw-Hill Companies, Inc./Lars A. Niki, photographer; **4.32:** © David M. Martin, M.D./Photo Researchers, Inc.; **Page**

116: © The McGraw-Hill Companies, Inc./Pat Watson, photographer; **Page 119 left:** © Wendy Schiff; **Page 119 right:** © Jonelle Weaver/Getty Images RF; **Page 120:** © Wendy Schiff

Chapter 5

Opener: © Photodisc/Getty Images RF; **Page 125 (Bee):** © Allan & Sandy Carey/Getty Images RF; **Page 126:** © Wendy Schiff; **Page 127 (Sugar):** © StockFood/SuperStock RF; **Page 127 (Honey):** © Brand X Pictures/Getty Images RF; **Page 127 bottom, Page 128 top, Page 128 bottom:** © Wendy Schiff; **5.6:** © Cole Group/Getty Images RF; **5.7:** © Wendy Schiff; **Page 131 (Carrots):** © C Squared Studios/Getty Images RF; **Page 131 (Lettuce), Page 131 (Raspberries):** © Burke/Triolo Productions/Getty Images RF; **Page 131 (Potato):** © The McGraw-Hill Companies, Inc./Christopher Kerrigan, photographer; **Page 131 (Banana):** © Stockdisc/PunchStock RF; **Page 131 (Apples):** © PhotoLink/Getty Images RF; **Page 133:** Scott Bauer/ARS/USDA, **Page 135 (Donut):** © Ingram Publishing/Fotosearch RF; **Page 135 (Cola), Page 137 top:** © Royalty Free/Corbis RF; **Page 137 bottom:** © PhotoLink/Getty Images RF; **5.13a,b:** © Wendy Schiff; **Page 140 both:** © PhotoLink/Getty Images RF; **Page 141:** © The McGraw-Hill Companies, Inc./Lars A. Niki, photographer; **Page 142:** © Wendy Schiff; **Page 143 right:** © The McGraw-Hill Companies, Inc./Bob Coyle, photographer; **5.14:** © Wendy Schiff; **Page 144 top:** © BananaStock/PunchStock RF; **5.15:** © Du Cane Medical Imaging Ltd/Photo Researchers, Inc.; **Page 145:** © Wendy Schiff; **5.17:** American Heart Association; **Page 147 top:** © Wendy Schiff; **Page 147 bottom left:** © Royalty Free/Corbis RF; **Page 147 right:** U.S. Air Force Photo by Master Sargent Michael A. Kaplan; **Page 148 top, Page 148 right:** © Photodisc/Getty Images RF; **Page 148 bottom:** © Comstock/PunchStock RF; **Page 149:** © Burke/Triolo Productions/Getty Images RF; **Page 150:** © Photodisc/Getty Images RF; **Page 151 top:** © C Squared Studios/Getty Images RF; **Page 151 middle:** © Kevin Sanchez/Cole Group/Getty Images RF; **Page 152:** © C Squared Studios/Getty Images RF; **Page 154:** © Royalty Free/Corbis RF; **Page 155:** © Burke/Triolo Productions/Getty Images RF

Chapter 6

Opener: © Fuse/Getty Images RF; **Page 158:** © Photodisc/Getty Images RF; **Page 159:** © John A. Rizzo/Getty Images RF; **Page 160:** © Photodisc/Getty Images RF; **6.5:** © The McGraw-Hill Companies, Inc./Elite Images, photographer; **Page 162:** © Wendy Schiff; **Page 164:** © The McGraw-Hill Companies, Inc./Bob Coyle, photographer; **Page 65:** © BananaStock/JupiterImages.com RF; **Page 169:** © The McGraw-Hill Companies, Inc./John

Flournoy, photographer; **6.18a,b:** © Ed Reschke; **Page 173:** © Photodisc/Getty Images RF; **Page 174:** © The McGraw-Hill Companies, Inc./Gary He, photographer; **Page 177 top, middle:** © Wendy Schiff; **Page 177 bottom:** © C Squared Studios/Getty Images RF; **Page 178 top:** © Adam Crowley/Getty Images RF; **Page 178 bottom:** © Royalty Free/Corbis RF; **Page 179 top:** © The McGraw-Hill Companies, Inc./Ken Cavanagh, photographer; **Page 179 bottom:** © The McGraw-Hill Companies, Inc./Elite Images, photographer; **Page 180 top:** © Ingram Publishing/Alamy RF; **Page 180 bottom, Page 181 top:** © Wendy Schiff; **Page 181 bottom:** © C Squared Studios/Getty Images RF; **Page 182:** © 2009 Oldways Preservation & Exchange Trust, http://oldwayspt.org; **Page 183:** © Photodisc/Punchstock RF; **Page 184:** © Ryan McVay/Getty Images RF; **6.26:** © The McGraw-Hill Companies, Inc./Jill Braaten, photographer; **Page 187 left:** © Allen Ross Photography; **Page 187 right:** Gwinnet County Police Department/Courtesy of the Centers for Disease Control; **6.30a,b:** © Arthur Glauberman/Photo Researchers, Inc.; **Page 191:** © Burke/Triolo Productions/Getty Images RF; **Page 192:** © Photodisc/PunchStock RF; **Page 193:** © Burke/Triolo Productions/Getty Images RF; **Page 194 left:** © Royalty Free/Corbis RF; **Page 194 right:** © Wendy Schiff; **Page 195:** © John A. Rizzo/Getty Images RF; **Page 196:** © The McGraw-Hill Companies, Inc./Elite Images, photographer; **Page 197:** © Spike Mafford/Getty Images RF; **Page 198, Page 199:** © Burke/Triolo Productions/Getty Images RF

Chapter 7

Opener: © Ingram Publishing/SuperStock RF; **Page 204 (Pizza), Page 204 (Tofu):** © C Squared Studios/Getty Images RF; **Page 204 (Ham):** © Burke/Triolo Productions/Getty Images RF; **Page 204 (Beans):** © Royalty Free/Corbis RF; **Page 204 (Peas):** © Getty Images RF; **Page 204 (Bagel):** © Photodisc/Getty Images RF; **Page 204 (Soup):** © John A. Rizzo/Getty Images RF; **7.3 left:** © C Squared Studios/Getty Images RF; **7.3 right:** © Photodisc/PunchStock RF; **Page 205 middle, Page 205 bottom:** © Wendy Schiff; **Page 206:** © Wendy Schiff; **7.8:** © Dr. Stanley Flegler/Visuals Unlimited/Getty Images; **Page 208 bottom:** © The McGraw-Hill Companies, Inc./Joe DeGrandis, photographer; **Page 210, Page 212 top:** © liquidllibrary/PictureQuest RF; **Page 212 bottom:** © Wendy Schiff; **Page 213:** © Ian Boddy/SPL/Photo Researchers, Inc.; **7.14, 7.15, Page 215 top:** © Wendy Schiff; **Page 215 bottom:** © Andrew Ward/Life File/Getty Images RF; **Page 217 top:** © & Courtesy of Sarah Clasen; **Page 217 right:** © Karl Weatherley/Getty Images RF; **Page 218 left:** Scott Bauer/ARS/USDA; **Page 218 (Roast), Page 218 (Fish):** © Photodisc/PunchStock RF; **Page 218 (Turkey):** © Paul Poplis/StockFood Creative/Getty Images; **Page 218 (Rice):**

© The McGraw-Hill Companies, Inc./Jacques Cornell, photographer; **Page 218 (Bread):** © C Squared Studios/Getty Images RF; **Page 218 (Beans):** © Burke/Triolo Productions/Getty Images RF; **Page 218 (Egg):** © Siede Preis/Getty Images RF; **Page 218 (Nuts):** © C Squared Studios/Getty Images RF; **Page 218 (Dairy):** © Photodisc/Getty Images RF; **7.17:** © Ingram Publishing/Alamy RF; **Page 220 top:** © PhotoLink/Getty Images RF; **Page 220 bottom right:** © Wendy Schiff; **Page 220 bottom left:** © Jonelle Weaver/Getty Images RF; **Page 221 top:** © Keith Ovregaard/Cole Group/Getty Images RF; **Page 221 bottom:** © Digital Vision/Getty Images RF; **7.18 left:** © C Squared Studios/Getty Images RF; **7.18 center:** © Royalty Free/Corbis RF; **7.18 right:** © C Squared Studios/Getty Images RF; **Page 222 bottom left:** © Mitch Hrdlicka/Getty Images RF; **Page 223:** © Jonelle Weaver/Getty Images RF; **Page 224:** © Wendy Schiff; **Page 225:** © Jonelle Weaver/Getty Images RF; **Page 226:** © Wendy Schiff; **7.19, 7.19 inset, 7.20:** Courtesy of the Centers for Disease Control/Dr. Lyle Conrad; **Page 229:** © Getty Images RF; **Page 230:** © Comstock/PunchStock RF; **7.21a-f, 7.22a,b, Page 232:** © Wendy Schiff; **Page 233 top:** © Rob Melynchuk/Getty Images RF; **Page 233 middle:** © Wendy Schiff; **Page 233 bottom:** © Keith Ovregaard/Cole Group/Getty Images RF; **Page 235 left:** © The McGraw-Hill Companies, Inc./Jacques Cornell, photographer; **Page 235 right:** © Wendy Schiff; **Page 236:** © Michael Lamotte/Cole Group/Getty Images RF; **Page 237 (Yoghurts):** © The McGraw-Hill Companies, Inc./Bob Coyle, photographer; **Page 237 (Salad):** © PhotoLink/Getty Images RF; **Page 237 (Bread):** © Digital Vision/Getty Images RF; **Page 238:** © Ingram Publishing/Alamy RF; **Page 239:** © Photodisc/Getty Images RF

Chapter 8

Opener: © The McGraw-Hill Companies, Inc.; **Page 241 both:** © C Squared Studios/Getty Images RF; **Page 243:** © Jules Frazier/Getty Images RF; **Page 244:** © Royalty Free/Corbis RF; **Page 246:** © Wendy Schiff; **Page 247:** USDA Photo by Bill Tarpening; **Page 248 top:** © Photodisc/Getty Images RF; **8.4:** © Wendy Schiff; **8.5:** © Ed Carey/Cole Group/Getty Images RF; **Page 250 (Oil):** © The McGraw-Hill Companies, Inc./Jacques Cornell, photographer; **Page 250 (Milk):** © The McGraw-Hill Companies, Inc./Ken Karp, photographer; **Page 250 (Broccoli):** © Stockdisc/PunchStock RF; **Page 250 (Nuts), Page 250 (Salmon):** © C Squared Studios/Getty Images RF; **Page 250 (Kale):** © Stockdisc/PunchStock RF; **8.6 (Oil):** © D. Hurst/Alamy RF; **8.6 (Mango):** © Stockdisc/PunchStock RF; **8.6 (Carrots):** © Comstock/JupiterImages RF; **8.6 (Milk):** © Judith Collins/Alamy RF; **8.6 (Cereal):** © Stockbyte/Getty Images RF; **8.6 (Almonds):** © Ingram Publishing/SuperStock RF; **Page 251 (Glasses):** © Photodisc/Getty Images RF; **Page 252:** © C Squared Studios/

Getty Images RF; **Page 254 top, Page 254 (Pumpkin):** © Ingram Publishing/Alamy RF; **Page 254 (Carrot):** © Photodisc/Getty Images RF; **Page 254 (Papaya):** © Burke/Triolo Productions/Getty Images RF; **Page 255 left:** © PhotoLink/Getty Images RF; **8.10:** Courtesy of the Centers for Disease Control; **8.11:** © Biophoto Associates/Photo Researchers, Inc.; **Page 257:** © Jackson Vereen/Cole Group/Getty Images RF; **Page 258 (Fish):** © Digital Vision/Getty Images RF; **Page 258 (Milk):** © The McGraw-Hill Companies, Inc./Ken Karp, photographer; **Page 258 (Mushrooms):** © C Squared Studios/Getty Images RF; **Page 259:** © Peter Cade/Getty Images RF; **8.16:** © Royalty Free/Corbis RF; **Page 261 (Mango):** © Stockdisc/PunchStock RF; **Page 261 (Asparagus), Page 261 (Sardines), Page 262:** © Burke/Triolo Productions/Getty Images RF; **8.18:** © Royalty Free/Corbis RF; **Page 263:** © Wendy Schiff; **Page 265 (Cornflakes):** © Photodisc/PunchStock RF; **Page 265 (Mushroom):** © Burke/Triolo Productions/Getty Images RF; **Page 265 (Orange):** © Dennis Gray/Cole Group/Getty Images RF; **Page 265 (Spinach):** © Royalty Free/Corbis RF; **8.21 (Mango):** © Stockdisc/PunchStock RF; **8.21 (Carrots):** © Comstock/JupiterImages RF; **8.21 (Milk):** © Judith Collins/Alamy RF; **8.21 (Cereal):** © Stockbyte/Getty Images RF; **8.21 (Almonds):** © Ingram Publishing/SuperStock RF; **8.22:** Courtesy of the Centers for Disease Control; **Page 267 (Ham):** © Royalty Free/Corbis RF; **Page 267 (Juice):** © Photodisc/Getty Images RF; **Page 267 (Peas):** © C Squared Studios/Getty Images RF; **Page 268 (Cereal):** © Photodisc/PunchStock RF; **Page 268 (Taco), Page 268 (Spinach):** © Royalty Free/Corbis RF; **Page 268 bottom:** © Mireille Vautier/Alamy; **Page 269 (Cereal):** © Comstock/PunchStock RF; **Page 269 (Chicken):** © Michael Lamotte/Cole Group/Getty Images RF; **Page 269 (Peanuts):** © C Squared Studios/Getty Images RF; **8.23:** Courtesy of the Centers for Disease Control; **Page 270 left:** © Wendy Schiff; **Page 270 right:** © C Squared Studios/Getty Images RF; **Page 271 (Potato):** © Royalty Free/Corbis RF; **Page 271 (Salmon):** © C Squared Studios/Getty Images RF; **Page 271 (Banana):** © Stockdisc/PunchStock RF; **Page 272 (Rice):** © Jules Frazier/Getty Images RF; **Page 272 (Asparagus):** © Burke/Triolo Productions/Getty Images RF; **Page 272 (Juice):** © Photodisc/Getty Images RF; **8.25 top:** © Dr. R. King/Photo Researchers, Inc.; **8.25 bottom:** © Dr. E. Walker/Photo Researchers, Inc.; **8.26a:** © Claude Edelmann/Photo Researchers, Inc.; **8.26b:** © Wellcome Trust/Custom Medical Stock Photo; **Page 276 (Sardines):** © Burke/Triolo Productions/Getty Images RF; **Page 276 (Soy Milk):** © Wendy Schiff; **Page 276 (Burger):** © Burke/Triolo Productions/Getty Images RF; **Page 277:** © Wendy Schiff; **Page 278:** Courtesy of the Centers for Disease Control; **Page 279 (Peppers):** © Jules Frazier/Getty Images RF; **Page 279 (Strawberries):** © Burke/Triolo Productions/Getty Images RF; **Page 279 (Kiwi):** ©

Ingram Publishing/Alamy RF; **Page 279 bottom:** © Wendy Schiff; **Page 281:** © The McGraw-Hill Companies, Inc./John Flournoy, photographer; **Page 284:** © Comstock Images/PictureQuest RF; **Page 287:** © Ingram Publishing/Alamy RF; **Page 289:** © C Squared Studios/Getty Images RF; **Page 290:** © Digital Vision/Getty Images RF; **Page 291:** © Wendy Schiff; **Page 292:** © Greg Kuchik/Getty Images RF; Page 294 left: © C Squared Studios/Getty Images RF; **Page 295:** © The McGraw-Hill Companies, Inc./Ken Karp, photographer

Chapter 9

Opener: SSGT Jason M. Carter, USMC/DoD Media; **Page 297:** © Comstock Images/PictureQuest RF; **Page 298:** © Royalty Free/Corbis RF; **Page 302 (Lettuce):** © Stockdisc/PunchStock RF; **Page 302 (Tomatoes):** © Burke/Triolo Productions/Getty Images RF; **9.6:** © Stephen J. Krasemann/Photo Researchers, Inc.; **Page 304:** © Photodisc/Getty Images RF; **Page 305 top:** © Comstock/PunchStock RF; **Page 305 bottom:** U.S. Navy photo by Seaman Aaron Shelley; **Page 306 top:** TSGT Lance Cheung, USAF/DoD Media; **Page 306 bottom left:** © Photodisc/PunchStock RF; **9.8:** © Royalty Free/Corbis RF; **9.9 (Mango):** © Stockdisc/PunchStock RF; **9.9 (Kale):** © Stockdisc/PunchStock RF; **9.9 (Milk):** © Ingram Publishing RF; **9.9 (Cereal):** © Stockbyte/Getty Images RF; **9.9 (Sardines):** © fStop/PunchStock RF; **Page 310:** © Comstock/Alamy RF; **Page 311 (Cereal):** © Photodisc/PunchStock RF; **Page 311 (Salad):** © Ingram Publishing/Alamy RF; **Page 311 (Oat Seeds):** © Siede Preis/Getty Images RF; **Page 311 (Peanut Butter):** © Burke/Triolo Productions/Getty Images RF; **9.12:** © Michael Klein/Peter Arnold, Inc.; **Page 312 bottom:** © Wendy Schiff; **Page 313 (Cereal):** © Photodisc/PunchStock RF; **Page 313 (Sardines):** © Burke/Triolo Productions/Getty Images RF; **Page 313 (Milk):** © The McGraw-Hill Companies, Inc./Ken Karp, photographer; **Page 313 bottom (all):** © Wendy Schiff; **9.14 (Broccoli):** © Burke/Triolo Productions/Getty Images RF; **9.14 (Orange Juice):** © Stockbyte/Getty Images RF; **9.14 (Cheese):** © Comstock/JupiterImages RF; **9.14 (Cereal):** © Stockbyte/Getty Images RF; **9.14 (Almonds):** © Stockbyte/Getty Images RF; **Page 314, Page 315 top:** © Wendy Schiff; **9.15:** © Yoav Levy/Phototake.com; **Page 317 top:** © Jonelle Weaver/Getty Images RF; **Page 317 bottom:** © Dynamic Graphics/JupiterImages RF; **Page 318 (Soup):** © John A. Rizzo/Getty Images RF; **Page 318 (Ham), Page 318 (Pickle):** © Burke/Triolo Productions/Getty Images RF; **Page 319:** © Wendy Schiff; **Page 320:** © Photodisc/Getty Images RF; **Page 322 top, Page 322 bottom:** © Wendy Schiff; **Page 323 left:** © Garry Davenport; **Page 323 right:** © The McGraw-Hill Companies, Inc./Ken Karp, photographer;

pher; **Page 324 (Potato):** © Royalty Free/Corbis RF; **Page 324 (Papaya):** © Burke/Triolo Productions/Getty Images RF; **Page 324 (Melon):** © C Squared Studios/Getty Images RF; **9.16 (Pear):** © Stockbyte/Getty Images RF; **9.16 (Squash):** © Burke/Triolo Productions/Getty Images RF; **9.16 (Yoghurt):** © Ingram Publishing/SuperStock RF; **9.16 (Bread):** © IT Stock/PunchStock RF; **9.16 (Shrimp):** © Comstock/JupiterImages RF; **Page 326 (Spinach):** © Burke/Triolo Productions/Getty Images RF; **Page 326 (Nuts):** © C Squared Studios/Getty Images RF; **Page 326 (Yam):** © Stockdisc/PunchStock RF; **9.17 (Berries):** © David Cook/blueshiftstudios/Alamy RF; **9.17 (Lima Beans):** © Brand Z Food/Alamy RF; **9.17 (Milk):** © Ingram Publishing RF; **9.17 (Cereal):** © The McGraw-Hill Companies, Inc./Jill Braaten, photographer; **9.17 (Kidney Beans):** © Royalty Free/Corbis RF; **Page 328:** © C Squared Studios/Getty Images RF; **Page 329 (Shrimp):** © John A. Rizzo/Getty Images RF; **Page 329 (Mushrooms):** © C Squared Studios/Getty Images RF; **Page 329 (Beans), Page 329 (Spinach):** © Royalty Free/Corbis RF; **Page 330 (Oatmeal):** © Comstock/PunchStock RF; **Page 330 (Beans):** © Wendy Schiff; **Page 330 (Chicken):** © Ernie Friedlander/Cole Group/Getty Images RF; **9.18 (Fruits):** © Stockbyte/Getty Images RF; **9.18 (Peas):** © Ingram Publishing/SuperStock RF; **9.18 (Oats):** © The McGraw-Hill Companies, Inc./Jacques Cornell, photographer; **9.18 (Beef):** © Comstock/JupiterImages RF; **9.19a:** © Dr. R. King/Photo Researchers, Inc.; **9.19b:** © Gladden Willis, M.D./Visuals Unlimited; **Page 332 top:** © liquidllibrary/PictureQuest RF; **Page 332 bottom:** © C Squared Studios/Getty Images RF; **Page 333 top, bottom:** © Wendy Schiff; **9.20:** Dr. Ananda S. Prasad/American Journal of Medicine; **Page 335 (Oysters):** © Wendy Schiff; **Page 335 (Crab), Page 335 (Pecans):** © C Squared Studios/Getty Images RF; **9.21 (Avocado):** © Ingram Publishing/SuperStock RF; **9.21 (Asparagus):** © Burke/Triolo Productions/Getty Images RF; **9.21 (Cheese):** © Burke/Triolo Productions/Getty Images RF; **9.21 (Bread):** © Everyday Images/Alamy RF; **9.21 (Chicken):** © Comstock/JupiterImages RF; **Page 336 top, Page 337 right:** © Wendy Schiff; **Page 337 (Milk):** © The McGraw-Hill Companies, Inc./Ken Karp, photographer; **Page 337 (Shrimp):** © Ingram Publishing/Alamy RF; **Page 337 (Egg):** © Siede Preis/Getty Images RF; **Page 338 (Broccoli):** © Burke/Triolo Productions/Getty Images RF; **Page 338 (Cauliflower), Page 338 (Brussels Sprouts):** © Burke/Triolo Productions/Getty Images RF; **Page 339 (Sunflower Seeds):** © The McGraw-Hill Companies, Inc./Jacques Cornell, photographer; **Page 339 (Egg):** © Burke/Triolo Productions/Getty Images RF; **Page 339 (Mushrooms):** © C Squared Studios/Getty Images RF; **Page 339 bottom:** © Wendy Schiff; **Page 340:** © Nancy R. Cohen/Getty Images RF; **Page 341:** © M. Freeman/PhotoLink/Getty Images RF; **Page 342:** © The McGraw-Hill

Companies, Inc./Gary He, photographer; **Page 343 (Glass of Water):** © John A. Rizzo/Getty Images RF; **Page 343 (Bottle of Water):** © Photodisc/Getty Images RF; **9.23, 9.24:** © Wendy Schiff; **Page 344 (Groceries):** © Burke/Triolo Productions/Getty Images RF; **Page 344 (Apple):** © C Squared Studios/ Getty Images RF; **Page 345:** © David Buffington/ Getty Images RF; **Page 346 (Smoothie):** © Jonelle Weaver/Getty Images RF; **Page 346 (Strawberries):** © Burke/Triolo Productions/Getty Images RF; **Page 347:** © Jonelle Weaver/Getty Images RF; **Page 348:** © Burke/Triolo Productions/Getty Images RF; **Page 349:** © Siede Preis/Getty Images RF

Chapter 10

Opener: © Wendy Schiff; **10.1a-c:** CDC/Office of Surveillance, Epidemiology, and Laboratory Services; **Page 352:** © Adam Crowley/Getty Images RF; **10.5a:** © The McGraw-Hill Companies, Inc./Dennis Strete, photographer; **10.5b:** © Gladden Willis, M.D./Visuals Unlimited; **10.6:** © University of Georgia Photographic Services. Photo by Paul Efland; **10.7:** Courtesy of Hologic; **10.8:** © Diana Linsley/ Linsley Photographics; **10.9:** © David Young-Wolf/ PhotoEdit Inc.; **10.10:** © FotoSearch Stock Photography RF; **Page 358:** © Photodisc/Getty Images RF; **Page 360:** © Steve Mason/Getty Images RF; **Page 361:** © Jules Frazier/Getty Images RF; **Page 362:** © Royalty Free/Corbis RF; **Page 363:** © Digital Vision/ PunchStock RF; **Page 366:** © The McGraw-Hill Companies, Inc./Lars A. Niki, photographer; **10.17:** © Science VU/Jackson/Visuals Unlimited; **Page 371, Page 372 left:** © Royalty Free/Corbis RF; **Page 372 right:** © Photodisc/Getty Images RF; **Page 373:** © The McGraw-Hill Companies, Inc./Lars A. Niki, photographer; **Page 375:** © Photodisc/PunchStock RF; **Page 376:** © The McGraw-Hill Companies, Inc./Andrew Resek, photographer; **Page 377 top, bottom:** © Wendy Schiff; **Page 378 (Bananas):** © Burke/Triolo Productions/Getty Images RF; **Page 378 (Apple):** © Photodisc/Getty Images RF; **Page 378 (Raisins):** © The McGraw-Hill Companies, Inc./ Jacques Cornell, photographer; **Page 378 bottom (both):** © Wendy Schiff; **Page 379 top:** © liquidllibrary/PictureQuest RF; **Page 379 bottom:** © David Buffington/Getty Images RF; **Page 380 left:** © Ryan McVay/Getty Images RF; **Page 380 right:** © Wendy Schiff; **Page 381:** © Royalty Free/Corbis RF; **10.21:** © Girishh/Alamy; **Page 386:** © The McGraw-Hill Companies, Inc./Lars A. Niki, photographer; **10.22:** © AP/Wide World Photos; **Page 389:** © Dynamic Images/JupiterImages RF; **Page 390:** © fStop/ Getty Images RF; **Page 391 top:** © The McGraw-Hill Companies, Inc./Lars A. Niki, photographer; **Page 391 bottom:** © Wendy Schiff; **Page 393:** © David Buffington/Getty Images RF; **Page 394 top:** © Digital Vision/Getty Images RF; **Page 394 bottom:** © Royalty Free/Corbis RF; **Page 395:** © Comstock/ PunchStock RF; **Page 396:** © PhotoLink/Getty Images RF; **Page 397:** © Photodisc/Getty Images

RF; **Page 398:** © Scott T. Baxter/Getty Images RF; **Page 399:** © Ryan McVay/Getty Images RF

Chapter 11

Opener: © AP/Wide World Photos; **11.1:** © Ingram Publishing RF; **Page 402:** © Sean Thompson/Photodisc/Getty Images RF; **11.2:** © Royalty Free/Corbis RF; **11.3:** © Wendy Schiff; **11.4 (Man at Desk):** © Stockdisc/PunchStock RF; **11.4 (Rollerblader):** © Ingram Publishing/Fotosearch RF; **11.4 (Man with Bike):** © Photodisc/Getty Images RF; **11.4 (Woman Exercising), 11.4 (Man in Gym):** © Ingram Publishing/Alamy RF; **11.4 (Woman with Flowers):** © Stockdisc/PunchStock RF; **11.4 (Woman with Stroller):** © Ingram Publishing/Fotosearch RF; **Page 404 bottom:** © Ryan McVay/Getty Images RF; **Page 408:** © Royalty Free/Corbis RF; **Page 410 right:** LCPL Richard A. Burkdall, USMC/DoD Media; **Page 410 left:** © Digital Vision/Punchstock RF; **Page 412:** U.S. Air Force photo by Tech. Sgt. Tracy L. DeMarco; **Page 413 (Bread):** © John A. Rizzo/Getty Images RF; **Page 413 (Lettuce):** © Burke/Triolo Productions/Getty Images RF; **Page 4.13 (Cookies):** © John A. Rizzo/Getty Images RF; **Page 413 (Pasta):** © Royalty Free/Corbis RF; **Page 413 (Oranges):** © Dennis Gray/Cole Group/Getty Images RF; **Page 413 (Celery):** © Burke/Triolo Productions/Getty Images RF; **Page 414 left:** © 1997 IMS Communications Ltd./Capstone Design. All Rights Reserved. RF; **Page 414 right:** © Wendy Schiff; **Page 415:** © Jonelle Weaver/Getty Images RF; **Page 416:** © Wendy Schiff; **Page 417:** © D. Fischer & P. Lyons/ Cole Group/Getty Images RF; **Page 418:** © Keith Ovregaard/Cole Group/Getty Images RF; **Page 419:** © Wendy Schiff; **Page 420:** LCPL Casey N. Thurston, USMC/DoD Media; **Page 421 top:** © Wendy Schiff; **Page 421 (Salt):** © C Squared Studios/Getty Images RF; **Page 421 (Juice):** © The McGraw-Hill Companies, Inc./Ken Karp, photographer; **Page 421 (Sugar):** © Royalty Free/Corbis RF; **Page 422:** © Javier Pierini/Getty Images RF; **Page 423:** © Comstock/Alamy RF; **Page 425 top:** © Nick Koudis/ Getty Images RF; **Page 425 (Tea), Page 425 (Coffee):** © John A. Rizzo/Getty Images RF; **Page 426:** © Royalty Free/Corbis RF; **Page 427 top:** © Jeff Maloney/Getty Images RF; **Page 427 bottom:** © Wendy Schiff; **Page 428:** © The McGraw-Hill Companies, Inc./Ken Cavanagh, photographer; **Page 429 top:** © Wendy Schiff; **Page 429 bottom:** © Ed Carey/ Cole Group/Getty Images RF; **Page 430 top:** © Royalty Free/Corbis RF; **Page 430 bottom:** © John A. Rizzo/Getty Images RF; **Page 431:** © Royalty Free/Corbis RF

Chapter 12

Opener (E. Coli): Courtesy of the Centers for Disease Control/National Escherichia, Shigella, Vibrio Reference Unit at CDC; **Opener (Salad):** © Wendy Schiff; **Page 433:** © The McGraw-Hill

Companies, Inc.; **Page 434:** © Wendy Schiff; **Page 435 top:** © PhotoAlto/PictureQuest RF; **Page 435 bottom:** © Dynamic Graphics Group/IT Stock Free/ Alamy RF; **Page 436 top, bottom:** Courtesy of the Centers for Disease Control; **Page 437 (Oysters):** © John A. Rizzo/Getty Images RF; **Page 437 (Cheese):** © J. Glenn/Cole Group/Getty Images RF; **Page 437 (Sausages):** © Burke/Triolo Productions/Getty Images RF; **Page 438 left:** © Eye of Science/Photo Researchers, Inc.; **Page 438 right:** © Burke/Triolo Productions/Getty Images RF; **Page 439:** © Royalty Free/Corbis RF; **12.1:** F.P. Williams, U.S. EPA; **Page 440 right:** Courtesy of the Centers for Disease Control; **Page 441 (Mushrooms):** © The McGraw-Hill Companies, Inc./Stephen P. Lynch, photographer; **Page 441 (Cheese):** © Stockbyte/PunchStock RF; **12.3:** © PhotoLink/Getty Images RF; **Page 442:** © Royalty Free/Corbis RF; **Page 443:** © The McGraw-Hill Companies, Inc./Rick Brady, photographer; **Page 444:** James Gathany/Courtesy of the Centers for Disease Control; **12.5, 12.6:** © Wendy Schiff; **Page 446 top:** © Royalty Free/Corbis RF; **Page 446 bottom:** USDA; **Page 447:** © C Squared Studios/ Getty Images RF; **12.7:** USDA, Be Food Safe Campaign; **Page 449 top:** © BananaStock/PunchStock RF; **Page 449 (Grapes):** © C Squared Studios/Getty Images RF; **Page 449 (Raisins):** © The McGraw-Hill Companies, Inc./Jacques Cornell, photographer; **Page 450 (Pickles):** © Kevin Sanchez/Cole Group/Getty Images RF; **Page 450 (Spam):** © The McGraw-Hill Companies, Inc./Elite Images, photographer; **Page 450 (Cheese):** © Burke/Triolo Productions/Getty Images RF; **Page 450 (Dried Fruits):** © C Squared Studios/Getty Images RF; **12.8:** Photo by Stephen Ausmus/ARS/USDA; **Page 452:** Photo by Jocelyn Augustino/FEMA; **Page 453:** © Wendy Schiff; **Page 455:** © Photodisc/Getty Images RF; **Page 456:** Photo by Tim McCabe, courtesy of the USDA Natural Resources Conservation Service; **12.10:** ARS/USDA; **Page 458:** © Brand X Pictures/ PunchStock RF; **12.13:** Courtesy of Katadyn North America; **Page 461:** © Steve Cole/Getty Images RF; **Page 463 top:** Courtesy of National Cancer Institute; **Page 463 bottom:** © Comstock Images/ PictureQuest RF; **Page 464:** © Kevin Sanchez/Cole Group/Getty Images RF; **Page 465:** Historicus/Library of Congress

Chapter 13

Opener: © Wendy Schiff; **Page 467:** © Brand X Pictures/PunchStock RF; **13.1 both:** © Lennart Nilsson/Albert Bonniers Forlag AB; **13.2, Page 470:** © Royalty Free/Corbis RF; **Page 472 (Cereal):** © The McGraw-Hill Companies, Inc./John Flournoy photographer; **Page 472 (Juice):** © The McGraw-Hill Companies, Inc./Emily & David Tietz, photographers; **Page 472 (Beans):** © Royalty Free/Corbis RF; **Page 473:** © Comstock/PunchStock RF; **Page 476, 13.5a:** © Photodisc/Getty Images RF; **13.5b:**

© Brand X Pictures/PunchStock RF; **Page 478:** USDA Photo by Ken Hammond; **13.6:** © Royalty Free/Corbis RF; **13.7:** © Keith Eng 2007 RF; **Page 481, 13.8:** © Wendy Schiff; **Page 482 bottom left:** © Photodisc/Getty Images RF; **Page 482 bottom right:** © Wendy Schiff; **Page 483 top:** © C Squared Studios/Getty Images RF; **Page 483 bottom:** © Creatas/PictureQuest RF; **Page 484 left & right:** © Wendy Schiff; **Page 485 left:** © Royalty Free/Corbis RF; **13.9:** © Creatas/PictureQuest RF; **Page 485 bottom:** © BananaStock/PictureQuest RF; **13.10:** © E. Gill/Custom Medical Stock Photo; **13.11:** USDA Photo by Ken Hammond; **13.12:** © BananaStock/PunchStock RF; **Page 488 top:** © Image Source/PunchStock RF; **Page 488 bottom:** © BananaStock/PunchStock RF; **Page 489:** © Pixtal/age fotostock RF; **Page 490:** © Photodisc/Getty Images RF; **Page 491 bottom:** © Rolf Bruderer/Getty Images RF; **Page 491 top, Page 493 top:** © BananaStock/PunchStock RF; **Page 493 bottom:** © The McGraw-Hill Companies, Inc./Ken Cavanagh, photographer;

13.14: © Purestock/Getty Images RF; **Page 496:** © Royalty Free/Corbis RF; **Page 497 top:** © Wendy Schiff; **Page 497 bottom:** © Ronnie Kaufman/Blend Images LLC RF; **13.16:** © Eric Fougére/Kipa/Corbis; **13.17:** © Steve Mason/Getty Images RF; **Page 500 bottom:** © Steve Cole/Getty Images RF; **Page 501, 13.18:** USDA Photo by Ken Hammond; **13.19:** Library of Congress, Prints and Photographs Division; **Page 505:** © Stockbyte RF; **Page 506:** © Royalty Free/Corbis RF; **Page 507 top & bottom:** © Wendy Schiff; **Page 509:** © Royalty-Free/Corbis RF

Chapter Icons

Food & Nutrition Tip Icon: © Jules Frazier/Getty Images RF; **Did You Know? Icon:** © Comstock/PunchStock RF; **Knowledge Checkpoint Icon:** © M. Lamotte/Cole Group/Getty Images RF; **Personal Dietary Analysis Icon:** © Digital Vision/Getty Images RF; **Chapter Highlight Icon:** © Photodisc/

PunchStock RF; **Recipe Box Icon:** © C Squared Studios/Getty Images RF; **Critical Thinking Icon:** © The McGraw-Hill Companies, Inc./Ken Karp, photographer; **Summary and Multiple Choice Icons:** © C Squared Studios/Getty Images RF; **Practice Test Icon:** © Stockdisc/PunchStock RF

Appendix

A-1: © Burke/Triolo Productions/Getty Images RF; **A-3:** © Ablestock/Alamy RF; **A-5:** © Burke/Triolo Productions/Getty Images RF; **A-14:** © C Squared Studios/Getty Images RF; **A-16:** © Royalty Free/Corbis RF; **A-21:** © The McGraw-Hill Companies, Inc./Ken Karp, photographer; **A-23 (Cheese):** © D. Hurst/Alamy RF; **A-23 (Ham):** © Royalty Free/Corbis RF; **A-23 (Eggs):** © The McGraw-Hill Companies, Inc./Ken Karp, photographer; **A-25:** © Royalty Free/Corbis RF; **A-42:** © Burke/Triolo Productions/Getty Images RF; **A-43:** © Wendy Schiff; **G-1:** © PhotoLink/Getty Images RF

Index

E

A

Dietary Reference Intakes (DRIs): Recommended Intakes for Individuals, Vitamins Food and Nutrition Board, Institute of Medicine, National Academies

Life Stage Group	Vitamin A (μg/d)[a]	Vitamin C (mg/d)	Vitamin D (μg/d)[b,c]	Vitamin E (mg/d)[d]	Vitamin K (μg/d)	Thiamin (mg/d)	Riboflavin (mg/d)	Niacin (mg/d)[e]	Vitamin B-6 (mg/d)	Folate (μg/d)[f]	Vitamin B-12 (μg/d)	Pantothenic Acid (mg/d)	Biotin (μg/d)	Choline (mg/d)[g]
Infants														
0–6 mo	400*	40*	10	4*	2.0*	0.2*	0.3*	2*	0.1*	65*	0.4*	1.7*	5*	125*
7–12 mo	500*	50*	10	5*	2.5*	0.3*	0.4*	4*	0.3*	80*	0.5*	1.8*	6*	150*
Children														
1–3 y	300	15	15	6	30*	0.5	0.5	6	0.5	150	0.9	2*	8*	200*
4–8 y	400	25	15	7	55*	0.6	0.6	8	0.6	200	1.2	3*	12*	250*
Males														
9–13 y	600	45	15	11	60*	0.9	0.9	12	1.0	300	1.8	4*	20*	375*
14–18 y	900	75	15	15	75*	1.2	1.3	16	1.3	400	2.4	5*	25*	550*
19–30 y	900	90	15	15	120*	1.2	1.3	16	1.3	400	2.4	5*	30*	550*
31–50 y	900	90	15	15	120*	1.2	1.3	16	1.3	400	2.4	5*	30*	550*
51–70 y	900	90	15	15	120*	1.2	1.3	16	1.7	400	2.4[h]	5*	30*	550*
>70 y	900	90	20	15	120*	1.2	1.3	16	1.7	400	2.4[h]	5*	30*	550*
Females														
9–13 y	600	45	15	11	60*	0.9	0.9	12	1.0	300	1.8	4*	20*	375*
14–18 y	700	65	15	15	75*	1.0	1.0	14	1.2	400[i]	2.4	5*	25*	400*
19–30 y	700	75	15	15	90*	1.1	1.1	14	1.3	400[i]	2.4	5*	30*	425*
31–50 y	700	75	15	15	90*	1.1	1.1	14	1.3	400[i]	2.4	5*	30*	425*
51–70 y	700	75	15	15	90*	1.1	1.1	14	1.5	400	2.4[h]	5*	30*	425*
>70 y	700	75	20	15	90*	1.1	1.1	14	1.5	400	2.4[h]	5*	30*	425*
Pregnancy														
≤18 y	750	80	15	15	75*	1.4	1.4	18	1.9	600[j]	2.6	6*	30*	450*
19–30 y	770	85	15	15	90*	1.4	1.4	18	1.9	600[j]	2.6	6*	30*	450*
31–50 y	770	85	15	15	90*	1.4	1.4	18	1.9	600[j]	2.6	6*	30*	450*
Lactation														
≤18 y	1200	115	15	19	75*	1.4	1.6	17	2.0	500	2.8	7*	35*	550*
19–30 y	1300	120	15	19	90*	1.4	1.6	17	2.0	500	2.8	7*	35*	550*
31–50 y	1300	120	15	19	90*	1.4	1.6	17	2.0	500	2.8	7*	35*	550*

mg = milligram, mg = microgram

NOTE: This table (taken from the DRI reports; see www.nap.edu) presents Recommended Dietary Allowances (RDAs) in **bold type** and Adequate Intakes (AIs) in ordinary type followed by an asterisk (*). RDAs and AIs may both be used as goals for individual intake. RDAs are set to meet the needs of almost all (97 to 98%) individuals in a group. For healthy breastfed infants, the AI is the mean intake. The AI for other life stage and gender groups is believed to cover needs of all individuals in the group, but lack of data or uncertainty in the data prevents being able to specify with confidence the percentage of individuals covered by this intake.

[a] As retinol activity equivalents (RAEs). 1 RAE = 1 μg retinol, 12 μg β-carotene, 24 μg α-carotene, or 24 μg β-cryptoxanthin. To calculate RAEs from REs of provitamin A carotenoids in foods, divide the REs by 2. For preformed vitamin A in foods or supplements and for provitamin A carotenoids in supplements, 1 RE = 1 RAE.

[b] cholecalciferol. 1 μg cholecalciferol = 40 IU vitamin D.

[c] In the absence of adequate exposure to sunlight.

[d] As α-tocopherol. α-Tocopherol includes RRR-α-tocopherol, the only form of α-tocopherol that occurs naturally in foods, and the 2R-stereoisomeric forms of α-tocopherol (RRR-, RSR-, RRS-, and RSS-α-tocopherol) that occur in fortified foods and supplements. It does not include the 2S-stereoisomeric forms of α-tocopherol (SRR-, SSR-, SRS-, and SSS-α-tocopherol), also found in fortified foods and supplements.

[e] As niacin equivalents (NE). 1 mg of niacin = 60 mg of tryptophan; 0–6 months = preformed niacin (not NE).

[f] As dietary folate equivalents (DFE). 1 DFE = 1 μg food folate = 0.6 μg of folic acid from fortified food or as a supplement consumed with food = 0.5 μg of a supplement taken on an empty stomach.

[g] Although AIs have been set for choline, there are few data to assess whether a dietary supply of choline is needed at all stages of the life cycle, and it may be that the choline requirement can be met by endogenous synthesis at some of these stages.

[h] Because 10 to 30% of older people may malabsorb food-bound B-12, it is advisable for those older than 50 years to meet their RDA mainly by consuming foods fortified with B-12 or a supplement containing B-12.

[i] In view of evidence linking folate intake with neural tube defects in the fetus, it is recommended that all women capable of becoming pregnant consume 400 μg from supplements or fortified foods in addition to intake of food folate from a varied diet.

[j] It is assumed that women will continue consuming 400 μg from supplements or fortified food until their pregnancy is confirmed and they enter prenatal care, which ordinarily occurs after the end of the periconceptional period—the critical time for formation of the neural tube.

Adapted from the Dietary Reference Intakes series, National Academies Press. Copyright 1997, 1998, 2000, 2001, 2011, by the National Academy of Sciences. The full reports are available from the National Academies Press at www.nap.edu.

B

Dietary Reference Intakes (DRIs): Recommended Intakes for Individuals, Elements
Food and Nutrition Board, Institute of Medicine, National Academies

Life Stage Group	Calcium (mg/d)	Chromium (μg/d)	Copper (μg/d)	Fluoride (mg/d)	Iodine (μg/d)	Iron (mg/d)	Magnesium (mg/d)	Manganese (mg/d)	Molybdenum (μg/d)	Phosphorus (mg/d)	Selenium (μg/d)	Zinc (mg/d)
Infants												
0–6 mo	200*	0.2*	200*	0.01*	110*	0.27*	30*	0.003*	2*	100*	15*	2*
7–12 mo	260*	5.5*	220*	0.5*	130*	11	75*	0.6*	3*	275*	20*	3
Children												
1–3 y	700	11*	340	0.7*	90	7	80	1.2*	17	460	20	3
4–8 y	1000	15*	440	1*	90	10	130	1.5*	22	500	30	5
Males												
9–13 y	1300	25*	700	2*	120	8	240	1.9*	34	1250	40	8
14–18 y	1300	35*	890	3*	150	11	410	2.2*	43	1250	55	11
19–30 y	1000	35*	900	4*	150	8	400	2.3*	45	700	55	11
31–50 y	1000	35*	900	4*	150	8	420	2.3*	45	700	55	11
51–70 y	1000	30*	900	4*	150	8	420	2.3*	45	700	55	11
>70 y	1200	30*	900	4*	150	8	420	2.3*	45	700	55	11
Females												
9–13 y	1300	21*	700	2*	120	8	240	1.6*	34	1250	40	8
14–18 y	1300	24*	890	3*	150	15	360	1.6*	43	1250	55	9
19–30 y	1000	25*	900	3*	150	18	310	1.8*	45	700	55	8
31–50 y	1000	25*	900	3*	150	18	320	1.8*	45	700	55	8
51–70 y	1200	20*	900	3*	150	8	320	1.8*	45	700	55	8
>70 y	1200	20*	900	3*	150	8	320	1.8*	45	700	55	8
Pregnancy												
≤18 y	1300	29*	1000	3*	220	27	400	2.0*	50	1250	60	12
19–30 y	1000	30*	1000	3*	220	27	350	2.0*	50	700	60	11
31–50 y	1000	30*	1000	3*	220	27	360	2.0*	50	700	60	11
Lactation												
≤18 y	1300	44*	1300	3*	290	10	360	2.6*	50	1250	70	13
19–30 y	1000	45*	1300	3*	290	9	310	2.6*	50	700	70	12
31–50 y	1000	45*	1300	3*	290	9	320	2.6*	50	700	70	12

NOTE: This table presents Recommended Dietary Allowances (RDAs) in **bold type** and Adequate Intakes (AIs) in ordinary type followed by an asterisk (*). RDAs and AIs may both be used as goals for individual intake. RDAs are set to meet the needs of almost all (97 to 98%) individuals in a group. For healthy breastfed infants, the AI is the mean intake. The AI for other life stage and gender groups is believed to cover needs of all individuals in the group, but lack of data or uncertainty in the data prevents being able to specify with confidence the percentage of individuals covered by this intake.

Sources: Dietary Reference Intakes for Calcium, Phosphorus, Magnesium, Vitamin D, and Fluoride (1997); Dietary Reference Intakes for Thiamin, Riboflavin, Niacin, Vitamin B-6, Folate, Vitamin B-12, Pantothenic Acid, Biotin, and Choline (1998); Dietary Reference Intakes for Vitamin C, Vitamin E, Selenium, and Carotenoids (2000); Dietary Reference Intakes for Vitamin A, Vitamin K, Arsenic, Boron, Chromium, Copper, Iodine, Iron, Manganese, Molybdenum, Nickel, Silicon, Vanadium, and Zinc (2001); and Dietary Reference Intakes for Calcium and Vitamin D (2011). These reports may be accessed via www.nap.edu.

Adapted from the Dietary Reference Intake series, National Academies Press. Copyright 1997, 1998, 2000, 2001, and 2011 by the National Academy of Sciences. The full reports are available from the National Academies Press at www.nap.edu.

C

Dietary Reference Intakes (DRIs): Recommended Intakes for Individuals, Macronutrients
Food and Nutrition Board, Institute of Medicine, National Academies

Life Stage Group	Carbohydrate (g/d)	Total Fiber (g/d)	Fat (g/d)	Linoleic Acid (g/d)	α-Linolenic Acid (g/d)	Protein[a] (g/d)
Infants						
0–6 mo	60*	ND	31*	4.4*	0.5*	9.1*
7–12 mo	95*	ND	30*	4.6*	0.5*	11.0
Children						
1–3 y	130	19*	ND[b]	7*	0.7*	13
4–8 y	130	25*	ND	10*	0.9*	19
Males						
9–13 y	130	31*	ND	12*	1.2*	34
14–18 y	130	38*	ND	16*	1.6*	52
19–30 y	130	38*	ND	17*	1.6*	56
31–50 y	130	38*	ND	17*	1.6*	56
51–70 y	130	30*	ND	14*	1.6*	56
>70 y	130	30*	ND	14*	1.6*	56
Females						
9–13 y	130	26*	ND	10*	1.0*	34
14–18 y	130	26*	ND	11*	1.1*	46
19–30 y	130	25*	ND	12*	1.1*	46
31–50 y	130	25*	ND	12*	1.1*	46
51–70 y	130	21*	ND	11*	1.1*	46
>70 y	130	21*	ND	11*	1.1*	46
Pregnancy						
14–18 y	175	28*	ND	13*	1.4*	71
19–30 y	175	28*	ND	13*	1.4*	71
31–50 y	175	28*	ND	13*	1.4*	71
Lactation						
14–18 y	210	29*	ND	13*	1.3*	71
19–30 y	210	29*	ND	13*	1.3*	71
31–50 y	210	29*	ND	13*	1.3*	71

NOTE: This table presents Recommended Dietary Allowances (RDAs) in **bold type** and Adequate Intakes (AIs) in ordinary type followed by an asterisk (*). RDAs and AIs may both be used as goals for individual intake. RDAs are set to meet the needs of almost all (97 to 98%) individuals in a group. For healthy breastfed infants, the AI is the mean intake. The AI for other life stage and gender groups is believed to cover needs of all individuals in the group, but lack of data or uncertainty in the data prevents being able to specify with confidence the percentage of individuals covered by this intake.

[a]Based on 0.8g protein/kg body weight for reference body weight.

[b]ND = not determinable at this time.

Sources: Dietary Reference Intakes for Energy, Carbohydrate, Fiber, Fat, Fatty Acids, Cholesterol, Protein, and Amino Acids (2002). This report may be accessed via www.nap.edu.

Adapted from the Dietary Reference Intake series, National Academies Press. Copyright 1997, 1998, 2000, 2001, by the National Academy of Sciences. The full reports are available from the National Academies Press at www.nap.edu.

Dietary Reference Intakes (DRIs): Recommended Intakes for Individuals, Electrolytes and Water
Food and Nutrition Board, Institute of Medicine, National Academies

Life Stage Group	Sodium (mg/d)	Potassium (mg/d)	Chloride (mg/d)	Water (L/d)
Infants				
0–6 mo	120*	400*	180*	0.7*
7–12 mo	370*	700*	570*	0.8*
Children				
1–3 y	1000*	3000*	1500*	1.3*
4–8 y	1200*	3800*	1900*	1.7*
Males				
9–13 y	1500*	4500*	2300*	2.4*
14–18 y	1500*	4700*	2300*	3.3*
19–30 y	1500*	4700*	2300*	3.7*
31–50 y	1500*	4700*	2300*	3.7*
51–70 y	1300*	4700*	2000*	3.7*
> 70 y	1200*	4700*	1800*	3.7*
Females				
9–13 y	1500*	4500*	2300*	2.1*
14–18 y	1500*	4700*	2300*	2.3*
19–30 y	1500*	4700*	2300*	2.7*
31–50 y	1500*	4700*	2300*	2.7*
51–70 y	1300*	4700*	2000*	2.7*
> 70 y	1200*	4700*	1800*	2.7*
Pregnancy				
14–18 y	1500*	4700*	2300*	3.0*
19–50 y	1500*	4700*	2300*	3.0*
Lactation				
14–18 y	1500*	5100*	2300*	3.8*
19–50 y	1500*	5100*	2300*	3.8*

NOTE: The table is adapted from the DRI reports. See www.nap.edu. Adequate Intakes (AIs) are followed by an asterisk (*). These may be used as a goal for individual intake. For healthy breastfed infants, the AI is the average intake. The AI for other life stage and gender groups is believed to cover the needs of all individuals in the group, but lack of data prevent being able to specify with confidence the percentage of individuals covered by this intake; therefore, no Recommended Dietary Allowance (RDA) was set.

Source: *Dietary Reference Intakes for Water, Potassium, Sodium, Chloride, and Sulfate* (2005). This report may be accessed via www.nap.edu.

Acceptable Macronutrient Distribution Ranges

	Range (percent of energy)		
Macronutrient	**Children, 1–3 y**	**Children, 4–18 y**	**Adults**
Fat	30–40	25–35	20–35
omega-6 polyunsaturated fats (linoleic acid)	5–10	5–10	5–10
omega-3 polyunsaturated fats[a] (α-linolenic acid)	0.6–1.2	0.6–1.2	0.6–1.2
Carbohydrate	45–65	45–65	45–65
Protein	5–20	10–30	10–35

[a]Approximately 10% of the total can come from longer-chain n-3 fatty acids.

SOURCE: *Dietary Reference Intakes for Energy, Carbohydrate, Fiber, Fat, Fatty Acids, Cholesterol, Protein, and Amino Acids* (2002). The report may be accessed via www.nap.edu.

Adapted from the Dietary Reference Intakes series, National Academies Press. Copyright 1997, 1998, 2000, 2001, 2011, by the National Academy of Sciences. The full reports are available from the National Academies Press at www.nap.edu.

E

Dietary Reference Intakes (DRIs): Tolerable Upper Intake Levels (UL[a]), Vitamins

Food and Nutrition Board, Institute of Medicine, National Academies

Life Stage Group	Vitamin A (µg/d)[b]	Vitamin C (mg/d)	Vitamin D (µg/d)	Vitamin E (mg/d)[c],d	Vitamin K	Thiamin	Riboflavin	Niacin (mg/d)[d]	Vitamin B-6 (mg/d)	Folate (µg/d)[d]	Vitamin B-12	Pantothenic Acid	Biotin	Choline (g/d)	Carotenoids[e]
Infants															
0–6 mo	600	ND	25	ND	ND	ND	ND	ND	ND	ND	ND	ND	ND	ND	ND
7–12 mo	600	ND	38	ND	ND	ND	ND	ND	ND	ND	ND	ND	ND	ND	ND
Children															
1–3 y	600	400	63	200	ND	ND	ND	10	30	300	ND	ND	ND	1.0	ND
4–8 y	900	650	75	300	ND	ND	ND	15	40	400	ND	ND	ND	1.0	ND
Males, Females															
9–13 y	1700	1200	100	600	ND	ND	ND	20	60	600	ND	ND	ND	2.0	ND
14–18 y	2800	1800	100	800	ND	ND	ND	30	80	800	ND	ND	ND	3.0	ND
19–70 y	3000	2000	100	1000	ND	ND	ND	35	100	1000	ND	ND	ND	3.5	ND
>70 y	3000	2000	100	1000	ND	ND	ND	35	100	1000	ND	ND	ND	3.5	ND
Pregnancy															
≤18 y	2800	1800	100	800	ND	ND	ND	30	80	800	ND	ND	ND	3.0	ND
19–50 y	3000	2000	100	1000	ND	ND	ND	35	100	1000	ND	ND	ND	3.5	ND
Lactation															
≤18 y	2800	1800	100	800	ND	ND	ND	30	80	800	ND	ND	ND	3.0	ND
19–50 y	3000	2000	100	1000	ND	ND	ND	35	100	1000	ND	ND	ND	3.5	ND

[a]UL = The maximum level of daily nutrient intake likely to pose no risk of adverse effects. Unless otherwise specified, the UL represents total intake from food, water, and supplements. Due to lack of suitable data, ULs could not be established for vitamin K, thiamin, riboflavin, vitamin B-12, pantothenic acid, biotin, or carotenoids. In the absence of ULs, extra caution may be warranted in consuming levels above recommended intakes.

[b]As preformed vitamin A only.

[c]As α-tocopherol; applies to any form of supplemental α-tocopherol.

[d]The ULs for vitamin E, niacin, and folate apply to synthetic forms obtained from supplements, fortified foods, or a combination of the two.

[e]β-Carotene supplements are advised only to serve as a provitamin A source for individuals at risk of vitamin A deficiency.

ND = Not determinable due to lack of data of adverse effects in this age group and concern with regard to lack of ability to handle excess amounts. Source of intake should be from food only to prevent high levels of intake.

SOURCES: Dietary Reference Intakes for Calcium, Phosphorus, Magnesium, Vitamin D (2011); Dietary Reference Intakes for Thiamin, Riboflavin, Niacin, Vitamin B-6, Folate, Vitamin B-12, Pantothenic Acid, Biotin, and Choline (1998); Dietary Reference Intakes for Vitamin C, Vitamin E, Selenium, and Carotenoids (2000); and Dietary Reference Intakes for Vitamin A, Vitamin K, Arsenic, Boron, Chromium, Copper, Iodine, Iron, Manganese, Molybdenum, Nickel, Silicon, Vanadium, and Zinc (2001). These reports may be accessed via www.nap.edu.

Adapted from the Dietary Reference Intakes series, National Academies Press. Copyright 1997, 1998, 2000, 2001, 2011, by the National Academy of Sciences. The full reports are available from the National Academies Press at www.nap.edu.